Anesthesia and Co-Existing Disease
SECOND EDITION

Anesthesia and Co-Existing Disease

SECOND EDITION

Robert K. Stoelting, M.D.

Professor and Chairman
Department of Anesthesia
Indiana University School of Medicine
Indianapolis, Indiana

Stephen F. Dierdorf, M.D.

Associate Professor
Department of Anesthesia
Indiana University School of Medicine
Indianapolis, Indiana

Richard L. McCammon, M.D.

Associate Professor
Department of Anesthesia
Indiana University School of Medicine
Indianapolis, Indiana

CHURCHILL LIVINGSTONE

New York, Edinburgh, London, Melbourne   1988

Library of Congress Cataloging in Publication Data

Anesthesia and co-existing disease / [edited by] Robert K. Stoelting,
Stephen F. Dierdorf, Richard L. McCammon.—2nd ed.
p.   cm.
Includes bibliographies and index.
ISBN 0-443-08555-2
1. Anesthesia—Complications and sequelae.   2. Therapeutics,
Surgical.   I. Stoelting, Robert K.   II. Dierdorf, Stephen F.
III. McCammon, Richard L.
[DNLM: 1. Anesthesia—adverse effects.   2. Anesthetics.   WO 245
A578]
RD82.5.A53   1988
610′.0024617—dc19
DNLM/DLC   88-2841
for Library of Congress   CIP

Second Edition © Churchill Livingstone Inc. 1988
First Edition © Churchill Livingstone Inc. 1983

Distributed in the United Kingdom by Churchill Livingstone.
Robert Stevenson House, 1-3 Baxter's Place, Leith Walk, Edinburgh
EH1 3AF, and by associated companies, branches, and representatives
throughout the world.

Accurate indications, adverse reactions, and dosage schedules for
drugs are provided in this book, but it is possible that they
may change. The reader is urged to review the package information
data of the manufacturers of the medications mentioned.

The Publishers have made every effort to trace the copyright holders
for borrowed material. If they have inadvertently overlooked any,
they will be pleased to make the necessary arrangements at the first
opportunity.

Acquisitions Editor: *Toni M. Tracy*
Copy Editor: *Ann Ruzycka*
Production Designer: *Gloria Brown*
Production Supervisor: *Jocelyn Eckstein*

Printed in the United States of America

First published in 1988
Second printing in 1988

PREFACE

Since its publication in 1983, the first edition of *Anesthesia and Co-Existing Disease* has found widespread acceptance as a source of information about the medical implications of co-existing pathophysiology on the management of anesthesia. Our stated goal in the first edition, to provide a concise description of the pathophysiology of disease states and their medical treatment that is relevant to care of patients in the perioperative period, has been further refined in this second edition. New developments and diseases (organ transplantation, lithotripsy, acquired immunodeficiency syndrome, Alzheimer's disease) are discussed in detail. The addition of a third editor, Richard L. McCammon, M.D., brings added expertise to this second edition.

This edition of *Anesthesia and Co-Existing Disease* is the product of the Editors. We believe we have provided a consistency of style that the reader will find useful. As with the first edition, we think that this book can serve both as an introductory source of information and as a reference book for review. Therefore, this book should be equally valuable to the physician trainee and the experienced anesthesiologist.

The Editors again wish to recognize the invaluable secretarial help of Deanna Walker in the preparation of the manuscript. The professionals at Churchill Livingstone have made invaluable contributions to the timely production of this second edition. In this regard, the Editors wish to specifically recognize the support and encouragement of Toni M. Tracy, President of Churchill Livingstone. Ann Ruzycka did a superb job with the copy editing and managed to keep the production schedule on course despite frequent additions of new material by the Editors. Finally, we are grateful to our families for their support during the many extra hours required to prepare this revision.

Robert K. Stoelting, M.D.
Stephen F. Dierdorf, M.D.
Richard L. McCammon, M.D.

PREFACE TO THE FIRST EDITION

Optimal management of anesthesia extends beyond an understanding of the pharmacology of drugs used during the intraoperative period and a dexterity in performance of technical procedures. Specifically, a knowledge of the pathophysiology of co-existing disease regardless of the reason for surgery and an understanding of the implications of concomitant drug therapy are mandatory for the optimal management of anesthesia in an individual patient. The goal of *Anesthesia and Co-Existing Disease* is to provide a concise description of the pathophysiology of disease states and their medical treatment that is relevant to the care of the patient in the perioperative period. Diseases or characteristics unique to the pediatric, geriatric, and pregnant patient are considered in separate chapters. There is a liberal use of illustrations and tables to reinforce written material. Discussions of disease states often include a section designated Management of Anesthesia. This section is designed to relate the impact of co-existing disease to the selection of drugs, techniques, and monitors to be employed in the perioperative period.

We feel that *Anesthesia and Co-Existing Disease* can serve both as an introductory source of information and as a reference for review. Therefore, this book should be equally valuable to the beginner or the individual with training and experience in the administration of anesthesia. Although several authors have contributed to this undertaking, a consistency in style is assured by virtue of the Editors' roles as the final "authors" so as to make the entire book read as if written by a single individual.

The Editors wish to recognize the invaluable secretarial help of Deanna Walker in preparation of manuscripts. We salute the contagious enthusiasm of Lewis Reines, President of Churchill Livingstone, in the initial formulation of the idea for this book. In addition, the superb cooperation of our copy editor, Donna Balopole, permitted us to continue to make important additions to the book as new information and references became available. As a result, we have been able to achieve our desire to provide a work which is current to within 6 months of publication. Finally, we are grateful to our colleagues and families for their understanding and support during the time the book was in preparation.

Robert K. Stoelting, M.D.
Stephen F. Dierdorf, M.D.

CONTENTS

Coronary Artery Disease

Coronary artery disease is estimated to be present in 10 million adults and is responsible for about one-third of all deaths in persons between 35 and 65 years of age.[1] Prognosis for patients with coronary artery disease is related to the number of coronary arteries involved, as well as the specific vessels that are diseased (Fig. 1-1).[1] It is likely that coronary artery disease is present in 5 percent to 10 percent of patients who undergo anesthesia and surgery. The presence of coronary artery disease is associated with increased postoperative morbidity and mortality.[2,3]

The history, review of current medications, physical examination, electrocardiogram, and radiograph of the chest are the five essential components of the preoperative cardiac evaluation.[4,5] More specialized procedures such as Holter monitoring (ambulatory electrocardiogram), exercise electrocardiography, echocardiography, radioisotope imaging, and cardiac catheterization and angiography are performed on the basis of these more fundamental evaluations. Consultation with the primary physician is helpful in understanding the significance of the patient's coronary artery disease and assuring that optimal preoperative preparation has been achieved. Ultimately, these data should determine whether patients are in the best possible medical condition before undergoing elective noncardiac surgery.

RISK FACTORS FOR THE DEVELOPMENT OF CORONARY ARTERY DISEASE

Risk factors for the development of coronary artery disease include (1) elevated plasma concentrations of cholesterol, specifically low-density lipoprotein cholesterol (LDL-C); (2) cigarette smoking; (3) hypertension; (4) diabetes mellitus; (5) advancing age; and (6) male sex (Table 1-1).[6] Family history as a risk factor is based on the presence or absence of these six characteristics. There is a linear correlation between plasma concentrations of cholesterol and the risk for development of coronary artery disease (Fig. 1-2).[6] Although rates of atherogenesis are variable among individuals with similar risk factors, it is possible to estimate an average rate of atherogenesis and how this rate will be modified at different plasma cholesterol concentrations. For example, when plasma cholesterol concentrations are below 200 mg·dl^{-1} and no other risk factors are present, a critical degree of atherosclerosis (about 60 percent of the surface of the coronary artery covered by a plaque) is reached in many by 70 years of age. With the addition of the risk factor of cigarette smoking, this critical stage is reached by 60 years of age, and by further addition of the risk factor of hypertension this decreases to 50 years of age.[6] Addition of the

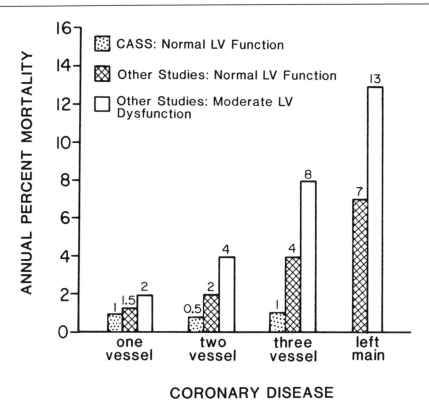

FIG. 1-1. Annual percent mortality among medically treated patients with coronary artery disease is increased in patients with left ventricular dysfunction, multiple diseased vessels or selective disease of the left main coronary artery. (Redrawn from Silverman KJ, Grossman W. Angina pectoris. N Engl J Med 1984;310:1712–7.)

risk factor of cigarette smoking is equivalent to increasing plasma cholesterol concentrations by 50 mg·dl^{-1} to 100 mg·dl^{-1}. It has been proposed that ideal plasma concentrations of cholesterol for individuals over 30 years of age are 200 mg·dl^{-1} or less and that attempts should be instituted to lower plasma concentrations

when they exceed the 75th percentile or about 240 mg·dl^{-1}.[7] Applying these criteria, 15 percent to 20 percent of the population has hypercholesterolemia. Diet (substitution of polyunsaturated fatty acids for saturated fatty acids) is the principal method for lowering plasma concentrations of cholesterol, although diets sufficiently palatable to achieve patient acceptance typically lower plasma cholesterol concentrations by only 10 percent or less. Hypocholesterolemic drugs, which act by inhibiting the rate-limiting enzyme step in the synthesis of cholesterol, may become useful in treatment of nonfamilial hypercholesterolemia.[8] It is estimated that maintaining plasma concentrations of cholesterol below 200 mg·dl^{-1} would lower the rate of coronary artery disease by 30 percent to 50 percent in individuals less than 65 years of age.[9]

TABLE 1-1.   Risk Factors for the
Development of Coronary Artery Disease

Hypercholesterolemia (above 200 mg·dl^{-1})
Cigarette smoking
Systemic hypertension
Diabetes mellitus
Advancing age
Male sex
Diet (excess cholesterol, saturated fatty acids, total calories)
Psychosocial characteristics

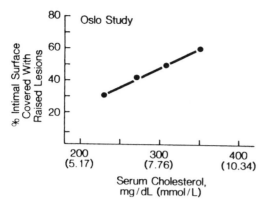

FIG. 1-2. Relation of premortem plasma (serum) cholesterol concentrations to severity of atherosclerosis (% intimal surface covered with raised lesions) discovered at autopsy. (Grundy SM. Cholesterol and coronary heart disease. A new era. JAMA 1986;256:2849–58. Copyright 1986, American Medical Association.)

Low-Density Lipoprotein Receptors

Receptors for LDL-C are present in liver cells and to a lesser extent in other tissues.[10] These receptors are the mechanism for removal of LDL-C, which are the principal cholesterol-carrying lipoproteins in plasma. Normally, two functional genes are inherited for LDL-C receptors, one from each parent. Individuals who inherit a single nonfunctional gene (i.e., heterozygotes) synthesize one-half the normal number of LDL-C receptors and their level of LDL-C is approximately twice normal. About 1 in every 500 persons has heterozygous familial hypercholesterolemia, and these individuals are prone to premature (before 65 years of age) coronary artery disease. Much less common is homozygous familial hypercholesterolemia in which abnormal genes for the LDL-C receptors are inherited from both parents; cholesterol levels are approximately four times normal, and very premature atherosclerosis is frequent. Genetic factors besides those involving the primary genes encoding for LDL-C receptors can also reduce the activity of these receptors. In this regard, it is presumed that events, such as increased hepatocyte concentrations of cholesterol or defective transport mechanisms for LDL-C receptors within cells, can result in decreases in the number of functioning LDL-C receptors.[6] Some patients may have abnormal LDL-C that has reduced affinity for receptors. Another cause of elevated LDL-C is increased production of very low density lipoproteins. In addition to genetic factors it is almost certain that diet (excess cholesterol, saturated fatty acids, total calories) often contributes to hypercholesterolemia.

HISTORY

An important goal of the history is to elicit the severity, progression, and functional limitations introduced by coronary artery disease. It must be appreciated that patients can remain asymptomatic despite 50 percent to 70 percent stenosis of a major coronary artery.

An accurate history requires a review of past and current medical records in addition to direct questioning of the patient. Specific areas to be explored in the history taken from patients with coronary artery disease before noncardiac surgery include determination of the (1) cardiac reserve, (2) characteristics of angina pectoris, (3) presence of a prior myocardial infarction, and (4) co-existence of noncardiac diseases. Finally, potential interactions of medications used in the treatment of coronary artery disease with drugs used to produce anesthesia must be considered.

Cardiac Reserve

Specific questions relating to exercise tolerance are essential for evaluating the patient's cardiac reserve. If patients can climb two or three flights of stairs without symptoms, it is likely that cardiac reserve is adequate. Conversely, limited exercise tolerance, in the absence of significant lung disease, is the most striking evidence of reduced cardiac reserve. Dyspnea following the onset of angina pectoris suggests the presence of acute left ventricular dysfunction due to myocardial ischemia. It is important to identify patients bordering on congestive heart failure, as the added stress of anesthesia, surgery, and fluid replacement may result in overt failure.

Angina Pectoris

Angina pectoris is the symptomatic manifestation of myocardial ischemia, which is caused by imbalances between myocardial oxygen supply and demand. Pain characterized as angina pectoris is typically (1) substernal chest pain that may radiate to the left neck and arm, (2) pain initiated by exercise, and (3) pain relieved by rest and/or sublingual nitroglycerin. Esophageal spasm can produce similar pain that is also relieved by the smooth muscle relaxant effects of nitroglycerin. In contrast to angina pectoris, however, pain produced by esophageal spasm rarely radiates to the left arm. Furthermore, pain due to esophageal spasm typically occurs with recumbency.

CHARACTERISTICS OF ANGINA PECTORIS

Preoperatively, it is important to determine the characteristics of angina pectoris. Angina pectoris is considered to be stable when there has been no change for at least 60 days in precipitating factors, frequency, and duration. Chest pain produced with less than normal activity or lasting for more prolonged periods than before is considered to be characteristic of unstable angina pectoris and may signal an impending myocardial infarction.

VASOSPASTIC ANGINA PECTORIS

Vasospastic angina pectoris due to spasm of coronary arteries (variant or Prinzmetal's angina) differs from classic angina pectoris in that it may occur at rest or with ordinary exercise but not during vigorous exertion. Cardiac dysrhythmias are common during chest pain due

to spasm of coronary arteries. Decreases in coronary blood flow during vasospastic angina pectoris seems to be caused by marked increases in tone of smooth muscles in large conduit epicardial coronary arteries. Events that trigger spasm of coronary arteries are not known. The majority of patients with vasospastic angina also have fixed atherosclerotic coronary artery stenoses of varying severity.

TREATMENT OF ANGINA PECTORIS

Treatment of angina pectoris should be based on the pathophysiologic mechanism of anginal syndromes.[11] The principal mechanism for angina pectoris associated with exercise seems to be an inadequate increase in myocardial oxygen delivery. Normally coronary blood flow can increase fourfold to fivefold, which is the principal mechanism to increase myocardial oxygen delivery since the heart already extracts nearly maximal amounts of oxygen. Atherosclerotic plaques interfere with the ability to increase coronary blood flow especially during exercise. Therapy of angina pectoris, therefore, should be directed toward reducing myocardial oxygen requirements. In this regard, nitroglycerin, beta-adrenergic antagonists and calcium entry blockers are effective. There is no conclusive evidence, however, that any particular beta-adrenergic antagonist is superior to the other for the management of angina pectoris associated with exercise.[11] Nitroglycerin or calcium entry blockers are indicated for the treatment of angina pectoris due to spasm of coronary arteries.

RATE-PRESSURE PRODUCT

It has not been documented that anginal thresholds during awake activity are identical to cardiac ischemic thresholds during anesthesia. Nevertheless, knowledge of the heart rate and/or systolic blood pressure at which angina pectoris or evidence of myocardial ischemia occurs on the electrocardiogram is important preoperative information. The product of heart rate and systolic blood pressure is known as the rate–pressure product. In awake

TABLE 1-2. Comparison of Two Patients with Identical Rate-Pressure Products

	Heart Rate (beats·min^{-1})	Systolic Blood Pressure (mmHg)	Rate-Pressure Product
Patient A	120	100	12,000
Patient B	75	160	12,000

Despite identical rate-pressure products, patient A is more likely to develop myocardial ischemia, since the rapid heart rate increases myocardial oxygen requirements and reduces the time for coronary blood flow to occur during diastole. In contrast, in patient B, elevated myocardial oxygen requirements produced by the increased systolic blood pressure are offset by improved perfusion through pressure-dependent coronary arteries, and the likelihood of ischemia is reduced.

patients, it has been demonstrated that angina pectoris occurs at a constant rate–pressure product.[12] It would seem logical not to exceed this product during anesthesia.

Although the rate–pressure product calls attention to the importance of myocardial oxygen requirements, it is more correct to consider the impact of heart rate and blood pressure on myocardial oxygen requirements independently (Table 1-2).[13] For example, an increased heart rate is more likely than hypertension to produce angina pectoris or signs of myocardial ischemia on the electrocardiogram (Fig. 1-3).[14] This is predictable, since rapid heart rates increase myocardial oxygen requirements and reduce the time during diastole for coronary blood flow and thus delivery of oxygen to occur. Conversely, elevated myocardial oxygen requirements produced by increased systolic blood pressure are offset by improved perfusion through pressure-dependent atherosclerotic coronary arteries.

Prior Myocardial Infarction

History of a prior myocardial infarction is important information in the preoperative evaluation. Two retrospective studies of large groups of adult patients have demonstrated that the incidence of myocardial reinfarctions in the perioperative period is related to the time elapsed since the previous myocardial infarctions (Table 1-3).[2,3] In these studies, the incidence of perioperative myocardial reinfarctions did not stabilize at 5 percent to 6 per-

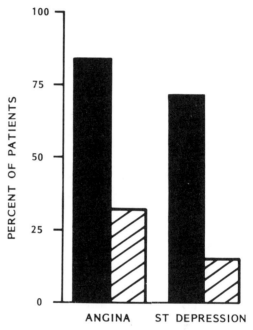

FIG. 1-3. Twenty patients with coronary artery disease were studied during atrial pacing to heart rates of 142 ± 4 beats·min^{-1} (Mean ± SE) and during intravenous infusion of methoxamine to increase systolic blood pressures to 196 ± 5 mmHg. Angina pectoris and depression of ST segments on the electrocardiogram developed in 85 percent and 70 percent of patients respectively during atrial pacing (solid bars). Similar changes developed in only 30 percent and 10 percent respectively during drug-induced hypertension (striped bars). These data demonstrate that stress of tachycardia results in more myocardial ischemia than does stress of increased left ventricular afterload produced by hypertension. (Data adapted from Loeb RP, Talano JV, Klodnycky ML, Gumnar RM. Effects of pharmacologically-induced hypertension or myocardial ischemia and coronary hemodynamics in patients with fixed coronary obstruction. Circulation 1978;57:41–6. By permission of the American Heart Association Inc.)

TABLE 1-3. Incidence of Perioperative Myocardial Reinfarction

Time Elapsed Since Prior Myocardial Infarction	Tarhan et al.[2]	Steen et al.[3]	Rao et al.[15]*
3 months	37%	27%	5.7%
3–6 months	16%	11%	2.3%
6 months	5%	6%	

* Values for Rao et al. are 0 to 3 months and 4 to 6 months, respectively.

cent until 6 months after the prior infarctions. This is the basis for the recommendation that elective operations, especially thoracic and upper abdominal procedures, be delayed for about 6 months after a myocardial infarction. Even after 6 months, the 5 percent to 6 percent incidence of myocardial reinfarctions was about 50 times greater than the 0.13 percent incidence of perioperative myocardial infarctions in patients undergoing similar operations but in the absence of a prior heart attack.

Mortality from myocardial reinfarctions in both these studies was greater than 50 percent, greatly exceeding the mortality of 10 percent to 20 percent observed with myocardial infarctions not associated with operative procedures. It is interesting to note that the incidence of myocardial infarction associated with coronary artery revascularization operations is substantial, but the mortality after these operations is usually less than 3 percent. Presumably, low mortality reflects increased myocardial oxygen delivery to the heart following revascularization. This contrasts with noncardiac surgery's lack of beneficial effects on the heart.

Close hemodynamic monitoring using intra-arterial and pulmonary artery catheters and prompt pharmacologic treatment or fluid infusion to treat hemodynamic alterations from normal ranges have been reported to reduce the risk of perioperative myocardial reinfarctions in high-risk patients.[9] For example, reinfarction rates in closely monitored and promptly treated patients were 5.7 percent and 2.3 percent, when the time elapsed since the prior infarction was up to 3 months and 4 months to 6 months, respectively (Table 1-3).[15] Corresponding mortality rates were 5.3 percent and zero. These myocardial reinfarction rates and mortality rates are substantially lower than those observed by other investigators (Table 1-3).[2,3]

FACTORS THAT INFLUENCE INCIDENCE OF MYOCARDIAL REINFARCTION

The incidence of myocardial reinfarction is increased in patients undergoing intrathoracic or intra-abdominal operations lasting longer than 3 hours (Table 1-4). Systolic blood pressure decreases greater than 30 percent lasting longer than 10 minutes are also associated with an increased incidence of myocardial reinfarction. Likewise, intraoperative hypertension and tachycardia are associated with an increased risk of myocardial reinfarction.[15] There is evidence that intraoperative myocardial ischemia, most often associated with tachycardia, increases the likelihood of postoperative myocardial infarction.[16] The risk of postoperative myocardial infarction following noncardiac surgery is increased in patients with known three-vessel coronary artery disease and in those with left main coronary artery disease.[17] Conversely, the risk of postoperative myocardial infarctions following noncardiac operations in patients with one-vessel or two-

TABLE 1-4. Incidence of Reinfarction

Duration of Operation	Upper Abdominal or Intrathoracic Operations	Other Operative Sites
<3 hours	5.9%	3.6%
>3 hours	15.9%*	3.8%

* P < 0.05 compared with other sites
(Data from Steen PA, Tinker JH, Tarhan S. Myocardial reinfarction after anesthesia and surgery. An update: Incidence, mortality, and predisposing factors. JAMA 1978; 239:2566–70.)

vessel coronary artery disease appears to be relatively low. Likewise, patients who have undergone prior coronary artery bypass graft operations are not at increased cardiac risk when subsequent noncardiac surgery is performed.[17] Factors that have not been shown to predispose to a myocardial reinfarction include the site of the previous myocardial infarction, the site of the operative procedure if the duration of the operation is less than 3 hours, and the drugs and/or techniques (regional vs. general) used to produce anesthesia. Attempts to develop a preoperative list of patient characteristics (age, prior myocardial infarction, aortic stenosis, evidence of congestive heart failure, cardiac dysrhythmias) that allows prediction of life-threatening postoperative complications has not been shown to be superior to the physical status classification of the American Society of Anesthesiologists.[18,19]

Co-Existing Noncardiac Disease

The history obtained from the patient should elicit symptoms and information relevant to co-existing noncardiac diseases. For example, patients with severe coronary artery disease are likely to manifest peripheral vascular disease. Indeed, the history of stroke or syncope should suggest the presence of significant cerebral vascular disease. Chronic obstructive airways disease should be suspected in patients with a history of chronic smoking. Renal dysfunction may be associated with chronic hypertension. Diabetes mellitus is the most likely endocrine disease encountered in patients with coronary artery disease.

CURRENT MEDICATIONS

Medical therapy of coronary artery disease is designed to reduce myocardial oxygen requirements and to improve coronary blood flow. Knowledge of the pharmacology of medications being used to achieve these goals, as well as of the potential adverse effects that can be produced by these drugs during anesthesia, is important information in the preoperative period. Indeed, drugs to be used during the intraoperative period may be determined by medications being administered to the patient preoperatively. Drugs most likely to be encountered in patients with coronary artery disease are beta-adrenergic antagonists and nitrates. In addition, patients with coronary artery disease may be receiving drugs classified as calcium entry blockers, antihypertensives, diuretics, and digitalis.

Beta-Adrenergic Antagonist Drugs

Beta-adrenergic antagonist drugs reduce myocardial oxygen requirements by decreasing heart rate and myocardial contractility (see the section Treatment of Angina Pectoris). Effective beta-adrenergic blockade is probably present when the resting heart rate is 50 beats·min^{-1} to 60 beats·min^{-1}. Routine physical activity should be expected to increase heart rate 10 percent to 20 percent. Patients on optimal doses of beta-adrenergic antagonist drugs have no evidence of congestive heart failure or atrioventricular heart block on the electrocardiogram.

ADVERSE EFFECTS DURING ANESTHESIA

Interactions between beta-adrenergic antagonist drugs and drugs likely to be used during anesthesia are predictable.[20] Knowledge of these interactions makes management of patients being treated with beta-adrenergic antagonist drugs safer. The greatest concern has been the possible exaggerated cardiac depressant effects produced by volatile anesthetics administered in the presence of beta-adrenergic blockade. Indeed, in dogs, cardiac depressant effects of halothane and propranolol are additive.[21] For example, cardiac depression in the presence of propranolol and 1 percent in-spired halothane is similar to that depression produced by 1.5 percent inspired halothane. This additive myocardial depression is not considered to be excessive or dangerous. Sim-ilar studies suggest that isoflurane is more compatible with beta-adrenergic blockade than halothane,[22] whereas cardiac depression pro-duced by enflurane plus propranolol[23] is greater than that observed during beta-adre-nergic blockade and halothane. Despite these differences, there is no clinical experience to support preferential selection of specific vol-atile anesthetics for administration to patients being treated with beta-adrenergic antagonist drugs. Indeed, the overwhelming evidence is that beta-adrenergic antagonist drugs (specifi-cally propranolol) do not increase the oper-ative risk and should not be discontinued preoperatively.[24] In fact, beta-adrenergic antagonist drugs being administered to pa-tients on a chronic basis are often included with the preoperative medication. Finally, there is no evidence of adverse interactions be-tween opioids and propranolol.[20]

The postoperative period is a time when inadvertent acute withdrawal of therapy with beta-adrenergic antagonist drugs may occur. Since adverse rebound phenomenon can occur within 24 hours after withdrawal of these drugs, it is important that postoperative pa-tients be returned to maintenance doses of beta-adrenergic antagonist drugs as soon as possible.

ANTAGONISM OF BRADYCARDIA AND HYPOTENSION DUE TO BETA-ADRENERGIC BLOCKADE

Several drugs can counteract the negative chronotropic and negative inotropic effects of beta-adrenergic blockade should these changes manifest in the perioperative period. Of these, atropine and beta-adrenergic agonists are the most effective and should be readily available for treatment of bradycardia or hypotension that may develop during administration of anesthesia to patients who are receiving beta-adrenergic antagonist drugs.

Atropine is the drug of choice when brady-cardia due to beta-adrenergic blockade devel-

ops. The dose is 0.4 mg to 0.6 mg administered intravenously up to a total dose of 2 mg to 3 mg. Atropine is effective because its vagolytic effects allow residual sympathetic nervous sys-tem innervation of the heart to emerge.

Isoproterenol is a pure beta-adrenergic agonist drug and, as such, is the specific phar-macologic antagonist for propranolol and re-lated beta-adrenergic antagonist drugs. Isopro-terenol must be given as a continuous intravenous infusion starting with 2 $\mu g \cdot min^{-1}$ to 5 $\mu g \cdot min^{-1}$ and adjusting the infusion rate to obtain the desired heart rate and blood pres-sure responses. Depending on the magnitude of beta-adrenergic blockade, large doses of iso-proterenol may be necessary. Dobutamine is also an effective catecholamine for reversal of adverse cardiac effects due to beta-adrenergic blockade. High doses of dopamine, as may be required to antagonize beta-adrenergic block-ade, could result in undesirable increases in systemic vascular resistance due to relatively unopposed alpha-adrenergic stimulation.

Calcium works at areas other than beta-adrenergic receptors to increase myocardial contractility in the presence of beta-adrenergic blockade. In contrast with isoproterenol, since calcium does not act on beta-adrenergic recep-tors, it is predictable that conventional doses of this drug (500 mg to 1000 mg of calcium chloride or gluconate administered intrave-nously over 10 minutes to 20 minutes) will be effective. Aminophylline (4 $mg \cdot kg^{-1}$ to 6 $mg \cdot kg^{-1}$ administered intravenously over 15 minutes) is effective in reversing beta-adrener-gic blockade, particularly when this drug is combined with beta-adrenergic agonist drugs. Digitalis may be administered to treat reduc-tions in myocardial contractility, assuming that bradycardia or atrioventricular heart block are not complicating beta-adrenergic blockade. Glucagon (5 mg to 10 mg) administered intra-venously followed by a continuous infusion of 1 $mg \cdot min^{-1}$ may be effective in some patients.

HYPOTENSION DUE TO OVERDOSE OF ANESTHETIC

Treatment of hypotension due to over-doses of anesthetic drugs has special impli-cations in patients who are also being treated with beta-adrenergic antagonist drugs. Theoretically, the beta-blocked and anesthetic-depressed myocardium might not tolerate increases in ventricular afterload due to drug-induced elevations in systemic vascular resistance (Fig. 1-4). Indeed, in healthy volunteers, the administration of phenylephrine to correct halothane-induced reductions in blood pressure results in decreases in cardiac output and elevations in pulmonary artery occlusion pressure.[25] Conceivably, this response would be even greater in the presence of co-existing beta-adrenergic blockade. Therefore, selection of sympathomimetic drugs with beta-agonist as well as alpha-agonist properties would seem to be the logical choice to treat reductions in perfusion pressure due to anesthetic-produced myocardial depression in the presence of beta-adrenergic blockade. With this goal in mind, ephedrine might be a more logical selection than either phenylephrine or methoxamine. Nevertheless, co-existing beta-adrenergic blockade would likely blunt beta agonist effects of ephedrine resulting in a predominance of alpha-adrenergic effects after administration of this drug.

Nitrates

The ability of nitroglycerin to reduce myocardial oxygen requirements is the most likely mechanism by which this drug relieves angina pectoris in patients with coronary artery disease. For example, nitroglycerin-induced venodilation and increased venous capacitance decreases venous return to the heart (e.g., preload), resulting in reduced ventricular end-diastolic pressures and volumes and, therefore, decreased myocardial oxygen requirements. The ability of nitroglycerin to dilate selectively large coronary arteries may be an important mechanism in the relief of vasospastic angina. Nitroglycerin, however, does not dilate coronary arterioles.

Calcium Entry Blockers

Calcium entry blockers are thought to act by interfering with calcium ion movement through channels present in excitable cell

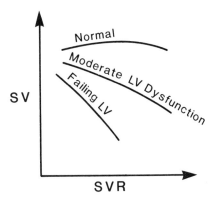

FIG. 1-4. Increasing vascular resistance to ejection of blood from the left ventricle (LV) into the systemic circulation (SVR or afterload) has little impact or stroke volume (SV) in patients with normal LV function. Conversely, increases in SVR occurring in the presence of moderate to severe (failing) LV dysfunction are accompanied by corresponding reductions in SV.

membranes. This ion movement is responsible for phase 2 of the action potential in excitable cell membranes, as well as phase 4 of the action potential in sinoatrial and atrioventricular nodal tissues (see Chapter 4). These ion channels through which calcium moves are referred to as slow channels in contrast to fast sodium channels, which are responsible for the rapid phase 0 and phase 1 depolarization: hence, the designation of calcium entry blockers as slow channel blockers.

Drugs that alter ion movement across slow channels predictably possess negative chronotropic, negative dromotropic (conduction velocity), negative inotropic, and vasodilating effects.[26] The relative potency of calcium entry blockers differs among the drugs tested. For example, verapamil decreases heart rate and conduction velocity of cardiac impulses more than it does contractile or smooth muscle function. Indeed, a major disadvantage of verapamil is the production of atrioventricular heart block. Nifedipine, in contrast to verapamil, is equally potent for all four pharmacologic effects produced by calcium entry blockers and is less likely to produce atrioventricular heart block. The negative inotropic and vasodilating effects of verapamil and nifedipine seem similar. Two indications for calcium entry blockers are treatment of supraventricular tachy-dysrhythmias (see Chapter 4) and management of ischemic heart disease, particularly angina pectoris, due to spasm of the coronary arteries.

Treatment of patients with calcium entry blockers may introduce the potential for adverse drug interactions during the perioperative period.[26] This prediction is based on the knowledge that calcium ions are necessary for functioning of myocardial, skeletal, and vascular smooth muscle. For example, myocardial depression and peripheral vasodilation produced by volatile anesthetics could be exaggerated by similar actions of calcium entry blockers. Despite these theoretical concerns, only additive, and not synergistic, cardiac depression seems to occur when patients with normal left ventricular function being treated chronically with calcium entry blockers and beta-adrenergic antagonist drugs receive volatile anesthetics.[27-29] Treatment of cardiac dysrhythmias with calcium entry blockers in patients anesthetized with halothane produces only transient reductions in blood pressure and infrequent prolongation of P–R intervals on the electrocardiogram. Because of the tendency to produce atrioventricular heart block, verapamil should be used cautiously in patients receiving digitalis or beta-adrenergic antagonist drugs. Nevertheless, in patients without preoperative evidence of cardiac conduction abnormalities, the chronic combined administration of calcium entry blockers and beta-adrenergic antagonist drugs is not associated with cardiac conduction abnormalities in the perioperative period.[30] It would seem prudent, however, to titrate doses of calcium entry blockers administered to patients with co-existing cardiac conduction abnormalities. Correction of hypotension or bradycardia due to calcium entry blockers includes the intravenous administration of atropine, isoproterenol, and calcium. Calcium entry blockers may potentiate the effects of depolarizing and nondepolarizing muscle relaxants and exaggerate disease states associated with skeletal muscle weakness.[31] Antagonism of neuromuscular blockade may be impaired because of diminished presynaptic release of acetylcholine in the presence of a calcium entry blocker.[32]

Antihypertensive Drugs

Antihypertensive drugs, like beta-adrenergic antagonists, should be maintained throughout the perioperative period. Nevertheless, it is important to be familiar with unique adverse effects produced by antihypertensive drugs, as well as with the impact of reduced sympathetic nervous system activity on cardiovascular compensatory responses in the perioperative period (see Chapter 6).

Diuretics

The major concern in patients receiving chronic diuretic therapy is hypokalemia. Elective operations are often discouraged when the preoperative plasma potassium concentrations are below 3.5 $mEq \cdot L^{-1}$ and some would recommend not performing surgery when the plasma potassium concentrations are below 3.0 $mEq \cdot L^{-1}$. This concern is based on the possibility of an increased incidence of cardiac dysrhythmias and unpredictable responses to nondepolarizing muscle relaxants in the presence of hypokalemia. Nevertheless, the incidence of cardiac dysrhythmias has not been documented to increase in chronically hypokalemic patients (plasma concentrations 2.6 $mEq \cdot L^{-1}$ to 3.4 $mEq \cdot L^{-1}$) undergoing elective operations[33] (see Chapter 22). It must be appreciated that reductions in total body potassium stores may not correlate with plasma potassium concentrations, nor can these stores be predictably corrected in 24 hours to 48 hours preceding surgery (see Chapter 22).

Diuretics, when given acutely, can reduce the intravascular fluid volume. This drug-induced hypovolemia has obvious implications for the management of anesthesia. Nevertheless, intravascular fluid volume is usually restored in the presence of chronic diuretic therapy, suggesting that perioperative responses consistent with hypovolemia are not necessarily due to this form of therapy.

Digitalis

Digitalis may be continued throughout the perioperative period, particularly if the drug is being administered for control of heart rate. It is mandatory, however, to elicit signs and symptoms of digitalis toxicity in the preoperative evaluation of any patient with a history of digitalis therapy (see Chapter 7). Furthermore, it must be appreciated that sympathetic nervous system stimulation and electrolyte shifts that accompany surgery and anesthesia will predispose to digitalis toxicity.

PHYSICAL EXAMINATION

The physical examination is frequently normal despite significant coronary artery disease. Nevertheless, signs of incipient left ventricular failure must be recognized (see Chapter 7). Carotid bruits may indicate previously unrecognized cerebral vascular disease. Orthostatic hypotension may reflect attenuated autonomic nervous system activity due to treatment with antihypertensive drugs. Evaluation of the upper airway and anticipated ease of tracheal intubation, accessibility of peripheral venous sites, and determination of collateral blood flow if cannulation of a peripheral artery for intraoperative monitoring is planned are important aspects of the preoperative physical examination.

ELECTROCARDIOGRAM

Review of the resting electrocardiogram is a fundamental aspect of the preoperative evaluation of patients with coronary artery disease. It is important to remember that a resting electrocardiogram, in the absence of chest pain, may be normal despite extensive coronary artery disease. Nevertheless, an electrocardiogram demonstrating ST segment depression greater than 1 mm, particularly during angina

pectoris, confirms the presence of subendocardial myocardial ischemia. Furthermore, the electrocardiogram lead demonstrating the changes of myocardial ischemia can help determine the specific coronary artery that is diseased (Table 1-5).

The most accepted criterion for an ischemic response on the exercise electrocardiogram is ST segment depression of 1 mm or more in patients in whom ST segments were isoelectric at rest. The exercise electrocardiogram of patients with narrowing of the left main coronary artery can show more than 2 mm of ST segment depression, often in association with angina pectoris, cardiac dysrhythmias, or hypotension. A decrease in blood pressure during exercise-induced ST segment depression suggests that a large portion of the myocardium is ischemic, and increases the likelihood that three-vessel or left main coronary artery disease is present. It is estimated that narrowing of a major coronary artery by more than 50 percent (flow is proportional to the fourth power of the radius) will be associated with inadequate oxygen delivery during periods of increased myocardial oxygen demand, as associated with exercise-induced hypertension and tachycardia. In this regard, the electrocardiogram during exercise simulates the sympathetic nervous stimulation that may accompany perioperative events such as laryngoscopy and surgical stimulation. Certainly, a normal electrocardiogram during exercise indicates that the coronary circulation is reasonably adequate. Nevertheless, approximately 10 percent of the adult population with normal coronary arteries can show ST segment changes on the electrocardiogram during exercise that resemble mild changes observed in patients with coronary artery disease. For this reason, use of exercise electrocardiography in asymptomatic patients is of doubtful value.

Vasospastic angina pectoris is characterized by ST segment elevation on the electrocardiogram during periods of myocardial ischemia. The presence of ST segment elevation implies extensive transmural myocardial ischemia in contrast to ST segment depression associated with subendocardial myocardial ischemia.

In addition to signs of myocardial ischemia, the preoperative electrocardiogram

TABLE 1-5. Relationship of Electrocardiogram Lead Reflecting Myocardial Ischemia to Area of Myocardium Involved

Electrocardiogram Lead	Coronary Artery Branch Responsible for Ischemia	Area of Myocardium that May Be Involved
II, III, aVF	Right coronary artery	Right atrium Interatrial septum Right ventricle Sinoatrial node Atrioventricular node Posterior fascicle of left bundle Posterior one-third of interventricular septum Posterior papillary muscle
V3–V5	Left anterior descending coronary artery	Anterolateral aspects of left ventricle Right bundle branch Anterior fascicle of left bundle Posterior fascicle of left bundle Anterior two-thirds of interventricular septum Anterior papillary muscle Posterior papillary muscle
I, aVL	Circumflex coronary artery	Lateral aspects of left ventricle Sinoatrial node Atrioventricular node Posterior fascicle of left bundle

should be examined for evidence of (1) a prior myocardial infarction, (2) cardiac hypertrophy, (3) abnormal cardiac rhythm and/or conduction disturbances, and (4) electrolyte abnormalities. It should be remembered that prior myocardial infarctions, especially if subendocardial, may not be accompanied by persistent changes on the electrocardiogram. The presence of premature ventricular beats may signal their likely occurrence intraoperatively. P-R intervals greater than 0.2 second are most often related to digitalis therapy. Blocks of conduction of the cardiac impulses that occur below the atrioventricular node most likely reflect pathologic changes rather than drug effect.

RADIOGRAPHS OF THE CHEST

Specific findings related to coronary artery disease are unlikely to be present on radiographs of the chest. Routinely, radiographs should be reviewed for evidence of cardiomegaly and congestive heart failure. Chronic pulmonary disease is suggested by the presence of hyperinflation of the lungs and a depressed diaphragm.

RADIOISOTOPE IMAGING

Radioisotope imaging requires intravenous injection of gamma-emitting radiopharmaceuticals that permit the imaging of blood within the heart and lungs. Scanning of myocardial perfusion using radioactive thallium provides a method for visualizing blood flow to the left ventricle. An area of decreased perfusion (cold spot) that appears only during exercise indicates ischemia, whereas a constant perfusion defect suggests an old myocardial infarction. Technetium, which accumulates in areas of acute myocardial necrosis, is a useful isotope test, especially when the diagnosis of myocardial infarction is equivocal. This preference for technetium is due to the abundance of free calcium in necrotic cells. Myocardial scintillation counting with thallium will detect a myocardial infarction almost immediately, but with technetium there will be a delay of 24 hours to 72 hours before detection of necrosis. Technetium scanning techniques can be used to measure left ventricular ejection fractions.

CARDIAC CATHETERIZATION AND ANGIOGRAPHY

Cardiac catheterization and angiography are highly specialized tests, which are not routinely performed or even indicated in most patients before noncardiac surgery. When available, however, these data provide objective evidence of left ventricular function and facilitate prediction of the patient's response to the stresses of anesthesia and operation. For example, left ventricular function can be classified as good or impaired based on the history, physical examination, and measurements obtained during cardiac catheterization (ejection fraction, left ventricular end-diastolic pressure, cardiac output, and assessment of ventricular wall motion) (Table 1-6).

Ejection Fraction

The ejection fraction equals the stroke volume divided by the end-diastolic volume. Stroke volume is the difference between the

end-diastolic volume and end-systolic volume. As such, ejection fractions may be useful indicators of ventricular function. Ejection fractions can be measured by isotope imaging angiography or echocardiography.

A normally contracting left ventricle will eject 55 percent to 75 percent (ejection fraction 0.55 to 0.75) of its end-diastolic volume as stroke volume with each cardiac contraction. Ejection fractions of 0.4 to 0.55 are common in patients with decreased myocardial contractility due to a prior myocardial infarction or increased left ventricular afterload in association with essential hypertension. Patients with ejection fractions in this range are usually asymptomatic. Symptoms of reduced cardiac reserve are likely to manifest during exercise when ejection fractions are 0.25 to 0.4. When ejection fractions are less than 0.25, it is likely that patients will be symptomatic at rest (New York Heart Association Class IV). It is predictable that the stress of anesthesia and operation will be poorly tolerated by patients with this degree of left ventricular dysfunction.

Left Ventricular End-Diastolic Pressure

A failing left ventricle is unable to empty adequately in systole, such that left ventricular end-diastolic volumes and pressures increase. In addition to end-diastolic volumes, end-diastolic pressures can be influenced by the compliance of the left ventricular muscle. Thus, elevated left ventricular end-diastolic pressures may reflect increased end-diastolic volumes, decreased compliance of the ventricle, or both. In the absence of mitral valve disease, mean left atrial pressures and pulmonary artery occlusion pressures reflect left ventricular end-diastolic pressures.

Normal left ventricular end-diastolic pressures are 12 mmHg or less. Corresponding normal values for the right ventricular end-diastolic pressures are 5 mmHg or less. Resting left ventricular end-diastolic pressures greater than 18 mmHg imply significantly reduced left ventricular contractility. However, with bed

TABLE 1-6. Evaluation of Left Ventricular Function

Good Function	Impaired Function
History and Physical Examination	
Angina pectoris	Prior myocardial infarction
Essential hypertension	
No evidence of congestive heart failure	Evidence of congestive heart failure
Cardiac Catheterization	
Ejection fraction > 0.55	Ejection fraction < 0.4
Left ventricular end-diastolic pressure < 12 mmHg	Left ventricular end-diastolic pressure > 18 mmHg
Cardiac index > 2.5 $L \cdot min^{-1} \cdot m^{-2}$	Cardiac index < 2 $L \cdot min^{-1} \cdot m^{-2}$
No areas of ventricular dyskinesia	Multiple areas of ventricular dyskinesia

rest, fluid restriction, and diuretics, this value may be normal despite the continued presence of severe left ventricular dysfunction. Under these circumstances, large increases in left ventricular end-diastolic pressures, following injection of the contrast medium during cardiac angiography, may indicate poor left ventricular responses to stress. Interpretation of left ventricular end-diastolic pressures must be made with the patient's exercise tolerance in mind.

Cardiac Index

A normal resting cardiac index is 2.5 $L \cdot min^{-1} \cdot m^{-2}$ to 3.5 $L \cdot min^{-1} \cdot m^{-2}$. Patients with left ventricular dysfunction can have normal resting cardiac outputs but be unable to increase flow in response to stress or exercise. A cardiac index below 2 $L \cdot min^{-1} \cdot m^{-2}$ in patients with coronary artery disease implies severe left ventricular dysfunction. Reductions in cardiac output may be associated with increased arterial to venous oxygen differences, as tissues continue to require the same amount of oxygen but must extract this oxygen from a reduced blood flow.

Angiography

The ventriculogram allows classification of left ventricular wall motion as normal, decreased (hypokinesia), absent (akinesia), or paradoxical (dyskinesia). A description of the filling of the coronary arteries during angiography should also be reviewed, keeping in mind the anatomy of the blood supply to certain special areas of the heart (Table 1-5). Patients with significant obstruction of the left anterior descending coronary artery are considered to be at increased risk during the perioperative period, since this vessel supplies a large portion of the left ventricle. Furthermore, the risk of myocardial infarction during and after noncardiac surgery is increased in patients with three-vessel coronary artery disease demonstrated on coronary angiography.[17] The

artery that supplies the atrioventricular node, as determined at cardiac catheterization, is designated the dominant artery.

ANATOMY AND PHYSIOLOGY OF THE CORONARY CIRCULATION

The arterial blood supply of the heart is derived from the left and right coronary arteries that arise from the sinuses of Valsalva located behind the cusps of the aortic valve at the root of the aorta (Fig. 1-5) (Table 1-5). Anatomically, these coronary arteries and their branches traverse the epicardial surface serving as conductance vessels offering little resistance to blood flow. Conversely, small coronary arterioles that ramify throughout cardiac muscle impose a highly variable resistance to blood flow and thus regulate distribution of coronary blood flow.[34] Coronary artery disease involves large epicardial coronary arteries and not arterioles. Furthermore, obstruction to blood flow in coronary arterioles may be fixed or dynamic changing with underlying smooth muscle tone in the blood vessels.

Resting coronary blood flow is about 80 $ml \cdot 100 \ g^{-1} \cdot min^{-1}$, which in an adult heart weighing 300 g is equivalent to 3 percent to 5 percent of the cardiac output. Most of the venous blood that has perfused the left ventricle enters the right atrium via the coronary sinus, whereas the majority of coronary blood flow to the right ventricle enters anterior cardiac veins that empty into the right atrium independent of the coronary sinus. Resting myocardial oxygen consumption is 8 $ml \cdot 100 \ g^{-1} \cdot min^{-1}$ to 10 $ml \cdot 100 \ g^{-1} \cdot min^{-1}$ or about 10 percent of the total body consumption of oxygen. Coronary arteries receive innervation from parasympathetic (vagus and cardiac plexus at the base of the aorta) and sympathetic fibers (stellate ganglion) and beta-1, beta-2, and alpha-2 receptors are present in vascular walls. Histamine receptors are also distributed in the coronary arteries with stimulation of histamine-1 receptors producing vasoconstriction and stimulation of histamine-2 receptors producing vasodila-

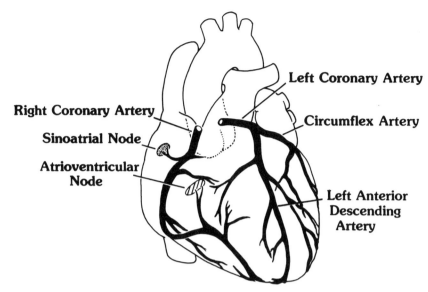

FIG. 1-5. Diagram of the arterial circulation of the heart. The right and left coronary arteries arise distal to the aortic valve in the sinus of Valsalva. The right coronary artery runs in the atrioventricular groove toward the posterior surface of the heart. The left coronary artery divides into the left anterior descending artery and the circumflex artery. The left anterior descending artery runs downward to the cardiac apex, and the circumflex artery winds around the left side of the heart in the atrioventricular groove.

tion.[35] Inclusion of H-2 antagonists in the preoperative medication would have the theoretical possibility of leaving histamine-1 receptor mediated coronary artery vasoconstriction unopposed. This is analogous to leaving histamine-1 receptor mediated bronchoconstriction unopposed when histamine-2 receptors in the airways are blocked.

His. Occlusion of the right coronary artery can lead to infarction of the sinoatrial node and atrial dysrhythmias. Third-degree atrioventricular heart block is a complication of infarction of the atrioventricular node. Ischemia of the atrioventricular node, however, is often transient, as its collateral blood supply is more adequate than that of the sinoatrial node.

Right Coronary Artery

The right coronary artery travels in the atrioventricular groove toward the posterior surface of the heart, giving off branches that supply the right atrium, interatrial septum, right ventricle, and posterior one-third of the interventricular septum. A branch of the right coronary artery supplies the sinoatrial node in 55 percent of individuals and another distal branch supplies the atrioventricular node in 90 percent. Branches of the proximal and distal right coronary artery also supply the bundle of

Left Coronary Artery

The left coronary artery divides into the left anterior descending coronary artery and the circumflex coronary artery. Branches of the left anterior descending coronary artery provide the blood supply to the anterolateral aspects of the left ventricle, the right bundle branch, the anterior fascicle of the left bundle branch, and the anterior two-thirds of the interventricular septum. Branches of the circumflex coronary artery supply blood to the lateral aspects of the left ventricle. A branch of the circumflex coronary artery also supplies the sinoatrial and atrioventricular nodes when these structures are not supplied by the right coronary artery. The posterior fascicle of the left bundle branch is supplied by branches from all three main coronary arteries.

Blood Supply to Papillary Muscles

Blood supply to papillary muscles deserves special consideration, since these muscles are vital to the competence of the mitral valve. The anterior papillary muscle is usually supplied by branches of the left coronary artery; the posterior papillary muscle typically receives blood flow from both the left and right coronary arteries. Nevertheless, collateral blood supply to the papillary muscles is well developed, so that occlusion of a single coronary artery does not usually cause infarction of a papillary muscle. Severe ischemia, however, may produce dysfunction of papillary muscles, leading to acute mitral regurgitation. Prompt treatment of ischemia, as with nitroglycerin, usually results in reversal of mitral valve dysfunction.

Unique Features of Coronary Blood Flow

Unique features of coronary blood flow include absence of anastomoses between the left and right coronary arteries and interruption of blood flow to the left ventricle during systole due to mechanical compression of vessels by myocardial contraction. Coronary blood flow to the right ventricle is less influenced by systole since pressures in the right ventricle are lower and less likely to compress intramyocardial vessels. Increased intracavitary pressures in the left ventricle, such as those due to elevations of ventricular end-diastolic volume or pressure, compresses subendocardial vessels and impairs blood flow to the subendocardium (Fig. 1-6). Indeed, the subendocardial region of the left ventricle is the most common site for myocardial infarction. An estimated 70 percent to 85 perecent of the coronary blood flow to the left ventricle occurs during diastole when compression of vessels by myocardial contraction is minimal. Tachycardia with associated decreases in the time for coronary blood flow to occur during diastole jeopardizes the adequacy of myocardial oxygen delivery, particularly if coronary arteries are narrowed by atherosclerosis. The impact of systole on coronary blood flow through the right ventricle

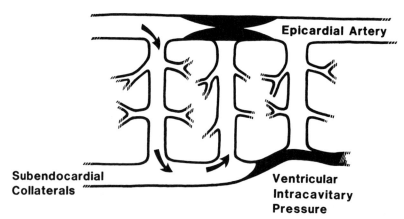

FIG. 1-6. Schematic diagram of a cross-section of the ventricular myocardium showing the impact of ventricular intracavitary pressures on subendocardial blood flow. An increase in pressure can compress subendocardial vessels and produce subendocardial ischemia. Likewise, compression of these vessels may eliminate collateral blood flow around an area of atherosclerosis in epicardial coronary arteries.

is minimal. This reflects the fact that pressure in the coronary arteries is greater than the intracavitary pressure developed in the right ventricle.

Coronary blood flow is determined almost entirely by vascular responses to local needs of cardiac muscle for nutrients, especially oxygen. Oxygen extraction by cardiac cells is nearly maximal, emphasizing that increased myocardial oxygen requirements are primarily met by increased coronary blood flow. Perfusion pressure is particularly important in maintaining coronary blood flow through atherosclerotic arteries that cannot dilate in response to autoregulatory mechanisms (e.g., pressure-dependent perfusion) (Fig. 1-7).[36]

Coronary Artery Steal

Coronary artery steal refers to diversion of blood flow from one area of myocardium to another area. Diversion of blood flow from one coronary artery branch to another represents intercoronary steal, whereas diversion of blood flow from subendocardial to subepicardial

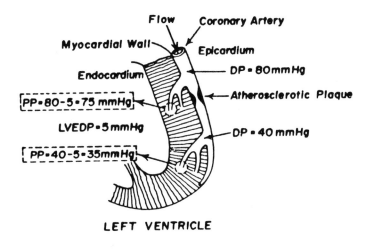

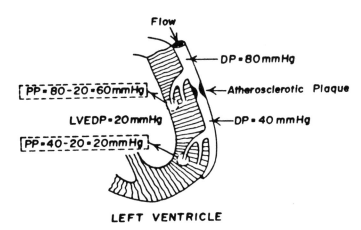

FIG. 1-7. Perfusion pressure (PP) in normal coronary arteries equals diastolic blood pressure (DP) minus left ventricular end-diastolic pressure (LVEDP). An atherosclerotic plaque decreases PP distal to the plaque (upper panel). Likewise, increases in LVEDP reduce PP (lower panel) (Shepherd JT, Vanhoutte PM. The human cardiovascular system: Facts and concepts. New York, Raven Press, 1979, p 222.)

areas is transmural steal. Conceptually, coronary arterioles in areas of myocardium vulnerable to myocardial ischemia (i.e., collateral flow-dependent areas) might be fully dilated to compensate for increased resistance to blood flow imposed by narrowed atherosclerotic vessels. Drug-induced vasodilation of normal coronary arterioles might then divert blood flow from fully dilated coronary arterioles served by arteriosclerotic vessels to these normal arterioles capable of vasodilation (i.e., coronary artery steal). Drugs capable of producing coronary artery steal and signs of regional myocardial ischemia include nitroprusside, papaverine, dipyridamole and adenosine. Among inhaled anesthetics, there is animal evidence that isoflurane, but not halothane, is a potent vasodilator of coronaryarterioles capable of producing coronary artery steal[37-39] (see the section Management of Anesthesia). The likelihood that drug-induced coronary artery steal and subsequent myocardial ischemia will occur in individual patients is dependent on a number of variables including (1) associated reductions in coronary perfusion pressure; (2) degree of coronary artery stenosis; (3) dynamic vs. fixed coronary artery stenosis; (4) single vs. multiple vessel disease; (5) immature vs. well-developed collaterals; and (6) co-existing myocardial oxygen requirements as determined by blood pressure, heart rate, preload, and afterload.[39] Factors that determine myocardial oxygen requirements and delivery may be influenced by concomitant use of beta-adrenergic antagonist drugs, inclusion of opioids in the drugs administered during anesthesia, and use of high inspired concentrations of oxygen made possible by avoiding the use of nitrous oxide.

MANAGEMENT OF ANESTHESIA

Management of anesthesia for patients with coronary artery disease undergoing noncardiac surgery can be considered from the aspects of preoperative medication and of the induction and maintenance of anesthesia. Optimal patient care in each of these areas is based on an understanding of the determinants of myocardial oxygen delivery relative to myocardial oxygen requirements (Table 1-7).

Myocardial Oxygen Delivery

Myocardial oxygen delivery is determined by coronary blood flow and oxygen content of the coronary artery blood. Coronary blood flow is directly proportional to the coronary perfusion pressure (diastolic blood pressure minus left ventricular end-diastolic pressure) and perfusion time (duration of diastole) and inversely related to coronary vascular resistance. Coronary vascular resistance is influenced by local metabolic factors such as oxygenation of myocardial muscle, viscosity of the blood, activity of the autonomic nervous system, and the patency of the coronary arteries. Autoregulation of coronary blood flow occurs by changes in coronary vascular resistance due to alterations in local metabolic requirements.

TABLE 1-7. Intraoperative Events that Influence Balance Between Myocardial Oxygen Delivery and Myocardial Oxygen Requirements

Decreased Oxygen Delivery	Increased Oxygen Requirements
Decreased coronary blood flow	Sympathetic nervous system stimulation
Tachycardia	Tachycardia
Diastolic hypotension	Systolic hypertension
Hypocapnia (coronary vasoconstriction)	Increased myocardial contractility
Coronary artery spasm	Increased afterload
Decreased oxygen content	
Anemia	
Arterial hypoxemia	
Shift of oxyhemoglobin dissociation curve to the left	
Increased preload (wall tension)	

In the presence of coronary atherosclerosis, however, changes in coronary vascular resistance cannot occur, and coronary blood flow becomes entirely pressure dependent (Fig. 1-7).[36] Oxygen content of arterial blood delivered to the heart is determined by the hemoglobin concentration and arterial oxygen saturation. Arterial oxygen saturation is influenced by arterial partial pressures of oxygen and the position of the oxyhemoglobin dissociation curve as reflected by the P-50. In the absence of arterial hypoxemia and anemia, it is difficult to increase delivery of oxygen to the myocardium via the oxygen-carrying capacity of the arterial blood. This is true because the heart maximally extracts the oxygen delivered to it by the coronary blood flow.

Myocardial Oxygen Requirements

Myocardial oxygen requirements are determined by heart rate, systemic blood pressure (afterload), ventricular volume (preload or venous return), and myocardial contractility. Activity of the sympathetic nervous system plays an important role in the regulation of those events that influence myocardial oxygen requirements. As stated earlier, increases in heart rate are more likely to produce myocardial ischemia than are elevations in systemic blood pressure (Table 1-2).[14] In contrast to determinants of myocardial oxygen delivery, factors that influence myocardial oxygen requirements can be predictably influenced by drugs administered in the perioperative period.

Preoperative Medication

The primary goal of preoperative medication for patients with coronary artery disease is to reduce anxiety. Anxiety can lead to secretion of catecholamines, manifested as elevations of blood pressure and heart rate. As a result of these changes, myocardial oxygen requirements are predictably increased. Indeed, patients with coronary artery disease often arrive in the operating room with evidence of myocardial ischemia on the electrocardiogram compared with the preoperative electrocardiogram.[16] It is not clear, however, whether these episodes of myocardial ischemia differ from those that may occur in these same patients during their daily lives unassociated with angina or hemodynamic changes.[40]

Anxiety reduction requires both psychologic and pharmacologic approaches. Patients arrive in the operating room in more relaxed states if they have been visited preoperatively and had the anesthetic sequence explained to them in detail. Pharmacologic sedation can be achieved with a wide variety of drugs or combinations of drugs; what is used often depends on the personal preference of the individual responsible for the management of anesthesia. The goal of drug administration is to produce maximum sedation and amnesia without undesirable degrees of circulatory and ventilatory depression. One useful approach to preoperative medication for patients with coronary artery disease is administration of intramuscular morphine (10 mg to 15 mg) plus scopolamine (0.4 mg to 0.6 mg), with or without benzodiazepines. Scopolamine is valuable because of its profound sedative and amnesic effects without producing undesirable changes in heart rate. Drugs used in the treatment of patients with coronary artery disease should be continued throughout the perioperative period including, in some instances, administration of these drugs with the preoperative medication (see the section Current Medications).[24,30] It is convincingly documented that abrupt withdrawal of beta-adrenergic antagonist drugs and antihypertensive drugs may result in excessive increases in sympathetic nervous system activity. This increased sympathetic nervous system activity is particularly undesirable in patients with coronary artery disease. It may also be appropriate to apply nitroglycerin ointment at the same time the preoperative medication is administered. Certainly, patients should have access to sublingual nitroglycerin in the period preceding the induction of anesthesia. Administration of H-2 receptor antagonists to elevate gastric fluid pH does not appear to produce adverse effects in patients with coronary artery disease, although these drugs have the theoretic ability to contribute to coronary artery vasoconstriction by virtue of leaving H1-mediated constricting effects relatively unopposed.

Intraoperative Management

The basic challenge during induction and maintenance of anesthesia for patients with coronary artery disease is to prevent myocardial ischemia. This goal is logically achieved by maintaining the balance between myocardial oxygen delivery and myocardial oxygen requirements. Intraoperative events associated with persistent tachycardia, systolic hypertension, sympathetic nervous system stimulation, arterial hypoxemia, or diastolic hypotension can adversely influence this delicate balance (Table 1-7). Iatrogenic hyperventilation of the lungs that greatly reduces arterial partial pressures of carbon dioxide are avoided, as hypocapnia has been stated to evoke coronary artery vasoconstriction. In the final analysis, maintenance of this balance is probably more important than the specific techniques and/or drugs chosen to produce anesthesia and skeletal muscle relaxation. It is critical that persistent and excessive changes in heart rate and blood pressure be avoided. A reasonable recommendation is to maintain heart rate and blood pressure within 20 percent of awake values. Nevertheless, an estimated one-half of the new ischemic episodes observed before cardiopulmonary bypass are not preceded by or associated with significant changes in blood pressure or heart rate.[40] In this regard, as many as one-half of all episodes of perioperative ischemia may not be preventable by providing optimal hemodynamic indices of myocardial oxygen supply and demand.[40] Furthermore, as many as 45 percent of patients show evidence of myocardial ischemia by thallium scan in the absence of hemodynamic changes during intubation of the trachea.[40,41] It is likely these episodes of silent myocardial ischemia are due to regional reductions in myocardial perfusion and oxygenation that are of questionable significance and identical to episodes that occur in these same patients during their daily activity unassociated with angina pectoris.

INDUCTION OF ANESTHESIA

Induction of anesthesia in patients with coronary artery disease can be acceptably accomplished with intravenous administration of barbiturates, benzodiazepine 3, opioids, or etomidate. Ketamine is not popular, since associated increases in heart rate and blood pressure would likely increase myocardial oxygen requirements. Intubation of the trachea is facilitated by the administration of succinylcholine or nondepolarizing muscle relaxants.

Myocardial ischemia can accompany sympathetic nervous system stimulation that results from direct laryngoscopy and intubation of the trachea.[42] A short duration of direct laryngoscopy (ideally less than 15 seconds) is important in minimizing the magnitude and duration of circulatory stimulation associated with intubation of the trachea. When duration of direct laryngoscopy is not likely to be short or when hypertension exists, it is reasonable to consider additional drugs and techniques to minimize pressor responses produced by the intubation sequence. For example, laryngotracheal lidocaine (2 mg·kg^{-1}), administered just before placing the tube in the trachea, minimizes the subsequent magnitude and duration of blood pressure increases evoked by tracheal stimulation. Likewise, intravenous lidocaine 1.5 mg·kg^{-1}, administered about 90 seconds before beginning direct laryngoscopy, may be efficacious in some patients. An alternative to lidocaine is intravenous administration of nitroprusside 1 µg·kg^{-1} to 2 µg·kg^{-1}, administered about 15 seconds before beginning direct laryngoscopy.[43] This dose of nitroprusside is effective in attenuating pressor responses (not heart rate responses) to laryngoscopy, as well as in treating hypertensive responses that can follow intubation of the trachea. These interventions are unlikely to alter heart rate increases often evoked by direct laryngoscopy. In this regard, continuous intravenous infusion of esmolol 100 µg·kg^{-1}·min^{-1} to 300 µg·kg^{-1}·min^{-1} before and during direct laryngoscopy may blunt increases in heart rate associated with intubation of the trachea (Fig. 1-8).[44] Small doses of short-acting opioids, such as fentanyl (1 μg·kg^{-1} to 3 μg·kg^{-1}) or sufentanil (0.1 μg·kg^{-1} to 0.3 μg·kg^{-1}) administered prior to direct laryngoscopy, may be useful in blunting circulatory responses evoked by intubation of the trachea.

Continuous intravenous infusion of nitroglycerin (0.25 μg·kg^{-1}·min^{-1} to 1 μg·kg^{-1}·min^{-1}) has been used as a prophylaxis against development of coronary vasospasm that can lead to myocardial ischemia in vulnerable patients. Despite the logic of this treatment, controlled studies have not consistently confirmed that this approach reduces the incidence of intraoperative myocardial ischemia.[45,46] The incidence of hypertension during noxious stimulation as produced by intubation of the trachea, however, is less in patients receiving continuous intravenous infusions of nitroglycerin.[46]

MAINTENANCE OF ANESTHESIA

Drugs chosen for the maintenance of anesthesia are often selected on the basis of the patient's left ventricular function, as determined by the history and physical examination with or without data from cardiac catheterization (Table 1-6). For example, patients with coronary artery disease but normal left ventricular function are likely to develop tachycardia and hypertension in response to intense stimulation, as during direct laryngoscopy or painful surgical stimulation. Controlled myocardial depression, using volatile anesthetics is appropriate in such patients, so as to prevent increased sympathetic nervous system activity

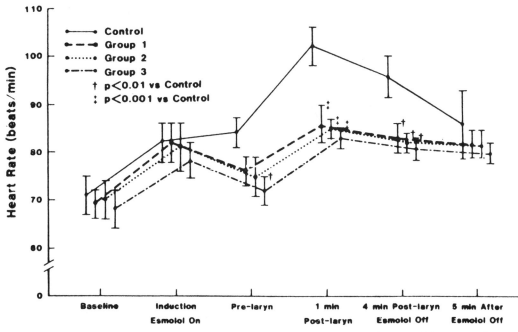

FIG. 1-8. Heart rate responses to laryngoscopy (larynx) in patients receiving esmolol as a continuous infusion in cumulative doses of 1,100 μg·kg^{-1} (group 1), 2,000 μg·kg^{-1} (group 2), and 2,700 μg·kg^{-1} (group 3). A control group did not receive esmolol. Esmolol infusion was initiated 3 minutes before and continued for 4 minutes after intubation of the trachea. (Menkhaus PG, Reves JG, Kissin I, et al. Cardiovascular effects of esmolol in anesthetized humans. Anesth Analg 1985;64:327–34. Reprinted with permission from IARS.)

and a subsequent elevation of myocardial oxygen requirements. Halothane, enflurane, or isoflurane are equally acceptable for use to produce controlled myocardial depression. Indeed, halothane and isoflurane produce similar changes in blood pressure and heart rate when administered to patients with coronary artery disease.[47] Volatile anesthetics can be used alone or in combination with nitrous oxide. Equally acceptable for maintenance of anesthesia is the use of a nitrous oxide–opioid technique, with addition of volatile anesthetics to treat undesirable increases in blood pressure that may accompany painful stimulation. When used to control intraoperative hypertension, both isoflurane and halothane are equally effective, but the mechanism for lowering blood pressure is different, reflecting peripheral vasodilation produced by isoflurane and

decreases in cardiac output produced by halothane (Fig. 1-9).[48]

Isoflurane is a more potent coronary arteriole vasodilator than halothane in patients with coronary artery disease.[49] Conceivably, isoflurane-induced coronary arteriole vasodilation, with or without associated reductions in coronary perfusion pressure, could result in coronary artery steal and regional myocardial ischemia (see the section Coronary Artery Steal). Evidence for isoflurane-induced coronary artery steal is the appearance of ischemic changes on the electrocardiogram and decreased myocardial lactate extraction in some patients anesthetized with isoflurane but not with halothane.[49] Nevertheless, most patients with coronary artery disease do not develop evidence of myocardial ischemia during administration of isoflurane, emphasizing the im-

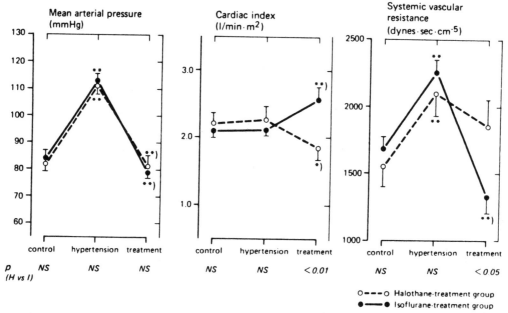

FIG. 1-9. Halothane (1 percent to 1.5 percent inspired) and isoflurane (1.5 percent to 2 percent inspired) were equally effective (treatment) in returning mean arterial pressure to near control levels in patients who became hypertensive during coronary artery bypass graft operations. Halothane lowers blood pressure principally by reductions in myocardial contractility (cardiac index), whereas reductions in blood pressure produced by isoflurane are due principally to reductions in systemic vascular resistance. (Hess W, Arnold B, Schulte-Sasse U, Tarnow J. Comparison of isoflurane and halothane when used to control intraoperative hypertension in patients undergoing coronary artery bypass surgery. Anesth Analg 1983;62:15–20. Reprinted with permission from IARS.)

portance of minimizing dose-related coronary arteriole vasodilation and/or reductions in coronary perfusion pressure.[48,50–51] Indeed, low concentrations of isoflurane (about 0.4 MAC) plus 50 percent nitrous oxide produce only modest declines in blood pressure and improve tolerance to pacing-induced myocardial ischemia in patients with coronary artery disease (Fig. 1-10).[52] Furthermore, administration of isoflurane to anesthetized hypertensive patients returns blood pressure to acceptable levels and results in disappearance of signs of myocardial ischemia on the electrocardiogram (Fig. 1-9).[48,50]

The multitude of diverse factors that determine whether isoflurane, or any drug capable of producing coronary arteriole vasodilation, will produce coronary artery steal and subsequent myocardial ischemia make it impossible to predict individual patient responses (see the section Coronary Artery Steal). In the final analysis, isoflurane (halothane and enflurane, too) may be beneficial in patients with coronary artery disease because it reduces myocardial oxygen requirements, or it may be detrimental because it lowers blood pressure and thus coronary perfusion pressure and, in addition, may produce coronary arteriole vasodilation with resulting coronary artery steal.

Patients with severely impaired left ventricular function, as associated with previous myocardial infarctions, may respond adversely to anesthetic-produced myocardial depression. In these patients, use of short-acting opioids may be selected rather than volatile anesthetic drugs. Indeed, high-dose fentanyl ($50~\mu g \cdot kg^{-1}$ to $100~\mu g \cdot kg^{-1}$) has been recommended for patients who cannot tolerate even minimal myocardial depression.[53] More traditional doses of opioids must be combined with other drugs, such as nitrous oxide, to assure complete amnesia. Although the combination of nitrous oxide with opioids has an impressive record of safety in patients with impaired ventricular function, nitrous oxide administered in the presence of opioids may be associated with significant circulatory

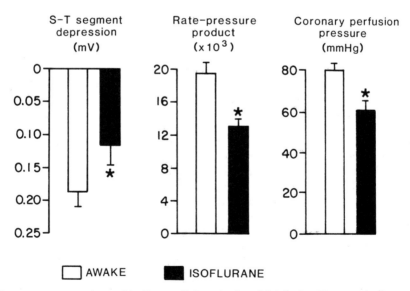

FIG. 1-10. Low concentrations of isoflurane (0.5 percent end-tidal) plus 50 percent nitrous oxide were associated with less ST segment depression on lead V5 of the electrocardiogram during electrical pacing (129 ± 5 beats min⁻¹, Mean ± SE) than during similar heart rates when awake. Rate-pressure products were less during inhalation of isoflurane than when awake. *P<0.01 isoflurane vs. awake. (Tarnow J, Narchies-Hornung A, Schulte-Sasse U. Isoflurane improves tolerance to pacing-induced myocardial ischemia. Anesthesiology 1986;64:147–56.)

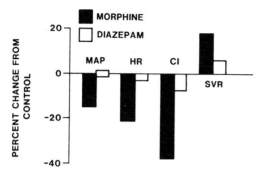

FIG. 1-11. Compared with control values, inhalation of 60 percent nitrous oxide after administration of morphine 1 mg·kg^{-1} to patients with coronary artery disease results in significant decreases (P < 0.05) in mean arterial pressure (MAP), heart rate (HR), cardiac index (CI), and increases in systemic vascular resistance (SVR). Conversely, inhalation of 60 percent nitrous oxide after administration of diazepam 0.5 mg·kg^{-1} does not produce significant circulatory changes. (Data adapted from Stoelting RK, Gibbs PS. Hemodynamic effects of morphine and morphine-nitrous oxide in valvular heart disease and coronary artery disease. Anesthesiology 1973;38:45–52; and from McCammon RL, Hilgenberg JC, Stoelting RK. Hemodynamic effects of diazepam and diazepam-nitrous oxide in patients with coronary artery disease. Anesth Analg 1980;59:438–41. Reprinted with permission from IARS.)

changes, including reductions in blood pressure and cardiac output (Fig. 1-11).[54,55] Indeed, cardiac depression produced by administration of nitrous oxide to patients who have previously received high doses of morphine (1 mg·kg^{-1}) is suggested by increases in pulmonary artery occlusion pressures when nitrous oxide is inhaled.[56] The combination of diazepam and fentanyl also produces reductions in blood pressure that are not seen when either drug is administered alone (Fig. 1-12).[57] Conversely, nitrous oxide added to background diazepam (Fig. 1-11)[54,55] or volatile anesthetic drugs does not produce signs of myocardial depression.[58] In animals, nitrous oxide produces dose-dependent constriction of epicardial coronary arteries in the absence of a detectable effect on coronary arterioles.[59]

Regional anesthesia is an acceptable technique in patients with coronary artery disease. Despite decreases in myocardial oxygen requirements produced by peripheral sympathetic nervous system blockade, it is important to realize that flow through coronary arteries narrowed by atherosclerosis is pressure-dependent. Therefore, reductions in blood pressure associated with regional anesthetic techniques should not be allowed to persist. Prompt treatment of blood pressure reductions that exceed 20 percent of the preblock value, with intravenous infusion of fluids and sympathomimetic drugs such as ephedrine, are indicated.

CHOICE OF MUSCLE RELAXANT

Choice of nondepolarizing muscle relaxants during maintenance of anesthesia for patients with coronary artery disease is dictated by the impact these drugs could have on the balance between myocardial oxygen delivery and requirements. For example, d-tubocurarine would be unlikely to increase myocardial oxygen requirements, since it does not alter heart rate or myocardial contractility. Reductions in diastolic blood pressure produced by d-tubocurarine, however, could reduce myocardial oxygen delivery. Gallamine is not a logical choice in patients with coronary artery disease, since increases in heart rate and blood pressure could adversely increase myocardial oxygen requirements. Pancuronium also increases heart rate and blood pressure, but the magnitude of these changes (about 10 percent to 15 percent above predrug values) would seem unlikely to alter adversely the balance between myocardial oxygen delivery and requirements. Nevertheless, there is evidence that myocardial ischemia may occasionally accompany even the modest increases in heart rate produced by pancuronium when administered to patients with coronary artery disease.[60] Circulatory changes produced by pancuronium can be used to offset negative inotropic and/or chronotropic effects of drugs being used for anesthesia. The presence of some degree of drug-induced beta-adrenergic blockade, as is so often present in patients with coronary artery disease, may attenuate increases in heart rate normally produced by pancuronium. Of note, however, is the observation that treatment with beta-adrenergic antagonist drugs does not prevent pancuronium-

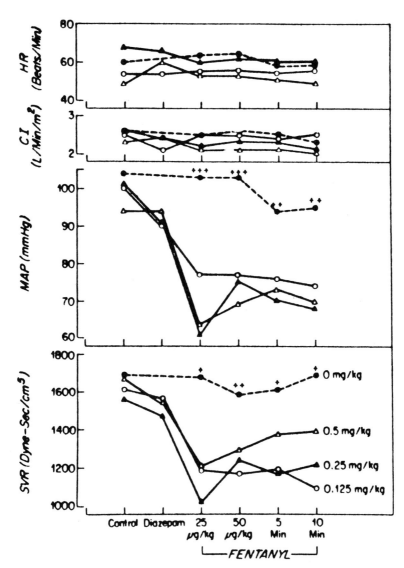

FIG. 1-12. Twenty patients undergoing coronary artery bypass graft operations received 0 to 0.5 mg·kg⁻¹ of diazepam administered intravenously followed by fentanyl administered at 400 μg·min⁻¹ to a total dose of 50 μg·kg⁻¹. Heart rate (HR) and cardiac index (CI) did not change in patients receiving fentanyl with or without previous diazepam. Prior treatment with diazepam was associated with reductions in mean arterial pressure (MAP) and systemic vascular resistance (SVR) when fentanyl was infused. + P < 0.05. + + P < 0.01. + + +P < 0.001. (Tomicheck RC, Rosow CE, Philbin DM, et al.Diazepam-fentanyl interaction—hemodynamic and hormonal effects in coronary artery surgery. Anesth Analg 1983;62:882–4. Reprinted with permission from IARS.)

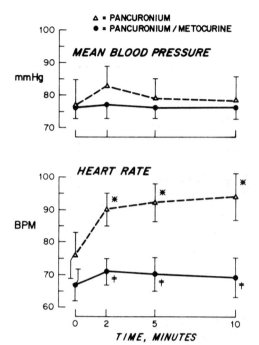

△ = PANCURONIUM
● = PANCURONIUM / METOCURINE

FIG. 1-13. Rapid intravenous administration of 2 × ED$_{95}$ for pancuronium during nitrous oxide-opioid-thiopental anesthesia produces slight increases in mean blood pressure and significant elevations of heart rate. Conversely, equally potent doses of pancuronium plus metocurine do not produce significant changes in blood pressure or heart rate. *P < 0.01 vs. control. #P < 0.02 vs. pancuronium plus metocurine. (Lebowitz PW, Ramsey FM, Savarese JJ, et al. Combination of pancuronium and metocurine. Neuromuscular and hemodynamic advantages over pancuronium alone. Anesth Analg 1981;60:12–7. Reprinted with permission from IARS.)

induced heart rate increases suggesting this response is more likely due to vagolytic than sympathomimetic effects of the muscle relaxant.[61] Metocurine does not alter heart rate and blood pressure reductions are modest when the dose does not exceed two times the ED$_{95}$. A combination of metocurine and pancuronium can also be used to provide neuromuscular blockade. The advantage of this combination is the use of smaller doses of pancuronium, which are not associated with increases in heart rate or blood pressure (Fig. 1-13).[62]

Intermediate-acting muscle relaxants lack significant cardiovascular effects and, there-fore, are unlikely to alter myocardial oxygen requirements or delivery. For example, blood pressure and heart rate are not altered by doses of vecuronium that exceed three times the ED$_{95}$.[61] Modest and transient declines in blood pressure may accompany rapid administration of doses of atracurium that exceed 2.5 times the ED$_{95}$ most likely reflecting drug-induced histamine release.[63] Administration of high doses of atracurium over 75 seconds is not associated with changes in blood pressure or heart rate.[64] Atracurium or vecuronium, in contrast to pancuronium, would not be expected to offset reductions in blood pressure or heart rate produced by drugs used for anesthesia.[65] This becomes particularly apparent when bradycardia accompanies administration of high doses of opioids. Indeed, profound heart rate slowing has been observed after administration of vecuronium to patients who have previously received high doses of sufentanil.[66] Although heart rate slowing may be desirable from the standpoint of myocardial oxygen requirements, excessive bradycardia may so reduce cardiac output that coronary perfusion pressure declines to unacceptable levels. Furthermore, abrupt bradycardia may increase the likelihood of cardiac dysrhythmias due to a reentry mechanism.

REVERSAL OF NEUROMUSCULAR BLOCKADE

Reversal of nondepolarizing neuromuscular blockade with anticholinesterase-anticholinergic drug combinations can be safely accomplished in patients with coronary artery disease. Glycopyrrolate, which is alleged to have less chronotropic effects than atropine, may be selected as the anticholinergic drug when excessive increases in heart rate are a possibility. Nevertheless, marked increases in heart rate rarely occur with reversal of nondepolarizing muscle relaxants, and atropine seems as acceptable as glycopyrrolate for inclusion with the anticholinesterase drug. Theoretically, it is possible that co-existing beta-adrenergic blockade could accentuate muscarinic effects of anticholinesterase drugs used to reverse muscle relaxants (see the section Adverse Effects during Anesthesia).

MONITORING

Perioperative monitoring is dictated by the complexity of the operative procedure and the severity of the coronary artery disease. An important goal in selecting monitors uniquely for patients with coronary artery disease is early detection of myocardial ischemia and/or reduced myocardial contractility.

Electrocardiogram. The electrocardiogram is a useful way to monitor the balance between myocardial oxygen delivery and requirements during general anesthesia. There is a predictable correlation between the lead of the electrocardiogram that reflects myocardial ischemia and the anatomic distribution of the diseased coronary artery (Table 1-5). For example, a V5 (precordial) lead (fifth interspace at the anterior anxillary line) will reflect myocardial ischemia present in that portion of the left ventricle supplied by the left anterior descending coronary artery.[67] Therefore, it would seem prudent to monitor this lead or its equivalent during the perioperative period in patients with known disease of the left coronary artery. Using a three-lead electrode system, one can obtain the equivalent of a V5 lead by placing the left arm lead in the V5 position and selecting aVL on the electrocardiogram monitor.[67] Lead II is a better choice for detection of myocardial ischemia that occurs in the distribution of the right coronary artery. Furthermore, lead II is ideal for the identification of P waves and the subsequent analysis of cardiac rhythm disturbances. Lead II, however, may not detect the more common occurrence of anterior or lateral wall myocardial ischemia that is specifically reflected by precordial leads. An esophageal electrocardiogram, by virtue of its position just posterior to the atrium and ventricle, results in augmented P waves and may facilitate intraoperative diagnosis of cardiac dysrhythmias or posterior wall myocardial ischemia.[68]

Significant myocardial ischemia is considered to be present when there is at least 1 mm of downsloping of ST segments from the baseline on the electrocardiogram. Cardiac dysrhythmias, cardiac conduction disturbances, digitalis therapy, electrolyte abnormalities, and hyperthermia can produce similar changes in the ST segment, in the absence of myocardial ischemia. Acute increases in pulmonary artery occlusion pressures associated with the appearance of abnormal wave forms (AV wave greater than 15 mmHg or a V wave greater than 30 mmHg) may reflect the presence of myocardial ischemia.[69] Indeed, abnormalities in tracings of pulmonary artery occlusion pressures may precede changes on the electrocardiogram that suggest myocardial ischemia.

Appearance of signs of myocardial ischemia on the electrocardiogram supports prompt and aggressive pharmacologic treatment of associated adverse changes in heart rate and/or blood pressure. Indeed, there is evidence that myocardial ischemia that occurs intraoperatively is a precursor to postoperative myocardial infarction.[16] Persistent elevations in heart rate are often treated with intravenous administration of beta-adrenergic antagonist drugs such as propranolol. Excessive increases in blood pressure without evidence of myocardial ischemia are often treated with nitroprusside. Nitroglycerin is a more appropriate choice when myocardial ischemia is associated with a normal to modestly elevated blood pressure. In this situation, nitroglycerin-induced reductions in preload will allow improvement is subendocardial blood flow, while not reducing blood pressure to the point that coronary perfusion pressure is jeopardized. Hypotension should be treated with sympathomimetic drugs to rapidly restore perfusion through pressure-dependent atherosclerotic coronary arteries. A drug that elevates blood pressure by increasing myocardial contractility, as well as systemic vascular resistance, is often chosen. In this regard, ephedrine may be superior to relatively pure alpha-agonist drugs such as phenylephrine. Nevertheless, co-existing beta-adrenergic blockade may convert ephedrine to a predominantly alpha-adrenergic agonist similar to phenylephrine. Furthermore, the dose of phenylephrine necessary to produce venoconstriction is less than the dose needed to constrict arteries, thus reducing the likelihood of drug-induced coronary artery vasoconstriction via stimulation of alpha-adrenergic receptors in coronary arteries. In addition to drugs, intravenous infusions of fluids to restore blood pressure is useful, since myocardial oxygen requirements for volume work of the heart are less than those for pressure work. A disadvantage of fluid infusions to correct hypotension is the time necessary for this treatment to be effective. Another risk of rapid fluid infusions may be increased preload leading to decreased subendocardial perfusion and ischemia. Regardless of the treatment, it is crucial to realize that prompt restoration of blood pressure is mandatory to maintain pressure-dependent blood flow through coronary arteries narrowed by atherosclerosis.

Pulmonary Artery Catheter. Monitoring pulmonary artery occlusion pressures as reflections of left ventricular filling pressures are helpful when large intravascular fluid volume shifts are expected intraoperatively. It is possible that patients with coronary artery disease may have large volume requirements, reflecting a co-existing decreased intravascular fluid volume due to high sympathetic nervous system activity. This volume deficit would be exaggerated by preoperative fasting. Maintenance of pulmonary artery occlusion pressures by intravenous infusions of crystalloid or colloid solutions may contribute to cardiovascular stability during the operative period. In addition to guiding volume replacement, a pulmonary artery catheter allows measurement of cardiac output and calculation of systemic and pulmonary vascular resistance, information essential for evaluating responses to inotropic or vasodilating drugs. Reproducibility of thermodilution cardiac outputs is improved by initiating these measurements at the same phase of the breathing cycle, preferably end-exhalation.[70] In addition, injectate temperature and volume may influence accuracy of thermodilution cardiac outputs.[71] For example, iced injectate solutions provide a better signal-to-noise ratio, but cold may be lost to the catheter wall or by rewarming of the syringe from handling before injection. For each degree of rewarming, an overestimation of cardiac output of 2.9 percent results and a 10 ml syringe held in a warm hand will increase 1 degree Celsius every 13 seconds.[71] A 10 ml injectate volume is commonly used as a larger volume improves the signal-to-noise ratio, especially when room temperature injectates are administered. If injectate volume is less than expected (e.g., 9 ml instead of 10 ml), the cal-

culated cardiac output will be falsely high, since the area under the curve is less. Even under optimal conditions, there must be a 10 percent to 15 percent change in cardiac output as measured by thermodilution before significant changes can be accepted to have occurred. Even measurements of cardiac output considered to be significant changes should be considered in the context of the clinical status of the patient as reflected by peripheral perfusion and urinary output. Sudden increases in pulmonary artery occlusion pressures may reflect acute myocardial ischemia. A V wave component of the pulmonary artery occlusion pressure tracing may reflect mitral regurgitation due to papillary muscle ischemia, whereas an A wave is most likely to develop when ventricular compliance is reduced by myocardial ischemia.

Indications for placement of pulmonary artery catheters continue to undergo scrutiny relative to information derived and financial cost. For example, central venous pressures and pulmonary artery occlusion pressures have been shown to correlate in patients with coronary artery disease when ejection fractions are above 0.5 and there is no evidence of left ventricular dyskinesia.[72] Conversely, when ejection fractions are below 0.5, there is no correlation and changes in filling pressures may even be in opposite directions. To further complicate interpretation of filling pressure measurements, it is apparent that changes in left ventricular compliance, such as commonly occur after coronary artery bypass graft operations, result in poor correlation between pulmonary artery occlusion pressures and left ventricular end-diastolic volumes (Fig. 1-14).[73,74]

Transesophageal Echocardiography. Transesophageal echocardiography is a monitoring technique that may provide a useful method for continuous intraoperative assessment of left ventricular function.[75] Global left ventricular function is evaluated by measurements of end-diastolic and end-systolic dimensions. From these dimensions estimates of ventricular volume, cardiac output, and ejection fraction are derived. As such, transesophageal echocardiography may become a useful monitor in the management of patients with coronary artery disease or those undergoing aortic cross-clamping who are at risk for acute

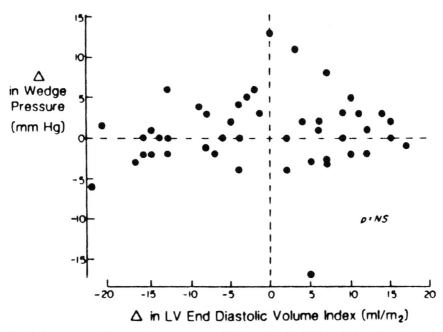

FIG. 1-14. Pulmonary capillary wedge pressure and left ventricular (LV) end-diastolic volume index (derived from determinations of ejection fraction and stroke volume) were measured in 12 surgical patients after coronary artery bypass graft operations to determine the usefulness of wedge pressures as indicators of left ventricular preload. Each dot represents hourly changes. The relationship between the two measured variables is random. (Hansen RM, Viquerat CE, Matthay MA, et al. Poor correlation between pulmonary artery wedge pressure and left ventricular end-diastolic volume after coronary artery bypass graft surgery. Anesthesiology 1986;64:764–70.)

ventricular dysfunction.[76,77] For example, regional deterioration in wall thickness or movement may allow early detection of myocardial ischemia, whereas reductions in myocardial contractility are reflected by decreases in the ejection fraction.[78]

Postoperative Period

Reductions in body temperature that occur intraoperatively may predispose to shivering on awakening leading to abrupt and excessive increases in myocardial oxygen requirements. Attempts to minimize reductions in body temperature and provision of supplemental oxygen are of obvious importance. Postoperative pain may result in activation of the sympathetic nervous system leading to increased myocardial oxygen requirements and myocar-

dial ischemia. This emphasizes the unique importance of providing adequate postoperative pain relief to patients with coronary artery disease. In this regard, it is of interest that postoperative myocardial reinfarction often occurs 48 hours to 72 hours postoperatively, a time that could correspond to discontinuation of supplemental oxygen and less aggressive treatment of pain.[2,3]

DIAGNOSIS OF PERIOPERATIVE MYOCARDIAL INFARCTIONS

Myocardial infarctions or reinfarctions that occur in the perioperative period can be difficult to recognize. Indeed, myocardial infarctions are often silent. Nevertheless, myocardial infarction must be considered in vulnerable patients who develop unexplained cardiac dysrhythmias, hypotension, or congestive heart failure in the perioperative period. Ventricular premature beats occur in over 90 percent of patients who experience acute myocardial infarctions. Likewise, sinus bradycardia and various degrees of atrioventricular heart block often accompany acute myocardial infarctions. Most deaths that occur in the first hours after myocardial infarction are due to cardiac tachydysrhythmias or bradydysrhythmias. Elevations of body temperature are frequently present. Pain typical of angina pectoris occurs in only about 25 percent of patients who experience myocardial infarctions in the postoperative period.[3]

Diagnosis of an acute myocardial infarction in the perioperative period is most often based on changes observed on the electrocardiogram and characteristic alterations in plasma concentrations of enzymes released from damaged cardiac cells. Cardiogenic shock is a feared and often fatal complication of acute myocardial infarctions.

Electrocardiogram

Almost all patients who develop acute myocardial infarctions in the perioperative period demonstrate serial changes on the electrocardiogram. These serial changes most likely reflect loss of normal myocardial cell membrane ion pumps. Alterations in ST segments are the first visible evidence. Typically, ST segments are characterized by convex elevations in those leads that overlie the damaged myocardium. Persistent elevations of ST segments beyond 2 days to 4 days should arouse suspicion of the presence of a left ventricular aneurysm. Elevation of ST segments on the electrocardiogram suggests a transmural myocardial infarction, whereas ST segment depression reflects ischemia or subendocardial infarction. T waves become symmetrically and often deeply inverted as ST segments begin to return to an isoelectric position. Q waves do not develop unless the acute myocardial infarction involves the entire thickness (i.e., transmural) of

the ventricular wall. Furthermore, Q waves do not develop immediately but become manifest only after sufficient time has passed for muscle necrosis to occur. For Q waves to be pathologic, they must be greater than 0.4 second in duration, and their depth must be more than 25 percent of the amplitude of the succeeding R waves.

SITE OF MYOCARDIAL INFARCTION

Focal myocardial infarctions are best reflected in specific leads of the electrocardiogram (Table 1-5). For example, inferior wall (diaphragmatic) myocardial infarctions are best seen on leads II, III and aVF of the electrocardiogram. Anterior wall myocardial infarctions manifest on leads I, aVL, and the precordial leads. Anteroseptal myocardial infarctions are best seen on leads V1–3, and anterolateral myocardial infarctions manifest on leads V4–6. Electrocardiographic localization of subendocardial myocardial infarctions is difficult because the electrocardiogram only poorly reflects subendocardial electrical activity.

Inferior or Anterior Wall Myocardial Infarctions. Inferior wall myocardial infarctions cannot be distinguished from anterior wall infarctions by the nature of the pain, incidence of cardiac dysrhythmias, or changes in plasma concentrations of cardiac enzymes. Symptoms of a myocardial infarction, however, are likely to reflect the principal distribution of the major coronary artery that is occluded. In this regard, it is not surprising that manifestations of inferior wall myocardial infarctions due to occlusion of the right coronary artery often differ from manifestations of left coronary artery occlusion that results in anterior wall myocardial infarctions (Table 1-5). For example, right ventricular dysfunction, bradycardia, and atrioventricular heart block are possible manifestations of inferior wall myocardial infarctions considering the distribution of the right coronary artery. Conversely, pulmonary edema with or without cardiogenic shock is a more likely manifestation of anterior wall myocardial infarctions due to occlusions of branches of the left main coronary artery. Temporary artificial cardiac pacemakers may be required if hemodynamically significant heart block accompanies myocardial infarctions.

Subendocardial Myocardial Infarction. Subendocardial myocardial infarction reflects damage to the inner third of the myocardium nearest the ventricular cavity. The subendocardium of the left ventricle is uniquely susceptible to myocardial ischemia because its nutrient vessels are completely occluded during systole by high intramuscular pressures generated by the contracting heart. Coronary atherosclerosis may predispose patients to subendocardial rather than transmural myocardial infarctions. Subendocardial myocardial infarctions are just as dangerous as transmural myocardial infarctions, and the incidence of cardiac dysrhythmias is similar.

Plasma Enzymes

Increases in plasma concentrations of myocardial-specific isoenzyme fractions of creatine kinase (CK-MB) are useful in confirming the diagnosis of an acute myocardial infarction. Increases in plasma concentrations of this isoenzyme are detectable within 3 hours after infarctions of cardiac muscle. Peak increases of CK-MB are reached in about 12 hours, with return of the plasma concentrations to near normal levels between 24 hours and 36 hours after the initial myocardial infarction. Plasma concentrations of the cardiac-specific isoenzyme fractions of lactic dehydrogenase begin to increase about 2 days after a myocardial infarction. Peak elevations of this isoenzyme occur after 3 days to 5 days and gradually return to normal concentrations in the plasma after 10 days to 14 days.

Cardiogenic Shock

Cardiogenic shock is present when hypotension and oliguria accompany an acute myocardial infarction and persist despite the dis-appearance of pain, correction of cardiac dysrhythmias, and restoration of intravascular fluid volume. Typically, mean arterial pressure is less than 60 mmHg, left ventricular end-diastolic pressure is above 18 mmHg, and the cardiac index is less than 2 $L \cdot min^{-1} \cdot m^{-2}$. Patients who develop cardiogenic shock have probably experienced infarction of more than 40 percent of the left ventricular muscle. Intravenous infusions of catecholamines such as dopamine or dobutamine may be tried in attempts to improve myocardial contractility and cardiac output. Digitalis is probably of no value in treatment of cardiogenic shock.

INTRA-AORTIC BALLOON COUNTERPULSATION

Intra-aortic balloon counterpulsation may be helpful in some patients who develop cardiogenic shock. The intra-aortic balloon is programmed to the electrocardiogram, so as to deflate just before systole and to inflate during diastole. Presystolic deflation of the balloon diminishes systemic blood pressure and afterload, which reduces cardiac work and myocardial oxygen requirements. Inflation of the balloon during diastole increases diastolic blood pressure and thus improves coronary blood flow and myocardial oxygen delivery. Intravenous infusions of combinations of catecholamines and vasodilators may serve as a pharmacologic alternative to mechanical counterpulsation with the intra-aortic balloon. Despite these aggressive forms of treatment, cardiogenic shock is often fatal.

Other Complications of Acute Myocardial Infarction

Rupture of the ventricular septum occurs in 0.5 percent to 1.0 percent of patients experiencing acute myocardial infarctions. A dramatic complication of such infarctions is acute mitral regurgitation due to rupture of infarcted papillary muscles. Cardiac rupture typically occurs 3 days to 10 days after the initial infarction. This complication usually leads to sudden death. An estimated 10 percent of deaths from myocardial infarction are due to cardiac rupture. Development of left ventricular aneurysms is usually a late complication, occurring months or even years after acute myocardial infarctions. Pericarditis, often manifested as pericardial friction rubs, occurs in a large proportion of patients who experience acute myocardial infarctions. Dressler's postmyocardial infarction syndrome is a delayed form of pericarditis that develops in about 3 percent of patients anywhere between the first week and many months after acute myocardial infarctions.

PERCUTANEOUS TRANSLUMINAL CORONARY ANGIOPLASTY

Percutaneous transluminal coronary angioplasty is performed by insertion of a small balloon into a diseased coronary artery by means of a catheter.[79] The balloon is inflated within the lumen of the coronary artery directly beneath the obstruction. The balloon flattens the atherosclerotic plaque into the vessel wall and restores vessel patency. Successful coronary angioplasty obviates the need for surgery, although there seems to be a tendency for lesions to recur after a few months. Unsuccessful coronary angioplasty may convert a previously narrowed coronary artery to an obstructed vessel associated with the need for urgent surgical myocardial revascularization.

CARDIAC TRANSPLANTATION

Cardiac transplantation is the only available treatment for returning patients with end-stage heart disease (most often due to coronary artery disease or cardiomyopathy) to functional life styles.[80,81] Organ damage related to heart disease must be reversible and the likelihood of long-term survival (patients less than

50 years to 60 years of age) must be good. Approximately 60 percent to 65 percent of patients survive for 3 years or longer after cardiac transplantation. Left ventricular ejection fractions are typically less than 0.2, and prognosis for survival is less than 12 months. Irreversible pulmonary hypertension as is often present in patients with congenital heart disease is a contraindication to cardiac transplantation.

Management of Anesthesia

Management of anesthesia for cardiac transplantation may include ketamine and/or benzodiazepines for induction of anesthesia plus opioids to provide analgesia during surgery.[82] Alternatively, opioids may be used for induction and maintenance of anesthesia. Volatile anesthetics have the potential to cause profound myocardial depression and vasodilation. Nitrous oxide is seldom used because of additive myocardial depressant effects in the presence of opioids and concern about enlargement of an accidental air embolus that may occur when large blood vessels are opened during the operation. Pancuronium or muscle relaxants with no blood pressure-lowering effects are useful. Airway equipment, including the anesthetic delivery tubing, is sterile and handled with sterile gloves. Bacterial filters are used on the inspired and exhaled limbs of the anesthetic delivery tubing. Many patients undergoing cardiac transplantation have abnormal coagulation reflecting passive congestion of the liver due to chronic heart failure.

Operative technique consists of cardiopulmonary bypass and anastomosis of the aorta, pulmonary artery, and left and right atria. Immunosuppressive drugs are usually initiated in the preoperative period. Intravascular catheters are placed using aseptic techniques. Monitors are those typically used during cardiopulmonary bypass except for the possible avoidance of a pulmonary artery catheter because of concern about infection and catheter-induced cardiac dysrhythmias. Furthermore, it is necessary to withdraw or remove the catheter when the recipient's heart is removed. Placement of a central venous pressure catheter via the left internal jugular vein leaves the right internal jugular vein available as an access site to perform cardiac biopsies in the postoperative period. Inotropic drugs, especially isoproterenol, may be required briefly to maintain myocardial contractility and heart rate of the donor heart following cardiopulmonary bypass. Therapeutic attempts to lower pulmonary vascular resistance may be necessary. Protamine to reverse heparin is administered cautiously, as it may induce exaggerated hypotension in heart transplant patients.[81]

The denervated transplanted heart assumes an intrinsic heart rate of about 110 beats·min^{-1}, reflecting the absence of normal vagal tone. Stroke volume responds to augmented preload by the Frank-Starling mechanism, emphasizing that these patients tolerate hypovolemia poorly. Likewise, sudden vasodilation, as that due to spinal or epidural anesthetics, is undesirable in patients with a cardiac transplant. The transplanted heart responds to direct acting catecholamines (may even be more sensitive than the normal heart), but drugs that act by indirect mechanisms (ephedrine) have less effect.[81]

Immunosuppression and Side Effects

Immunosuppression regimens vary but usually include prednisone, azathioprine, and cyclosporine. Transvenous right ventricular endomyocardial biopsies are performed at weekly intervals in the first 6 weeks postoperatively to provide early warning of allograft rejection. Decreased voltage on the electrocardiogram and signs of cardiac failure provide late signs of graft rejection. The most frequent cause of death in cardiac transplant patients is the development of opportunistic infections, emphasizing the importance of adherence to aseptic techniques in the perioperative period. An increased incidence of cancer, particularly of the lymphoproliferative type, appears to be inherent in any type of long-term immunosuppression. A premature and rapidly pro-

gressive form of coronary artery disease occurs in nearly 50 percent of patients within 2 years to 5 years after transplantation.[80] This form of coronary artery disease is not associated with angina pectoris because of the lack of afferent reinnervation of the graft. Nephrotoxicity and hypertension may accompany cyclosporine therapy, leukopenia is an accompaniment of azathioprine, and osteoporosis and glucose intolerance are well recognized side effects of long-term administration of corticosteroids.

REFERENCES

1. Silverman KJ, Grossman W. Angina pectoris. N Engl J Med 1984;310:1712–7
2. Tarhan S, Moffitt EA, Taylor WF, Guiliani ER. Myocardial infarction after general anesthesia. JAMA 1972;220:1451–4
3. Steen PA, Tinker JH, Tarhan S. Myocardial reinfarction after anesthesia and surgery. An update: Incidence, mortality, and predisposing factors. JAMA 1978;239:2566–70
4. Goldberg AH. The patient with heart disease. Preoperative evaluation and preparation. Anesth Analg 1976;55:618–21
5. Foex P. Preoperative assessment of patients with cardiac disease. Br J Anaesth 1978;50:15–23
6. Grundy SM. Cholesterol and coronary heart disease. A new era. JAMA 1986;256:2849–58
7. Lowering blood cholesterol to prevent heart disease. Consensus Conference. JAMA 1;985;253:2080–90
8. Therapeutic response to lovastatin (Mevinolin) in nonfamilial hypercholesterolemia. A multicenter study. JAMA 1986;256:2829–34
9. Stamler J, Wentworth D, Neaton J. Is the relationship between serum cholesterol and risk of death from coronary heart disease continuous and graded? JAMA 1986;256:2823–8
10. Kovanen PT, Bilheimer DW, Goldstein JL, et al. Regulatory role for hepatic low density lipoprotein receptors in vivo in the dog. Proc Natl Acad Sci USA 1981;78:1194–8
11. Chatterjee K, Rouleau J-L, Parmley WW. Medical management of patients with angina. Has first-line management changed? JAMA 1984;252:1170–7
12. Cokkinos DV, Voridis EM. Constancy of pressure rate product in pacing-induced angina pectoris. Br Heart J 1976;38:39–42
13. Barash PG, Kopriva CJ. The rate-pressure product

in clinical anesthesia: boon or bane? (Editorial). Anesth Analg 1980;59:229–31

14. Loeb HS, Saudye A, Croke RP, et al. Effects of pharmacologically-induced hypertension on myocardial ischemia and coronary hemodynamics in patients with fixed coronary obstruction. Circulation 1978;57:41–6

15. Rao TLK, Jacobs KH, El-Etr AA. Reinfarction following anesthesia in patients with myocardial infarction. Anesthesiology 1983;59:499–505

16. Slogoff S, Keats AS. Does perioperative myocardial ischemia lead to postoperative myocardial infarction? Anesthesiology 1985;62:107–14

17. Mahar LJ, Steen PA, Tinker JH, et al. Perioperative myocardial infarction in patients with coronary artery disease with and without aorto-coronary artery bypass grafts. J Thorac Cardiovasc Surg 1978;76:533–7

18. Goldman L, Caldera DL, Nussbaum SR, et al. Multifactorial index of cardiac risk in noncardiac surgical procedures. N Engl J Med 1977;297:845–50

19. Jeffrey CC, Kunsman J, Cullen DJ, Brewster DC. A prospective evaluation of cardiac risk index. Anesthesiology 1983;58:462–4

20. Chung DC. Anaesthetic problems associated with the treatment of cardiovascular disease. II. Beta-adrenergic antagonists. Can Anaesth Soc J 1981;28:105–13

21. Roberts JG, Foex P, Clarke NS, Bennett MJ. Haemodynamic interactions of high-dose propranolol pretreatment and anaesthesia in the dog. I. Halothane dose-response studies. Br J Anaesth 1976;48:315–25

22. Philbin DM, Lowenstein E. Lack of beta-adrenergic activity of isoflurane in the dogs: A comparison of circulatory effects of halothane and isoflurane after propranolol administration. Br J Anaesth 1976;48:1165–70

23. Horan BF, Prys-Roberts C, Hamilton WK, Roberts JG. Haemodynamic responses to enflurane anaesthesia and hypovolaemia in the dog and their modification by propranolol. Br J Anaesth 1977;49:1189–97

24. Slogoff S, Keats AS, Ott E. Preoperative propranolol therapy and aorto-coronary bypass operation. JAMA 1978;240:1487–90

25. Filner BE, Karliner JS. Alterations of normal left ventricular performance by general anesthesia. Anesthesiology 1976;45:610–21

26. Reves JG, Kissin I, Lell WA, Tosone S. Calcium entry blockers: Uses and implications for anesthesiologists. Anesthesiology 1982;57:504–18

27. Schulte-Sasse U, Hess W, Markschies-Harnung A, Tarnow J. Combined effects of halothane anesthesia and verapamil on systemic hemodynamics and left ventricular myocardial contractility in patients with ischemic heart disease. Anesth Analg 1984;63:791–8

28. Kapur PA, Bloor BC, Flacke WE, Olewine SK. Comparison of cardiovascular responses to verapamil during enflurane, isoflurane, or halothane anesthesia in the dog. Anesthesiology 1984;61:156–60

29. Merin RG. Calcium channel blocking drugs and anesthetics: Is the drug interaction beneficial or detrimental? Anesthesiology 1987;66:111–3

30. Henling CE, Slogoff S, Kodali SV, Arlund C. Heart block after coronary artery bypass—effect of chronic administration of calcium-entry blockers and beta-blockers. Anesth Analg 1984;63:515–20

31. Durant NN, Nguyen N, Katz R. Potentiation of neuromuscular blockade by verapamil. Anesthesiology 1984;60:298–303

32. Lawson NW, Kraynack BJ, Gintautas J. Neuromuscular and electrocardiographic responses to verapamil in dogs. Anesth Analg 1983;62:50–4

33. Vitez TS, Soper LE, Soper PC. Chronic hypokalemia and intraoperative dysrhythmias. Anesthesiology 1985;63:130–3

34. Sethna DH, Moffitt EA. An appreciation of the coronary circulation. Anesth Analg 1986;65:294–305

35. Bristow MR, Ginsberg R, Harrison DC. Histamine and the human heart: The other receptor system. Am J Cardiol 1982;49:249–51

36. Shepherd JT, Vanhoutte PM. The Human Cardiovascular System: Facts and Concepts. New York. Raven Press 1979:1–375.

37. Sill JC, Bove AA, Nugent M, et al. Effects of isoflurane on coronary arterioles in the intact dog. Anesthesiology 1987;66:273–9

38. Buffington CW, Romson JL, Levine A, Duttlinger NC, Huang AH. Isoflurane induces coronary steal in a canine model of chronic coronary occlusion. Anesthesiology 1987;66:280–92

39. Priebe H-J, Foex P. Isoflurane causes regional myocardial dysfunction in dogs with critical coronary artery stenoses. Anesthesiology 1987;66:293–300

40. Slogoff S, Keats AS. Further observations on perioperative myocardial ischemia. Anesthesiology 1986;65:539–42

41. Kleinman B, Henkin RE, Glisson SN, et al. Qualitative evaluation of coronary flow during anesthetic induction using thallium-201 perfusion scans. Anesthesiology 1986;64:157–64

42. Roy WL, Edelist G, Gilbert B. Myocardial ischemia during noncardiac surgical procedures in patients with coronary artery disease. Anesthesiology 1979;51:393–7

43. Stoelting RK. Attenuation of blood pressure response to laryngoscopy and tracheal intubation

with sodium nitroprusside. Anesth Analg 1979;58:116–9

44. Menkhaus PG, Reves JG, Kisson I, et al. Cardiovascular effects of esmolol in anesthetized humans. Anesth Analg 1985;64:327–34
45. Thomson IR, Mutch WAC, Culligan JD. Failure of intravenous nitroglycerin to prevent intraoperative myocardial ischemia during fentanyl-pancuronium anesthesia. Anesthesiology 1984;61:385–93
46. Gallagher JD, Moore RA, Jose AB, Botros SB, Clark DL. Prophylactic nitroglycerin infusions during coronary artery bypass surgery. Anesthesiology 1986;64:785–9
47. Bastard OG, Carter JG, Moyers JR, Bross BA. Circulatory effects of isoflurane in patients with ischemic heart disease: A comparison with halothane. Anesth Analg 1984;63:635–9
48. Hess W, Arnold B, Schulte-Sasse U, Tarnow J. Comparison of isoflurane and halothane when used to control intraoperative hypertension in patients undergoing coronary artery bypass surgery. Anesth Analg 1983;62:15–20
49. Reiz S, Balfors E, Sorensen MD, et al. Isoflurane-a powerful coronary vasodilator in patients with ischemic disease. Anesthhesiology 1983;59:91–7
50. O'Young J, Mastrocostopoulos G, Hilgenberg A, et al. Myocardial circulatory and metabolic effects of isoflurane and sufentanil during coronary artery surgery. Anesthesiology 1987;66:653–8
51. Smith JS, Cahalan MK, Benefiel DJ, et al. Fentanyl versus fentanyl and isoflurane in patients with impaired left ventricular function. Anesthesiology 1985;63:A18
52. Tarnow J, Markschies-Hornung A, Schulte-Sasse U. Isoflurane improves the tolerance to pacing induced myocardial ischemia. Anesthesiology 1986;64:147–56
53. Lunn JK, Stanley TH, Eisele J, et al. High dose fentanyl anesthesia for coronary artery surgery: Plasma fentanyl concentrations and influence of nitrous oxide on cardiovascular responses. Anesth Analg 1979;58:390–5
54. Stoelting RK, Gibbs PS. Hemodynamic effects of morphine and morphine-nitrous oxide in valvular heart disease and coronary artery disease. Anesthesiology 1973;38:45–52
55. McCammon RL, Hilgenberg JC, Stoelting RK. Hemodynamic effects of diazepam and diazepam-nitrous oxide in patients with coronary artery disease. Anesth Analg 1980;59:438–41
56. Lappas DG, Buckley MJ, Laver MB, et al. Left ventricular performance and pulmonary circulation following addition of nitrous oxide to morphine during coronary-artery surgery. Anesthesiology 1975;43:61–9
57. Tomicheck RC, Rosow CE, Philbin DM, et al. Diazepam-fentanyl interaction-hemodynamic and hormonal effects in coronary artery surgery. Anesth Analg 1983;62:881–4
58. Smith NT, Calverley RK, Prys-Roberts C, et al. Impact of nitrous oxide on the circulation during enflurane anesthesia in man. Anesthesiology 1978;48:345–9
59. Wilkowski DAW, Sill JC, Bonta W, Owen R, Bove AA. Nitrous oxide constricts epicardial coronary arteries without effect on coronary arterioles. Anesthesiology 1987;66:659–65
60. Thomson IR, Putnins CL. Adverse effects of pancuronium during high-dose fentanyl anesthesia for coronary artery bypass grafting. Anesthesiology 1985;62:708–13
61. Morris RB, Cahalan MK, Miller RD, et al. The cardiovascular effects of vecuronium (ORG NC45) and pancuronium in patients undergoing coronary artery bypass grafting. Anesthesiology 1983;58:438–40
62. Lebowitz PW, Ramsey FM, Savarese JJ, et al. Combination of pancuronium and metocurine: Neuromuscular and hemodynamic advantages over pancuronium alone. Anesth Analg 1981;60:12–7
63. Basta SJ, Ali HH, Savarese JJ, et al. Clinical pharmacology of atracurium besylate (BW33A): A new non-depolarizing muscle relaxant. Anesth Analg 1982;61:723–9
64. Scott RPF, Savarese JJ, Basta SJ, et al. Clinical pharmacology of atracurium given in high doses. Br J Anaesth 1986;58:834–8
65. Salmenpera M, Peltola K, Takkumen O, Heinonen J. Cardiovascular effects of pancuronium and vecuronium during high-dose fentanyl anesthesia. Anesth Analg 1983;62:1059–64
66. Starr NJ, Sethna DH, Estafanous FG. Bradycardia and asystole following rapid administration of sufentanil with vecuronium. Anesthesiology 1986;64:521–3
67. Kaplan JA, King SB. The precordial electrocardiographic lead (V_5) in patients who have coronary-artery disease. Anesthesiology 1976;45:570–4
68. Kates RA, Zaidan JR, Kaplan JA. Esophageal lead for intraoperative electrocardiographic monitoring. Anesth Analg 1982;61:781–5
69. Kaplan JA, Wells PH. Early diagnosis of myocardial ischemia using the pulmonary arterial catheter. Anesth Analg 1981;60:789–93
70. Stevens JH, Raffin TA, Mihm FG, Rosenthal MH, Stetz CW. Thermodilution cardiac output measurement. Effects of the respiratory cycle on its reproducibility. JAMA 1985;253:2240–42
71. Nadeau S, Noble WH. Limitations of cardiac out-

put measurements by thermodilution. Can Anaesth Soc J 1986;33:780–4

72. Mangano DT. Monitoring pulmonary artery pressure in coronary-artery disease. Anesthesiology 1980;53:364–70

73. Hansen RM, Viquerat CE, Matthay MA, et al. Poor correlation between pulmonary arterial wedge pressure and left ventricular end-diastolic volume after coronary artery bypass graft surgery. Anesthesiology 1986;64:764–70

74. Calvin JE, Dreidger AA, Sibbald E. Does the pulmonary capillary wedge pressure predict left ventricular preload in critically ill patients? Crit Care Med 1981;9:437–43

75. Clements FM, deBruijn NP. Perioperative evaluation or regional wall motion by transesophageal two-dimensional echocardiography. Anesth Analg 1987;66:249–61

76. Konstadt SN, Thys D, Mindich BP, Kaplan JA, Goldman M. Validation of quantitative intraoperative transesophageal echocardiography. Anesthesiology 1986;65:418–21

77. LaMantia K, Lehmann K, Barash P. Echocardiography in the perioperative period. Acute Care 1985;11:106–16

78. Smith JS, Cahalan MK, Benefiel DJ. Intraoperative detection of myocardial ischemia in high risk patients. Circulation 1985;72:1015–21

79. Rentrop KP, Cohen M, Blanke H, Phillips RA. Changes in collateral filling after controlled coronary artery occlusion by an angioplasty balloon in human subjects. J Am Coll Cardiol 1985;5:587–93

80. Schroeder JS, Hunt SA. Cardiac transplantation: Where are we? N Engl J Med 1986;315:961–5

81. Borland LM, Cook DR. Anesthesia for organ transplantation. In:Stoelting RK, Barash PG, Gallagher TJ, eds. Advances in Anesthesia. Chicago. Year Book Medical Publishers 1986:1–36

82. Demas K, Wyner J, Mihm FG, Samuels S. Anesthesia for heart transplantation. A retrospective study and review. Br J Anaesth 1986;58:1357–64

2

Valvular Heart Disease

Management of patients with valvular heart disease in the perioperative period requires an understanding of the hemodynamic alterations that accompany dysfunction of cardiac valves. The most frequently encountered cardiac valvular lesions produce pressure (mitral stenosis, aortic stenosis) or volume (mitral regurgitation, aortic regurgitation) overload on the left ventricle. Drug selections for patients with valvular heart disease are based on the likely effects that drug-induced changes in cardiac rhythm, heart rate, blood pressure, systemic vascular resistance, and pulmonary vascular resistance will have relative to the pathophysiology of the heart disease.

PREOPERATIVE EVALUATION

Preoperative evaluation of patients with valvular heart disease includes assessment of the severity of the cardiac disease, the degree of impaired myocardial contractility, and the presence of associated major organ disease (pulmonary, renal, hepatic). Recognition of compensatory mechanisms for maintaining cardiac output (increased sympathetic nervous system activity, cardiac hypertrophy) and of the role of drug therapy is needed. This information can be obtained from the history and physical examination and from a review of current laboratory data.

History and Physical Examination

Questions designed to define exercise tolerance of patients with known valvular heart disease are essential for evaluating cardiac reserve. In this regard, it is useful to classify patients according to the criteria of the New York Heart Association (Table 2-1). Congestive heart failure is a frequent companion of chronic valvular heart disease. When myocardial contractility is impaired, patients may complain of dyspnea, orthopnea, and fatigability. Compensatory increases in sympathetic nervous system activity can manifest as anxiety, diaphoresis, and resting tachycardia. In support of the diagnosis of congestive heart failure would be, on physical examination, the findings of basilar chest rales, jugular venous distention, and the presence of third heart sounds (see Chapter 7). Ideally, elective surgery is deferred until congestive heart failure can be treated and myocardial contractility optimized.

Disease of heart valves rarely presents without an accompanying murmur reflecting turbulent blood flow across the valves. The character, location, intensity, and direction of radiation of a cardiac murmur provide clues as to the location and severity of the lesion (Fig. 2-1).[1] During systole, the aortic and pulmonic valves are open and the mitral and tricuspid valves are closed. Therefore, cardiac murmurs

37

TABLE 2-1. New York Heart Association Classification of Patients with Heart Disease

Class	Description
1	Asymptomatic
2	Symptoms with ordinary activity but comfortable at rest
3	Symptoms with minimal activity but comfortable at rest
4	Symptoms at rest

occurring in systole are due either to stenosis of the aortic or pulmonic valves or to incompetence of the mitral or tricuspid valves. During diastole, the aortic and pulmonic valves are closed, and the mitral and tricuspid valves are open. Therefore, cardiac murmurs occurring in diastole are due either to stenosis of the mitral or tricuspid valves or incompetence of the aortic or pulmonic valves.

Atrial dysrhythmias are seen in all types of valvular heart disease. Atrial fibrillation is most common with rheumatic mitral valve disease associated with enlargement of the left atrium. An irregular heart rate plus differences between the precordial and peripheral heart rates suggests the presence of atrial fibrillation. Initially, atrial fibrillation is paroxysmal, but after several years, this cardiac rhythm becomes persistent.

Angina pectoris can occur in patients with valvular disease even in the absence of coronary artery disease. This reflects an increased myocardial oxygen demand due to increased cardiac muscle mass that exceeds the ability of even normal coronary arteries to deliver adequate amounts of oxygen. Furthermore, valvular heart disease and coronary artery disease frequently co-exist. Indeed, 50 percent of patients over 50 years of age with aortic stenosis have associated coronary artery disease.

Likely drug therapy in patients with valvular heart disease includes digitalis and diuretics. Digitalis, most often used to improve myocardial contractility and to slow the ventricular heart rate response in patients with atrial fibrillation, has been shown to improve left ventricular filling in these patients by prolonging the duration of diastole. Adequate digitalis effect for heart rate control is indicated by a resting ventricular rate of less that 80 beats·min^{-1}, which increases no more than 15 beats·min^{-1} with mild physical activity. Without adequate preoperative heart rate control, stimulation of the sympathetic nervous system, as during intubation of the trachea or during maximum surgical manipulation, will very likely adversely increase heart rate, with subsequent reductions in diastolic filling times and stroke volume. Signs of digitalis toxicity (prolonged P-R intervals and ventricular premature beats on the electrocardiogram and patient complaints related to gastrointestinal dysfunction) must be appreciated. Vulnerability to the development of digitalis toxicity is increased when concomitant diuretic therapy has led to total body depletion of potassium.

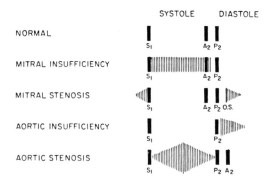

FIG. 2-1. Position and characteristics of heart sounds and murmurs in the presence of valvular heart disease. (Fishman MC, Hoffman AR, Klausner RD, Rockson SG, Thaler MS. Medicine. Philadelphia. JB Lippincott Co. 1981;42.)

Laboratory Measurements

The electrocardiogram often reflects characteristic changes due to valvular heart disease. For example, broad and notched P waves suggest the presence of left atrial enlargement typical of mitral stenosis. Ventricular hypertrophy is mirrored by the presence of left or right axis deviation.

Radiographs of the chest should be reviewed for the size and shape of the heart and great vessels and vascular markings in the lungs. On a posterior-anterior radiograph of the chest, heart size should not exceed 50 percent of the internal diameter of the thoracic cage. The shadow of the left heart border from above downward represents the aorta, pulmonary artery, left atrium, and left ventricle; on the right side the shadow is due to the superior vena cava and right atrium. Enlargement of the left atrium can result in elevation of the left bronchus and an increase in the angle of the carina to greater than 90 degrees. Vascular markings in the peripheral lung fields may be sparse in the presence of severe pulmonary hypertension.

Severe valvular heart disease can interfere with oxygenation and ventilation, as reflected by measurement of the arterial blood gases. For example, prolonged increases in left atrial pressures will be reflected back into the pulmonary veins and eventually into pulmonary parenchymal tissues. These changes can produce alterations in the relation of ventilation to perfusion, as well as the development of pulmonary edema, leading to reductions in arterial oxygen partial pressures.

Transvalvular pressure gradients determined at cardiac catheterization provide useful information as to the severity of cardiac valvular disease. Mitral and aortic stenosis are considered to be present when transvalvular pressure gradients are greater than 10 mmHg and 50 mmHg, respectively.[2] These limits are

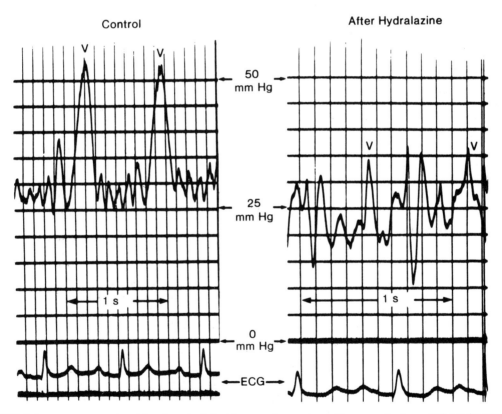

FIG. 2-2. Regurgitant blood flow into the left atrium produces a large V wave on the trace of the pulmonary artery occlusion pressure obtained from a patient with mitral regurgitation. The administration of a vasodilator drug (hydralazine) reduces impedance to forward ejection of the left ventricular stroke volume. As a result, the volume of regurgitant flow into the left atrium is less, and the magnitude of the V wave on the recording of the pulmonary artery occlusion pressure is reduced. (Greenberg BH, Rahimtoola SH. Vasodilator therapy for valvular heart disease. JAMA 1981;246:269–72. Copyright 1981, American Medical Association.)

valid only in the absence of congestive heart failure. For example, when cardiac failure accompanies aortic stenosis, transvalvular gradients of only 20 mmHg signify severe valvular disease. Severity of valvular regurgitation can be estimated by visualizing the amount of angiographic dye that regurgitates back into the cardiac chamber distal to the diseased valve. Monitoring the magnitude of V waves on tracings obtained during recording of pulmonary artery occlusion pressures can be a clinically useful measure of the severity of mitral regurgitation (Fig. 2-2).[3] In patients with mitral stenosis or mitral regurgitation, measurement of pulmonary artery pressures and right ventricular filling pressures may reveal evidence of pulmonary hypertension and right ventricular failure. Coronary artery angiography may provide evidence of coronary artery disease in patients with valvular disease. Indeed, mitral regurgitation secondary to papillary muscle dysfunction may reflect myocardial ischemia or prior myocardial infarctions.

Echocardiography is a noninvasive technique that uses ultrasonic waves to analyze cardiac valves and left ventricular wall function in patients with valvular disease.[4] This technique is particularly valuable in detecting mitral stenosis and in evaluating the severity of aortic stenosis.

MITRAL STENOSIS

Mitral stenosis is almost always due to fusion of the mitral valve leaflets at the commissures during the healing process of acute rheumatic carditis. Symptoms due to progressive reductions in the size of the mitral valve orifice do not usually develop until about 20 years after the initial episode of rheumatic fever. Patients are likely to be symptomatic when the size of the mitral valve orifice (normally 4 cm^2 to 6 cm^2) has decreased at least 50 percent. When the mitral valve area is less than 1.0 cm^2, mean left atrial pressures of 25 mmHg are necessary to maintain an adequate resting cardiac output. An average of 7 years separates the onset of symptoms from complete incapacity.

Clinically, this valvular lesion is recognized by the characteristic opening snap that occurs early in diastole, and by a rumbling diastolic murmur best heard at the apex of the heart. The opening snap is caused by vibrations set in motion when the mobile but stenosed valve initially opens. Calcification of the valve may result in disappearance of the opening snap. Left atrial enlargement is visible on radiographs of the chest as straightening of the left heart border, widening of the carinal angle, and displacement of a barium-filled esophagus on a lateral view. In the absence of atrial fibrillation, large biphasic P waves on the electrocardiogram suggest left atrial enlargement. Surgical replacement of the diseased valve may ultimately become necessary. Catheter balloon valvuloplasty using a percutaneous venous introduction and transseptal approach to the mitral valve may be used to reduce obstruction to flow in selected patients.[5]

Pathophysiology

Mitral stenosis is characterized by mechanical obstruction to left ventricular diastolic filling secondary to progressive decreases in the orifice of the mitral valve. Valvular obstruction produces increases in left atrial pressures and chamber size. Left ventricular filling and stroke volume in the presence of mild mitral stenosis are usually maintained at rest by increased left atrial pressures. Stroke volume, however, may decrease during stress-induced tachycardia or when effective atrial contraction is lost, as during junctional rhythm or atrial fibrillation.

Pulmonary venous pressure is elevated in association with increased left atrial pressures. Pulmonary edema is likely when pulmonary venous pressures exceed the oncotic pressure of plasma proteins. If the rise in this pressure is gradual, however, there is an increase in lymphatic drainage from the lungs and a thickening of capillary basement membranes that permits patients to tolerate increased pressures without the development of pulmonary edema. For unknown reasons, in about 30 percent of patients there is an accelerated increase in pulmonary artery pressures and elevated pulmonary vascular resistance leading to persistent pulmonary hypertension. Furthermore, pulmonary arteriolar constriction with an associated increase in pulmonary vascular resistance is likely when left atrial pressures are chronically elevated above 25 mmHg. Changes in the pulmonary vasculature also result in decreased compliance of the lungs and increased work of breathing.

Despite the impediment to diastolic filling of the left ventricle imposed by stenotic mitral valves, left ventricular end-diastolic volumes and pressures usually remain normal. High volumes or pressures suggest the presence of mitral regurgitation, aortic regurgitation, or primary myocardial disease.

Stasis of blood in the distended left atrium predisposes to the formation of thrombi, which can be displaced as systemic emboli, especially with the onset of atrial fibrillation. Likewise, venous thrombosis is encouraged by the low cardiac output and decreased mobility of these patients. For these reasons, patients with mitral stenosis may be receiving chronic anticoagulant therapy. Dyspnea, orthopnea, and pulmonary edema may accompany exercise, pregnancy, or abrupt onset of atrial fibrillation.

Management of Anesthesia for Noncardiac Surgery

Prophylactic antibiotics instituted in the preoperative period for protection against the development of infective endocarditis are usually recommended for patients with mitral stenosis who are scheduled for noncardiac surgery. Patients taking digitalis for control of ventricular rate responses during atrial fibrillation should have this drug continued until the time of surgery. Since diuretic therapy is frequent, plasma potassium concentrations should be measured preoperatively. In addition, the presence of orthostatic hypotenison may be evidence of diuretic-induced hypovolemia. Advisability of discontinuing anticoagulant medication before elective surgery is unclear. In one report, the incidence of thromboembolism was not increased when anticoagulant medication was gradually discontinued 1 day to 3 days preoperatively, allowing prothrombin time to return to within 20 percent of normal.[6] A prudent approach would seem to be gradual reductions in doses of anticoagulant drugs in the preoperative period, so as to maintain tests of coagulation (prothrombin time, activated partial thromboplastin time) near normal levels.

Small valve orifices associated with mitral stenosis impair left ventricular filling such that heart rate responses must be considered with drugs administered to patients with this abnormality. Indeed, excessive increases in heart rate can so shorten diastolic filling times of the left ventricle that stroke volume, cardiac output, and blood pressure are reduced. For example, increased heart rates due to preoperative anxiety may be responsible for detrimental effects on stroke volume.

Effects of drugs on systemic and pulmonary vascular resistance must be considered in patients with mitral stenosis. For example, sudden drug-induced reductions in systemic vascular resistance in the presence of a fixed left ventricular stroke volume or co-existing reductions of intravascular fluid volume can lead to undesirable degrees of hypotension. Likewise, arterial hypoxemia, acidosis, or administration of alpha-adrenergic agonist drugs can further increase an already elevated pulmonary vascular resistance.

Preoperative preparation of patients with mitral stenosis should be designed to reduce anxiety and the likelihood of adverse circulatory responses produced by increased heart rate. During the preoperative interview, in addition to detailing with the patient the events that will take place in the perioperative period, it is also reasonable to consider pharmacologic attempts to reduce anxiety. The best drug or drug combination for reducing anxiety is not known, but it must be appreciated that these patients can be more susceptible than normal individuals to ventilatory depressant effects of sedative drugs. Furthermore, use of anticholinergic drugs is controversial because of concern that adverse increases in heart rate could occur. Therefore, when anticholinergic drugs are included in the preoperative medication, it is prudent to choose scopolamine or glycopyrrolate, as these drugs have fewer chronotropic effects than atropine.

Induction of anesthesia in the presence of mitral stenosis can be achieved with intravenous administration of barbiturates, benzodiazepines, or etomidate followed by succinylcholine to facilitate intubation of the trachea. An increased incidence of ventricular dysrhythmias after administration of succinylcholine to patients taking digitalis has not been a consistent observation.[7] Ketamine is probably not a good choice for induction of anesthesia because of its propensity to increase heart rate.

Drugs used for maintenance of anesthesia should be associated with minimal changes in heart rate and in systemic and pulmonary vascular resistance. Furthermore, these drugs should not greatly reduce myocardial contractility. These goals can be achieved with combinations of nitrous oxide and opioids or low concentrations of volatile drugs. Although nitrous oxide can increase pulmonary vascular resistance, it is unlikely that the magnitude of this change would justify avoiding this drug in patients with mitral stenosis (Fig. 2-3).[8] Controlled ventilation of the lungs and normocapnia are ideal, remembering that respiratory alkalosis and concomitant reductions in plasma potassium concentrations are particularly undesirable in patients receiving digitalis.

Choice of nondepolarizing muscle relaxants is determined by the circulatory effects these drugs are likely to produce. Peripheral vasodilation after administration of d-tubocurarine could result in undesirable degrees of hypotension. Pancuronium is avoided because of its ability to increase the speed of transmission of cardiac impulses through the atrioventricular node, which could lead to excessive increases in heart rate.[9] Such increases would seem particularly likely in the presence of atrial fibrillation, since the ventricular response to atrial impulses is determined by the degree of atrioventricular conduction. Therefore, muscle relaxants with minimal circulatory effects (metocurine, atracurium, vecuronium) are useful in patients with mitral stenosis. There is no reason to avoid pharmacologic reversal of nondepolarizing muscle relaxants,

but the adverse effects of drug-induced tachycardia should be considered. Theoretically, glycopyrrolate would be a better choice than atropine to combine with anticholinesterase drugs. This recommendation is based on the suggestion that glycopyrrolate has less chronotropic effects than atropine.

Use of invasive monitoring depends on the complexity of the operative procedure and the magnitude of physiologic impairment produced by mitral stenosis. Continuous monitoring of intra-arterial blood pressure and atrial filling pressures in indicated when major operative procedures are planned, particularly in patients with mitral stenosis who are symptomatic at rest or who have persistent pulmonary hypertension. These monitors are helpful in confirming the adequacy of ventilation, oxygenation, and intravascular fluid volume replacement and for assessing the efficacy of drug therapy on cardiac contractility. An increase in right atrial pressures could reflect nitrous oxide-induced pulmonary vasoconstriction, suggesting the need to discontinue this drug. Intraoperative fluid replacement must be carefully titrated as these patients are susceptible to volume overload and to the development of left ventricular failure and pulmonary edema. Likewise, the head-down position is not well tolerated by these patients, since pulmonary blood volume is already increased.

Light anesthesia and surgical stimulation can lead to systemic hypertension plus reductions in cardiac output due to elevations in systemic and pulmonary vascular resistance. When this occurs, intravenous infusions of nitroprusside ($0.2 \ \mu g \cdot kg^{-1} \cdot min^{-1}$ to 4 $\mu g \cdot kg^{-1} \cdot min^{-1}$) may be effective in reducing systemic vascular resistance, pulmonary artery pressures, and left atrial pressures.[10] Furthermore, nitroprusside-induced reductions in systemic vascular resistance are also associated with increases in left ventricular stroke volume, particularly when co-existing pulmonary hypertension is severe or mitral regurgitation co-exists with mitral stenosis (Fig. 2-4).[10]

Correction of intraoperative hypotension with sympathomimetic drugs can be achieved with ephedrine or phenylephrine. Advantages of ephedrine include its beta-adrenergic activ-

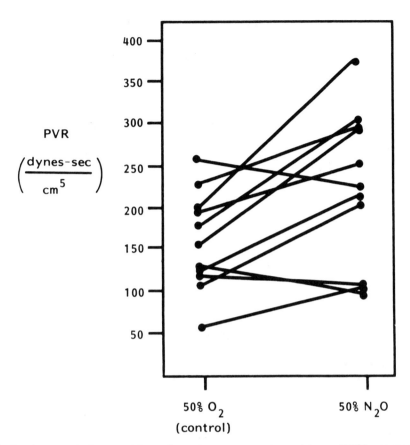

FIG. 2-3. The impact of nitrous oxide on the pulmonary vascular resistance (PVR) was measured in 11 patients with co-existing pulmonary hypertension due to mitral valve disease. Each solid circle represents an individual patient. Compared with PVR while breathing 50 percent O_2 (control), the inhalation of 50 percent nitrous oxide for 10 minutes increased the calculated PVR in 8 of 11 patients. Nevertheless, the magnitude of increase in PVR was not sufficient to recommend the routine avoidance of nitrous oxide in patients with co-existing pulmonary hypertension. (Hilgenberg JC, McCammon RL, Stoelting RK. Pulmonary and systemic vascular responses to nitrous oxide in patients with mitral stenosis and pulmonary hypertension. Anesth Analg 1980;59:323–6. Reprinted with permission from IARS.)

ity, which results in increases in myocardial contractility and cardiac output even though ventricular afterload is increased. The disadvantage of ephedrine is its ability to increase heart rate. Phenylephrine eliminates the concern regarding heart rate, but increases in ventricular afterload that follow the administration of this predominantly alpha-adrenergic agonist drug can decrease left ventricular stroke volume.[11]

Intraoperative tachycardia that is hemodynamically significant can be treated with small intravenous doses of propranolol (0.1 mg·min⁻¹ not to exceed 50 μg·kg⁻¹) or with digoxin (0.25 mg to 0.75 mg). Addition of low doses of volatile anesthetics to deepen anesthesia may be effective in reducing heart rates that are elevated in response to surgical stimulation. Marked increases in heart rate that produce life-threatening decreases in stroke volume, cardiac output, and blood pressure are best treated with electrical cardioversion.

Postoperatively, patients with mitral stenosis are at high risk for developing pulmonary

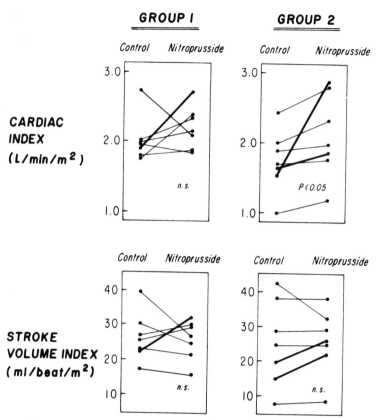

FIG. 2-4. The cardiovascular effects of an intravenous infusion of nitroprusside (range 0.2 μg·kg^{-1}·min^{-1} to 4 μg·kg^{-1}·min^{-1}) were evaluated intraoperatively in seven patients with pure mitral stenosis (Group 1) and seven patients with mixed mitral stenosis and mitral regurgitation (Group 2). The infusion of nitroprusside did not produce adverse effects on cardiac function in any patient. Furthermore, in patients with severe pulmonary hypertension (thick lines) the infusion of nitroprusside led to substantial increases in cardiac index and stroke volume index. These data confirm that nitroprusside-induced reductions in systemic vascular resistance are not detrimental to cardiac function in patients with pure mitral stenosis. Indeed, when associated pulmonary hypertension is severe, drug-induced reductions in afterload may even be beneficial. (Stone JG, Hoar PF, Faltas AN, Khambatta HJ. Nitroprusside and mitral stenosis. Anesth Analg 1980;59:662–5. Reprinted with permission from IARS.)

edema and right heart failure. Pain, respiratory acidosis, and arterial hypoxemia may be the responsible events for increasing heart rate or pulmonary vascular resistance. This again emphasizes the importance of continuing cardiac monitoring in the postoperative period. Decreased pulmonary compliance and increased oxygen cost of breathing often accompany chronic mitral stenosis. These changes may necessitate mechanical support of ventilation in the postoperative period, particularly following major thoracic or abdominal surgery.

MITRAL REGURGITATION

Mitral regurgitation is usually due to rheumatic fever and is almost always associated with mitral stenosis. Isolated mitral regurgitation in the absence of prior rheumatic fever is often acute. For example, acute mitral regurgitation may be due to papillary muscle dysfunction following a myocardial infarction or rupture of a chordae tendineae secondary to infective endocarditis. Another cause of mitral regurgitation is dilation of the mitral valve due to left ventricular hypertrophy. A systolic murmur, best heard at the apex of the heart, is a constant feature of this type of valvular disease. Surgical replacement of the diseased valve may ultimately become necessary.

Pathophysiology

Left atrial volume overload is the major pathophysiologic change produced by mitral regurgitation. Indeed, the basic hemodynamic problem in mitral regurgitation is a decrease in the forward left ventricular stroke volume because part of the stroke volume is regurgitated through the incompetent mitral valve into the left atrium. Patients with regurgitant fractions greater than 0.6 are considered to have severe mitral regurgitation. This regurgitant flow is responsible for V waves seen on recordings of the pulmonary artery occlusion pressures obtained from these patients (Fig. 2-2).[3] The size of the V waves correlates with the magnitude of the regurgitant flow.

The fraction of the left ventricular stroke volume that enters the left atrium depends on the (1) size of the mitral valve orifice; (2) heart rate, which determines the duration of ventricular ejection; and (3) pressure gradient across the mitral valve. For example, mild increases in heart rate can improve forward left ventricular stroke volume, and bradycardia could result in acute volume overload of the left atrium. Pressure gradients across the mitral valve depend on the compliance of the left ventricle and on the impedance to left ventricular ejection into the aorta. Pharmacologic interventions that alter this impedance have a major impact on the distribution of the left ventricular stroke volume. For example, reductions in systemic vascular resistance in response to the administration of hydralazine or nitroprusside can greatly improve forward left ventricular stroke volume in patients with mitral regurgitation.[3] Vasodilator therapy is particularly effective for increasing cardiac output when acute mitral regurgitation results in rapid increases in left atrial pressures that lead to pulmonary edema. When this regurgitation is due to papillary muscle dysfunction following myocardial infarctions, use of vasodilator therapy may improve cardiac output to the extent that surgery for replacement of the mitral valve can be deferred until patients have stabilized.

Patients with isolated mitral regurgitation are less dependent on properly timed left atrial contractions for left ventricular filling than are patients with mitral or aortic stenosis. Indeed, conversion from atrial fibrillation to normal sinus rhythm produces minimal changes in cardiac output. Myocardial ischemia is unlikely in the presence of mitral regurgitation because the increased ventricular wall tension is quickly dissipated as the stroke volume is rapidly ejected into both the aorta and left atrium. Furthermore, when mitral regurgitation develops gradually, the compliant left atrium is able to accommodate increased regurgitant volumes without increases in atrial pressures.

The frequent combination of mitral regurgitation and mitral stenosis results in increased volume and pressure work by the heart. In this situation, increased flow rates across the stenotic valve secondary to regurgitation markedly increase left atrial pressures. These patients develop atrial fibrillation, pulmonary edema, and pulmonary hypertension earlier than do patients with isolated mitral regurgitation.

Management of Anesthesia for Noncardiac Surgery

Patients with mitral regurgitation should receive prophylactic antibiotics before surgery to protect against the development of infective endocarditis. Preoperative medication requirements are not critical in these patients. Management of anesthesia should be designed to reduce the likelihood of reductions in heart rate or increases in systemic vascular resistance that would lead to decreases in forward left ventricular stroke volume. Conversely, cardiac output can be improved by modest increases in heart rate and reductions in systemic vascular resistance.

General anesthesia is the usual choice for

patients with mitral regurgitation. Although reductions in systemic vascular resistance are theoretically beneficial, the uncontrolled nature of this response with regional anesthesia detracts from the use of these techniques. Induction of anesthesia can be accomplished with intravenous administration of barbiturates, benzodiazepines, or etomidate followed by succinylcholine to facilitate intubation of the trachea. Theoretically, pharmacologic effects of drugs administered intravenously could be reduced by dilution effects of regurgitant flow. For example, the duration of action of succinylcholine could be shortened by this dilution effect plus increased metabolism, since the drug is exposed to plasma cholinesterase for a longer time. Measurements to support these speculations, however, are not available.

In the absence of severe left ventricular dysfunction, maintenance of anesthesia can be provided with nitrous oxide plus volatile drugs. Volatile drugs can also be used to attenuate undesirable increases in blood pressure and systemic vascular resistance that can accompany surgical stimulation. When myocardial function is severely compromised, nitrous oxide-opioid techniques, which minimize depression of myocardial contractility, may be better choices. Choice of nondepolarizing muscle relaxants is based on the circulatory effects likely to be associated with these drugs. Although d-tubocurarine reduces systemic vascular resistance, the magnitude of this response is not predictable. Therefore, the most useful selections are drugs with minimal to no circulatory effects, such as metocurine, atracurium or vecuronium. Pancuronium is also acceptable, as modest increases in heart rate produced by this drug would very likely increase foward left ventricular stroke volume.

Ventilation of the lungs is ideally controlled and adjusted to maintain near normal arterial carbon dioxide partial pressures. Patterns of ventilation should provide sufficient time between breaths for venous return to occur. Maintenance of intravascular fluid volume with prompt replacement of blood loss is important for maintaining cardiac filling volumes and ejection of an optimal forward left ventricular stroke volume.

Minor operations performed on patients with asymptomatic mitral regurgitation do not require invasive monitoring. In the presence of severe mitral regurgitation, the use of invasive monitoring is helpful for detecting the onset of undesirable degrees of depression of myocardial contractility and for facilitating intravenous fluid replacement. Certainly, a pulmonary artery catheter is indicated when peripheral vasodilating drugs are administered in attempts to increase forward left ventricular stroke volume. Measurements of cardiac output by thermodilution confirms the response to reductions in systemic vascular resistance produced by drugs such as nitroprusside. It should be remembered that regurgitation of blood into the left atrium produces V waves on recordings of the pulmonary artery occlusion pressures. Changes in the amplitude of V waves can assist in estimating the magnitude of mitral regurgitation (Fig. 2-2).[3]

AORTIC STENOSIS

Isolated nonrheumatic aortic stenosis usually results from progressive calcification and stenosis of a congenitally abnormal (usually bicuspid) valve (see Chapter 3). In contrast, aortic stenosis due to rheumatic fever almost always occurs in association with mitral valve disease. In either situation, the natural history of aortic valve disease includes a long latent period, often 30 years or more before symptoms occur.

Clinically, aortic stenosis is recognized by its characteristic systolic murmur best heard in the second right interspace. Since many patients with aortic stenosis are asymptomatic, it is important to listen for this cardiac murmur in all patients scheduled for surgery. Radiographs of the chest may show a prominent ascending aorta due to poststenotic dilation. The characteristic triad of symptoms associated with aortic stenosis includes angina pectoris, dyspnea on exertion, and a history of syncope. Syncope characteristically occurs with effort, presumably reflecting inability of the heart to maintain an adequate cardiac output and systemic blood pressure in the presence of peripheral vasodilation associated with exercise.

The incidence of sudden death is increased in patients with aortic stenosis. Indeed, when any of the triad of symptoms is present, the patient's life expectancy without surgery is less than 5 years, and 15 percent to 20 percent of these patients experience sudden death. Co-existing aortic stenosis is a significant risk factor in the development of postoperative cardiac morbidity following elective noncardiac surgery.[12] Surgical replacement of the diseased valve may ultimately become necessary. Percutaneous transluminal valvuloplasty may be an alternative to surgery in selected patients.[5]

Pathophysiology

Obstruction to ejection of blood into the aorta due to reductions in the orifice of the aortic valve necessitates an increase in left ventricular systolic pressures so as to maintain forward stroke volume. Aortic valve area is usually decreased to about 25 percent of its normal 2.5 cm^2 to 3.5 cm^2 size when increased left ventricular systolic pressures are present. These pressures are associated with compensatory increases in the thickness of the left ventricular wall with little change in chamber size, referred to as concentric hypertrophy. Eventually, dilation of the left ventricular chamber occurs, and myocardial contractility diminishes.

The magnitude of the pressure gradient across the aortic valve serves as an estimate of the severity of aortic stenosis. Hemodynamically significant aortic stenosis is associated with pressure gradients of greater than 50 mmHg. Furthermore, aortic stenosis is almost always associated with some degree of aortic regurgitation.

Angina pectoris often occurs in patients with aortic stenosis, despite the absence of coronary artery disease. This reflects increased myocardial oxygen needs due to the increased amounts of ventricular muscle associated with concentric myocardial hypertrophy. Furthermore, myocardial oxygen delivery is decreased, due to compression of subendocardial coronary blood vessels by increased left ventricular systolic pressures.

Left ventricular filling in patients with aortic stenosis is very dependent on atrial contractions, heart rate, and a normal intravascular fluid volume. Indeed, loss of normal atrial contractions, as during junctional rhythm or atrial fibrillation, may produce significant decreases in stroke volume and blood pressure. Heart rate is important, as this determines time available for filling of the ventricles and ejection of forward left ventricular stroke volume. For example, marked increases in heart rate can reduce the time for left ventricular filling and ejection, leading to undesirable decreases in stroke volume. Likewise, sudden reductions in heart rate can lead to acute overdistention of the left ventricle.

Management of Anesthesia for Noncardiac Surgery

Goals during the management of anesthesia for noncardiac surgery in patients with aortic stenosis are maintenance of normal sinus rhythm and avoidance of extreme and prolonged alterations in heart rate, systemic vascular resistance, and intravascular fluid volume. Preservation of normal sinus rhythm is critical, since the left ventricle is dependent on properly timed atrial contractions to assure optimal left ventricular end-diastolic volumes. Modest increases in heart rate and blood pressure are acceptable, but the implications in terms of myocardial oxygen requirements must be considered. In view of the obstruction to left ventricular ejection, it must be appreciated that decreases in systemic vascular resistance may be associated with large reductions in blood pressure and subsequent reductions in coronary blood flow. Conversely, increases in systemic vascular resistance and blood pressure can lead to reductions in stroke volume. A direct current defibrillator should be immediately available whenever anesthesia is administered to patients with aortic stenosis. External cardiac massage is unlikely to be effective should cardiac arrest occur, since it is difficult to create an adequate stroke volume across a stenotic aortic valve using mechanical compression of the sternum.

Administration of antibiotics before surgery is recommended to provide protection against development of infective endocarditis, particularly when aortic stenosis is associated with rheumatic heart disease. Preoperative medication must be tailored to minimize the likelihood of reductions in systemic vascular resistance. General anesthesia is preferable to regional techniques, since peripheral sympathetic nervous system blockade produced by the latter can lead to undesirable reductions in systemic vascular resistance. If regional techniques are selected, it should be remembered that onset of peripheral sympathetic nervous system blockade is more rapid after subarachnoid anesthetics than after epidural techniques.

Induction of anesthesia in the presence of aortic stenosis can be accomplished with intravenous administration of barbiturates, benzodiazepines, or etomidate. Succinylcholine is useful for the facilitation of tracheal intubation.

Maintenance of anesthesia is accomplished with combinations of nitrous oxide plus volatile or injected drugs. A disadvantage of volatile drugs (especially halothane) is depression of sinoatrial node automaticity, which may lead to a junctional rhythm and loss of properly timed atrial contractions. Furthermore, when left ventricular function is severely impaired by aortic stenosis, it is important to avoid additional depression of myocardial contractility with excessive concentrations of volatile anesthetics. Maintenance of anesthesia with nitrous oxide plus opioids or with opioids alone in high doses (50 $\mu g \cdot kg^{-1}$ to 100 $\mu g \cdot kg^{-1}$ of fentanyl) has been recommended for patients with marked left ventricular dysfunction due to aortic stenosis.[13]

Nondepolarizing muscle relaxants with minimal effects on the circulation are useful, although the modest increases in blood pressure and heart rate typically produced by pancuronium are acceptable. Controlled ventilation of the lungs is acceptable, but the ventilator should be set to minimize reductions in stroke volume produced by positive intrathoracic pressure. This is often achieved by a slow cycling rate, so as to assure sufficient time for venous return between breaths. Intravascular fluid volume must be maintained by prompt replacement of blood loss and liberal administration (5 $ml \cdot kg^{-1} \cdot hr^{-1}$) of intravenous fluids.

Intraoperative monitoring of patients with aortic stenosis should include an electrocardiogram lead that will reflect left ventricular ischemia. Use of arterial and pulmonary artery catheters depends on the magnitude of the surgery and the severity of the aortic stenosis. These monitors are invaluable in helping to determine if intraoperative hypotension is due to hypovolemia or to cardiac failure. It should be remembered that pulmonary artery occlusion pressures may overestimate left ventricular end-diastolic pressures because of decreased compliance of the left ventricle that accompanies chronic aortic stenosis.

Intraoperatively, the onset of junctional rhythm or bradycardia should be treated promptly with intravenous administration of atropine. Persistent elevations in heart rate can be treated with intravenous administration of propranolol. Large doses of propranolol, however, must be avoided, since these patients may be dependent on endogenous beta-adrenergic activity to maintain stroke volume, particularly in the presence of increased systemic vascular resistance that occurs in response to surgical stimulation. Supraventricular tachycardia should be promptly terminated with electrical cardioversion. Lidocaine should be immediately available, as these patients have a propensity to develop ventricular cardiac dysrhythmias.

AORTIC REGURGITATION

Aortic regurgitation may be acute or chronic. Acute aortic regurgitation is most often due to infective endocarditis, trauma, or dissection of a thoracic aneurysm. Treatment is prompt surgical replacement of the aortic valve. Chronic aortic regurgitation is usually due to prior rheumatic fever or persistent systemic hypertension. A diastolic murmur best heard in the second right interspace plus evidence of left ventricular enlargement on radiographs of the chest and the electrocardiogram are characteristic of aortic regurgitation. In contrast to aortic stenosis, occurrence of sudden death with aortic regurgitation is rare. Surgical replacement of the diseased valve may ultimately become necessary.

Pathophysiology

The basic hemodynamic problem in aortic regurgitation is a decrease in forward left ventricular stroke volume because of regurgitation of part of the ejected stroke volume from the aorta back into the left ventricle. The magnitude of the regurgitant volume depends on the (1) duration for regurgitant flow to occur, which is determined by the heart rate; and (2) pressure gradient across the aortic valve, which is dependent on systemic vascular resistance. The magnitude of aortic regurgitation will be reduced by increases in heart rate and decreases in systemic vascular resistance. Indeed, increasing the heart rate with an artificial cardiac pacemaker or reducing systemic vascular resistance with exercise leads to decreases in the magnitude of regurgitant flow and increased forward left ventricular stroke volume. This is consistent with the observation that patients with aortic regurgitation often tolerate exercise but can develop pulmonary edema at rest.

A gradual onset of aortic regurgitation is associated with marked increases in left ventricular muscle mass. Increased myocardial oxygen requirements secondary to left ventricular hypertrophy, plus characteristic decreases in aortic diastolic pressure, which reduces coronary blood flow, can manifest as angina pectoris due to subendocardial ischemia in the absence of coronary artery disease. When aortic regurgitation is acute, sudden increases in ventricular volume occur before ventricular hypertrophy can develop. This limits the effectiveness of such compensatory mechanisms as increased heart rate and increased myocardial

contractility in maintaining an adequate cardiac output.

Compared to patients with chronic aortic regurgitation, patients who develop acute regurgitation are more likely to manifest reductions in cardiac output and blood pressure following changes in heart rate, cardiac rhythm, and myocardial contractility. Infusions of nitroprusside may be effective in improving forward stroke volume when acute aortic regurgitation results in left ventricular volume overload and a decreased cardiac output.

Management of Anesthesia for Noncardiac Surgery

Management of anesthesia for noncardiac surgery in patients with aortic regurgitation is designed to maintain forward left ventricular stroke volume by minimizing the occurrence of abrupt and excessive changes in heart rate, systemic vascular resistance, myocardial contractility, and intravascular fluid volume. Ideally, heart rate is slightly increased with modest reductions in systemic vascular resistance, so as to reduce impedance to forward ejection of the left ventricular stroke volume. Still, it should be remembered that these patients may be exquisitely sensitive to peripheral vasodilation. Preoperative administration of antibiotics to protect against the development of infective endocarditis is indicated. There are no special recommendations regarding preoperative medication.

General anesthesia is usually chosen. Although regional anesthesia produces desirable decreases in systemic vascular resistance, it is difficult to control reliably the magnitude of this change. Induction of anesthesia may be accomplished with intravenous administration of barbiturates, benzodiazepines, or etomidate. Ketamine would be advantageous by virtue of its ability to accelerate heart rate, but the accompanying elevation in the resistance to ejection of forward left ventricular stroke volume due to increased systemic vascular resistance could be undesirable. Nevertheless, when intravascular fluid volume is judged to be decreased, use of ketamine for induction of anesthesia is an acceptable choice. Succinylcholine is often administered for facilitation of intubation of the trachea, remembering that drug-induced bradycardia could produce acute left ventricular volume overload.

Maintenance of anesthesia in the presence of mild aortic regurgitation and minimal cardiac dysfunction can be accomplished with combinations of nitrous oxide plus opioids or volatile anesthetics. Drug-induced reductions in systemic vascular resistance may facilitate forward left ventricular stroke volume. This response, however, should not be achieved at the expense of drug-induced myocardial depression and hypotension. Indeed, patients with severe left ventricular dysfunction may not tolerate even minimal additional reductions in myocardial contractility. In these patients, nitrous oxide–opioid combinations are preferable to the use of volatile anesthetics. Low concentrations of volatile drugs, however, are not likely to be associated with extreme reductions in myocardial contractility. Furthermore, it must be remembered that nitrous oxide added to opioids or benzodiazepines added to opioids can produce circulatory depression that is not apparent when opioids or nitrous oxide are used alone.[14,15] In extreme instances of cardiac dysfunction, the use of short-acting opioids such as fentanyl in high doses (50 μg·kg^{-1} to 100 μg·kg^{-1}) as the sole drug for maintenance of anesthesia may be the best choice for providing adequate amnesia without producing additional cardiac depression.[13]

Nondepolarizing muscle relaxants are chosen on the basis of associated circulatory effects. The magnitude of reductions in systemic vascular resistance produced by d-tubocurarine is not controllable, making this drug an unlikely choice. Absence of significant circulatory changes following administration of metocurine, atracurium, or vecuronium, or the modest increases in heart rate produced by pancuronium, make these drugs useful choices. The potential, however, for increased myocardial oxygen requirements following pancuronium-induced increases in heart rate should be appreciated. Cardiac output is optimized by providing sufficient time for venous return during controlled ventilation of the lungs (i.e., slow breathing rate) and by maintaining intravascular fluid volume near or slightly above preoperative levels.

Bradycardia or junctional rhythms are undesirable in patients with aortic regurgitation, particularly in those individuals with a noncompliant left ventricle that is highly dependent on atrial contractions for diastolic filling. Should these cardiac rhythm changes occur intraoperatively, they should be treated promptly with intravenous administration of atropine.

In patients with severe aortic regurgitation, decreases in cardiac output due to increased systemic vascular resistance associated with systemic hypertension can be treated with continuous intravenous infusions of nitroprusside. Combinations of preoperative fluid loading and intravenous infusions of nitroprusside during surgery for cardiac valve replacement have been shown to produce more favorable changes in systemic vascular resistance and cardiac output than does vasodilator therapy alone (Fig. 2-5).[16]

Intraoperative monitoring should include the use of electrocardiogram leads that will reflect left ventricular ischemia. When the magnitude of the surgical procedure and the degree of aortic regurgitation are substantial, the use of invasive monitoring is a consideration. Pulmonary artery catheters are helpful in guiding intravenous volume replacement and for judging responses of cardiac output to peripheral vasodilating drugs.

TRICUSPID REGURGITATION

Tricuspid regurgitation is usually functional, reflecting dilation of the right ventricle due to pulmonary hypertension. Indeed, such regurgitation often accompanies pulmonary hypertension and right ventricular volume overloading due to left ventricular failure produced by aortic or mitral valve disease. There is also a significant incidence of tricuspid regurgitation secondary to infective endocarditis associated with intravenous injection of drugs for nonmedical purposes. Tricuspid regurgitation is invariably associated with tricuspid

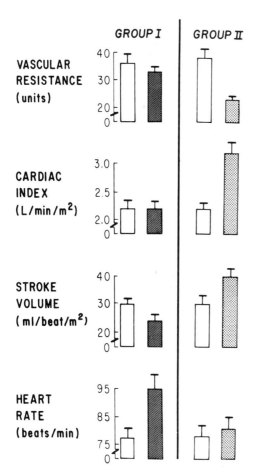

FIG. 2-5. Data (Mean ± SE) were collected before induction of anesthesia (clear bars) and during surgical stimulation (shaded bars) in 17 patients with cardiac valvular regurgitation (7 with mitral regurgitation, 7 with aortic regurgitation, 3 with both). All patients were undergoing prosthetic replacement of the diseased cardiac valve. Following awake measurements, both groups received continuous intravenous infusions of nitroprusside (range 1.3 $\mu g \cdot kg^{-1} \cdot min^{-1}$ to 3.7 $\mu g \cdot kg^{-1} \cdot min^{-1}$). Group II patients also received preoperative fluid loading with approximately 2 liters of lactated Ringer's solution. These data demonstrate that the combination of afterload reduction and preload augmentation (Group II) produced more desirable circulatory responses than afterload reduction alone (Group 1). (Stone JG, Hoar PF, Calabro JR, et al. Afterload reductions and preload augmentation of patients with cardiac failure and valvular regurgitation. Anesth Analg 1980;59:737–42. Reprinted with permission from IARS.)

stenosis when valve dysfunction is the result of prior rheumatic fever.

Pathophysiology

The basic hemodynamic consequence of tricuspid regurgitation is right atrial volume overload that is well tolerated. The high compliance of the right atrium and vena cavae results in minimal increases in right atrial pressure, even in the presence of large regurgitant volumes. Even surgical removal of the tricuspid valve, as in patients with infective endocarditis, is usually well tolerated.

Although pure tricuspid regurgitation is relatively benign, the addition of a right ventricular pressure overload, as produced by left ventricular failure or pulmonary hypertension, will often lead to right ventricular failure. Right ventricular failure causes increased regurgitation through the incompetent tricuspid valve, with further decreases in left ventricular stroke volume due to decreased pulmonary blood flow. Combinations of right ventricular failure and left ventricular underloading can cause right atrial pressures to exceed left atrial pressures, leading in some patients to right-to-left intracardiac shunts through an incompletely closed foramen ovale.

Management of Anesthesia for Noncardiac Surgery

Management of anesthesia in patients with tricuspid regurgitation will be similar whether regurgitation is isolated or associated with aortic or mitral valve disease. Intravascular fluid volume and central venous pressure must be maintained in a high normal range, to assure adequate right ventricular stroke volume and left ventricular filling. High intrathoracic pressures due to positive pressure ventilation of the lungs or drug-induced venodilation will reduce venous return and eventually compromise left ventricular stroke volume. Likewise, events known to increase pulmonary vascular resistance, such as arterial hypoxemia and hypercarbia, should be avoided.

No specific anesthetic drugs or techniques can be advocated for management of patients with tricuspid regurgitation. Nevertheless, halothane has been recommended because of its alleged vasodilating effects on the pulmonary vasculature. Likewise, ketamine is a reasonable choice, as it maintains venous return. Nitrous oxide is a weak pulmonary vasoconstrictor when combined with opioids and could increase the magnitude of tricuspid regurgitation by this mechanism. If nitrous oxide is used, the prudent approach would be to monitor central venous pressures and consider the possible role of nitrous oxide should undesirable elevations in right atrial pressures occur.

Intraoperative monitors should include measurement of right atrial filling pressures to guide intravenous fluid replacement and to detect adverse effects of anesthetic drugs or techniques on the magnitude of tricuspid regurgitation. Intravenous infusion of air via tubing used to deliver intravenous solutions must be guarded against, in view of the possibility of a right-to-left intracardiac shunt through an incompletely closed foramen ovale.

MITRAL VALVE PROLAPSE

Mitral valve prolapse (click-murmur syndrome, Barlow's syndrome) is characterized by prolapse of the mitral valve leaflets into the left atrium during systole.[17] Presence of this valvular abnormality is suggested by the auscultatory finding of a nonejection click best heard at the apex, which may or may not be associated with a late systolic murmur of mitral regurgitation. This auscultatory finding is present in about 5 percent of the population, which makes mitral valve prolapse one of the most common of all cardiac abnormalities. In the absence of a nonejection click, echocardiographic or angiographic studies are prerequisites for the diagnosis of mitral valve prolapse. Histologic and anatomic abnormalities of the mitral valve in patients with this syndrome include redundancy and myxomatous

degeneration of the leaflets, dilation of the mitral valve annulus, and elongation and thinning of the chordae tendineae.

The etiology of mitral valve prolapse is unclear, although there is a definite familial occurrence.[18] On physical examination, individuals with mitral valve prolapse are often tall and thin and may have associated findings such as high arched palate, pectus excavatum, kyphoscoliosis, or hyperextensible joints. Indeed, the classic occurrence of this abnormality is in Marfan's syndrome. There is an increased incidence of this cardiac abnormality in patients with von Willebrand's syndrome.[19] Poor left ventricular contractility due to muscular dystrophy, cardiomyopathy or coronary artery disease is associated with mitral valve prolapse. This valvular abnormality may occur in patients with atrial septal defects or tricuspid regurgitation. Damage to the mitral valve from rheumatic heart disease can also result in mitral valve prolapse.

Complications

Despite the prevalence of mitral valve prolapse, the majority of patients are asymptomatic, emphasizing the usual benign course of this abnormality. Nevertheless, potentially serious complications can result from mitral valve prolapse (Table 2-2).[17] For example, mitral valve prolapse is probably the most common cause of pure mitral regurgitation, which may progress to the need for surgical intervention. Infective endocarditis is an important potential complication of mitral valve prolapse

TABLE 2-2.   Complications Associated with Mitral Valve Prolapse

Mitral regurgitation
Infective endocarditis
Ruptured chordae tendineae
Transient ischemic attacks
Cardiac dysrhythmias—ventricular premature beats
Atrioventricular heart block
ST segment and T wave changes on the electrocardiogram
Sudden death (extremely rare)

accounting for 10 percent to 15 percent of cases. Mitral valve prolapse without superimposed endocarditis is the underlying pathologic abnormality in the majority of patients with ruptured chordae tendineae. This valvular abnormality is responsible for about 40 percent of the transient ischemic attacks that occur in individuals less than 45 years of age. These patients may be subsequently treated with drugs to decrease platelet aggregation (aspirin, dipyridamole) or to produce anticoagulation (coumarin). It is postulated that a clot originates from the rough surface of the prolapsed mitral valve or the traumatized adjacent left atrial surface. Atrial and ventricular dysrhythmias are not uncommon, with premature ventricular beats being the most frequent. Beta-adrenergic antagonist drugs are the most effective therapy for control of cardiac dysrhythmias in these patients. This may reflect nonspecific antidysrhythmic effects or drug-induced increases in left ventricular end-diastolic volumes that serve to reduce the degree of mitral valve prolapse. Supraventricular tachydysrhythmias may occur and are consistent with the occasional association of mitral valve prolapse with preexcitation syndromes. Bradycardia associated with atrioventricular heart block may be resistant to atropine and may require intravenous infusions of isoproterenol or use of artificial cardiac pacemakers. The electrocardiogram, although usually normal, may reflect T-wave flattening or inversion with or without ST segment depression.[18] Sudden death is an extremely rare complication that is assumed to be due to ventricular cardiac dysrhythmias. Indeed, this complication is so rare that it need not be mentioned to patients or their families as undue anxiety may occur.[17]

Management of Anesthesia for Noncardiac Surgery

The important principle in the management of anesthesia for patients known to have mitral valve prolapse is the recognition that increased left ventricular emptying can accentuate prolapse leading to cardiac dysrhythmias and/or acute mitral regurgitation.[19] Perioperative events that can increase left ventricular emptying include (1) increased sympathetic nervous system activity, (2) reductions in systemic vascular resistance, and (3) assumption of the upright posture. Reductions in anxiety are important goals of the preanesthetic interview and premedication of these patients. Nevertheless, the possibility of undesirable drug-induced increases in heart rate (atropine) or reductions in systemic vascular resistance (opioids) should be considered when selecting the dose for premedication of these patients. Antibiotics should be administered for protection against the development of infective endocarditis.

Intravenous induction of anesthesia is acceptably accomplished with an intravenous administration of barbiturates, benzodiazepines, or etomidate, remembering that excessive reductions in systemic vascular resistance are undesirable. With this in mind, it is important to optimize intravascular fluid volume in the preoperative period. Ketamine is not recommended for administration to patients with mitral valve prolapse because of its ability to stimulate the sympathetic nervous system.

Maintenance of anesthesia is designed to minimize sympathetic nervous system activation secondary to noxious intraoperative stimulation. Volatile anesthetics, combined with nitrous oxide and/or opioids, are useful for attenuating sympathetic nervous system activity keeping in mind the importance of titrating doses to avoid reductions in systemic vascular resistance. Provision of anesthesia with regional techniques is not encouraged because of the potential adverse effects of uncontrolled peripheral vasodilation.

Skeletal muscle relaxation is acceptably produced by drugs such as metocurine, atracurium and vecuronium since these muscle relaxants produce limited to no circulatory changes. Pancuronium would not be a likely selection in view of its stimulant effects on heart rate and cardiac contractility. Likewise, peripheral vasodilation following administration of d-tubocurarine would be undesirable.

Unexpected cardiac dysrhythmias may occur during anesthesia, emphasizing the need to monitor the electrocardiogram in these patients.[20] Ventricular cardiac dysrhythmias are particularly likely to occur during operations performed in the head-up or sitting position, presumably reflecting increased left ventricular emptying and accentuation of mitral valve prolapse. Lidocaine and propranolol should be immediately available to treat intraoperative cardiac dysrhythmias. Prompt replacement of blood loss and generous intravenous fluid maintenance (5 ml·kg^{-1}·hr^{-1}) will most likely optimize intravascular fluid volume and reduce potential adverse effects of positive pressure ventilation of the lungs. Furthermore, a high normal intravascular fluid volume helps maintain forward left ventricular stroke volume should acute intraoperative mitral regurgitation occur. If vasopressors are required, an alpha-adrenergic agonist such as phenylephrine is appropriate. Production of controlled hypotension with peripheral vasodilator drugs is an unlikely approach as associated reductions in systemic vascular resistance would likely increase the magnitude of mitral valve prolapse.

CARDIAC MYXOMAS

Cardiac myxomas account for about one-half of all primary cardiac tumors.[21] Typically, these tumors are benign with 75 percent originating in the left atrium and 20 percent from the right atrium. Most often cardiac myxomas arise from the fossa ovalis and are attached to it by a pedicle.

Manifestations of cardiac myxomas reflect interference with filling and emptying of the involved cardiac chamber and release of emboli composed either of myxomatous material or thrombi that have formed on the tumors. Left atrial myxomas mimic mitral valve disease and are associated with pulmonary venous obstruction and pulmonary edema. Conversely, right atrial myxomas mimic tricuspid valve disease and are associated with impaired venous return and signs of right heart failure or constrictive pericarditis. A right atrial myxoma should be suspected in patients with isolated tricuspid stenosis. Likewise, any surgically removed emboli should be examined microscopically for myxomatous material. Syncope is a common

event in these patients. Anemia is present in about one-third of patients.

Cardiac murmurs that change with position provide suggestive evidence of the presence of intracavitary cardiac tumors. Echocardiography is a useful technique for noninvasive diagnosis of myxomas. Radionuclide scans may also be useful.

Treatment of cardiac myxomas is surgical excision using cardiopulmonary bypass. Occasionally, damage to heart valves may be so extensive that replacement is necessary. Because of occasional local recurrences, resection of that portion of the atrial septum from which the tumor arises may be indicated.

SURGERY IN PATIENTS WITH PROSTHETIC HEART VALVES

Preoperative evaluation of patients with prosthetic heart valves includes (1) evaluation for paravalvular leak or other mechanical dysfunctions, as well as underlying congestive heart failure; and (2) management of anticoagulation (see the section Mitral Stenosis). Preoperative measurements of plasma concentrations of bilirubin and the reticulocyte count may be helpful in detecting occult hemolysis due to prosthetic valve dysfunction. Changes in valve sounds or appearance of new cardiac murmurs must be appreciated. Echocardiography and occasionally cardiac catheterization may be performed in assessing the patient's heart valve function. Antibiotic prophylaxis is mandatory in patients with prosthetic valves.

Mitral valve prostheses have an average valve area of 2.1 cm^2 to 2.6 cm^2 and have average transprosthesis diastolic pressure gradients of 4 mmHg to 7 mmHg as normal cardiac outputs. In most patients, elevated pulmonary vascular resistance declines to normal after mitral valve replacement.

Aortic valve prostheses have an average valve area of 1.3 cm^2 to 2 cm^2. The systolic pressure gradients across these valves range from 7 mmHg to 19 mmHg.

REFERENCES

1. Fishman MC, Hoffmsn AR, Klausner RD, Rockson SG, Thaler MS. Medicine. Philadelphia. J.B. Lippincott Co. 1981:42
2. Rapaport E. Natural history of aortic and mitral valve disease. Am J Cardiol 1975;35:221–7
3. Greenberg BH, Rahimtoola SH. Vasodilator therapy for valvular heart disease. JAMA 1981;246:269–72
4. Clements FM, deBruijn NP. Perioperative evaluation of regional wall motion by transesophageal two-dimensional echocardiography. Anesth Analg 1987;66:249–61
5. McKay CR, Kawanishi DT, Rahimtoola SH. Catheter balloon valvuloplasty of the mitral valve in adults using a double-balloon technique. JAMA 1987;257:1753–61
6. Tinker JH, Tarhan S. Discontinuing anticoagulant therapy in surgical patients with cardiac prosthesis. JAMA 1978;239:738–9
7. Perez HR. Cardiac arrhythmias after succinylcholine. Anesth Analg 1970;49:33–8
8. Hilgenberg JC, McCammon RL, Stoelting RK. Pulmonary and systemic vascular responses to nitrous oxide in patients with mitral stenosis and pulmonary hypertension. Anesth Analg 1980;59:323–6
9. Geha DG, Rozelle BC, Raessler KL, et al. Pancuronium bromide enhances atrioventricular conduction in halothane-anesthetized dogs. Anesthesiology 1977;46:342–5
10. Stone JG, Hoar PF, Faltas AN, Khambatta HJ. Nitroprusside and mitral stenosis. Anesth Analg 1980;59:662–5
11. Bolen JL, Lopes MG, Harrison DC, Alderman EL. Analysis of left ventricular function in response to afterload changes in patients with mitral stenosis. Circulation 1975;52:894–900
12. Goldman L, Caldera DL, Nussbaum SR, et al. Multifactorial index of cardiac risk in noncardiac surgical procedures. N Engl J Med 1977;297:845–50
13. Stanley TH, Webster LR. Anesthetic requirements and cardiovascular effects of fentanyl-oxygen and fentanyl-diazepam-oxygen anesthesia in man. Anesth Analg 1978;57:411–6
14. Stoelting RK, Gibbs PS. Hemodynamic effects of morphine and morphine-nitrous oxide in valvular heart disease and coronary-artery disease. Anesthesiology 1973;38:45–52
15. Tomicheck RC, Rosow CE, Philbin DM, Moss J, Teplick RS, Schneider RC. Diazepam-fentanyl interaction-hemodynamic and hormonal effects in coronary artery surgery. Anesth Analg 1983;62:881–4
16. Stone JG, Hoar PF, Calabro JR, Khambatta HJ. Afterload reduction and preload augmentation improve the anesthetic management of patients with cardiac failure and valvular regurgitation. Anesth Analg 1980;59:737–42
17. Jeresaty RM. Mitral valve prolapse: An update. JAMA 1985;254:793–5
18. Kowalski SE. Mitral valve prolapse. Can Anaesth Soc J 1985;32:138–41
19. Krantz EM, Viljoen JF, Schermer R, Canas MS. Mitral valve prolapse. Anesth Analg 1980;59:379–83
20. Berry FA, Lake CL, Johns RA, Rogers BM. Mitral valve prolapse—another cause of intraoperative dysrhythmias in the pediatric patient. Anesthesiology 1985;62:662–4
21. Harvey WP. Clinical aspects of cardiac tumors. Am J Cardiol 1968;21:328–36

3

Congenital Heart Disease

Approximately 8 of every 1,000 live births are associated with some form of congenital heart disease.[1] Causes of such disease are most often unknown but can include maternal infections (rubella in the first trimester of gestation) and maternal drug ingestion. The presence of congenital heart defects in either parents or siblings is associated with a fourfold increase in the incidence of congenital heart disease in the newborn. Prematurity, multiple gestations, and the presence of noncardiac congenital anomalies are also associated with an increased incidence of cardiac defects.

Although more than 100 different congenital heart lesions are known, nearly 90 percent of all cardiac defects can be placed in 1 of 10 categories (Table 3-1). Signs and symptoms of congenital heart disease most often include dyspnea and slow physical development (Table 3-2). Management of anesthesia for patients with congenital heart disease requires thorough knowledge of the pathophysiology of each cardiac defect. In this respect, it is convenient to categorize congenital heart defects as those lesions that result in (1) left-to-right intracardiac shunts, (2) right-to-left intracardiac shunts, (3) separation of the pulmonary and systemic circulations, (4) mixing of blood between the pulmonary and systemic circulations, (5) increased myocardial work, and (6) mechanical obstruction of the airways.

LEFT-TO-RIGHT INTRACARDIAC SHUNTS

Left-to-right intracardiac shunts or their equivalent can occur at the atrial, ventricular, or arterial level (Table 3-3). The ultimate result of these shunts, regardless of their location, is increased pulmonary blood flow with pulmonary hypertension, right ventricular hypertrophy, and eventually congestive heart failure. The younger the patient at the time of operation, the greater the likelihood that pulmonary vascular resistance will normalize. In older patients, if pulmonary vascular resistance is one-third or less of systemic vascular resistance, progressive pulmonary vascular disease after operation is unlikely.[2] The onset and severity of clinical symptoms vary with the site and magnitude of the vascular shunt.

Secundum Atrial Septal Defects

Secundum atrial septal defects are most often located in the center of the interatrial septum and can vary from a single opening to a fenestrated septum (Fig. 3-1). Isolated defects are usually well tolerated in childhood and

57

TABLE 3-1.   Common Congenital Heart Defects

Defect	Percent of Total Defects
Ventricular septal defect	28
Secundum atrial septal defect	10
Patent ductus arteriosus	10
Tetralogy of Fallot	10
Pulmonary stenosis	10
Aortic stenosis	7
Coarctation of the aorta	5
Transposition of the great arteries	5
Primum atrial septal defect	3
Total anomalous pulmonary venous return	1

often produce symptoms only after the second or third decade of life.

CLINICAL MANIFESTATIONS

The presence of secundum atrial septal defects are occasionally first suspected when there is a history of frequent pulmonary infections or when a systolic murmur is noted over the area of the pulmonary valve during a routine physical examination. For example, less than 20 percent of newborns with atrial septal defects have a characteristic cardiac murmur. The incidence of systolic ejection murmurs over the pulmonary valve area, however, increases to 80 percent by 5 years of age. The second heart sound in the presence of atrial septal defects is widely split. Increased pulmonary blood flow associated with these de-

TABLE 3-2.   Signs and Symptoms of Congenital Heart Disease

Infants	Children
Tachypnea	Dyspnea
Failure to gain weight	Slow physical development
Heart rate above 200 beats·min^{-1}	Decreased exercise tolerance
Heart murmur	Heart murmur
Congestive heart failure	Congestive heart failure
Cyanosis	Cyanosis
	Clubbing of digits
	Squatting
	Elevated blood pressure

TABLE 3-3.   Congenital Heart Defects Resulting in a Left-to-Right Intracardiac Shunt or Its Equivalent

Secundum atrial septal defect
Primum atrial septal defect (endocardial cushion defect)
Ventricular septal defect
Aorticopulmonary fenestration

fects leads to increased right ventricular work, pulmonary hypertension, and right ventricular failure. Radiographs of the chest reveal signs of increased pulmonary blood flow, characterized by an enlarged pulmonary artery trunk and hypertrophy of the right atrium and ventricle. The electrocardiogram typically shows a pattern of right bundle branch block and right

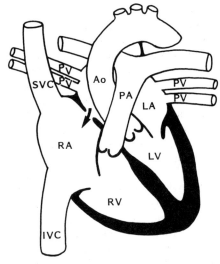

FIG. 3-1.   Schematic diagram of a secundum atrial septal defect located in the center of the interatrial septum. Blood flows along a pressure gradient from the left atrium (LA) to the right atrium (RA). The resulting left-to-right intracardiac shunt is associated with increased flow through the pulmonary artery (PA). Surgical closure of the defect is indicated when the pulmonary artery blood flow is double the flow into the aorta (Ao). Decreases in systemic vascular resistance or increases in pulmonary vascular resistance will decrease the pressure gradient across the defect leading to a reduction in the magnitude of the shunt. RV = right ventricle; LV = left ventricle; SVC = superior vena cava; IVC = inferior vena cava; PV = pulmonary vein.

axis deviation. First-degree atrioventricular heart block may be present. Echocardiography often demonstrates an increased right ventricular dimension and paradoxical motion of the atrial septum. Mitral valve prolapse, which occurs in about 30 percent of patients with this cardiac defect, can also be detected with echocardiography. Cardiac catheterization usually reveals increases in venous oxygen saturations at the right atrial level. These increases in oxygen saturations may not be apparent until the ventricular level if streaming of the shunted blood occurs.

TREATMENT

Surgical closure of secundum atrial septal defects is indicated when pulmonary blood flow is at least twice systemic blood flow. Surgery is not indicated when pulmonary hypertension has progressed to the point that pulmonary vascular pressures are near systemic vascular pressures, as closure of the defect under these circumstances is associated with high mortality.

Primum Atrial Septal Defects (Endocardial Cushion Defects)

Primum atrial septal defects are characterized by large openings low in the interatrial septum. These defects frequently involve the mitral and tricuspid valves; mitral regurgitation in association with a cleft anterior leaflet of the mitral valve is present in about one-half of patients. Physiologically, primum and secundum atrial septal defects are similar.

CLINICAL MANIFESTATIONS

Clinical presentations of primum atrial septal defects are usually in infancy or early childhood and are characterized by frequent pulmonary infections, failure to thrive, tachycardia, and congestive heart failure. Physical findings differ from those observed in the presence of secundum atrial septal defects only if mitral and/or tricuspid regurgitation are present. Findings on radiographs of the chest and the electrocardiogram are similar to those observed in the presence of secundum defects. Echocardiography and angiocardiography are important for defining the placement of the mitral and tricuspid valves. Cardiac catheterization usually reveals increases in venous oxygen saturation at both atrial and ventricular levels, as well as the presence of pulmonary hypertension.

TREATMENT

Surgical repair of primum atrial septal defects is usually necessary in the first decade of life to prevent pulmonary hypertension from becoming irreversible. Initially, palliative banding of the pulmonary artery may be selected in attempts to reduce the magnitude of the left-to-right intracardiac shunts. Mortality with banding, however, remains high, and for this reason, some favor a complete repair even at a very young age.[3] Nevertheless, complete surgical repair is often unsuccessful because of the inability to produce adequately functioning mitral and tricuspid valves from the rudimentary leaflets that are present. A residual cleft mitral valve might be vulnerable to infective endocarditis. Residual pulmonary hypertension occurring after surgical correction of this defect assumes importance in the postoperative period, since this may lead to tricuspid regurgitation and right ventricular failure. Surgical repair also carries the risk of third-degree atrioventricular heart block, since these defects are often near the conduction system necessary for propagation of cardiac impulses. Sinoatrial node or atrioventricular node dysfunction or atrial fibrillation may manifest years after successful surgical repair.

MANAGEMENT OF ANESTHESIA

Atrial septal defects associated with left-to-right intracardiac shunts have only minor implications for the management of anesthesia. For example, as long as systemic blood flow remains normal, pharmacokinetics of inhaled drugs will not be significantly altered despite increased pulmonary blood flow.[4] Conversely, increased pulmonary blood flow could dilute drugs that are injected intravenously. It is unlikely, however, that this potential dilution will alter clinical responses to these drugs, since pulmonary circulation time is very short. Another effect of increased pulmonary blood flow is that positive pressure ventilation of the lungs is well tolerated.

Changes in systemic vascular resistance during the perioperative period have important implications for patients with atrial septal defects. For example, drugs or events that produce prolonged increases in systemic vascular resistance should be avoided, as this change will favor an increase in the magnitude of left-to-right shunts at the atrial level. This is particularly true with primum defects associated with mitral regurgitation. Conversely, decreases in systemic vascular resistance, as produced by volatile anesthetics, or increases in pulmonary vascular resistance due to positive pressure ventilation of the lungs, will tend to decrease the magnitude of the shunts.

Other considerations for the management of anesthesia in the presence of atrial septal defects include the need to provide antibiotics in the preoperative period to protect against the development of infective endocarditis. In addition, it is imperative to avoid meticulously the entrance of air into the circulation, as can occur via the tubing used to deliver intravenous solutions. Transient supraventricular dysrhythmias and atrioventricular conduction defects are common in the early postoperative period after surgical repair of atrial septal defects.

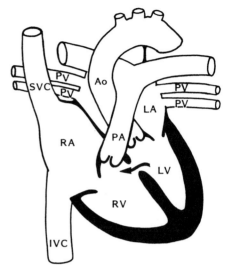

FIG. 3-2. Schematic diagram of a ventricular septal defect located just below the muscular ridge that separates the body of the right ventricle (RV) from the pulmonary artery (PA) outflow tract. Blood flow is along a pressure gradient from the left ventricle (LV) to the RV. The resulting left-to-right intracardiac shunt is associated with a pulmonary blood flow that exceeds the volume of LV ejection into the aorta (Ao). Decreases in systemic vascular resistance decrease the pressure gradient across the defect and reduce the magnitude of the shunt.

Ventricular Septal Defects

Ventricular septal defects are the most common congenital heart defect (Table 3-1). The incidence of these defects in premature births is four times that in term infants. About 90 percent of these defects are located below the crista supraventricularis, a muscular ridge that separates the body of the right ventricle from the pulmonary artery outflow tract (Fig. 3-2). These defects may be single openings in the muscular portion of the ventricular septum or multiple lesions giving rise to a fenestrated septum.

CLINICAL MANIFESTATIONS

Clinical manifestations of ventricular septal defects depend on the size of the defects and on the pulmonary vascular resistance. Patients with small defects are usually asymptomatic but have loud pansystolic murmurs that are of maximum intensity along the left sternal border. Radiographs of the chest and the electrocardiogram are typically normal. The magnitude of the left-to-right intracardiac shunts is usually minimal, such that the ratio of pulmonary to systemic blood flow is less than 1.5 to 1.

Patients with moderate-sized ventricular septal defects may be asymptomatic, but radiographs of the chest typically demonstrate biventricular enlargement and evidence of increased pulmonary blood flow. Cardiac catheterization usually reveals that pulmonary blood flow exceeds systemic blood flow by 1.5 to 3 times. Pulmonary vascular resistance may be moderately elevated. A 15 mmHg to 20 mmHg gradient across the pulmonary artery outflow tract may develop as right ventricular hypertrophy results in obstruction to blood flow at this position.

A large ventricular septal defect is characterized by a left-to-right intracardiac shunt that results in a pulmonary blood flow that exceeds systemic blood flow by 3 to 5 times. Symptoms appear early in life (often at about 4 weeks of age) and are characterized by tachypnea, failure to gain weight, recurrent pulmonary infections, and congestive heart failure. Radiographs of the chest and the electrocardiogram reveal evidence of biventricular hypertrophy and pulmonary hypertension.

Ventricular septal defects that open into the pulmonary outflow portion of the right ventricle may be complicated by aortic regurgitation due to prolapse of an aortic cusp into the defect. Left ventricular-to-right atrial septal defects (Gerbode defects) are associated with cardiac conduction disturbances and tricuspid regurgitation.

TREATMENT

About 25 percent of all ventricular septal defects will close spontaneously without surgical intervention. Furthermore, about one-half of infants who develop congestive heart failure due to ventricular septal defects will improve with medical management. When medical management is not successful, it is necessary to consider palliative surgical procedures such as pulmonary artery banding. Placement of a constricting band around the pulmonary artery serves to increase resistance to right ventricular ejection. This increased resistance serves to reduce the magnitude of the left-to-right shunts at the ventricular level. This procedure may also prevent development of irreversible pulmonary hypertension. Elevations of pulmonary vascular resistance seem to be reversible when banding is performed before 2 years of age.

MANAGEMENT OF ANESTHESIA

Administration of antibiotics to provide prophylaxis against bacterial endocarditis is indicated when noncardiac surgery is planned in patients with ventricular septal defects. Pharmacokinetics of inhaled and injected drugs are not significantly altered by these defects. As with atrial septal defects, acute and persistent elevations in systemic vascular resistance or reductions in pulmonary vascular resistance are undesirable, as these changes could accentuate the magnitude of left-to-right shunts at the ventricular level. In this regard, volatile anesthetics that decrease systemic vascular resistance and positive pressure ventilation of the lungs, which increases pulmonary vascular resistance are well tolerated. However, there may be increased delivery of depressant drugs to the heart if coronary blood flow is increased to supply the hypertrophied ventricles. Conceivably, increasing the inspired concentrations of volatile anesthetics to high levels to achieve rapid inductions of anesthesia, as is often done in normal children, could result in excessive depression of the heart before the central nervous system is anesthetized.

Right ventricular infundibular hypertrophy may be present in some patients with ventricular septal defects. Normally, this is a beneficial change, as it increases the resistance to right ventricular ejection, leading to reductions in the magnitude of left-to-right intracardiac shunts. Nevertheless, perioperative events that exaggerate this obstruction to right ventricular outflow, such as increased myocardial contractility or hypovolemia, must be minimized. Therefore, these patients are often anesthetized with volatile anesthetics. In addition, intravascular fluid volume should be maintained by prompt replacement of blood loss.

Anesthesia for placement of pulmonary artery bands is best achieved with drugs that provide minimum cardiac depression. Muscle relaxants are used to prevent patient movement.

If bradycardia or hypotension develop during surgery, it may be necessary to remove the pulmonary artery band rapidly. Continuous monitoring of blood pressure via an intra-arterial catheter is helpful. Positive end-expiratory pressure may be useful in the presence of congestive heart failure but should be discontinued when the pulmonary artery band is in place. High mortality associated with pulmonary artery banding has led to attempts at complete surgical correction at an early age using cardiopulmonary bypass. Third-degree atrioventricular heart block may follow surgical closure if the cardiac conduction system is near the septal defect. Premature ventricular beats may reflect electrical instability of the ventricle due to surgical ventriculotomy. The risk of ventricular tachycardia, however, is low if postoperative ventricular filling pressures are normal.

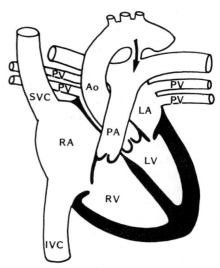

FIG. 3-3. Schematic diagram of a patent ductus arteriosus connecting the arch of the aorta (Ao) with the pulmonary artery (PA). Blood flow is from the high pressure Ao into the PA. The resulting systemic-to-pulmonary shunt (left-to-right shunt) leads to increased pulmonary blood flow. Reductions in systemic vascular resistance or increases in pulmonary vascular resistance will decrease the magnitude of the shunt through the ductus arteriosus.

Patent Ductus Arteriosus

Failure of the ductus arteriosus to close after birth results in passage of oxygenated blood from the aorta into the pulmonary artery (Fig. 3-3). The ratio of pulmonary to systemic blood flow depends on the (1) pressure gradient from the aorta to the pulmonary artery, (2) ratio of pulmonary to systemic vascular resistance, and (3) diameter and length of the ductus arteriosus.

CLINICAL MANIFESTATIONS

Most patients with a patent ductus arteriosus are asymptomatic and have only moderate left-to-right shunts. This cardiac defect is often detected during a routine physical examination, when characteristic continuous systolic and diastolic murmurs are heard. When the magnitude of the left-to-right shunt is large, there may be evidence of left ventricular hypertrophy and increased pulmonary blood flow on radiographs of the chest and the electrocardiogram.

TREATMENT

Treatment is by surgical ligation of the ductus arteriosus through a left thoracotomy incision. Ideally, surgery is performed after the patient is 2 years of age. Without surgical correction, most patients remain asymptomatic until adolescence, when pulmonary hypertension and congestive heart failure can intervene. Administration of indomethacin may result in closure of a patent ductus arteriosus present in premature infants with respiratory distress syndrome.[5]

MANAGEMENT OF ANESTHESIA

Antibiotics for protection against the development of infective endocarditis should be administered to patients with a patent ductus arteriosus who are scheduled for noncardiac surgery. When surgical closure of the ductus arteriosus is planned, appropriate preparations must be taken in anticipation of the possibility of a large blood loss should control of the ductus arteriosus be lost during attempted ligation. Anesthesia with volatile drugs is useful, as these drugs tend to lower blood pressure, so there is less danger of the ductus arteriosus escaping from the vascular clamp or tearing, as it is being divided. Furthermore, reductions in systemic vascular resistance produced by volatile anesthetics may improve systemic blood flow by decreasing the magnitude of the left-to-right shunt. Likewise, positive pressure ventilation of the lungs is well tolerated, as increased airway pressure elevates pulmonary vascular resistance and thus reduces the pressure gradient across the ductus arteriosus. Conversely, increases in systemic vascular resistance or reductions in pulmonary vascular resistance should be avoided, as these changes would increase the magnitude of the shunt. Continuous monitoring of blood pressure via a catheter placed in a peripheral artery is helpful during the intraoperative period.

Ligation of the ductus arteriosus is often associated with significant systemic hypertension in the early postoperative period. Management of this hypertension is with the continuous infusion of vasodilator drugs such as nitroprusside. Longer acting antihypertensive drugs, such as hydralazine, can be gradually substituted for nitroprusside if hypertension persists.

Aorticopulmonary Fenestration

Aorticopulmonary fenestration is characterized by a communication between the left side of the ascending aorta and the right wall of the main pulmonary artery, just anterior to the origin of the right pulmonary artery. This communication is due to a failure of the spiral aorticopulmonary septum to fuse and separate completely the aorta from the pulmonary artery. Clinical and hemodynamic manifestations of an aorticopulmonary communication are similar to a large patent ductus arteriosus. The correct diagnosis is made by angiocar-

diography. Treatment is surgical and requires the use of cardiopulmonary bypass. Management of anesthesia entails the same principles as outlined for patients with patent ductus arteriosus.

RIGHT-TO-LEFT INTRACARDIAC SHUNTS

A variety of congenital heart defects result in right-to-left intracardiac shunts, with associated reductions in pulmonary blood flow and the development of arterial hypoxemia (Table 3-4). Survival in the presence of right-to-left shunts requires communications between the systemic and pulmonary circulations and obstruction to blood flow from the right ventricle. The time of onset and severity of symptoms usually depend on the degree of obstruction.

Tetralogy of Fallot is the prototype of these defects. Principles for management of anesthesia are the same for all defects in this group.

Tetralogy of Fallot

Tetralogy of Fallot is the most common congenital heart defect producing right-to-left intracardiac shunts with reduced pulmonary blood flow and arterial hypoxemia. Anatomic defects, which characterize this tetralogy, are a ventricular septal defect, an aorta that overrides the pulmonary outflow tract, obstruction

TABLE 3-4. Congenital Heart Defects Resulting in a Right-to-Left Intracardiac Shunt

Tetralogy of Fallot
Eisenmenger's syndrome
Ebstein malformation of the tricuspid valve
Pulmonary atresia with a ventricular septal defect (pseudotruncus)
Tricuspid atresia
Foramen ovale

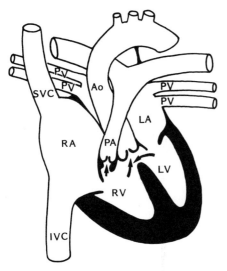

FIG. 3-4. Schematic diagram of the anatomic cardiac defects associated with tetralogy of Fallot. Defects include (1) a ventricular septal defect, (2) an aorta (Ao) that overrides the pulmonary artery (PA) outflow tract, (3) obstruction to blood flow through a narrowed PA or stenotic pulmonary valve, and (4) right ventricular hypertrophy. Obstruction to PA outflow results in a pressure gradient that favors blood flow across the ventricular septal defect from the right ventricle (RV) to the left ventricle (LV). The resulting right-to-left intracardiac shunt combined with obstruction to ejection of the right ventricular stroke volume leads to marked reductions in pulmonary blood flow and the development of arterial hypoxemia. Events that increase pulmonary vascular resistance or decrease systemic vascular resistance will increase the magnitude of the shunt and accentuate arterial hypoxemia.

of the pulmonary artery outflow tract, and right ventricular hypertrophy (Fig. 3-4). The ventricular septal defect is typically large and single. Infundibular pulmonary artery stenosis is prominent, and about 70 percent of patients have bicuspid aortic valves. The distal pulmonary artery may be hypoplastic or even absent. In general, the greater the stenosis of the pulmonary artery, the greater the overriding of the aorta. Right ventricular hypertrophy occurs because the large ventricular septal defect allows the right ventricle to be continuously exposed to high pressures present in the left ventricle.

CLINICAL MANIFESTATIONS

Clinical manifestations of tetralogy of Fallot depend on the size of the right ventricular outflow tract. In general, cyanosis due to arterial hypoxemia will be apparent by 6 months of age. Clubbing of the distal ends of the digits is rarely seen before 6 months of age. The most common auscultatory finding is an ejection murmur heard along the left sternal border, resulting from blood flow across the infundibular pulmonary stenosis. Congestive heart failure rarely develops because the large ventricular septal defect allows equilibration of intraventricular pressures and cardiac workload. Radiographs of the chest typically show reductions in the vascularity of the lungs. The electrocardiogram is characterized by changes of right axis deviation and right ventricular hypertrophy. Arterial blood gases and pH are likely to reveal normal carbon dioxide partial pressures and pH and markedly reduced arterial oxygen partial pressures (usually below 50 mmHg) even when breathing 100 percent oxygen.

Squatting is a common feature of children with tetralogy of Fallot. It is speculated that squatting increases systemic vascular resistance by kinking large arteries in the inguinal area.[6] The resulting increase in systemic vascular resistance tends to reduce the magnitude of the right-to-left intracardiac shunts leading to increased pulmonary blood flow with a subsequent improvement in arterial oxygenation and carbon dioxide elimination.

Hypercyanotic Attacks. About 35 percent of children with tetralogy of Fallot develop hypercyanotic attacks or tet spells. These attacks can occur without obvious provocation but are often associated with crying or exercise. Hyperventilation and syncope may accompany these periods of increased arterial hypoxemia. The mechanism for the attacks is not known. The most likely explanation, however, is a sudden reduction in pulmonary blood flow due to either spasm of the infundibular cardiac muscle or decrease in systemic vascular resistance. Morphine, propranolol, and phenylephrine have been used to treat hypercyanotic attacks, with the best responses being observed after the administration of phenylephrine. Presumably phyenylephrine, by increasing systemic vascular resistance, forces more blood through the lungs. Propranolol is most likely to be effective when the hypercyanotic attack is due to spasm of the infundibular cardiac muscle. Indeed, chronic oral propranolol therapy is indicated in patients who have recurrent hypercyanotic attacks due to spasm of this muscle. Recurrent hypercyanotic attacks are an indication for surgical correction of abnormalities associated with tetralogy of Fallot.

Cerebrovascular Accidents. Cerebrovascular accidents are common in children with severe tetralogy of Fallot. Cerebral vascular thrombosis or severe arterial hypoxemia may be the explanations for these adverse responses. Dehydration and polycythemia may contribute to thrombosis. Hemoglobin concentrations exceeding 20 $g \cdot dl^{-1}$ are common in these patients.

Cerebral Abscesses. A cerebral abscess is suggested by the abrupt onset of headache, fever, and lethargy, followed by persistent emesis and the appearance of seizure activity. The most likely cause is bacterial seeding into areas of prior cerebral infarction.

Infective Endocarditis. Infective endocarditis is a constant danger in patients with tetralogy of Fallot. This complication is associated with a high mortality. Antibiotics should be administered to protect against this whenever dental or surgical procedures are planned in these patients.

TREATMENT

Surgical treatment of tetralogy of Fallot is initially with palliative procedures designed to increase pulmonary blood flow by virtue of the anastomosis of a systemic artery to a pulmonary artery. After successful systemic-to-pulmonary artery shunt procedures, the pulmonary vasculature usually enlarges, arterial oxygen partial pressures increase, and polycythemia regresses. Complete correction of the cardiac defects is subsequently accomplished using cardiopulmonary bypass when patients are 3 years to 6 years old.

Palliative surgical procedures designed to increase pulmonary blood flow include the (1) Potts' operation, (2) Waterston shunt, and (3) Blalock-Taussig shunt. Potts' operation consists of a direct anastomosis between the descending thoracic aorta and the left pulmonary artery. This operation is no longer popular because excessive increases in pulmonary blood flow may result in pulmonary hypertension and congestive heart failure. Furthermore, takedown of this anastomosis during subsequent complete surgical correction is difficult.

The Waterson shunt is a direct anastomosis between the ascending thoracic aorta and the right pulmonary artery. Takedown of this anastomosis at the time of complete surgical correction is easier than with the Potts' operation. The proper sizing, however, of the anastomosis produced by a Waterson shunt is difficult. As a result, excessive increases in pulmonary blood flow and pulmonary hypertension can result. Furthermore, the right pulmonary artery may thrombose after this procedure in occasional patients.

The Blalock-Taussig shunt consists of an anastomosis between a branch of the thoracic aorta and one of the pulmonary arteries. A popular approach is an end-to-side anastomosis between the subclavian artery and the pulmonary artery on the side opposite the aortic arch. The long length of the subclavian artery limits pulmonary blood flow through the shunt and minimizes the incidence of excessive increases in pulmonary blood flow and development of pulmonary hypertension. The major complications of this vascular anastomosis include thrombosis of the shunt and the development of subclavian steal syndrome.

Complete surgical repair of tetralogy of Fallot typically consists of closure of the ventricular septal defect with a Dacron patch and enlargement of the pulmonary artery outflow tract by placement of synthetic grafts. Pulmonary regurgitation due to an incompetent pulmonary valve usually results from surgical correction of the cardiac defects but poses no major hazard unless the distal pulmonary arteries are hypoplastic, in which case volume overload of the right ventricle secondary to regurgitant blood flow may result. Major complications of complete surgical repair include third-degree atrioventricular heart block and difficulty in achieving hemostasis. Platelet dysfunction and hypofibrinogenemia are common in these patients and may contribute to postoperative bleeding problems. Right-to-left intracardiac shunting often develops through the foramen ovale in the postoperative period. Shunting through the foramen ovale acts as a safety valve should the right ventricle not be able to function at the same efficiency as the left ventricle.

MANAGEMENT OF ANESTHESIA

Management of anesthesia for patients with tetralogy of Fallot requires a thorough understanding of those events and drugs that can alter the magnitude of right-to-left intracardiac shunts. For example, when shunt magnitude is acutely increased, there are associated reductions in pulmonary blood flow and arterial oxygen partial pressures. Furthermore, the magnitude of the shunt alters pharmacokinetics of both inhaled and injected drugs.

The magnitude of right-to-left intracardiac shunts can be increased by (1) reductions in systemic vascular resistance, (2) increases in the pulmonary vascular resistance, and (3) increases in myocardial contractility that accentuate infundibular obstruction to ejection of blood by the right ventricle. In many respects, resistance to ejection of blood into the pulmonary artery outflow tract is relatively fixed, and hence the magnitude of the shunts is inversely proportional to the systemic vascular resistance. Pharmacologic-induced responses that decrease systemic vascular resistance (volatile anesthetics, histamine release, ganglionic blockade, alpha-adrenergic blockade, and direct peripheral vasodilation) will increase the magnitude of the shunts and accentuate arterial hypoxemia. Pulmonary blood flow can be reduced by increases in pulmonary vascular resistance that accompany such intraoperative ventilatory maneuvers as intermittent positive airway pressure or positive end-expiratory pressure. Furthermore, loss of negative intrapleural pressure upon opening the chest will increase pulmonary vascular resistance and the magnitude of the shunts. Nevertheless, advantages of controlled ventilation of the lungs during operations offset this potential hazard. Indeed, arterial oxygenation does not predictably deteriorate in patients with tetralogy of Fallot, either with the institution of positive pressure ventilation of the lungs or after the opening of the chest.

Preoperatively, it is important to avoid dehydration by maintaining oral feedings in the very young or by providing intravenous fluids before arriving in the operating room. Crying associated with intramuscular administration of drugs used for preoperative medication can lead to hypercyanotic attacks. For this reason, it may be prudent to avoid administration of drugs by this route until patients are in highly supervised environments where alpha-adrenergic agonist drugs such as phenylephrine or methoxamine are immediately available for treatment of hypercyanotic attacks. Sympathomimetic drugs with beta-adrenergic agonist properties are not chosen, as they may accentuate spasm of the infundibular cardiac muscle. Beta-adrenergic antagonist drugs should be continued until the induction of anesthesia in patients receiving these drugs for prophylaxis against hypercyanotic attacks.

Induction of anesthesia in patients with tetralogy of Fallot is often accomplished with intramuscular (3 mg·kg^{-1} to 4 mg·kg^{-1}) or intravenous (1 mg·kg^{-1} to 2 mg·kg^{-1}) administration of ketamine. The onset of anesthesia after injection of ketamine may be associated with an improvement in arterial oxygenation, which presumably reflects increased pulmonary blood flow due to ketamine-induced elevations in systemic vascular resistance, that lead to decreases in the magnitude of the right-to-left intracardiac shunts. Ketamine has also been alleged to increase pulmonary vascular resistance, which would be undesirable in patients with right-to-left shunts. The efficacious response to ketamine of patients with tetralogy of Fallot, however, suggests this concern is not clinically significant. Intubation of the trachea is facilitated by administration of muscle relaxants. It should be remembered that the onset of action of drugs administered intravenously may be more rapid in the presence of right-to-left shunts, since the dilutional effect in the lungs is not present. For this reason, it may be prudent to reduce the rate of intravenous injection of depressant drugs in these patients.

Induction of anesthesia with volatile anesthetics in patients with tetralogy of Fallot is not recommended. Although reduced pulmonary blood flow will slow achievement of anesthetic concentrations, the hazards of reductions in blood pressure and systemic vascular resistance are great. Indeed, hypercyanotic attacks can occur during administration of low concentrations of volatile anesthetics.

Maintenance of anesthesia is often achieved with nitrous oxide combined with ketamine. The advantage of this combination is the preservation of the systemic vascular resistance. Nitrous oxide may also increase pulmonary vascular resistance, but this potential adverse effect is more than offset by the beneficial effects of this inhaled anesthetic on the systemic circulation. The principal disadvantage of using nitrous oxide is the associated reduction in inspired oxygen concentrations. Theoretically, increased inspired oxygen concentrations could decrease pulmonary vascular resistance, leading to increased pulmonary blood flow and improved arterial oxygen partial pressures. Therefore, it would seem prudent to limit the inspired concentrations of nitrous oxide to 50 percent. Opioids or benzodiazepines may also be considered for use during the maintenance of anesthesia, but doses and rates of administration must be adjusted to minimize reductions in blood pressure or systemic vascular resistance.

Intraoperative skeletal muscle paralysis is often provided by pancuronium, as this drug maintains blood pressure and systemic vascular resistance. Mild increases in heart rate associated with administration of pancuronium are helpful in maintaining left ventricular cardiac output. Vecuronium and atracurium would also be acceptable but could not be expected to produce beneficial hemodynamic stimulation. d-Tubocurarine would not be a logical choice, as this drug could increase the magnitude of right-to-left intracardiac shunts, by virtue of its ability to decrease systemic vascular resistance secondary to histamine release and block of impulse transmission through peripheral autonomic ganglia.

Ventilation of the lungs should be controlled, but it must be appreciated that excessive positive airway pressures may adversely increase resistance to blood flow through the lungs. Intravascular fluid volume must be maintained with intravenous fluid administration, since acute hypovolemia will tend to increase the magnitude of right-to-left intracardiac shunts. In view of co-existing polycythemia, it is probably not necessary to consider replacement of erythrocytes until about 20 percent of the blood volume has been lost. It is crucial that meticulous care be taken to avoid infusion of air via the tubing used to deliver intravenous solutions, since this could lead to systemic embolization of air. Alpha-adrenergic agonist drugs such as phenylephrine must be immediately available to treat undesirable reductions in systemic blood pressure due to decreases in systemic vascular resistance.

Eisenmenger's Syndrome

Eisenmenger's syndrome describes situations in which left-to-right intracardiac shunts are reversed due to elevations in pulmonary vascular resistance to levels that equal or exceed the systemic vascular resistance. Shunt reversal occurs in about 50 percent of untreated patients with large ventricular septal defects but in only about 10 percent of patients with atrial septal defects. Manifestations of intracardiac shunt reversal reflect decreases in pulmonary blood flow with resulting arterial hypoxemia. The presence of this syndrome contraindicates surgical correction of the congenital cardiac defects, as pulmonary vascular resistance is irreversibly elevated.

Management of anesthesia for noncardiac surgery in patients with Eisenmenger's syndrome is as outlined for tetralogy of Fallot.[7] Despite the potential for undesirable reductions in blood pressure and systemic vascular resistance, the successful management of anesthesia using epidural techniques has been described in patients undergoing tubal ligation and cesarean section.[8] Should epidural techniques be selected, however, it would seem prudent not to add epinephrine to the local anesthetic solutions injected into the epidural space. This recommendation is based on the observation that peripheral beta-adrenergic effects produced by the epinephrine absorbed from the epidural space into the systemic circulation greatly exaggerate reductions in blood pressure and systemic vascular resistance that are associated with epidural blocks.

Ebstein Malformation of the Tricuspid Valve

Ebstein malformation of the tricuspid valve occurs in less than 1 percent of patients with congenital heart disease. The major anatomic abnormality of this malformation is the downward displacement of the tricuspid valve into the right ventricle. The mitral valve may also have abnormal placement of leaflets. The right atrium is almost always enlarged. Frequently, there are right-to-left shunts through patent foramen ovales or associated atrial septal defects. Malformation of the tricuspid valve causes obstruction to right ventricular filling, decrease in the size of the right ventricle, and tricuspid regurgitation, leading to right heart failure. Enlargement of the right atrium can be so massive that the apical portions of the lungs are compressed, resulting in restrictive pulmonary disease. Fatigue, dyspnea, and cardiac tachydysrhythmias are frequently observed in these patients. Hazards during anesthesia include development of cardiac tachydysrhythmias and arterial hypoxemia due to increases in the magnitude of the right-to-left intracardiac shunts.[9] Elevated right atrial pressures may indicate the presence of right ventricular failure. Delayed onset of effects after intravenous administration of drugs most likely reflects pooling and dilution in an enlarged right atrium.

Tricuspid Atresia

Tricuspid atresia is characterized by arterial hypoxemia, a small right ventricle, a large left ventricle, and markedly reduced pulmonary blood flow. Poorly oxygenated blood from the right atrium passes through an atrial septal defect into the left atrium, mixes with oxygenated blood, and then enters the left ventricle for ejection into the systemic circulation. Pulmonary blood flow is via a ventricular septal defect, patent ductus arteriosus, or bronchial vessels.

TREATMENT

Fontan procedures (anastomosis of the right atrial appendage to the right pulmonary artery so as to bypass the right ventricle and provide a direct aortopulmonary communication) are used for treatment of tricuspid atresia. This operation is also used for treatment of transposition of the great vessels and pulmonary artery atresia. Management of anesthesia for patients undergoing Fontan procedures has been successfully achieved with opioids or volatile anesthetics.[10] Immediately after cardiopulmonary bypass and continuing into the early postoperative period it is important to maintain elevated right atrial pressures (16 mmHg to 20 mmHg) to facilitate pulmonary blood flow. Increases in pulmonary vascular resistance due to acidosis, hypothermia, peak airway pressures above 15 cmH2O, or a reaction to the tracheal tube may cause right-sided heart failure. Early extubation of the trachea and spontaneous ventilation are desirable. Positive inotropic drugs (dopamine) with or without vasodilators (nitroprusside) are often required to optimize cardiac output and maintain low pulmonary vascular resistance. Pleural effusions, ascites, and lower extremity edema are not uncommon postoperatively but usually resolve within a few weeks.

Foramen Ovale

The foramen ovale is mechanically closed by left atrial pressures that exceed pressures in the right atrium. Eventually, the foramen ovale becomes permanently closed. In about 30 percent of normal patients, however, the foramen ovale remains probe patent.[11] In these individuals, elevations of right atrial pressures above pressures in the left atrium can lead to right-to-left intracardiac shunts through the foramen ovale. Unexplained arterial hypoxemia or paradoxical air embolism during the perioperative period may be due to the shunting of blood or air through a previously closed foramen ovale.[12]

SEPARATION OF THE PULMONARY AND SYSTEMIC CIRCULATIONS

Transposition of the great arteries is an example of a cardiac defect that results in separation of the pulmonary and systemic circulations.

Transposition of the Great Arteries

Transposition of the great arteries results from failure of the truncus arteriosus to spiral (Fig. 3-5). As a result, the aorta arises from the right ventricle and the pulmonary artery arises from the left ventricle. Anatomically, transposition means the left and right ventricles are not connected in series. As a result, the pulmonary and systemic circulations function independently, which results in profound arterial hypoxemia. Survival is not possible unless there is intermixing of blood between the two circulations through an atrial septal defect, ventricular septal defect, or patent ductus arteriosus. About 10 percent of infants with preductal types of coarctation of the aorta also have transportation of the great arteries.

CLINICAL MANIFESTATIONS

Persistent cyanosis at birth is often the first clue to the presence of transposition of the great arteries. Congestive heart failure appears early in life. The electrocardiogram is normal at birth, but in the presence of transposition of the great arteries, neonatal patterns of right

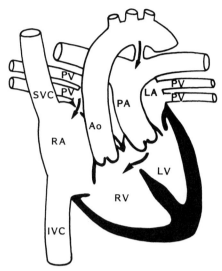

FIG. 3-5. Schematic diagram of transposition of the great arteries. The right ventricle (RV) and left ventricle (LV) are not connected in series. Instead, the two ventricles function as parallel and independent circulations, with the aorta (Ao) arising from the RV and the pulmonary artery (PA) arising from the LV. Survival is not possible unless mixing of blood between the two circulations occurs through an atrial septal defect, ventricular septal defect, or patent ductus arteriosus. Initial treatment of patients with transposition of the great arteries is to create an atrial septal defect, or to enlarge a coexisting one.

ventricular hypertrophy persist beyond the newborn period. Cardiac catheterization reveals normal systemic and pulmonary artery pressures and severe arterial hypoxemia. Echocardiography may demonstrate the pulmonary valve opening earlier and closing later than the aortic valve, which is the reverse of the normal situation.

TREATMENT

Initial treatment of transposition of the great arteries includes palliative procedures designed to increase intermixing of blood between the two circulations so as to improve systemic oxygenation. Such a procedure is performed at cardiac catheterization as soon as the diagnosis of transposition of the great arteries is confirmed. Complete surgical correction is then performed at 6 months to 9 months of age, using cardiopulmonary bypass. The most common palliative procedure is creation of an atrial septal defect by passing a ballooned catheter across the foramen ovale, inflating the balloon, and then pulling the entire catheter through the foramen ovale to enlarge the opening. This balloon atrial septostomy is known as the Rashkind procedure.[13] Third-degree atrioventricular heart block may follow a balloon septostomy. Therefore, chronotropic drugs such as atropine and isoproterenol must be available for immediate intravenous infusion.

It may be necessary to perform pulmonary artery banding to prevent intractable congestive heart failure from developing when large ventricular septal defects accompany transposition of the great arteries. Patients with transposition of the great arteries plus left ventricular outflow obstruction may require a Blalock-Taussig shunt to permit survival until complete surgical correction can be performed.

Complete surgical correction of transposition of the great arteries is most often accomplished by removing the atrial septum and replacing it with a baffle made of pericardium. This baffle is placed so as to redirect superior and inferior vena caval blood toward the mitral valve, whereas pulmonary venous return is directed toward the tricuspid valve. This surgically produced reversal of flow at the atrial level is known as the Mustard procedure.[14] Complications of this operation include third-degree atrioventricular heart block and obstruction of the vena cava. In addition, long-term ability of the right ventricle to perform as a left ventricle in terms of coronary perfusion, as well as the function of the tricuspid valve, is unknown.

Patients with transposition of the great arteries plus left ventricular outlet obstruction have been treated by closing the ventricular septal defect and creating pulmonary outflow tracts with Dacron conduits that contain an artificial valve. This operation is known as the Rastelli procedure.[15] Unlike the Mustard procedure, the Rastelli operation restores the normal anatomic relationship, with the left ventricle pumping systemic blood and the right ventricle pumping pulmonary blood. Fontan procedures may also be used in treatment of these patients (see the section Tricuspid Atresia).

MANAGEMENT OF ANESTHESIA

Management of anesthesia in the presence of transposition of the great arteries must take into account separation of the pulmonary and systemic circulations. Drugs administered intravenously will be distributed with minimal dilution to organs such as the heart and brain. Therefore, doses and rates of injection of intravenously administered drugs may need to be reduced. Conversely, onset of anesthesia produced by inhaled drugs will be delayed, as only small portions of the inhaled drugs reach the systemic circulation. In the final analysis, induction and maintenance of anesthesia are often accomplished with ketamine, combined with muscle relaxants to facilitate intubation of the trachea. Ketamine can be supplemented with opioids or benzodiazepines for maintenance of anesthesia. Nitrous oxide has limited application, since it is important to administer high inspired oxygen concentrations to these patients. Potential cardiac depressant effects of volatile anesthetics detract from use of these drugs. Pancuronium is useful if intraoperative skeletal muscle paralysis is indicated.

Dehydration must be avoided in the perioperative period. These patients may have hematocrits in excess of 70 percent, which may contribute to the high incidence of cerebral venous thrombosis. This suggests that these patients should not have oral fluids withheld for prolonged periods. If fluids cannot be ingested orally, intravenous infusion of fluids should be started in the operative period. Atrial dysrhythmias and conduction disturbances may occur postoperatively.

MIXING OF BLOOD BETWEEN THE PULMONARY AND SYSTEMIC CIRCULATIONS

Several uncommon congenital heart defects result in mixing of oxygenated and unoxygenated blood. As a result of this mixing, pulmonary arterial blood has higher oxygen saturations than systemic venous blood, and systemic arterial blood has lower oxygen saturations than pulmonary venous blood. Arterial hypoxemia varies in severity, depending on the magnitude of pulmonary blood flow.

Truncus Arteriosus

Truncus arteriosus refers to the situation in which a single arterial trunk gives rise to the aorta and pulmonary artery (Fig. 3-6). This single arterial trunk overrides both ventricles, which are connected through a ventricular septal defect. Mortality is high, with the median age of survival being about 5 weeks to 6 weeks.

CLINICAL MANIFESTATIONS

Presenting signs and symptoms of truncus arteriosus include failure to thrive, arterial hypoxemia, and congestive heart failure soon

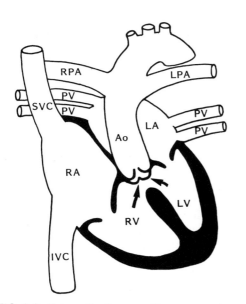

FIG. 3-6. Schematic diagram of truncus arteriosus in which the pulmonary artery (RPA = right pulmonary artery, LPA = left pulmonary artery) and aorta (Ao) arise from a single trunk that overrides the left ventricle (LV) and right ventricle (RV). This trunk receives blood from both ventricles by virtue of a ventricular septal defect.

after birth. Peripheral pulses may be accentuated due to rapid diastolic runoff of blood into the pulmonary bed. Auscultation of the chest and evaluation of the electrocardiogram do not give predictable information and are not diagnostic. Radiographs of the chest reveal cardiomegaly and increased vascularity of the lung fields. The diagnosis is confirmed by angiocardiography performed during cardiac catheterization.

TREATMENT

Surgical treatment of truncus arteriosus includes banding of the right and left pulmonary arteries if pulmonary blood flow is excessive. In addition, associated ventricular septal defects can be closed, so only left ventricular output enters the truncus arteriosus. When this is done, Dacron conduits with a valve are also placed between the right ventricle and pulmonary artery.

MANAGEMENT OF ANESTHESIA

Management of anesthesia in the presence of truncus arteriosus is determined by the magnitude of pulmonary blood flow. When pulmonary blood flow is increased, the use of positive end-expiratory pressure is beneficial and may serve to decrease symptoms of congestive heart failure. Patients with a reduced pulmonary blood flow and arterial hypoxemia should be managed as described for tetralogy of Fallot.

Partial Anomalous Pulmonary Venous Return

Partial anomalous pulmonary venous return is characterized by the presence of left or right pulmonary veins that empty into the right side of the circulation rather than the left atrium. In about one-half of the cases, the aberrant pulmonary veins drain into the superior vena cava. In the remaining cases, pulmonary veins enter the right atrium, inferior vena cava, azygous vein, or coronary sinus. Partial anomalous pulmonary venous return may be more common than appreciated, as suggested by the presence of this anomaly in about 0.5 percent of routine autopsies.

Onset and severity of symptoms produced by this abnormality depend on the amount of pulmonary blood flow routed through the right side of the heart. Fatigue and exertional dyspnea are the most frequent initial manifestations, usually appearing in early adulthood. Cyanosis and congestive heart failure are likely if more than 50 percent of the pulmonary venous flow enters the right side of the circulation.

Angiography is the most useful technique for confirming the diagnosis of partial anomalous pulmonary venous return. Cardiac catheterization usually reveals normal intracardiac pressures and increased oxygen saturations of blood in the right side of the heart. Treatment is by surgical repair.

Total Anomalous Pulmonary Venous Return

Total anomalous pulmonary venous return is characterized by drainage of all four of the pulmonary veins into the systemic venous system. The most common presentation of this defect, accounting for about one-half the cases, is drainage of the four pulmonary veins into the left innominate vein, in association with a left-sided superior vena cava. Oxygenated blood reaches the left atrium by way of atrial septal defects. A patent ductus arteriosus is present in about one-third of cases.

CLINICAL MANIFESTATIONS

Total anomalous pulmonary venous return presents clinically as congestive heart failure in 50 percent of patients by 1 month of age and in 90 percent by 1 year. The definitive diagnosis is by angiocardiography. Mortality is about 80 percent by 1 year of age, unless surgical correction using cardiopulmonary bypass is performed.

MANAGEMENT OF ANESTHESIA

Management of anesthesia in the presence of total anomalous pulmonary venous return may include positive end-expiratory pressure applied to the airways in attempts to reduce excessive pulmonary blood flow. Patients who present with pulmonary edema should be given positive pressure ventilation to the lungs through a tube placed in the trachea before cardiac catheterization. Operative manipulations of the right atrium, which would be tolerated by normal patients, may result in obstruction to flow into the right atrium, manifesting as prompt reductions in blood pressure and the onset of bradycardia. Intravenous transfusions are hazardous, as increases in right atrial pressures are transmitted to the pulmonary veins, leading to the possibility of pulmonary edema.

Hypoplastic Left Heart Syndrome

Hypoplastic left heart syndrome occurs in about 7.5 percent of infants with congenital heart disease and is characterized by left ventricular hypoplasia, mitral valve hypoplasia, aortic valve atresia, and hypoplasia of the ascending aorta.[16] Extracardiac congenital anomalies do not usually accompany this syndrome. There is complete mixing of pulmonary venous and systemic venous blood in a single ventricle which is connected in parallel to both the pulmonary and systemic circulation. Systemic blood flow is dependent on a patent ductus arteriosus. In addition to ductal patency, infant survival is also dependent on a balance between systemic vascular resistance and pulmonary vascular resistance, since both circulations are supplied from a single ventricle in a parallel fashion. Abrupt decreases in pulmonary vascular resistance after delivery results in increased pulmonary blood flow at the expense of systemic blood flow (pulmonary steal phenomenon). When this occurs, coronary and systemic blood flow are inadequate leading to metabolic acidosis, high output cardiac failure, and ventricular fibrillation despite increasingly high levels of arterial oxygen partial pressures due to the high pulmonary blood flow (Fig. 3-7).[16] Alternatively, postnatal events that lead to elevations of pulmonary vascular resistance can reduce pulmonary blood flow so severely that arterial hypoxemia worsens leading to progressive metabolic acidosis and circulatory collapse (Fig. 3-7).[16] Because rapid changes in pulmonary vascular resistance occur in the postnatal period, the necessary fine balance between pulmonary vascular resistance and systemic vascular resistance is unstable and difficult to maintain.

TREATMENT

Treatment of hypoplastic left heart syndrome is surgical, beginning with palliative procedures that eliminate the need for continued patency of the ductus arteriosus. Preoperatively, continuous intravenous infusions of prostaglandin E-1 may be necessary to prevent physiologic closure of the ductus arteriosus. In

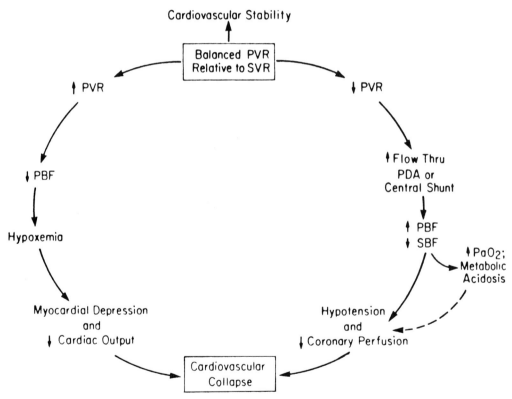

FIG. 3-7. Cardiovascular stability in the presence of hypoplastic left heart syndrome requires a balance between pulmonary vascular resistance (PVR) relative to systemic vascular resistance (SVR). Abrupt decreases in PVR after delivery can result in excessive pulmonary blood flow (PBF) relative to systemic blood flow (SBF) with cardiovascular collapse despite the absence of arterial hypoxemia. Conversely, postnatal changes that elevate PVR can lead to cardiovascular collapse in the presence of arterial hypoxemia. (Hansen DD, Hickey PR. Anesthesia for hypoplastic left heart syndrome: Use of high-dose fentanyl in 30 neonates. Anesth Analg 1986;65:127–32. Reprinted with permission from IARS.)

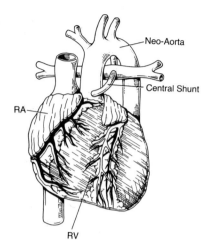

FIG. 3-8. Anatomy after first-stage palliative procedure for hypoplastic left heart syndrome in the neonatal period. The ascending aorta has been reconstructed from the proximal pulmonary artery to form a neoaorta. (Hansen DD, Hickey PR. Anesthesia for hypoplastic left heart syndrome: Use of high-dose fentanyl in 30 neonates. Anesth Analg 1986;65:127–32. Reprinted with permission from IARS.)

addition, inotropes and sodium bicarbonate may be necessary.

The palliative procedure consists of reconstruction of the ascending aorta using the proximal pulmonary artery (Fig. 3-8).[16] A systemic-to-pulmonary shunt to provide pulmonary blood flow is placed between the reconstructed aorta and distal pulmonary artery. Typically, infants are placed on cardiopulmonary bypass to allow production of whole body hypothermia and reconstruction of the aorta is then accomplished during 40 minutes to 60 minutes of circulatory arrest. The central shunt is placed after reinstitution of cardiopulmonary bypass and during rewarming. The completed palliative procedure leaves the single right ventricle connected in parallel to the systemic circulation and pulmonary circulations. The stage is set, however, for later correction with Fontan procedures when pulmonary vascular resistance has decreased to adult levels (see the section Tricuspid Atresia). Fontan procedures, plus elimination of systemic-to-pulmonary shunts, separates the two circulations and facilitates development of normal arterial oxygen saturations.

MANAGEMENT OF ANESTHESIA

Umbilical artery and intravenous catheters are usually placed before the arrival of infants in the operating room. After institution of monitoring (blood pressure, electrocardiogram, and temperature), induction of anesthesia is often accomplished with fentanyl 50 $\mu g \cdot kg^{-1}$ to 75 $\mu g \cdot kg^{-1}$ administered simultaneously with pancuronium, 0.1 $mg \cdot kg^{-1}$ to 0.15 $mg \cdot kg^{-1}$.[16] These infants are vulnerable to the development of ventricular fibrillation due to inadequate coronary blood flow before the palliative procedure. The danger of ventricular fibrillation and borderline cardiac status argues against use of volatile anesthetics in these infants. The lungs are ventilated with 100 percent oxygen and the trachea intubated. Crystalloid solutions, 10 $ml \cdot kg^{-1}$ to 15 $ml \cdot kg^{-1}$, are often infused before cardiopulmonary bypass is performed. After induction of anesthesia and intubation of the trachea, ventilation of the lungs is adjusted on the basis of arterial blood gas measurements. High arterial partial pressures of oxygen imply high pulmonary blood flow at the expense of the systemic circulation. Indeed, if initial arterial oxygen partial pressures are greater than 100 mmHg, maneuvers to increase pulmonary vascular resistance and decrease pulmonary blood flow are instituted. For example, reductions in the volume of ventilation lead to increases in arterial carbon dioxide partial pressures and decreases in pH, resulting in increased pulmonary vascular resistance and reductions in pulmonary blood flow. If arterial oxygen partial pressures still remain unacceptably elevated, institution of positive end-expiratory pressure leads to increased lung volumes and a further elevation in pulmonary vascular resistance. In extreme cases, temporary occlusion of one pulmonary artery serves to reduce the arterial partial pressures of oxygen.

Dopamine or isoproterenol are administered when necessary for inotropic support at the conclusion of cardiopulmonary bypass. Selection of specific inotropic drugs is influenced by the pulmonary vascular resistance. The most frequent problem after cardiopulmonary bypass is too little pulmonary blood flow with associated arterial hypoxemia (arterial oxygen partial pressures less than 20 mmHg).[16] Attempts directed at improving arterial oxygenation include hyperventilation of the lungs to produce low arterial partial pressures of carbon dioxide (20 mmHg to 25 mmHg) and elevated pH and infusions of isoproterenol to decrease pulmonary vascular resistance. Arterial oxygen partial pressures above 50 mmHg after cardiopulmonary bypass may indicate inadequate systemic blood flow and the likely occurrence of progressive metabolic acidosis unless steps are taken to decrease pulmonary blood flow.

Double Outlet Right Ventricle

Double outlet right ventricle is characterized by the origin of the aorta from the posterior wall of the right ventricle. Left ventricular outflow is via a ventricular septal defect that permits blood flow into the right ventricle. Arterial hypoxemia does not occur unless there is obstruction to pulmonary outflow. This cardiac defect is rare, accounting for only about 0.5 percent of patients with congenital heart disease.

Clinically, most of these patients present with congestive heart failure. Presentation is indistinguishable from that of patients with large ventricular septal defects. Angiocardiography performed at cardiac catheterization is usually required to establish the diagnosis, since radiographs of the chest and the electrocardiogram are nonspecific.

Surgical treatment may include banding of the pulmonary artery or a Blalock-Taussig shunt, depending on the magnitude of the pulmonary blood flow. Complete repair may be attempted by placing a tunnel of synthetic material from the ventricular septal defect to the aorta. Management of anesthesia is dependent on the magnitude of pulmonary blood flow.

INCREASED MYOCARDIAL WORK

Aortic stenosis, coarctation of the aorta, and pulmonary stenosis are examples of congenital cardiac defects characterized by increased cardiac work due to obstruction to ejection of blood from the left or right ventricle. These lesions require the myocardium to produce considerably more hydraulic work than normal.

Aortic Stenosis

Aortic stenosis is the most common cause of obstruction to ejection of the left ventricular stroke volume. The site of this obstruction can be valvular, subvalvular (hypertrophic cardiomyopathy), or supravalvular (see Chapters 2 and 8). Cardiac catheterization is necessary to determine the site of obstruction, as well as the pressure gradients across the aortic valve. Regardless of the type of aortic stenosis, the myocardium must generate intraventricular pressures that are two to three times normal, while pressures in the aorta remain in physiologic ranges. Resulting concentric myocardial hypertrophy leads to increased myocardial oxygen requirements. Furthermore, the high velocity of blood flow through the stenotic area predisposes to the development of infective endocarditis and is associated with poststenotic dilation of the aorta.

CLINICAL MANIFESTATIONS

Auscultation of the chest in the presence of aortic stenosis reveals systolic ejection murmurs best heard at the second right intercostal space and radiating to the neck. Most patients with congenital aortic stenosis are asymptomatic until adulthood. Infants with severe aortic stenosis, however, may present with signs of congestive heart failure. Most infants with aortic stenosis severe enough to produce symptoms will also have endocardial fibroelastosis involving the left side of the heart. Subvalvular aortic stenosis rarely presents in infancy. The electrocardiogram in the presence of congenital aortic stenosis typically shows left ventricular hypertrophy. Depression of the ST segment is likely during exercise, particularly if pressure gradients across the aortic valve are greater than 50 mmHg. Radiographs of the chest reveal left ventricular hypertrophy, with or without poststenotic dilation of the aorta. Calcification of the aortic valve will not usually be apparent before 15 years of age.

Sudden death, rare in children with aortic stenosis, can occur in adult patients and is presumably due to cardiac dysrhythmias. Likewise, angina pectoris is uncommon in the very young but reaches an incidence of about 20 percent between the ages of 15 years and 30 years. Angina pectoris in the absence of coronary artery disease reflects inability of coronary blood flow to meet increased myocardial oxygen requirements of the hypertrophied left ventricle. Syncope can occur when pressure gradients across the aortic valve exceeds 50 mmHg.

Findings in patients with supravalvular stenosis may include a characteristic appearance in which the facial bones are prominent, the forehead rounded, and the upper lip pursed. Strabismus, inguinal hernias, dental abnormalities, and moderate mental retardation are commonly present. Blood pressure readings taken in the upper extremities may be unequal, depending on how the high-velocity jet stream of blood ejected through the stenotic aortic valve strikes the innominate artery.

TREATMENT

Medical treatment is not predictably successful in management of patients with congenital aortic stenosis. The exception is patients with subvalvular stenosis, in whom reductions in myocardial contractility with beta-adrenergic antagonist drugs may be useful until surgical correction can be undertaken.

Surgical treatment is indicated in patients with pressure gradients greater than 50 mmHg across the aortic valve at rest or in whom syncope or angina pectoris have occurred. Pressure gradients of 40 mmHg due to supravalvular aortic stenosis are considered indications for surgery, since high pressures in the coronary arteries may lead to premature development of atherosclerosis. Children with congenital aortic stenosis at the level of the valve are usually treated with valvulotomy performed during cardiopulmonary bypass. Aortic valve replacement is often necessary at a later age.

Subvalvular aortic stenosis is treated by resection of the abnormal musculature. Supravalvular aortic stenosis is corrected by widening the lumen of the aorta with an artificial patch.

MANAGEMENT OF ANESTHESIA

Management of anesthesia is outlined in Chapters 2 and 8.

Coarctation of the Aorta

Coarctation of the aorta accounts for about 5 percent of patients with congenital heart disease. Depending on the position of the narrowing in the aorta in relation to the ductus arteriosus, this abnormality is designated as preductal (infantile) or postductal (adult).

PREDUCTAL

Anatomically, the preductal form of coarctation of the aorta is most often characterized by a localized constriction, just proximal to the ductus arteriosus, or diffuse narrowing of the arch of the aorta. Associated cardiac defects include patent ductus arteriosus in about two-thirds, ventricular septal defects in one-third, and bicuspid aortic valves in about one-fourth of patients. Transposition of the great arteries is present in about 10 percent of cases. Cardiac catheterization is necessary to detect associated defects. Radiographs of the chest reveal biventricular enlargement. A prominent fluctuation in the quality of the femoral pulse is characteristic.

Congestive heart failure as a result of this cardiac defect is usually manifest within the first weeks of life. Treatment is initially with digitalis and diuretics. If rapid improvement does not occur, surgical repair should be undertaken. Surgical treatment includes resection of the stenotic portion of the aorta and closure of the ductus arteriosus if it has remained patent. The pulmonary artery may need to be banded at the same operation if a ventricular septal defect is also present.

Management of anesthesia in patients with the preductal form of coarctation of the aorta may be mainly resuscitative, as these infants are often critically ill. Positive end-expiratory pressure can be helpful in the presence of left ventricular failure and at the same time can serve to decrease excessive pulmonary blood flow if there is an associated ventricular septal defect. Surgically, a patent ductus arteriosus must be ligated before repairing the coarctation. This initial ligation can eliminate the majority of blood flow to the lower half of the body until the repair of the narrowed portion of the aorta is completed. As a result, metabolic acidosis, requiring therapy with sodium bicarbonate, may develop during this phase of the operation. Monitoring of arterial blood pressure is best achieved by a catheter in the right radial artery, as the left subclavian artery may be clamped during the operation.

POSTDUCTAL

Coarctation of the aorta that manifests in young adults characteristically involves that portion of the aorta immediately distal to the left subclavian artery. Diagnosis is often a chance finding on routine physical examination, when either hypertension or systolic murmurs are detected. Characteristically, there is hypertension present in the upper extremities, reduced blood pressure in the legs, and a palpable delay in the femoral pulse. Hypertension presumably reflects ejection of the left ventricular stroke volume into the fixed resistance created by the narrowed artery. Arterial pulses are prominent in the upper extremities and weak or absent in the legs. Systolic murmurs are best heard over the stenotic area of the aorta in the left paravertebral area. If obstruction to blood flow is severe, blood reaches the lower part of the body through development of extensive collateral systems involving the internal mammary and intercostal arteries. Continuous murmurs over these enlarged collateral vessels may be audible.

Radiographs of the chest may reveal left ventricular hypertrophy and notching along the lower borders of the ribs, reflecting development of collateral circulation via the intercostal arteries. The electrocardiogram usually reveals changes associated with left ventricular hypertrophy. Cardiac catheterization and angiocardiography are necessary to determine pressure gradients across the coarctation and to define the anatomic characteristics of the narrowing. Echocardiography is also helpful in defining the site and severity of the coarctation. About one-half of these patients also have a bicuspid aortic valve.

Complications associated with a postductal coarctation of the aorta include cerebral hemorrhage, cerebral thrombosis, rupture of the aorta, and necrotizing arteritis. Bicuspid aortic valves are vulnerable to the development of infective endocarditis. Therefore, these patients should be treated with antibiotics before undergoing dental or surgical procedures.

Surgical intervention is indicated when systolic hypertension exceeds 180 mmHg or when there are resting pressure gradients greater than 40 mmHg across the coarctation. Surgical repair is accomplished by resection of the stenotic portion of the aorta and end-to-end anastomosis. Synthetic grafts may be necessary to approximate the aorta if the resected stenotic portion is unusually long.

Management of anesthesia for correction of coarctation of the aorta must consider the (1) adequacy of perfusion of the lower portion of the body during cross-clamping of the aorta, (2) propensity for systemic hypertension during cross-clamping of the aorta, and (3) danger of neurologic sequelae due to ischemia of the spinal cord. Continuous monitoring of arterial blood pressure both above and below the level of the coarctation is achieved by placement of catheters in the right radial artery and right femoral artery. By monitoring these pressures simultaneously, it is possible to evaluate the adequacy of collateral circulation during periods of aortic cross-clamping. Mean arterial pressures in the lower extremities should be at least 40 mmHg to assure adequate blood flow to the kidneys and spinal cord. If blood pressure in the lower portion of the body cannot be maintained above this level, it may be necessary to use partial circulatory bypass.

Excessive increases in systolic blood pressure during cross-clamping of the aorta may adversely increase the work of the heart and make surgical repair more difficult. In this situation, use of volatile anesthetics is helpful in maintaining a normal blood pressure. If hypertension persists, continuous intravenous infusions of nitroprusside or trimethaphan should be considered. Although both drugs are effective, reductions in cardiac output produced by trimethaphan make this drug an attractive choice. Disadvantages of lowering blood pressure to normal levels may be excessive reductions in blood pressure in the lower part of the body and subsequent ischemia of the spinal cord or kidneys. In this regard, somatosensory evoked cortical potentials are useful to monitor spinal cord function and the adequacy of its blood flow during cross-clamping of the aorta.

Postoperatively, there may be paradoxical increases in blood pressure. Baroreceptor reflexes, activation of the renin-angiotensin-aldosterone system, and excessive release of catecholamines have all been implicated as possible causes. Regardless of the etiology, intravenous administration of nitroprusside or trimethaphan, with or without propranolol, work well to control systemic hypertension in the early postoperative period. Longer-acting antihypertensive drugs, such as hydralazine or labetalol can be instituted if hypertension persists. Abdominal pain may occur in the postoperative period and is presumably due to sudden increases in blood flow to the gastrointestinal tract, leading to increased vasoactivity. Intraoperative damage to the spinal cord due to prolonged hypotension or ligation of collateral vessels will manifest in the postoperative period as paraplegia.

Hypertension may persist chronically even after successful correction of the coarctation. In this regard, the younger the patient at the time of surgical correction, the more likely is blood pressure to normalize.[2] Premature coronary artery disease may reflect effects of hypertension before surgery. The risks of a bicuspid aortic valve persist after the surgery and include infective endocarditis and development of aortic regurgitation.

Pulmonary Stenosis

Pulmonary stenosis accounts for about 10 percent of all patients with congenital heart disease. Congenital pulmonary stenosis is valvular in 90 percent of the cases and infundibular in the remainder. About three-fourths of these patients will have a probe-patent foramen ovale, and 10 percent will have an associated atrial septal defect. Infundibular pulmonary stenosis is often associated with ventricular septal defects.

CLINICAL MANIFESTATIONS

Clinical manifestations of congenital pulmonary stenosis vary with the degree of obstruction to ejection of right ventricular stroke volume. Mild to moderate degrees of pulmonary stenosis are usually not associated with symptoms. Detection of systolic ejection murmurs, best heard at the second left intercostal space, is often the first clue that this stenosis is present. The intensity and duration of cardiac murmurs parallel the severity of the stenosis. Right atrial and ventricular hypertrophy and right ventricular failure can occur when pulmonary stenosis is severe. Arterial hypoxemia and congestive heart failure may be manifestations of severe pulmonary stenosis in neonates. Onset of symptoms in neonates may correspond to closure of the ductus arteriosus. Patients presenting at older ages may have episodes of syncope and angina pectoris. Sudden death can also occur and is thought to be due to infarction of the right ventricle. Radiographs of the chest and the electrocardiogram show evidence of right atrial and ventricular enlargement. Pulmonary stenosis is considered to be severe when gradients measured across the valve during cardiac catheterization are greater than 50 mmHg.

TREATMENT

Surgical treatment of congenital pulmonary stenosis is often a valvulotomy performed during cardiopulmonary bypass. Alternatively, catheter balloon valvuloplasty may be effective therapy. Infundibular pulmonary stenosis is treated by resection of excess ventricular muscle.

MANAGEMENT OF ANESTHESIA

Management of anesthesia is designed to avoid increases in right ventricular oxygen requirements. Therefore, excessive increases in heart rate and myocardial contractility are undesirable. The impact of changes in pulmonary vascular resistance is minimized by the presence of the fixed obstruction at the pulmonary valve. As a result, elevations in pulmonary vascular resistance due to positive pressure ventilation of the lungs are unlikely to produce significant increases in right ventricular afterload and oxygen requirements. These patients are extremely difficult to resuscitate if cardiac arrest occurs because cardiac massage is not highly effective in forcing blood across stenotic pulmonary valves. Therefore, reductions in blood pressure should be promptly treated with sympathomimetic drugs. Likewise, cardiac dysrhythmias or increases in heart rate that become hemodynamically significant should be rapidly corrected, using drugs such as lidocaine or propranolol. In addition, an electrical defibrillator should be available when anesthesia is administered to patients with pulmonary stenosis.

MECHANICAL OBSTRUCTION OF THE TRACHEA

The trachea can be obstructed by circulatory anomalies that produce a vascular ring, or by dilation of the pulmonary artery secondary to the absence of the pulmonary valve. These lesions must be considered when evaluating children with unexplained stridor or other evidence of upper airway obstruction. The possibility of an undiagnosed vascular ring should always be considered in the differential diagnosis of airway obstruction that follows placement of a nasogastric tube or an esophageal stethoscope.

Double Aortic Arch

Double aortic arch results in a vascular ring that can produce pressure on the trachea and esophagus. Compression resulting from this pressure can manifest as inspiratory stridor, difficulty mobilizing secretions, and dysphagia. Individuals with this cardiac defect usually prefer to lie with the neck extended, as flexion of the neck often accentuates compression of the trachea.

Surgical transection of the smaller aortic arch is the treatment of choice in symptomatic patients. During surgery, the tube in the trachea should be placed beyond the area of tracheal compression if this can be safely accomplished without producing an endobronchial intubation. It must be appreciated that an esophageal stethoscope or nasogastric tube can cause occlusion of the trachea, if the tracheal tube remains above the level of vascular compression. Clinical improvement after surgical transection is often immediate. Tracheomalacia from prolonged compression of the trachea, however, can jeopardize the patency of the trachea.

Aberrant Left Pulmonary Artery

Tracheal or bronchial obstruction can occur when the left pulmonary artery is absent and the arterial supply to the left lung is derived from a branch of the right pulmonary artery passing between the trachea and esophagus. This anatomic arrangement has been referred to as a vascular sling, since a complete ring is not present. The sling can cause obstruction of the right mainstem bronchus, the distal trachea, or rarely the left mainstem bronchus.

Clinical manifestations of an aberrant pulmonary artery include stridor, wheezing, and occasionally arterial hypoxemia. In contrast to true vascular rings, esophageal obstruction is rare, and stridor produced by this defect is usually during exhalation rather than inspiration. Radiographs of the chest may reveal abnormal separations between the esophagus and trachea. Hyperinflation or atelectasis of either lung may be present. Angiography is the most accurate approach for confirming the diagnosis.

Surgical division of the aberrant left pulmonary artery at its origin and redirection of its course anterior to the trachea, with anastomosis to the main pulmonary artery, is the treatment of choice. In the first months of life, surgical correction using deep hypothermia without cardiopulmonary bypass has been described.[17] Theoretically, continuous positive airway pressure or positive end-expiratory pressure should relieve airway obstruction and associated stridor in these cases.

Absent Pulmonary Valve

Absence of the pulmonary valve results in dilation of the pulmonary artery, which can result in compression of the trachea and left mainstem bronchus. This lesion can occur as an isolated defect or in conjunction with tetralogy of Fallot. Symptoms include signs of tracheal obstruction and occasionally the development of arterial hypoxemia and congestive heart failure. Any increase in pulmonary vascular resistance, as may occur with arterial hypoxemia or hypercarbia, will accentuate airway obstruction. Intubation of the trachea and maintenance of 4 mmHg to 6 mmHg of continuous positive airway pressure can be used to keep the trachea distended and thus reduce the magnitude of airway obstruction. Definitive treatment is insertion of a tubular graft with an artificial pulmonary valve.[18]

REFERENCES

1. Keith JD. Prevalance, incidence, and epidemiology. In: Keith JD, Rowe RD, Vlad P, eds. Heart disease in infancy and childhood. New York: Macmillan, 1978;1–13
2. Perloff JK. Adults with surgically treated congenital heart disease. JAMA 1983;250:2033–6
3. McCabe JC, Engle MA, Gay WA, Ebert PA. Surgical treatment of endocardial cushion defects. Am J Cardiol 1977;39:72–7
4. Eger II EI. Effect of ventilation/perfusion abnormalities. In: Eger II EI. Anesthetic uptake and action. Baltimore: Williams & Wilkins, 1974;146–59
5. Brash AR, Hickey DE, Graham TP, et al. Pharmacokinetics of indomethacin in the neonate: relation of plasma indomethacin levels to response of the ductus arteriosus. N Engl J Med 1981;305:62–62
6. O'Donnell TV, McIlroy MB. The circulatory effects of squatting. Am Heart J 1962;64:347–56
7. Lumley J, Whitwam JG, Morgan M. General anesthesia in the presence of Eisenmenger's syndrome. Anesth Analg 1977;56:543–7
8. Spinnato JA, Kraynack BJ, Cooper MW. Eisenmenger's syndrome in pregnancy: epidural anesthesia for elective cesarean section. N Engl J Med 1981;304–1215–6
9. Elsten JL, Kim YD, Hanowell ST, Macnamara TE. Prolonged induction with exaggerated chamber enlargement in Ebstein's anomaly. Anesth Analg 1981;60:909–10
10. Fyman PN, Goodman K, Casthely PA, et al. Anesthetic management of patients undergoing Fontan procedure. Anesth Analg 1986;65:516–9
11. Hagen PT, Scholtz DG, Edwards WD. Incidence and size of patent foramen ovale during the first 10 decades of life: An autopsy study of 965 normal hearts. Mayo Clin Proc 1984;59:17–20
12. Moorthy SS, LoSasso AM. Patency of the foramen ovale in the critically ill patient. Anesthesiology 1974;41:405–7
13. Rashkind WJ, Miller WW. Creation of an atrial septal defect without thoracotomy. JAMA 1966;196:991–2
14. Mustard WT, Keith JD, Trusler GA, et al. The surgical management of transposition of the great vessels. J Thorac Cardiovasc Surg 1964;48:953–8
15. Rastelli GC, McGoon DC, Wallace RB. Anatomic correction of the great arteries with ventricular septal defect and subpulmonary stenosis. J Thorac Cardiovasc Surg 1969;58:545–52
16. Hansen DD, Hickey PR. Anesthesia for hypoplastic left heart syndrome: Use of high-dose fentanyl in 30 neonates. Anesth Analg 1986;65:127–32
17. McLeskey CH, Martin WE. Anesthesia for repair of a pulmonary-artery sling in an infant with severe tracheal stenosis. Anesthesiology 1977;46:368–70
18. Litwin SB, Rosenthal A, Fellows K. Surgical management of young infants with tetralogy of Fallot, absence of the pulmonary valve, and respiratory distress. J Thorac Cardiovasc Surg 1973;65:552–8

4

Abnormalities of Cardiac Conduction and Cardiac Rhythm

Cardiac dysrhythmias that occur in the perioperative period can usually be explained on the basis of abnormalities of cardiac impulse conduction (reentry) or impulse formation (automaticity). Reentry excitation is the mechanism for most cardiac dysrhythmias and reflects reexcitation of tissues by return of the same cardiac impulses in a circuitous fashion (Fig. 4-1).[1] For cardiac impulses to complete a reentry circuit, they must be initially unidirectionally blocked. This contrasts with automaticity in which new cardiac impulses are generated each time to excite the heart. Enhanced automaticity leads to cardiac dysrhythmias by facilitating repetitive firing from a single focus.

Events that accompany the perioperative period are often associated with changes in cardiac automaticity or conditions that favor reentry pathways (Table 4-1). For example, increased blood pressure, as in response to intubation of the trachea or surgical stimulation, can stretch Purkinje fibers, which both enhances automaticity and at the same time slows conduction velocity of cardiac impulses, which favors a reentry pathway. Cardiac dysrhythmias associated with halothane are most likely due to a reentry mechanism. For example, halothane has been shown to slow conduction of cardiac impulses through the atrioventricular node and His-Purkinje system in a dose-related manner.[2] In addition, halothane depresses cardiac impulse formation in the sinoatrial node. As a result, wandering atrial pacemakers and junctional rhythms are common during administration of halothane. These responses reflect suppression of sinoatrial node activity and the appearance of cardiac pacemakers nearer the atrioventricular node. Enflurane also slows conduction of cardiac impulses through the atrioventricular node but, unlike halothane, does not slow conduction of impulses through the His-Purkinje system.[3] This may be at least a partial explanation for the reduced incidence of epinephrine-associated cardiac dysrhythmias during administration of enflurane as compared with halothane. Isoflurane resembles enflurane in that the occurrence of epinephrine-induced cardiac dysrhythmias is unlikely.[4] Pancuronium has also been shown to speed conduction of cardiac impulses through the atrioventricular node (Fig. 4-2).[5] This is consistent with increases in heart rate that accompany administration of this muscle relaxant.

The importance of cardiac dysrhythmias in the management of anesthesia relates to the effects of the specific rhythm disturbance on cardiac output and possible interactions of antidysrhythmic drugs with those drugs administered to produce anesthesia. A knowledge of the electrophysiology of cardiac cells and the

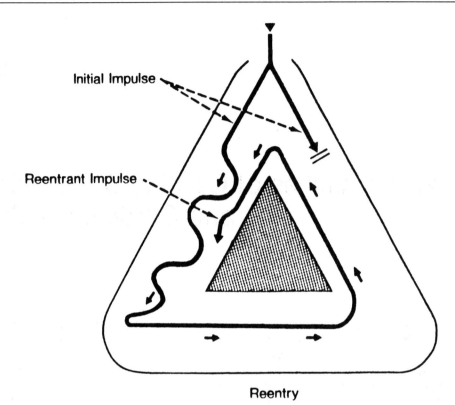

Reentry

FIG. 4-1. The essential requirement for initiation of reentry excitation is a unilateral block that prevents uniform anterograde propagation of the initial cardiac impulse. This same cardiac impulse can, under appropriate conditions, traverse the area of blockade in a retrograde direction and become a reentrant cardiac impulse. (Akhtar M. Management of ventricular tachyarrhythmias. JAMA 1982;247:671–4. Copyright 1982, American Medical Association.)

anatomy of the conduction system for the transmission of cardiac impulses permits a better understanding of why abnormal cardiac rhythms develop and why antidysrhythmic drugs are effective in suppressing these rhythms.

TABLE 4-1. Events Associated with Cardiac Dysrhythmias in the Perioperative Period

Volatile anesthetics
Arterial hypoxemia
Hypercarbia
Systemic hypertension
Endogenous or exogenous catecholamines
Electrolyte imbalance
Intubation of the trachea
Co-existing cardiac disease

ELECTROPHYSIOLOGY OF CARDIAC CELLS

Electrophysiology of cardiac cells is depicted by the cardiac action potential, which is divided into five phases for descriptive purposes (Fig. 4-3). These phases reflect movement of ions through channels in cardiac cell membranes. Channels have been characterized as fast sodium, slow calcium, chloride, and potassium channels. Phase 0 represents rapid depolarization of cardiac cell membranes due to inward movement of sodium ions through specific channels that are activated when spontaneous phase 4 depolarization reaches threshold potential of about −70 mV. This phase parallels QRS complexes on the electrocardi-

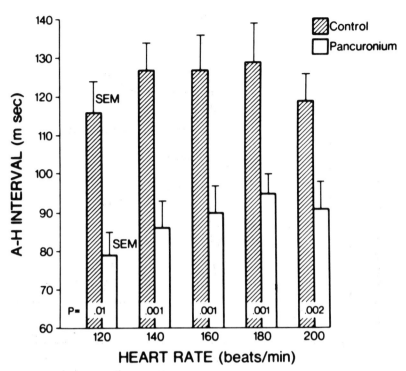

FIG. 4-2. The A-H interval was determined before and after the intravenous administration of pancuronium to dogs anesthetized with halothane. Heart rate was controlled by an atrial pacemaker. Pancuronium decreased the A-H interval at every paced heart rate, confirming that this muscle relaxant speeds conduction of cardiac impulses through the atrioventricular node. (Ghea DG, Rozelle BC, Raessler KL, et al. Pancuronium bromide enhances atrioventricular conduction in halothane-anesthetized dogs. Anesthesiology 1977;46:342–5.)

ogram. Phases 1 through 3 represent repolarization with phase 3 corresponding to T waves on the electrocardiogram. Phase 2 lasts 150 msec to 200 msec and is due to closure of fast sodium channels and inward movement of calcium ions through slow calcium channels. Simultaneously, there is a decrease in permeability of potassium channels that prevents rapid outflow of potassium ions further prolonging phase 2. The sustained plateau of phase 2 provides the prolonged period of contraction necessary for the ventricles to eject blood and distinguishes cardiac action potentials from those developed by skeletal muscle cells. Phase 3 is due principally to a return to normal of cardiac cell membrane permeability to sodium ions and an abrupt increase in permeability to potassium ions allowing loss of these ions so as to restore transmembrane potential to -90 mV. Phase 4 is the resting diastolic potential. The effective (absolute) refractory period is the time during the action potential when cardiac impulses cannot be conducted regardless of the intensity of the stimulus. During the relative refractory period, a stronger than normal stimulus can initiate propagation of cardiac impulses. Automatic cardiac pacemaker cells differ from nonautomatic contractile cells in that phase 4 is not stable but undergoes spontaneous depolarization until reaching threshold potential, when another cardiac action potential occurs. Pacemaker cells in the sinoatrial node have the highest intrinsic rate of phase 4 depolarization and thus predominate over pacemaker cells at other sites (atria, atrioventricular node, ventricles) that have slower intrinsic rates of depolarization.

Automaticity refers to the slope of phase 4 depolarization. Increasing this slope leads to

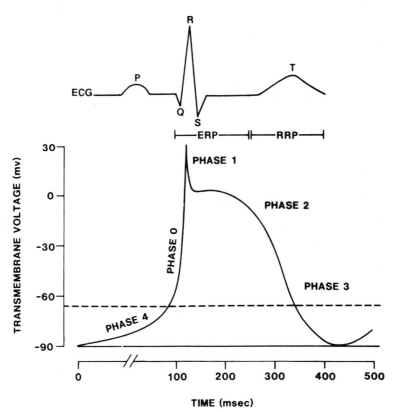

FIG. 4-3. Schematic diagram of a transmembrane action potential generated by an automatic cardiac cell and of the relationship of this action potential to events depicted on the electrocardiogram (ECG). Phase 4 undergoes spontaneous depolarization from the resting membrane potential (-90 mV) until the threshold potential (broken line) is reached. Depolarization (phase 0) occurs when the threshold potential is reached and corresponds to the QRS complex on the ECG. Phases 1 through 3 represent repolarization, with phase 3 corresponding to the T wave on the ECG. The effective refractory period (ERP) is that time during which cardiac impulses cannot be conducted regardless of the intensity of the stimulus. During the relative refractory period (RRP) a stronger than normal stimulus can initiate an action potential. The action potential from a contractile cardiac cell differs from an automatic cell in that phase 4 does not undergo spontaneous depolarization.

enhanced automaticity, which is manifested as an accelerated heart rate and ventricular irritability. Events that increase the slope of phase 4 depolarization include beta-adrenergic stimulation (arterial hypoxemia, hypercarbia, endogenous release of catecholamines, sympathomimetic drugs, exogenous administration of epinephrine), acute hypokalemia, and hyperthermia. In addition, increased stretch of myocardial fibers and cells due to hypertension or increased ventricular volumes, such as accompany congestive heart failure, leads to acceleration of phase 4 depolarization. Ventricular cardiac dysrhythmias associated with hypertension during painful stimulation in anesthetized patients are likely to be due to this mechanism. Increased automaticity can also be caused by decreases in the negativity of the resting membrane potential or increases in the negativity of the threshold potential (Fig. 4-3). For example, hyperkalemia decreases the negativity of the resting membrane potential and thus increases membrane excitability (see Fig. 22-4).

Factors that decrease the slope of phase 4 depolarization include vagal stimulation, positive airway pressure, sudden elevations of plasma potassium concentrations, and hypothermia. Vagal innervation is predominantly limited to atrial cardiac cells. Therefore, changes in vagal tone do not greatly influence automaticity of the ventricle. The less the slope of phase 4 depolarization, the longer it takes to reach threshold potential. Therefore, heart rate slows and cardiac pacemaker cells near the atrioventricular node or in the ventricles are likely to become dominant.

CONDUCTION OF CARDIAC IMPULSES

Cardiac impulses originate in the sinoatrial node and travel rapidly across the atria to the atrioventricular node (Fig. 4-4). The major delay in transmission of cardiac impulses from the atria to the ventricles occur at the atrioventricular node. This delay is normally 60 msec to 140 msec and corresponds to the A-H interval on the His bundle electrocardiogram. Knowledge of the blood supply to the sinoatrial and atrioventricular nodes can help one understand and predict cardiac rhythm disturbances that are associated with atherosclerosis of the major coronary arteries. For example, the right coronary artery supplies the sinoatrial node in about 55 percent of patients, whereas the blood supply in the remaining patients is from the circumflex coronary artery. Therefore, it is predictable that atherosclerotic disease of the right coronary artery is likely to be associated with dysfunction of the sinoatrial node and/or impaired conduction of cardiac impulses through the atrioventricular node.

After cardiac impulses cross the atrioventricular node, they enter the bundle of His, which subsequently divides into right and left bundles (Fig. 4-4). The right bundle is a thin structure that crosses over the right ventricle. The left bundle divides into an anterior fascicle activating the anterior portion of the left ventricle, and a larger posterior fascicle activating the remainder of the left ventricle. Transmission of cardiac impulses along the right and left bundles activates the right and left ventri-

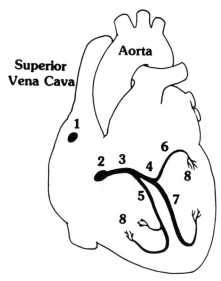

FIG. 4-4. Schematic diagram of the electrical conduction system of the heart. The cardiac impulse originates in the sinoatrial node (1) and rapidly passes to the atrioventricular node (2). After passing through the atrioventricular node, the impulse enters the bundle of His (3). The bundle of His divides into a thick left bundle branch (4) and a thin right bundle branch (5). The left bundle branch subsequently divides into an anterior (6) and thicker posterior (7) fascicle. The bundle branches terminate in the His-Purkinje system (8), which covers the surfaces of both ventricles.

cles by way of the His-Purkinje system, which covers the subendocardial surfaces of both ventricles. The H-V interval on the His bundle electrocardiogram (normally 30 msec to 55 msec) reflects the time necessary for conduction of cardiac impulses through the His-Purkinje system.

ANTIDYSRHYTHMIC DRUGS

Antidysrhythmic drugs are administered when correction of identifiable precipitating events (Table 4-1) is not sufficient to suppress cardiac dysrhythmias. These drugs act by altering electrophysiologic characteristics of the myocardial cells (Table 4-2). For example, most antidysrhythmic drugs suppress automaticity in pacemaker cells by decreasing the slope of phase 4 depolarization. Quinidine, procainamide, and propranolol slow conduction of cardiac impulses and prolong the effective refractory period of cardiac action potentials. Prolongation of the effective refractory period serves to eliminate reentry circuits by converting unidirectional block to total bidirectional block. Conversely, lidocaine and phenytoin facilitate conduction of cardiac impulses, which eliminates unidirectional block and thus prevents the occurrence of cardiac dysrhythmias due to a reentry circuit. Antidysrhythmic drugs also produce characteristic changes on the electrocardiogram (Table 4-2).

Quinidine

Quinidine is an effective drug for control of atrial and ventricular tachydysrhythmias and for the conversion of atrial flutter or fibrillation to normal sinus rhythm. It is common to administer digitalis before treating atrial fibrillation with quinidine since occasional patients will manifest paradoxical increases in the rate of ventricular response when quinidine is administered. Quinidine is administered intravenously at a rate of 50 mg·hr^{-1} to 75 mg·hr^{-1}. Therapeutic blood levels are 2 μg·ml^{-1} to 4 μg·ml^{-1}. Quinidine can produce direct myocardial depression, peripheral vasodilation, and hypotension, especially when administered intravenously. Monitoring of the electrocardiogram is useful to detect prolongation of the time for conduction of cardiac impulses. Thrombocytopenia is rare but may be severe and can result in clinically significant bleeding. Quinidine interferes with normal neuromuscular transmission and may accentuate the effects of nondepolarizing muscle relaxants.[6,7]

Procainamide

Procainamide is as effective as quinidine for treatment of ventricular tachydysrhythmias and premature ventricular beats. The effectiveness of procainamide against atrial dysrhythmias is comparable to that of quinidine. The initial dose can be given intravenously but the rate of administration should not exceed 100 mg every 5 minutes. Infusion is continued until the desired effect is achieved or a total dose of 700 mg to 1,000 mg is reached. Therapeutic blood levels of procainamide are 4 μg·ml^{-1} to 8 μg·ml^{-1}. Flecainide is a fluorinated local anesthetic analog of procainamide that is effective, when administered orally, in suppression of nonsustained ventricular dysrhythmias.

Procainamide depresses the myocardium more than quinidine but peripheral vasodilation is less. Therefore, hypotension during treatment with procainamide is most likely due to direct myocardial depression. Excessive

TABLE 4-2. Electrophysiologic and Electrocardiographic Characteristics of Antidysrhythmic Drugs

	Automaticity	Excitability	Effective Refractory Period	Duration of Action Potential	P-R Interval	QRS Duration
Quinidine	Decreased	Decreased	Increased	Increased	Increased	Increased
Procainamide	Decreased	Decreased	Increased	Increased	Increased	Increased
Propranolol	Decreased	Decreased	Increased	Increased	Increased	Increased
Lidocaine	Decreased	Decreased	Decreased	Decreased	No change	No change
Phenytoin	Decreased	Decreased	Decreased	Decreased	No change	No change
Disopyramide	Decreased	Decreased	Increased	Increased	No change	No change
Bretylium	No change	No change	Increased	Increased	No change	No change
Amiodarone	No change	No change	Increased	Increased	Increased	Increased
Verapamil	Decreased	No change	Decreased	Decreased	No change	No change

plasma concentrations of procainamide can slow conduction of cardiac impulses through the atrioventricular node and intraventricular conduction system. Chronic administration of procainamide can result in a lupus-erythematosus-like syndrome manifesting most often as arthralgia and hepatomegaly. In animals, large doses of procainamide (5 mg·kg^{-1}) potentiate nondepolarizing muscle relaxants [6,7]

Propranolol

Propranolol is effective in slowing ventricular responses during atrial fibrillation and for the treatment of ventricular dysrhythmias. It is a useful drug for conversion of atrial flutter or paroxysmal atrial tachycardia to normal sinus rhythm. Propranolol and quinidine may be used in combination, since they have synergistic effects in the suppression of atrial tachydysrhythmias. The antidysrhythmic action of propranolol is presumed to reflect antagonism of beta-adrenergic activity on the excitable and conducting tissues of the heart. Direct membrane effects are relatively unimportant with the usual therapeutic concentrations of the drug. The intravenous dose of propranolol for the treatment of acute cardiac dysrhythmias is 0.1 mg·min^{-1} to 0.2 mg·min^{-1} usually not to exceed a total dose of about 50 µg·kg^{-1}.

Disadvantages of propranolol in the treatment of digitalis-induced supraventricular or ventricular dysrhythmias are depression of myocardial contractility and a further prolongation of conduction of cardiac impulses through the atrioventricular node. Therefore, propranolol is not the drug of first choice in the treatment of cardiac dysrhythmias due to digitalis. Certainly propranolol is not a logical choice when digitalis toxicity is associated with atrioventricular heart block. Propranolol should not be administered to patients with histories of bronchial asthma, as beta-adrenergic blockade can precipitate bronchospasm in susceptible patients. When treating cardiac dysrhythmias during the intraoperative period, it must be remembered that cardiac depression produced by propranolol can be additive, with reductions in myocardial contractility produced by volatile anesthetics (see Chapter 1).

Lidocaine

Lidocaine is effective in the treatment and suppression of ventricular dysrhythmias and is the drug of choice in the treatment of digitalis-induced ventricular irritability. Therapeutic blood concentrations of lidocaine (2 µg·ml^{-1} to 5 µg·ml^{-1}) reduce automaticity of subsidiary cardiac pacemakers without affecting myocardial contractility or conduction of cardiac impulses through the atrioventricular node. The threshold for ventricular fibrillation is elevated by lidocaine. Lidocaine is not predictably effective in the treatment of supraventricular dysrhythmias. Tocainide is an orally effective amine analog of lidocaine that is used for suppression of symptomatic ventricular dysrhythmias.

Lidocaine is inactivated to a large extent in the liver, such that hepatic function and blood flow to the liver influence the doses needed to achieve antidysrhythmic concentrations. In awake patients with normal hepatic function, an initial intravenous dose of 1 mg·kg^{-1} to 2 mg·kg^{-1}, followed by continuous infusions of 30 µg·kg^{-1}·min^{-1} to 60 µg·kg^{-1}·min^{-1} (2 mg·min^{-1} to 4 mg·min^{-1} to 70 kg patients), should provide therapeutic blood levels. When decreased hepatic blood flow is secondary to reductions in cardiac output (acute myocardial infarctions, congestive heart failure, general anesthesia), the initial intravenous dose should be reduced to 1 mg·kg^{-1} to 1.5 mg·kg^{-1}, followed by continuous infusion rates of about 30 µg·kg^{-1}·min^{-1}. In the presence of decreased lidocaine delivery to the liver for metabolism, these reduced doses should be associated with blood levels similar to those achieved with higher doses administered to patients with normal hepatic blood flow. The potential need to reduce doses of lidocaine during general anesthesia, so as to achieve the same therapeutic blood levels as produced by higher doses administered to awake patients, is an important concept. Large doses of lidocaine (5 mg·kg^{-1}) administered to animals increase the intensity and duration of neuromuscular blockade produced by d-tubocurarine.[7]

Phenytoin

Phenytoin is highly effective in the treatment of supraventricular and ventricular dysrhythmias associated with digitalis toxicity. This drug is not effective in the suppression of atrial tachydysrhythmias. Phenytoin does not alter myocardial contractility and has the added advantage of enhancing conduction of cardiac impulses through the atrioventricular node. As such, phenytoin is a useful drug for the treatment of digitalis-induced cardiac dysrhythmias with or without atrioventricular heart block. The usual intravenous dose of phenytoin is 20 mg·min^{-1}, administered until cardiac dysrhythmias disappear or a total dose of 1,000 mg is reached. Cardiac depression is uncommon when phenytoin is administered slowly in incremental doses. Profound hypotension, bradycardia, and atrioventricular heart block, however, have been observed after rapid intravenous administration of bolus doses exceeding 300 mg. Symptoms of central nervous system toxicity include nystagmus, sedation, and ataxia. It should be appreciated that phenytoin will precipitate in 5 percent glucose in water.

Ecainide

Ecainide is a unique antidysrhythmic drug that combines the electrophysiologic effects of quinidine and lidocaine so as to suppress ventricular cardiac dysrhythmias. In contrast to quinidine, encainide has no consistent effect on peripheral vasculature so alterations in blood pressure are uncommon after oral or intravenous administration.

Disopyramide

Disopyramide produces electrophysiologic effects on cardiac cells similar to those of quinidine. Atrial and ventricular dysrhythmias are effectively suppressed by this drug. Therapeutic blood levels are 2 μg·ml^{-1} to 4 μg·ml^{-1}. The most common side effects are dry mouth and urinary hesitancy, which reflect anticholinergic effects produced by this drug. Dependence on renal clearance is evidenced by prolongation of drug effects in patients with severe kidney dysfunction. This drug may increase the sensitivity of the neuromuscular junction to the effects of nondepolarizing muscle relaxants.[8]

Bretylium

Bretylium is uniquely effective in treating ventricular tachycardia and fibrillation that are unresponsive to other forms of therapy, including lidocaine, procainamide, and repeated electrical shocks. Doses of bretylium for treatment of refractory or recurrent ventricular tachycardia are 5 mg·kg^{-1} to 10 mg·kg^{-1}, administered intravenously over 5 minutes to 10 minutes. Continuous intravenous infusions of bretylium at rates of 1 mg·min^{-1} to 2 mg·min^{-1} may be necessary following the loading doses. It must be appreciated that hypotension can accompany administration of this drug. In refractory ventricular fibrillation, 5 mg·kg^{-1} of bretylium is given rapidly as an intravenous injection. If ventricular fibrillation persists, the dose can be increased to 10 mg·kg^{-1} and repeated at 15 minute to 20 minute intervals until a maximum dose of 30 mg·kg^{-1} has been given.

Antidysrhythmic actions of bretylium are thought to be due to its action on adrenergic receptors, which includes initial stimulation of neurotransmitter release followed by prevention of the release of norepinephrine. Bretylium is not recommended for treatment of digitalis toxicity because the initial release of catecholamines caused by this drug may aggravate co-existing toxic effects of digitalis.

Amiodarone

Amiodarone is a benzofurane derivative that resembles thyroxine structurally and is effective in suppression of recurrent supraventricular and ventricular tachydysrhythmias. Administered intravenously over 2 minutes to 5 minutes, a dose of 5 mg·kg^{-1} produces prompt antidysrhythmic effects. Chronic oral administration of amiodarone is associated with prolonged therapeutic effects even after the drug is discontinued as reflected by elimination half-times of 29 days.

Antiadrenergic effects of amiodarone may be enhanced in the presence of general anesthesia manifesting as atropine-resistant bradycardia and hypotension.[9] The potential need for a temporary artificial cardiac pacemaker and administration of sympathomimetics, such as isoproterenol, should be considered in patients being treated with this drug and scheduled to undergo surgery. Diffuse pulmonary fibrosis and neurologic abnormalities including proximal skeletal muscle weakness and peripheral neuropathies may occur. Transient elevations of transaminase enzymes are common. Chronic amiodarone therapy is associated with alterations in thyroid function causing either hyperthyroidism or hypothyroidism. Rarely, there may be cyanotic discoloration of the face that persists even after the drug is discontinued.

Verapamil

Verapamil 50 μg·kg^{-1} to 150 μg·kg^{-1} infused intravenously over 1 minute to 3 minutes is uniquely effective in suppression of reentrant supraventricular tachydysrhythmias.[10] The mechanism for this success is presumed to be the ability of verapamil to reduce the entry of calcium into cells (see Chapter 1). This makes the atrioventricular node relatively refractory to stimulation, so that fewer cardiac impulses from the rapidly firing sinoatrial node are conducted to activate subsequently the ventricular conduction system. Verapamil has also been shown to reduce the heart rate to a greater extent than digoxin in patients with chronic atrial fibrillation. Calcium entry blockers are relatively ineffective in suppressing ectopic pacemakers in the ventricles.

Calcium entry blockers, by interfering with calcium kinetics, could potentiate myocardial depressant effects of volatile anesthetics. Indeed, verapamil produces reductions in cardiac output when administered to anesthetized patients with co-existing left ventricular dysfunction.[11] Conversely, the interaction with volatile anesthetics is minimal in the absence of co-existing heart disease.[12] Verapamil potentiates the effects of depolarizing and nondepolarizing muscle relaxants similar to that produced by mycin antibiotics.[13] Antagonism of neuromuscular blockade may be impaired because of diminished presynaptic release of acetylcholine.[14] The possibility of drug-induced third degree atrioventricular heart block must be appreciated when considering the acute intravenous administration of verapamil to patients being treated chronically with beta-adrenergic antagonist drugs.

Digitalis

Vagomimetic effects of digitalis on the sinoatrial and atrioventricular nodes make this class of drugs an excellent choice for slowing heart rate, particularly in the presence of supraventricular tachycardia or atrial fibrillation. Intravenous digoxin, 0.25 mg every 20 minutes to 30 minutes to a total dose of 0.5 mg to 0.75 mg, can be given intraoperatively to slow the ventricular response, especially in patients who manifest rapid atrial fibrillation. Intraoperative use of digoxin must be tempered with the realization that this drug is almost entirely dependent on renal excretion for its elimination. In addition, it should be appreciated that geriatric patients are sensitive to the effects of digitalis. This may be reflected by decreased skeletal muscle mass, such that more drug is available for action on cardiac receptors.[15]

DISTURBANCES OF CARDIAC CONDUCTION AND RHYTHM

The electrocardiogram is the cornerstone for diagnosing and treating disturbances of cardiac conduction and rhythm. It is recorded at a paper speed of 25 mm·sec^{-1} and a calibration of 1 mV·cm^{-1}. The normal electrocardiogram consists of three waves, designated the P wave, QRS complex, and T wave. The P wave is due to atrial depolarization, and the QRS complex reflects depolarization of the ventricles (Fig. 4-3). The T wave is due to repolarization of the ventricles. The P-R interval is the time necessary for cardiac impulses to pass through the atrioventricular node. Transmission of cardiac impulses is via specialized conduction systems present in the atria and ventricles (Fig. 4-4). The following questions should be asked when interpreting the electrocardiogram:

1. What is the heart rate?
2. Are P waves present and what is their relationship to the QRS complexes?
3. What is the duration of the P-R interval?
4. What is the duration of the QRS complex?
5. Is the ventricular rhythm regular?
6. Are there early cardiac beats or abnormal pauses after a QRS complex?

The heart rate can be calculated from the electrocardiogram, remembering that the paper speed is 25 mm·sec^{-1} and that each thin line on the paper represents 0.04 second. Therefore, each thick line on the paper is 0.2 second. P waves are normally upright except in lead aVR. Inverted P waves are present when an abnormal pathway exists for the conduction of cardiac impulses or when atrial sites other than the sinoatrial node exist. Amplitude of P waves should not exceed 2.5 mm, and the duration should not exceed 0.11 second. Atrial hypertrophy is evidenced by increased amplitude or width of P waves. It must be ascertained that there is one P wave for each QRS complex. Lead II reflects P waves most predictably and is thus the lead most often selected for analysis of cardiac dysrhythmias in the perioperative period.

The P-R interval is 0.12 second to 0.2 second at normal heart rates. This interval is prolonged when there is increased delay of conduction of cardiac impulses through the atrioventricular node and is shortened in junctional rhythms. The QRS complex is normally 0.05 second to 0.1 second in duration. Abnormal intraventricular conduction of cardiac impulses is suggested by QRS complexes that exceed 0.12 second. Pathologic Q waves exceed 0.04 second in width. ST segments are normally isoelectric but can be elevated up to 1 mm in standard and precordial leads in the absence of any cardiac abnormality. ST segments, however, are never normally depressed. T waves are in the same direction as QRS complexes and should not exceed 5 mm in amplitude in standard leads or 10 mm in precordial leads. Q-T intervals must be corrected for heart rate but normally should be less than one-half of the preceding P-R interval.

Disturbances of conduction of cardiac impulses can be classified according to the site of the conduction block relative to the atrioventricular node (Table 4-3). Heart block occurring above the atrioventricular node is usually benign and transient, whereas heart block below this node tends to be progressive and permanent.

TABLE 4-3. Classification of Heart Block

First-Degree Atrioventricular Heart Block

Second-Degree Atrioventricular Heart Block
   Mobitz type I (Wenckebach)
   Mobitz type II

Unifascicular Heart Block
   Left anterior hemiblock
   Left posterior hemiblock

Right Bundle Branch Block

Left Bundle Branch Block

Bifascicular Heart Block
   Right bundle branch block plus left anterior hemiblock
   Right bundle branch block plus left posterior hemiblock

Third-Degree (Trifascicular, complete) Atrioventricular Heart Block
   Nodal
   Infranodal

First-Degree Atrioventricular Heart Block

First-degree atrioventricular heart block is a delay in the passage of cardiac impulses through the atrioventricular node. The diagnostic feature is a P-R interval greater than 0.2 second in the presence of a normal heart rate. Prolonged P-R intervals may reflect degenerative changes in the atrioventricular conduction system caused by aging. Other causes of this block include increased vagal tone (halothane, digitalis), ischemia of the atrioventricular node, myocarditis, cardiomyopathy, and aortic regurgitation. This form of heart block is usually asymptomatic. Intravenous administration of atropine is effective in speeding transmission of cardiac impulses through the atrioventricular node.

Second-Degree Atrioventricular Heart Block

Second-degree atrioventricular heart block is categorized as Mobitz type I block (Wenckebach) or Mobitz type II block. Mobitz type I block is caused by delayed conduction of cardiac impulses through the atrioventricular node. There is a progressive prolongation of the P-R intervals until a beat is entirely blocked (dropped beat), followed by a repeat of this sequence. In contrast, Mobitz type II block reflects disease of the His-Purkinje conduction system and is characterized by sudden interruption of the conduction of cardiac impulses below the atrioventricular node without prior prolongation of the P-R intervals. Type II block has a more serious prognosis than type I, as it frequently progresses to third-degree atrioventricular heart block. An artificial cardiac pacemaker is justified in patients manifesting Mobitz type II block, even in the absence of symptoms such as syncope.[16]

Unifascicular Heart Block

Block of conduction of cardiac impulses over the left anterior or posterior fascicle of the left bundle branch is characterized as unifas-cicular heart block (Fig. 4-4). Hemiblock is also a term used to designate block of conduction in one of the two fascicles of the left bundle branch.

LEFT ANTERIOR HEMIBLOCK

Block of the left anterior fascicle of the left bundle branch is designated as left anterior hemiblock. Left axis deviation greater than minus 60 degrees is the characteristic abnormality present on the electrocardiogram. Even though hemiblock is a form of intraventricular block, the duration of the QRS complexes is normal or only minimally prolonged.

LEFT POSTERIOR HEMIBLOCK

The posterior fascicle of the left bundle branch is larger and better perfused than the anterior fascicle. Therefore, the posterior fascicle is resistant to damage, and left posterior hemiblock is uncommon. Right axis deviation greater than plus 120 degrees on the electrocardiogram is characteristic of left posterior hemiblock. The duration of the QRS complexes is normal or only minimally prolonged.

Right Bundle Branch Block

Block of conduction of cardiac impulses over the right bundle branch is present in about 1 percent of hospitalized adult patients.[17] Right bundle branch block does not always imply cardiac disease and is often of no clinical significance. On the electrocardiogram this block is recognized by QRS complexes that exceed 0.1 second in duration and broad RSR complexes in leads V1 and V3. Incomplete right bundle branch block (QRS complex duration 0.09 second to 0.1 second) is frequently present in patients with elevated right ventricular pressures, as produced by chronic pulmonary disease or atrial septal defects.

Left Bundle Branch Block

The essential feature of left bundle branch block on the electrocardiogram are QRS complexes greater than 0.12 second in duration and wide notched R waves in all leads. A similar pattern, but with a QRS complex duration of 0.1 second to 0.12 second, is due to incomplete left bundle branch block. Left bundle branch block, in contrast to right bundle branch block, is often associated with coronary artery disease. In addition, this block is frequently indicative of left ventricular hypertrophy that accompanies chronic hypertension or cardiac valve disease.

The presence of left bundle branch block may have special implications for the insertion of a pulmonary artery catheter.[18] Right bundle branch block occurs during insertion of pulmonary artery catheters in about 5 percent of patients with coronary artery disease. Theoretically, third-degree atrioventricular heart block could occur during insertion of such a catheter into patients with co-existing left bundle branch block. Nevertheless, clinical experience has not confirmed an increased incidence of third-degree heart block in these patients during insertion of pulmonary artery catheters.

Intermittent Bundle Branch Block

Intermittent right or left bundle branch block may be related to heart rate or blood pressure. For example, the acute onset of left bundle branch block has been observed during anesthesia when the heart rate exceeds 115 beats·min[-1][19,20] or during episodes of hypertension. Intermittent left bundle branch block may also develop during surgery in the absence of associated tachycardia or hypertension.[21] The onset of left bundle branch block during surgery is important, as it may signal an acute myocardial infarction. It should be remembered that it is difficult to diagnose a myocardial infarction on the electrocardiogram in the presence of a left bundle branch block and rapid heart rates when associated widening of the QRS complexes can be mistaken for ventricular tachycardia.

Bifascicular Heart Block

Bifascicular heart block is present when right bundle branch block is associated with block of one of the fascicles of the left bundle branch. Block of the right bundle branch and the anterior fascicle of the left bundle branch (left anterior hemiblock) is the most frequent combination. On the electrocardiogram this type of bifascicular heart block appears as right bundle branch block with marked left axis deviation. This pattern is seen in about 1 percent of all electrocardiograms recorded from adults.[22] Each year about 1 percent to 2 percent of those individuals with this pattern progress to third-degree atrioventricular heart block.[16] The combination of right bundle branch block and block of the posterior fascicle of the left bundle branch (left posterior hemiblock) is infrequent. In contrast to left anterior hemiblock, however, this form of block often progresses to third-degree atrioventricular heart block.

A theoretical concern in patients with bifascicular heart block is that perioperative events such as alterations in blood pressure, arterial oxygenation, or electrolyte concentrations might compromise conduction of cardiac impulses in the one remaining intact fascicle, leading to the acute onset of third-degree atrioventricular heart block. There is no evidence, however, that surgery performed during general anesthesia or with regional techniques predisposes the patient with co-existing bifascicular block to the development of third-degree atrioventricular heart block.[22–24] Therefore, placement of prophylactic artificial cardiac pacemakers is not recommended before administration of regional or general anesthesia in patients with bifascicular block.[22–24] This recommendation is based on the intraoperative courses of patients with bifascicular block who had normal P-R intervals on the preoperative electrocardiogram and who denied a history of unexplained syncope that might suggest the prior occurrence of transient third-degree atrioventricular heart block. Conceivably, a temporary transvenous cardiac pacemaker should be placed before major surgical procedures when the P-R intervals are prolonged on the preoperative electrocardiogram or when there is a history of syncope, particularly in patients with block of the right bundle branch and the left posterior fascicle. Nevertheless, even symptomatic patients have undergone uneventful surgery without the presence of prophylactic artificial cardiac pacemakers.[25]

TABLE 4-4. Causes of Third-degree Atrioventricular Heart Block

Primary fibrous degeneration of the cardiac conduction system (Lenegre's disease, Lev's disease)
Coronary artery disease (acute myocardial infarction)
Cardiomyopathy
Myocarditis
Iatrogenic following cardiac surgery
Congenital
Increased parasympathetic tone
Drugs (digitalis, beta-adrenergic antagonists, quinidine)
Electrolyte derangements (hyperkalemia)

Third-Degree (Trifascicular, Complete) Atrioventricular Heart Block

Third-degree atrioventricular heart block is characterized by complete absence of conduction of cardiac impulses from the atria to the ventricles. Continued activity of the ventricle is due to stimulation from a cardiac pacemaker distal to the site of the conduction block. When conduction block is near the atrioventricular node, the heart rate is 45 beats·min^{-1} to 55 beats·min^{-1}, and the QRS complexes on the electrocardiogram appear normal. When conduction block is well below the atrioventricular node, the heart rate is 30 beats·min^{-1} to 40 beats·min^{-1} and the QRS complexes are wide.

The most frequent cause of third-degree atrioventricular heart block in adults is primary fibrous degeneration of the cardiac conduction system associated with aging (Lenegre's disease).[26] Degenerative changes in tissues adjacent to the mitral annulus can also interrupt the cardiac conduction system (Lev's disease).[27] Other causes of third-degree atrioventricular heart block are detailed in Table 4-4.

The onset of third-degree atrioventricular heart block may be signaled by episodes of vertigo and syncope. Syncope associated with seizures is designated Adams-Stokes attacks. Congestive heart failure can occur when stroke volume is unable to offset the reduced cardiac output produced by slow heart rates associated with third-degree atrioventricular heart block.

Treatment of third-degree atrioventricular heart block is with permanently implanted artificial cardiac pacemakers. A temporary transvenous cardiac pacemaker should be placed before the induction of anesthesia for placement of a permanent pacemaker. This recommendation is based on the clinical impression that the likelihood of cardiac arrest is increased during induction of anesthesia in patients with third-degree atrioventricular heart block. In some situations, the continuous intravenous infusion of isoproterenol (1 μg·min^{-1} to 4 μg·min^{-1}) may be necessary to maintain adequate ventricular rates until the pacemaker can be placed. It must be appreciated that antidysrhythmic drugs may suppress cardiac pacemaker sites in the ventricle and probably should not be administered to patients with third-degree atrioventricular heart block in the absence of artificial cardiac pacemakers.

Sinus Tachycardia

Sinus tachycardia is present when heart rate exceeds 120 beats·min^{-1}. Increased heart rate is common in the perioperative period and may reflect anxiety, pain, sepsis, hypovolemia, fever, light anesthesia, or congestive heart failure. Treatment is determined by the cause for the increased heart rate. When sinus tachycardia results in myocardial ischemia, it is appropriate to slow the heart rate with beta-adrenergic antagonist drugs, such as propranolol.

Sinus Bradycardia

Sinus bradycardia is defined as heart rates less than 60 beats·min^{-1}. This can be a normal finding in physically active people with high degrees of parasympathetic nervous system activity. An acute diaphragmatic myocardial infarction or the presence of severe pain represent conditions in which discharge of the sinoatrial node can be normally slow. Halothane may decrease heart rate by decreasing the automaticity of the sinoatrial node.[1] Other factors that slow heart rate by depression of sinoatrial node automaticity rather than by vagal stimulation include beta-adrenergic antagonist drugs, hypothermia, hypothyroidism, and icterus. In the presence of carotid sinus hypersensitivity, prolonged asystole can follow even minimal pressure on the carotid sinus. Intravenous administration of atropine is the treatment of choice when heart rate slowing becomes hemodynamically significant.

Sick Sinus Syndrome

Inappropriate sinus bradycardia associated with degenerative changes in the sinoatrial node has been designated as the sick sinus syndrome. Frequently, bradycardia due to this cause is complicated by episodes of supraventricular tachycardia. Patients can be asymptomatic but often complain of palpitations and syncopal episodes. Diminished automaticity of the sinoatrial node is emphasized by the attenuated heart rate response that occurs during physical exercise or after intravenous administration of atropine.

Artificial cardiac pacemakers are often inappropriately inserted in patients with sick sinus syndrome in anticipation of severe bradycardia if antidysrhythmic drugs are employed.[16] This treatment is justified only when symptomatic bradycardia is demonstrated to be caused by therapeutic plasma concentrations of the drugs necessary to control tachycardia. In many patients, drugs used for suppression of atrial tachydysrhythmias are well tolerated without impairing sinoatrial node function. The high incidence of pulmonary embolism in these patients is the rationale for anticoagulation.

Atrial Premature Beats

Atrial premature beats arise from ectopic cardiac pacemakers in the atria. They are recognized on the electrocardiogram by the presence of early and abnormally shaped P waves. Duration of the QRS complexes is normal because activation of the ventricle occurs by normal conduction pathways. When aberrant conduction of cardiac impulses occur, however, the configuration of the QRS complexes are widened and can mimic premature ventricular beats. A distinguishing feature is that an atrial premature beat, unlike a ventricular premature beat, is not usually followed by a compensatory pause. Atrial premature beats can occur in patients with or without heart disease and are usually insignificant except when they precede the onset of a tachydysrhythmia. Acceleration of the heart rate with intravenous administration of atropine usually abolishes premature atrial beats.

Paroxysmal Atrial Tachycardia

Paroxysmal atrial tachycardia is the rapid repetition of atrial premature beats that originate from a cardiac pacemaker outside the sinoatrial node. This tachydysrhythmia is characterized by a sudden onset that is immediately preceded by an atrial premature beat. Cardiac rhythm is absolutely regular at a rate of 150 beats·min^{-1} to 200 beats·min^{-1}. A reentry mechanism is responsible for most instances of this tachycardia.[28]

Initial therapy is manually applied pressure over the area of the carotid sinus in attempts to increase vagal tone.[29] The carotid sinus is located at the site of maximum pulsation of the carotid artery in the neck, which is usually immediately lateral to the thyroid cartilage. Pressure is applied for 10 seconds to 20 seconds, during constant monitoring of the electrocardiogram. Application of pressure over the area of the right carotid sinus is more likely to be successful than is compression applied over the left carotid sinus. Under no circumstances should both carotid sinuses be compressed simultaneously. If unilateral pressure fails to terminate the tachycardia, certain drugs can be administered intravenously in attempts to slow heart rate. For example, verapamil is highly effective in treatment of this dysrhythmia (see the section Verapamil). Alternative drugs include phenylephrine (0.1 mg to 0.5mg), propranolol (0.1 mg·min^{-1} to a maximum dose of 50 μg·kg^{-1}) and digoxin (0.25 mg to 0.75 mg). Electrical cardioversion may be necessary if all other measures fail.

When paroxysmal atrial tachycardia is due to digitalis toxicity, plasma potassium concentrations should be normalized and phenytoin (20 mg·min^{-1}) administered intravenously until the heart rate slows or the total dose of phenytoin reaches 1,000 mg. Intravenous administration of propranolol may also be effective. Treatment of this tachycardia with electrical cardioversion can lead to the development of ventricular dysrhythmias.[30]

Atrial Flutter

Atrial flutter exhibits a regular atrial rate of 250 beats·min^{-1} to 350 beats·min^{-1}, with varying degrees of conduction block through the atrioventricular node. Typically, the conduction block at the atrioventricular node is 2:1. The baseline of the electrocardiogram reveals flutter waves (F waves), resulting in a "sawtooth" pattern. Initial treatment of atrial flutter is with intravenous administration of digoxin (0.25 mg to 0.75 mg), often combined with propranolol. Electrical cardioversion may be necessary if this dysrhythmia remains hemodynamically significant. Prophylaxis against recurrent flutter is provided by chronic administration of digitalis preparations combined, if necessary, with quinidine or propranolol.

Atrial Fibrillation

Atrial fibrillation is characterized by chaotic atrial activity (350 beats·min^{-1} to 500 beats·min^{-1}), with an irregular but slower ventricular response. No distinct P waves are discernible on the electrocardiogram. In the absence of treatment designed to slow conduction of cardiac impulses through the atrioventricular node, the ventricular response can be greater than 140 beats·min^{-1}. Absence of synchronized atrial contractions combined with rapid ventricular responses can greatly reduce cardiac output and in some patients produce congestive heart failure.

Initial treatment of atrial fibrillation in adults is with intravenous administration of verapamil or digoxin (see the sections Verapamil and Digitalis). Ventricular rates of 70 beats·min^{-1} to 90 beats·min^{-1} are considered to reflect adequate therapeutic effects of digitalis. Propranolol (0.25 mg to 0.5 mg administered intravenously) can have additive effects with digitalis and can be used in combination with digoxin for both acute and chronic control of heart rate. Atrial fibrillation is particularly common after cardiac or thoracic surgery and has been attributed to pericardial and/or myocardial inflammation that develops after the surgical procedure. Although controversial, prophylactic use of digoxin may be considered preoperatively for patients considered vulnerable to development of atrial fibrillation after thoracic or cardiac surgery.[31] Electrical cardioversion may be required to treat atrial fibrillation that manifests for the first time after cardiac or thoracic surgery.

Systemic embolization is a serious problem in patients with atrial fibrillation and may require chronic anticoagulation. Thrombi typically form in the atria, reflecting stasis of blood in these cardiac chambers associated with loss of coordinated atrial contractions.

Junctional (Nodal) Rhythm

Junctional rhythm is due to the activity of ectopic cardiac pacemakers in tissues surrounding the atrioventricular node. Impulses initiated by these pacemakers travel to the ventricles in a normal fashion and are also conducted retrograde into the atrium. Depending on the site of the pacemaker, P waves (1) precede the QRS complexes, but the P-R intervals are shortened (less than 0.1 second); (2) follow the QRS complexes; or (3) are lost in the QRS complexes. Junctional rhythm leading to a decrease in blood pressure and cardiac output occurs frequently during general anesthesia, particularly when halothane is being administered. Treatment with atropine is indicated when junctional rhythm becomes hemodynamically significant.

Wandering Atrial Pacemaker

Wandering atrial pacemaker is characterized by the presence of numerous sites in the atria acting as cardiac pacemakers. The electrocardiogram reveals P waves with different configurations and P-R intervals that vary with each QRS complex. Treatment of this condition is usually not necessary unless loss of coordinated atrial contractions leads to reductions in blood pressure; when this occurs, atropine may be administered intravenously.

Ventricular Premature Beats

Ventricular premature beats arise from ectopic cardiac pacemakers located below the atrioventricular node. On the electrocardiogram, these beats are identified by (1) their premature occurrence, (2) absence of a P wave preceding the QRS complex, (3) a wide and often bizarre QRS complex, (4) an ST segment that slopes in the opposite direction from the QRS complex, (5) an inverted T wave, and (6)

a compensatory pause that follows the premature beat. The compensatory pause occurs because the ventricle is still refractory from the preceding premature beat when the next cardiac impulse arrives. Premature ventricular beats are associated with coronary artery disease, digitalis toxicity, arterial hypoxemia, hypercarbia, hypertension, and mechanical irritation of the ventricles as can occur from insertion of a pulmonary artery catheter.

Ventricular premature beats should be treated when they are frequent (more than 6 min^{-1}), multifocal, occur in salvos of three or more, or take place during the ascending limb of the T wave (R on T phenomenon), which corresponds to the relative refractory period of the ventricle (Fig. 4-3). These characteristics are associated with an increased incidence of ventricular tachycardia and fibrillation. The first step in treatment is elimination of the underlying cause, such as arterial hypoxemia or other events associated with excessive sympathetic nervous system activity. If premature beats persist, the drug of choice for suppression, regardless of etiology, is lidocaine, administered as an initial intravenous dose of 1 mg·kg^{-1} to 2 mg·kg^{-1}. This initial dose can be followed with continuous intravenous infusions of lidocaine (30 μg·kg^{-1}·min^{-1} to 60 μg·kg^{-1}·min^{-1}), to maintain therapeutic blood levels and continued suppression of premature beats. Oral administration of quinidine or procainamide may be useful for chronic suppression of ectopic ventricular pacemakers that are responsible for these beats.

Ventricular Tachycardia

Ventricular tachycardia is defined as three or more consecutive premature ventricular beats at a calculated heart rate greater than 120 beats·min^{-1}. QRS complexes on the electrocardiogram are widened, reflecting aberrant intraventricular conduction of cardiac impulses, and there are no identifiable P waves. It should be appreciated that ventricular tachycardia can resemble paroxysmal atrial tachycardia with aberrant conduction.

Ventricular tachycardia is common following acute myocardial infarctions and in the presence of inflammatory or infectious diseases of the heart. Electrical cardioversion is the treatment of choice when ventricular tachycardia becomes hemodynamically significant. If this dysrhythmia is well tolerated, initial treatment can be with the intravenous injection of 1 mg·kg^{-1} to 2 mg·kg^{-1} of lidocaine. Intravenous administration of bretylium may be effective when ventricular tachycardia persists despite treatment with lidocaine or the use of electrical cardioversion (see the section Bretylium).

Ventricular Fibrillation

Ventricular fibrillation is characterized by chaotic and asynchronous contraction of the ventricles with no visible QRS complexes on the electrocardiogram. There is no associated stroke volume with this cardiac rhythm, emphasizing the need to institute immediate cardiopulmonary resuscitation. Conditions that predispose the patient to ventricular fibrillation include myocardial ischemia, electrolyte imbalance, arterial hypoxemia, hypothermia, and drugs that increase cardiac automaticity. Electrical defibrillation is the only effective treatment. When ventricular fibrillation is refractory to treatment, the intravenous injection of bretylium may improve the response to electrical defibrillation (see the section Bretylium).

PREEXCITATION SYNDROMES

Preexcitation syndromes are characterized by activation of a portion of the ventricles by cardiac impulses that travel from the atria via accessory (anomalous) atrioventricular conduction pathways.[32] These accessory pathways are thought to result from a developmental failure to eradicate remnants of atrioventricular connections present during cardiogenesis. The three accessory pathways responsible for preexcitation syndromes have been designated as the Kent fibers, James fibers, and Mahaim fibers (Table 4-5; Fig. 4-5).[32] The most common

TABLE 4-5. Electrocardiographic Abnormalities Associated with Preexcitation Syndromes

Kent fibers or accessory atrioventricular pathway (Wolff-Parkinson-White syndrome)
  Short P-R interval (<0.12 sec)
  Wide QRS complex (>0.12 sec)
  Delta wave

James fibers or intranodal bypass tract (Lown-Ganong-Levine syndrome)
  Short P-R interval (<0.12 sec)
  Normal QRS complex duration
  No delta wave

Mahaim fibers or nodoventricula, nodofascicular, or fasciculoventricular pathway
  Normal to slightly short P-R interval
  Wide QRS complex (>0.12 sec)
  Delta wave

type of accessory pathways leading to early (i.e., preexcitation) activation of the ventricles are Kent fibers; the other connections are rare and require sophisticated intracardiac stimulation techniques and recordings to be demonstrated. These preexcitation pathways bypass the atrioventricular node so that activation of the ventricles occurs earlier than it would if cardiac impulses reached the ventricles by the usual internodal pathways. For example, conduction of cardiac impulses through the atrioventricular node is normally delayed so that P-R intervals on the electrocardiogram are 0.12 second to 0.2 second. Electrocardiographic manifestations associated with preexcitation syndromes depend on the specific accessory pathway responsible for the early activation of the ventricle and the amount of ventricular muscle activated by accessory pathways (Table 4-5).[32] Furthermore, the pattern of preexcitation present on the electrocardiogram may be intermittent. Any factor that changes the balance of conduction between normal and accessory pathways can either augment or abolish the pattern seen on the electrocardiogram.

Cardiac dysrhythmias associated with preexcitation syndromes are most often paroxysmal supraventricular tachycardias and only occasionally atrial fibrillation or flutter. Supraventricular tachycardia is due to retrograde conduction (i.e., circus movement) of cardiac impulses over accessory pathways. A prema-

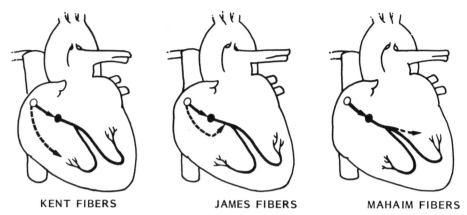

KENT FIBERS   JAMES FIBERS   MAHAIM FIBERS

FIG. 4-5. Schematic diagram of the three most common accessory atrioventricular conduction pathways associated with preexcitation syndromes. Kent fibers typically bridge the atrium and ventricle without passing through the atrioventricular node. James fibers bypass the atrioventricular node and attach to the bundle of His. Mahaim fibers shunt cardiac impulses from the bundle of His or either bundle branch into the intraventricular septal myocardium. ○, sinoatrial node; ●, atrioventricular node.

ture beat exposing the different properties of the multiple atrioventricular connections is the usual initiating mechanism. Occasional atrial fibrillation or flutter is most likely due to antegrade conduction of cardiac impulses over accessory pathways. Usually these cardiac dysrhythmias are sporadic and well tolerated, as affected patients are typically young and coronary artery disease is absent; but serious ventricular dysrhythmias can result. Indeed, presence of accessory pathways with short antegrade refractory periods may lead to life-threatening ventricular response rates if atrial fibrillation occurs. Examples of preexcitation syndromes include the Wolff-Parkinson-White syndrome, Lown-Ganong-Levine syndrome, and abnormalities due to conduction via the Mahaim pathway.

Wolff-Parkinson-White Syndrome

The Wolff-Parkinson-White syndrome is the most frequent of the preexcitation syndromes, with an incidence that may approach 0.3 percent of the general population.[32] The

incidence may be even higher in first-degree relatives of patients with this syndrome.[33] In this syndrome, cardiac impulses from the sinoatrial node travel simultaneously down normal conduction pathways and the accessory Kent fibers (Fig. 4-5). Lack of a physiologic delay in the transmission of cardiac impulses along the Kent fibers results in characteristic short P-R intervals on the electrocardiogram. Wide QRS complexes and delta waves reflect the fact that ventricular excitation is a composite of cardiac impulses conducted by normal and accessory pathways. For example, delta waves are the initial components of the QRS complexes caused by early activation of the ventricle by cardiac impulses traveling via accessory pathways. Paroxysmal atrial tachycardia (120 beats·min^{-1} to 140 beats·min^{-1}) is the most frequent cardiac dysrhythmia associated with this syndrome. The onset of this dysrhythmia is most likely due to a reentry mechanism. In extreme cases, syncope and/or congestive heart failure result from rapid heart rates.

TREATMENT

Initial treatment of supraventricular tachycardia in patients with preexcitation syndromes characterized as Wolff-Parkinson-

TABLE 4-6. Treatment of Supraventricular Tachycardia in Patients with Preexcitation Syndromes

Vagal Stimulation	Intravenous Drug Administration	Electrical Pacing	Cardioversion
Valsalva maneuver	Verapamil 0.05 to 0.15 mg·kg^{-1}		
Gag reflex	Diltiazem 0.25 mg·kg^{-1}		
Immersion of face in cold water (diving reflex)	Propranolol 0.025 to 0.05 mg·kg^{-1}		
	Ajmaline 1 mg·kg^{-1}		
	Procainamide 10 mg·kg^{-1}		

White syndrome should consider the effectiveness of vagal maneuvers (Table 4-6).[32] These maneuvers must be performed promptly after the onset of supraventricular tachycardia, as any delay is likely to be associated with increasing sympathetic nervous system activity and decreased likelihood vagal stimulation will be successful. If vagal stimulation fails, the intravenous injection of drugs that abruptly prolong the refractory period of the atrioventricular node (verapamil, diltiazem, propranolol) or that lengthen the refractory period of accessory pathways (ajmaline, procainamide) should be administered to interrupt supraventricular tachycardia (Table 4-6).[32,34] Electrical pacing or cardioversion is rarely required to interrupt supraventricular tachycardia in these patients. To prevent supraventricular tachycardia, drugs such as amiodarone, ecainide or sotalol are often effective.[32] These drugs depress conduction of cardiac impulses and increase the relative refractory period in both the atrioventricular node and accessory pathways. Quinidine and procainamide are also acceptable considerations. The most effective drug for prophylaxis in individual patients may be based on trial and error responses in each patient.

Initial treatment of atrial fibrillation in patients with preexcitation syndromes characterized as Wolff-Parkinson-White syndrome is influenced by the ventricular response rate and hemodynamic consequences of the cardiac dysrhythmia (Table 4-7).[32] Cardioversion is necessary if a rapid ventricular rhythm during atrial fibrillation leads to life-threatening hypotension. If atrial fibrillation is tolerated, drugs that prolong the refractory period of accessory pathways (procainamide, ajmaline, disopyramide) should be administered. Digitalis and verapamil may decrease the refractory period of accessory pathways responsible for atrial fibrillation resulting in an increase in ventricular response during this dysrhythmia.[32,34] Likewise, increased sympathetic nervous system activity after the onset of atrial fibrillation tends to decrease the refractory period of accessory pathways. Prophylaxis against occurrence of paroxysmal atrial fibrillation in these patients is with drugs that lengthen the refractory period of accessory pathways (amiodarone, quinidine) often combined with beta-adrenergic antagonists.[32]

In patients resistant to medical management, surgical transection of accessory pathways may be attempted.[32] Surgical treatment includes division of accessory pathways by an endocardial approach using cardiopulmonary bypass or, alternatively, an epicardial (external) closed heart approach for division and/or cryoablation of accessory pathways. The external approach avoids the need for atriotomy, cardiopulmonary bypass, and induced cardiac arrest. Because this approach does not require opening the heart, atrioventricular conduction can be monitored continuously, thus reducing the likelihood of unrecognized heart block during transection of the accessory pathways. Intracardiac recordings during electrically induced supraventricular tachycardia at the time of surgery, as well as epicardial mapping, have shown the most common accessory pathways are those connecting the left atrium with the left ventricle.[32]

TABLE 4-7. Treatment of Atrial Fibrillation in Patients with Preexcitation Syndromes

Cardioversion
Procainamide 10 mg·kg^{-1}
Ajmaline 1 mg·kg^{-1}
Disopyramide 5 to 10 mg·kg^{-1} orally

MANAGEMENT OF ANESTHESIA

The goal during management of anesthesia in patients with preexcitation syndromes characterized as Wolff-Parkinson-White syndrome is to avoid events that would alter the balance of conduction of cardiac impulses through the normal and accessory pathways and thus predispose the patient to the development of acute tachydysrhythmias.[35,36] Specifically, events predictably associated with increased sympathetic nervous system activity should be avoided. All antidysrhythmic drugs should be continued through the perioperative period. Logic would suggest avoidance of drugs in the preoperative medication that are known to increase heart rate. Although atropine has been used in preoperative medication without adverse heart rate responses,[36] scopolamine or glycopyrrolate would seem to be more logical choices if administration of anticholinergic drugs is deemed necessary. Reduction of anxiety with preoperative medication is desirable, but no specific drug has proven superior.

Induction of anesthesia can be safely accomplished with intravenous administration of barbiturates, benzodiazepines, or etomidate. Thiopental has been said to increase aberrant conduction of cardiac impulses, but this has not been substantiated by clinical use of the drug.[36] Sympathomimetic stimulating effects of ketamine would detract from its use in patients with this syndrome. Intubation of the trachea and maintenance of anesthesia should be accomplished with drugs selected to minimize the likelihood of increased activity of the sympathetic nervous system, as may occur in response to direct laryngoscopy or surgical stimulation. Nitrous oxide combined with volatile anesthetics has been successfully used for maintenance of anesthesia in these patients.[36] Theoretically, halothane, which slows conduction of cardiac impulses through the atrioventricular node and His-Purkinje system, would be more likely to be associated with cardiac dysrhythmias due to reentry mechanisms than enflurane, which slows conduction only through the atrioventricular node.[2,3] These drug effects on normal conduction pathways, however, do not mean that similar effects occur on accessory pathways. In this regard, thiopental, diazepam, and fentanyl have been

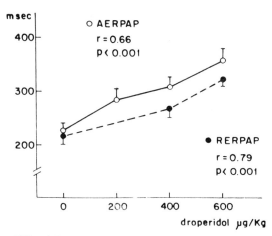

FIG. 4-6. Droperidol produces dose-dependent prolongation of the antegrade and retrograde effective refractory period of accessory pathways. (Gomez-Arnau J, Marquez-Montes J, Avello F. Fentanyl and droperidol effects on the refractoriness of the accessory pathway in the Wolff-Parkinson-White syndrome. Anesthesiology 1983;58:307–13.)

shown to lack effects on conduction of cardiac impulses over accessory pathways in these patients. Concentrations of volatile anesthetics sufficient to prevent sympathetic nervous system responses produced by intense stimulation are recommended.

It would seem logical to establish an adequate depth of anesthesia with volatile drugs and/or opioids before attempting intubation of the trachea. Large doses of droperidol (200 $\mu g \cdot kg^{-1}$ to 600 $\mu g \cdot kg^{-1}$) increase the antegrade and retrograde effective refractory period of accessory pathways, which would reduce the likelihood of tachydysrhythmias in these patients (Fig. 4-6).[37] Nondepolarizing muscle relaxants with minimal effects on heart rate and blood pressure are useful to provide skeletal muscle relaxation for intubation of the trachea and, if necessary, during surgery. Pancuronium should probably be avoided, as it can increase the speed of conduction of cardiac impulses through the atrioventricular node (Fig. 4-2).[5] Nevertheless, this effect of pancuronium has not been demonstrated to occur on conduction of cardiac impulses via accessory pathways in these patients. Neostigmine, as used for reversal of nondepolarizing neuromuscular blockade, has been alleged to predispose to cardiac dysrhythmias in these patients,[38] but this has not been substantiated by subsequent clinical experience.[36] Abrupt onset of hemodynamically significant tachydysrhythmias in the perioperative period is effectively treated by electrical cardioversion.

An increasing number of patients with Wolff-Parkinson-White syndrome are being treated with surgical transection of the accessory pathways identified by intraoperative endocardial mapping. Although experience is limited, it would seem logical to avoid drugs during the intraoperative period that could alter conduction of cardiac impulses over accessory pathways. Induction and maintenance of anesthesia with benzodiazepines and opioids plus muscle relaxants with minimal circulatory effects would seem logical. Avoidance of administration of antidysrhythmic or sympathomimetic drugs that might have residual effects on accessory pathways and their identification by endocardial mapping seems prudent but cannot be supported by specific data. Electrical cardioversion and artificial cardiac pacing are useful in treating hemodynamically significant tachydysrhythmias that may occur during identification of the accessory pathways.

Lown-Ganong-Levine Syndrome

The Lown-Ganong-Levine syndrome is due to accessory conduction pathways designated as the James fibers. These fibers bypass the atrioventricular node and insert directly into the bundle of His (Fig. 4-5). As a result, the normal physiologic delay in conduction of cardiac impulses at the atrioventricular node is lost. This syndrome is characterized on the electrocardiogram by short P-R intervals and normal appearing QRS complexes, without associated delta waves. Atrial flutter-fibrillation is the cardiac dysrhythmia most frequently associated with this syndrome. Treatment and management of anesthesia is the same as detailed for patients with the Wolff-Parkinson-White syndrome.

Mahaim Pathway

This variant of the preexcitation syndrome is characterized by normal to slightly short P-R intervals, wide QRS complexes, and delta waves on the electrocardiogram. This syndrome results from accessory conduction pathways known as Mahaim fibers, which arise below the atrioventricular node and insert directly into ventricular muscle (Fig. 4-5). Treatment and management of anesthesia is the same as detailed for patients with the Wolff-Parkinson-White syndrome.

PROLONGED Q-T INTERVAL SYNDROMES

Prolonged Q-T interval syndromes are rare inherited abnormalities with important implications for management of anesthesia.[39,40] The diagnostic feature is prolonged Q-T intervals (greater than 0.44 second) on the electrocardiogram even when corrected for heart rate. It is important to rule out bundle branch block (i.e., wide QRS complexes) as a cause of prolonged Q-T intervals. Prolonged Q-T intervals on the electrocardiogram in the presence of congenital neural deafness are designated as Jervell–Lange-Nielsen syndrome. An estimated 0.25 percent to 1 percent of patients with congenital deafness have prolonged Q-T intervals on the electrocardiogram. Prolonged Q-T intervals on the electrocardiogram in the absence of congenital deafness are designated as Romano-Ward syndrome. Right radical neck dissections may result in increases in the Q-T intervals and cardiac dysrhythmias in the postoperative period (Fig. 4-7).[41] Similar changes do not follow left radical neck dissections (Fig. 4-7).[41] The most common type of acquired prolonged Q-T interval syndromes are due to antidysrhythmic drugs including quinidine and disopyramide. In this regard, previously undiagnosed patients may be at increased risk should they be treated with certain antidysrhythmic drugs. Phenothiazines, lithium, tricyclic antidepressants, direutic-induced hy-

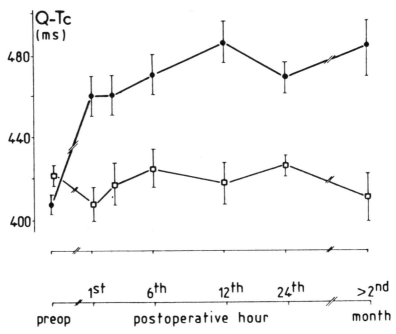

FIG. 4-7. Corrected Q-T intervals (Q-T$_c$) in milliseconds (ms) were prolonged after right radical neck dissections (solid symbols) but not after left radical neck dissections (clear symbols). Mean ± SE (Otteni JC, Pottecher T, Bronner G, Flesch H, Diebolt JR. Prolongation of the Q-T interval and sudden cardiac arrest following right radical neck dissection. Anesthesiology 1983;59:358–61.)

pokalemia, and hypocalcemia may also prolong Q-T intervals on the electrocardiogram. Avoidance of electrolyte disturbances in the postoperative period after right radical neck dissections becomes particularly important should surgically induced prolongation of Q-T intervals on the electrocardiogram appear.

Syncope associated with inherited prolonged Q-T interval syndromes manifest in infancy or early childhood and may be confused with seizure disorders if an electrocardiogram is not obtained. Syncopal attacks are often triggered by sympathetic nervous system stimulation as produced by exercise or fright. Indeed, prolonged Q-T intervals on the electrocardiogram may be present only after exercise or only intermittently. Syncope and occasional sudden death in these patients is presumed to be due to ventricular cardiac dysrhythmias. A preoperative electrocardiogram to rule out prolonged Q-T interval syndromes is useful in children with congenital deafness or family histories of sudden death, as the physical examination is likely to be otherwise

unremarkable. Likewise, members of the family of afflicted individuals should be evaluated with electrocardiograms.

Delayed repolarization of the ventricles as reflected by prolonged Q-T intervals on the electrocardiogram increases susceptibility of the heart to dysrhythmias. The most accepted mechanism for Q-T interval syndromes is a congenital asymmetrical sympathetic innervation of the heart due to increases in left cardiac sympathetic nerve activity or decreases in right cardiac sympathetic nerve activity. A second hypothesis is that the primary abnormality is an inherited defect in the mechanism necessary for outward movement of potassium during phase 3 of the cardiac action potential.

Treatment

Treatment of prolonged Q-T interval syndromes is empiric and directed at pharmacologic and surgical attempts to reduce cardiac sympathetic nervous system activity. In this regard, initial treatment is often drug-induced, beta-adrenergic blockade. Indeed, mortality in untreated patients decreases from over 70 percent to less than 10 percent in treated patients. Beta-adrenergic antagonist drugs shorten Q-T intervals in affected patients, reduce sympathetic nervous system activity, and increase the threshold for ventricular fibrillation. In unresponsive patients, other drugs including phenytoin, primidone, verapamil, or bretylium may be substituted. If there is no response to medical therapy, a left stellate ganglion block may be considered to abolish temporarily the sympathetic nervous system imbalance that exists between left and right cardiac nerves. A successful block is best indicated by shortening of the Q-T intervals on the electrocardiogram. The effect of a left stellate ganglion block is only transient; therefore, it is used only to control acute cardiac dysrhythmias, to assess whether surgical ganglionectomy will be successful, and as preoperative preparation of patients not on medical treatment requiring emergency surgery. Indeed, patients not diagnosed and treated preoperatively tend to develop life-threatening cardiac dysrhythias during anesthesia. An artificial cardiac pacemaker may be necessary in occasional patients who develop symptomatic bradycardia due to treatment with beta-adrenergic antagonist drugs.

Management of Anesthesia

Management of anesthesia in patients with prolonged Q-T interval syndromes is based on prior production of beta-adrenergic blockade or performance of prophylactic left stellate ganglion block. Events known to prolong Q-T intervals, such as abrupt increases in sympathetic nervous system activity associated with preoperative anxiety or with noxious stimulation than can occur intraoperatively and acute hypokalemia due to iatrogenic hyperventilation of the lungs, must be minimized. In this regard, it seems logical to provide pharmacologic preoperative medication to reduce anxiety. Inclusion of anticholinergic drugs in the preoperative medication is questionable in view of the possible alteration in the balance of sympathetic and parasympathetic nervous system activity that can accompany administration of these drugs. Reductions in plasma concentrations of calcium, potassium, or magnesium are also undesirable, as these electrolyte alterations can prolong Q-T intervals.

Induction of anesthesia has been safely accomplished with thiopental despite the ability of this drug to prolong Q-T intervals of normal patients. Ketamine is not selected because of its sympathetic nervous system-stimulating effects. Intubation of the trachea should be considered only after establishment of a depth of anesthesia with volatile anesthetics considered sufficient to minimize effects of noxious stimulation. The choice of volatile drugs should be designed to provide suppression of sympathetic nervous system responses to painful stimulation, as well as avoidance of sensitization of the heart to the arrhythmogenic effects of catecholamines. In this regard, isoflurane or enflurane with or without nitrous oxide are acceptable.[39,42] Because of its association with cardiac dysrhythmias in the presence of increased plasma concentrations of catecholamines halothane is a less attractive selection. Opioids are acceptable but often must be supplemented with volatile anesthetics to blunt sympathetic nervous system responses to painful stimulation. Extubation of the trachea may be considered while patients are still adequately anesthetized to minimize sympathetic nervous system stimulation associated with this event.

Choice of muscle relaxants is guided by avoidance of drugs that could stimulate directly or indirectly the sympathetic nervous system. For example, succinylcholine prolongs Q-T intervals of normal patients and has been associated with ventricular fibrillation in these patients.[42] Conversely, succinylcholine has been administered to these patients without incident. Likewise, pancuronium has been used to provide muscle relaxation without incident despite its sympathomimetic activity. Vecuronium or atracurium would be acceptable drugs to facilitate intubation of the trachea or to provide intraoperative skeletal muscle relaxation.[42] Pharmacologic reversal of nondepolarizing neuromuscular blockade does not seem to alter adversely Q-T intervals in these patients.

An electrical defibrillator should be immediately available, as the likelihood of perioperative ventricular fibrillation is increased. Propranolol is often chosen for treatment of acute ventricular dysrhythmias that develop intraoperatively. Lidocaine, procainamide, and quinidine are not recommended for management of acute cardiac dysrhythmias, as these drugs can prolong Q-T intervals on the electrocardiogram.[41] Nevertheless, lidocaine has been reported to be effective in reversing intraoperative ventricular tachycardia in a patient with this syndrome. The ability of phenytoin to shorten Q-T intervals on the electrocardiogram is the rationale for administering this drug orally in the postoperative period.

REFERENCES

1. Akhtar M. Management of ventricular tachyarrhythmias. JAMA 1982;247:671–4
2. Atlee JL, Rusy BF. Halothane depression of A-V conduction studied by electrograms of the bundle of His in dogs. Anesthesiology 1972;36:112–8
3. Atlee JL, Rusy BF. Atrioventricular conduction times and atrioventricular nodal conductivity during enflurane anesthesia in dogs. Anesthesiology 1977;47:498–503
4. Johnston RR, Eger EI, Wilson C. A comparative interaction of epinephrine with enflurane, isoflurane, and halothane in man. Anesth Analg 1976;55:709–12
5. Geha DG, Rozelle BC, Raessler KL, et al. Pancuronium bromide enhances atrioventricular conduction in halothane-anesthetized dogs. Anesthesiology 1977;46:342–5
6. Miller RD, Way WL, Katzung BG. The potentiation of neuromuscular blocking agents by quinidine. Anesthesiology 1967;28:1036–41
7. Harrah MD, Way WL, Katzung BG. The interaction of d-tubocurarine with antiarrhythmic drugs. Anesthesiology 1970;33:406–10
8. Healy TEJ, O'Shea MD, Massey J. Disopyramide and neuromuscular transmission. Br J Anaesth 1981;53:495–8
9. Liberman BA, Teasdale SJ. Anaesthesia and amiodarone. Can Anaesth Soc J 1985;32:629–38
10. Wu D. Supraventricular tachycardias. JAMA 1983;249:3357–60
11. Chew CYC, Hecht HS, Collett JT, McAllister RG, Singh BN. Influence of severity of ventricular dysfunction on hemodynamic responses to intravenously administered verapamil in ischemic heart disease. Am J Cardiol 1981;47:917–22
12. Schulte-Sasse U, Hess W, Markschies-Harnung A, Tarnow J. Combined effects of halothane anesthesia and verapamil on systemic hemodynamics and left ventricular myocardial contractility in patients with ischemic heart disease. Anesth Analg 1984;63:791–8
13. Durant NN, Nguyen N, Katz R. Potentiation of neuromuscular blockade by verapamil. Anesthesiology 1984;60:298–303
14. Lawson NW, Kraynack BJ, Gintautas J. Neuromuscular and electrocardiographic responses to verapamil in dogs. Anesth Analg 1983;62:50–4
15. Chung DC. Anaesthetic problems associated with the treatment of cardiovascular disease. I. Digitalis toxicity. Can Anaesth Soc J 1981;28:6–16
16. Phibbs B, Friedman HS, Graboys TB, et al. Indications for pacing in the treatment of bradyarrhythmias. Report of an independent study group. JAMA 1984;252:1307–11
17. Mulcahy R, Hickey N, Mauser B. An etiology of bundle branch block. Br Heart J 1968;30:34–7
18. Thomson IR, Dalton BC, Lappas DG, Lowenstein E. Right bundle-branch block and complete heart block caused by the Swan-Ganz catheter. Anesthesiology 1979;51:359–62
19. Rorie DK, Muldoon SM, Krabill DR. Transient bundle branch block occurring during anesthesia. Anesth Analg 1972;51:633–7
20. Pratila M, Pratilas V, Dimich I. Transient left-bundle branch block during anesthesia. Anesthesiology 1979;51:461–3
21. Edelman JD, Hurlbert BJ. Intermittent left bundle branch block during anesthesia. Anesth Analg 1981;59:628–30
22. Rooney S-M, Goldiner PL, Muss E. Relationship of right bundle-branch block and marked left axis deviation to complete heart block during general anesthesia. Anesthesiology 1976;44:64–6
23. Venkataraman K, Madias JE, Hood WB. Indications for prophylactic preoperative insertion of pacemaker in patients with right bundle branch block and left anterior hemiblock. Chest 1975;68:501–6
24. Coriat P, Harari A, Ducardonet A, et al. Risk of advanced heart block during extradural anaesthesia in patients with right bundle branch block and left anterior hemiblock. Br J Anaesth 1981;53:545–8
25. Bellocci F, Santarelli P, Di-Gennaro M, et al. The risk of cardiac complications in surgical patients with bifascicular block: A clinical and electrophysiologic study in 98 patients. Chest 1980;77:343–8

26. Davies M, Harris A. Pathological basis of primary heart block. Br Heart J 1966;31:219–26
27. Lev M. Anatomic basis for atrioventricular block. Am J Med 1964;37:742–8
28. Jones RM, Broadbent MP, Adams AP. Anaesthetic considerations in patients with paroxysmal supraventricular tachycardia. A review and report of cases. Anaesthesia 1984;39:307–13
29. Sprague DH, Mandel SD. Paroxysmal supraventricular tachycardia during anesthesia. Anesthesiology 1977;46:75–7
30. Kleiger R, Lown B. Cardioversion and digitalis. II. Clinical studies. Circulation 1966;33:878–87
31. Chee TP, Prakash NS, Desser KB, Benchimil A. Postoperative supraventricular arrhythmias and the role of prophylactic digoxin in cardiac surgery. Am Heart J 1982;104:941–7
32. Wellens HJJ, Brugada P, Penn OC. The management of preexcitation syndromes. JAMA 1987;257:2325–33
33. Vidaillet HJ, Pressley JC, Henke E, Harrell FE, German LD. Familial occurrence of accessory atrioventricular pathways (preexcitation syndrome). N Engl J Med 1987;317:65–9
34. Prystowsky EN. Pharmacologic therapy of tachyarrhythmias in patients with Wolff-Parkinson-White syndrome. Herz 1983;8:133–43
35. vanderStarre PJA. Wolff-Parkinson-White syndrome during anesthesia. Anesthesiology 1978;48:369–72
36. Sadowski AR, Moyers JR. Anesthetic management of the Wolff-Parkinson-White syndrome. Anesthesiology 1979;51:553–6
37. Gomez-Arnau J, Marques-Montes J, Avello F. Fentanyl and droperidol effects on the refractoriness of the accessory pathway in the Wolff-Parkinson-White syndrome. Anesthesiology 1983;58:307–13
38. Hannington-Kiff JG. The Wolff-Parkinson-White syndrome and general anesthesia. Br J Anaesth 1968;40:791–5
39. Galloway PA, Glass PSA. Anesthetic implications of prolonged QT interval syndromes. Anesth Analg 1985;64:612–20
40. Moss AJ. Prolonged QT interval syndromes. JAMA 1986;256:2985–8
41. Otteni JC, Pottecher T, Bronner G, Flesch H, Diebold JR. Prolongation of the Q-T interval and sudden cardiac arrest following right radical neck dissection. Anesthesiology 1983;59:358–61
42. Wilton NCT, Hantler CB. Congenital long QT syndrome: Changes in QT interval during anesthesia with thiopental, vecuronium, fentanyl and isoflurane. Anesth Analg 1987;66:357–60

5

Artificial Cardiac Pacemakers

Each year in the United States about 100,000 new patients receive permanent artificial cardiac pacemakers[1]. When this number is added to the existing 500,000 previously implanted cardiac pacemakers, it is apparent that perioperative management of these patients may be a frequent consideration. About one-half of these patients are over 70 years of age. An additional problem is that an increasing number of different types of pacemakers requires a frequent updating of knowledge in this area.

The physiologic basis for the effectiveness of artificial cardiac pacemakers is the fact that the myocardium will contract when stimulated by an electrical current. Although considerable controversy exists as to the specific indications for implantation of artificial cardiac pacemakers, a clinical history of bradycardia associated with syncope or congestive heart failure should suggest that such indications are needed. Appearance of changes in conduction of cardiac impulses (bundle branch block, Mobitz type II block) in association with acute myocardial infarctions may be an indication for temporary artificial cardiac pacing. If third-degree atrioventricular heart block is caused by overdoses of drugs, use of temporary transvenous pacemakers may be all that is required. Likewise, temporary artificial cardiac pacing will be required when transient third-degree atrioventricular heart block follows cardiopulmonary bypass. Bifascicular heart block or sick sinus syndrome are not indications for pro-

phylactic insertion of artificial cardiac pacemakers (see Chapter 4). Asymptomatic patients with congenital third-degree atrioventricular heart block do not require artificial cardiac pacing, as the lack of symptoms confirms the underlying heart rate is responsive to changing physiologic needs. A pulmonary artery catheter with a pacing electrode may be used if simultaneous pressure monitoring and pacing capabilities are required. Patient movement, however, may result in sufficient changes in catheter position to lose pacing.

TYPES OF ARTIFICIAL CARDIAC PACEMAKERS

Once the need for an artificial cardiac pacemaker has been established, the selection of the pacemaker system is based on (1) the specific indication for the pacemaker, (2) the emergent nature of the procedure, and (3) the life expectancy of the patients. Pacemakers can be inserted intravenously (endocardial lead) or by the subcostal approach (epicardial or myocardial leads). All pacemakers consist of two components designated as the pulse generator and pacing electrode leads (Table 5-1).[2] Electrical impulses are formed in the pulse generator and transmitted to the endocardial or myocardial surface of the heart resulting in mechanical contractions. The pulse generator is a

TABLE 5-1. Definition of Terms Used in Describing Artificial Cardiac Pacemakers

Term	Definition
Pulse generator	Consists of the energy source (battery) and electrical circuits necessary for pacing and sensing functions
Implanted or external	Anatomic placement of the pulse generator relative to the skin
Lead	Insulated wire connecting the pulse generator with the electrode
Electrode	Exposed metal end of electrode in contact with endocardium or epicardium (myocardium)
Endocardial pacing	Right atrium or right ventricle are stimulated by contact of electrode with the endocardium following transvenous insertion of the lead
Epicardial pacing	Right atrium or right ventricle are stimulated by insertion of electrode through the epicardium into the myocardium under direct vision
Unipolar pacing	Describes placement of the negative (stimulating) electrode in the atrium or ventricle and the positive (ground) electrode distant from the heart (metallic portion of the pulse generator or subcutaneous tissue)
Bipolar pacing	Describes placement of the negative and positive electrodes in the cardiac chamber being paced as characteristic of temporary ventricular pacing
Stimulation threshold	Minimal amount of current (amperes) or voltage (volts) necessary to cause contraction of the chamber that is being paced
Resistance	Measure of the combined resistance of the electrode-lead-myocardial interface as calculated using Ohm's law with values for current and voltage thresholds. Normal value is 350 ohms to 1,000 ohms.
R-wave sensitivity	Minimal voltage of intrinsic R-wave necessary to activate the sensing circuit of the pulse generator and thus inhibit or trigger the pacing circuit. An R-wave sensitivity of about 3 mV on an external pulse generator will maintain ventricle-inhibited pacing.
Hysteresis	Difference between intrinsic heart rate at which pacing begins (about 60 beats·min^{-1}) and pacing rate (72 beats·min^{-1})

hermetically sealed metal can weighing 30 g to 130 g most often powered by a lithium battery. Modern pulse generators are noninvasively (transcutaneously) programmable for multiple functions (Table 5-2).[1] A five letter generic code has simplified the identification and description of types of pacemaker function (Table 5-3).[1,2] Several different types of pulse generators are available (Table 5-4) (Fig. 5-1).[1,2]

Ventricular Asynchronous (Fixed Rate) Pulse Generators

Ventricular asynchronous pulse generators (VOO) deliver electrical impulses to the cardiac ventricle at regular and preset intervals (usually an effective heart rate of 70 beats·min^{-1} to 72 beats·min^{-1}) that is independent of the patient's intrinsic heart rate (Fig. 5-1).[1] Therefore, these electrical impulses can occur in random fashion relative to the intrinsic cardiac rhythm of the patient. An artificially produced contraction of the ventricle occurs when the impulse from the pulse generator is of sufficient energy and does not occur during the refractory period of the ventricle. This type of pulse generator finds its greatest usefulness in the management of bradycardia due to sudden onset of third-degree atrioventricular heart block. Permanent VOO pulse generators are rarely, if ever, used.[2]

Advantages of VOO pulse generators are their simplicity and reliability. Problems associated with their use include (1) energy wastage as the generator continues to emit impulses even when the patient has a physiologic

TABLE 5-2. Programmable Functions of Cardiac Pacemaker Generators

Discharge rate

Electrical output delivered to myocardium

Refractory period

R-wave sensitivity

Hysteresis

Mode of generator function (designed by first three letters of generic code; see Tables 5-3 and 5-4)

Lower rate limit

Upper rate limit

Atrioventricular delay (P-R interval)

heart rate, and (2) competition with the patient's instrinsic conduction system for control of ventricular activation. For example, pacemaker-induced ventricular tachycardia or fibrillation could occur if the myocardium sur-

rounding a pacing electrode is repolarizing (R on T phenomenon) just when an impulse from the pulse generator arrives. In reality, this rarely occurs since relatively low energy levels are required for capture of the ventricle as compared to the ventricular fibrillation threshold. In fact, the minimum energy capable of causing ventricular fibrillation during the vulnerable period is about 100 times greater than the maximum output of the pulse generator.[3] Therefore, the risk of iatrogenic ventricular fibrillation is minimal.

Atrial Asynchronous (Fixed-Rate) Pulse Generators

Atrial asynchronous pulse generators (AOO) are identical to VOO pulse generators except that the stimulating lead is placed on

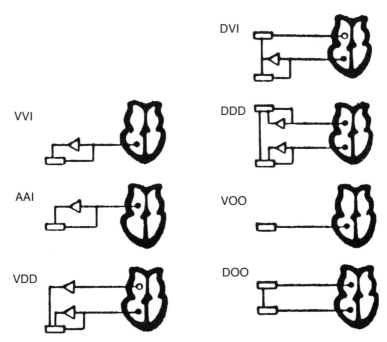

FIG. 5.1 Basic circuitry design of various pacing modes. See Table 5-4 for definition of three-letter identification code. □, output oscillator; ◁, sensing amplifer. (Ludmer PL, Goldschlager N. Cardiac pacing in the 1980's. N Engl J Med 1986;311:1671–80.)

TABLE 5-3. Generic Code for Identification and Description of Pacemaker Function

First Letter	Second Letter	Third Letter	Fourth Letter	Fifth Letter
Cardiac chamber paced	Cardiac chamber in which electrical activity is sensed	Response of generator to sensed R-waves and P-waves	Programmable functions of the generator	Antitachycardia functions of the generator
V-Ventricle	V-Ventricle	T-Triggered	P-Programmable (rate and/or output only)	B-Bursts
A-Atrium	A-Atrium	I-Inhibited	M-Multiprogrammable (see Table 5-2)	N-Normal rate competition*
D-Dual (atrium and ventricle)	D-Dual	D-Dual	C-Communicating†	S-Scanning
	0-None (Asynchronous)	0-None (Asynchronous)	0-None (fixed function)	E-External

* Stimuli delivered at normal rates upon sensing of tachycardia (underdrive pacing).
† Capability of being noninvasively interrogated.

TABLE 5-4. Types of Artificial Cardiac Pulse Generators

Letter Number*			Description
I	II	III	
A	O	O	Asynchronous (fixed rate) atrial pacing
V	O	O	Asynchronous (fixed rate) ventricular pacing
A	A	I	Noncompetitive (demand) atrial pacing, electrical output inhibited by intrinsic atrial depolarizations (P-waves)
V	V	I	Noncompetitive (demand) ventricular pacing, electrical output inhibited by intrinsic ventricular depolarizations (R-waves)
A	A	T	Triggered atrial pacing, electrical output triggered by intrinsic atrial depolarizations (P-waves)
V	V	T	Triggered ventricular pacing, electrical output triggered by intrinsic ventricular depolarizations (R-waves)
D	V	I	Paces (sequential) in atrium and ventricle, does not sense P-waves, does sense R-waves
D	D	D	Paces and senses in atrium and ventricle
V	D	D	Paces in ventricle, senses in atrium and ventricle, synchronized with atrial activity and paces ventricle after a present atrioventricular interval preset

* See Table 5-3 for definition of letter numbers.

the right atrium (Fig. 5-1).[1] An AOO pulse generator is of no value if atrioventricular heart block is present. These pulse generators are of greatest value when bradycardia is present and conduction of cardiac impulses through the atrioventricular node is normal.

Ventricular Noncompetitive (Demand or Synchronous) Pulse Generators

Ventricular noncompetitive pulse generators are designed (synchronized) to deliver electrical stimuli to the ventricle only when spontaneous cardiac impulses do not occur in a preselected time interval (Fig. 5-1).[1] As a result, competition between the patient's intrinsic cardiac rhythm and electrical impulses from the pulse generator cannot occur, thus eliminating the potential for iatrogenic ventricular fibrillation.[1,2] Furthermore, in contrast to asynchronous pulse generators, these artificial cardiac pacemakers are energy sparing. Ventricular noncompetitive pulse generators are indicated in patients with (1) chronic atrial flutter and fibrillation with persistent or episodic atrioventricular heart block and (2) atrial standstill or bradycardia in the absence of a need for the hemodynamic benefit of atrial systole.

Electromagnetic waves may be interpreted as spontaneous cardiac activity leading to suppression of ventricular noncompetitive pulse generators (see the section, Electrocautery). These pulse generators can be converted to the ventricular asynchronous mode by application of an external converter magnet, which closes a switch, thus inactivating the sensing mechanism. Asynchronous pacing permits preoperative assessment of the pacing (capture) function of a pulse generator, which is inhibited by a faster intrinsic heart rate. The magnet rate may be the same as or different from the programmed automatic rate and will decrease as an indication of battery power depletion.

Ventricular noncompetitive pulse generators are categorized as ventricular inhibited (VVI) or ventricular triggered (VVT), depending on the response of the pulse generator to intrinsic cardiac depolarizations (i.e., R-waves) (Table 5-3).[1,2]

VENTRICULAR-INHIBITED

Activity of VVI pulse generators is inhibited when the patient's intrinsic heart rate (R-wave frequency) remains above the preset rate of the pulse generator. When the patient's heart rate declines below the preset rate, the absence of R-waves results in activation of the pulse generator. VVI pulse generators are the most common type of permanently implanted pacemakers.

VENTRICULAR-TRIGGERED

VVT pulse generators sense every intrinsic depolarization of the heart, thus firing an electrical impulse during the absolute refractory period. If normal electrical activity of the heart does not occur, this pulse generator is designed to deliver an electrical impulse at a preset interval. This type of pulse generator is rarely used since it is energy wasting, being triggered by every intrinsic R-wave.

Atrial Noncompetitive (Demand or Synchronous) Pulse Generators

Atrial noncompetitive pulse generators resemble ventricular noncompetitive pulse generators, except that the electrical signal is delivered to the atrium rather than to the ventricle (Fig. 5-1).[1] These atrial pulse generators may be atrial inhibited (AAI) or atrial triggered (AAT), depending on the response of the pulse generator to intrinsic atrial depolarizations (P-waves) (Table 5-3).[1,2] The atrium is paced and the ventricle is depolarized by conduction of the paced atrial impulse through the atrioventricular node and His-Purkinje system. Atrial noncompetitive pacing is useful in patients with symptomatic sinus bradycardia in

the presence of normal conduction of cardiac impulses through the atrioventricular node.

Sequential Pulse Generators

Sequential pulse generators (DVI, DDD, VDD) are designed to preserve the atrioventricular contraction sequence (Table 5-3).[1,2] An atrial contribution to ventricular filling may result in a 20 percent to 30 percent increase in cardiac output for a given heart rate compared with ventricular pacing (see the section Hemodynamic Effects of Pacing). Electrodes for these pulse generators are present in the atrium and ventricle and the P-R interval is adjustable (Fig. 5-1).[1] An important advantage of these pulse generators is the ability to increase the ventricular rate in response to increases in the intrinsic rate of atrial depolarization such as those that accompany exercise and thus mimic the normal physiologic state.

VDD pulse generators have been largely replaced by DDD systems that have the VDD function incorporated in their design.[1] DDD pulse generators are the most sophisticated pacing systems available, as both atrial and ventricular circuits are capable of sensing and pacing their respective chambers (Table 5-3) (Fig. 5-1).[1] As a result, these pulse generators will pace atria on demand in patients with atrial bradycardia and intact atrioventricular conduction, will pace atria and ventricles sequentially in patients with atrial bradycardia and atrioventricular block, and will pace ventricles in response to intrinsic atrial activity. Most functions are programmable for each chamber individually (Table 5-1). Disadvantages of dual-chamber pulse generators compared with single-chamber pulse generators include shorter battery life spans, since more energy is required, and the potential for pacemaker-induced tachycardia due to retrograde ventriculoatrial conduction of cardiac impulses.[1] DDD multiprogrammable pulse generators may become the predominant type of pulse generators inserted when dual-chamber devices are selected.[1]

Antitachycardia Functions of Pulse Generators

Continuing evolution of pulse generators may allow insertion of devices that are patient activated to terminate reentrant tachydysrhythmias. Scanning pulse generators may possess a memory for termination of supraventricular tachycardias. Implantable defibrillators in pulse generators may provide a mechanism for termination of recurrent rapid ventricular tachycardia or ventricular fibrillation. Such implantable devices deliver 25 joules per defibrillation with enough stored energy for about 100 defibrillations.[2]

HEMODYNAMIC EFFECTS OF PACING

Optimal cardiac output depends on myocardial contractility, heart rate, and appropriate relationships between atrial and ventricular contractions. Artificial cardiac pacemaker-induced elevations in heart rate from bradycardia levels will increase cardiac output in the presence of normal myocardial contractility. In this regard, ventricular pacing may be life-saving in establishing a physiologic heart rate but may not always result in the highest cardiac output possible at that heart rate. This emphasizes the importance of atrial contractions, as well as the temporal relationships between atrial and ventricular contractions. In the presence of the normal conduction of cardiac impulses through the atrioventricular node, atrial pacing produces 20 percent to 30 percent increases in cardiac output compared with that produced by ventricular pacing.[2]

Atrioventricular sequential pacing is necessary to assure proper timing of atrial and ventricular contractions in the presence of atrioventricular heart block. Sequential pacing produces improvements in cardiac output as compared with ventricular pacing. The contribution of atrial contractions to ventricular filling is reduced when left ventricular end-diastolic pressures exceed 20 mmHg.[2] Often cardiac output measurements must be performed to establish optimal atrial pacing rates.

COMPONENTS OF ARTIFICIAL CARDIAC PACEMAKER PULSE GENERATORS

An understanding of artificial cardiac pacemaker pulse generators is particularly important when employing temporary external cardiac pacing as may be necessary immediately after cardiopulmonary bypass. A typical external pulse generator for ventricular pacing consists of (1) an off-on switch, (2) a setting for the energy output delivered in milliamperes to the ventricle, (3) an R-wave sensitivity setting in millivolts that controls the ease with which the pulse generator is inhibited by intrinsic R-waves, and (4) a setting for heart rate in beats·min^{-1}. Depending on the setting of the sensitivity dial, this becomes either a VOO (asynchronous) or VVI (demand) pulse generator. A typical external pulse generator (DDD or DVI) for atrioventricular sequential pacing consists of (1) an off-on switch, (2) separate settings for the energy output delivered in milliamperes to the atrium and ventricle, (3) a setting for the A-V interval in milliseconds, (4) an R-wave sensitivity setting in millivolts that controls the ease with which the pulse generator is inhibited by intrinsic R-waves, and (5) a setting for heart rate in beats·min^{-1}. The A-V interval is usually set initially at 150 ms. The typical heart rate setting for the external pulse generator in 70 beats·min^{-1} to 90 beats·min^{-1}. If a pulmonary artery catheter is in place, the optimum heart rate can be determined by measuring thermodilution cardiac outputs.

Internal pulse generators with properly placed electrodes typically have stimulation thresholds of 0.3 mA to 1 mA. Stimulation threshold will usually increase for several days after placement of artificial cardiac pacemakers. Therefore, stimulation thresholds are often set at about twice the initial capture thresholds. Permanent artificial cardiac pulse generators use mercury-zinc batteries, lithium batteries, or nuclear powered units. The expected longevity of the various power sources ranges from 4 years to 6 years for mercury-zinc batteries, 7 years to 10 years for lithium batteries, and 10 years to 20 years for nuclear units.

PREOPERATIVE EVALUATION OF PATIENTS WITH ARTIFICIAL CARDIAC PACEMAKERS

Preoperative evaluation of patients with artificial cardiac pacemakers includes determination of the reason for placing the pacemaker, type of generator and date the pulse generator was placed, and adequacy of present pacemaker function. A knowledge of the three to five letter code for the implanted pulse generator permits an understanding of how the pacemaker is supposed to work (Table 5-3).[1,2] A preoperative history of vertigo or syncope may reflect dysfunction of the artificial cardiac pacemaker. The rate of discharge of atrial or ventricular asynchronous pacemakers is the most important indicator of pulse generator function. A regular peripheral heart rate of 70 beats·min^{-1} to 72 beats·min^{-1} indicates that a VOO or uninhibited VVI generator is pacing the heart. A regular heart rate greater than 70 beats·min^{-1} to 72 beats·min^{-1} could mean that the patient has a functioning but inhibited VVI pacemaker. Alternatively, it could reflect a nonfunctioning VVI or VOO pacemaker. A 10 percent decrease in heart rate from the initial fixed discharge rate is a sign of battery failure. An irregular heart rate may reflect competition of a VOO pulse generator with the patient's intrinsic heart rate or a VVI pulse generator that is not sensing R-waves.

The electrocardiogram is evaluated in pacemaker patients to confirm one-to-one capture as evidenced by pacemaker spikes for every palpated peripheral pulse. This evaluation is not helpful in patients with VVI pulse generators and heart rates greater than the preset pacemaker rate. In these patients, Valsalva maneuvers may sufficiently lower intrinsic heart rate to permit confirmation of pacemaker function. Alternatively, proper function of ventricular synchronous and sequential car-

diac pacemakers can be confirmed by demonstrating appearance of captured beats on the electrocardiogram when the pacemaker is converted to the asynchronous mode by placement of an external converter magnet over the pulse generator. Attempts to slow heart rate in patients with angina pectoris or by massage of the carotid sinus that could dislodge atherosclerotic plaques are not recommended. Radiographs of the chest are useful to confirm the absence of breaks in pacemaker electrodes.

MANAGEMENT OF ANESTHESIA

Management of anesthesia in patients with artificial cardiac pacemakers includes monitoring to confirm continued function of pulse generators and ready availability of equipment and drugs to maintain an acceptable intrinsic heart rate if necessary (Table 5-5). If electrocautery interferes with the electrocardiogram, a finger on a peripheral pulse and/or auscultation through an esophageal stethoscope confirms continued cardiac activity. Insertion of pulmonary artery catheters will not disturb epicardial electrodes but might become entangled in or dislodge recently placed transvenous (endocardial) electrodes. Dislodgement of endocardial electrodes, however, has not been observed when these electrodes have been in place for greater than 4 weeks.[2] Choice of drugs used for anesthesia is not altered by the presence of functioning artificial cardiac pacemakers. Artificial cardiac pacemakers that are functioning normally preoperatively should continue to function intraoperatively without

TABLE 5-5. Adjuncts for Administration of Anesthesia to Patients with Artificial Cardiac Pacemakers

Continuous monitoring of the electrocardiogram

Continuous monitoring of a peripheral pulse

Electrical defibrillator

External converter magnet

Drugs—atropine, isoproterenol

incident. Nevertheless, intraoperative use of electrocautery or events that alter stimulation thresholds could result in pacemaker dysfunction.

Electrocautery

Electromagnetic interference from electrocautery may cause an electrical artifact that is sensed by VVI pulse generators as intrinsic R-waves. The pulse generator will be inhibited if the artifact that is sensed exceeds the R-wave sensitivity of the pulse generator. Most VVI pulse generators can be inhibited for one impulse during reversion to VOO pacing.[2] Therefore, multiple artifacts produced by repeated intermittent uses of electrocautery within short time periods could shut off VVI pulse generators leading to decreases in heart rate and cardiac output.[2] If the electrocautery artifact suppresses the R-wave sensitivity for a longer period of time, these pulse generators revert to asynchronous modes (VVO) for as long as electrocautery is being used. When use of electrocautery is discontinued, these pulse generators should return to their normal VVI modes. More important, newer pulse generators have complex circuitry designed to minimize problems from external electrical interference.

Applying an external converter magnet over VVI pulse generators may be used to convert them to VOO pulse generators, thus almost eliminating the possibility of inhibition by electrocautery. Unlike standard VVI pulse generators, however, application of an external converter magnet to some programmable pacemakers should be avoided during electrocautery use because the chance for reprogramming occurs.[4] Even the external converter magnet may fail if electrocautery current is of sufficiently high density. Therefore, it would seem prudent to have drugs such as atropine and isoproterenol (4 $\mu g \cdot ml^{-1}$) prepared for intravenous infusion, should artificial cardiac pacemaker failure occur and third-degree atrioventricular heart block become hemodynamically significant. VOO pulse generators should not be affected by electrocautery since they do not depend on intrinsic atrial or ventricular activ-

ity for initiation of their electrical impulses. For all pulse generators, however, it is recommended that the (1) ground plate for the electrocautery be placed as far as possible from the pulse generator to minimize detection of the current by the pulse generator; (2) electrocautery be used in short bursts no more frequent than every 10 seconds, especially when being used close to the pulse generator; and (3) electrocautery current be as low as possible.[5] Ventricular fibrillation in patients who have permanent artificial cardiac pacemakers should be managed in the conventional way with the exception that defibrillator paddles should not be placed directly over the pulse generator.

Stimulation Thresholds

Stimulation thresholds are not static values but may be altered by a number of physiologic and pharmacologic events (Table 5-6). Increases in stimulation thresholds could result in failure of artificial cardiac pacemakers to sense or capture, whereas decreases in stimulation thresholds may make patients vulnerable to ventricular fibrillation. For example, potassium equilibrium across cell membranes determines resting membrane potentials. Acute decreases in plasma potassium concentrations moves the resting membrane potential further from the threshold potential (i.e., becomes more negative) and could result in a loss of pacing due to increased stimulation thresholds. Conversely, acute increases in plasma potassium concentrations brings the resting membrane potentials nearer the threshold potentials (i.e., becomes less negative). As a re-

TABLE 5-6. Factors That Can Alter Stimulation Thresholds of Artificial Cardiac Pacemakers

Hyperkalemia
Hypokalemia
Arterial hypoxemia
Myocardial ischemia
Myocardial infarction
Catecholamines

sult, less current density at the electrode-tissue interface is necessary to initiate an action potential, making capture by artificial cardiac pacemakers easier (i.e., stimulation thresholds are decreased). Artificial cardiac pacemakers thus continue to function in the presence of acute hyperkalemia, but ventricular tachycardia or ventricular fibrillation are hazards if pacing impulses are emitted into repolarizing myocardial tissue.[2] Despite these concerns, there is no evidence that intraoperative artificial cardiac pacemaker function is altered by events that may result in changes in stimulation thresholds. Nevertheless, it would seem prudent to avoid events that acutely increase or decrease (hyperventilation of the lungs, diuretic therapy) plasma potassium concentrations. In this regard, neurosurgical patients are at a greater risk for acute hypokalemia during anesthesia and surgery than other patients because they receive intraoperative diuretic therapy and hyperventilation of the lungs. Conceivably, succinylcholine could adversely increase plasma potassium concentrations but, more important could inhibit otherwise normally functioning artificial cardiac pacemakers by causing contraction of muscle groups (myopotential inhibition) that are interpreted as intrinsic R-waves by pulse generators. Therefore, it may be prudent to administer defasciculating doses of nondepolarizing muscle relaxants before injection of succinylcholine. No anesthetic drugs, including halothane, enflurane, and isoflurane, or techniques have been shown to alter adversely stimulation thresholds and subsequent responses to artificial cardiac pacemakers. A rare occurrence is transvenous pacemaker failure associated with positive pressure ventilation of the lungs, which may reflect abrupt volume changes in the heart and cardiac septal deviation that causes loss of electrode contact with the endocardial surface of the myocardium.[6]

Anesthesia for Insertion of Permanent Artificial Cardiac Pacemakers

Anesthesia for insertion of permanent artificial cardiac pacemakers in the presence of third-degree atrioventricular heart block has been associated with a high incidence of cardiac arrest.[5] Therefore, it is recommended that transvenous cardiac pacemakers be inserted before the induction of anesthesia. The patient's arm should not be placed in hyperextension when the brachial vein has been used for insertion of transvenous pacemakers. It must be remembered that the presence of transvenous pacemakers creates a situation in which there is a direct connection between external electrical sources and the endocardium. This predisposes patients to hazards of ventricular fibrillation from microshock levels of electrical current.

REFERENCES

1. Ludmer PL, Goldschlager N. Cardiac pacing in the 1980's. N Engl J Med 1984;311:1671–80
2. Zaidan JR. Pacemakers. Anesthesiology 1984;60:319–34
3. Lown B, Kosowsky B. Artificial cardiac pacemakers. I. N Engl J Med 1970;283:907–16
4. Domino KB, Smith TC. Electrocautery—induced reprogramming of a pacemaker using a precordial magnet. Anesth Analg 1983;62:609–12
5. Simon AB. Perioperative management of the pacemaker patient. Anesthesiology 1977;46:127–31
6. Thiagarajah S, Azar I, Agres M, Lear E. Pacemaker malfunction associated with positive-pressure ventilation. Anesthesiology 1983;58:565–6

6

Essential Hypertension

Essential hypertension is defined as sustained elevations of arterial blood pressure independent of known causes. As such, essential hypertension accounts for 80 percent to 85 percent of all individuals between the ages of 30 years and 55 years with elevated blood pressure. Renal disease is responsible for hypertension in about 10 percent of patients. Rare causes of hypertension include excess adrenocortical function, primary aldosteronism, and pheochromocytoma.

There are no precise physiologic guidelines for classifying individuals as hypertensive. Recognizing that any classification is arbitrary, the World Health Organization has defined hypertension as systolic blood pressures above 160 mmHg and/or diastolic blood pressures greater than 95 mmHg. By this definition, it is estimated that 35 million adults in the United States have essential hypertension.[1] More than 10 million hypertensive patients are currently receiving antihypertensive drugs at a cost that exceeds that for any other single disease. Benefits of therapy in preventing stroke, congestive heart failure, left ventricular hypertrophy and increasingly severe hypertension have been clearly established. In contrast, there is no convincing evidence that either overall mortality or the clinical complications of coronary artery disease are significantly reduced by treatment of patients with diastolic blood pressures between 90 mmHg and 99 mmHg.[1]

PROGRESSION OF ESSENTIAL HYPERTENSION

Progression of essential hypertension can be divided into three stages: (1) borderline hypertension, (2) sustained diastolic hypertension, and (3) hypertension associated with deleterious changes in major organs. Progression through these changes often takes 15 years to 20 years. Accelerated hypertension is present when all three stages are passed through rapidly.

Borderline Hypertension

Borderline hypertension is characterized by detection of occasional systolic blood pressures above 160 mmHg or diastolic blood pressures above 95 mmHg. These patients are normotensive at other times. A consistent physiologic change during borderline hypertension is an elevation of cardiac output of

117

about 15 percent. Systemic vascular resistance is variably altered but is consistently elevated during exercise.

Sustained Diastolic Hypertension

After prolonged periods of borderline hypertension, the stage characterized by a persistent elevation of the diastolic blood pressure above 95 mmHg is entered. Sustained diastolic hypertension is further subdivided as mild, moderate (105 mmHg to 115 mmHg), and severe. Cardiac output is normal to slightly decreased, and systemic vascular resistance is consistently elevated during this stage.

Detectable Organ Involvement

Detectable organ involvement, particularly as manifested in the brain, heart, and kidneys, follows prolonged periods of sustained elevations in systemic vascular resistance. Major organ complications associated with hypertension include cerebral hemorrhage, renal dysfunction, and congestive heart failure (Fig. 6-1). Hypertension also acts as a coronary risk factor in the sense that persistently elevated systemic blood pressures are associated with accelerated development of atherosclerosis. It is speculated that hypertension results in an increased physical stress on the vascular walls of arteries. This physical stress is presumed to result in injury that initiates proliferation of smooth muscle cells in arterial walls (response-to-injury hypothesis). The preponderance of atherosclerotic disease in high pressure systemic arteries compared with the low pressure pulmonary arteries is consistent with this hypothesis. Uneven blood flow patterns produce additional stresses, which may account for the frequent localization of atherosclerotic lesions at sites such as arterial bifurcations. In addition, hypertension enhances clinical manifestations of coronary artery disease by increasing left ventricular pressure work and by producing ventricular hypertrophy (Fig. 6-1). Both of these changes increase myocardial oxygen requirements in the presence of reduced coronary blood flow and oxygen delivery produced by narrowed lumens of diseased coronary arteries. Furthermore, subendocardial blood flow is reduced by increased left ventricular end-diastolic pressures acting to compress arterioles in this region.

Accelerated Hypertension

Accelerated hypertension occurs in about 1 percent of patients with essential hypertension and appears to be associated with activation of the renin-angiotensin system. Patients with renovascular hypertension are most likely to develop accelerated hypertension.

Typically, accelerated hypertension is characterized by rapid increases in diastolic blood pressure, usually to above 130 mmHg, and by the appearance of retinopathy. Left ventricular failure and renal dysfunction (proteinuria, azotemia, oliguria) are inevitable if blood pressure is not aggressively lowered. It may be acceptable to distinguish between accelerated hypertension and malignant hypertension by diagnosing the latter only when papilledema is present.

PATHOPHYSIOLOGY OF ESSENTIAL HYPERTENSION

Pathophysiologic hallmarks of essential hypertension are edema and hypertrophy of arteriolar smooth muscles.[2] These changes lead to reductions in the lumens of blood vessels and increased resistance to blood flow. As a result, blood pressure must be increased to maintain an unchanged blood flow through these narrowed arteries. These blood vessels

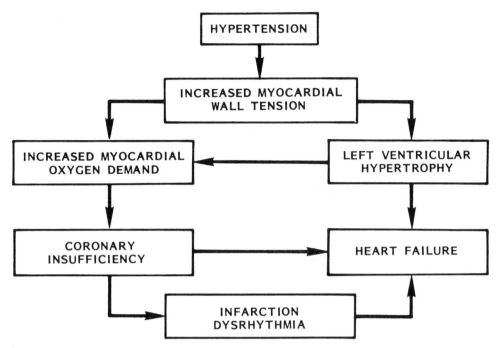

FIG. 6-1. Chronic elevations in systemic blood pressure initiate a series of pathophysiologic changes that may culminate in left ventricular heart failure.

respond normally to vasoconstricting impulses from the sympathetic nervous system. Since the lumen size is reduced by hypertrophy, however, even a normal degree of vasoconstriction in response to sympathetic nervous system stimulation is associated with a relatiively greater reduction in lumen size than that which occurs in normal blood vessels exposed to the same stimuli. As a result, increases in resistance to flow through diseased vessels are exaggerated by vasoconstriction. This explains the exaggerated pressor responses exhibited by patients with essential hypertension during painful stimulation such as direct laryngoscopy for intubation of the trachea or in response to noxious surgical stimulation.[3,4]

Blood volume in hypertensive patients is normal to reduced, but there is central redistribution of this volume, presumably as a result of altered tone in capacitance vessels.[3] This redistribution is necessary for maintenance of cardiac output as left ventricular hypertrophy severely limits diastolic compliance and thus ventricular filling. Hypertensive patients are vulnerable to dilation of capacitance vessels with associated decreases in venous return.

TREATMENT OF ESSENTIAL HYPERTENSION

Antihypertensive drugs used for treatment of essential hypertension are classified as diuretics, sympatholytics, and vasodilators.[5] The frequent use of combination drug therapy is based on the observation that efficacy of single drugs is often offset by homeostatic compensation. For example, diuretics cause compensatory increases in renin activity, presumably reflecting depletion of intravascular fluid volume. Conversely, drugs that reduce sympathetic nervous system activity often lead to increases in intravascular fluid volume. Vasodilators, which do not attenuate baroreceptor reflex activity, typically produce increased heart rates that can offset the blood pressure lowering effects of these drugs. With these responses in mind, one can prescribe combinations of antihypertensive drugs that both lower blood pressure and offset undesirable compensatory responses associated with individual drugs (Table 6-1). Furthermore, combination drug therapy permits maximum therapeutic effects with reduced doses of single drugs, thus reducing the likelihood of dose-related side effects. Nevertheless, it is estimated that half or more of all patients with mild hypertension can achieve blood pressure levels of less than 140/90 mmHg with only one of several drugs and more than 90 percent can be controlled with two drugs.[1]

A frequently neglected aspect of drug selection for treatment of hypertension is the effect of this drug or drugs on the quality of the patient's life. In this regard, drugs that act on the central and/or peripheral sympathetic nervous system are less well tolerated than drugs that lack these effects.[6]

MANAGEMENT OF ANTIHYPERTENSIVE DRUGS IN THE PERIOPERATIVE PERIOD

The question as to whether antihypertensive drugs should be discontinued preoperatively has been extensively discussed.[7,8] This question is based on the fact that many drugs used for the treatment of essential hypertension interfere with autonomic nervous system function. Since a properly functioning autonomic nervous system is necessary for homeostatic responses, patients being treated with antihypertensive drugs might conceivably be at increased risk during anesthesia.

Data collected from patients receiving antihypertensive drugs have resulted in conflicting conclusions. Hypotension that responded poorly to sympathomimetic drugs during induction or maintenance of anesthesia has been attributed to therapy with antihypertensive drugs and was the basis for recommendations that these drugs be discontinued before elective operation. Conversely, others observed a greater incidence of hypotension during anesthesia in untreated hypertensive patients.[9] Furthermore, ephedrine was always effective in restoring blood pressure to normal levels in these patients.[9] Still other studies have demonstrated that hypertensive patients, with or without antihypertensive drug therapy, are more likely to have marked fluctuations in blood pressure during anesthesia.[4,8] These extremes of blood pressure are often associated with signs of myocardial ischemia on the electrocardiogram.[8] Based on available information, the inescapable conclusion is that antihypertensive drugs should be continued throughout the perioperative period, so as to assure optimum medical control of blood pressure.

Rational perioperative management of patients receiving antihypertensive drugs requires an understanding of the possible adverse interactions of these medications with drugs used to produce anesthesia. Specific concerns during administration of anesthesia to these patients include (1) attenuation of sympathetic nervous system activity, (2) modification of responses to sympathomimetic drugs, (3) predominance of parasympathetic nervous system activity, and (4) sedation. Plasma potassium concentrations below 3.5 $mEq \cdot L^{-1}$ occur in 20 percent to 40 percent of patients with essential hypertension receiving diuretic therapy despite potassium supplementation.[10] Nevertheless, this drug-induced hypokalemia has not been documented to increase the incidence of cardiac dysrhythmias in awake or anesthetized patients.[10,11]

Attenuation of Sympathetic Nervous System Activity

Attenuation of sympathetic nervous system activity as a result of therapy with antihypertensive drugs is manifest on the heart and peripheral vasculature. Preoperatively, this attenuation is reflected by orthostatic hypoten-

TABLE 6-1. Combinations of Antihypertensive Drugs Used to Treat Essential Hypertension

Primary Drug	Diuretic	Alpha-Methyldopa	Clonidine	Guanethidine, Guanabenz, Guanadrel	Hydralazine	Prazosin	Minoxidil	Captopril	Beta-Blocker	Labetalol
Diuretic		Yes	Yes	Yes	Yes	Yes	Yes	Yes	Yes	Usually
Alpha-Methyldopa	Yes		No	Yes	Yes	Yes	Yes	Possible	Yes	Unknown
Clonidine	Yes	No		Unknown	Yes	No	Yes	Unknown	No	Unknown
Guanethidine	Yes	Yes	Unknown		Yes	No	Yes	Unknown	Possible	Unknown
Guanabenz	Yes	Yes	Unknown		Yes	No	Yes	Unknown	Possible	Unknown
Guanadrel	Yes	Yes	Unknown		Yes	No	Yes	Unknown	Possible	Unknown
Hydralazine	Usually	Yes	Yes	Yes		Possible	No	Possible	Usually	Unknown
Prazosin	Yes	Yes	No	No	Possible		Unknown	Yes	Yes	Unknown
Minoxidil	Always	Yes	Yes	Yes	No	Unknown		Possible	Always	Unknown
Captopril	Yes	Possible	Unknown	Unknown	Possible	Yes	Possible		Yes	Unknown
Beta-Blocker	Yes	Yes	No	Possible	Yes	Yes	Yes	Yes		No
Labetalol	Yes	Unknown	Unknown	Unknown	Unknown	Unknown	Unknown	Unknown	No	

sion. During anesthesia, exaggerated reductions in blood pressure, as associated with minor blood loss, positive airway pressure, or sudden changes in body position, may reflect impaired degrees of compensatory peripheral vascular vasoconstriction due to inhibitory effects of antihypertensive drugs on the sympathetic nervous system. Theoretically, reduced cardiac sympathetic activity due to antihypertensive drugs could decrease myocardial contractility to the extent that pulmonary edema might occur as a result of aggressive expansion of the intravascular fluid volume.

Modification of Responses to Sympathomimetic Drugs

Responses to sympathomimetic drugs (vasopressors) in the presence of therapy with antihypertensive drugs depend on the mechanism of action of both classes of drugs. To evoke responses, sympathomimetic drugs must stimulate alpha-adrenergic receptors directly (direct-acting vasopressors), or evoke release of norepinephrine (indirect-acting vasopressors). Most sympathomimetic drugs exert combinations of direct and indirect effects, but one of these mechanisms usually predominates. Antihypertensive drugs that deplete norepinephrine or that act on peripheral vascular smooth muscle decrease the sensitivity to predominantly indirect-acting sympathomimetic drugs such as ephedrine.[12] Conversely, sympathetic nervous system blockade that deprives alpha-adrenergic receptors of tonic impulses results in an increased sensitivity of these sites to norepinephrine. As a result, exaggerated blood pressure increases can follow administration of direct-acting sympathomimetic drugs.[12]

Predominance of Parasympathetic Nervous System Activity

Selective impairment of sympathetic nervous system activity by antihypertensive drugs results in predominance of parasympathetic nervous system tone, as reflected by nasal stuffiness, bradycardia, increased gastric hydrogen ion secretion, and diarrhea. Conceivably, bradycardia could limit heart rate responses to intraoperative reductions in blood pressure. Furthermore, drug-induced bradycardia may obscure the usual increases in heart rate associated with inadequate concentrations of anesthetic drugs relative to the surgical stimulus. Likewise, heart rate increases that normally occur with acute reductions in intravascular fluid volume or carbon dioxide accumulation due to hypoventilation may be absent. Although not documented, it is conceivable that exaggerated reductions in heart rate could occur when drugs that normally increase vagal activity, such as anticholinesterase drugs, are administered during anesthesia to patients receiving antihypertensive drugs.

Sedation

Antihypertensive drugs that lower blood pressure in association with reductions in central nervous system concentrations of catecholamines are frequently associated with sedation. Sedative effects are consistent with reductions in anesthetic requirements in the presence of antihypertensive drugs that act on the central nervous system.

PHARMACOLOGY OF ANTIHYPERTENSIVE DRUGS

The usual doses (Table 6-1) and unique pharmacology of each antihypertensive drug must be considered when planning management of anesthesia. In addition to diuretics, drugs that may be encountered in patients being treated for essential hypertension include alpha-methyldopa, clonidine, guanethidine, hydralazine, prazosin, minoxidil, captopril, beta-adrenergic antagonists and combined alpha- and beta-adrenergic antagonists (Table 6-2).

TABLE 6-2. Drugs Used to Treat Essential Hypertension

Generic Name	Trade Name	Oral Dose for Maintenance Therapy in Adults $(mg \cdot day^{-1})$
Alpha-Methyldopa	Aldomet	250–300
Clonidine	Catapres	0.2–2.4
Guanethidine	Ismelin	10–300
Guanabenz	Wytensin	8–64
Guanadrel	Hylorel	25–75
Hydralazine	Apresoline	40–300
Prazosin	Minipress	3–20
Minoxidil	Loniten	5–40
Captopril	Capoten	100–450
Propranolol	Inderal	40–960
Metoprolol	Lopressor	100–400
Nadolol	Corgard	40–320
Atenolol	Tenormin	50–200
Labetalol	Trandate	400–1,600

Alpha-Methyldopa

The most likely explanation for the antihypertensive effects of alpha-methyldopa is the accumulation of alpha-methylated amines, which stimulate inhibitory alpha-2 receptors in the central nervous system, resulting in a reduced outflow of sympathetic nervous system impulses.[13] As a result, systemic vascular resistance and blood pressure are reduced. Alpha-methyldopa may also act as a false neurotransmitter in place of norepinephrine. In this regard, it is thought that alpha-methyldopa enters postganglionic sympathetic nerve endings, where it is converted to alpha-methyldopamine. Alpha-methyldopamine is then converted to alpha-methylnorepinephrine, which is released in response to stimulation of the sympathetic nervous system. Alpha-methylnorepinephrine has weaker sympathomimetic effects than does the usual endogenous neurotransmitter, norepinephrine.

Orthostatic hypotension is rarely a result of treatment with alpha-methyldopa. Predominance of parasympathetic nervous system activity, however, may be manifested as bradycardia. Sedation associated with alpha-methyldopa therapy is consistent with the observation in animals that anesthetic requirements are reduced by this drug (Fig. 6-2).[14] Decreased blood pressure responses after administration of ephedrine have also been documented in animals pretreated with alpha-methyldopa, but the significance, if any, in patients is not known (Table 6-3).[14] Alpha-methyldopa is a logical choice in patients with renal disease, since this drug maintains or increases renal blood flow.

About 20 percent of patients treated with alpha-methyldopa develop positive Coombs' tests, which should suggest the possibility of difficulty in cross-matching whole blood for that patient. A rare but important side effect of treatment with this drug is hepatic dysfunction. Preoperatively, elevated plasma transaminase enzyme concentrations in patients receiving alpha-methyldopa should suggest drug-induced hepatic dysfunction. Patients who are receiving alpha-methyldopa could manifest marked increases in blood pressure after administration of propranolol.[15] This hypertensive response presumably reflects the ability of propranolol to block the usual vasodilating effects of alpha-methylnorepinephrine. As a result, only the potent alpha-stimulating effects of this metabolite are apparent. Therefore, blood pressure responses resemble that which would be anticipated after release of norepinephrine. Naloxone has also been observed to interfere with the antihypertensive effects of alpha-methyldopa.[16]

Sudden withdrawal of alpha-methyldopa therapy can result in rebound hypertension.[17] The incidence, however, of this complication seems to be less than that observed after discontinuation of other centrally acting antihypertensive drugs.

Dementia has been observed in patients treated with alpha-methyldopa who subsequently receive butyrophenone drugs such as haloperidol.[18] This dementia may be caused by the ability of both drugs to prevent dopamine from acting at specific receptors in the central nervous system. Logic would suggest caution in the use of Innovar, since this drug combination contains a butyrophenone derivative, droperidol.

TABLE 6-3. Effects of Antihypertensive Drugs on the Blood Pressure Response Produced by Ephedrine Administered to Dogs During Halothane Anesthesia

Drug	Systolic Blood Pressure Increase (Mean ± SD) Following Intravenous Administration of Ephedrine (0.5 mg·kg^{-1})	
	Before Antihypertensive Drug	After Antihypertensive Drug
Alpha-Methyldopa (50 mg·kg^{-1}·day^{-1} for 3 days)	86 ± 14	30 ± 14
Alpha-Methyldopa (100 mg·kg^{-1}·day^{-1} for 3 days)	86 ± 14	23 ± 7
Alpha-Methyldopa (200 mg·kg^{-1}·day^{-1} for 3 days)	86 ± 14	14 ± 6
Guanethidine (15 mg·kg^{-1}·day^{-1} for 3 days)	78 ± 21	19 ± 7

(Data from Miller RD, Way WL, Eger EI. The effects of alpha-methyldopa, reserpine, guanethidine, and iproniazid on minimum alveolar anesthetic requirement (MAC). Anesthesiology 1969;29:1153–8)

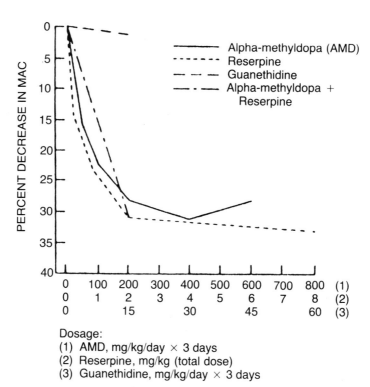

Dosage:
(1) AMD, mg/kg/day × 3 days
(2) Reserpine, mg/kg (total dose)
(3) Guanethidine, mg/kg/day × 3 days

FIG. 6-2. Antihypertensive drugs that cross the blood-brain barrier, deplete central nervous system catecholamines, and produce sedation are associated with reductions in anesthetic requirements (MAC) for halothane. Guanethidine does not cross the blood-brain barrier and anesthetic requirements are not altered. (Miller RD, Way WL, Eger EI. The effects of alpha-methyldopa, reserpine, guanethidine, and iproniazid on minimum alveolar anesthetic requirement (MAC). Anesthesiology 1969;29:1153–8)

Clonidine

Clonidine is thought to stimulate inhibitory alpha-2 receptors in the central nervous system. This stimulation results in decreased outflow of sympathetic nervous system impulses to the periphery, with subsequent reductions in systemic vascular resistance and blood pressure. Clonidine is particularly effective in patients with hypertension due to excess presence of renin. Orthostatic hypotension is rare, since homeostatic compensatory reflex responses are maintained. Bradycardia and dry mouth may accompany treatment with clonidine. Sedation may be prominent and is consistent with the nearly 50 percent reduction in halothane anesthetic requirements in animals produced by either 5 $\mu g \cdot kg^{-1}$ or 20 $\mu g \cdot kg^{-1}$ clonidine administered intravenously (Fig. 6-3).[19] In patients, orally administered clonidine reduces fentanyl anesthetic requirements.[20] As with other antihypertensives, retention of sodium and water often occurs such that com-

binations of clonidine with diuretics are often necessary.

Rebound hypertension has been observed when therapy with clonidine is discontinued. Indeed, discontinuation of treatment with clonidine before elective surgery has been associated with development of adverse increases in blood pressure before the induction of anesthesia, as well as after surgery, while still in the postanesthesia recovery room.[21,22] Rebound hypertension is most likely to occur in patients who are receiving greater than 1.2 mg of clonidine daily. The speculated mechanism for this rebound hypertension is an abrupt increase in systemic vascular resistance due to release of catecholamines. Beta-adrenergic blockade may exaggerate the degree of rebound hypertension by blocking vasodilating effects and leaving unopposed the vasoconstricting actions of catecholamines. Continuation of clonidine throughout the perioperative period is difficult, since a parenteral form of this drug is not available. Therefore, consideration should be given to replacing clonidine before elective surgery with alternative anti-

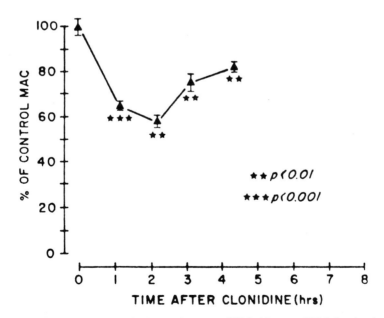

FIG. 6-3. Changes in halothane anesthetic requirements (MAC, Mean ± SE) following intravenous administration of clonidine, 5 $\mu g \cdot kg^{-1}$, to dogs. (Bloor BC, Flacke WE. Reduction in halothane anesthetic requirement by clonidine, an alpha-adrenergic agonist. Anesth Analg 1982;61:741–5 Reprinted with permission from IARS.)

hypertensive drugs such as hydralazine. Alternatively, transdermal clonidine may provide sustained therapeutic effects for as long as 7 days.[23] It should be appreciated that rebound hypertension is not unique to clonidine and may occur following abrupt discontinuation of antihypertensive drugs that act on the central nervous system. Antihypertensive drugs that act independently of the autonomic nervous system (hydralazine, captopril) do not seem to be associated with rebound hypertension.

Naloxone 0.4 mg administered intravenously has been observed to reverse hypotensive and heart rate slowing effects of clonidine in over one-half of treated patients.[24] Therefore, it may be prudent to avoid administration of opioid antagonists to patients who are also receiving clonidine. Clonidine has been shown to be effective in suppressing signs and symptoms of withdrawal from opioids. It is thought that clonidine replaces opioid-mediated inhibition with alpha-2 mediated inhibition of central nervous system sympathetic activity.[25] Clonidine is also useful as an aid in the differential diagnosis of hypertension, which may be due to pheochromocytoma (see Chapter 23). Administered intrathecally, clonidine acts as an analgesic and can be substituted for morphine when tolerance to the opioid develops.[26]

Guanethidine

Guanethidine acts selectively on the peripheral sympathetic nervous system to depress function of postganglionic sympathetic nerves. This selective action occurs because guanethidine uses the same uptake mechanism that transports norepinephrine into postganglionic nerve endings. Once in storage vesicles, guanethidine causes the release of norepinephrine by direct actions and also inhibits depolarization produced by nerve stimulation. Resulting reductions in sympathetic nervous system activity at peripheral alpha- and beta-adrenergic receptors leads to vasodilation. As a result, venous return and cardiac output are decreased, leading to predictable reductions in blood pressure. Guanethidine is used in the treatment of hypertension that is resistant to less potent drugs.

Reductions in peripheral sympathetic nervous system activity produced by guanethidine are also responsible for side effects produced by this drug. Orthostatic hypotension is the most frequent adverse effect, reflecting decreased responsiveness of resistance and capacitance blood vessels to sympathetic nervous system stimulation. Predominance of parasympathetic nervous system activity is often manifested as bradycardia and diarrhea. Fluid retention can lead to resistance to antihypertensive effects if diuretics are not administered concurrently.

Guanethidine, like alpha-methyldopa, sensitizes postsynaptic receptors to norepinephrine and direct-acting sympathomimetics. Therefore, administration of guanethidine to patients with pheochromocytomas is not appropriate. Conversely, responses to indirect-acting sympathomimetic drugs are impaired by guanethidine (Table 6-3).[14]

Guanethidine, unlike alpha-methyldopa, does not enter the central nervous system. As a result, sedation and reductions in anesthetic requirements do not occur (Fig. 6-2). Skeletal muscle weakness, presumably due to decreased neuromuscular transmission, occasionally results, but sensitivity to muscle relaxants has not been observed.

Antihypertensive effects of guanethidine may be lost in patients receiving drugs that block the mechanism for norepinephrine uptake into postganglionic sympathetic nerve endings because guanethidine uses the same mechanism for entrance into these nerve endings. Indeed, recurrence of hypertension, previously controlled with guanethidine, has been observed after initiation of treatment of mental depression with tricyclic antidepressant drugs.[27] Since these drugs block uptake of norepinephrine into postganglionic sympathetic nerve endings, it is presumed that access of guanethidine to nerve endings is also prevented. Other drugs that block uptake of norepinephrine, and presumably guanethidine, into postganglionic nerve endings include ephedrine (present in over-the-counter cold remedies), ketamine, cocaine, alpha-adrenergic antagonist drugs, and possibly pancuronium.

Guanabenz

Guanabenz lowers blood pressure by reducing sympathetic nervous system outflow from the central nervous system similar to clonidine. Sedation and dryness of the mouth are the most common side effects; orthostatic hypotension is less likely than in patients treated with guanethidine. Rebound hypertension occurs with abrupt discontinuation of this drug, but its prolonged elimination half-time delays the appearance of this response.

Guanadrel

Guanadrel resembles guanethidine but has a more rapid onset and shorter duration of action and produces less orthostatic hypotension.

Hydralazine

Hydralazine probably interferes with calcium transport at arterial vascular smooth muscle and thus lowers blood pressure by arterial vasodilation. Activity of baroreceptor reflexes remains intact, leading to increased outflow of sympathetic nervous system impulses to the heart and peripheral vasculature in response to hydralazine-induced reductions in blood pressure. This increased sympathetic nervous system activity may offset the desired antihypertensive effects of hydralazine. Baroreceptor reflex stimulation can be prevented by combining hydralazine with other antihypertensive drugs, such as guanethidine, or beta-adrenergic antagonist drugs, such as propranolol. Indeed, hydralazine is most frequently used as a third drug in combination with beta-adrenergic antagonist drugs plus diuretics to offset sodium and water retention.

Hydralazine, in contrast to other antihypertensive drugs, does not produce orthostatic hypotension, which reflects continued func-tion of baroreceptors and the preferential dilation of arterioles compared to veins. Hydralazine is a frequent choice for patients with renal disease, since this drug either maintains or increases renal blood flow. A lupus erythematosus-like syndrome occurs in 10 percent to 20 percent of patients treated for more than 6 months, especially if the daily dose of hydralazine exceeds 400 mg.[28] This response occurs predominantly in patients who are slow acetylators. Symptoms of rheumatoid arthritis can also accompany prolonged treatment with hydralazine. Although unproven, it is conceivable that exaggerated hypotension in the intraoperative period could occur in the presence of vasodilating drugs used to produce anesthesia.

Prazosin

Prazosin lowers blood pressure by reducing systemic vascular resistance via selective postsynaptic alpha-1 receptor blockade. Absence of presynaptic alpha-2 blockade leaves the normal inhibition of norepinephrine release intact. In contrast to hydralazine, prazosin does not cause reflex tachycardia. Also unlike hydralazine, this drug preferentially acts on alpha receptors in veins and may cause orthostatic hypotension. Fluid retention requires concomitant administration of diuretics. Syncope may occur early in treatment, especially if patients are hypovolemic.

Minoxidil

Minoxidil lowers blood pressure by direct relaxation of arteriolar smooth muscle with little effect on venous capacitance vessels. This drug causes marked fluid retention and tachycardia, necessitating its use with diuretics and beta-adrenergic antagonist drugs. Orthostatic hypotension is not prominent in patients treated with this drug. Pericardial effusions and cardiac tamponade develop in about 3 percent of patients, especially if severe renal dysfunction is present.[17] Hypertrichosis, most notable around the face and arms, occurs in nearly all patients treated for more than 1 month.

Captopril

Captopril acts by competitive inhibition of angiotensin I-converting enzyme, which is necessary for conversion of inactive angiotensin I to angiotensin II (Fig. 6-4). Angiotensin II is also responsible for stimulating secretion of aldosterone by the adrenal cortex. As a result of inhibition of this enzyme, there are decreases in plasma concentrations of angiotensin II and aldosterone. Renin levels often increase due to loss of the negative feedback control normally provided by angiotensin II, whereas decreases in aldosterone secretion result in slight increases in plasma potassium concentrations.[29] It is presumed that reductions in angiotensin II activity lead to decreased sodium and water retention with subsequent reductions in systemic vascular resistance and blood pressure. Vasodilating effects of kinins may also play a role in the production of decreases in blood pressure since converting enzyme inhibited by captopril is also responsible for the metabolism of bradykinin.

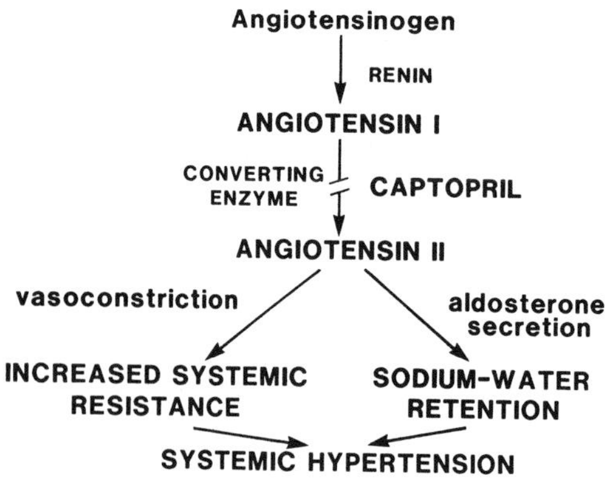

The most common side effect of captopril therapy occurring in about 10 percent of patients is a skin rash sometimes accompanied by fever and arthritis. Proteinuria has been observed with prolonged treatment of patients with chronic renal disease. Captopril may cause marked elevations in plasma creatinine concentrations when administered to volume-depleted patients or those with renal disease. Hyperkalemia may occur in patients with impaired renal function, particularly if potassium-sparing diuretics are combined with captopril.[30] Inhibition of kinin metabolism may exacerbate wheezing in patients with chronic obstructive airways disease who are treated with captopril.[31] Neutropenia has been observed in about 0.3 percent of patients, emphasizing the need to monitor white blood cell counts during the first few months of captopril treatment. Compared with alpha-methyldopa and propranolol, captopril produces less alteration in general well being (cognitive function, work performance, physical symptoms) and thus achieves better patient acceptance than drugs acting on the central nervous system.[6]

Beta-Adrenergic Antagonist Drugs

Beta-adrenergic antagonist drugs effective in treatment of hypertension include propranolol, metoprolol, nadolol, atenolol, and timolol (Table 6-2). Inhibition of the release of renin from the kidneys may contribute to the antihypertensive effects of drugs that produce beta-adrenergic blockade, particularly in patients with high plasma renin activity. Since reductions in secretion of renin will lead to decreased release of aldosterone, beta-adrenergic antagonist drugs will prevent compensatory sodium and water retention that accompanies treatment with vasodilator drugs. Furthermore, beta-adrenergic blockage attenuates baroreceptor-mediated increases in heart rate associated with vasodilator therapy. One of the main ad-

FIG. 6-4. Captopril competitively inhibits the activity of the converting enzyme that normally converts angiotensin I to angiotensin II. As a result, the formation of angiotensin II and subsequent events that can contribute to increased blood pressure are attenuated.

vantages of beta-adrenergic antagonist drugs, as used for the treatment of essential hypertension, is the absence of postural hypotension. These drugs are also less likely than centrally acting drugs to produce sedation. It must be recognized that abrupt discontinuation of beta-adrenergic drugs can be associated with excessive increases in sympathetic nervous system activity. Treatment with these drugs, or equivalent medications, should be continued throughout the perioperative period. Knowledge of the pharmacology of beta-adrenergic antagonist drugs and the potential adverse interactions of these drugs with medications used during anesthesia is important (see Chapter 1).

Labetalol

Labetalol is a selective alpha-1 receptor antagonist and nonselective beta receptor antagonist.[32] Chronic oral administration of labetalol lowers blood pressure principally by reductions in systemic vascular resistance, as cardiac output and heart rate does not change. This drug is about one-half as potent as phentolamine in its ability to block alpha receptors and one-fourth as potent as propranolol as an antagonist at beta receptors. Antianginal effects of labetalol are less than those produced by propranolol and bronchospasm is less likely. The most common side effect produced by labetalol is orthostatic hypotension. Fluid retention is the reason for often administering labetalol with diuretics. Bradycardia may occur in the presence of excessive plasma concentrations of labetalol.

MANAGEMENT OF ANESTHESIA

Considerations for the perioperative management of patients with essential hypertension who are scheduled for elective or emergency operations are outlined in Table 6-4.

TABLE 6-4. Management of Anesthesia for Patients with Essential Hypertension

Preoperative Evaluation
    Determine adequacy of blood pressure control
    Review pharmacology of antihypertensive drugs
    Detect associated organ dysfunction
        Orthostatic hypotension
        Coronary artery disease
        Cerebral vascular disease
        Peripheral vascular disease
        Renal dysfunction

Induction of Anesthesia and Intubation of the Trachea
    Expect exaggerated blood pressure changes
    Minimize the blood pressure response with short duration laryngoscopy

Maintenance of Anesthesia
    For control of blood pressure elevations use volatile anesthetics
    Monitor electrocardiogram for evidence of myocardial ischemia

Postoperative Management
    Anticipate excessive increases in blood pressure
    Maintain monitoring established intraoperatively

Emergency surgery in patients with uncontrolled hypertension introduces the added question of the safe level for maintenance of blood pressure during the perioperative period. In this situation, systemic blood pressure may be safely lowered to about 140/90 mmHg, assuming the absence of central nervous system disease or renal dysfunction (see the section Hypertensive Crises). Reductions of blood pressure to this level are associated with adequate renal blood flow and reduced systemic vascular resistance such that myocardial performance is likely to improve.

Preoperative Evaluation

Preoperative evaluation of patients with essential hypertension should determine the adequacy of blood pressure control. It is important to review the pharmacology of the drugs being used to treat essential hypertension. Detection of orthostatic hypotension during the preoperative evaluation may be evidence that antihypertensive drugs are interfering with normal function of the sympathetic nervous system. Evidence of major organ dysfunction, particularly the presence of incipient congestive heart failure, must be sought.

Patients with essential hypertension are assumed to have coronary artery disease until proven otherwise. In addition, hypertensive patients may manifest left ventricular hypertrophy, which is most likely due to the excess work load imposed on the heart by increased systemic vascular resistance. Potential adverse effects introduced by the presence of coronary artery disease and left ventricular hypertrophy include decreased myocardial oxygen delivery and increased myocardial oxygen requirements. Therefore, the margin of safety, which is substantial in normotensive patients, may be greatly reduced in patients with essential hypertension.

Evidence of peripheral vascular disease must be recognized, particularly when placement of intra-arterial catheters in the perioperative period is anticipated. Manifestations of cerebral vascular disease must be appreciated. Essential hypertension is associated with shifts to the right of curves for the autoregulation of cerebral blood flow. This shift suggests that cerebral blood flow in these patients is more dependent on perfusion pressure than in normotensive patients. Renal dysfunction, secondary to longstanding hypertension, places patients at increased risk and signals that the hypertensive disease process is widespread.

Ideally, all patients with essential hypertension should be rendered normotensive before performance of elective surgery. This recommendation is based on the observation that the incidence of hypotension and evidence of myocardial ischemia on the electrocardiogram during the maintenance of anesthesia is increased in patients who remain hypertensive before induction of anesthesia.[3,8] Furthermore, blood pressure reductions during anesthesia are greater in hypertensive than in normotensive patients.[4] Blood pressure elevations during the intraoperative period are more likely to occur in patients with histories of essential hypertension, regardless of the degree of blood pressure control present before the induction

of anesthesia (Table 6-5).[4] There is no evidence, however, that the incidence of postoperative cardiac complications is increased when hypertensive patients undergo elective operations, as long as preoperative diastolic blood pressures do not exceed 110 mmHg (Table 6-5).[4] Nevertheless, in specific areas of surgery such as carotid endarterectomy, co-existence of inadequately controlled hypertension has been shown to be associated with increased frequency of both transient and permanent neurologic deficits.[33] Furthermore, co-existing hypertension may increase the occurrence of postoperative myocardial reinfarctions in patients with histories of previous myocardial infarctions.[34]

Antihypertensive drugs that have rendered patients normotensive preoperatively should be continued throughout the perioperative period. There is no evidence that therapy with antihypertensive drugs adversely influences the conduct of anesthesia. Conversely, there is convincing evidence that absence of blood pressure control before surgery results in undesirable responses during the conduct of anesthesia.[3,4,8]

Induction of Anesthesia and Intubation of the Trachea

Induction of anesthesia with intravenous administration of barbiturates, benzodiazepines, or etomidate is acceptable. Exaggerated reductions in blood pressure, however, may occur, particularly if hypertension is present preoperatively. This most likely reflects drug-induced peripheral vasodilation in the presence of a reduced intravascular fluid volume. Indeed, plasma volume may be reduced in the presence of diastolic hypertension.[35] Ketamine is rarely selected for induction of anesthesia, as its circulatory stimulant effects could adversely increase blood pressure, particularly in patients with co-existing hypertension.

Intubation of the trachea is a hazardous event in these patients. It must be appreciated that patients with essential hypertension, even when rendered normotensive before surgery,

TABLE 6-5. Risks of General Anesthesia and Elective Operations in Hypertensive Patients

Blood Pressure Status Before Operation	Incidence of Perioperative Hypertensive Episodes	Incidence of Postoperative Cardiac Complications
Normotensive	8%*	11%
Treated and rendered normotensive	27%	24%
Treated but remain hypertensive	25%	7%
Untreated and hypertensive	20%	12%

* P < 0.05 compared with other groups in same column.

(Data from Goldman L, Caldera DL. Risks of general anesthesia and elective operation in the hypertensive patient. Anesthesiology 1979;50:285–92)

manifest exaggerated blood pressure responses to events that stimulate the sympathetic nervous system.[10] Appearance of evidence of myocardial ischemia on the electrocardiogram often accompanies increases in blood pressure and/or heart rate produced by direct laryngoscopy and intubation of the trachea.[36]

A frequent concern is that drugs used for the intravenous induction of anesthesia do not provide sufficient depression to prevent circulatory responses produced by intubation of the trachea. For this reason, it may seem prudent to increase the depth of anesthesia with additional drugs, such as intravenous administration of opioids or inhalation of volatile anesthetics, before intubation of the trachea is attempted. Indeed, it is a clinical impression that prior intravenous administration of fentanyl (50 µg to 150 µg) or sufentanil (10 µg to 30 µg) reduces blood pressure responses produced by direct laryngoscopy. In addition, it has been demonstrated that 1.5 MAC enflurane or halothane will block sympathetic nervous system responses to surgical skin incision in 50 percent of patients.[37] The relevance of this MAC concentration to responses elicited by intubation of the trachea is not known. Regardless of the drugs administered before intubation of the trachea is attempted, it must be appreciated that an excessive depth of anes-

thesia can produce reductions in blood pressure that may be as undesirable as hypertension.

An important concept for limiting pressor responses elicited by intubation of the trachea is to minimize the duration of direct laryngoscopy to 15 seconds or less.[38] In addition, administration of laryngotracheal lidocaine (2 mg·kg^{-1}) immediately before placement of the tube in the trachea may minimize additional pressor responses produced by this stimulus.[39] When the duration of direct laryngoscopy cannot be limited to less than 15 seconds, it may be reasonable to consider intravenous administration of nitroprusside (1 µg·kg^{-1} to 2 µg·kg^{-1})[40] or lidocaine (1.5 mg·kg^{-1})[39] injected just before beginning direct laryngoscopy in an attempt to attenuate blood pressure responses produced by intubation of the trachea.

Maintenance of Anesthesia

The goal during maintenance of anesthesia is to adjust the depth of anesthesia in appropriate directions to minimize wide fluctuations of blood pressure. In this regard, techniques using volatile anesthetics are useful for permitting rapid adjustments in depth in response to changes in blood pressure. Indeed, management of intraoperative blood pressure lability with the anesthetic technique may be more important than preoperative control of hypertension.[4]

The most likely intraoperative changes in blood pressure are hypertensive episodes produced by noxious surgical stimulation. Remember that the incidence of perioperative hypertensive episodes is increased in patients with a diagnosis of essential hypertension, even if they have been previously rendered normotensive with antihypertensive drugs (Table 6-5).[4] Volatile anesthetics are ideal for attenuating activity of the sympathetic nervous system, which is responsible for pressor responses. Halothane, enflurane, and isoflurane produce dose-dependent reductions in blood pressure. Although each drug lowers blood pressure by different primary mechanisms, there is no evidence that a specific volatile anesthetic is a more appropriate choice for control of intraoperative hypertension (see Fig. 1-9).[41] A nitrous oxide-opioid technique is also acceptable for the maintenance of anesthesia. If this approach is selected, however, it should be appreciated that addition of volatile drugs is often necessary to control undesirable elevations in blood pressure, particularly during periods of maximal surgical stimulation. Continuous intravenous infusions of nitroprusside are alternatives to the use of volatile anesthetics for maintaining normotension during the intraoperative period.

Hypotension that occurs during the maintenance of anesthesia is often treated by decreasing the concentrations of anesthetic drugs plus infusing fluids intravenously to increase intravascular fluid volume. Sympathomimetic drugs, such as ephedrine, may be necessary to maintain perfusion pressure until the underlying cause of the hypotension can be corrected. Another cause of acute reductions in blood pressure may be the sudden onset of junctional cardiac rhythms. Avoidance of extreme reductions in the arterial carbon dioxide partial pressures and of excessive concentrations of volatile anesthetic drugs (particularly halothane) will reduce the incidence of this cardiac rhythm. Intravenous administration of atropine is the treatment if hemodynamically significant junctional rhythm persists.

Perioperative monitors for patients with co-existing essential hypertension are determined by the complexity of the surgery. The electrocardiogram is monitored with the goal of recognizing changes suggestive of myocardial ischemia, as this is one of the major problems encountered. The high incidence of myocardial ischemia most likely reflects the fact that increased diastolic intracavitary pressures in the left ventricle compress subendocardial coronary arteries, leading to subendocardial ischemia. Invasive monitoring, using intra-arterial and pulmonary artery catheters, is often indicated if major surgery is planned and there is evidence of left ventricular dysfunction at the preoperative evaluation. Invasive monitoring is also necessary when emergency surgery in the presence of uncontrolled hypertension is required.

There is no evidence that a specific muscle relaxant is the best selection in patients with essential hypertension, although drugs such as atracurium or vecuronium would seem logical selections in view of their minimal-to-absent effects on blood pressure. Theoretically, gallamine, and d-tubocurarine would be unattractive choices because of their effects on the heart rate and blood pressure respectively. Although pancuronium can increase blood pressure, there is no evidence that this pressor response is exaggerated by co-existing hypertension.

Regional anesthesia is a questionable choice when high levels of sympathetic nervous system blockade would be associated with the sensory levels necessary for the planned operative procedures. This caution is based on the possibility of excessive or unpredictable reductions in blood pressure when vasodilation unmasks a decreased intravascular fluid volume. It must be appreciated that essential hypertension may be associated with not only a decreased intravascular fluid volume but also with a high incidence of coronary artery disease, which means that reductions in blood pressure are more likely to result in myocardial ischemia.

Postoperative Management

Hypertension in the early postoperative period is a frequent response in patients with histories of co-existing hypertension. The mechanism is not known but most likely reflects exaggerated responses these patients manifest to any form of sympathetic nervous system stimulation. If hypertension persists despite adequate analgesia, it may be necessary to administer peripherally acting smooth muscle vasodilator drugs (see the section Hypertensive Crises). It is also important to monitor the electrocardiogram for signs of myocardial ischemia in the postoperative period.

HYPERTENSIVE CRISES

The most frequently chosen drugs for the management of abrupt and persistent elevations in blood pressure in the perioperative period are nitroprusside, trimethaphan, diazoxide, hydralazine, and labetalol.

Nitroprusside

Nitroprusside is effective for producing rapid reductions of blood pressure to normal levels. Potency of nitroprusside, however, requires careful titration of doses, using devices to maintain constant rates of intravenous infusion of the drug. Continuous monitoring of blood pressure via an intra-arterial catheter is useful during its infusion. Occasionally, use of noninvasive techniques, such as a Doppler sensor may be acceptable for monitoring blood pressure. During anesthesia and in the early postoperative period, nitroprusside infusion rates of 0.5 $\mu g \cdot kg^{-1} \cdot min^{-1}$ to 5.0 $\mu g \cdot kg^{-1} \cdot min^{-1}$ are usually adequate for returning blood pressure to normotensive levels. When chronically administered, doses should not exceed 0.5 $mg \cdot kg^{-1} \cdot hr^{-1}$ (8 $\mu g \cdot kg^{-1} \cdot min^{-1}$).[42]

Since nitroprusside has no effect on the myocardium or the autonomic nervous system, cardiac output is usually unchanged or increased when the blood pressure is lowered. Increases in heart rate may accompany administration of nitroprusside and offset blood pressure-lowering effects of this drug. This response reflects intact baroreceptor reflexes, which sense drug-induced reductions in blood pressure. Propranolol, administered intravenously, is effective for slowing the heart rate and allowing reductions in the infusion rate of nitroprusside.

Cyanide toxicity due to nitroprusside should be suspected in patients who develop (1) resistance to the blood pressure-lowering effects of nitroprusside (require greater than 8 $\mu g \cdot kg^{-1} \cdot min^{-1}$), (2) tachyphylaxis, or (3) metabolic acidosis. Nitroprusside should be immediately discontinued in such patients. If symptoms of cyanide toxicity persist, specific cyanide antagonists such as thiosulfate (150 $mg \cdot kg^{-1}$ intravenously over 15 minutes) should be administered.[42,43]

Trimethaphan

Trimethaphan is a ganglionic blocking drug that acts rapidly but so briefly that it must be given by continuous intravenous infusions. Infusion rates of 0.5 $mg \cdot min^{-1}$ to 2 $mg \cdot min^{-1}$ are usually sufficient to return the blood pressure to normal levels. As with nitroprusside, constant blood pressure monitoring via an intra-arterial catheter or Doppler sensor is necessary.

Trimethaphan lowers blood pressure by arteriolar vasodilation and by reducing cardiac output. Reflex tachycardia may offset reductions in blood pressure and may contribute to occasional resistance to the blood pressure-lowering effects of this drug. Propranolol, administered intravenously, may be effective in slowing the heart rate and thus improving effectiveness of trimethaphan for lowering blood pressure. Histamine release secondary to the administration of trimethaphan makes this drug inappropriate in the managment of hypertension due to pheochromocytoma. Large doses of trimethaphan may potentiate nondepolarizing muscle relaxants by an unknown mechanism.[44]

Diazoxide

Diazoxide is a nondiuretic thiazide derivative that reduces systolic and diastolic blood pressure by direct relaxant actions on arteriolar smooth muscle. Baroreceptor reflexes are not depressed, so that decreases in systemic vascular resistance are accompanied by reflex increases in heart rate and cardiac output.

Intravenous injection of diazoxide (2.5 $mg \cdot kg^{-1}$ to 5 $mg \cdot kg^{-1}$) rapidly lowers an abnormally elevated blood pressure to normal levels in 2 minutes to 5 minutes. Duration of action is 6 hours to 12 hours. Previous recommendations that the drug had to be injected rapidly (less than 20 seconds) to offset the high degree of protein binding (90 percent) and thus produce a blood pressure-lowering effect are probably erroneous. Uninterrupted (i.e., continuous) monitoring of blood pressure is probably not mandatory when administering diazoxide to hypertensive patients.

Although excessive reductions in blood pressure after administration of diazoxide are unlikely, a disadvantage of this drug compared with nitroprusside or trimethaphan is the inability to adjust doses in accordance with blood pressure responses. Blood pressure-lowering effects of diazoxide may be accentuated in patients who are also receiving beta-adrenergic antagonist drugs. This occurs because baroreceptor-mediated increases in heart rate that normally occur during reductions in blood pressure are blocked. When used in patients with eclampsia, diazoxide acts as a powerful uterine relaxant; uterine contractions can be reestablished with oxytocin. Diazoxide inhibits the release of insulin from the pancreas, but hypoglycemia is not a factor with the administration of single doses. Stimulation of catecholamine release contraindicates use of this drug in patients with pheochromocytoma.

Hydralazine

Hydralazine is a vascular smooth muscle vasodilator that is particularly effective for treating postoperative elevations in diastolic blood pressure. For example, in adults intravenous injection of hydralazine, 5 mg to 10 mg, can be repeated every 10 minutes to 20 minutes until diastolic blood pressures are reduced to below 110 mmHg. Hydralazine is not as effective in lowering elevations in systolic blood pressure that occur in the absence of diastolic hypertension.

Labetalol

Intravenous administration of labetalol (20 mg to 40 mg over 2 minutes) produces reductions in blood pressure because of simultaneous decreases in cardiac output and peripheral vascular resistance. Prompt reductions in blood pressure produced by intravenous administration of labetalol make this a useful drug in the treatment of hypertensive emergencies.[45]

REFERENCES

1. Chobanian AV. Antihypertensive therapy in evolution. N Engl J Med 1986;314:1701–2
2. Folkow B. Cardiovascular structural adaptation; its role in the initiation and maintenance of primary hypertension. Clin Sci Mol Med 1978;55:3–22
3. Prys-Roberts C. Anaesthesia and hypertension. Br J Anaesth 1984;56:711–24
4. Goldman L, Caldera DL. Risks of general anesthesia and elective operation in the hypertensive patient. Anesthesiology 1979;50:285–92
5. Gottlieb TR, Chidsey CA. The clinicians' guide to pharmacology of antihypertensive agents. Geriatrics 1976;31:99–110
6. Croog SH, Levine S, Testa MA, et al. The effects of antihypertensive therapy on the quality of life. N Engl J Med 1986;314:1657–64
7. Dingle HR. Antihypertensive drugs and anaesthesia. Anaesthesia 1966;21:151–72
8. Prys-Roberts C, Meloche R, Foex P. Studies of anesthesia in relation to hypertension. I. Cardiovascular responses to treated and untreated patients. Br J Anaesth 1971;43:122–37
9. Katz RL, Weintraub HD, Papper EM. Anesthesia, surgery, and rauwolfia. Anesthesiology 1964;25:142–7
10. Papademetrious V, Burris J, Kukich S, Freis ED. Effectiveness of potassium chloride or triamterene in thiazide hypokalemia. Arch Intern Med 1985;145:1986–90
11. Vitez TS, Soper LE, Wong KC, Soper P. Chronic hypokalemia and intraoperative dysrhythmias. Anesthesiology 1985;63:130–3
12. Eger EI, Hamilton WK. The effect of reserpine on the action of various vasopressors. Anesthesiology 1959;20:641–5
13. Frohlich ED. Methyldopa: Mechanisms and treatment 25 years later. Arch Intern Med 1980;140:954–9
14. Miller RD, Way WL, Eger EI. The effects of alphamethyldopa, reserpine, guanethidine, and iproniazid on minimum alveolar anesthetic requirement (MAC). Anesthesiology 1969;29:1153–8
15. Nies AS, Shand DG. Hypertensive responses to propranolol in a patient treated with methyldopa-a proposed mechanism. Clin Pharmacol Ther 1973;14:823–6
16. Kunos G, Farsang C, Ramirez-Gonzolez MD. Beta-endorphin: Possible involvement in the antihypertensive effect of central alpha-receptor activation. Science 1981;211:82–3
17. Husserl FE, Messerli FH. Adverse effects of antihypertensive drugs. Drugs 1981;22:188–210

18. Thornton WE. Dementia induced by methyldopa with haloperidol. N Engl J Med 1976;294:1222
19. Bloor BC, Flacke WE. Reduction in halothane anesthetic requirements by clonidine, an alpha-adrenergic agonist. Anesth Analg 1982;61:741–5
20. Ghignone M, Quintin L, Duke PC et al. Effects of clonidine on narcotic requirements and hemodynamic response during induction of fentanyl anesthesia and endotracheal intubation. Anesthesiology 1986;64:36–42
21. Bruce DL, Croley TF, Lee JS. Preoperative clonidine withdrawal syndrome. Anesthesiology 1979;51:90–2
22. Brodsky JB, Bravo JJ. Acute postoperative clonidine withdrawal syndrome. Anesthesiology 1976;44:519–20
23. Weber MA, Drayer JIM, McMahon FG, et al. Transdermal administration of clonidine for treatment of high blood pressure. Arch Intern Med 1984;144:1211–3
24. Farsang C, Kapocsi J, Vajda L, et al. Reversal by naloxone of the antihypertensive action of clonidine: Involvement of the sympathetic nervous system. Circulation 1984;69:461–7
25. Gold MS, Pottash AC, Sweeney DR, Kleber HD. Opiate withdrawal using clonidine. A safe, effective, and rapid nonopiate treatment. JAMA 1980;243:343–6
26. Milne B, Cervenko FW, Jhamandas K, Sutak M. Local clonidine: Analgesia and effect on opiate withdrawal in the rat. Anesthesiology 1985;62:34–8
27. Mitchell JR, Oates JA. Guanethidine and related agents. I. Mechanism of the selective blockade of adrenergic neurons and its antagonism by drugs. J Pharmacol Exp Ther 1970;172:100–7
28. Lee SL, Chase PH. Drug-induced systemic lupus erythematosus: A critical review. Semin Arthritis Rheum 1975;5:83–103
29. Johnston CI, Millar JA, McGrath BP, Matthews PG. Long-term effects of captopril (SQ14225) on blood-pressure and hormone levels in essential hypertension. Lancet 1979;2:493–6
30. Vidt DG, Bravo EL, Fouad FM. Captopril. N Engl J Med 1982;214–9
31. Semple PF, Herd GW. Cough and wheeze caused by inhibitors of angiotensin-converting enzyme. N Engl J Med 1986;314:61
32. Wallin JD, O'Neill WM. Labetalol. Current research and therapeutic status. Arch Intern Med 1983;143:485–90
33. Asiddas CB, Donegan JH, Whitesell RC, Kalbfleisch JH. Factors associated with perioperative complications during carotid endarterectomy. Anesth Analg 1982;61:631–7
34. Steen PA, Tinker JH, Tarhan S. Myocardial reinfarction after anesthesia and surgery. An update, incidence, mortality and predisposing factors. JAMA 1978;239:2566–70
35. Tarazi RC, Frohlich ED, Dustan HP. Plasma volume in men with essential hypertension. N Engl J Med 1968;278:762–5
36. Roy WL, Edelist G, Gilbert B. Myocardial ischemia during noncardiac surgical procedures in patients with coronary artery disease. Anesthesiology 1979;51:393–7
37. Roizen MF, Horrigan RW, Frazer BM. Anesthetic doses blocking adrenergic (stress) and cardiovascular responses to incision-MAC BAR. Anesthesiology 1981;54:390–8
38. Stoelting RK. Blood pressure and heart rate changes during short duration laryngoscopy for tracheal intubation: Influence of viscous or intravenous lidocaine. Anesth Analg 1978;57:197–9
39. Stoelting RK. Circulatory changes during direct laryngoscopy and tracheal intubation: Influence of duration of laryngoscopy with or without prior lidocaine. Anesthesiology 1977;47:381–3
40. Stoelting RK: Attenuation of blood pressure response to laryngoscopy and tracheal intubation with sodium nitroprusside. Anesth Analg 1979;58:116–9
41. Hess W, Arnold B, Schulte-Sasse UWE, Tarnow J. Comparison of isoflurane and halothane when used to control intraoperative hypertension in patients undergoing coronary artery bypass surgery. Anesth Analg 1983;62:15–20
42. Michenfelder JD, Tinker JH. Cyanide toxicity and thiosulfate protection during chronic administration of sodium nitroprusside in the dog: Correlation with a human case. Anesthesiology 1977;47:441–8
43. Perschau RA, Modell JH, Bright RW, Shirley PD. Suspected sodium-nitroprusside-induced cyanide intoxication. Anesth Analg 1977;56:533–7
44. Wilson SL, Miller RN, Wright C, Hasse D. Prolonged neuromuscular blockade associated with trimethaphan: A case report. Anesth Analg 1976;55:353–6
45. Morel DR, Forster A, Suter PM. I.V. Labetalol in the treatment of hypertension following coronary-artery surgery. Br J Anaesth 1982;54:1191–6

7

Congestive Heart Failure

Congestive heart failure is most often due to cardiac valve abnormalities or impaired myocardial contractility secondary to coronary artery disease or cardiomyopathy. The hallmark of congestive heart failure is decreased myocardial contractility. It is useful to describe congestive heart failure as left-sided, right-sided, or biventricular. Left ventricular failure results in symptoms and signs of pulmonary congestion, while right ventricular failure leads to symptoms and signs of systemic venous hypertension. It is important to remember that the most frequent cause of right ventricular failure is left ventricular failure. The presence of congestive heart failure in the preoperative period is the most important single abnormality that has been shown to contribute to postoperative cardiac morbidity and mortality.[1]

COMPENSATORY MECHANISMS AND CONGESTIVE HEART FAILURE

The heart has a number of adaptive physiologic mechanisms that assist in meeting increased demands placed on it by diseased valves or poor myocardial contractility. These mechanisms include (1) the Frank-Starling principle, (2) the inotropic state, (3) heart rate, and (4) myocardial hypertrophy and dilation.

Frank-Starling Principle

The Frank-Starling principle is illustrated by increased left ventricular stroke volume that accompanies elevations of left ventricular end-diastolic pressures (Fig. 7-1). Increased stroke volume occurs because the tension developed by contracting muscle is greater when the resting length of that muscle is increased. Resting muscle length is determined by end-diastolic volumes, which are closely related to end-diastolic filling pressures. The magnitude of stroke volume increase produced by increased resting lengths of the ventricular muscle fibers depends on the state of myocardial contractility. For example, when myocardial contractility is reduced, as in congestive heart failure, a lower stroke volume is achieved relative to any given left ventricular end-diastolic filling pressure (Fig. 7-1). Constriction of venous capacitance vessels shifts blood centrally, which helps maintain cardiac output by the Frank-Starling principle.

Inotropic State

Inotropic state describes the velocity with which myocardial muscles contract relative to the tension developed by the muscles. At

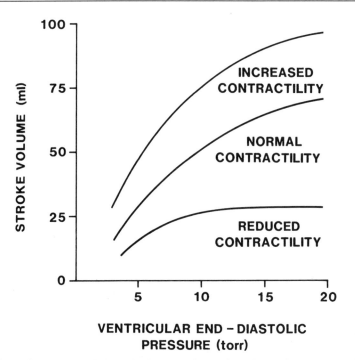

Fig. 7-1. The Frank-Starling principle is the increase in stroke volume that accompanies progressive elevations in left or right ventricular end-diastolic pressures. These schematic cardiac function curves illustrate the Frank-Starling principle for three different states of myocardial contractility. When myocardial contractility is enhanced, a greater stroke volume can be achieved for any given ventricular end-diastolic pressure. Conversely, when myocardial contractility is reduced, as in congestive heart failure, a lower stroke volume is achieved relative to any given left ventricular end-diastolic pressure.

higher inotropic states, as during stimulation of the sympathetic nervous system, myocardial muscles contract faster and develop more tension. Maximum velocity of contraction is referred to as V_{max}. When inotropic states of the heart are increased, as in the presence of catecholamines, V_{max} is increased. Conversely, V_{max} is depressed when myocardial contractility is impaired. Volatile anesthetics have been demonstrated to reduce V_{max} (Fig. 7-2).[2] In clinical practice, the rate of rise of intraventricular pressures (dp/dt) simulates V_{max} and is used as an approximation of inotropic states of the heart.

Congestive heart failure is associated with a depletion of catecholamines in the heart, with subsequent reductions in inotropic capability. This depletion is probably due to reductions of tyrosine hydroxylase activity. This enzyme is the rate-limiting enzyme in the conversion of tyrosine to DOPA and the subsequent formation of the neurotransmitter nor-

epinephrine (Fig. 7-3). In contrast to depletion of myocardial catecholamines, plasma concentrations, as well as urinary excretion of catecholamines, are invariably increased in patients with congestive heart failure.[3] Furthermore, there is a decrease in the density of beta-adrenergic receptors in the muscle of failing hearts and decreased inotropic responses to beta-agonist stimulation.[4]

Heart Rate

Because of compensatory changes in stroke volume, changes in heart rate do not greatly alter cardiac output when cardiac function is normal. Nevertheless, increased heart rates are associated with increased inotropic states of the myocardium. Increases in myocardial contractility that accompany elevations in heart rate are known as the rate-treppe phe-

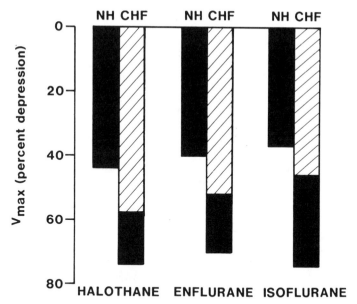

Fig. 7-2. The effect of equipotent concentrations (1 MAC) of halothane, enflurane, and isoflurane on the maximal velocity of shortening (V_{max}) of isolated papillary muscles taken from adult cats with normal hearts (NH) or experimentally-induced congestive heart failure (CHF) was studied. Depression of papillary muscle contractility (V_{max}) in muscle taken from the NH and exposed only to the anesthetic (solid bars) was less than the depression of V_{max} produced by the combination of CHF (hashed bars) and anesthetic (solid bars). (Data adapted from Kemmotsu O, Hashimoto Y, Shimosato S. The effects of fluroxene and enflurane on contractile performance of isolated papillary muscles from failing hearts. Anesthesiology 1974;40:252–60)

nomenon. In the presence of congestive heart failure, the stroke volume is relatively fixed, and cardiac output varies directly with heart rate. Tachycardia is an expected finding in the presence of congestive heart failure reflecting activation of the sympathetic nervous system.

Myocardial Hypertrophy and Dilation

Myocardial hypertrophy and dilation represent compensatory mechanisms that develop in response to chronic pressure and/or volume overloading of the heart. Chronic pressure overload and hypertrophy of the heart occur in the presence of systemic hypertension, pulmonary hypertension, and mitral and aortic stenosis. Myocardial hypertrophy helps overcome pressure loads on the heart but has limitations, since hypertrophied cardiac muscles

function at a lower inotropic states than non-hypertrophied muscles.

Chronic volume overload and dilation of the heart occurs in the presence of mitral and aortic regurgitation. Cardiac dilation leads to compensatory increases in cardiac output by the Frank-Starling principle. Increased cardiac wall tensions, however, produced by the enlarged ventricular radius are also associated with elevated myocardial oxygen requirements and decreased cardiac efficiency.

MANIFESTATIONS OF LEFT VENTRICULAR FAILURE

History

Dyspnea is the most frequent and often the earliest symptom of left ventricular failure. Dyspnea reflects interstitial pulmonary edema,

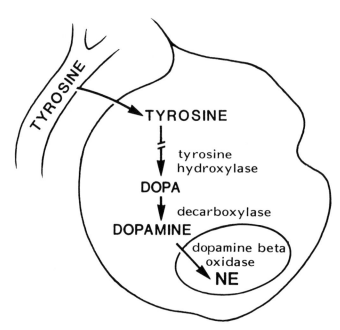

Fig. 7-3. Synthesis of the neurotransmitter norepinephrine (NE) begins with passage of tyrosine from the circulation into varicosities of postganglionic sympathetic nerve endings. A series of enzyme-controlled steps determines the conversion of tyrosine to DOPA to dopamine and eventually to NE in vesicles of the nerve endings. Tyrosine hydroxylase is the rate-limiting enzyme, and its depletion from the myocardium in the presence of chronic congestive heart failure results in decreased production of NE.

which causes increased stiffness of the lungs and thereby necessitates a greater work of breathing. Orthopnea is exaggerated dyspnea that develops when patients assume a supine position. This reflects mobilization of fluid from previously dependent areas and inability of the failing left ventricle to handle this increased intravascular fluid volume. Cough associated with orthopnea is differentiated from that due to chronic bronchitis by the fact that the latter is more productive of sputum. Insomnia and unexplained fatigue may also be due to left ventricular failure. Indeed, the hallmark of decreased cardiac reserve and low cardiac output is fatigue at rest or with minimal exertion.

Physical Examination

In the presence of left ventricular failure, there are compensatory increases in sympathetic nervous system activity, which manifest as resting tachycardia and peripheral vasoconstriction. Unexplained resting tachycardia in the preoperative period should suggest congestive heart failure, particularly if patients are elderly or are known to have co-existing heart disease. Vasoconstriction helps maintain blood pressure and flow to the brain and heart despite reductions in cardiac output. Blood flow to the kidneys, splanchnic viscera, and skeletal muscles is reduced by vasoconstriction; renal blood flow may be decreased to 25 percent of normal. Decreased renal blood flow can manifest as increased blood urea nitrogen concentrations and oliguria.

A prominent physical finding of left ventricular failure is the detection of rales during auscultation of the chest. Rales may be confined to the bases of the lungs when congestive heart failure is mild. Tachypnea and accentuation of the pulmonary component of the second heart sound are early indications of interstitial pulmonary edema. A third heart sound (ventricular diastolic gallop) indicates significant left ventricular dysfunction and may be the first sign of serious heart disease or congestive heart failure. This sound is due to blood entering and distending a relatively noncompliant left ventricle. A fourth heart sound (atrial gallop) is often associated with ventricular hypertrophy and does not necessarily signify the presence of heart disease.

Chest Radiograph

The earliest radiographic sign of left ventricular failure and associated pulmonary venous hypertension is evidence of distention of the pulmonary veins in the upper lobes of the lung. Interstitial pulmonary edema appears as thickening of intralobular septa (Kerley's lines) due to increased venous pressure, and as perivascular edema, which manifests on radiographs of the chest as both a hilar and perihilar haze. In later stages of congestive heart failure, alveolar pulmonary edema produces large homogeneous densities in the lungs. These densities often manifest as a central distribution, resulting in a "butterfly" appearance.

Radiographic changes of pulmonary congestion may lag behind acute elevations of left atrial pressure by up to 12 hours. Likewise, radiographic patterns of pulmonary congestion may persist for 1 day to 4 days after normalization of cardiac filling pressures.

MANIFESTATIONS OF RIGHT VENTRICULAR FAILURE

Venous Congestion

The hallmark of right ventricular failure is venous congestion, which is best appreciated by examination of the jugular veins. For example, distention of the external jugular veins above the clavicles of patients in the sitting position suggests the presence of right ventricular failure. With inspiration, the intrathoracic negative pressure increases such that venous return is enhanced and jugular venous pressure falls. If the right ventricle is failing, however, any increased venous return causes a further rise rather than the normal fall in jugular venous pressure with inspiration. Therefore, distention of the neck veins may increase with inspiration (Kussmaul's sign). A similar pattern may be observed in the presence of cardiac tamponade.

Edema and Organ Involvement

Pitting dependent edema, particularly of the ankles, is an early manifestation of right ventricular failure. The liver also becomes engorged. Rapid enlargement distends the liver against its capsule and produces right upper quadrant pain. Moderate congestion is associated with abnormal liver function tests, including elevation of plasma concentrations of bilirubin and transaminase enzymes. Severe liver engorgement may be associated with prolonged prothrombin times. Ascites is a late manifestation of right ventricular failure and is most likely to occur in patients with heart failure due to constrictive pericarditis or tricuspid stenosis.

TREATMENT OF CONGESTIVE HEART FAILURE

Pharmacologic treatment of congestive heart failure is with digitalis preparations plus diuretics. Vasodilator drugs can also be used to improve cardiac output in the presence of acute and chronic congestive heart failure.[5,6]

Digitalis

Digitalis is the single most important drug for increasing myocardial contractility and cardiac output in patients with congestive heart failure. The mechanism of positive inotropic effects produced by digitalis includes direct effects on the heart, which modify its mechanical and electrical activity, and indirect effects due to reflex alterations in autonomic nervous system activity. At the heart, digitalis inhibits the sodium pump, which increases intracellular concentrations of calcium and improves contractility of myocardial fibrils. Enhanced parasympathetic activity produced by therapeutic concentrations of digitalis is useful in slowing rapid heart rates, especially in patients with atrial fibrillation. Several preparations of digitalis are available, but the most frequently used is digoxin (Table 7-1).

It is important to remember that digoxin is excreted by the kidneys. Renal elimination of digoxin parallels creatinine clearance. Patients with normal renal function excrete about 40 percent of the digoxin administered. Therefore, daily doses of digoxin should be adjusted to replace that which is eliminated by the kidneys. Sensitivity to digoxin can be increased in the perioperative period if there are associated decreases in renal function.

PROPHYLACTIC USE OF DIGITALIS

Prophylactic administration of digitalis to patients scheduled for elective operations without evidence of congestive heart failure is controversial. The disadvantage of such prophylaxis is administration of a drug with a small therapeutic-to-toxic dose difference to patients with no clinical indication for the drug. Furthermore, differentiation of anesthetic-induced cardiac dysrhythmias from those due to digitalis toxicity may be difficult.[7] Indeed, such events as increases in sympathetic nervous system activity, decreases in plasma potassium concentrations, and reductions in renal function are likely to occur intraoperatively and thus enhance the chances of increased pharmacologic effects from circulating digitalis. Despite these theoretical disadvantages, there is evidence that patients with limited cardiac reserve may benefit from prophylactic administration of digitalis. For example, preoperative administration of oral digoxin (0.75 mg in divided doses the day before

TABLE 7-1. Characteristics of Frequently Used Digitalis Preparations

Description	Digoxin	Digitoxin
Absorption from the gastrointestinal tract	Good	Excellent
Onset of action after intravenous administration (minutes)	5–30	30–120
Peak effect (hours)	1.5–5	4–12
Elimination half-time (hours)	31–33	120–168
Route of elimination	Renal	Hepatic
Average digitalizing dose (mg)		
Intravenous	0.5–1	0.8–1.2
Oral	0.75–1.5	0.8–1.2
Average daily maintenance dose (oral, mg)	0.125–0.5	0.05–0.2
Therapeutic plasma concentrations $(ng \cdot ml^{-1})$	0.5–2	10–35

surgery and 0.25 mg before the induction of anesthesia) reduces the incidence of atrial fibrillation in geriatric patients undergoing thoracic or abdominal surgery.[8] Prophylactic digoxin also reduces evidence of impaired cardiac function in patients with coronary artery disease recovering from anesthesia (Fig. 7-4).[9] For these reasons, it may be reasonable to conclude that beneficial effects of prophylactic digitalis administered to selected patients in the preoperative period outweighs any potential risks of digitalis toxicity. Certainly, there are no data to support discontinuing digitalis preoperatively, especially if the drug is being administered for control of heart rate.

DIGITALIS TOXICITY

Digitalis toxicity is always a hazard in patients being treated with this drug. In the preoperative period, the possibility of digitalis toxicity should be considered when patients complain of anorexia or nausea. Digitalis toxicity should be particularly suspect in the presence of hypokalemia.

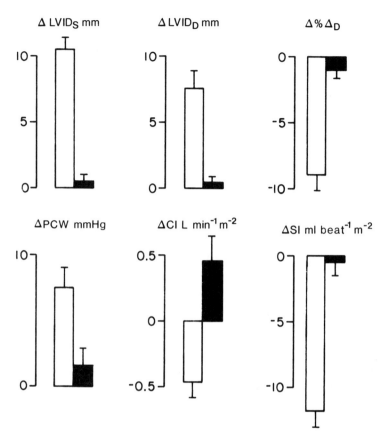

Fig. 7-4. M-mode echocardiograms and systemic hemodynamics were measured in patients with coronary artery disease and receiving intravenous digoxin (10 μg·kg^{-1}) 48, 24, and 3 hours before surgery (solid bars) or not receiving digoxin (clear bars). Values are differences in preoperative and postoperative measurements. Postoperatively, there were significant differences among groups with respect to left ventricular dimension (LVID), pulmonary capillary wedge pressure (PCW), cardiac index (CI) and stroke index (SI). In these patients with coronary artery disease, prophylactic preoperative intravenous digoxin attenuates postoperative cardiac dysfunction. (Redrawn from Pinaud MLJ, Blanloeil YAG, Souron RJ. Preoperative prophylactic digitalization of patients with coronary artery disease—a randomized echocardiographic and hemodynamic study. Anesth Analg 1983;62:865–9. Reprinted with permission from IARS.)

Cardiac Manifestations of Digitalis Toxicity. Cardiac dysrhythmias are the first evidence of digitalis toxicity in about one-third of patients. Although no specific cardiac dysrhythmia is pathognomonic for digitalis toxicity, ventricular premature beats (particularly bigeminal) and various forms of atrioventricular heart block are common. Depression of ST segments and T-waves on the electrocardiogram are nonspecific changes that do not necessarily indicate digitalis toxicity. Ventricular fibrillation is the most frequent cause of death from digitalis toxicity.

Plasma Digitalis Concentrations. The wide range of overlap between therapeutic and toxic plasma concentrations of digitalis preparations has cast doubt on the usefulness of plasma concentrations as the sole indicator of digitalis toxicity (Table 7-1). Nevertheless, plasma digoxin concentrations above 3 ng·ml^{-1} usually reflect toxic levels of drug.[10]

Treatment of Digitalis-Induced Cardiac Dysrhythmias. Treatment of digitalis toxicity includes correction of predisposing events (hypokalemia, arterial hypoxemia), administration of drugs (lidocaine, pheyntoin, atropine) to treat cardiac dysrhythmias, and insertion of a temporary transvenous cardiac pacemaker if complete heart block is present.[11] Potassium decreases binding of digitalis to cardiac tissue and thus directly antagonizes cardiotoxic effects of these drugs. Conversely, potassium will intensify digitalis-induced heart block and depress automaticity of ectopic pacemakers in the ventricle leading to complete heart block, emphasizing the importance of measuring plasma potassium concentrations before administration of supplemental potassium. If renal function is normal and heart block is not present, it is acceptable to administer 0.025 $mEq \cdot kg^{-1}$ to 0.05 $mEq \cdot kg^{-1}$ of potassium intravenously to suppress life-threatening cardiac dysrhythmias associated with digitalis toxicity.

Lidocaine 0.5 $mg \cdot kg^{-1}$ to 1 $mg \cdot kg^{-1}$ administered intravenously is useful as the initial treatment of digitalis-induced ventricular irritability[7] that is not accompanied by hypokalemia. Therapeutic plasma concentrations of lidocaine suppress ectopic ventricular cardiac pacemakers without affecting myocardial contractility or prolonging conduction of cardiac impulses through the atrioventricular node. Lidocaine is not highly effective in management of digitalis-induced supraventricular dysrhythmias. For treatment of these cardiac dysrhythmias, the drug of choice is phenytoin administered intravenously at a rate of 20 $mg \cdot min^{-1}$ until cardiac dysrhythmias disappear or a total dose of 1,000 mg is reached.[7] Atropine can be used to increase heart rate by offsetting excessive parasympathetic nervous system activity produced by toxic plasma concentrations of digitalis. Propranolol is effective in suppressing increased cardiac automaticity produced by digitalis toxicity, but its tendency to slow conduction of cardiac impulses through the atrioventricular node limits its usefulness when conduction block is present. When heart rate remains slow despite appropriate drug therapy, it may be necessary to insert a temporary transvenous cardiac pacemaker.

Life-threatening digitalis toxicity can be treated by administering antibodies (Fab fragments) to the drug, thus decreasing plasma concentrations of digitalis available to attach to cardiac cell membranes.[12] External electrical cardioversion must be used with caution to treat digitalis-induced supraventricular cardiac dysrhythmias as even more severe cardiac dysrhythmias, including ventricular fibrillation, have occurred following this mode of therapy in the presence of digitalis toxicity.[13]

Diuretics

Diuretics are effective in the treatment of congestive heart failure by virtue of facilitating excretion of excess total body water by the kidneys. Thiazide diuretics (chlorothiazide, hydrochlorothiazide) produce diuretic effects by inhibiting reabsorption of sodium and chloride in distal convoluted renal tubules. These drugs also cause increased renal tubular secretion and subsequent urinary excretion of potassium. Indeed, the most frequent adverse side effect of thiazide diuretic therapy is hypokalemia, which is often associated with hypochloremic alkalosis. These changes are particularly undesirable in patients who are also receiving digitalis preparations, as the likelihood of digitalis toxicity is increased by hypokalemia and metabolic alkalosis. Acute hypovolemia produced by diuretic-induced diuresis may be reflected by orthostatic hypotension.

Loop diuretics (furosemide, ethacrynic acid) act by inhibition of sodium reabsorption at the loop of Henle. Adverse effects produced by loop diuretics are similar to those produced by thiazide diuretics. Spironolactone and triamterene are potassium-sparing diuretics that work by inhibiting effects of aldosterone on distal renal tubules. These drugs counter kaliuretic effects of thiazide and loop diuretics and, therefore, are useful in combination with potassium-losing diuretics.

Vasodilators

Peripheral vasodilating drugs may be useful for the management of acute and chronic congestive heart failure.[5] Drugs that have been successfully used include nitroprusside, nitroglycerin, trimethaphan, phentolamine, and hydralazine. Under most circumstances, administration of these drugs requires devices to regulate their continuous intravenous infusion. Furthermore, invasive monitoring, including arterial and pulmonary artery catheters, is essential to determine changes in cardiac filling pressures, stroke volume, and systemic and pulmonary vascular resistance produced by the drug. Vasodilators increase cardiac output by reducing impedance to the forward ejection of ventricular stroke volume. As a result, forward stroke volume produced by each ventricular contraction is increased and cardiac output is elevated.

Vasodilator therapy is particularly effective in treating congestive heart failure due to the sudden onset of mechanical abnormalities. Examples of mechanical lesions include (1) acute mitral regurgitation from myocardial infarctions, ruptured chordae tendineae, or infective endocarditis; (2) acute aortic regurgitation from dissection of the aorta or infective endocarditis; and (3) acute perforation of the ventricular septum secondary to myocardial infarctions. The limiting factor in the treatment of acute congestive heart failure with vasodilator drugs is a fall in systemic blood pressure. It is unlikely that treatment with vasodilator drugs can be continued if mean arterial pressure decreases more than 20 percent below the predrug value.

SURGERY IN THE PRESENCE OF CONGESTIVE HEART FAILURE

Elective operations should not be performed in patients who manifest evidence of congestive heart failure. In fact, presence of congestive heart failure has been shown to be the single most important factor for predicting postoperative cardiac morbidity.[1] If surgery cannot be deferred, drugs and techniques chosen to provide anesthesia must be selected with the goal of optimizing cardiac output.

General Anesthesia

Ketamine is a useful drug for induction of anesthesia in the presence of congestive heart failure. Use of volatile anesthetics for maintenance of anesthesia is questionable in view of the dose-dependent cardiac depressant effects produced by these drugs. Cardiac depression produced by the combined effects of volatile anesthetics and congestive heart failure is greater than that produced by anesthetics in the absence of congestive heart failure (Fig. 7-2).[2] Opioids or benzodiazepines are attractive choices, since they do not produce direct myocardial depression. It must be remembered, however, that the addition of nitrous oxide to opioids or the combination of benzodiazepines and opioids is associated with significant depression of cardiac output and blood pressure.[14,15] Conversely, nitrous oxide added to diazepam does not produce cardiac depression.[16] In the presence of severe congestive heart failure, use of opioids as the only drug for maintenance of anesthesia may be justified. Positive-pressure ventilation of the lungs may be beneficial by decreasing pulmonary congestion and improving arterial oxygenation. Monitoring is adjusted to the complexity of the operation. Invasive monitoring of arterial pressures, as well as cardiac filling pressures, is justified when major operations are necessary in the presence of congestive heart failure. Support of the cardiac output with drugs such as dopamine or dobutamine may be necessary in the perioperative period.

Drug interactions in patients treated with digitalis should be anticipated. For example, succinylcholine, or any other drug that can abruptly increase parasympathetic nervous system activity, could theoretically have additive effects with digitalis. Nevertheless, clinical experience does not support the occurrence of an increased incidence of cardiac dysrhythmias in patients treated with digitalis and receiving succinylcholine.[17] Sympathomimetics with beta-adrenergic agonist effects, as well as pancuronium, may increase the likelihood of cardiac dysrhythmias in patients being treated with digitalis. Calcium may accentuate the effects of previously therapeutic plasma concentrations of digitalis. Hyperventilation of the lungs, which acutely lowers plasma concentrations of potassium, must be avoided in patients treated with digitalis. Although of questionable clinical significance, simultaneous administration of oral antacids and digitalis may decrease gastrointestinal absorption of digitalis.[18]

Regional Anesthesia

Regional anesthesia is an acceptable selection to provide anesthesia for peripheral operations in the presence of congestive heart failure. In fact, mild reductions in systemic vascular resistance secondary to peripheral sympathetic nervous system blockade may permit increased cardiac output. Nevertheless, reductions in systemic vascular resistance produced by epidural or subarachnoid anesthetics are not easy to control. Therefore, regional anesthesia should probably not be selected over general anesthesia if the only reason is the belief that regional blocks will reliably improve cardiac output.

SURGERY IN THE PRESENCE OF DIGITALIS TOXICITY

Proceeding with anesthesia and surgery in the presence of suspected or confirmed digitalis toxicity depends entirely on the urgency of the surgery. Certainly elective operations should be delayed until digitalis toxicity subsides. When the surgical disease is life-threatening, it will be necessary to proceed with the operative procedure despite digitalis toxicity. In this situation, events or drugs, such as ketamine, that stimulate the autonomic nervous system should be avoided. Halothane (and by inference other volatile anesthetics) has been shown to antagonize cardiac effects of digitalis in animals.[19] This suggests that volatile anesthetics would be reasonable choices in the presence of digitalis toxicity. Hyperventilation of the lungs, which can acutely lower plasma

potassium concentrations, must be avoided. Drugs to treat digitalis-induced cardiac dysrhythmias must be readily available (see the section Treatment of Digitalis-induced Cardiac Dysrhythmias).

REFERENCES

1. Goldman L, Caldera DL, Nussbaum SR, et al. Multifactorial index of cardiac risk in noncardiac surgical procedures. N Engl J Med 1977;297:845–50
2. Kemmotsu O, Hashimoto Y, Shimosato S. The effects of fluroxene and enflurane on contractile performance of isolated papillary muscles from failing hearts. Anesthesiology 1974;40:252–60
3. Francis GS, Goldsmith SR, Ziesche SM, Cohn JN. Response of plasma norepinephrine and epinephrine to dynamic exercise in patients with congestive heart failure. Am J Cardiol 1982;49:1152–6
4. Bristox MR, Ginsburg R, Monobe W, et al. Decreased catecholamine sensitivity and B-adrenergic-receptor density in failing human hearts. N Engl J Med 1982;307:205–11
5. Rubin SA, Swan HJC. Vasodilator therapy for heart failure. Concepts, applications, and challenges. JAMA 1981;245:761–3
6. Sodums MT, Walsh RA, O'Rourke RA. Digitalis in heart failure. Farewell to the foxglove? JAMA 1981;246:158–60
7. Chung DC. Anesthetic problems associated with the treatment of cardiovascular disease. I. Digitalis toxicity. Can Anaesth Soc J 1981;28:6–16
8. Chee TP, Prakash NS, Desser KB, Benchimol A. Postoperative supraventricular arrhythmias and the role of prophylactic digoxin in cardiac surgery. Am Heart J 1982;104:974–7
9. Pinaud MLJ, Blanloeil YAG, Souron RJ. Preoperative prophylactic digitalization of patients with coronary artery disease—a randomized echocardiographic and hemodynamic study. Anesth Analg 1983;62:865–9
10. Doherty JA. How and when to use digitalis serum levels. JAMA 1978;239:2594–6
11. Mason DT, Zelis R, Lee G, et al. Currrent concepts and treatment of digitalis toxicity. Am J Cardiol 1971;27:546–59
12. Ochs HR, Smith TW. Reversal of advanced digitoxin toxicity and modification of pharmacokinetics by specific antibodies and Fab fragments. J Clin Invest 1977;60:1303–13

13. Lown B. Electrical reversion of cardiac arrhythmias. Br Heart J 1967;29:469–89

14. Stoelting RK, Gibbs PS. Hemodynamic effects of morphine and morphine-nitrous oxide in valvular heart disease and coronary artery disease. Anesthesiology 1973;38:45–52

15. Tomicheck RC, Rosow CE, Philbin DM, et al. Diazepam-fentanyl interaction-hemodynamic and hormonal effects in coronary artery surgery. Anesth Analg 1983;62:881–4

16. McCammon RL, Hilgenberg JC, Stoelting RK. Hemodynamic effects of diazepam and diazepam-nitrous oxide in patients with coronary artery disease. Anesth Analg 1980;59:438–41

17. Bartolone RS, Rao TLK. Dysrhythmias following muscle relaxant administration in patients receiving digitalis. Anesthesiology 1983;58:567–9.

18. Brown DD, Juhl RP. Decreased bioavailability of digoxin due to antacids and kaolin-pectin. N Engl J Med 1976;295:1034–7

19. Morrow DH, Townley NT. Anesthesia and digitalis toxicity: An experimental study. Anesth Analg 1964;43:510–19

8

Cardiomyopathies

Cardiomyopathies refer to disorders that directly affect one or both cardiac ventricles in a diffuse fashion that may result in congestive heart failure.[1] Congestive heart failure in these patients often cannot be attributed to coronary artery disease, valvular heart disease, pericardial disease or hypertension. Classification of cardiomyopathies is as dilated (congestive), nondilated (restrictive), and hypertrophic (Table 8-1). This classification is based principally on the left ventricular ejection fraction and ventricular volume as depicted by echocardiography or radionuclide ventriculography.

DILATED CARDIOMYOPATHY

Dilated cardiomyopathy is characterized by profound reductions in left ventricular ejection fractions (often less than 0.4) and left ventricular dilation (Table 8-1). Cardiac output may be normal or low, and left atrial pressures may be normal or high. Left ventricular failure exists in most patients at some time and biventricular failure develops in many. Ventricular dilation may be so marked that functional mitral and/or tricuspid regurgitation occurs.

Common electrocardiographic patterns include left bundle branch block and evidence of left ventricular hypertrophy. ST-segment and T-wave abnormalities are invariably present. Premature ventricular beats or atrial fibrillation are common. Unexplained Q-waves mimic previous myocardial infarctions. Radiographs of the chest often show evidence of pulmonary hypertension and biventricular cardiac enlargement.

Mural thrombi are likely to form in dilated and hypokinetic chambers. Indeed, there is a high incidence of systemic embolization in these patients.

The course of dilated cardiomyopathy is characterized by intermittent congestive heart failure and systemic embolism. Angina pectoris may be prominent. Prognosis is poor with only 25 percent to 40 percent of patients surviving 5 years after angiographic diagnosis. Sudden death is presumed to reflect acute cardiac dysrhythmias. The most common cause of death, however, is irreversible congestive heart failure.

Etiology

Multiple myocardial infarctions due to diffuse coronary artery disease are the most common cause of dilated cardiomyopathy.[1] There is a striking association of this cardiomyopathy with chronic alcohol abuse. Dilated cardiomyopathy may occur in peripartum pa-

149

TABLE 8-1.   Classification and Hemodynamic Characteristics of Cardiomyopathies

Type of Cardiomyopathy	Left Ventricular Ejection Fraction	Ventricular Volume	Ventricular Filling Pressures	Stroke Volume
Dilated (congestive) cardiomyopathy	Marked decrease	Marked increase	Normal to increased	Normal to decreased
Nondilated (restrictive) cardiomyopathy	Normal to decreased	Normal to decreased	Marked increase	Normal to decreased
Hypertrophic cardiomyopathy	Marked increase	Marked decrease	Normal to increased	Normal to increased

tients most often manifesting 1 week to 6 weeks after delivery. Collagen vascular diseases and sarcoidosis have been associated with dilated cardiomyopathy. On occasion, cancer chemotherapeutic drugs may produce this type of cardiomyopathy (see Chapter 30).[2] Many cases of dilated cardiomyopathy are idiopathic, but a viral etiology is suggested by the frequent occurrence of a febrile-illness preceding the onset of cardiac dysfunction.

Treatment

Treatment of congestive heart failure due to this form of cardiomyopathy is with digitalis and diuretics. If the failure is intractable, administration of peripheral vasodilating drugs may be considered. Corticosteroids may be of some benefit when congestive cardiomyopathy is due to collagen vascular diseases or sarcoidosis. Anticoagulant therapy may be instituted because of the high incidence of systemic embolism, although the benefits of this prophylactic therapy have not been documented.[1] Beta-adrenergic antagonist drugs are not recommended since these drugs could precipitate congestive heart failure.

Management of Anesthesia

Goals during the management of anesthesia in patients with congestive cardiomyopathy include (1) avoidance of drug-induced myocardial depression, (2) maintenance of normovolemia, and (3) prevention of increases in ventricular afterload. Theoretically, the vasodilating properties of enflurane or isoflurane would be desirable, but the ability of these drugs to produce direct myocardial depression must be considered. Halothane probably should not be selected because of its myocardial depressant properties. Ketamine may further reduce cardiac output if activation of the sympathetic nervous system and increased systemic vascular resistance accompany administration of this drug. A technique using opioids would seem logical for minimizing the likelihood of anesthetic-induced myocardial depression. If nitrous oxide is included, the interaction between this drug and opioids, as well as between benzodiazepines and opioids, to produce unexpected myocardial depression must be appreciated. Low doses of volatile anesthetics can be added to inspired gases should surgical stimulation produce undesirable increases in heart rate or systemic vascular resistance. Beta-adrenergic antagonist drugs to slow the heart rate, like volatile anesthetics, must be used with caution, in view of the potential for these drugs to produce myocardial depression. Skeletal muscle paralysis is often provided with nondepolarizing muscle relaxants that have minimal cardiovascular effects. Intravenous infusion of crystalloid solutions or blood should be guided by cardiac filling pressures, to reduce the likelihood of volume overload. A pulmonary artery catheter, by permitting determination of cardiac output and cardiac filling pressures, facilitates early recognition of the need for inotropic support or administration of peripheral vasodilating drugs. Intraoperative hypotension is best treated with drugs, such as ephedrine, which provide some degree of beta-adrenergic stimulation. Conversely, predominant alpha-adrenergic stimulation, as produced by phenylephrine, could produce adverse increases in ventricular afterload due to elevation of systemic vascular resistance.

Regional anesthesia may be an attractive alternative to general anesthesia in selected patients with dilated cardiomyopathy.[3] For example, epidural anesthesia produces changes in preload and afterload that mimic pharmacologic goals in treatment of this disease. Nevertheless, clinical experience is limited and caution is indicated for avoiding an abrupt onset of a high blockade of the sympathetic nervous system.

NONDILATED CARDIOMYOPATHY

Nondilated cardiomyopathy resembles constrictive pericarditis being characterized by marked increases in ventricular filling pressures, often in association with reductions in cardiac output (Table 8-1). Signs of right heart failure (hepatosplenomegaly and ascites) predominate. The myocardium is noncompliant and diastolic filling is impeded, reflecting infiltration of the myocardium by abnormal material. Indeed, nondilated cardiomyopathy most often results from such infiltrative diseases as amyloidosis, hemochromatosis or glycogen storage diseases. There is no effective treatment for nondilated cardiomyopathy, and death is usually due to cardiac dysrhythmias or irreversible congestive heart failure. Management of anesthesia invokes the same principles as outlined for patients with cardiac tamponade (see Chapter 10).

HYPERTROPHIC CARDIOMYOPATHY

Hypertrophic cardiomyopathy (also known as idiopathic hypertrophic subaortic stenosis or asymmetric septal hypertrophy) is characterized by obstruction to left ventricular outflow produced by an asymmetric hypertrophy of intraventricular septal muscle. In addition, obstruction to ejection of left ventricular stroke volume can be accentuated by the septal leaflet of the mitral valve, which is pulled into the outflow tract during rapid systolic ejection.

Echocardiography or cardiac catheterization usually establishes the diagnosis of hypertrophic cardiomyopathy. Echocardiography should identify an interventricular septum that is more than 1.3 times as thick as the posterior left ventricular wall, a decreased luminal diameter of the left ventricular outflow tract, and systolic anterior motion of the septal leaflet of the mitral valve. Cardiac catheterization may disclose a pressure gradient within the left ventricular outflow tract with a normal aortic valve pressure gradient. Provocative measures such as the Valsalva maneuver may be required to elicit evidence of left ventricular outflow obstruction during echocardiography or cardiac catheterization, emphasizing the dynamic nature of this obstruction. In some patients, cardiac catheterization reveals obliteration of the left ventricular cavity or evidence of mitral regurgitation.

Increased left ventricular muscle mass is necessary to overcome obstruction to ejection of the stroke volume. This left ventricular hypertrophy may be so massive that the volume of the left ventricular chamber is reduced. Despite these adverse changes, the stroke volume remains normal due to the hypercontractile state of the myocardium (Table 8-1). Indeed, left ventricular ejection fractions may approach 80 percent.

Hypertrophic cardiomyopathy is often familial, being transmitted as an autosomal dominant characteristic.[4] The age distribution at diagnosis of this disease is bimodal with a peak incidence early in the fifth decade and a second peak early in the seventh decade. Most geriatric patients are female. Sporadic cases of hypertrophic cardiomyopathy may be related to chronic hypertension or to abnormal responses by cardiac muscle to prolonged catecholamine stimulation. It has been suggested that hypertrophic cardiomyopathy should be considered in otherwise asymptomatic geriatric patients in whom systolic murmurs develop during long-standing hypertension.[5] Furthermore, previously unrecognized hypertrophic cardiomyopathy may manifest intraoperatively as hypotension and sudden increases in the intensity of systolic murmurs typically in association with acute hemorrhage or drug-induced vasodilation.[6,7]

The major symptoms of hypertrophic cardiomyopathy are syncope, angina pectoris, and congestive heart failure. Marked left ventricular hypertrophy makes these patients particularly vulnerable to myocardial ischemia, especially when subendocardial blood flow is reduced due to excessive pressures in the left ventricle. Furthermore, the incidence of coronary artery disease is increased in these patients and this may subsequently increase the risk of anesthesia and surgery.[8] Sudden death is the most unpredictable and devastating complication of hypertrophic cardiomyopathy and occurs most commonly in patients 10 years to 30 years of age.[4] Cardiac dysrhythmias, especially ventricular tachycardia, are the most likely causes of sudden death.

The electrocardiogram often shows changes consistent with left ventricle hypertrophy. Nevertheless, as many as 15 percent of patients manifest no evidence of left ventricular hypertrophy on the electrocardiogram despite increased cardiac muscle mass. Q-waves seen on the electrocardiogram mimic those seen in patients with prior myocardial infarctions. However, Q-waves in patients with hypertrophic cardiomyopathy are most likely due to septal hypertrophy. Ventricular premature beats and atrial fibrillation are common in these patients.

Treatment

Treatment of hypertrophic cardiomyopathy is directed at relieving the obstruction, which can be either intermittent or fixed, to ejection of the left ventricular stroke volume. The crucial concept in the treatment of these patients is the realization that the obstruction is dynamic. For example, drugs or events that alter myocardial contractility, preload, and af-

TABLE 8-2. Hypertrophic Cardiomyopathy and Obstruction to Ejection of Left Ventricular Stroke Volume

Factors that Increase Obstruction
  Increased myocardial contractility
    Sympathetic nervous system stimulation
      (drugs or noxious stimulatioon)
    Digitalis
    Tachycardia
  Decreased preload
    Decreased intravascular fluid volume
    Vasodilator drugs (nitroprusside)
  Decreased afterload
    Decreased systemic vascular resistance
      (hypotension)
    Vasodilator drugs (nitroprusside)

Factors that Decrease Obstruction
  Decreased myocardial contractility
    Beta-adrenergic blockade (propranolol)
    Volatile anesthetics (halothane)
  Increased preload
    Increased intravascular fluid volume
    Bradycardia
  Increased afterload
    Alpha-adrenergic stimulation (phenylephrine)
    Increased intravascular fluid volume

terload can influence the magnitude of obstruction to left ventricular outflow (Table 8-2).

Reductions in heart rate and myocardial contractility produced by beta-adrenergic antagonist drugs such as propranolol are useful for reducing obstruction to left ventricular outflow and improving stroke volume. Amiodarone may reduce the likelihood of cardiac dysrhythmias in these patients. Diuretics could exacerbate outflow obstruction by decreasing preload but in reality reduce symptoms of pulmonary congestion when administered in combination with beta-adrenergic antagonist drugs or verapamil. Chronic atrial fibrillation represents a condition where drugs such as verapamil may be administered to these patients without exacerbation of obstruction to left ventricular ejection.

Surgical therapy of hypertrophic cardiomyopathy is most often septal myectomy in which 2 g to 5 g of the basal septum is resected through an aortotomy. Alternatively, a septal myotomy without removal of tissue may be performed. The objective of surgical therapy is relief of the obstruction to left ventricular ejection with concomitant reductions in left ventricular systolic pressures. Mortality may approach 8 percent, and for this reason surgical therapy is usually reserved for symptomatic patients with outflow gradients that exceed 50 mmHg.[4] Mitral valve replacement may be indicated in patients who develop mitral regurgitation due to intrinsic abnormality of the mitral valve.

Management of Anesthesia

Management of anesthesia in patients with hypertrophic cardiomyopathy is directed towards minimizing the pressure gradient across the left ventricular outflow obstruction.[8] It must be appreciated that reductions in myocardial contractility and increases in preload and afterload will decrease the magnitude of left ventricular obstruction (Table 8-2). For example, mild cardiac depression produced by volatile anesthetics and expansion of the intravascular fluid volume will distend the left ventricle and increase stroke volume. Intraoperative events associated with increased myocardial contractility (beta-adrenergic stimulation from drugs or activation of the sympathetic nervous system by noxious surgical stimulation), reductions in preload (positive pressure ventilation of the lungs), and decreases in afterload (acute hypovolemia, drug-induced reductions in systemic vascular resistance) must be avoided, as these events increase obstruction to left ventricular ejection.

PREOPERATIVE PREPARATION

Preoperative medication should ideally reduce apprehension and associated activation of the sympathetic nervous system. Use of atropine is questionable, since increases in heart rate may reduce cardiac output. In contrast, scopolamine produces desirable sedation when used in conjunction with other central nervous system depressant drugs. Changes in heart rate are unlikely after the administration of scopolamine. Expansion of intravascular fluid volume in the preoperative period is important for maintaining intraoperative stroke volume and minimizing adverse effects of positive pressure ventilation of the lungs.

INDUCTION OF ANESTHESIA

Induction of anesthesia may be accomplished with barbiturates, benzodiazepines, or etomidate. Ketamine is not a good choice, since increases in myocardial contractility will accentuate obstruction to left ventricular outflow and reduce stroke volume. The duration of direct laryngoscopy should be brief to minimize activation of the sympathetic nervous system. Administration of volatile anesthetics before intubation of the trachea may be useful.

MAINTENANCE OF ANESTHESIA

Maintenance of anesthesia is designed to produce mild depression of myocardial contractility and at the same time preserve a normal systemic vascular resistance. Nitrous oxide, combined with volatile anesthetics such as halothane, is acceptable. Theoretically, enflurane and isoflurane would be less ideal choices than halothane, as these drugs decrease systemic vascular resistance more than halothane.[9,10] Nevertheless, enflurane has been administered to these patients without apparent detrimental effects.[8] Opioids are not likely choices, as they do not produce myocardial depression and at the same time can reduce systemic vascular resistance. Regional anesthesia is not recommended for these patients as sympathetic nervous system blockade reduces systemic vascular resistance and increases venous capacitance, which may contribute to left ventricular outflow obstruction.

Nondepolarizing muscle relaxants (metocurine, vecuronium, atracurium), which have minimal to no effect on the circulation, are useful choices for production of skeletal muscle paralysis. Pancuronium is not a good selection because of its ability to increase heart rate and myocardial contractility. Likewise, sudden reductions of systemic vascular resistance produced by d-tubocurarine are unacceptable.

Invasive monitoring of arterial and cardiac filling pressures is helpful. When intraoperative hypotension occurs due to decreases in ventricular filling or systemic vascular resistance, drugs with predominant alpha-adrenergic agonist activity, such as phenylephrine, will reliably increase blood pressure and decrease obstruction to left ventricular outflow. Drugs with beta-adrenergic agonist activity (isoproterenol, dopamine, dobutamine, ephedrine) are not recommended for treatment of hypotension, as drug-induced increases in cardiac contractility and heart rate can increase obstruction to ejection of the left ventricular stroke volume.[7] Prompt replacement of blood loss and generous intravenous fluid administration, as guided by measurement of cardiac filling pressures, is indicated to maintain intravascular fluid volume and normal blood pressures. Increased inspired concentrations of volatile anesthetics are useful for treatment of persistent hypertension. Vasodilating drugs such as nitroprusside or nitroglycerin are not good choices for lowering blood pressure, since reductions in systemic vascular resistance can increase the obstruction to left ventricular outflow.[7]

Maintenance of normal sinus rhythm is critical, as ventricular filling is dependent on left atrial contractions. Changes from sinus to junctional rhythm should be treated by reducing the inhaled concentrations of volatile anesthetics. If this dysrhythmia persists, the intravenous administration of atropine is indicated. Propranolol is useful for slowing persistently elevated heart rates. Overall, the risk of general anesthesia in these patients seems acceptable.[8]

REFERENCES

1. Johnson RA, Palacios I. Dilated cardiomyopathies of the adult. N Engl J Med 1982;307: 1051–8
2. Appelbaum FR, Strauchen JA, Craw RG, et al. Acute lethal carditis caused by high-dose combination chemotherapy: A unique clinical and pathological entity. Lancet 1976;1:56–62
3. Amaranath L, Eskandiari S, Lockrem J, Rollins M. Epidural analgesia for total hip replacement in a patient with dilated cardiomyopathy. Can Anaesth Soc J 1986;33:84–8
4. Maron BJ, Bonow RO, Canon RO, et al. Hypertrophic cardiomyopathy. Interrelations of clinical manifestations, pathophysiology and therapy. N Engl J Med 1987;316:780–90;844–51
5. Petrin TJ, Tavel ME. Idiopathic hypertrophic subaortic stenosis as observed in a large community hospital. Relation to age and history of hypertension. J Am Geriatr Soc 1979;27:43–6
6. Lanier W, Prough DS. Intraoperative diagnosis of hypertrophic obstructive cardiomyopathy. Anesthesiology 1984;60:61–3
7. Pearson J, Reves JG. Unusual cause of hypotension after coronary artery bypass grafting: Idiopathic hypertrophic subaortic stenosis. Anesthesiology 1984;60:592–4
8. Thompson RC, Liberthson RR, Lowenstein E. Perioperative anesthetic risk of noncardiac surgery in hypertrophic obstructive cardiomyopathy. JAMA 1985;254:2419–21
9. Calverley RK, Smith NT, Prys-Roberts C, et al. Cardiovascular effects of enflurane anesthesia during controlled ventilation in man. Anesth Analg 1978;57:619–28
10. Eger EI, Smith NT, Stoelting RK, et al. Cardiovascular effects of halothane in man. Anesthesiology 1970;32:396–409

9

Cor Pulmonale

Cor pulmonale is the designation for right ventricular hypertrophy and eventual cardiac dysfunction that occurs secondary to chronic pulmonary artery hypertension.[1,2] The most frequent causes of cor pulmonale are chronic bronchitis and pulmonary emphysema. Males are affected five times more often than females. About 75 percent of patients are over 50 years of age. It is estimated that 10 percent to 30 percent of patients admitted to the hospital with congestive heart failure exhibit evidence of cor pulmonale.

Prognosis for patients with cor pulmonale is determined by the pulmonary disease responsible for initiating increases in pulmonary vascular resistance. Prognosis for longevity is favorable in patients with chronic obstructive airways disease in whom arterial oxygenation can be maintained at near normal levels. Prognosis is poor in those patients in whom cor pulmonale is the result of gradual destruction of pulmonary vessels by intrinsic vascular disease or pulmonary fibrosis. These anatomic changes produce irreversible alterations in the pulmonary vasculature, resulting in fixed elevations of pulmonary vascular resistance.

PATHOPHYSIOLOGY

The normal pulmonary circulation is a highly distensible, low resistance, and low pressure system; the mean pulmonary artery pressure is typically below 20 mmHg. Furthermore, the pulmonary circulation can normally accept substantial increases in blood flow with only small changes in pulmonary artery pressures. Ultimately, however, increases in pulmonary artery pressure due to elevations in pulmonary vascular resistance are responsible for the manifestations of cor pulmonale. Pulmonary artery hypertension is considered to be moderate when mean pulmonary artery pressures exceed 35 mmHg.

Increased pulmonary vascular resistance may be due to anatomic and/or vasomotor mechanisms. Anatomic reductions in the size of the pulmonary vascular bed result from destruction of pulmonary capillaries by such disease processes as chronic obstructive airways disease, pulmonary thromboembolism, pulmonary vasculitis, and pulmonary fibrosis. Vasomotor-mediated increases in pulmonary vascular resistance are most often due to arterial hypoxemia. For example, arterial hypoxemia induces vasoconstriction of pulmonary precapillary arteries and arterioles. If this vasoconstriction is sustained, it produces hypertrophy of vascular smooth muscle and irreversible elevations of pulmonary vascular resistance. Systemic acidosis also promotes pulmonary vasoconstriction and acts synergistically with arterial hypoxemia.

155

CLINICAL MANIFESTATIONS

Clinical manifestations of cor pulmonale are often nonspecific and tend to be obscured by co-existing chronic obstructive airways disease. Increases in pulmonary artery pressures are usually associated with initial complaints of easy fatigability and chest discomfort. As right ventricular function becomes more impaired, there is increasing dyspnea during exercise, and effort-related syncope can occur. Accentuation of the pulmonic component of the second heart sound and a diastolic murmur due to incompetence of the pulmonary valve connote severe pulmonary artery hypertension. Right heart catheterization reveals elevated pressures in the pulmonary artery and normal pulmonary artery occlusion pressures. Overt right ventricular failure is evidenced by the presence of a third heart sound, elevated jugular venous pressures, hepatosplenomegaly, and peripheral dependent edema.

The rate at which right ventricular dysfunction develops depends on the magnitude of pressure increases in the pulmonary circulation and the rapidity with which these elevations occur. For example, pulmonary embolism may produce right ventricular failure, with mean pulmonary artery pressures as low as 30 mmHg. In contrast, when pulmonary hypertension develops gradually, as with chronic obstructive airways disease, and the right ventricle has time to compensate, cardiac failure rarely occurs until mean pulmonary artery pressures exceed 50 mmHg.[2]

Patients with chronic obstructive airways disease may develop acute right ventricular failure during pulmonary infections. This failure may reverse spontaneously with successful treatment of pulmonary infections, presumably reflecting a concomitant reduction of pulmonary vascular resistance.

Chest Radiography

Radiographs of the chest in the presence of cor pulmonale typically demonstrate signs of chronic obstructive airways disease and evidence of right ventricular hypertrophy. A decrease in the retrosternal space seen on the lateral projection of the radiograph is consistent with right ventricular hypertrophy. Prominent pulmonary artery shadows and decreased pulmonary vascular markings are suggestive of pulmonary hypertension. In patients with chronic obstructive airways disease, dramatic changes in heart size may characteristically occur between episodes of acute pulmonary dysfunction and recovery.

Electrocardiogram

The electrocardiogram in the presence of cor pulmonale may show signs of right atrial and ventricular hypertrophy. Right atrial hypertrophy is suggested by peaked P-waves in leads II, III, or aVF. Right axis deviation and a partial or complete right bundle branch block are often seen on the electrocardiogram when right ventricular hypertrophy is present.

TREATMENT OF COR PULMONALE

The goal in treatment of cor pulmonale is to decrease the workload of the right ventricle by decreasing pulmonary vascular resistance. This goal is best achieved by returning the arterial oxygen partial pressures, carbon dioxide partial pressures, and pH to a normal range, assuming that pulmonary artery and arteriole vasoconstriction are reversible. This assumption is likely to be valid in the presence of chronic obstructive airways disease, particularly during exacerbations caused by acute pulmonary infections. In contrast, pulmonary vascular resistance is unlikely to be responsive to treatment when anatomic occlusive lesions are responsible for pulmonary artery hypertension. Treatment of cor pulmonale includes administration of supplemental oxygen, antibiotics, bronchodilators, digitalis, and diuretics.

Oxygen

The most important initial treatment in patients with cor pulmonale is administration of supplemental oxygen designed to increase the arterial oxygen partial pressures to about 60 mmHg.[3] This degree of arterial oxygenation is sufficient to relax pulmonary arteries and arterioles and to reduce pulmonary vascular resistance, with a subsequent improvement in right ventricular function. In addition, there is usually an improvement in cerebration and a decrease in the hematocrit. Nevertheless, in some patients, the entire stimulus to ventilation is mediated by an hypoxic drive from the carotid bodies. In these patients, an increase in the arterial oxygen partial pressures above 50 mmHg to 60 mmHg can suppress the hypoxic drive to ventilation and lead to hypoventilation. Indeed, if respiratory acidosis worsens in the presence of appropriate oxygen therapy, it will be necessary to institute mechanical support of ventilation. An alternative to mechanical ventilation of the lungs is the continuous intravenous infusion of doxapram (2 mg·min^{-1} to 3 mg·min^{-1}), which serves to maintain ventilation and thus permit the continued administration of supplemental oxygen.[4]

Antibiotics

Prompt treatment with antibiotics will minimize additional increases in pulmonary vascular resistance associated with acute pulmonary infections. The patient's sputum should be cultured so as to determine the causative organism and its sensitivity to specific antibiotics. Treatment with antibiotics, however, should not be delayed for the results of these studies. Invading organisms are most often strains of *Hemophilus* or pneumococcus, which are usually sensitive to ampicillin. A cephalosporin antibiotic is an acceptable alternative to treatment with ampicillin.

Bronchodilators

Any reversible component of bronchoconstriction can be treated with aminophylline or beta-adrenergic agonist drugs such as terbutaline or albuterol. Doses of aminophylline may require careful adjustment to compensate for decreased hepatic clearance of this drug in the presence of congestive heart failure.

Digitalis

A digitalis preparation will improve right and left ventricular function when congestive heart failure is present. Digitalis, however, must be used cautiously, since the risk of drug toxicity is increased in the presence of arterial hypoxemia, acidosis, and electrolyte imbalances common in patients with cor pulmonale.

Diuretics

Diuretics offer significant benefit in treating congestive heart failure due to increased pulmonary vascular resistance.[5] For example, excess fluid accumulation in the lungs interferes with optimal matching of alveolar ventilation to pulmonary blood flow. In addition, this excess fluid can contribute to the elevation in pulmonary vascular resistance.

Careful monitoring of plasma electrolyte concentrations during treatment with diuretics is important. For example, hypokalemia and metabolic alkalosis are potential complications of therapy with diuretics. Severe metabolic alkalosis is undesirable, as this change depresses the effectiveness of carbon dioxide as a ventilatory stimulant. Furthermore, metabolic alkalosis, associated with hypochloremia, impairs renal excretion of bicarbonate, which can aggravate co-existing acid-base disturbances. Diuretic-induced depletion of intravascular fluid volume can produce undesirable reductions in cardiac output.

MANAGEMENT OF ANESTHESIA

It is mandatory that elective operations in patients with cor pulmonale not be performed until reversible components of co-existing chronic obstructive airways disease is treated. Preoperative preparation is directed toward (1) elimination and control of acute and/or chronic pulmonary infections, (2) reversal of bronchospasm, (3) improvement of secretion clearance, (4) expansion of collapsed or poorly ventilated alveoli, (5) hydration, and (6) correction of electrolyte imbalance. Arterial blood gases and pH should be determined to provide guidelines for management of the patient in the intraoperative and postoperative period.

Preoperative Medication

Preoperative medication should avoid drugs likely to produce depression of ventilation. Although opioids are the most potent in this regard, any medication that produces sedation can result in depression of ventilation. Often, a preoperative interview will serve to allay the patient's apprehension and eliminate the need for pharmacologic premedication.

Depressant effects of anticholinergic drugs on mucociliary activity and possible impairment of clearance of secretions often outweigh the advantages of including these drugs as part of the preoperative medication. If it is concluded that anticholinergic drugs are necessary, an alternative is to administer these drugs intravenously just before induction of anesthesia.

Induction of Anesthesia

Induction of anesthesia is most often accomplished with an intravenous administration of barbiturates, benzodiazepines, or etom-idate. An adequate depth of anesthesia should be present before placement of a tube in the trachea, as this stimulus in lightly anesthetized patients can elicit reflex bronchospasm. Furthermore, elevations in systemic and pulmonary vascular resistance may accompany intubation of the trachea when the concentration of anesthetic drugs is minimal.[6]

Maintenance of Anesthesia

Maintenance of anesthesia is usually with combinations of nitrous oxide and volatile drugs or short-acting opioids. Enflurane and isoflurane are as effective as halothane in reversing allergic bronchoconstriction in a dog model.[7] If similar effects occur in humans, these drugs would be logical selections in the presence of increased airway resistance due to reversible bronchospasm (see Chapter 16). Large doses of opioids in the intraoperative period should be avoided, as they could contribute to prolonged depression of ventilation in the postoperative period. Nitrous oxide has been shown to increase pulmonary vascular resistance in the presence of large doses of opioids but not in the presence of diazepam or volatile drugs.[8–10] Nitrous oxide can be safely administered to these patients as long as the effect of this drug on pulmonary vascular resistance is monitored by measurement of right atrial pressures. Choice of nondepolarizing muscle relaxants is not critical, although histamine release associated with administration of certain of these drugs could have adverse effects on pulmonary vascular and airway resistance.

Regional anesthetic techniques are appropriate considerations for superficial surgery or operations on the extremities of patients with cor pulmonale. Operations that would require high sensory levels are not optimally performed with regional anesthesia in patients with pulmonary hypertension, since reductions in systemic vascular resistance and systemic blood pressure can produce undesirable decreases in right ventricular stroke volume.

MONITORING

Intraoperative monitoring of patients with cor pulmonale is dependent on the magnitude of the surgery. An intra-arterial catheter is desirable for invasive operations, as this allows frequent determinations of arterial blood gases and subsequent adjustments in inspired oxygen concentrations and minute ventilation. It should be remembered that many drugs, including vasodilators, barbiturates, nitrous oxide, and volatile anesthetics, can inhibit hypoxic pulmonary vasoconstriction, which could further impair the relation of ventilation to perfusion and impair arterial oxygenation.[11]

A right atrial catheter gives important information regarding right ventricular function and the safety of intravenous infusion of fluids. Abrupt increases in right atrial pressures during the intraoperative period signal right ventricular dysfunction and mandate a search for causes of sudden increases in pulmonary vascular resistance, as can be produced by unrecognized arterial hypoxemia, hypoventilation, or drugs such as nitrous oxide. Furthermore, maintenance of an adequate right heart filling pressure is necessary to insure an optimal right ventricular stroke volume. Adequate hydration is also crucial for liquifying secretions and facilitating their removal from small bronchioles.

When left ventricular dysfunction accompanies cor pulmonale and the magnitude of the surgery includes the likelihood of large volume replacement, it is helpful to place a pulmonary artery catheter, which permits optimal regulation of intravascular fluid volume and cardiac output with volume infusion and inotropic drugs.

VENTILATION

Intermittent positive pressure breathing is most often selected for the intraoperative management of ventilation in patients with cor pulmonale. Although positive pressure applied to the airways and alveoli can increase pulmonary vascular resistance, this potential adverse effect is usually more than offset by improved arterial oxygenation. Improved arterial oxygenation during positive pressure ventilation of the lungs presumably reflects better distribution of ventilation to perfusion. Excessive reductions in the arterial carbon dioxide partial pressures during controlled ventilation of the lungs should be avoided, since metabolic alkalosis could produce hypokalemia. This is particularly important in patients who are being treated with digitalis, since acute reductions in plasma potassium concentrations can predispose to digitalis toxicity. Humidification of the inhaled gases helps maintain hydration and liquefaction of secretions.

PRIMARY PULMONARY HYPERTENSION

Primary pulmonary hypertension is a diagnosis of exclusion based on ruling out secondary causes of elevations in pulmonary artery pressures such as pulmonary embolism and chronic obstructive airways disease.[12] Conditions associated with primary pulmonary hypertension include cirrhosis of the liver, collagen vascular diseases, and Raynaud's disease. The association with advanced liver disease implicates vasoactive compounds that bypass liver degradation; the association with collagen vascular diseases implicates an underlying vasculitis, and the association with Raynaud's disease indicates the presence of vasospasm. Familial cases of primary pulmonary hypertension are well documented.

The natural history of primary pulmonary hypertension is not well defined. Although average survival after the diagnosis is 2 years, occasional patients survive 15 years to 20 years. Medical therapy has included anticoagulation and vasodilator therapy. Presence of thrombi in the small pulmonary vessels in many patients dying of primary pulmonary hypertension is the rationale for prophylactic anticoagulation. A small pulmonary embolism, which might have little effect on normal patients, could have catastrophic consequences in patients with pulmonary hypertension. Favorable initial responses to administration of vasodilators may not persist, and normalization of pulmonary artery pressures rarely occurs in these patients. In an animal model of pulmonary hypertension, nitroglycerin but not nitroprusside lowered pulmonary artery pressure and pulmonary vascular resistance.[13]

REFERENCES

1. Fishman AP. Chronic cor pulmonale. Am Rev Respir Dis 1976;114:775–94
2. Robotham JL. Cardiovascular disturbance in chronic respiratory insufficiency. Am J Cardiol 1981;47:941–9
3. Flick MR, Block AJ. Chronic oxygen therapy. Med Clin North Am 1977;61:1397–1408
4. Moser KM, Luchsinger PC, Adamson JS, et al. Respiratory stimulation with intravenous doxapram in respiratory failure. A double blind cooperative study. N Engl J Med 1973;288:427–31
5. Heinemann HO. Right-side heart failure and the use of diuretics. Am J Med 1978;64:367–70
6. Sorensen MB, Jacobsen E. Pulmonary hemodynamics during induction of anesthesia. Anesthesiology 1977;46:246–51
7. Hirshman CA, Edelstein G, Peetz S, et al. Mechanism of action of inhalational anesthesia on airways. Anesthesiology 1982;56:107–11
8. Hilgenberg JC, McCammon RL, Stoelting RK. Pulmonary and systemic vascular responses to nitrous oxide in patients with mitral stenosis and pulmonary hypertension. Anesth Analg 1980;59:323–6
9. McCammon RL, Hilgenberg JC, Stoelting RK. Hemodynamic effects of diazepam and diazepam-nitrous oxide in patients with coronary artery disease. Anesth Analg 1980;59:438–41
10. Stoelting RK, Reis RR, Longnecker DE. Hemodynamic responses to nitrous oxide-halothane and halothane in patients with valvular heart disease. Anesthesiology 1972;37:430–5
11. Mathers J, Benumof JL, Wahrenbrock EA. General anesthetics and regional hypoxic pulmonary vasconstriction. Anesthesiology 1977;46:111–4
12. Rich S, Brundage BH. Primary pulmonary hypertension. JAMA 1984;251:2252–4
13. Pearl RG, Rosenthal MH, Ashton JPA. Pulmonary vasodilator effects of nitroglycerin and sodium nitroprusside in canine oleic acid-induced pulmonary hypertension. Anesthesiology 1983;58:514–8.

10

Diseases of the Pericardium

Diseases of the pericardium include cardiac tamponade, acute pericarditis, and chronic constrictive pericarditis. Management of anesthesia in patients with one of these diagnoses requires an understanding of alterations in cardiovascular function produced by specific pericardial diseases. Improper management of anesthesia in the presence of pericardial disease may accentuate the degree of associated cardiovascular dysfunction.[1]

Pericardial fluid is an ultrafiltrate of plasma. Normally, the pericardial space contains 20 ml to 25 ml of this fluid. Intrapericardial pressure is subatmospheric, decreasing on inspiration and increasing on exhalation. Although the pericardium is not essential to life, it serves to isolate the heart from other structures preventing adhesions and inward spread of infection while keeping the heart in an optimal functional position and shape. Pericardium also provides for lymph drainage of the myocardium.

CARDIAC TAMPONADE

Cardiac tamponade is characterized by reductions in stroke volume and blood pressure due to increased intrapericardial pressures. Elevated intrapericardial pressures are due to accumulation of fluid in the pericardial space. Accumulation of pericardial fluid may be due to chest trauma, postoperative bleeding after cardiac surgery, perforation of the ventricle by artificial cardiac pacemakers or central venous pressure catheters, metastases from malignant disease, infections, or chronic renal failure. The incidence of cardiac tamponade after cardiac surgery ranges from 3 percent to 6 percent.[1] Cardiac tamponade has been observed in up to 6 percent of patients in renal failure and in 15 percent to 55 percent of patients with uremic pericarditis.[2]

Pathophysiology

Cardiac tamponade results from impaired diastolic filling of the heart due to continuous elevation of intrapericardial pressures. Hemodynamic alterations depend on the amount and rapidity of accumulation of pericardial fluid. A large volume of pericardial fluid (80 ml to 100 ml) may be tolerated if the accumulation is gradual, allowing stretching of the pericardium. Conversely, acute accumulation of small volumes of pericardial fluid can produce cardiac tamponade.

Stroke volume is decreased due to sustained elevations of intrapericardial pressure, which limits diastolic filling of the left and right ventricles. Activation of the sympathetic nervous system occurs in an attempt to maintain cardiac output and blood pressure by virtue of tachycardia and peripheral vasoconstriction. Indeed, cardiac output and blood pressure are maintained as long as pressures in central veins exceed right ventricular end-diastolic pressures. As intrapericardial pressure increases further, compensatory mechanisms fail and profound cardiovascular collapse occurs. Myocardial ischemia is a possibility as coronary blood flow is decreased due to tachycardia, hypotension, and elevated transmural pressures on the ventricles, causing increased coronary artery resistance.

Diagnosis

A high index of suspicion is necessary for the prompt diagnosis of cardiac tamponade (Table 10-1). Patients may complain of dyspnea and manifest diaphoresis. Peripheral vasoconstriction, tachycardia, hypotension, and elevated central venous pressure may be present. Heart sounds may be distant. Many of these findings mimic pulmonary embolism.

Pulsus paradoxus is an exaggerated decrease in systolic blood pressure during inspiration in the presence of elevated intrapericardial pressures. Normally, systolic blood pressure decreases less than 6 mmHg during inspiration reflecting a concomitant increase in the capacity of the pulmonary vascular bed that transiently reduces venous return and subsequent left ventricular stroke volume. A decline in systolic blood pressure by more than 10 mmHg during inspiration is a classic sign of increased intrapericardial pressures (Fig. 10-1).[3] In the absence of a continuous recording of intra-arterial blood pressure, pulsus paradoxus is determined by auscultation of the blood pressure until the first heart sound is heard intermittently. The blood pressure cuff is deflated until all beats are audible, and the difference between the two auscultated blood pressures is the paradoxical pulse. Pulsus paradoxus may be absent when acute tamponade occurs in the presence of an atrial septal defect or left ventricular dysfunction.[4] Distention of

neck veins, which increases with inspiration (Kussmaul's venous sign), reflects increased intrapericardial pressures but is rarely seen in the presence of cardiac tamponade.

Progressive elevations in right atrial pressures, right ventricular end-diastolic pressures, and pulmonary artery occlusion pressures reflect increased intrapericardial pressures. Eventually, these cardiac filling pressures, as measured from a pulmonary artery catheter, equalize at a value of about 20 mmHg.[5] It should be remembered that accumulation of blood and blood clots over the right ventricle, as often occurs following cardiac surgery, may result in elevation of right atrial pressures, although the pulmonary artery occlusion pressures remain normal.

The electrocardiogram in the presence of cardiac tamponade may show decreased voltage of the QRS complexes and T-waves due to a short-circuiting effect of pericardial fluid. Evidence of myocardial ischemia may also be present. Electrical alternans, due to changes in cardiac position, resulting from the rotational pendular movement of the heart, occurs in 10 percent to 15 percent of patients with pericardial effusions.[1]

The echocardiogram is a reliable and clinically useful method for documenting the presence of even small amounts of fluid in the pericardial space. The cardiac silhouette on radiographs of the chest does not change until about 250 ml of fluid are present in the pericardial space. Other radiologic signs include

TABLE 10-1. Clinical Features of Cardiac Tamponade

Sympathetic nervous system stimulation

Hypotension

Elevated venous pressures

Distant heart sounds

Pulsus paradoxus

Kussmaul's venous sign*

Equalization of atrial filling pressures and pulmonary artery end-diastolic pressures

* More likely to be present in patients with chronic constrictive pericarditis.

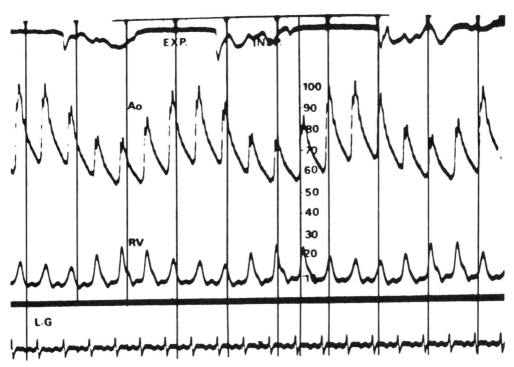

FIG. 10-1. Pulses paradoxus in the presence of constrictive pericarditis is indicated by marked decreases in systolic blood pressure (Ao) during inspiration (INSP). (Shabetal R, Fowler NO, Guntheroth WG. The hemodynamics of cardiac tamponade and constrictive pericarditis. Am J Cardiol 1970;26:480–9)

sudden and nonspecific cardiac enlargement and diminished cardiac pulsation on fluoroscopy.

Treatment

Definitive therapy of cardiac tamponade due to nontraumatic causes is drainage of pericardial fluid via a percutaneous pericardiocentesis through a subxiphoid or subcostal approach using local anesthesia (1 percent to 1.5 percent lidocaine) and with continuous monitoring of the electrocardiogram. Removal of only small amounts of pericardial fluid often results in significant decreases in intrapericardial pressures. A pericardiotomy performed in the operating room under local or general anesthesia is the recommended therapy when car-

diac tamponade results from trauma or develops after thoracic surgery.

Temporary measures designed to maintain stroke volume until definitive treatment of cardiac tamponade can be instituted include expansion of intravascular fluid volume, administration of catecholamines to increase myocardial contractility, and correction of metabolic acidosis.[1] Expansion of intravascular fluid volume can be achieved by intravenous infusion of colloid or crystalloid solutions (500 ml over 5 minutes to 10 minutes). Volume infusion that increases right atrial pressures to 25 mmHg to 30 mmHg may be necessary to offset effects of increased intrapericardial pressures and thus to favor venous return to the right atrium. Left ventricular stroke volume is likely to increase as a result of this increased venous return.[6] Despite the time-honored acceptance of intravascular volume expansion for the emergency therapy of cardiac tamponade, improvement in hemodynamic function may be limited and pericardiocentesis should not be delayed (Table 10-2).[7]

Continuous intravenous infusion of isoproterenol or other catecholamines may be an effective temporizing measure for increasing myocardial contractility and heart rate, although the beneficial effects of these drugs in animals with experimentally induced cardiac tamponade has not been reproducible in patients.[8] Digitalis is not of proven value for treatment of low cardiac output associated with cardiac tamponade, emphasizing the large increase in systemic vascular resistance that may accompany administration of this drug. A similar undesirable effect on systemic vascular resistance could accompany administration of alpha-adrenergic agonist drugs including high doses of dopamine. Vasodilator drugs, such as nitroprusside or hydralazine, could theoretically improve cardiac output, but their use can be considered only when intravascular fluid volume is optimal. As with intravascular fluid replacement, it is clear that drug therapy should never delay definitive treatment (i.e., pericardiocentesis) of cardiac tamponade.[7]

Metabolic acidosis due to low cardiac output is appropriately treated with intravenous administration of sodium bicarbonate, 0.5 $mEq \cdot kg^{-1}$ to 1 $mEq \cdot kg^{-1}$. Correction of metabolic acidosis is important as increased hydrogen ion concentrations can depress myocardial contractility and attenuate positive inotropic effects of catecholamines. Atropine may be necessary to treat bradycardia that results from depressor vagal reflexes as intrapericardial pressures increase.[9]

Management of Anesthesia

Institution of general anesthesia and positive pressure ventilation of the lungs in the presence of cardiac tamponade that is hemodynamically significant can lead to profound hypotension and even cardiac arrest. Reasons for hypotension include anesthetic-induced peripheral vasodilation, direct myocardial depression, and decreased venous return. Therefore, pericardiocentesis performed with local anesthesia is the preferred approach for the initial management of patients who are hypotensive due to a low cardiac output produced by cardiac tamponade.[10] In most patients, a subxiphoid pericardial window can be accomplished under local anesthesia with lidocaine. Ketamine, administered intravenously, can be used to provide sedation in selected patients.[1] After hemodynamic status has been improved by removal of some of the accumulated pericardial fluid, it is acceptable to induce general anesthesia and institute positive pressure ventilation of the lungs to permit surgical exploration of the chest and more definitive treatment of cardiac tamponade. Induction and maintenance of anesthesia are often with ketamine or benzodiazepines plus nitrous oxide. Circulatory effects of pancuron-

TABLE 10-2. Effects of Volume Expansion and Pericardiocentesis in Patients with Acute Cardiac Tamponade

	Cardiac Tamponade	Cardiac Tamponade Plus Volume Expansion with 500 ml Normal Saline	After Pericardiocentesis
Mean arterial pressure (mmHg)	83 ± 16	82 ± 19	80 ± 13
Right atrial pressure (mmHg)	15 ± 3	17 ± 4	8 ± 4*
Pulsus paradoxus (mmHg)	25 ± 12	25 ± 15	8 ± 4*
Cardiac output (L·min^{-1})	5.1 ± 2.6	5.5 ± 2.6	9.1 ± 3*
Heart rate (beats·min^{-1})	118 ± 11	112 ± 11	121 ± 16

$P < 0.05$ vs. other conditions.

(Data from Kerber RE, Gascho JA, Litchfield R, et al. Hemodynamic effects of volume expansion and nitroprusside compared with pericardiocentesis in patients with acute cardiac tamponade. N Engl J Med 1982;307:929–31).

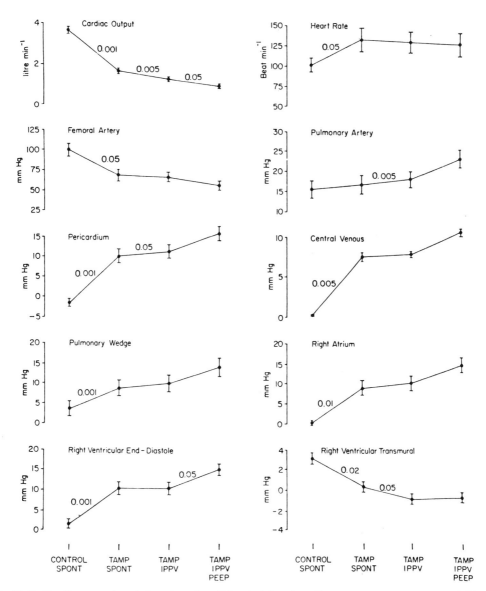

FIG. 10-2. Cardiac output and pleural, pericardial, arterial and cardiac pressures were measured (Mean ± SE) in animals during different modes of ventilation in the presence of acute cardiac tamponade. SPONT = spontaneous breathing; TAMP = cardiac tamponade; IPPV = intermittent positive pressure ventilation; PEEP = positive end-expiratory pressure. (Moller CT, Schoonbee CG, Rosendorff C. Haemodynamics of cardiac tamponade during various modes of ventilation. Br J Anaesth 1979;51:409–15. Copyright © Macmillan Magazines Ltd.)

ium make this a useful drug for production of skeletal muscle paralysis in these patients. Monitors should include intra-arterial and central venous pressure catheters.

If it is not possible to relieve increased intrapericardial pressures causing cardiac tamponade before the induction of anesthesia, the goal must be to maintain the cardiac output. Anesthetic-induced reductions in myocardial contractility, systemic vascular resistance, and heart rate must be avoided. Increased intrathoracic pressures due to straining or coughing during induction of anesthesia or to controlled ventilation of the lungs may further reduce venous return in the presence of increased intrapericardial pressures (Fig. 10-2).[11] In this regard, it may be prudent to avoid vigorous positive pressure ventilation of the lungs until the chest is opened and drainage of the pericardial space is imminent. Ketamine is useful for induction and maintenance of anesthesia, as this drug tends to increase myocardial contractility, systemic vascular resistance, and heart rate. Induction of anesthesia with diazepam, followed by maintenance of anesthesia with nitrous oxide plus fentanyl and pancuronium for skeletal muscle relaxation, has also been successfully used in these patients.[12] Continuous monitoring of central venous and systemic blood pressures should be instituted before the induction of anesthesia. Maintenance of elevated central venous pressures with liberal administration of intravenous fluids is necessary to maintain venous return. Continuous infusion of catecholamines such as isoproterenol, dopamine, or dobutamine may be required to maintain myocardial contractility until the pericardial space can be surgically drained. In addition, personnel and equipment must be available to perform an emergency pericardiocentesis or rapidly open the chest, should circulatory collapse occur after induction of anesthesia.

ACUTE PERICARDITIS

Acute pericarditis designates an inflammatory process of the pericardium, which may result from a variety of causes (Table 10-3).

TABLE 10-3. Causes of Acute Pericarditis

Infectious
  Viral
  Bacterial
  Fungal
  Tuberculosis
Idiopathic—acute benign pericarditis

Postmyocardial infarction
  Rapid onset
  Delayed onset (Dressler's syndrome)

Systemic disease
  Rheumatoid arthritis
  Systemic lupus erythematosus
  Scleroderma

Post-traumatic

Metastatic disease

Chronic renal failure

Drugs

Radiation

Acute benign pericarditis is its most frequent form and is presumed to be due to viral infections.[13] Pericarditis is a frequent complication of acute myocardial infarctions. Dressler's syndrome is a delayed form of acute pericarditis, which may follow myocardial infarctions.

Diagnosis

Diagnosis of acute pericarditis is based on the sudden onset of severe chest pain, which is exaggerated by inspiration or assuming the supine position. Pain can be lessened by sitting up. Absence of changes in the plasma concentrations of creatine kinase and the relationship of chest discomfort to inspiration help rule out coronary artery disease. In uremic pericarditis, chest pain is sometimes conspicuously absent. In some instances, pain of acute pericarditis can radiate to the abdomen and mimic surgical disease.

A low-grade fever and sinus tachycardia are frequent findings in the presence of acute pericarditis. Auscultation of the chest often reveals a friction rub, which is described as to-and-fro, leathery in quality, and of increased intensity during exhalation. There is concave elevation of ST segments on the electrocardiogram, which presumably reflects extension of the inflammatory reaction from the pericardium to the surface of the heart. Acute pericarditis does not alter cardiac function in the absence of an associated pericardial effusion.

Pericardial Effusion

The inflammatory reaction characteristic of acute pericarditis may be associated with the accumulation of fluid in the pericardial space. Echocardiography is the most accurate and easily applicable method for detection of pericardial effusions. Symptoms produced by pericardial effusions depend on the amount and speed of accumulation of fluid. As stated earlier, if effusions have developed gradually, the pericardium can stretch and accommodate a large volume of fluid with no significant increase in intrapericardial pressures; a smaller volume of fluid that accumulates rapidly can produce cardiac tamponade.

CHRONIC CONSTRICTIVE PERICARDITIS

Chronic constrictive pericarditis resembles cardiac tamponade in that both processes impede diastolic filling of the ventricles and reduce stroke volume. Most cases of chronic constrictive pericarditis are idiopathic. Known causes of constrictive pericarditis include radiation therapy, chronic renal failure, rheumatoid arthritis, neoplasms, and tuberculosis.

Diagnosis

Constrictive pericarditis involves both sides of the heart, but the dominant manifestations are often those of right ventricular failure with venous congestion, hepatosplenomegaly, and ascites. Elevation and eventual equalization of right atrial pressures, pulmonary artery diastolic pressures, and pulmonary artery occlusion pressures occur in the presence of both chronic constrictive pericarditis and cardiac tamponade. Atrial dysrhythmias are common in patients with chronic constrictive pericarditis, presumably reflecting involvement of the superficial sinoatrial node by the disease process. Atrial fibrillation or flutter is present in one-fourth of patients. Exaggerated distention of neck veins during inspiration (Kussmaul's sign) is seen more frequently in patients with chronic constrictive pericarditis than in patients with cardiac tamponade; accentuated decreases in systolic blood pressure during inspiration (pulsus paradoxus) are seen more frequently in patients with cardiac tamponade. Radiographs of the chest reveal a normal to small heart, and calcium is often visible in the pericardium. Echocardiography, although more useful in the diagnosis of cardiac tamponade, may demonstrate findings (separation of the pericardium and epicardium with a small echo-free space and thickened echoes from anterior and posterior pericardium) characteristic of constrictive pericarditis. Computed tomography has also proved useful in diagnosing constrictive pericarditis or pericardial effusions. The electrocardiogram is usually not diagnostic; but low voltage QRS complexes, inversion of T-waves, and notched P-waves may occur. Unlike cardiac tamponade, electrical alternans is absent on the electrocardiogram of patients with constrictive pericarditis. Systolic time intervals are normal, serving to differentiate constrictive pericarditis from cardiac disease.

Treatment

Treatment of chronic constrictive pericarditis is surgical removal of the pericardium. A pericardectomy is usually performed with the cardiopulmonary bypass machine in a "standby mode" should tearing of atrial or ventricular myocardium during removal of adherent pericardium from the heart necessitate institution of cardiopulmonary bypass. Bleeding from raw cardiac surfaces may necessitate massive blood replacement. Unlike cardiac tamponade in which hemodynamic improvement occurs promptly, surgical removal of only the parietal pericardium in the presence of constrictive pericarditis is not associated with immediate decreases in right atrial pressures or increases in cardiac output. Typically, right atrial pressures decline by 2 days to 5 days postoperatively, suggesting that decreased myocardial compliance secondary to chronic constriction is at least partially reversible. Absence of immediate hemodynamic improvement may reflect disuse atrophy from prolonged constriction of myocardial muscle fibers, underlying cardiac disease, or persistent constrictive effects from sclerotic epicardium, which is not removed with the parietal pericardium.

Management of Anesthesia

In the absence of hypotension due to increased intrapericardial pressures, anesthetic drugs or techniques that do not greatly decrease venous return, produce bradycardia, or directly depress the myocardium can be used. Combinations of benzodiazepines, opioids, and nitrous oxide have been used successfully in patients undergoing pericardectomy. Circulatory responses evoked by pancuronium are acceptable in these patients, although exaggerated increases in heart rate are undesirable. Muscle relaxants with minimal to no circulatory effects, such as metocurine, atracurium, or vecuronium, are alternatives to the administration of pancuronium. When hemodynamic compromise from elevated intrapericardial pressures is severe, treatment and management of anesthesia is as described for cardiac tamponade (see the section Cardiac Tamponade).

Invasive monitoring of arterial and venous pressures is useful, as removal of adherent pericardium may be tedious and associated with decreases in blood pressure and cardiac output. Cardiac dysrhythmias are common, emphasizing the importance of the immediate presence of antidysrhythmic drugs and a defibrillator. Venous access and appropriate fluids are necessary to treat occasional massive blood loss associated with pericardectomy. Postoperative ventilatory insufficiency may necessitate continued mechanical ventilation of the lungs. Cardiac dysrhythmias and low cardiac output may persist in the postoperative period. An unusual complication of subtotal pericardectomy is pneumopericardium.

REFERENCES

1. Lake CL. Anesthesia and pericardial disease. Anesth Analg 1983;62:431–43
2. Singh S, Newmark K, Ishikawa I. Pericardectomy in uremia, treatment of choice for cardiac tamponade in chronic renal failure. JAMA 1974;228:1132–5
3. Shabetai R, Fowler NO, Guntheroth WG. The hemodynamics of cardiac tamponade and constrictive pericarditis. Am J Cardiol 1970;26:480–9
4. Winer HL, Kronzon I Absence of paradoxical pulse in patients with cardiac tamponade and atrial septal defect. Am J Cardiol 1979;44:378–9
5. Weeks KR, Chatterjee K, Block S, et al. Bedside hemodynamic monitoring: Its value in the diagnosis of tamponade complicating cardiac surgery. J Thorac Cardiovasc Surg 1976;71:250–2
6. DeCrestofaro D, Liu CK. The hemodynamics of cardiac tamponade and blood volume overload in dogs. Cardiovasc Res 1969;3:292–8
7. Kerber RE, Gascho JA, Litchfield R, et al. Hemodynamic effects of volume expansion and nitroprusside compared with pericardiocentesis in patients with acute cardiac tamponade. N Engl J Med 1982;307:929–31
8. Martins JB, Manuel JB, Marcus ML, Kerber RE. Comparative effects of catecholamines in cardiac tamponade: Experimental and clinical studies. Am J Cardiol 1980;46:59–66
9. Friedman HS, Lajam F, Gomes JA, et al. Demonstration of a depressor reflex in acute cardiac tamponade. J Thorac Cardiovasc Surg 1977;73:278–86
10. Stanley TH, Weidauer HE. Anesthesia for the patient with cardiac tamponade. Anesth Analg 1973;52:110–4
11. Moller CT, Schoonbee CG, Rosendorff C. Haemodynamics of cardiac tamponade during various modes of ventilation. Br J Anaesth 1979;51:409–15
12. Konchigeri HN, Levitsky S. Anesthetic considerations for pericardectomy in uremic pericardial effusion. Anesth Analg 1976;55:378–82
13. Fowler NO, Manitsas GT. Infectious pericarditis. Prog Cardiovasc Dis 1973;16:323–36

11

Aneurysms of the Thoracic and Abdominal Aorta

Aneurysms of the aorta may involve the ascending or descending portions of the thoracic aorta or the portion of the aorta below the diaphragm. A dissecting aneurysm denotes a tear in the intima of the aorta, which allows blood to enter and permeate between the walls of the vessel, producing a false lumen, which extends for various distances, occluding side branches. Ultimately, the dissection may reenter the lumen through another tear in the intima or rupture through the adventitia.

Three major anatomic types of dissecting aneurysms of the thoracic aorta have been described.[1] Type I dissections arise from the ascending aorta and extend retrograde around the arch of the aorta and/or anterograde toward the abdominal aorta (Fig. 11-1). They account for about 70 percent of all patients with aneurysms of the thoracic aorta. Type II dissections also arise in the ascending aorta. Type III dissections typically begin just distal to the left subclavian artery and extend anterograde as far as the iliac arteries (Fig. 11-1). About 20 percent of aortic dissections are classified as type III.

Many mechanisms have been proposed as causes for the development of aneurysms of the aorta. A majority of patients are hypertensive, and many of them have associated atherosclerosis. It is generally believed that degeneration of the media of the aorta (cystic medial necrosis) is the primary mechanism for dissection of

the aorta. Deceleration injuries, as occur from automobile accidents, are another cause for dissection.

ANEURYSMS OF THE ASCENDING THORACIC AORTA

Aneurysms of the ascending thoracic aorta (type I and II dissections) are usually fusiform rather than saccular and are most often due to atherosclerosis.[2] Patients who develop these aneurysms are usually middle-aged and are not always hypertensive. Less than 5 percent of these aneurysms are caused by lues. Individuals afflicted with Marfan's syndrome are particularly prone to develop type II dissections.

Signs and Symptoms

Clinical symptoms resulting from aneurysms of the ascending thoracic aorta reflect their close proximity to the trachea, esophagus, and laryngeal nerves. Inspiratory stridor, dysphagia, and hoarseness may occur. Retrograde dissection of these aneurysms can result in ob-

169

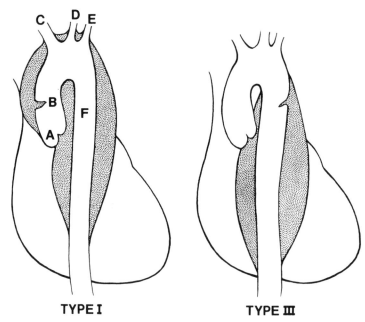

TYPE I   **TYPE III**

FIG. 11-1. Schematic diagrams of type I and type III dissections of the thoracic aorta. Type I dissections arise from a tear in the intima of the ascending aorta. The resulting dissection (shaded area) can extend retrograde to involve the aortic valve or produce cardiac tamponade. Likewise, type I dissections can extend anterograde and involve side branches of the aorta. Type II dissections differ from type I only in the limitation of the extension to the arch of the aorta. Type III dissections arise from a tear in the intima of the descending thoracic aorta, usually just distal to the left subclavian artery. Type III dissections (shaded area) extend anterograde and in extreme cases can involve the iliac arteries. A = aortic valve, B = ascending thoracic aorta, C = innominate artery, D = left common carotid artery, E = left subclavian artery, F = descending thoracic aorta.

struction of the carotid and coronary arteries or in cardiac tamponade. This emphasizes the importance of evaluating cerebral and cardiac function before surgery. The most important complication of these aneurysms is retrograde dissection producing acute aortic regurgitation.[3] About one-half of patients with type I dissections have involvement of the aortic valve.

Radiographs of the chest usually show a widened aortomediastinal shadow. Echocardiography may be helpful in diagnosing pericardial effusions due to retrograde dissection of the aorta. Contrast aortography will define the origin and extent of the dissection. This knowledge is essential in the perioperative period for determining the proper site for intra-arterial monitoring of blood pressure (left or right radial artery) and the need to monitor cerebral perfusion pressures (aortic arch vessel involvement).

Treatment

Medical therapy of dissections of aneurysms of the ascending thoracic aorta is directed at reducing pressures on the aortic wall so as to prevent further extension or rupture of the hematoma and to facilitate healing of the wall. Reductions in blood pressure and myocardial contractility can be achieved with either trimethaphan or nitroprusside combined with propranolol.

Surgical intervention is indicated to prevent retrograde dissection of aneurysms, which could lead to fatal aortic regurgitation or cardiac tamponade. Indeed, aortic regurgitation is often the indication for surgery. Specific surgical therapy usually involves resection of the diseased aorta and replacement with a synthetic graft. Occasionally, surgical obliteration of the false lumen may be adequate treatment. When aortic regurgitation occurs, either valve annuloplasty or replacement with a prosthetic valve is necessary. It may also be necessary to reimplant the coronary arteries if their ostia are narrowed by extension of the dissection into the sinus of Valsalva. Composite graft repair has been recommended for any patient with Marfan's syndrome in whom the diameter of the ascending aorta exceeds 6 cm, regardless of symptoms or the presence of aortic regurgitation.[4]

Cardiopulmonary bypass, with cannulation of the right atrium and femoral artery to provide retrograde perfusion, may be necessary for resection of aneurysms of the ascending thoracic aorta. Occasionally, cannulation of the individual aortic arch vessels is necessary to maintain cerebral perfusion.[5] Heparin-coated shunts circumventing the aneurysm remove the need for systemic heparinization and cardiopulmonary bypass.[6] Furthermore, a shunt minimizes the increase in systemic blood pressure that often accompanies cross-clamping of the aorta.

Management of Anesthesia

Placement of the intra-arterial catheter for monitoring of intraoperative blood pressure depends on the location of the aortic aneurysm. Since dissection of the aorta frequently involves the innominate artery, a left artery catheter is often indicated. A pulmonary artery catheter is helpful in ascertaining the presence or absence of left ventricular failure. A precordial electrocardiogram lead is useful for the early detection of myocardial ischemia involving the left ventricle. Monitoring of carotid blood flow with a Doppler sensor and continuous recording of the electroencephalogram is helpful in assessing the adequacy of cerebral

perfusion. Measurement of somatosensory-evoked potentials is likewise useful for monitoring adequacy of blood flow to the brain and spinal cord. Constant monitoring of urine output, and if necessary stimulation of urine output with furosemide or mannitol, assure that reapproximation of the aortic walls did not compromise renal blood flow.

Induction of anesthesia and intubation of the trachea must minimize undesirable increases in blood pressure that could exacerbate aortic dissections. Likewise, during maintenance of anesthesia, it is important to use appropriate drugs (volatile anesthetics, peripheral vasodilators) to minimize elevations in blood pressure in response to surgical stimulation or cross-clamping of the aorta. Ideally, mean arterial pressure is maintained in the range of 70 mmHg to 80 mmHg. General anesthesia also provides the potential for producing additional cerebral metabolic depression with barbiturates during surgery involving vessels of the arch of the aorta.

Postoperative Management

The postoperative course after resection of an aneurysm of the ascending thoracic aorta can be complicated by hypertension, tachycardia, and central nervous system dysfunction.[7] Elevated blood pressure is undesirable, since it increases the risk of myocardial ischemia and breakdown of the surgical vascular anastomosis of the aorta. Therefore, vasodilator and/or beta-adrenergic antagonist drugs may be necessary to maintain an acceptable blood pressure. Furthermore, postoperative monitoring of the electrocardiogram is helpful in the early recognition of cardiac dysrhythmias or changes in ST segments that suggest myocardial ischemia. Cerebrovascular accidents may be produced by air or thrombotic emboli that occur during surgical resection of diseased aorta.[8] Patients with co-existing cerebrovascular disease are particularly prone to develop this complication. This emphasizes the importance of performing a neurologic examination both preoperatively and postoperatively.

ANEURYSMS OF THE DESCENDING THORACIC AORTA

Aneurysms of the descending thoracic aorta (type III dissections) are usually asymptomatic and show little tendency to rupture. Deceleration chest injuries, as can occur from automobile accidents, can result in such aneurysms.[9] Presumably this is due to the fact that the aorta is fixed at a point just distal to the origin of the left subclavian artery. Trauma at this site can tear the intima of the aortic wall, which allows blood to dissect into the media of the vessel. When type III dissections occur, they are most commonly anterograde to below the diaphragm. Therefore, acute aortic regurgitation or cardiac tamponade are unlikely complications. Such dissections most often develop in geriatric patients with atherosclerosis.

Myocardial Contusion

In addition to causing aneurysms of the descending thoracic aorta, deceleration injuries involving the anterior chest wall are also the most frequent cause of myocardial contusion.[10] Sudden deceleration from speeds as low as 20 miles·hr^{-1} may produce injury to the heart without obvious external signs of trauma. The right ventricle, because of its immediate substernal location, is most likely to be injured. Selective right ventricular dysfunction may occur if concussive injury is severe. Chest pain resembling angina pectoris and unrelieved by nitrates occurs in a large percentage of patients. Thrombosis of a coronary artery may result from blunt chest trauma. The presence of chest pain and changes on the electrocardiogram resembling myocardial infarction, especially in young persons, should prompt questions about recent chest trauma.

This trauma may have seemed trivial at the time.

Any change on the electrocardiogram in the presence of blunt chest trauma must arouse suspicion for contusion. Nevertheless, the sensitivity of the electrocardiogram is variable, as numerous abnormalities may occur including supraventricular and ventricular dysrhythmias, sinus and atrioventricular node dysfunction, right and left bundle branch blocks, and prolongation of Q-T intervals.[10] The value of radiographs of the chest in the diagnosis of myocardial contusion is limited to recognizing associated injuries. In this regard, sternal fractures are associated with cardiac damage in a substantial percentage of cases. Elevation of the myocardial band of creatine kinase may mirror cardiac damage from myocardial contusion, although normal levels have been present in patients with autopsy-proven myocardial contusion. Radionuclide angiography and 2-D echocardiography are useful in demonstrating functional abnormalities (changes in systolic and diastolic volumes, wall motion, and ejection fraction) associated with myocardial contusion.

Serial electrocardiograms should be recorded in accident victims with chest trauma. If patients are hemodynamically stable, myocardial contusion tends to be a benign process and treatment is supportive. Fluid replacement is guided by monitoring atrial filling pressures, cardiac output, and urine output.

Treatment

Treatment of type III dissections is generally conservative. Vasodilator drugs, such as trimethaphan or nitroprusside, are used to maintain a mean arterial pressure of 70 mmHg to 80 mmHg. Propranolol is frequently added to the vasodilator regimen in an attempt to reduce velocity of blood ejection from the left ventricle. Administration of these drugs should be accompanied by continuous monitoring of arterial and left atrial filling pressures. Urinary output is constantly monitored and a diuretic is administered when necessary to maintain adequate urine output.

Type III dissections that remain confined to the thoracic aorta are amenable to surgical resection. Dissections that extend below the diaphragm or that extend to the arch of the aorta are usually too extensive for resection. Aneurysms of the descending thoracic aorta due to trauma should be surgically resected as an elective procedure, as it is likely that these aneurysms will eventually dissect. Surgical access to this type of aneurysm is through a left thoracotomy.

Management of Anesthesia

Proper monitoring is more important than the actual drugs selected for anesthesia in patients undergoing resection of aneurysms of the descending thoracic aorta. Specifically, it is important to monitor arterial blood pressure above (right radial artery) and below (femoral artery) the aneurysm. This allows assessment of the adequacy of cerebral perfusion as well as blood flow to the kidneys and spinal cord during cross-clamping of the aorta. Measurement of somatosensory-evoked potentials is another method to monitor the adequacy of blood flow to the brain and spinal cord. Sympathomimetic and/or vasodilator drugs may be required to adjust perfusion pressures above and below the aortic dissection. Mean arterial pressure in the upper part of the body should be maintained near 100 mmHg, and mean arterial pressure distal to the aneurysm should be maintained above 50 mmHg. Use of nitroprusside to treat blood pressure elevations above the aortic cross-clamp must be balanced against likely deleterious reductions in renal blood flow and perfusion of the spinal cord should vasodilator therapy concomitantly lower perfusion pressure below the cross-clamp.[11] The use of a temporary external bypass shunt (left atrium to femoral artery) with pump outputs in the range of 35 ml·kg^{-1} has been suggested as a measure that will assure adequate blood flow and pressure in the distal aorta.[12] The disadvantage of these shunts is increased resistance to blood flow. Left ventricular function should be monitored using a pulmonary artery catheter. Diuresis should be established preoperatively and maintained during the operation with osmotic diuretics as well as furosemide if necessary.

Selective endobronchial intubation allowing collapse of the left lung facilitates surgical exposure during resection of these aneurysms.[13] Nevertheless, use of an endobronchial tube for these operations is not considered mandatory.[14] Indeed, a disadvantage of one lung ventilation is the production of an iatrogenic intrapulmonary shunt that can lead to arterial hypoxemia despite high inspired concentrations of oxygen. The magnitude of this iatrogenic shunt can be reduced by minimizing pulmonary blood flow through the collapsed left lung. Also, application of 5 cmH$_2$O to 10 cmH$_2$O continuous positive airway pressure to the nondependent unventilated lung may improve arterial oxygenation.[15] If this does not improve arterial oxygenation, it may be beneficial to apply 5 cmH$_2$O to 10 cmH$_2$O positive end-expiratory pressure to the dependent ventilated lung.

Postoperative Course

Neurologic deficits, particularly in the lower extremities, can follow extensive thoracoabdominal aortic surgery. This complication most likely results from ischemia of the spinal cord due to hypotension and surgical interruption of arteries supplying the anterior spinal artery. The incidence of acute renal tubular necrosis seems to be less when diuresis is maintained in the presence of adequate blood flow and pressure in the distal aorta.

ANEURYSMS OF THE ABDOMINAL AORTA

Aneurysms of the abdominal aorta are most often due to atherosclerosis and usually occur in men over 60 years of age. Widespread arteriosclerosis is frequently present. There may be a familial tendency for abdominal aortic aneurysms as evidenced by more than an 11-fold increase in the incidence of these aneurysms among patients with an affected first-degree relative.[16] Because early diagnosis and elective management of abdominal aneurysms significantly prolongs life, noninvasive screening to detect early abdominal aneurysm formation may be warranted in relatives of patients with this disease.

Symptoms

Clinical presentation of aneurysms of the abdominal aorta is usually as a painless and pulsating abdominal mass. The size of the aneurysm parallels the incidence of rupture. For example, the incidence of spontaneous rupture is about 5 percent when the aneurysm is less than 5 cm in diameter.[17] The incidence of spontaneous rupture increases to more than 70 percent when the diameter exceeds 7 cm. Therefore, elective surgical resection is indicated when the estimated diameter of the aneurysm exceeds 5 cm. Extension of the abdominal aneurysm to include the renal arteries, which occurs in about 5 percent of patients, is a serious problem.

Management of Anesthesia

Anesthesia for resection of aneurysms of the abdominal aorta is usually general rather than regional. The potential for sudden and large blood loss intraoperatively detracts from the use of regional techniques. Invasive monitoring of arterial and left atrial filling pressures is indicated. Measurement of pulmonary artery occlusion pressures via a pulmonary artery catheter is helpful in detecting patients who develop left ventricular dysfunction during hypertension produced by cross-clamping of the abdominal aorta.[18] Patients with coronary artery disease are more likely than patients without it to develop myocardial ischemia during increases in blood pressure produced by cross-clamping of the aorta. Increases of 7 mmHg or greater in pulmonary artery occlusion pressures or appearance of V-waves on the pulmonary artery occlusion pressure tracings are often associated with myocardial ischemia (Fig. 11-2).[18] Presumably, these elevated pressures during cross-clamping of the aorta reflect acute left ventricular dysfunction due to myocardial ischemia. Monitoring of a precordial lead of the electrocardiogram is also helpful in the early detection of myocardial ischemia. Monitoring central venous pressures in the presence of coronary artery disease does not reliably reflect left ventricular function and cannot be used as a substitute for a pulmonary artery catheter. Treatment of intraoperative myocardial ischemia is by reducing blood pressure and heart rate to acceptable levels with pharmacologic interventions, using volatile anesthetics, peripheral vasodilating drugs, and/or beta-adrenergic antagonist drugs. Urine output should be maintained with intravenous volume infusion and diuretics if oliguria persists in the absence of hypovolemia.

Myocardial ischemia can also accompany hypotension associated with uncontrolled blood loss or sudden unclamping of the abdominal aorta. The mechanism for hypotension after removal of the aortic cross-clamp is unclear, but most likely reflects a sudden increase in venous capacitance. Furthermore, the release of acid metabolites that have accumulated in the ischemic extremity can produce myocardial depression and peripheral vasodilation. Reductions in blood pressure associated with removal of the aortic cross-clamp can be minimized by infusing intravenous fluids to maintain pulmonary artery occlusion pressures between 10 mmHg to 20 mmHg before unclamping.[19] Furthermore, gradual removal of the aortic cross-clamp minimizes reductions in blood pressure by allowing time for the return of pooled venous blood to the central circulation. Intravenous administration of sodium bicarbonate may be useful if arterial pH is decreased below about 7.2 after unclamping of the abdominal aorta.

Postoperative Course

Patients undergoing resections of abdominal aortic aneurysms are at increased risk for developing acute renal failure postoperatively.

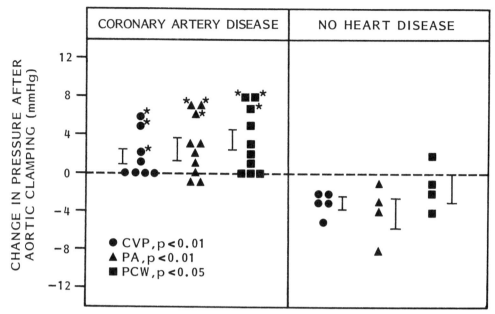

FIG. 11-2. Central venous pressure (CVP), pulmonary artery pressure (PA), and pulmonary capillary wedge pressure (PCW), were measured following infrarenal cross-clamping of the abdominal aorta in patients with or without coronary artery disease. Asterisks represent values associated with signs of myocardial ischemia on the electrocardiogram. Note that increases of 7 mmHg or greater in the PCW were associated with evidence of myocardial ischemia. The significant values refer to comparison of the two groups of patients. (Attia RR, Murphy JD, Snider M, et al. Myocardial ischemia due to infrarenal aortic cross-clamping during aortic surgery in patients with severe coronary artery disease. Circulation 1976;53:961–5. By permission of the American Heart Association, Inc.)

The mechanism for this response is not clear but may involve alterations in the distribution of intrarenal blood flow, caused by hypotension or emboli to the renal artery.[20] The incidence of acute renal failure has declined with aggressive intraoperative fluid therapy, blood pressure control, and maintenance of urine output during the perioperative period.[21]

REFERENCES

1. Anagnostopoulos CE, Prabhakar MJS, Kittle CF. Aortic dissections and dissecting aneurysms. Am J Cardiol 1972;30:263–73
2. Liddicoat JE, Bekassy SM, Rubio PA, et al. Ascending aortic aneurysms: Review of 100 consecutive cases. Circulation 1975;51:202–9
3. Najafi H, Dye WS, Hushang J, et al. Aortic insufficiency secondary to aortic root aneurysm dissection. Arch Surg 1975;110:1401–7
4. Gott VL, Pyeritz RE, Magovern GJ, et al. Surgical treatment of aneurysms of the ascending aorta in the Marfan syndrome. Results of composite-graft repair in 50 patients. N Engl J Med 1986;314:1070–4
5. Ruben JC. Dissecting aneurysms of the ascending aorta. J Cardiovasc Surg 1977;18:267–72
6. Wolfe WG, Kleinman LH, Wechsler AS, Sabiston DC. Heparin-coated shunts for lesions of the descending thoracic aorta. Arch Surg 1977;112:1481–7
7. Sabawala PB, Strong MJ, Keats AS. Surgery of the aorta and its branches. Anesthesiology 1970;33:229–59
8. Crawford ES, Salwa AS, Schuessler JS. Treatment of aneurysm of transverse aortic arch. J Thorac Cardiovasc Surg 1979;78:383–93
9. Schwartz ML, Fisher R, Sako Y, et al. Posttraumatic aneurysms of the thoracic aorta. Surgery 1975;78:589–93
10. Rothstein RJ. Myocardial contusion. JAMA 1983;250:2189–91
11. Gelman S, Reves JG, Fowler K, et al. Regional blood flow during cross-clamping of the thoracic

aorta and infusion of sodium nitroprusside. J Thorac Cardiovasc Surg 1983;85:287–91

12. Kopman EA, Ferguson TB. Intraoperative monitoring of femoral artery pressure during replacement of aneurysm of descending thoracic aorta. Anesth Analg 1977;56:603–5

13. Das BB, Fenstermacher JM, Keats AS. Endobronchial anesthesia resection of aneurysms of the descending aorta. Anesthesiology 1970;32:152–5

14. Romagnoli A, Cooper JR. Anesthesia for aortic operations. Cleve Clin Q 1981;48:147–52

15. Alfery DD, Benumof JL, Trousdale FR. Improving oxygenation during one lung ventilation: The effects of PEEP and blood flow restriction to the nonventilated lung. Anesthesiology 1981;55:381–5

16. Johansen K, Loepsell T. Familial tendency for abdominal aortic aneurysms. JAMA 1986;256:1934–6

17. Thompson JE, Garrett WV. Peripheral-arterial surgery. N Engl J Med 1980;302:491–503

18. Attia RR, Murphy JD, Snider MT, et al. Myocardial ischemia due to infrarenal aortic cross-clamping during aortic surgery in patients with severe coronary artery disease. Circulation 1976;53:961–5

19. Silverstein PR, Caldera DI, Cullen DJ, et al. Avoiding the hemodynamic consequences of aortic cross-clamping and unclamping. Anesthesiology 1979;50:462–6

20. Berkowitz HD, Shantharam S. Renin release and renal cortical ischemia following aortic cross-clamping. Arch Surg 1974;109:612–7

21. Thompson JE, Hollier LH, Patman RD, Pearson AV. Surgical management of abdominal aortic aneurysm. Factors influencing mortality and morbidity—a 20 year experience. Ann Surg 1975;181:654–61

12

Peripheral Vascular Disease

Peripheral vascular disease affects arteries and arterioles more often than veins. Involvement of blood vessels may be localized or generalized. A common feature of diseases classified as vasculitis syndromes is necrotizing vasculitis (Table 12-1).

TAKAYASHU'S SYNDROME

Takayashu's syndrome or pulseless disease is a collective term given to a group of diseases in which there is minimal or no palpable arterial pulsation in the extremities (most often upper) and neck.[1] The lack of peripheral pulses reflects chronic inflammation of the aorta and its major branches. Veins are spared from the inflammatory process. Involved vessels are characteristically shortened and thickened and are subject to thrombus formation and luminal obstruction. The cause of this necrotizing vasculitis of the arteries is not known. Women between 20 years and 50 years of age are affected in over 85 percent of the cases. Many of these patients are of Asian or Mexican descent.[2]

Signs and Symptoms

Signs and symptoms of Takayashu's syndrome manifest on multiple organ systems (Table 12-2). Decreased perfusion to the brain due to involvement of the carotid arteries by the occlusive inflammatory and thrombotic processes can manifest as vertigo, visual disturbances, seizures, and cerebral vascular accidents, with hemiparesis or hemiplegia. Bruits can be heard over the stenosed carotid or subclavian vessels. Hyperextension of the neck may reduce carotid blood flow by stretching the shortened arteries. Indeed, patients often hold their heads in a flexed (drooping) position to prevent syncope.

Involvement of the pulmonary arteries by necrotizing vasculitis occurs in about 50 percent of patients and can manifest as pulmonary hypertension. Ventilation-perfusion abnormalities and associated increases in the alveolar-to-arterial partial pressure differences for oxygen most likely reflect occlusion of small pulmonary arteries by the inflammatory process. Myocardial ischemia can be due to inflammation of the coronary arteries. There may be involvement of the cardiac valves and cardiac conduction system. Renal artery stenosis can lead to reduced renal function as well as initiation of events leading to renal hypertension. Ankylosing spondylitis and rheumatoid arthritis can accompany this syndrome.

Treatment

Treatment of Takayashu's syndrome is usually with corticosteroids. Anticoagulation is instituted in some patients. Life-threatening

TABLE 12-1. Classification of Vasculitis Syndromes

Takayashu's syndrome (aortic arch arteritis, pulseless disease)

Thromboangitis obliterans (Buerger's disease)

Wegner's granulomatosis (lymphomatoid rheumatica)

Polyarteritis nodosa

Henoch-Schönlein purpura

or incapacitating arterial occlusions are sometimes amenable to surgical intervention.[2]

Management of Anesthesia

Takayashu's syndrome may be encountered in patients presenting for obstetrical anesthesia, incidental surgery, or such corrective vascular procedures as carotid endarterectomy. Formulation of a plan for the management of anesthesia must take into account the drugs used for treatment of this syndrome, as

TABLE 12-2. Signs and Symptoms of Takayashu's Syndrome

Central Nervous System
  Vertigo
  Visual disturbances
  Syncope
  Seizures
  Cerebral vascular accidents
  Shortened and stenosed carotid arteries

Cardiovascular System
  Multiple occlusions of peripheral arteries
  Coronary artery disease
  Cardiac valve dysfunction
  Cardiac conduction defects

Pulmonary
  Pulmonary hypertension
  Ventilation-perfusion mismatch

Renal
  Renal artery stenosis
  Renal dysfunction
  Renal hypertension

Musculoskeletal
  Ankylosing spondylitis
  Rheumatoid arthritis

well as multiple organ system involvement with necrotizing vasculitis.[3,4] For example, chronic corticosteroid therapy may result in suppression of adrenocortical function such that supplemental exogenous corticosteroids are indicated in the perioperative period. Regional anesthesia may not be a prudent selection in the presence of anticoagulation. Associated musculoskeletal changes can make performance of a lumbar epidural block or subarachnoid block technically difficult.

Blood pressure may be difficult to measure by classic methods. The Doppler sensor is effective, however, for determining blood pressure, since this device detects flow velocity rather than movement of the arterial wall. Nevertheless, blood pressure determined by the Doppler sensor may be less than central aortic pressure. Indeed, blood pressure is predictably decreased in the upper extremities because of narrowing of the arterial lumen.

There is a theoretical but undocumented concern regarding cannulation of arteries that may be involved by the inflammatory process characteristic of this syndrome. Nevertheless, a catheter placed in the radial artery is useful for confirming the presence of an adequate perfusion pressure during major operations. Monitoring blood pressure from a catheter placed in the femoral artery is acceptable, but it should be appreciated that blood pressure in the legs may be higher than the actual coronary or cerebral perfusion pressure. In addition, constant monitoring of the electrocardiogram and urine output provides an index of the adequacy of perfusion of the heart and kidneys respectively. Placement of a pulmonary artery catheter is acceptable if the magnitude of the surgery dictates.[4] In patients with known compromise of carotid blood flow, intraoperative monitoring of the electroencephalogram may be useful for detecting cerebral ischemia.

It must be remembered that hyperextension of the neck, as during direct laryngoscopy for intubation of the trachea, can compromise blood flow through carotid arteries that are shortened because of the inflammatory process that accompanies this disease. Indeed, the significance of changes in head position on cerebral function should be established during the preoperative interview.

Regardless of the drugs selected to produce anesthesia, the most important goal is the maintenance of adequate perfusion pressures during the intraoperative period. Therefore, anesthetic-induced reductions in blood pressure due to decreases in cardiac output or systemic vascular resistance must be recognized promptly and treated by decreasing the concentration of anesthetic drug or expanding the intravascular fluid volume. The use of sympathomimetic drugs is indicated to maintain perfusion pressures until the underlying cause for the reduction in blood pressure can be corrected. Avoidance of excessive hyperventilation of the lungs and use of volatile anesthetics may favor maintenance of cerebral blood flow in patients in whom the disease process involves the carotid arteries.[4]

THROMBOANGIITIS OBLITERANS

Thromboangiitis obliterans (Buerger's disease) is an inflammatory and occlusive disease that involves arteries and veins.[5] This disease has its greatest incidence in men, often of Jewish extraction, between 20 years and 40 years of age. Although the cause of this disease is not known, there is an undeniable association with cigarette smoking. Cold and trauma are also associated with an exacerbation of the disease process.

Signs and Symptoms

The lumens of arteries and veins are compromised early by characteristic inflammatory infiltrates. These focal lesions are usually interspersed with areas of normal vessel wall. In many respects, it is difficult to distinguish this disease from atherosclerosis. Diagnosis of thromboangiitis obliterans can be confirmed only by the biopsy of an active vascular lesion.

The most prominent early clinical finding is vasospasm that alternates with periods of quiescence. Vascular changes are typically present in the extremities, although cerebral, coronary, and mesenteric vessels can be involved on rare occasions. Intermittent claudication reflects accumulation of pain-producing metabolites due to poor skeletal muscle blood flow. Migratory thrombophlebitis, usually involving the lower extremities, occurs in a high percentage of patients.

Treatment

Treatment of thromboangiitis obliterans consists of discontinuing smoking and avoidance of trauma to ischemic extremities. Cold ambient temperature is undesirable, as this can accentuate vasospasm. Corticosteroids and peripheral vasodilating drugs have been used with unpredictable success. A surgical sympathectomy (removal of L1–3 ganglia of the sympathetic chain) can be considered if medical treatment is not satisfactory.

Management of Anesthesia

Management of anesthesia in the presence of thromboangiitis obliterans requires avoidance of events that could damage already ischemic extremities. Positioning during surgery must insure the absence of unnecessary pressure on the extremities. It would seem prudent to increase the ambient temperature of the operating room and to warm and humidify the inspired gases so as to maintain body temperature. Monitoring of blood pressure is ideally accomplished using a Doppler sensor. Arterial catheterization for purposes of monitoring blood pressure or arterial blood gases is not recommended, in view of the likely presence of an already compromised circulation to the extremities. The presence of pulmonary disease must be considered, since these patients are frequently cigarette smokers. If cigarette smoking is excessive, levels of carboxyhemoglobin may be elevated, reducing the amounts of oxygen that can be carried by hemoglobin. In addition, the oxyhemoglobin dissociation curve may be shifted to the left in cigarette smokers, further compromising the delivery of oxygen to tissues (see Chapter 14). For these reasons, it may be prudent to increase inspired concentrations of oxygen during the perioperative period.

The possible interaction of anesthetic drugs with peripheral vasodilators used to treat thromboangiitis obliterans, as well as the potential need for supplemental corticosteroids, must be considered preoperatively. In the final analysis, regional or general anesthesia can be administered to these patients. If a regional anesthetic technique is selected, it is best not to include epinephrine with the local anesthetic, so as to avoid any possibility of accentuating co-existing vasospasm.

WEGENER'S GRANULOMATOSIS

Wegener's granulomatosis is characterized by the formation of granulomas in the vicinity of inflamed vessels. Necrotizing vasculitis is widespread and involves both small arteries and veins. The etiology of this disease is uncertain, although immunologic dysfunction and hypersensitivity to an unidentified antigen are possibilities.[6]

Signs and Symptoms

Signs and symptoms of Wegener's granulomatosis depend on the organ involved by the necrotizing vasculitis. The respiratory tract, cardiovascular system, nervous system, and kidneys are often affected by the disease process.

RESPIRATORY TRACT

The nose, maxillary sinus, hard palate, larynx, and upper trachea may be infiltrated by necrotizing granulomas. Sinusitis may be the presenting complaint. Laryngeal mucosa may be replaced by granulation tissue, resulting in a narrowing of the glottic opening. Destructive lesions of the epiglottis are common. Vasculitis may result in occlusion of pulmonary vessels, leading to ventilation-perfusion abnormalities. There may be a random interstitial distribution of pulmonary granulomas, with surrounding infection, effusion, and hemorrhage. Indeed, pneumonia and pulmonary hemorrhage are complications of this disease process. Central necrosis of the granulomas can result in the presence of thick-walled cavities in various regions of the lung. Bronchi may be eroded by inflammatory exudate, leading to obstruction of the airways with associated increases in intrapulmonary shunting.

CARDIOVASCULAR SYSTEM

Cardiovascular effects of Wegener's granulomatosis include vasculitis involving peripheral arteries and veins and necrotizing changes in the walls of the coronary arteries. Distortion of cardiac valves and impairment of conduction of the cardiac impulse reflect infiltration of these areas by the necrotizing process. Left ventricular hypertrophy may be present. Infarction of the tips of digits reflects arteritis involving peripheral vessels.

NERVOUS SYSTEM

Granulomatous lesions may involve the cranial nerves, cerebrum, or skull. Cerebral arterial aneurysms and cerebrovascular accidents due to arteritis of the cerebral vessels may occur. Arteritis often involves the vasa nervorum of peripheral nerves, producing a peripheral neuropathy. Skeletal muscle wasting may reflect neuritis or necrotizing myopathy.

KIDNEYS

Wegener's granulomatosis of the kidney can cause complete destruction of the renal glomeruli. Hematuria and azotemia are common findings. Progressive renal failure is the most frequent cause of death in patients with Wegener's granulomatosis.

Treatment

Cyclophosphamide is the drug of choice in the treatment of Wegener's granulomatosis. This drug produces dramatic remissions in nearly every patient. Corticosteroids have also been used in the treatment of this disease.

Management of Anesthesia

Management of anesthesia in patients with Wegener's granulomatosis requires an appreciation of the widespread organ involvement associated with this disease. The potential adverse effects of drugs used in its treatment must be considered. For example, cyclophosphamide produces profound suppression of the immune system. In addition, this drug is associated with leukopenia, hemolytic anemia, and decreased activity of plasma cholinesterase enzyme. Drug-induced decreases in plasma cholinesterase activity have been associated with variable responses to succinylcholine, but prolonged duration of neuromuscular blockade, as may occur in patients with atypical cholinesterase enzyme, has not occurred.[7] Supplemental corticosteroids in the perioperative period may be indicated for patients being treated chronically with these drugs.

Gentleness during direct laryngoscopy is important, as bleeding from granulomas and dislodgement of friable ulcerated tissues can occur. A smaller than expected endotracheal tube may be required if the glottic opening is narrowed by granulomatous changes. Suctioning of the airway may be needed to remove necrotic debris. Administration of high inspired concentrations of oxygen should be considered in view of the likely presence of pulmonary disease. Indwelling arterial catheters should be used infrequently and arterial punctures should be limited, since arteritis is likely to involve peripheral vessels. A careful neurologic examination to detect the presence of peripheral neuropathies should be performed before the decision is made to use regional anesthetic techniques. The choice and doses of muscle relaxants may be influenced by the effect of cyclophosphamide on plasma cholinesterase activity and the magnitude of renal dysfunction produced by the disease. Implications for the use of succinylcholine in the presence of skeletal muscle atrophy due to neuritis should also be considered. Conceivably, volatile anesthetic drugs could be associated with exaggerated myocardial depression when the disease process involves the myocardium and cardiac valves. Monitoring of the electrocardiogram is helpful in detecting disturbances of cardiac conduction. Ultimately, the rational administration of anesthesia to patients with Wegener's granulomatosis is based on the magnitude and type of organ system dysfunction produced by the disease.

TEMPORAL ARTERITIS

Temporal arteritis is a vasculitis that can lead to a sudden unilateral blindness. Blindness reflects occlusive arteritis in the branches of the ophthalmic artery. Any patient over 60 years of age complaining of a unilateral headache is suspect for this diagnosis. Evidence of arteritis on a biopsy of the temporal artery is present in about 90 percent of patients. The cause of this arteritis is not known. High doses of corticosteroids (usually prednisone) are mandatory to control symptoms and to prevent permanent blindness.

POLYARTERITIS NODOSA

Polyarteritis nodosa is a multisystem disease of unknown etiology characterized by acute inflammation and fibrinoid necrosis of small arteries. Renal involvement occurs in about 75 percent of patients and is the most common cause of death. This involvement is typically a necrotizing glomerulitis that manifests as hematuria, proteinuria, and azotemia. Hypertension is frequent and presumably reflects renal disease. Myocardial ischemia and infarction may occur secondary to coronary arteritis. Treatment of polyarteritis nodosa is nonspecific but often includes the administration of corticosteroids.

Management of anesthesia in patients with polyarteritis nodosa should take into consideration the likelihood of renal and cardiac disease and the implications of co-existing hypertension. Supplemental corticosteroids are appropriate if patients have been receiving these drugs preoperatively for treatment of their underlying disease.

HENOCH-SCHÖNLEIN PURPURA

Henoch-Schönlein purpura is a vasculitis presumed to be due to an immune-mediated hypersensitivity reaction. This disease primarily affects children. Target organs include joints, kidneys, and the gastrointestinal tract. Kidney involvement can progress to renal failure. Corticosteroids are frequently used in the treatment of this disease process.

RAYNAUD'S PHENOMENON

Raynaud's phenomenon is an abnormal sensitivity of small arteries and arterioles to vasoconstrictive stimuli. The etiology of this disease is not known, but overactivity of the sympathetic nervous system with excess production of neurotransmitter or interference with the inactivation of norepinephrine are possible explanations. Exposure to cold ambient temperatures is a well-recognized cause of severe arterial spasm in these patients. Women are affected most often and emotional instability is often present.

Raynaud's phenomenon is nearly always associated with an underlying disease, most often scleroderma or systemic lupus erythe-

matosus. Primary pulmonary hypertension may also accompany Raynaud's phenomenon. Ultimately, the prognosis depends on the progression of the associated underlying disease. Often Raynaud's phenomenon is characterized by a slow progression that may consist of stationary periods lasting years.

Signs and Symptoms

The initial clinical manifestations of Raynaud's phenomenon are pallor and cyanosis of the digits, followed by erythema and edema. Arterial vasoconstriction of the digital arteries is responsible for the initial pallor, and stasis of blood leads to cyanosis. Erythema and edema occur when the arteries suddenly reopen. These initial attacks are most often precipitated by exposure to cold ambient temperatures, and only one digit may be affected. Eventually additional fingers are involved and in some instances fingers and toes may become ischemic. Numbness and diaphoresis often occur during the attacks. Burning and throbbing pain typically follow the ischemic episode.

Treatment

The treatment of Raynaud's phenomenon consists of avoiding such precipitating causes as exposure to cold ambient temperatures and abstaining from cigarette smoking. Arterial spasm and pain may be relieved on occasion by the intravenous administration of reserpine[8] or guanethidine[9] into a tourniquet-isolated extremity. In severe cases with trophic changes, surgical interruption of the sympathetic nerve supply to the hand (transection of preganglionic fibers in the sympathetic chain at T2 and T3) may be considered but has not produced consistently predictable or good results.

Management of Anesthesia

There are no specific recommendations as to choices of drugs to produce general anesthesia in patients with Raynaud's phenomenon. Maintenance of body temperature and increasing the ambient temperature of the operating room would seem logical. Blood pressure is best monitored by a noninvasive technique such as the Doppler sensor. The hazards of placing a catheter in a peripheral artery of a potentially ischemic extremity must be weighed against the advantages that continuous monitoring of blood pressure would provide.

Regional anesthesia is acceptable for peripheral operations in patients with Raynaud's phenomenon. Indeed, regional anesthetic techniques that block the sympathetic nervous system innervation to an extremity are often used for diagnostic purposes. If a regional anesthetic technique is selected, it is best not to include epinephrine with the local anesthetic, as the catecholamine could provoke undesirable vasoconstriction.

MOYAMOYA DISEASE

Moyamoya disease is a rare neurovascular disease characterized by narrowing or occlusion of both internal carotid arteries. Children and adults are affected and a familial tendency may be present. The most common presentation in children is transient ischemic attacks, whereas in adults the most common presentation is intracerebral hemorrhage. The incidence of intracranial aneurysms associated with Moyamoya disease has been estimated to be 14 percent in adults but is rare in childhood.[10]

Medical management of these patients includes use of antiplatelet (aspirin) and cerebral vasodilating (verapamil) drugs. Surgical treatment has included bypass (superficial temporal to middle cerebral artery anastomosis) and revascularization procedures. Management of anesthesia must recognize the impor-

tance of preserving a proper balance between cerebral blood flow and cerebral oxygen consumption. Isoflurane has been recommended because of its mild cerebral vasodilating effects and ability to greatly reduce cerebral metabolic rate.[11] Normocapnia is maintained to avoid any possible detrimental effect of altered arterial partial pressures of carbon dioxide on cerebral blood flow. The presence of neurologic changes may preclude the use of succinylcholine. Increased intraoperative bleeding may reflect effects of therapy with antiplatelet drugs. Cardiac rhythm disturbances have been reported in these patients during anesthesia and surgery. Patients with a history of seizures should be maintained on anticonvulsant medications.

ACUTE ARTERIAL OCCLUSIVE DISEASE

Acute arterial occlusion in the extremities usually results from an embolus originating from the heart. These types of emboli can originate from (1) thrombi in the akinetic portion of the left ventricle in patients with a prior myocardial infarction, (2) an enlarged and often fibrillating left atrium, (3) prosthetic heart valves, (4) vegetations of infective endocarditis, and (5) left atrial myxomas. Emboli usually lodge at the bifurcations of large arteries.

Signs and Symptoms

The clinical picture of acute arterial occlusion is characterized by evidence of ischemia below the site of vascular obstruction. The involved extremity shows sharply demarcated color changes, and the skin feels cool below the site of the obstruction. Furthermore, veins are collapsed and distal arterial pulses are not palpable. Patients most often complain of the sudden onset of pain in the ischemia area. Paresthesias and muscle weakness of the involved extremity can also occur.

Treatment

The prognosis after an acute arterial occlusion depends on the size of the artery involved and the presence of collateral circulation. Surgical removal of the embolus is indicated if conservative measures fail to improve blood flow to the ischemic area within about 2 hours. All surgically removed emboli should be examined microscopically for myxomatous material to detect the presence of a previously unsuspected atrial myxoma (see Chapter 2).

CHRONIC ARTERIAL OCCLUSIVE DISEASE

Chronic arterial occlusive disease is nearly always due to atherosclerosis. The majority of these patients also have clinical evidence of coronary and/or cerebral atherosclerotic disease. Aortoiliac occlusive disease can be treated surgically by endarterectomy or aortofemoral bypass. Vascular bypass surgery for arterial occlusive disease distal to the popliteal artery is not highly successful.

VENOUS THROMBUS FORMATION

Venous thrombus formation that does not elicit a local reaction or overt symptoms is referred to as phlebothrombosis. Thrombophlebitis is present when venous thrombus formation is associated with a local inflammatory reaction. It is commonly believed that phlebothrombosis precedes thrombophlebitis. Venous thrombus formation may involve superficial or deep veins. Thrombi developing in

superficial veins as follows intravenous infusions or injections of drugs are rarely associated with detectable pulmonary embolism. This likely reflects intense inflammation that accompanies superficial venous thrombosis leading to rapid total occlusion of the vein. Pulmonary embolism is a risk of deep vein thrombosis (see Chapter 13).

Predisposing Factors

Predisposing factors for venous thrombus formation are (1) venous stasis, (2) abnormality of the venous wall, and (3) altered coagulation states (Table 12-3). Venous stasis is the most important and is most likely to occur (1) after surgical procedures that impose prolonged immobility, (2) during pregnancy, and (3) in the presence of a low cardiac output associated with congestive heart failure or an acute myocardial infarction. Venous stasis results in failure to rapidly clear activated clotting factors from veins predisposing to thrombus formation. Co-existing endothelial wall damage and hypercoagulable states (oral contraceptives, carcinoma particularly of the lung) predispose to thrombus formation. It is not known whether surgery predisposes patients to hypercoagula-

TABLE 12-3. Predisposing Factors for Venous Thrombus Formation

Venous Stasis
   Surgical procedures
   Pregnancy
   Congestive heart failure
   Myocardial infarction

Abnormality of Venous Wall
   Varicose veins
   Drug-induced irritation

Altered Coagulation States
   Oral contraceptives
   Carcinoma

Orthopedic Surgery on Lower Extremity
   Hip surgery
   Knee reconstruction

Morbid Obesity

Elderly

ble states, although certain forms of surgery (especially orthopedic surgery on the lower extremity and prostatectomy) are associated with an increased incidence of deep vein thrombosis. For example, it is estimated that 45 percent to 70 percent of patients undergoing lower extremity orthopedic surgery develop deep vein thrombosis.[12] Morbidly obese individuals and geriatric patients seem predisposed to the formation of venous thrombi.

Signs and Symptoms

Local elevations in venous pressure and inflammatory reactions are responsible for the initial signs and symptoms of venous thrombus formation. Phlebothrombosis is associated with minimal symptoms. Nevertheless, phlebothrombosis may be associated with pain in response to stimulation that would not produce discomfort in normal extremities. When thrombophlebitis involves superficial veins, the area around the vessel is warm, erythematous, and painful. The thrombosed vein is felt as a firm cordlike structure. Thrombophlebitis involving deep veins is characterized by throbbing pain that may be continuous. There may be edema and associated muscle spasm. An increased erythrocyte sedimentation rate and leukocytosis are often present.

Ultimately, the diagnosis of deep vein thrombosis depends on laboratory tests, as clinical signs and symptoms are inconsistent and nonspecific. For example, only about 50 percent of patients with tenderness and swelling of the calf are demonstrated to have deep vein thrombosis on a venogram. Venography is the most invasive but also most reliable method for documenting deep vein thrombosis. Impedence plethysmography and Doppler ultrasonography are useful in detecting thrombi above the knees. Radioactive fibrinogen scanning is sensitive for detecting thrombi in veins below the knees, but soft tissue above the knees often shields radioactivity. Furthermore, deposition of fibrinogen in areas of inflammation or hemorrhage outside veins, as occur after hip surgery, may yield false-positive results.

Prophylaxis

Small subcutaneous doses of heparin reduce the incidence of venous thrombus formation and subsequent pulmonary embolism in the postoperative period (see Chapter 13). The typical heparin regimen is 5,000 U administered subcutaneously 2 hours preoperatively and then every 8 hours to 12 hours postoperatively for 4 days to 5 days.[13]

Treatment

Treatment of superficial venous thrombosis is with the application of local heat to, continual elevation of, and restricted use of the extremity involved. Medical management of deep vein thrombosis is with systemic anticoagulation using heparin, complete bed rest, elevation of the involved extremity, and the continuous application of heat. Anticoagulation is necessary to reduce the likelihood of propagation of the venous thrombus or the occurrence of pulmonary embolism. Intensive medical treatment is continued until local tenderness and edema have subsided. Surgical removal of the venous thrombus may be necessary when large veins are involved, as with iliofemoral thrombophlebitis. Ligation of the inferior vena cava may be considered in patients who do not tolerate anticoagulation or in whom pulmonary embolism occurs despite anticoagulation.

REFERENCES

1. Nasu T. Pathology of pulseless disease: A systematic study and critical review of twenty-one cases reported in Japan. Angiology 1963;16:225–42
2. Gupta S. Surgical and immunological aspects of Takayashu's disease. Ann R Coll Surg Engl 1982;63:325–32
3. Ramanathan S, Gupta U, Chalon J, Turndorf H.

Anesthetic considerations in Takayashu arteritis. Anesth Analg 1979;58:247–9

4. Warner MA, Hughes DR, Messick JM, Anesthetic management of a patient with pulseless disease. Anesth Analg 1983;62:532–5

5. Williams G. Recent view of Buerger's disease. J Clin Pathol 1969;22:573–8

6. Lake CL. Anesthesia and Wegener's granulomatosis: Case report and review of the literature. Anesth Analg 1978;57:353–9

7. Dillman JF. Safe use of succinylcholine during repeated anesthetics in a patient treated with cyclophosphamide. Anesth Analg 1987;66:351–3

8. Gorsky BH. Intravenous perfusion with reserpine for Raynaud's phenomenon. Regional Anesth 1977;2:5

9. Holland AJC, Davies KH, Wallace DH. Sympathetic blockade of isolated limbs by intravenous guanethidine. Can Anaesth Soc J 1977;24:597–602

10. Waga S, Tochio H. Intracranial aneurysm associated with Moyamoya disease in childhood. Surg Neurol 1985;23:237–43

11. Brown SC, Lam AM. Moyamoya disease—a review of clinical experience and anesthetic management. Can J Anaesth 1987;34:71–5

12. Hirsh J, Gallus AS. ^{125}I-labelled fibrinogen scanning. JAMA 1975;233:970–3

13. Sherry S. Low dose heparin prophylaxis for postoperative venous thromboembolism. N Engl J Med 1975;293:300–2

Pulmonary Embolism

Deep vein thrombosis with subsequent pulmonary embolism is one of the most frequent causes of postoperative morbidity and mortality. Although the true incidence of pulmonary embolism is not known, it is estimated that deep vein thrombosis and pulmonary embolism are associated with 300,000 to 600,000 hospitalizations annually and that as many as 50,000 individuals die each year as a result of pulmonary embolism.[1] It is uncommon for pulmonary embolism to develop in patients without the presence of one or more risk factors that usually predispose to venous stasis (see Table 13-1). The usual sites for formation of venous thrombi that lead to pulmonary embolism are the deep veins of the legs, the pelvic veins, and the right atrium of patients with atrial fibrillation. Venous thrombi formed below the knees or in the upper extremities rarely give rise to significant pulmonary embolism. In addition to thrombi from veins, pulmonary embolism may be due to fat, air, amniotic fluid, and, on rare occasions, cells from neoplasms.

PATHOPHYSIOLOGY

Pulmonary embolism produces complex alterations in pulmonary mechanics and circulatory function.[1] For example, alveolar dead space increases acutely when perfusion to a segment of the lung ceases, but ventilation to that portion of the lung continues. Compensatory mechanisms, such as bronchoconstriction, may serve to reduce ventilation to the unperfused area of the lung and thus return ventilation-to-perfusion ratios toward normal. After 12 hours to 24 hours, unperfused alveoli become deficient in surfactant, leading to atelectasis. Pulmonary compliance and lung volumes are subsequently decreased and airway resistance increases. These changes in pulmonary mechanics play important roles in the development of arterial hypoxemia, which often accompanies pulmonary embolism. Occlusion of a pulmonary artery by an embolus

TABLE 13-1. Signs and Symptoms of Pulmonary Embolism

Sign/Symptom	Percent of Patients
Acute dyspnea	80–85
Tachypnea ($>$20 breaths·min^{-1})	75–85
Pleuritic chest pain	65–70
Nonproductive cough	50–60
Accentuation of pulmonary valve closure sound	50–60
Rales	50–60
Tachycardia ($>$100 beats·min^{-1})	45–65
Fever (38–39 degrees Celsius)	40–50
Hemoptysis	30

often leads to the development of tissue necrosis distal to the vascular obstruction.

Obstruction to blood flow through the lungs by an embolus acutely increases pulmonary vascular resistance. In addition, local release of vasoactive substances such as serotonin may contribute to constriction of pulmonary vasculature. Indeed, pulmonary hypertension is the most significant pathophysiologic change affecting the cardiovascular system. Right ventricular failure develops when elevations in pulmonary vascular resistance are extreme.

CLINICAL MANIFESTATIONS

Clinical manifestations of pulmonary embolism are nonspecific, and the diagnosis is often difficult to establish on clinical grounds alone (Table 13-1).[1] Nevertheless, history and physical examination constitute the only basis for initially suspecting pulmonary embolism. Often these findings overlap with other cardiopulmonary diseases, emphasizing the importance of a high index of suspicion in recognizing patients with pulmonary embolism. The most consistent manifestation is an acute onset of dyspnea,[2] which most likely reflects a suddenly increased alveolar dead space and a decreased pulmonary compliance. Stimulation of pulmonary receptors and local release of serotonin from the embolus may also contribute to dyspnea. Often dyspnea and associated apprehension seem out of proportion to the degree and extent of objective abnormal findings. Typically, respiration is rapid (30 breaths·min^{-1} to 50 breaths·min^{-1}) and shallow. Substernal chest pain, which may be indistinguishable from angina pectoris, often accompanies a large pulmonary embolus. Hypotension and increased central venous pressures are consistent with the diagnosis of pulmonary embolus. Nevertheless, pulmonary artery pressures are not significantly elevated in normal patients until at least 50 percent of the pulmonary circulation has been occluded by clot. Conversely, in patients with co-existing cardiopulmonary disease, a relatively small volume of clot may abruptly elevate pulmonary artery pressures. Wheezing may be heard on auscultation of the lungs. Tachycardia is frequently present.

Blood Gases

Arterial blood gases may or may not reflect arterial hypoxemia. Changes in ventilation–perfusion relationships are the most likely explanation for reductions in arterial oxygenation that accompany pulmonary embolism. Mild hyperventilation is frequently confirmed by low arterial carbon dioxide partial pressures.

Electrocardiogram

The principal usefulness of the electrocardiogram in the presence of a pulmonary embolism is to rule out myocardial ischemia or infarction as causes of chest pain. Changes on the electrocardiogram reflecting acute cor pulmonale are usually transient unless the pulmonary embolism is large. Nevertheless, abrupt appearance of right axis deviation on the electrocardiogram, associated with incomplete or complete right bundle branch block and tall peaked T-waves, suggests a pulmonary embolus in a previously asymptomatic patient. Additional findings consistent with acute cor pulmonale include a systolic ejection murmur best heard over the area of the pulmonary valve, wide and fixed splitting of the second heart sound, and enlargement of the pulmonary artery and right ventricle on radiographs of the chest.

Pulmonary Infarction

Occlusion of a pulmonary artery by an embolus can lead to the development of infarction and necrosis of distal lung tissue. It is estimated that pulmonary infarction develops in

10 percent to 15 percent of patients after occurrence of a pulmonary embolism. If the infarcted area extends to the surface of the lung, a reactive pleuritis develops. The triad of cough, hemoptysis, and pleuritic chest pain is suggestive of the development of a pulmonary infarction. This triad typically does not manifest for several hours or even days after the initial pulmonary embolism. Radiographs of the chest in the presence of pulmonary infarction may reveal a wedge-shaped density associated with a pleural effusion and elevated hemidiaphragm on the same side reflecting decreased lung volumes, which result from atelectasis accompanying pulmonary embolism. An isolated pulmonary infiltrate may be interpreted as pneumonia but, together with an associated evaluation of the corresponding hemidiaphragm, should also suggest pulmonary embolism. Frequently, pulmonary infarction is silent, manifesting only as low-grade temperature elevations. Body temperature elevations make it difficult to distinguish pulmonary infarctions from pulmonary infections.

Pulmonary Embolism During Anesthesia

Manifestations of pulmonary embolism during anesthesia are nonspecific and often transient.[3] Changes suggestive of pulmonary embolism include unexplained arterial hypoxemia, hypotension, tachycardia, and bronchospasm. The electrocardiogram and central venous pressure may reflect abrupt onset of pulmonary hypertension and right ventricular dysfunction. Monitoring the end-tidal carbon dioxide concentrations will reveal increased arterial to alveolar differences for carbon dioxide due to ventilation of unperfused alveoli.

LABORATORY DIAGNOSIS

Standard laboratory determinations are of minimial help. The triad of increased plasma levels of lactic dehydrogenase and of bilirubin in the presence of normal glutamic oxaloacetic transaminase concentrations has not proved to be a reliable indication of pulmonary embolism. Measurements of plasma enzyme concentrations, however, may facilitate differentiation of pulmonary embolism from acute myocardial infarctions. For example, delayed and nonspecific elevations of plasma concentrations of the isoenzyme-3 fraction of lactic dehydrogenase suggests pulmonary embolism. In contrast, elevation of the plasma concentrations of glutamic oxaloacetic transaminase and of the cardiac-specific isoenzyme fraction of creatine kinase suggests an acute myocardial infarction rather than a pulmonary embolism. Leukocytosis and an elevated erythrocyte sedimentation rate are frequent changes associated with pulmonary infarctions.

DEFINITIVE DIAGNOSIS

Definitive diagnosis of pulmonary embolism may require both invasive and noninvasive diagnostic tests, including pulmonary perfusion scans, pulmonary ventilation scans, and pulmonary arteriography.

Pulmonary Perfusion-Ventilation Scan

Pulmonary perfusion-ventilation scan is a valuable noninvasive test, which utilizes gamma-emitting isotopes to delineate pulmonary blood flow.[4] This test is sensitive and is almost always abnormal when clinically significant pulmonary embolism is present. For example, a normal ventilation scan over an area that shows a perfusion defect is highly suggestive of pulmonary embolism. Pulmonary perfusion scans that are matched for poor ventilation and perfusion are indicative of other diseases such as chronic obstructive airways disease.

Pulmonary Angiography

Selective pulmonary angiography is the most definitive test for demonstrating the presence of a pulmonary embolism. An intravascular filling defect and an arterial vessel cutoff are considered diagnostic of pulmonary embolism. Decreased pulmonary vascularity and asymmetric pulmonary blood flow are suggestive of pulmonary embolism but may also reflect other disease processes involving the lungs. Serial angiography studies may demonstrate dissolution of the pulmonary embolism over several days.

Angiography is an invasive procedure, associated with significant risks related to (1) right heart catheterization, (2) development of cardiac dysrhythmias, and (3) allergic reactions to the contrast media. Therefore, this diagnostic test should be reserved for those instances when a significant pulmonary embolism is suspected but the pulmonary perfusion-ventilation scan is not diagnostic. Should suspected pulmonary embolism occur in patients being monitored with pulmonary artery catheters, it is permissible to use this catheter for pulmonary angiography.[5] Contrast medium is injected through the distal port with the catheter placed in a proximal pulmonary artery.

TREATMENT

Treatment of pulmonary embolism is designed to support cardiopulmonary function and to prevent extension or recurrence of the pulmonary embolism by institution of systemic anticoagulation. Surgical intervention may be indicated in selected cases. The importance of prompt diagnosis and treatment is emphasized by the reduction in mortality from 18 percent to 35 percent in patients with unrecognized pulmonary embolism to about 8 percent in treated patients.[1]

Supportive Treatment

Increased inspired concentrations of oxygen are administered to correct arterial hypoxemia associated with pulmonary embolism. Cardiac dysrhythmias usually respond to intravenous administration of lidocaine. Hypotension due to a low cardiac output may require treatment with catecholamines such as isoproterenol, dopamine, or dobutamine. Isoproterenol is an attractive choice, as it is more likely than other catecholamines to reduce pulmonary vascular resistance. Nevertheless, the value of pulmonary vasodilators in the management of pulmonary embolism is not well defined. Digitalis may be considered if a low cardiac output persists. Aminophylline, administered intravenously, is helpful when bronchospasm is present. Intubation of the trachea and institution of controlled ventilation of the lungs with positive end-expiratory pressure is indicated should pulmonary edema complicate pulmonary embolism. Analgesic therapy to treat pain associated with pulmonary embolism is important but must be prescribed with the underlying stability of the cardiovascular system in mind.

Systemic Anticoagulation

Systemic anticoagulation with intravenous administration of heparin is indicated in patients with the diagnosis of pulmonary embolism. Heparin works almost immediately to prevent extension of venous thrombus or recurrence of additional embolization to the lungs. Furthermore, heparin serves to block the local release of serotonin, which is felt to accentuate pulmonary vasoconstriction that accompanies pulmonary embolism. Therapy should begin with the intravenous injection of heparin (5,000 U) followed by a continuous infusion of heparin (usually 1,200 $U \cdot hr^{-1}$ to 1,800 $U \cdot hr^{-1}$) so as to maintain activated partial thromboplastin time 2 times to 2.5 times the control levels for that patient. Plasma concentrations of platelets should be monitored, as 5 percent to 30 percent of patients manifest heparin-induced thrombocytopenia 2 days to 10 days after initiation of anticoagulant therapy.[6] The incidence of thrombocytopenia is higher in patients receiving bovine-lung heparin compared with intestinal mucosa preparations.[6]

The major hazard of systemic anticoagulation is spontaneous hemorrhage. Indeed, bleeding due to heparin anticoagulation occurs in about 10 percent of patients. The incidence of spontaneous hemorrhage is even greater when heparin-induced thrombocytopenia is present.[6] Intracranial hemorrhage is a feared complication of heparin therapy. Nevertheless, the only absolute contraindication to the use of heparin is the presence of a known coagulation disorder or active hemorrhage. Hemoptysis from pulmonary infarction is not a contraindication to therapy with heparin.

Animal data demonstrating that it takes 7 days to 12 days for a thrombus to become firmly adherent to the vein wall is the rationale for continuing heparin therapy for this period of time. Subsequently, oral anticoagulants such as warfarin are necessary to maintain the antithrombotic state on a long-term basis. Although there is no unanimity concerning the optimal duration of long-term oral anticoagulant therapy, there is a concensus that 3 months to 6 months is often adequate. Serial determinations of prothrombin time are used to measure the adequacy of the oral anticoagulant dose. Anticoagulation is judged adequate when prothrombin times are prolonged 2 times to 2.5 times the normal values.

PROPHYLAXIS

Low-dose heparin therapy (5,000 U 2 hours before surgery and every 8 hours to 12 hours thereafter until patients are ambulatory) reduces the incidence of deep vein thrombosis after thoracoabdominal surgery from greater than 30 percent to less than 10 percent.[9] Nevertheless, prevention of pulmonary embolism and reduction in mortality produced by low-dose heparin in these patients is not certain.[10] The frequency of deep vein thrombosis is re-duced by low-dose heparin prophylaxis in patients undergoing total hip replacement but not in those undergoing open prostatectomy.[11] Aspirin, dextran (10 ml·kg^{-1} during surgery and for several days postoperatively) and warfarin have also been shown to be effective prophylaxis for reducing the incidence of deep vein thrombosis in patients undergoing hip surgery. The pneumatic compression boot that compresses the lower extremities to promote venous blood flow dramatically reduces the incidence of deep vein thrombosis in neurosurgical patients.[12] Electrical stimulation of calf muscles increases venous flow and reduces the incidence of deep vein thrombosis almost as well as low-dose heparin.[13] Early ambulation is the best prophylaxis against venous stasis with resultant deep vein thrombosis and the risk of subsequent pulmonary embolism.

Thrombolytic Agents

Thrombolytic drugs such as urokinase and streptokinase may accelerate the lysis of the pulmonary embolus.[7] Spontaneous hemorrhage is the most significant risk of these drugs. Therefore, treatment with thrombolytic drugs is not indicated unless the pulmonary embolism is massive (involvement of more than 50 percent of the pulmonary circulation as reflected by pulmonary angiography), or profound cardiovascular collapse is present. Because thrombolytic drugs may lyse previously formed clots, recent postoperative patients and individuals who have sustained significant traumatic injuries probably should not be treated with these drugs.

Surgical Intervention

Surgical intervention is indicated when recurrent pulmonary embolism occurs despite systemic anticoagulation or in those patients in whom anticoagulation is not tolerated or is contraindicated. Since more than 90 percent of pulmonary emboli originate from thrombi in lower extremities, surgical maneuvers are often directed toward interruption of the inferior vena cava. Placement of an umbrella filter in the inferior vena cava below the renal veins, using fluorscopy, is associated with less morbidity and mortality than surgical ligation of the inferior vena cava. Migration of this umbrella filter is a serious hazard and occurs in about 5 percent of patients treated in this manner.

Pulmonary artery embolectomy using cardiopulmonary bypass is restricted to patients with a massive pulmonary embolism documented by pulmonary arteriography who are unresponsive to medical treatment. Transvenous removal of pulmonary emboli has been successfully accomplished in a few patients using a suction cup catheter that is floated into the pulmonary artery via a peripheral vein.[8]

MANAGEMENT OF ANESTHESIA

Management of anesthesia for the surgical treatment of life-threatening pulmonary embolism is designed to support vital organ function and minimize anesthetic-induced myocardial depression. The majority of patients will arrive in the operating room with a tube in the trachea and ventilation of the lungs being controlled with high inspired concentrations of oxygen. Monitoring of arterial and cardiac filling pressures is essential. It is important to monitor right atrial filling pressures and to adjust the rate of intravenous fluid administration so as to optimize right ventricular stroke volume in the presence of marked increases in afterload. It may be necessary to support cardiac output with continuous intravenous infusions of catecholamines during the operative procedure. In this regard, isoproterenol increases myocardial contractility and decreases pulmonary vascular resistance. The disadvantage of isoproterenol is a reduction in diastolic blood pressure, which may jeopardize coronary blood flow. Dopamine or dobutamine are acceptable alternative drugs to isopro-

terenol, but neither of these drugs is known to produce decreases in pulmonary vascular resistance. In fact, dopamine in high doses, may increase pulmonary vascular resistance.

Induction and maintenance of anesthesia should avoid accentuation of co-existing arterial hypoxemia, hypotension, and pulmonary hypertension. Induction of anesthesia is often accomplished with benzodiazepines. Ketamine is a possible choice, but its potential adverse effects on pulmonary vascular resistance must be considered. Maintenance of anesthesia can be achieved with any drug or drug combination that does not produce excessive myocardial depression. Nitrous oxide can be used, but it should be discontinued if evidence of increased pulmonary vascular resistance accompanies its administration. Likewise, the need for high inspired concentrations of oxygen may limit the use of nitrous oxide. Pancuronium would be a useful selection for production of skeletal muscle paralysis. Intermediate-acting muscle relaxants with minimal to no circulatory effects would also be acceptable choices.

Removal of embolic fragments from the distal pulmonary arteries may be facilitated by the application of positive pressure ventilation of the lungs when the surgeon applies suction through the arteriotomy placed in the pulmonary trunk. Although the cardiopulmonary status of these patients is perilous before surgery, significant hemodynamic improvement usually results postoperatively.

FAT EMBOLISM

Fat embolism should be considered in patients who develop dyspnea, tachycardia, mental confusion, fever, and often petechial rashes over the upper part of the body 12 hours to 72 hours after trauma that includes multiple fractures or major fracture to long bones.[14] The source of fat is controversial but may represent disruption of the adipose architecture of bone marrow. Intravascular fat deposits may cause organ ischemia and pulmonary hypertension. Often, there is diffuse alveolar capillary leak that resembles acute respiratory failure. Arterial hypoxemia is an invariable component of fat embolism. Circulating fat may also cause platelet aggregation. Sometimes fat droplets are seen in retinal vessels.

Laboratory data may reveal mild to severe thrombocytopenia and mild anemia. Elevated plasma lipase concentrations or the presence of lipiduria are suggestive of fat embolism but may also occur after trauma in the absence of this problem. Development of fat embolism more than 72 hours after trauma is unlikely.

Treatment of fat embolism is supportive including intubation of the trachea and mechanical ventilation of the lungs in patients who develop acute respiratory failure. Large doses of corticosteroids (methylprednisolone 10 mg·kg^{-1} to 15 mg·kg^{-1} for 4 days to 5 days) may be beneficial.[14] Heparin and intravenous administration of ethanol are not useful.

REFERENCES

1. Sasahara AA, Sharma GVRK, Barsamian EM, et al. Pulmonary thromboembolism. Diagnosis and treatment. JAMA 1983;249:2945–9
2. Stein PD, Willis PW, DeMets DL. History and physical examination in acute pulmonary embolism in patients without preexisting cardiac or pulmonary disease. Am J Cardiol 1981;47:218–23
3. Divekan VM, Kamdar BM, Pansare SN. Pulmonary embolism during anaesthesia: Case report. Can Anaesth Soc J 1981;28:277–9
4. McNell BJ. Ventilation-perfusion studies and the diagnosis of pulmonary embolism: Concise communication. J Nucl Med 1980;21:319–23
5. Berry AJ. Pulmonary embolism during spinal anesthesia: Angiographic diagnosis via a flow-directed pulmonary artery catheter. Anesthesiology 1982;57:57–9
6. Bell WR, Royall RM. Heparin-associated thrombocytopenia: A comparison of three heparin preparations. N Engl J Med 1980;303:902–7
7. Sasahara AA, Sharma GVRK, Tow DE, et al. Clinical use of thrombolytic agents in venous thromboembolism. Arch Intern Med 1982;142:684–8
8. Greenfield LJ, Peyton MD, Brown PP, Elkins RC. Transvenous management of pulmonary embolic diseases. Ann Surg 1974;1980:461–8
9. Kakkar VV, Spindler J, Plute PT, et al. Efficacy of low doses of heparin in prevention of deep vein thrombosis after major surgery: A double-blind randomized trial. Lancet 1972;2:101–4
10. International Multi-centre trial: Prevention of fatal postoperative pulmonary embolism by low doses of heparin. Lancet 1975;2:45–8
11. Leyvraz PF, Richard J, Bachman F, et al. Adjusted versus fixed-dose subcutaneous heparin in the prevention of deep-vein thrombosis after total hip replacement. N Engl J Med 1983;309:954–8
12. Skellman JJ, Collins RCC, Coe NP, et al. Prevention of deep vein thrombosis in neurosurgical patients: A controlled randomized trial of external pneumatic compression boots. Surgery 1978;83:354–60
13. Sasahara AA, Sharma GVRK, Parisi AF. New developments in detection and prevention of venous thromboembolism. Am J Cardiol 1979;43:1214–9
14. Gossling HR, Donahue TA. The fat embolism syndrome. JAMA 1979;241:2740–6

14

Obstructive Airways Disease

Obstructive airways disease is the most frequent cause of pulmonary dysfunction. The common pathophysiologic characteristic of all of these disorders is an increased resistance to the flow of gases in the airways. This increased airway resistance can be due to a variety of different pathogenic mechanisms, can be acute or chronic, can be reversible or irreversible, and can arise in different segments of the airway. Regional differences in airway resistance lead to areas of mismatch of ventilation to perfusion. As a result, there is abnormal regional oxygen exchange, and arterial hypoxemia is likely to develop while breathing room air. Retention of carbon dioxide with the development of respiratory acidosis can also occur when regional hypoventilation is severe. In addition to increased airway resistance, obstructive airways disease is characterized by dyspnea, reflecting the increased work of breathing introduced by the elevated resistance to gas flow.

Physical examination of patients with obstructive airways disease reveals evidence of increased intrathoracic gas volumes. For example, the anterior-to-posterior diameter of the chest is increased, the diaphragm is depressed, the thorax is hyper-resonant to percussion, and the intercostal spaces are widened. Auscultation of the chest will likely reveal wheezing during exhalation. Wheezing is the term used to describe the sound produced by turbulent gas flow through narrow airways. As obstruc-

tion becomes more severe, wheezing becomes more prominent and is audible during earlier phases of exhalation. Forced exhalation may reveal wheezing that was not audible during quiet breathing.

Radiographs of the chest reveal hyperinflated lungs with increased radiolucency due to decreased pulmonary blood flow. The diaphragm is depressed, particularly on lateral views of the thorax. Heart size, as viewed on the radiograph, appears to be reduced, unless pulmonary hypertension has led to right ventricular enlargement.

Pulmonary function studies in the presence of obstructive airways disease reveal reductions in expiratory flow rates due to increased airway resistance. For example, the forced exhaled volume in 1 second (FEV_1) is typically less than 80 percent of the vital capacity in the presence of obstructive airways disease (Fig. 14-1).[1] Measurement of the FEV_1 alone can be misleading, as this value may be low if vital capacity is also reduced or patients are uncooperative. The maximum midexpiratory flow rate (MEFR 25 percent to 75 percent) is also decreased in the presence of obstructive airways disease. In contrast to measurement of FEV_1, the MEFR is not influenced by patient effort. The FEV_1 is primarily sensitive to large airways obstruction and does not measure subtle changes in more peripheral airways. Conversely, MEFR is a better indicator of small airways involvement than measurement of FEV_1.

195

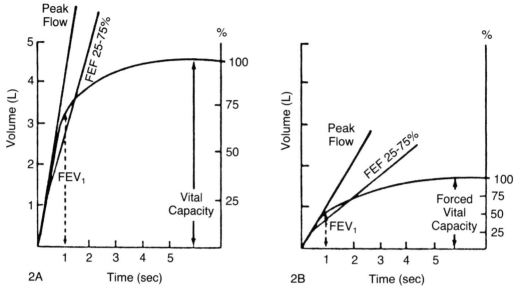

FIG. 14-1. Spirogram changes of a normal subject (2a) and a patient in bronchospasm (2b). The forced exhaled volume in 1 second (FEV_1) is typically less than 80 percent of the vital capacity in the presence of obstructive airways disease. Peak flow and maximum midexpiratory flow rate (FEF 25% to 75%) are also decreased in these patients (2b). (Kingston HGG, Hirshman CA. Perioperative management of the patient with asthma. Anesth Analg 1984;63:844–55. Reprinted with permission from IARS.)

All abnormal findings relating to expiratory flow rates should be repeated after administration of bronchodilator drugs, so as to define the presence of reversible components contributing to increased airway resistance. An increase in the FEV_1 of at least 15 percent is considered evidence of significant reversibility of airway obstruction and should encourage further drug therapy directed at reduction of airway constriction. In addition to decreased expiratory flow rates, patients with obstructive airways disease manifest increased total lung capacities, which are most likely due to enlarged residual volumes. An elevated ratio of residual volume to total lung capacity is suggestive of obstructive airways disease. Vital capacity is typically normal in the presence of increased airway resistance. The presence of a normal vital capacity and reduced expiratory flow rates serves to distinguish patients with obstructive airways disease from those with restrictive pulmonary disease.

When considering the common features of obstructive airways disease, it is possible to categorize these processes as reversible and irreversible conditions. Bronchial asthma is the classic example of obstructive airways disease that is characterized by acute and reversible elevations of airway resistance. Irreversible conditions, characterized by progressive and persistent increases in airway resistance despite treatment, include pulmonary emphysema, chronic bronchitis, bronchiectasis, cystic fibrosis, and Kartagener's syndrome. Regardless of the presence or absence of coexisting obstructive airways disease, it is important to appreciate the impact of surgery on pulmonary function, anticipate likely postoperative pulmonary complications, and institute prophylaxis against postoperative pulmonary complications.

BRONCHIAL ASTHMA

Bronchial asthma is a common form of obstructive airways disease affecting 3 percent to 5 percent of the population.[2] Sixty-five percent of patients develop symptoms before 5 years of age, and males outnumber female patients by about two to one. It is estimated that approximately 5,000 deaths occur from bronchial asthma each year in the United States.[3]

Manifestations

Active bronchial asthma is characterized by diffuse and usually reversible narrowing of the airways recognized as audible wheezing during auscultation of the chest. Airway hyperreactivity in response to chemical, pharmacologic, and mechanical (intubation of the trachea) stimuli is an important component of bronchial asthma. The degree of airway narrowing and hence the severity of symptoms can change abruptly. The parasympathetic nervous system promotes constriction of airway smooth muscle and appears to mediate sudden changes in airway caliber considered characteristic of bronchial asthma. In addition to airway hyper-reactivity, there is often increased mucous secretion and edema of the airways that further contribute to increased airway resistance. Obstruction to airflow due to airway hyper-reactivity, excess mucus secretion and edema of the airways leads to changes in lung volumes, peak flow rates, and chest wall mechanics and is associated with altered distribution of ventilation and perfusion, which may lead to arterial hypoxemia, hypercarbia, and altered cardiovascular function. These changes reflect the severity of airways obstruction and may persist even when patients are asymptomatic (Table 14-1).[1,4] The ratio of FEV_1 to vital capacity is likely to be less than 80 percent, whereas total lung capacity and ratio of residual volume to total lung capacity will be increased. Mild bronchial asthma is usually accompanied by normal arterial partial pressures

of oxygen and carbon dioxide. As severity of bronchial asthma increases, both partial pressures are likely to decrease. Further progression of bronchial asthma is associated with additional reductions in the partial pressures of oxygen, and the partial pressures of carbon dioxide begin to increase.

Active bronchial asthma is often associated with elevated eosinophil counts (above 300 mm^3). Adequately treated patients with bronchial asthma will usually have eosinophil counts below 50 mm^3, although rising counts often precede the appearance of worsening clinical symptoms.

Radiographs of the chest may reveal hyperinflation of the lungs but are more useful in ruling out pneumonia or congestive heart failure that may be associated with bronchial asthma. Electrocardiograms may show evidence of acute right heart failure and ventricular irritability during acute attacks.

Classification

Bronchial asthma is not a single disease but rather comprises a group of disorders with various pathologic mechanisms. Principal classifications of bronchial asthma include (1) immunoglobulin E-mediated asthma, (2) exercise-induced asthma, (3) aspirin-induced asthma, (4) occupational asthma, and (5) infectious asthma.

IMMUNOGLOBULIN E-MEDIATED ASTHMA

Immunoglobulin E-mediated bronchial asthma is the most common form of reversible obstructive airways disease. This disorder is

TABLE 14-1. Severity of Airways Obstruction

	FEV_1 (% predicted)	$MEFR_{25-75}$ (% predicted)	PaO_2	$PaCO_2$
Asymptomatic or mild	65–80	60–75	Normal	Normal
Moderate	50–64	45–59		
Marked	35–49	30–44		
Severe (status asthmaticus)	Unobtainable	Unobtainable		

(Data from Kingston HGG, Hirshman CA. Perioperative management of the patient with asthma. Anesth Analg 1984; 63:844–55)

believed to be an inherited condition because of the frequent presence of a family history of either bronchial asthma or some other immunoglobulin E-mediated disorder.

Increased airway resistance in the presence of immunoglobulin E-mediated asthma is due to (1) increased muscle tone of bronchial smooth muscles manifesting as bronchoconstriction, (2) edema of the bronchial mucosa, and (3) secretion of viscous mucus. These changes are initiated by release of vasoactive substances, including histamine, from mast cells in the lungs. Presumably, inhalation of antigens causes elaboration of antibodies of the immunoglobulin E class. Following reexposure to these inhaled antigens, an antigen-antibody complex forms on the surfaces of mast cells, leading to degranulation and release of vasoactive substances. The subsequent increase in large airway resistance also initiates a vagus-mediated reflex, which causes alveolar ducts to constrict.

EXERCISE-INDUCED ASTHMA

Exercise-induced bronchial asthma is characterized by bronchoconstriction that accompanies increased physical activity.[5] The pathogenesis of this form of asthma is not clear but may be related to alterations in transmucosal temperature gradients associated with inhalation of cold and dry air.

ASPIRIN-INDUCED ASTHMA

Aspirin-induced bronchial asthma is characterized by acute episodes of bronchoconstriction related to the ingestion of aspirin. Nasal polyps are frequently associated with this form of asthma. These patients are often sensitive to derivatives of benzoic acid, suggesting the need for caution in the use of ester local anesthetics.

OCCUPATIONAL ASTHMA

Occupational bronchial asthma is bronchoconstriction associated with inhalation of substances ranging from animal dander to fumes from grains, plastics, and metals. These agents produce their symptoms by direct effects on airways and not by immunologic means.

INFECTIOUS ASTHMA

Infectious asthma is increased airway resistance due to acute inflammatory disease of the bronchi. Causative agents can be viruses, bacteria, or *Mycoplasma* organisms. Eradication of the infectious organisms results in a rapid subsidence of bronchoconstriction.

Treatment

Rising total blood eosinophil counts confirm the onset of acute exacerbations of bronchial asthma and the need to introduce specific pharmacologic treatment designed to produce bronchodilation. In addition, oral and/or intravenous hydration plus humidification of inspired gases is important, so as to minimize production of viscous mucus, which can obstruct already narrowed airways. If arterial blood gases reveal increasing arterial partial pressures of carbon dioxide, it may be necessary to intubate the trachea and institute mechanical ventilation of the lungs.[6] Elevation of the arterial partial pressures of carbon dioxide above 50 mmHg in patients with acute attacks of bronchial asthma warns of impending exhaustion and the imminent likelihood of the need for mechanical support of ventilation.

Drug therapy designed to treat bronchial asthma most often includes beta-adrenergic agonist drugs, aminophylline, and corticosteroids. Other potentially useful regimens include anticholinergic drugs and mast cell stabilizers such as cromolyn. Aerosol administration of drugs permits delivery of high concentrations to the airways with less likelihood of systemic effects. Energy for production of aerosols is provided by fluorocarbon propellant generators or jet nebulizers. During anesthesia, T-piece adaptors and connectors allow delivery of aerosol drugs directly into the anesthesia circuit for delivery to airways during inspiration.[7]

BETA-ADRENERGIC AGONIST DRUGS

Beta-adrenergic agonist drugs most likely produce bronchodilation by stimulating the enzyme adenylate cyclase, which is responsible for the conversion of adenosine triphosphate to cyclic adenosine monophosphate. Increases in intracellular concentrations of cyclic adenosine monophosphate reduce smooth muscle tone and thus produce bronchodilation.

Epinephrine and isoproterenol are useful beta-adrenergic agonist drugs for producing bronchodilation, but their stimulation of beta-1 cardiac receptors can result in cardiac dysrhythmias, particularly in the presence of arterial hypoxemia and/or hypercarbia. Drugs that selectively stimulate beta-2 receptors in bronchial smooth muscle are less likely to produce these undesirable cardiac effects. Examples of beta-2 adrenergic agonist drugs that can be administered by aerosol inhalation include isoetharine, metaproterenol, albuterol (salbutamol), and terbutaline (Table 14-2). Isoetharine and metaproterenol are shorter acting and less specific for beta-2 receptors than are albuterol or terbutaline.

An adverse response to treatment with these drugs is hypokalemia due to beta-2 adrenergic stimulation that causes an intracellular redistribution of potassium. Hypokalemia could result in dangerous cardiac dysrhythmias, especially in the presence of active bronchial asthma and associated derangement of arterial blood gases. Indeed, asthma-related deaths have been attributed to abuse of bronchodilator aerosols.[3]

Isoetharine. Isoetharine is as effective as isoproterenol as a bronchodilator and has a low incidence of side effects. A typical adult dose is 5 mg inhaled over 15 minutes to 20 minuutes.

Metaproterenol. Metaproterenol 0.65 mg produces prompt and sustained reductions in airway resistance. Tolerance may occur with repeated administration of this drug.

Albuterol. Albuterol is a potent bronchodilator that promptly reduces airway resistance for 4 hours to 6 hours when administered to adults as an aerosol. The metered aerosol device delivers about 100 μg of drug per puff and 1 puff to 4 puffs is the usual adult dose. This aerosol dose is unlikely to produce cardiac effects. As with other beta-adrenergic agonist drugs, chronic use leads to tolerance.

Terbutaline. Terbutaline can be administered as an aerosol (0.75 mg to 1.5 mg in 2 ml of saline) or subcutaneously (0.25 mg). This drug and other beta-2 adrenergic agonist drugs must be used with caution in parturients, as they may inhibit labor.

AMINOPHYLLINE

Aminophylline is considered to be standard therapy in every patient with bronchospasm. Bronchodilation produced by aminophylline is often attributed to drug-induced inhibition of phosphodiesterase enzyme with subsequent increases in intracellular concentrations of cyclic adenosine monophosphate

TABLE 14-2. Beta-Adrenergic Agonist Drugs for Inhalation

	Beta-2 Receptor Selectivity	Peak Effect (minutes)	Duration of Effect (hours)
Isoproterenol	0	5–15	1–2
Isoetharine	+	15–60	1–2
Metaproterenol	+ +	30–60	3–4
Albuterol (salbutamol)	+ + +	30–60	4–6
Terbutaline	+ + +	30–60	4–6

and resulting relaxation of bronchial smooth muscle. Perhaps more important than this enzyme inhibition are aminophylline's antiadenosine effects, which facilitate endogenous release of catecholamines.[8] In the absence of prior treatment, the dose of aminophylline is 5 mg·kg^{-1} administered intravenously over about 15 minutes, followed by 0.5 mg^{-1}·kg^{-1}·hr^{-1} to 1 mg·kg^{-1}·hr^{-1}. During treatment, it is necessary to maintain blood concentrations of theophylline between 10 mg·L^{-1} to 20 mg·L^{-1}. Blood levels in excess of 20 mg·L^{-1} are associated with seizures and adverse cardiac effects, including cardiac dysrhythmias. Acute, but not chronic, administration of aminophylline reduces the dose of epinephrine necessary to produce cardiac dysrhythmias in animals anesthetized with halothane.[9] Alterations in hepatic function or total hepatic blood flow can also influence blood levels of theophylline produced by given infusion rates, emphasizing the importance of frequent measurements of plasma concentrations of this drug. Aminophylline readily crosses the placenta and may produce toxicity in infants of mothers receiving this drug during labor. This risk is accentuated in premature infants, as a greater proportion of aminophylline is converted to caffeine.[1] In animals, aminophylline reverses barbiturate anesthesia, presumably by its ability to antagonize adenosine receptors, which facilitates release of norepinephrine. A change in the depth of anesthesia may be an important consideration in asthmatic patients because of the risk of provoking bronchospasm in lightly anesthetized patients. This potential drug interaction may deserve consideration when determining the dose of drugs, especially barbiturates, to be administered for induction of anesthesia in patients being treated with aminophylline. Likewise, aminophylline-induced reductions in anesthetic requirements for volatile anesthetics could result in unexpected light levels of anesthesia. Nevertheless, halothane anesthetic requirements (MAC) are not altered in animals acutely treated with aminophylline.[10]

CORTICOSTEROIDS

Corticosteroids are extensively used in the management of acute exacerbations of bronchial asthma, as well as in maintenance of sta-

ble asymptomatic states of the disease. Indeed, treatment of acute bronchial asthma with intravenous methylprednisolone reduces the subsequent need to admit patients to the hospital.[11] There is no difference in effect among cortisol, methylprednisolone, and dexamethasone as used for the treatment of asthma.[12] Presumably, anti-inflammatory effects of these drugs, plus their membrane-stabilizing effects that reduce the release of histamine from mast cells, contribute to their therapeutic effects. In addition, corticosteroids used in combination therapy seem to potentiate effects of beta-adrenergic agonist drugs.

The major adverse effect of chronic treatment with corticosteroids is suppression of adrenal cortex function. Adrenal cortex suppression is related to the dose of administered corticosteroid. Administration of the lowest effective dose of corticosteroid early in the morning, when endogenous secretion is low, or use of alternative day schedules for corticosteroid therapy should minimize this adverse effect. Systemic effects of corticosteroids can also be minimized by administering drugs by inhalation as metered aerosols. For example, beclomethasone, administered as an aerosol, is often as effective as an orally administered corticosteroid. Nevertheless, suppression of adrenal cortex activity must still be suspected, as substantial amounts of inhaled drugs can be deposited in the mouth and swallowed, with subsequent systemic absorption.

ANTICHOLINERGIC DRUGS

Anticholinergic drugs, including atropine and glycopyrrolate, have been shown to decrease airway resistance in normal patients.[13] Presumably, this response reflects inhibition of the effects of acetylcholine on postganglionic cholinergic receptors in airway smooth muscle, leading to decreased intracellular concentrations of cyclic guanosine monophosphate. Indeed, bronchoconstriction produced by stimulation of the parasympathetic nervous system is most likely due to increased intracellular concentrations of cyclic guanosine monophosphate.

Use of anticholinergic drugs to treat bronchial asthma is limited by cardiovascular effects of these drugs. Furthermore, viscosity of secretions may be increased by anticholinergic drugs, making it difficult to clear them from the airways. The selectivity of anticholinergic effects on the airways can be improved by administering these drugs by inhalation. Ipratropium is a derivative of atropine, which can be administered as a metered aerosol in the presence of bronchospasm.[13] This drug is poorly absorbed from the gastrointestinal tract, reducing the incidence of systemic side effects should it be swallowed during administration as an aerosol.

CROMOLYN

Cromolyn is a membrane stabilizer that prevents degranulation of mast cells and subsequent release of vasoactive substances responsible for bronchoconstriction. Use of this drug is entirely for prophylaxis against development of acute attacks of bronchial asthma. Cromolyn is of no value in management of coexisting bronchoconstriction, since this drug does not counter effects of vasoactive substances that have already been released. Furthermore, cromolyn does not produce bronchodilation by any direct mechanism. Since absorption from the gastrointestinal tract is poor, it is administered as a metered aerosol.

Management of Anesthesia

Management of anesthesia for patients with bronchial asthma requires an understanding of the pathophysiology of the disease process and of the pharmacology of drugs being used for its treatment.[1] Preoperative evaluation, preanesthetic medication, and induction and maintenance of anesthesia are all based on an appreciation of the abnormalities associated with the presence of bronchial asthma.

PREOPERATIVE EVALUATION

Preoperative evaluation of the current status of bronchial asthma includes auscultation of the chest and measurement of total blood

eosinophil counts. Absence of wheezing during quiet breathing and total blood eosinophil counts below 50 mm^3 suggest that patients are not experiencing acute exacerbations of their disease. Performance of pulmonary function studies before and after bronchodilator therapy may be indicated in patients with known bronchial asthma who are scheduled for major elective operations. Chest physiotherapy, systemic hydration, appropriate antibiotics, and bronchodilator therapy in the preoperative period will often improve reversible components of bronchial asthma, as evidenced by pulmonary function tests. Comparison of radiographs of the chest with previous radiographs is helpful in evaluating the status of the disease process. Measurement of arterial blood gases before undertaking elective surgery is indicated if there are any questions about the adequacy of ventilation or arterial oxygenation.

PREANESTHETIC MEDICATION

No studies confirm a preferred drug or combination of drugs for use as preanesthetic medication in patients with bronchial asthma. Additionally, no evidence shows that opioids, in doses used for preanesthetic medication, produce direct or reflex bronchoconstriction or stimulate release of vasoactive substances from mast cells. More important to consider is the possible ventilatory depressant effects of opioids. Use of anticholinergic drugs should be individualized, remembering that these drugs can increase the viscosity of secretions, making it difficult to remove them from the airways. Furthermore, achievement of reductions in airway resistance by inhibition of postganglionic cholinergic receptors is unlikely with intramuscular doses of anticholinergic drugs used for preanesthetic medication. Use of H-2 receptor antagonists, such as cimetidine, in patients with bronchial asthma is questionable. This concern is based on the evidence that histamine mediates bronchoconstriction via H-1 receptors, during which bronchodilation is mediated by H-2 receptors.[14] Conceivably, antagonism of H-2 receptors by antagonist drugs would unmask histamine mediated H-1 receptor bronchoconstriction, leading to acute increases in airway resistance in patients with bronchial asthma.

Bronchodilator drugs used in the treatment of bronchial asthma should be continued to the time of induction of anesthesia. For example, cromolyn does not interact adversely with drugs used during anesthesia and thus can be safely continued in the immediate preoperative period. Supplementation with exogenous corticosteroids may be indicated before major surgery if adrenal cortex suppression from drugs used to treat bronchial asthma is a possibility.

INDUCTION AND MAINTENANCE OF ANESTHESIA

The goal during induction and maintenance of anesthesia in patients with bronchial asthma is to depress airway reflexes with anesthetic drugs so as to avoid bronchoconstriction of the hyper-reactive airways in response to mechanical stimulation. Indeed, stimuli that do not cause problems in the absence of bronchial asthma can precipitate life-threatening bronchoconstriction in patients with this disease.

Regional anesthesia is an attractive choice when the site of operation is superficial or on the extremities or when avoidance of intubation of the trachea is considered to be desirable. In the majority of patients, however, a general anesthetic will be necessary. Induction of anesthesia with barbiturates, benzodiazepines, or etomidate is acceptable; but it must be remembered that these drugs are unlikely to depress adequately airway reflexes, allowing precipitation of bronchospasm should intubation of the trachea be attempted. Ketamine, presumably reflecting its sympathomimetic effects, has been shown to be superior to thiopental for preventing increases in airway resistance (Fig. 14-2).[15] Therefore, ketamine, 1 mg·kg^{-1} to 2 mg·kg^{-1}, may be a useful drug for induction of anesthesia. Increased secretions associated with administration of ketamine may detract from the use of this drug in patients with bronchial asthma.

After unconsciousness is produced by intravenous injection of drugs, the lungs are often ventilated with a gas mixture that contains vol-atile anesthetics. The goal is to establish a depth of anesthesia that will depress hyperreactive airway reflexes sufficiently to permit intubation of the trachea without precipitating bronchoconstriction. Indeed, the one factor that has been shown to precipitate bronchoconstriction in patients with asthma is the introduction of a tube into the trachea without previously establishing a sufficient depth of anesthesia to suppress airway reflexes.[16] Halothane is most often selected because of its ability to produuce bronchodilation of the constricted airway. Nevertheless, halothane is not an ideal drug, since it sensitizes the myocardium to the dysrhythmic effects of beta-adrenergic stimulation as produced by beta-adrenergic agonist drugs and aminophylline (see the section Aminophylline). Cardiac dysrhythmias during administration of aminophylline would seem even less likely with other volatile anesthetics, such as enflurane or isoflurane, which do not sensitize the myocardium. Consistent with this speculation is the report that induction of enflurane anesthesia in animals treated with aminophylline does not cause cardiac dysrhythmias.[17] It is likely that enflurane or isoflurane are equally acceptable alternatives to halothane for administration to patients with increased airway resistance due to bronchial asthma. Indeed, enflurane and isoflurane have been observed to produce beneficial airway effects in patients with status asthmaticus.[18] Furthermore, enflurane and isoflurane are as effective as halothane in reversing allergic bronchoconstriction in a dog model (Fig. 14-3).[19]

Rates of intravenous infusion of aminophylline may need to be decreased during the intraoperative period because of decreased inactivation of aminophylline by the liver due to decreased hepatic blood flow. Indeed, infusion rates (0.5 ml·kg^{-1}·hr^{-1} to 1 ml·kg^{-1}·hr^{-1}) associated with therapeutic plasma concentrations of aminophylline in awake states may result in toxic plasma concentrations when hepatic blood flow is reduced during anesthesia. Therefore, it would seem prudent to reduce infusion rates by approximately 30 percent to offset a similar reduction in hepatic blood flow predictable during anesthesia and surgical stimulation, particularly during upper abdominal operations.

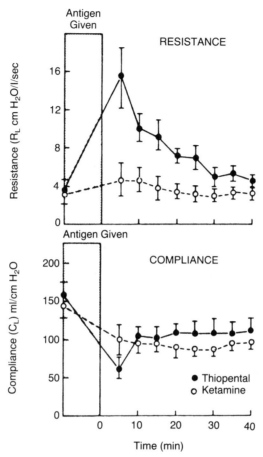

FIG. 14-2. Pulmonary resistance (R_L) and dynamic compliance (C_L) before and after Ascaris antigen aerosol challenge during thiopental and ketamine anesthesia in dogs. (Hirshman CA, Downes H, Farbood A, Bergman NA. Ketamine block of bronchospasm in experimental canine asthma. Br J Anaesth 1979;51:713–8)

An alternative to the administration of volatile anesthetics to suppress airway reflexes before intubation of the trachea may be the intravenous injection of lidocaine.[20] Lidocaine, 1 mg·kg^{-1} to 2 mg·kg^{-1} intravenously, given immediately before intubation of the trachea, is useful for preventing reflex bronchoconstriction provoked by instrumentation of the airway. Furthermore, the continuous intravenous administration of lidocaine 1 mg·kg^{-1}·hr^{-1} to 3 mg·kg^{-1}·hr^{-1} can be used in place of volatile anesthetics in patients with limited cardiac reserve, in whom deep anesthesia may be needed to suppress reflex activity of hyper-reactive airways. The decision to administer intratracheal lidocaine just before placement of a tube in the trachea must consider both the beneficial effect of topical anesthesia and the possible initiation of bronchospasm by placement of the solution into hyper-reactive airways. Although speciific data are not available to support a recommendation for use of intratracheal lidocaine in patients with bronchial asthma, clinical experience suggests that, in the presence of adequate anesthesia, bronchospasm does not follow intratracheal administration of lidocaine.

Skeletal muscle relaxation during maintenance of anesthesia is often provided with nondepolarizing muscle relaxants. In this regard, drugs with limited ability to evoke the

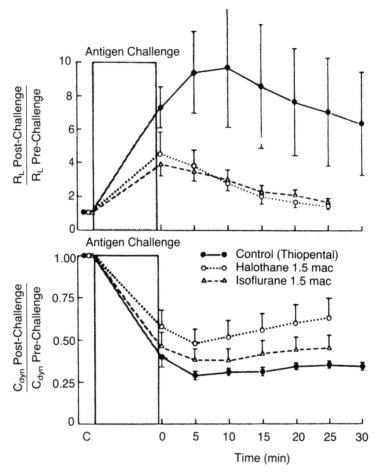

FIG. 14-3. Pulmonary resistance (R_L) and dynamic compliance (C_{dyn}) in dogs before and after Ascaris antigen challenge during thiopental, halothane or isoflurane anesthesia in dogs. Halothane and isoflurane are equally effective in attenuating antigen-induced elevations in R_L. (Hirshman CA, Edelstein G, Peetz S, et al. Mechanism of action of inhalation anesthesia on airways. Anesthesiology 1982;56:107–11)

release of histamine, such as vecuronium, pancuronium, or atracurium are useful. If atracurium is selected, it is prudent to slow its rate of injection to minimize the unlikely potential for drug-induced histamine release. Although histamine release has been attributed to succinylcholine, there is no evidence that this drug is associated with the onset of increased airway resistance in patients with bronchial asthma.[21] Conversely, d-tubocurarine can stimulate the release of histamine and increase airway resistance. Theoretically, reversal of nondepolarizing neuromuscular blockade with anticholinesterase drugs could precipitate

bronchospasm secondary to stimulation of postganglionic cholinergic receptors in airway smooth muscle. The fact that bronchospasm does not predictably occur after administration of anticholinesterase drugs may reflect protective effects provided by the simultaneous administration of anticholinergic drugs.

Intraoperatively, the best arterial oxygenation and ventilation are provided by mechanical ventilation of the lungs. A slow inspiratory flow rate provides optimal distribution of ventilation. A sufficient time for passive exhalation to occur is necessary to prevent air trapping in the presence of increased airway resistance. In this respect, positive end-expiratory pressure may not be ideal because of the likelihood that it would impair adequate exhalation in the presence of narrowed airways. Humidification and warming of inspired gases would seem logical, particularly in patients with histories of exercise-induced asthma, in which bronchoconstriction is presumed to be due to transmucosal loss of heat. Nevertheless, it must be appreciated that particulate humidification, as produced by ultrasonic nebulizers and pneumatic aerosols, can produce bronchoconstriction.[22] Liberal intravenous administration of crystalloid solutions during the perioperative period is important for maintaining adequate hydration and insuring the presence of less viscous secretions, which can be more easily expelled from the airways.

At the conclusion of anesthesia for elective surgery, it is prudent to remove the tube from the trachea while anesthesia is still sufficient to suppress hyperactive airway reflexes. When it is deemed unwise to remove the tube from the trachea until the patient is awake, it would seem reasonable to attempt to minimize the likelihood of airway stimulation due to the tracheal tube. Therefore, continuous intravenous infusion of lidocaine, 1 $mg \cdot kg^{-1} \cdot hr^{-1}$ to 3 $mg \cdot kg^{-1} \cdot hr^{-1}$ may be useful.

In rare circumstances where life-threatening status asthmaticus persists despite aggressive pharmacologic therapy, it may be acceptable to consider general anesthesia in an attempt to produce bronchodilation. In this regard, halothane, enflurane, and isofurane have been described as an effective therapy in selected patients.[18,23] Clearly, this is a hazardous approach in desperately ill patients and can only be considered when the potential benefits are judged to merit the risks.

Etiology and Treatment of Intraoperative Bronchospasm

Bronchospasm that occurs intraoperatively can be due to factors other than bronchial asthma. It is imperative that treatment using drugs appropriate for the management of bronchoconstriction due to bronchial asthma not be instituted until more likely causes for expiratory wheezing associated with increased peak airway pressures are considered. Causes of wheezing not due to bronchial asthma include (1) mechanical obstruction of the tracheal tube by secretions, kinking, or overinflation of the tracheal tube cuff; (2) inadequate anesthesia for the surgical stimulus, resulting in active expiratory efforts with associated reductions in the functional residual capacity and narrowing of the airways; (3) endobronchical intubation; (4) pulmonary edema; (5) inhalation of gastric fluid; and (6) pneumothorax.[7]

Increased airway resistance that occurs intraoperatively and is unrelated to bronchial asthma is treated by optimizing the depth of anesthesia with volatile anesthetics and/or administration of muscle relaxants. Conversely, true bronchospasm may respond to deepening of anesthesia with volatile anesthetics but not administration of muscle relaxants. The efficacy of volatile anesthetics in reducing airway resistance may reflect direct relaxant effects on bronchial smooth muscle, depression of parasympathetic-mediated constrictive reflexes, or attenuation of release of bronchoactive mediators such as histamine, although experimental evidence does not support the latter mechanism.[24] Bronchospasm in patients with bronchial asthma that does not respond to adjustments in the depth of anesthesia is treated with drugs. For example, the cornerstone of pharmacologic treatment of acute bronchospasm is with intravenous administration of aminophylline at rates of 0.5 $mg \cdot kg^{-1} \cdot hr^{-1}$ to 1 $mg \cdot kg^{-1} \cdot hr^{-1}$, after administration of loading doses of 5 $mg \cdot kg^{-1}$ administered over about 15 minutes. Aminophylline is often combined with the metered aerosol administration of beta-2 adrenergic agonist drugs such as albuterol. Albuterol can be administered via devices placed in the inspiratory limbs of anesthesia delivery circuits (see the section Beta-Adrenergic Agonist Drugs). When bronchospasm is severe, or persists despite intravenous administration of aminophylline and inhalation of albuterol, the use of intravenous corticosteroids should be considered (see the section Corticosteroids).

PULMONARY EMPHYSEMA

Pulmonary emphysema is characterized by irreversible enlargement of the alveolar air ducts accompanied by destruction of the walls of these air spaces. The principal pathophysiologic change is the loss of elastic recoil of the lungs, which results in collapse of airways during exhalation, leading to increased airway resistance (Table 14-3). Obstruction to expiratory flow can also lead to formation of bullae, with compression of adjacent lung tissue. Severe dyspnea is characteristic of pulmonary emphysema, reflecting increased work of breathing due to loss of elastic recoil of the lungs. The cause of this loss is not known, but the major predisposing factor for the development of pulmonary emphysema is cigarette smoking. In some patients, an inherited deficiency of alpha-1-antitrypsin globulin may allow increased activity of proteolytic enzymes, leading to lung destruction. Nevertheless, this inherited defect probably accounts for less than 15 percent of pulmonary emphysema patients. Exposure to environmental pollutants also has a positive correlation with the development of pulmonary emphysema in some patients.

Preoperative Evaluation

Preoperative evaluation of patients with pulmonary emphysema should determine the severity of the disease and elucidate any reversible components, such as infection or bronchospasm. It is firmly established that preoperative recognition and treatment of chronic obstructive airways disease, including pulmonary emphysema and chronic bronchitis, will lessen the incidence of postoperative pulmonary complications.[25,26] The history, pulmonary function studies, and measurement of arterial blood gases and pH are most important in evaluating the severity and significance of pulmonary emphysema before elective surgery.

Presence of dyspnea, cough, sputum production, and decreased exercise tolerance suggest the need for pulmonary function studies. Measurement of the ratio of the FEV_1 to the vital capacity may be helpful in predicting the severity of pulmonary disease. For example, the risk of postoperative respiratory failure is increased if the measured ratio is less than 50 percent.[25] Furthermore, this ratio is an excellent predictor of the ability to cough and clear secretions from the airways.

Measurement of arterial blood gases and pH should be performed before major elective surgery in patients with complaints of severe dyspnea and reduced exercise tolerance. It is unusual for carbon dioxide retention to occur until the ratio of FEV_1-to-vital capacity is less than 0.35. Characteristically, patients with pulmonary emphysema maintain normal arterial blood gases, reflecting a high minute ventilation in an attempt to overcome increased airway resistance. Indeed, these patients are often described as *pink puffers*. Detection of arterial partial pressures of carbon dioxide above 50 mmHg cautions against performance of elec-

TABLE 14-3. Comparison of Features of Pulmonary Emphysema and Chronic Bronchitis

Feature	Pulmonary Emphysema	Chronic Bronchitis
Mechanism of airway obstruction	Loss of elastic recoil	Decreased airway lumen due to mucus and inflammation
Forced exhaled volume in 1 sec (FEV_1)	Decreased	Decreased
Total lung capacity	Marked increase	Marked increase
Dyspnea	Severe	Moderate
Arterial hypoxemia and carbon dioxide retention	Late	Early
Cor pulmonale	Late	Early
Prognosis	Good	Poor

tive surgery, as the risk of postoperative respiratory failure is increased.[27]

Preoperative detection and treatment of cor pulmonale is essential (see Chapter 9). It should be appreciated that chronic obstructive airways disease is the most frequent cause of cor pulmonale. Pulmonary hypertension that can predispose to development of cor pulmonale is present when mean pulmonary artery pressure exceeds 20 mmHg. The primary treatment of cor pulmonale is relief of pulmonary vascular vasospasm by improved arterial oxygenation and correction of acidemia. Diuretic therapy and positive inotropic drugs may improve cardiac function, but it must be remembered that cor pulmonale is not due to intrinsic dysfunction of the heart but instead reflects pulmonary disease that leads to increased pulmonary vascular resistance.

Eradication of acute infection with appropriate antibiotics before elective surgery is important, particularly if infection is contributing to respiratory failure, as evidenced by carbon dioxide retention. Production of purulent sputum suggests active infection and is an indication for the administration of antibiotics. Use of antibiotics, however, to sterilize the sputum is to be avoided, as this practice can lead to an overgrowth of resistant bacteria or fungi. Chest physiotherapy combined with adequate hydration of patients is a useful approach for facilitating removal of secretions from the airways.

Steps to improve preoperative respiratory muscle power include good nutrition and treatment of hypokalemia, which can predispose the patient to skeletal muscle weakness. Familiarization in the preoperative period with respiratory therapy equipment and techniques to be used in the postoperative period is important for optimal patient cooperation after surgery. Preoperative use of intermittent positive pressure breathing has not been shown to reduce the incidence of postoperative pulmonary complications.[28]

Pulmonary function studies and arterial blood gases should be repeated after antibiotic and bronchodilator therapy. Ideally, previously prolonged expiratory flow rates and elevated partial pressures of carbon dioxide should return to normal and sputum production decrease. Wheezing should be reduced or absent. These changes suggest a beneficial response to therapy and should place patients with chronic obstructive airways disease at decreased risks for development of postoperative pulmonary complications.

CESSATION OF CIGARETTE SMOKING

Postoperative pulmonary complications are increased in those who smoke cigarettes.[29] Therefore, cessation of cigarette smoking in the perioperative period would seem prudent, although sufficient time for reversible changes to occur may not always be available. Nevertheless, adverse effects of carbon monoxide on oxygen-carrying capacity and of nicotine on the cardiovascular system are short-lived.[29] For example, elimination half-times of carbon monoxide are about 4 hours to 6 hours, such that smoke-free intervals of 12 hours to 18 hours should result in substantial declines in carboxyhemoglobin levels, reversal of tissue hypoxia, and normalization of the oxyhemoglobin dissociation curve. Indeed, within 12 hours after cessation of smoking, the P_{50} increases from 22.9 mmHg to 26.4 mmHg, and plasma levels of carboxyhemoglobin decrease from 6.5 percent to 1.1 percent.[30] Elevated plasma concentrations of carboxyhemoglobin, as may accompany smoke inhalation, can cause the pulse oximeter to overestimate hemoglobin saturations with oxygen (see Chapters 33 and 35). It seems unlikely, however, that low plasma carboxyhemoglobin concentrations associated with cigarette smoking would produce clinically significant overestimations. Carbon monoxide may also cause negative inotropic effects. Sympathomimetic effects of nicotine on the heart are transient, lasting only 20 minutes to 30 minutes. Despite these favorable responses, short-term abstinence from cigarettes has not been proven to decrease the incidence of postoperative pulmonary complications.

Cigarette smoking causes mucous hypersecretion, impairment of mucociliary transport activity, and narrowing of small airways. In contrast to favorable effects of short-term abstinence from smoking on levels of carboxyhemoglobin, improvement in ciliary and small airway function and decreases in sputum production occur slowly over periods of weeks after cigarette smoking is stopped. Indeed, the incidence of postoperative pulmonary complications after coronary artery surgery decreases only when abstinence from cigarette smoking is greater than 8 weeks (Fig. 14-4).[31]

Cigarette smoke may interfere with normal immune responses and could exaggerate suppression of these responses associated with anesthesia and surgery. Return of normal immune function may require at least 6 weeks of abstinence from smoking.[27] Some components of smoke may stimulate hepatic enzymes, which could influence perioperative analgesic requirements. Again, a period of 6 weeks to 8 weeks of abstinence is necessary before hepatic enzyme activity returns to normal. Paradoxically, the incidence of deep vein thrombosis after myocardial infarction and lower abdominal surgery is dramatically reduced in smokers compared with nonsmokers.[32,33] This is even more surprising considering that chronic cigarette smoking is often associated with elevated hematocrits and associated increases in blood viscosity. Although evidence is not available, it is possible that deprived smokers are more restless and move about more than nonsmokers and thus minimize venous stasis.[33]

Logic supports a strong recommendation to patients to cease cigarette smoking before undergoing elective surgery. Even brief periods of abstinence will improve oxygen-carrying capacity of the blood. Arguments that the time available is too brief to be useful are unconvincing. It seems illogical to sacrifice proven advantages for theoretical concerns that sputum may become more viscous and difficult to clear if patients abruptly stop smoking.

Management of Anesthesia

Presence of pulmonary emphysema does not dictate the use of specific drugs or techniques for management of anesthesia. Regional anesthesia is most suited for operations that do not invade the peritoneum or surgical procedures performed on the extremities.[26,34] Lower abdominal surgery can be performed using regional techniques, but general anesthesia is equally acceptable.[34] General anesthesia is the usual choice for upper abdominal and intrathoracic operations.

More important than the drugs or techniques selected is the realization that these patients are susceptible to the development of acute respiratory failure in the postoperative

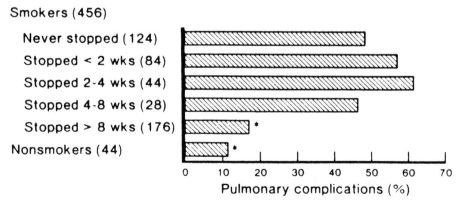

FIG. 14-4. Preoperative duration of smoking cessation and pulmonary complication rates after coronary artery bypass graft operations. The incidence of pulmonary complications after this type of surgery decreases only when abstinence from cigarette smoking is greater than 8 weeks. (Warner MA, Divertie MB, Tinker JH. Preoperative cessation of smoking and pulmonary complications in coronary artery bypass patients. Anesthesiology 1984;60:380–3)

period. Therefore, continued intubation of the trachea and mechanical ventilation of the lungs may be necessary, particularly after major surgery.

REGIONAL ANESTHESIA

Regional anesthesia remains a useful selection in patients with co-existing pulmonary disease only when sedative drugs are not needed. For example, it must be appreciated that these patients may be extremely sensitive to depressant effects of sedative drugs used for systemic medication. If patient anxiety is substantial, however, small doses of intravenous benzodiazepines, such as midazolam, in increments of 1 mg to 2 mg can be administered with minimal likelihood of producing undesirable degrees of ventilatory depression. Regional anesthetic techniques that produce sensory anesthesia above T-6 are not recommended, as this level can lead to decreases in expiratory reserve volumes. The most important adverse effect produced by these decreases is gas flow inadequate to produce an effective cough and leading to reduced clearance of secretions from airways.

GENERAL ANESTHESIA

In patients with co-existing pulmonary disease, general anesthesia is often provided with volatile anesthetic drugs, using humidification of the inspired gases and mechanical ventilation of the lungs. Volatile drugs are useful because of the body's ability to eliminate them rapidly via the lungs and thus minimize residual ventilatory depression in the early postoperative period. Furthermore, volatile anesthetics may produce beneficial effects secondary to drug-induced bronchodilation. Halothane, enflurane, and isoflurane would seem to be equally acceptable selections for administration to patients with pulmonary emphysema.

Nitrous oxide is frequently administered in combination with volatile anesthetics. When using nitrous oxide, one should consider the potential passage of this gas into pulmonary bullae associated with pulmonary em-physema. Conceivably, nitrous oxide could lead to enlargement and rupture of bullae, resulting in development of tension pneumothorax.[35] Another potential disadvantage of nitrous oxide is the limitation on the inspired concentrations of oxygen introduced by the use of this anesthetic. In this regard, it is important to remember that inhaled anesthetics may attenuate regional hypoxic pulmonary vasoconstriction, leading to increased degrees of right-to-left intrapulmonary shunting. It is conceivable that increased inspired concentrations of oxygen would be necessary to offset the potential adverse consequences of this anesthetic-induced change.

Opioids, although acceptable, are less ideal for the maintenance of anesthesia in these patients. For example, opioids can be associated with prolonged depression of ventilation, reflecting their slow rate of inactivation by the liver and/or elimination by the kidneys. Even the duration of depression of ventilation produced by drugs such as thiopental and midazolam is prolonged in patients with chronic obstructive airways disease as compared with normal patients.[36] High inspired concentrations of nitrous oxide may be required to insure amnesia when opioids are used for the maintenance of anesthesia. Administration of adequate inspired concentrations of oxygen may be compromised by the need to administer high concentrations of nitrous oxide.

Humidification of inspired gases during anesthesia is important to prevent drying of secretions in the airways. It should be remembered that placement of a tube in the trachea results in bypass of nearly all the airway humidification system. Furthermore, high flows of dry anesthetic gases intensify the need for humidification of inhaled gases. Systemic dehydration due to inadequate fluid administration during the perioperative period can result in excessive drying of secretions in the airways, despite humidification of inhaled gases.

Controlled ventilation of the lungs is useful for optimizing arterial oxygenation in patients with pulmonary emphysema who are undergoing prolonged operations.[27] Large tidal volumes (10 ml·kg^{-1} to 15 ml·kg^{-1}) combined with slow inspiratory flow rates minimize the likelihood of turbulent air flow through airways and maintain an optimal matching of ventilation to perfusion. Slow rates of breathing (6 breaths·min^{-1} to 10 breaths·min^{-1}) allow sufficient time for venous return to the heart and are less likely to be associated with undesirable degrees of hyperventilation, as reflected by the arterial partial pressures of carbon dioxide. Furthermore, slow rates of breathing provide sufficient time for complete exhalation to occur, which is particularly important if air trapping is to be prevented in patients with chronic obstructive airways disease. The hazard of pulmonary barotrauma in the presence of pulmonary bullae should be appreciated, particularly if high positive airway pressures are required to provide adequate ventilation of the lungs. Overall, the intraoperative use of large tidal volumes and slow breathing rates is as efficacious as positive end-expiratory pressure with respect to arterial oxygenation, without the detrimental cardiovascular effects produced by sustained positive airway pressure. If spontaneous ventilation is permitted during anesthesia, it should be appreciated that depression of ventilation produced by halothane, and presumably other volatile anesthetics, is greater in patients with chronic obstructive airways disease as compared to patients with normal lungs.[27] Regardless of the method of ventilation of the lungs selected during surgery, objective adjustments in the mode of ventilation or in ventilator settings can be made only on the basis of measurements of arterial blood gases and pH.

Impairment of gas exchange across the alveolar-capillary membrane is an inevitable accompaniment of general anesthesia. The magnitude of this impairment depends on a number of factors, which include (1) co-existing pulmonary disease, (2) cardiac output, (3) functional residual capacity, (4) patient age, and (5) position necessitated by the surgical procedure. The unifying pathway through which all these factors express themselves on gas exchange relates to the impact of these events on the distribution of ventilation and pulmonary blood flow. Optimum gas exchange occurs when alveoli share inspired gas and pulmonary blood flows equally. Evidence for mismatch of ventilation to perfusion is an increase in the alveolar-to-arterial difference for oxygen and carbon dioxide. There is some ventilation-to-perfusion inequality in normal lungs, but this inequality is increased by pulmonary disease and is further exaggerated by changes that occur during the perioperative period.

Normal distribution of ventilation and perfusion is characterized by a relative overventilation of nondependent lung zones and relative overperfusion of dependent lung regions. This physiologic mismatch is increased when more pulmonary blood flow is directed to dependent portions of the lung or when ventilation is redistributed to nondependent regions. Distribution of pulmonary blood flow is gravity dependent and is influenced by the interrelationships between pulmonary artery pressure, pulmonary venous pressure, and pressures present in the alveoli. For example, an unperfused but ventilated area of the lungs can be created by increasing alveolar pressures above pulmonary venous pressures with the application of positive pressure to the airways. Likewise, decreases in pulmonary artery pressures due to reductions in cardiac output, secondary to anesthetic-induced myocardial depression or reductions in the intravascular fluid volume, will lead to underperfusion of alveoli relative to ventilation. Evidence for anesthetic-induced changes in pulmonary blood flow leading to impaired gas exchange is an increase in the arterial-to-alveolar difference for carbon dioxide during anesthesia. For example, this gradient is normally less than 1 mmHg in the awake state but can reach 5 mmHg to 6 mmHg during general anesthesia. The possibility of a carbon dioxide gradient must be remembered when monitoring exhaled (end-tidal) concentrations of carbon dioxide as reflections of the arterial concentrations of this gas.

Normally, some modification of the distribution of pulmonary blood flow is possible by initiation of regional vasoconstriction of pulmonary arterioles supplying alveoli with low partial pressures of oxygen. This hypoxic pulmonary vasoconstriction diverts pulmonary blood flow from underventilated alveoli and thus improves matching of ventilation to perfusion and serves to optimize arterial oxygenation. Some, but not all studies, suggest that inhaled anesthetics may attenuate or abolish this protective response. The impact of this anesthetic-induced effect is offset by increased inspired concentrations of oxygen administered intraoperatively.

Distribution of ventilation depends on the (1) elastic properties of alveoli, (2) preinspiratory volume of alveoli, and (3) method of expansion of the chest wall. For example, distribution of ventilation is influenced by whether the diaphragm is an actively contracting or a passively displaced muscle. During spontaneous ventilation in the supine or lateral decubitus position, contraction of the diaphragm results in preferential inflation of dependent lung regions. Furthermore, halothane and possibly other inhaled anesthetics preferentially depress activity of intercostal muscles, which interferes with stabilization of the rib cage.[37] As a result, the chest wall tends to collapse inward as the diaphragm contracts, making patients vulnerable to hypoventilation during anesthesia and in the early postoperative period, if residual effects of anesthetics persist. When the diaphragm is made passive by muscle relaxants, distribution of ventilation becomes dependent on intra-abdominal pressures. A uniform inflating pressure applied on the thoracic side of the diaphragm will result in the greatest displacement of the diaphragm along nondependent regions of the lung. This increases distribution of ventilation to these nondependent regions, whereas gravity-dependent pulmonary blood flow is still predominantly distributed to dependent regions. The result is an accentuation of the mismatch of ventilation to perfusion, which can manifest as impairment of gas exchange across alveolar capillary membranes.

Gas exchange across alveolar capillary membranes during anesthesia is also influenced by changes in the functional residual capacity. Induction of general anesthesia plus skeletal muscle paralysis can be associated with decreases in the functional residual capacity, leading to a tendency for airways with diameters of 1 mm or less to collapse. As a result, mismatch of ventilation to perfusion is accentuated, as reflected by increases in the alveolar-to-arterial difference for oxygen. Lung volume, at which small airways begin to close, is defined as the closing volume (Fig. 14-5).[38] Closing volume is not altered by anesthesia. Maintenance of the functional residual capacity and prevention of small airways closure is facilitated by mechanical ventilation of the lungs, using large tidal volumes with or without positive end-expiratory pressure.

Management of Ventilation in the Postoperative Period

Management of ventilation of the lungs in the postoperative period in patients with co-existing pulmonary disease ranges from observation in highly monitored environments to mechanical ventilation of the lungs for several days.[39] Continued intubation of the trachea and mechanical ventilation of the lungs in the immediate postoperative period is likely to be necessary for patients with significant co-existing pulmonary disease. For example, it is likely that patients with a preoperative ratio of FEV_1 to vital capacity that is less than 0.50 will need continued mechanical support of ventilation of the lungs in the early postoperative period, especially if upper abdominal or thoracic surgery has been performed.[25] Presence of preoperative arterial partial pressures of carbon dioxide that exceed 50 mmHg is likely to be associated with the need for postoperative mechanical ventilation. It should be appreciated that measured arterial partial pressures of carbon dioxide in the preoperative period may be falsely low if the arterial puncture was painful and produced an increased volume of ventilation. Elevated plasma concentrations of bicarbonate in the presence of normal arterial partial pressures of carbon dioxide suggest that acute hyperventilation was masking chronic carbon dioxide retention. When the arterial partial pressures of carbon dioxide have been chronically elevated, it is important not to correct the hypercarbia abruptly. Sudden reductions can result in profound alkalemia, since bicarbonate cannot be rapidly excreted by the kidneys. This alkalemia can be associated with cardiac dysrhythmias and central nervous system stimulation, culminating in seizures.

When continued mechanical ventilation of the lungs is necessary in the postoperative period, it is recommended that inspired con-

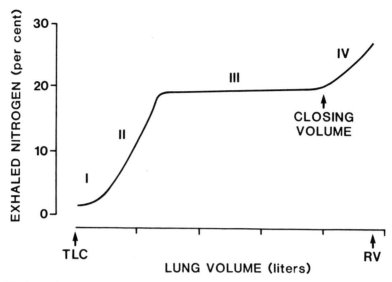

FIG. 14-5. Closing volume is determined by plotting the nitrogen concentration during exhalation to residual volume (RV). Exhalation is preceded by inhalation of a single breath of pure oxygen to total lung capacity (TLC). This initial breath contains dead space gas rich in nitrogen. This gas enters alveoli in the upper lung zones; the remainder of the breath, consisting of pure oxygen, goes to the lower lung zones. As a result, the concentration of nitrogen is higher in the upper lung zone alveoli. Phase I is exhalation of dead space gas containing only oxygen. This phase is followed by an abrupt increase in the exhaled concentration of nitrogen (phase II), reflecting a mixing of dead space and alveolar gas. Phase III is alveolar gas from alveoli throughout the lungs. As exhalation continues, the airways at the bases of the lungs begin to collapse and there is an abrupt increase in the slope of the nitrogen concentration (phase IV), since alveolar gas is now predominantly from upper lung zones. The lung volume at which the nitrogen concentration abruptly increases represents the beginning of airway closure and is designated the closing volume. Phase III will reflect a stable concentration of nitrogen only if the distribution of ventilation is uniform. When distribution of ventilation is not uniform, gas coming from alveoli during exhalation will contain differing concentrations of nitrogen, and phase III will continue to rise.

centrations of oxygen and ventilator settings be adjusted to maintain the arterial partial pressures of oxygen between 60 mmHg to 100 mmHg and the arterial partial pressures of carbon dioxide in a range that maintains the arterial pH between 7.36 and 7.44. Until these values can be confirmed in the postoperative period, it is customary to administer at least 50 percent oxygen, using tidal volumes of 10 ml·kg^{-1} to 15 ml·kg^{-1} and ventilatory rates of 6 breaths·min^{-1} to 10 breaths·min^{-1}. Positive end-expiratory pressure may be necessary if the arterial partial pressures of oxygen cannot be maintained above 60 mmHg, breathing 50 percent oxygen (see Chapter 16). It must be remembered that positive end-expiratory pressure may be associated with increased air trap-ping in patients with chronic obstructive airways disease.

In addition to measuring arterial blood gases and pH, an indication of airway resistance can be derived by determining the difference between dynamic and static lung compliance. Dynamic lung compliance is the ratio of the exhaled tidal volume to peak measured airway pressure. This ratio reflects resistance to gas flow through airways, as well as compliance of the lungs and thorax. Conversely, static lung compliance is measured by dividing the exhaled tidal volume by the plateau airway pressure present when inspiration is held for 1 seconds to 1.5 seconds. Static lung compliance reflects only lung and thoracic compliance. Therefore, the difference between dynamic and static lung compliance and the trend of these measurements is an indicator of airway resistance. Decisions to discontinue mechanical support of ventilation of the lungs and remove the tracheal tube are based on the clinical status and measurements of indices of pulmonary function (see Chapter 16).

CHRONIC BRONCHITIS

Chronic bronchitis is characterized by chronic or recurrent secretion of excess mucus into the bronchi. Enlarged mucous glands, combined with excess secretion of mucus, result in reductions in lumens of airways and associated increases in resistance to gas flow through these airways. Nevertheless, many patients have excess secretion of mucus without evidence of obstructive airways disease. Conversely, other patients have severe obstructive airways disease, but mucus secretion is not particularly prominent. Finally, some patients with chronic bronchitis manifest eosinophilia, and often the obstructive component of the pulmonary disease in these patients can be reduced with bronchodilator therapy, as used for the treatment of bronchial asthma.

Cigarette smoking is the major predisposing factor to the development of chronic bronchitis. Environmental pollution appears to play some role, but its effects are minor compared with those of cigarette smoke. Many patients with chronic bronchitis experience recurrent bronchial infections. Organisms responsible for bronchial infections are bacteria (*Diplococcus pneumoniae, Hemophilus influenzae*), viruses, and Mycoplasma organisms. In some instances, infection in the airways may be the result of chronic bronchitis rather than its cause. Infection produces inflammation and fibrosis that contribute to narrowing of airways.

Clinical features of chronic bronchitis can resemble or contrast with findings present in patients with pulmonary emphysema (Table 14-3). Patients with chronic bronchitis are often termed *blue bloaters* because arterial hypoxemia and carbon dioxide retention tend to occur early in the course of the disease, which contrasts with pulmonary emphysema. On the other hand, because small airways account for only a small proportion of total airway resistance, chronic bronchitis must be advanced before dyspnea becomes apparent, which again contrasts with pulmonary emphysema. Expiratory flow rates in chronic bronchitis show an obstructive pattern. Total lung capacity is less elevated than in patients with pulmonary emphysema, and the lungs contain more blood. As a result, the lungs are less radiolucent, and radiographs of the chest may not be characteristic of obstructive airways disease. Cor pulmonale occurs relatively early in patients with chronic bronchitis (seee Chapter 9). Although the primary impairment of the heart involves the right ventricle, there can also be associated left ventricular dysfunction in about one-half of patients. Pulmonary artery occlusion pressures are often elevated in these patients, most likely reflecting decreased left ventricular compliance as the expanding right ventricle causes the interventricular septum to encroach on the left side of the heart.

Prognosis of chronic bronchitis is poor, with death often occurring within 5 years after the first episode of acute respiratory failure. Preoperative evaluation and management of anesthesia are as described for patients with pulmonary emphysema.

BRONCHIECTASIS

Bronchiectasis is characterized by permanent abnormal dilation of the bronchi. Dilation of various parts of the airways occurs in many lung diseases, including pulmonary emphysema and chronic bronchitis. Definitive diagnosis of bronchiectasis depends on demonstrating persistent and widespread bronchodilation by bronchography during all phases of ventilation.

Any process that causes recurrent bronchial infections is capable of producing bronchiectasis. Affected bronchi frequently contain purulent secretions, which predictably leads to purulent sputum production. In addition, affected bronchi often contain highly vascularized granulation tissue, which may be the source of recurrent hemoptysis. Extensive collateral circulation can arise from bronchial and intercostal arteries. If these vessels connect with the pulmonary circulation, there is transmission of systemic pressure, and pulmonary hypertension and cor pulmonale are possible. If these collateral vessels connect to branches of the pulmonary veins, the subsequent transmission of systemic pressures can lead to pulmonary edema. Recurrent sinus infections are common. Chronic bronchiectasis may be accompanied by clubbing, pulmonary osteoarthropathy, or amyloidosis. Pulmonary function changes are unpredictable, ranging from no change to alterations characteristic of obstructive or restrictive pulmonary disease.

Treatment

Treatment of bronchiectasis includes chest physiotherapy and postural drainage to facilitate elimination of secretions from the airways. Prophylactic antibiotic therapy is recommended with prompt and specific antibiotic treatment being added to the protocol for intercurrent bronchopulmonary infections. Surgical resection of diseased portions of the lungs is recommended when there are recurrent infections in localized areas of lung or recurrent hemoptysis.

Management of Anesthesia

Management of anesthesia in patients with chronic bronchiectasis should include consideration of the use of double lumen endotracheal tubes to prevent spillage of purulent sputum into normal areas of the lungs. Instrumentation of the nares may not be prudent, in view of the high incidence of chronic sinusitis in these patients.

CYSTIC FIBROSIS

Cystic fibrosis is a genetic disease, which is transmitted as an autosomal recessive trait. The disease affects exocrine glands, leading to secretion of chemically abnormal sweat and a highly viscous mucus. Indeed, the diagnosis of cystic fibrosis is based on demonstration of increased concentrations of sodium, potassium, and chloride (about 60 $mEq \cdot L^{-1}$) in the sweat, which are present at birth and remain elevated throughout life. Availability of antibiotics and improved supportive treatment, including postural drainage and physiotherapy, has increased the number of patients who survive to adulthood. In addition, mild clinical variants of cystic fibrosis are characterized by frequent pulmonary infections.

Clinical Manifestations

Pulmonary involvement characterized by obstruction of airways with viscous mucus is the most consistent clinical manifestation of cystic fibrosis. There is persistent bronchial infection and irreversible fibrotic changes in the airways. Frequent pulmonary complications include abscess formation, empyema, and hemoptysis. Copious amounts of thick, greenish, and purulent sputum are common. Nasal polyps occur frequently. Late pulmonary changes include development of bronchiectasis and diffuse parenchymal fibrosis. Expiratory flow rates are decreased, airway resistance and residual volumes are increased, and there is an exaggerated mismatch of ventilation to perfusion. Spontaneous pneumothorax is common in older children and adults. Arterial hypoxemia, hypoventilation, and respiratory acidosis are frequently terminal events.

Pancreatic insufficiency reflects mucous obstruction of ducts in this organ. Hepatic cirrhosis and portal hypertension develop, with progressive obstruction of bile ducts by viscous mucus. Gastrointestinal obstruction manifesting as meconium ileus may be a manifestation of cystic fibrosis at birth. Infants with cystic fibrosis are at increased risk for hemorrhage, arising from vitamin K deficiency related to malabsorption of fat-soluble vitamins.

Management of Anesthesia

Management of anesthesia in patients with cystic fibrosis invokes the same principles as outlined for patients with pulmonary emphysema. Elective surgical procedures should be delayed until optimal pulmonary function can be assured by control of bronchial infections and facilitation of the removal of secretions from the airways. Vitamin K treatment may be necessary if hepatic function is poor or absorption of fat-soluble vitamins from the gastrointestinal tract is impaired. Preoperative medication is probably not necessary, as sedation may lead to undesirable ventilatory depression, and anticholinergic drugs may further increase viscosity of secretions. Maintenance of anesthesia with volatile anesthetics allows use of high inspired concentrations of oxygen and can reduce airway resistance by decreasing the tone of bronchial smooth muscles. Furthermore, volatile anesthetics are helpful in reducing responsiveness of hyperreactive airways characteristic of cystic fibrosis. Humidification of inspired gases is important for maintaining secretions in a less viscous state. Frequent suctioning of the trachea is often necessary during the operative period.

KARTAGENER'S SYNDROME

Kartagener's syndrome consists of situs inversus, chronic sinusitis, and bronchiectasis.[40] This syndrome is inherited as an autosomal recessive trait and accounts for about 0.5 percent of patients with dextrocardia. These patients experience repeated pulmonary infections and chronic otitis media beginning in childhood. A productive cough and hemoptysis are common. Bronchiectasis is the most prominent feature of the syndrome. Isolated dextrocardia is almost always associated with congenital heart disease, whereas the incidence of cardiac defects is low when accompanied by situs inversus.

The principal defect in patients with this syndrome is a generalized abnormality of ciliary function with failure to transport mucus towards the glottic opening at normal rates. This defect in ciliary motility extends to spermatozoa, and most males with this disease are sterile.

TRACHEAL STENOSIS

Tracheal stenosis is an extreme example of obstructive airways disease that typically develops after mechanical ventilation of the lungs requiring prolonged translaryngeal intubation of the trachea or tracheostomy. Tracheal mucosal ischemia that may progress to destruction of cartilaginous rings and subsequent circumferential constricting scar formation is minimized by use of high residual volume cuffs on tracheal tubes so as not to produce excessive pressure on underlying mucosa. Infection and systemic hypotension may contribute to events that culminate in tracheal stenosis.

Tracheal stenosis becomes symptomatic when the lumen of the adult trachea is reduced to less than 5 mm. Symptoms may not develop until several weeks after extubation of the trachea. Dyspnea is prominent even at rest, as these patients must use accessory muscles of respiration during all phases of the breathing cycle. Ineffective cough is present and stridor may be audible. Patients with tracheal stenosis breathe slowly because they cannot increase their tidal volumes despite additional muscular efforts. Peak flow rates are reduced during exhalation. Flow volume plots of forced exhaled vital capacity and inspiratory vital capacity may be useful in detecting tracheal stenosis. Tomograms of the trachea demonstrate tracheal narrowing in these patients.

Tracheal dilation may be useful in some patients, but often surgical resection of the stenotic tracheal segment with primary anastomosis is required.[41] Anesthesia for tracheal resection may be complicated by total airway obstruction during surgical mobilization of the trachea. Initially, a translaryngeal tube is placed in the trachea. After surgical exposure, the distal normal trachea is opened and a sterile cuffed tube inserted and attached to the anesthetic breathing system. Maintenance of anesthesia with volatile anesthetics is useful for assuring maximum inspired concentrations of oxygen. In selected patients, high frequency ventilation may be useful. Addition of helium (50 percent to 75 percent) to inspired gases reduces density of these gases and may improve flow through the area of tracheal narrowing.

IMPACT OF SURGERY ON PULMONARY FUNCTION

Nearness of the operation to the diaphragm is the most important factor in producing mechanical abnormalities of the lung and alterations in gas exchange at alveolar capillary membranes during the early postoperative period.[39] For example, changes in pulmonary mechanics and gas exchange are greatest after upper abdominal operations, less after thoracic and lower abdominal procedures, and least after superficial procedures and operations performed on the extremities. These postoperative pulmonary changes include reductions in tidal volume, vital capacity, functional residual capacity, FEV_1, and arterial partial pressure of oxygen, as well as increases in the respiratory rate. These changes are maximal 24 hours to 48 hours after surgery.

Mechanical Abnormalities

Vital capacity is reduced to about 40 percent of the preoperative value on the day of upper abdominal surgery. Even 7 days after operation, vital capacity is only 60 percent to 70 percent of the preoperative level. Vital capacity has returned to near preoperative levels by 10 days to 14 days after upper abdominal operations.

Effects of lower abdominal surgery and intrathoracic operations not involving resection of lung tissue on pulmonary mechanics are similar. For example, vital capacity is reduced to about 60 percent of preoperative values on the day of surgery. Vital capacity gradually improves and by 7 days postoperatively is about 80 percent of the preoperative value.

After upper abdominal surgery, the FEV_1 is reduced to the same extent as the vital capacity. Therefore, the ratio of FEV_1 to vital capacity is not altered after surgery. This unchanged ratio suggests the absence of large airways obstruction after upper abdominal surgery. Nevertheless, it is likely that more sensitive tests would demonstrate increased airway resistance after upper abdominal surgery.

In contrast to vital capacity, functional residual capacity remains unchanged from preoperative levels until about 16 hours after upper abdominal surgery.[39] By 16 hours to 24 hours after operation, functional residual capacity has decreased to about 70 percent of preoperative levels. It then gradually returns to preoperative levels between 7 days and 10 days after surgery. This delayed reduction in functional residual capacity suggests that alterations in breathing patterns in the postoperative period are responsible for this later change. The usual explanation is that incisional pain leads to reduced tidal volumes and vital capacity, which ultimately manifests as reductions in functional residual capacity. Complete relief of postoperative pain, however, using intercostal nerve blocks or epidural analgesia, results in only partial restoration of vital capacity, whereas functional residual capacity is only minimally changed.[39] Furthermore, vital capacity is still decreased after upper abdominal surgery when epidural analgesia is present on awakening from anesthesia.[42] This suggests that changes in addition to breathing patterns contribute to decreases in functional residual capacity in the postoperative period. Failure of complete analgesia to prevent such decreases suggests that trauma from the surgical procedure interferes with normal function of the chest wall by changing the normal relationship of the diaphragm, intercostal muscles, and abdominal muscles.

Reduction in functional residual capacity in the postoperative period is important because of its effect on the patency of small airways, particularly those less than 1 mm in diameter. These small airways are not supported by cartilage and thus are influenced by transmitted pleural pressures. Normally, pleural pressures are less than atmospheric pressure, resulting in positive transpulmonary pressures, which distend the lungs, including small airways. When the functional residual capacity is reduced, it is likely that pleural pressures will exceed atmospheric pressures in gravity-dependent areas of the lungs, causing small airways to be narrowed or closed. The net effect of small airway closure is a decrease in the arterial partial pressures of oxygen, reflecting reductions in ventilation to affected lung regions despite continued pulmonary blood flow.

Gas Exchange

Gas exchange at alveolar capillary membranes in the postoperative period is characterized by reductions in the arterial partial pressures of oxygen without predictable alterations in the arterial partial pressures of carbon dioxide or pH. Decreases in the arterial partial pressures of oxygen can be categorized as immediate and delayed reductions in arterial oxygenation.

IMMEDIATE REDUCTIONS IN ARTERIAL OXYGENATION

Reductions in the arterial partial pressures of oxygen that occur immediately after surgery most likely reflect the impact of anesthetic drugs and events occurring intraoperatively. For example, residual effects of anesthetic drugs may impair regional hypoxic pulmonary vasoconstriction. Absence of this vasoconstriction will exaggerate the impact of poorly ven-

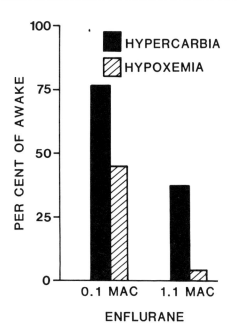

FIG. 14-6. The ventilatory response to normoxic hypercarbia and isocapnic hypoxemia was determined in healthy volunteers awake, during sedation with 0.1 MAC enflurane, and during anesthesia with 1.1 MAC enflurane. Enflurane produces dose-related decreases in the ventilatory response to hypercarbia and hypoxemia. The greatest impact of enflurane is on the ventilatory response to hypoxemia, which is dependent on the peripheral carotid bodies. In contrast, the ventilatory response to carbon dioxide, which is mediated by medullary chemoreceptors in the central nervous system, is depressed less by enflurane. (Data adapted from Knill RL, Manninen PH, Clement JL. Ventilation and chemoreflexes during enflurane sedation and anesthesia in man. Can Anaesth Soc J 1979;26:353–60)

tilated areas of the lungs on arterial oxygenation by preventing compensatory reductions in pulmonary blood flow to these regions. Volatile anesthetics also cause decreased ventilatory responses to carbon dioxide, arterial hypoxemia, and acidemia. Indeed, subanesthetic concentrations (0.1 MAC) of halothane and enflurane (Fig. 14-6)[43] nearly eliminate ventilatory responses normally produced by reductions in the arterial partial pressures of oxygen below 60 mmHg. These subanesthetic concentrations also reduce by more than one-half ventilatory responses to acidemia. Likewise, small doses of opioids depress ventilatory responses to increased concentrations of carbon dioxide or reduced amounts of oxygen in arterial blood.[44] These observations emphasize the decreased ability of patients to compensate for arterial hypoxemia that accompanies the early postoperative period. Other factors that may contribute to less than optimal arterial oxygenation in this period include depletion of carbon dioxide stores by intraoperative hyperventilation, leading to reduced minute ventilation in the postoperative period;[45] decreased cardiac output; and increased total body oxygen consumption due to increased activity of skeletal muscles manifesting as shivering. In the absence of co-existing abnormalities of lung function, arterial partial pressures of oxygen have usually returned to preoperative levels by 2 hours after uncomplicated general anesthesia for minor operations.

DELAYED REDUCTIONS IN ARTERIAL OXYGENATION

Reductions in the arterial partial pressures of oxygen that persist beyond the early postoperative period most likely reflect mechanical abnormalities of the lungs, as reflected by decreases in the functional residual capacity.[39] For example, alveoli collapse as functional residual capacity decreases, resulting in venous admixture due to continued perfusion of these unventilated alveoli. Arterial oxygenation may not return to preoperative levels until 10 days to 14 days after surgery associated with reductions in functional residual capacity. Upper abdominal surgery has the greatest effect on functional residual capacity and is followed by the greatest reductions in the arterial partial pressures of oxygen. The magnitude of reductions in arterial oxygenation in the postoperative period is accentuated by the increasing age of patients. Decreased arterial oxygenation due to mismatch of ventilation to perfusion is often remedied by modest increases in inspired concentrations of oxygen. Conversely, reductions in the arterial partial pressures of oxygen due to perfusion of unventilated alveoli are refractory to oxygen therapy.

POSTOPERATIVE PULMONARY COMPLICATIONS

The incidence of postoperative pulmonary complications is difficult to determine because there is no general agreement as to what represents pulmonary morbidity. Postoperative pulmonary complications are most often characterized as atelectasis followed by pneumonia. The severity of these complications parallels the magnitude of reductions in lung volumes. Presumably, decreases in vital capacity and functional residual capacity interfere with the generation of an effective cough, as well as contributing to the collapse of alveoli. The net effect is decreased clearance of secretions from the airways and atelectasis, leading to pneumonia and reductions in the arterial partial pressures of oxygen (Fig. 14-7).

As would be expected from changes in pulmonary mechanics, the frequency of postoperative pulmonary complications is greatest after upper abdominal surgery.[39] In addition to sites of operation, other factors that influence the incidence of postoperative pulmonary complications include co-existing pulmonary disease, obesity, increasing age, and cigarette smoking (see the section Cessation of Cigarette Smoking). For example, the likelihood of postoperative pulmonary complications is increased in patients with co-existing pulmonary disease associated with sputum production, decreased vital capacity, or decreased FEV_1, as documented in the preoperative period. A 30 percent or greater increase in body weight above normal increases the risk of such complications. Presumably, the diaphragm is displaced cephalad, which tends to decrease lung volumes of the lower lobes, resulting in mismatch of ventilation to perfusion. Relationships between the duration of anesthesia and the incidence of postoperative pulmonary complications are not clear, although some reports describe positive correlations between duration of surgery and subsequent development of pulmonary complications.[39] The role of the type of upper abdominal incision in development of these complications is also controversial. Many feel that transverse upper abdominal incisions produce fewer adverse changes on pulmonary mechanics than do ver-

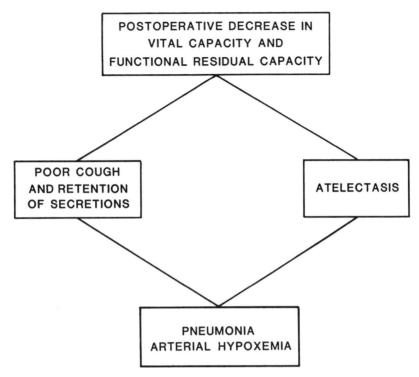

FIG. 14-7. Pathogenesis of postoperative pulmonary complications.

tical abdominal incisions. Indeed, in one study patients with subcostal incisions for cholecystectomy had less decrease in vital capacity and the arterial partial pressures of oxygen than did patients who underwent the same operation via midline abdominal incisions.[46] Presumably, less pain associated with transverse upper abdominal incisions would also facilitate deep breathing and clearing of secretions from the airways. Nevertheless, in another report there was no difference between the two incisions and subsequent postoperative reductions in tidal volume, vital capacity, functional residual capacity, and arterial partial pressures of oxygen.[47] In view of these findings, it is probable that the incidence of postoperative pulmonary complications is also comparable.

Choice of drugs or techniques used to produce anesthesia does not seem to alter predictably the incidence of postoperative pulmonary infections. For example, repeated studies in patients with normal pulmonary function have not demonstrated any differences in the incidence of pulmonary complications in those receiving general anesthesia compared with regional anesthesia.[39] Similar studies performed in patients with chronic obstructive airways disease reveal a higher incidence of postoperative respiratory failure in patients who receive general anesthesia.[26] This difference, however, may reflect the fact that operative sites rather than regional techniques dictated selection of general anesthesia.

PROPHYLAXIS AGAINST POSTOPERATIVE PULMONARY COMPLICATIONS

Prophylaxis against development of postoperative pulmonary complications is based on restoring decreased lung volumes and facilitating the production of an effective cough so as to remove secretions from the airways. Identification of functional residual capacity as the most important lung volume in the postoperative period provides a specific goal of therapy. Indeed, treatment regimens that maintain or improve the functional residual capacity can be expected to improve both pulmonary mechanics and gas exchange. The large number of therapeutic approaches designed to provide prophylaxis against development of postoperative pulmonary infections suggests that no single treatment has been widely accepted. Often the best clinical response is obtained using a combination of treatments.

Voluntary Deep Breathing

Voluntary deep breathing with slow inspiration and maintenance of inspiration at peak inflation for 3 seconds to 5 seconds creates large transpulmonary pressure gradients and facilitates reexpansion of collapsed alveoli and restoration of lung volumes.[48] This mode of treatment requires motivated patients and relief of pain to permit maximal inspirations.

Ambulation has great therapeutic benefit in the prevention of postoperative pulmonary complications. For example, changing from the supine to sitting position increases the functional residual capacity. A change from sitting in bed to sitting in a chair, with the associated ambulation necessary to reach the chair, produces a greater increase in functional residual capacity than that associated with assuming the sitting position in bed. In addition, arterial oxygenation following upper abdominal surgery is improved by assuming the sitting position. Presumably, the increased functional residual capacity improves the matching of ventilation to perfusion. There is evidence that voluntary deep breathing plus ambulation is as effective as, and in some instances better than, the use of intermittent positive pressure breathing to prevent postoperative pulmonary complications.[49]

Intermittent Positive Pressure Breathing

Intermittent positive pressure breathing as a method to reduce the incidence of postoperative pulmonary complications is controversial. It is speculated that positive airway pressure will expand collapsed alveoli, leading to a restoration of lung volumes with improvement in the elimination of secretions from the airways and an increase in the arterial partial pressures of oxygen. Nevertheless, studies on the efficacy of this therapy have been inconclusive.[50] Part of the failure of intermittent positive pressure breathing may be due to emphasis on peak pressures achieved at the apparatus used to deliver the treatment rather than insisting on achievement of optimal tidal volumes. Particularly in uncooperative patients, peak pressures and tidal volumes do not correlate. Ideally, patients should inhale three times to six times the predicted tidal volume for the positive pressure breathing treatment to be effective. This inhaled tidal volume should be monitored with a spirometer placed on the exhalation valve.

Incentive Spirometry

Incentive spirometry is a type of voluntary deep breathing in which patients are given inspired volumes as a goal to achieve. This treatment also emphasizes holding the inhaled volumes to provide sustained inflations important for expanding collapsed alveoli. The major disadvantage is the need for patient cooperation to accomplish the treatment.

Expiratory Maneuvers

Expiratory maneuvers, such as inflating balloons, the use of blow-bottles, or performing a forced vital capacity, are not recommended, since performance of these events causes patients to exhale to below the functional residual capacity. For example, to inflate a balloon, patients must generate pleural pressures that exceed airway pressures, causing alveoli to become smaller or to collapse. Indeed, the only therapeutic benefit elicited by expiratory maneuvers is the deep breath that must be taken initially.

Analgesia with Opioids

Relief of postoperative pain using opioids should be viewed as a method to allow such other therapeutic regimens as changes in posture and ambulation to be better accepted by patients. Psychological factors can influence postoperative pain and the need for opioids. Furthermore, preoperative instruction of patients combined with reassurance can reduce the need for opioids in the postoperative period. Patient controlled analgesia, in which patients control the rate of intravenous opioid infusions, minimizes pharmacokinetic and pharmacodynamic differences among individuals.[51] Using this technique, patients are able to maintain near optimal levels of analgesia with minimal sedation or side effects.

Analgesia with Nerve Blocks

The role of intercostal nerve blocks or epidural techniques to provide postoperative analgesia is controversial. There is no doubt that these techniques provide analgesia, but their role in reducing the incidence of postoperative pulmonary complications is not confirmed.

INTERCOSTAL NERVE BLOCKS

Direct intrathoracic block of intercostal nerves at the conclusion of surgery is an effective technique for limiting changes in the vital capacity after thoracotomy.[52] Decreases in blood pressure[53] and the production of total spinal anesthesia[54] have been observed after direct intrathoracic block. The mechanism for the reduction in blood pressure is not clear; total spinal anesthesia most likely reflects passage of local anesthetics along nerve sheaths into the subarachnoid space. The picture resulting from a total spinal anesthetic is difficult to distinguish from unrecognized cerebral hypoxia, as patients are flaccid and apneic and their pupils are widely dilated and unreactive to light in the postoperative period. It is possible that bilateral intercostal nerve blocks could impair the ability to cough and effectively clear secretions from the airways.

EPIDURAL NERVE BLOCK

Postoperative analgesia provided by injection of local anesthetics into the epidural space partially restores the vital capacity, but functional residual capacity is unchanged.[39] Nevertheless, pain relief provided by epidural block has been reported to be superior to intravenous opioids for reducing the incidence of postoperative pulmonary complications.[55] In view of the complexity of performing epidural analgesia, most reserve this technique for patients with high risks for developing complications that could lead to respiratory failure. In addition to the complexity of the technique, associated sympathetic and sensory nerve blocks can produce orthostatic hypotension and interfere with ambulation in the early postoperative period.

Analgesia with Epidural Opioids

Opioids placed in the epidural space produce prolonged and intense postoperative relief of pain.[56] Analgesia provided by epidural opioids is free from sympathetic and proprioceptive nerve blockade associated with local anesthetics placed in the epidural space. Therefore, early ambulation is possible in patients treated with epidural opioids. In one study, epidural opioids administered after abdominal surgery were more than twice as effective for restoring the FEV_1 than intravenously administered drugs.[56] In the same study, improvement in FEV_1 provided by epidural opioids was similar to that seen in patients who received epidural local anesthetics (Fig. 14-8).[56] Enthusiasm for epidural opioids must be tempered by observations that sedation is frequently produced by this treatment. More important, profound ventilatory depression may occur 6 hours to 12 hours after placement of opioids into the epidural space. Presumably, opioids are absorbed into the subarachnoid space and ultimately diffuse into the area of the fourth cerebral ventricle, where they can depress the medullary ventilatory center. Use of lipid soluble opioids, injection with the patient in the sitting position, avoidance of vigorous diaphragmatic movements shortly after the injection, and utilization of minimal drug doses should minimize the likelihood of cephalad migration of large amounts of opioids and subsequent depression of ventilation.

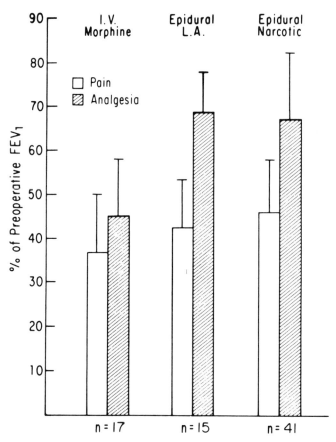

FIG. 14-8. The forced exhaled volume in 1 second (FEV_1) was measured as a percent of the preoperative value in adult patients (n = number of patients studied) after upper abdominal surgery. Production of analgesia with intravenous morphine does not significantly increase the FEV_1. Conversely, production of analgesia with local anesthetics or opioids placed in the epidural space returns the FEV_1 to about 70 percent of the preoperative value. (Bromage PR, Comporesi E, Chestnut D. Epidural narcotics for postoperative analgesia. Anesth Analg 1980;59:473–80. Reprinted with permission from IARS.)

Chest Physiotherapy and Postural Drainage

Combinations of chest physiotherapy and postural drainage plus deep breathing exercises taught in the preoperative period have been reported to reduce the incidence of radiographic findings of atelectasis after performance of cholecystectomy.[39] Presumably, vibrations produced on the chest wall by physiotherapy result in displacement of mucus plugs from peripheral airways. Appropriate positioning facilitates elimination of loosened mucus from the airways. Close observation by the therapist is necessary to see how much sputum is produced and to assure that patients are taking deep breaths.

Ultrasonic Nebulizer

Ultrasonic nebulizers produce a dense aerosol of distilled water that is irritating to the larynx and upper trachea. This creates involuntary coughing and helps to clear secretions from the airways. Patients must have an intact cough mechanism to benefit from this treatment. Furthermore, the aerosol produced can cause bronchoconstriction in patients with hyper-reactive airways. Some patients are refractory and do not cough even during the first treatment, and others become resistant to the treatment.

Transcutaneous Electrical Nerve Stimulation

Transcutaneous electrical nerve stimulation, as a method for providing postoperative analgesia and reducing the incidence of pulmonary complications, is attractive because of its simplicity. This form of analgesia attenuates reductions in vital capacity and functional re-sidual capacity that develop after upper abdominal surgery.[57]

REFERENCES

1. Kingston HGG, Hirshman CA. Perioperative management of the patient with asthma. Anesth Analg 1984;63:844–55
2. Cockcroft DW, Berscheid BA, Murdoch KY. Unimodal distribution of bronchial responsiveness to inhaled histamine in a random human population. Chest 1983;751–4
3. Benatar SR. Fatal asthma. N Engl J Med 1986;314:423–8
4. McFadden ER, Kiser R, deGroot WJ. Acute bronchial asthma: Relations between clinical and physiologic manifestations. N Engl J Med 1973;288:221–5
5. Deal EC, McFadden ER, Ingram RH, et al. Airway responsiveness to cold air and hyperpnea in normal subjects and in those with hay fever and asthma. Am Rev Respir Dis 1980;121:621–8
6. Bernstein IL, Raghuprasad PK. Status asthmaticus: Treat aggressively for best result. J Respir Dis 1980;1:64–72
7. Sprague DH. Treatment of intraoperative bronchospasm with nebulized isoetharine. Anesthesiology 1977;46:222–4
8. Fredholm BB. Are methylxanthine's effects due to the antagonism of endogenous adenosine? Trends Pharm Sci 1980;1:129–32
9. Prokocimer PG, Nichols E, Gaga DM, Maze M. Epinephrine arrhythmogenicity is enhanced by acute, but not by chronic aminophylline administration during halothane anesthesia in dogs. Anesthesiology 1986;65:13–8
10. Nichols EA, Louie GL, Prokocimer PG, Maze M. Halothane anesthetic requirements are not affected by aminophylline treatment in rats and dogs. Anesthesiology 1986;65:637–41
11. Littenberg IB, Gluck EH. A controlled trial of methylprednisolone in the emergency treatment of acute asthma. N Engl J Med 1973;289:600–3
12. Sue MA, Kwong FK, Klaustermeyer WB. A comparison of intravenous hydrocortisone, methylprednisolone, and dexamethasone in acute bronchial asthma. Ann Allergy 1986;56:406–9
13. Gal TJ, Suratt PM. Atropine and glycopyrrolate effects on lung mechanics in normal man. Anesth Analg 1981;60:85–90
14. Nathan R, Segall N, Schocket A. A comparison of the actions of H-1 and H-2 antihistamine on

histamine-induced bronchoconstriction and cutaneous wheal response in asthmatic patients. J Allergy Clin Immunol 1981;67:171–7

15. Hirshman CA, Downes H, Farbood A, Bergman NA. Ketamine block of bronchospasm in experimental canine asthma. Br J Anaesth 1979;51:713–8

16. Shnider SM, Papper EM. Anesthesia for the asthmatic patient. Anesthesiology 1961;22:886–92

17. Stirt JA, Berger JM, Roe SD, et al. Safety of enflurane following administration of aminophylline in experimental animals. Anesth Analg 1981;60:871–3

18. Parnass SM, Feld JM, Chamberlin WH, Segil LJ. Status asthmaticus treated with isoflurane and enflurane. Anesth Analg 1987;66:193–5

19. Hirshman CA, Edelstein G, Peetz S, et al. Mechanism of action of inhalational anesthesia on airways. Anesthesiology 1982;56:107–11

20. Downes H, Gerber N, Hirshman CA, I.V. lignocaine in reflex and allergic bronchoconstriction. Br J Anaesth 1980;52:873–8

21. Koga Y, Downes H, Leon D, Hirshman CA. Mechanism of tracheal constriction by succinylcholine. Anesthesiology 1981;55:138–42

22. Cheney FU, Hornbein TF, Crawford EW. The effects of ultrasonically-produced aerosols on airway resistance in man. Anesthesiology 1968;29:1099–1106

23. Schwartz SH. Treatment of status asthmaticus with halothane. JAMA 1984;151:2688–9

24. Hermens JM, Edelstein G, Hanifin JM, et al. Inhalational anesthesia and histamine release during bronchospasm. Anesthesiology 1984; 61:69–72

25. Stein M, Cassara EL. Preoperative pulmonary evaluation and therapy for surgery patients. JAMA 1970;211:878–90

26. Tarhan S, Moffitt EA, Sessler AD, et al. Risk of anesthesia and surgery in patients with chronic bronchitis and chronic obstructive pulmonary disease. Surgery 1973;74:720–6

27. Pietak S, Weenig CS, Hickey RF, Fairley HB. Anesthetic effects on ventilation in patients with chronic obstructive pulmonary disease. Anesthesiology 1975;42:160–6

28. Cottrell JE, Siker ES. Preoperative intermittent positive pressure breathing therapy in patients with chronic obstructive lung disease: Effect on postoperative pulmonary complications. Anesth Analg 1973;52:258–62

29. Pearce AC, Jones RM. Smoking and anesthesia: Preoperative abstinence and perioperative morbidity. Anesthesiology 1984;61:576–84

30. Kambam JR, Chen LH, Hyman SA. Effect of short-term smoking halt on carboxyhemoglobin levels and P_{50} values. Anesth Analg 1986;65:1186–8

31. Warner MA, Divertie MB, Tinker JH. Preoperative cessation of smoking and pulmonary complications in coronary artery bypass patients. Anesthesiology 1984;60:380–3

32. Clayton JK, Anderson JA, McNicol GP. Effect of cigarette smoking on subsequent postoperative thromboembolic disease in gynaecological patients. Br Med J 1978;2:402–3

33. Bucknall TE, Bowker T, Leaper DJ. Does increased movement protect smokers from postoperative deep vein thrombosis? Br Med J 1980;1:447–8

34. Ravin MB. Comparison of spinal and general anesthesia for lower abdominal surgery in patients with chronic obstructive pulmonary disease. Anesthesiology 1971;35:319–22

35. Gold MI, Joseph SI. Bilateral tension pneumothorax following induction of anesthesia in two patients with chronic obstructive airway disease. Anesthesiology 1973;38:93–6

36. Gross JB, Zebrowski ME, Carel WD, et al. Time course of ventilatory depression after thiopental and midazolam in normal subjects and in patients with chronic obstructive pulmonary disease. Anesthesiology 1983;58:540–4

37. Tusiewicz K, Bryan AC, Froese AB. Contributions of changing rib cage-diaphragm interactions to the ventilatory depression of halothane anesthesia. Anesthesiology 1977;47:327–37

38. Rehder K, Marsh HM, Rodarte JR, Hyatt RE. Airway closure. Anesthesiology 1977;47:40–52

39. Craig DB. Postoperative recovery of pulmonary function. Anesth Analg 1981;60:46–52

40. Woodring JH, Royer JM, McDonagh D. Kartagener's syndrome. JAMA 1982;247:2814–6

41. Boyan CP, Privitera PA. Resection of stenotic trachea: A case presentation. Anesth Analg 1976;55:191–4

42. Spence AA, Smith G. Postoperative analgesia and lung function: A comparison of morphine with extradural block. Br J Anaesth 1971; 43:144–8

43. Knill RL, Manninen PH, Clement JL. Ventilation and chemoreflexes during enflurane sedation and anesthesia in man. Can Anaesth Soc J 1979;26:353–60

44. Weil JV, McCullough RE, Kline JS, Sodal IE. Diminished ventilatory response to hypoxia and hypercapnia after morphine in normal man. N Engl J Med 1975;292:1103–6

45. Sullivan SF, Patterson RW. Posthyperventilation hypoxia: Theoretical considerations in man. Anesthesiology 1968;29:981–6

46. Ali J, Kahn TA. The comparative effects of muscle transection and median upper abdominal incisions on postoperative pulmonary function. Surg Gynecol Obstet 1979;148:863–6.

47. Williams CD, Brenowitz JB. Ventilatory patterns after vertical and transverse upper abdominal incisions. Am J Surg 1975;130:725–8

48. Bartlett RH, Gazzaniga AB, Geraghty TR. Respiratory maneuvers to prevent postoperative pulmonary complications. JAMA 1973;224:1017–21

49. Ali J. The effects of intermittent positive pressure breathing (IPPB) on postoperative pulmonary function (abstract). Ann R Coll Phys Surg (Can) 1979;12:36

50. McConnell DH, Maloney JV, Buckberg GD. Postoperative intermittent positive-pressure breathing treatments. J Thorac Cardiovasc Surg 1974;68:944–52

51. White PF. Postoperative pain management with patient controlled analgesia. Semin Anes 1986;4:116–22

52. Toledo-Pereyra LH, DeMeester TR. Prospective randomized evaluation of intrathoracic nerve block with bupivacaine on postoperative ventilatory function. Ann Thorac Surg 1979;27:203–5

53. Brodsky JB, James MBD. Hypotension from intraoperative intercostal nerve blocks. Regional Anes 1979;4:17–8.

54. Benumof JL, Semenza J. Total spinal anesthesia following intrathoracic intercostal nerve blocks. Anesthesiology 1975;43:124–5

55. Modig J. Lumbar epidural nerve blockade versus parenteral analgesics. Acta Anaesthesiol Scand (Suppl) 1978;70:30–5

56. Bromage PR, Camporesi E, Chestnut D. Epidural narcotics for postoperative analgesia. Anesth Analg 1980;59:473–80

57. Ali J, Yaffe C, Serrette C. The effect of transcutaneous electric nerve stimulation on postoperative pain and pulmonary function. Surgery 1981;89:507–12

15

Restrictive Pulmonary Disease

Restrictive pulmonary disease is most often due to processes that reduce the inherent elasticity of the lungs. Despite many different etiologies, it is useful to classify pulmonary dysfunction due to decreased elasticity of the lungs as acute and chronic intrinsic restrictive pulmonary disease. On occasion, the lungs are normal, and restrictive pulmonary disease is due to abnormalities of the thoracic cage, pleura, or abdominal contents. The nonpulmonary causes are categorized as chronic extrinsic restrictive pulmonary disease.

Intrinsic and extrinsic restrictive pulmonary disease is characterized by reductions in lung compliance. Loss of inherent elastic properties and development of pulmonary fibrosis is responsible for decreased lung compliance characteristic of intrinsic disease. Furthermore, intrinsic disease can result in obliteration of pulmonary vasculature, leading to pulmonary hypertension and cor pulmonale. Lung compliance may also be decreased by extrapulmonary changes. Regardless of the mechanism for decreased compliance, the net effect is reduction in total lung volume (Fig. 15-1). Indeed, reductions in vital capacity (normal 70 ml·kg^{-1}) are the classic evidence of restrictive pulmonary disease. In contrast to obstructive airways disease, expiratory flow rates are normal in these patients.

Patients with restrictive pulmonary disease complain of dyspnea, reflecting the increased work of breathing necessary to expand the poorly compliant lungs. A rapid and shallow pattern of breathing is characteristic, since this minimizes the work of breathing in the presence of decreased lung compliance. A reduction in the arterial partial pressures of carbon dioxide reflects hyperventilation produced by the rapid and shallow pattern of breathing. Indeed, the arterial partial pressures of carbon dioxide are usually maintained at decreased to normal values until restrictive pulmonary disease is far advanced.

ACUTE INTRINSIC RESTRICTIVE PULMONARY DISEASE

Acute intrinsic restrictive pulmonary disease is most often due to leakage of intravascular fluid into the interstitium of the lungs and into alveoli, manifesting as pulmonary edema. Loss of intravascular fluid into the lungs can reflect damage to pulmonary capillary endothelium or increased pulmonary vascular pressures due to left ventricular dysfunction. Examples of acute disease include adult respiratory distress syndrome, aspiration pneumonitis, neurogenic pulmonary edema, opioid-induced pulmonary edema, and high-altitude pulmonary edema.

227

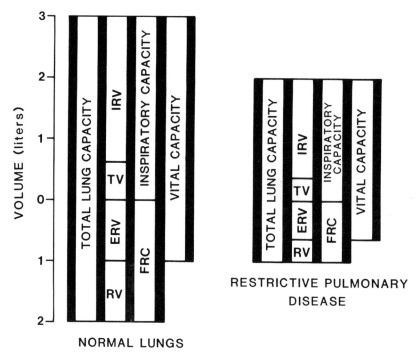

FIG. 15-1. Schematic depiction of total lung capacity and the components that comprise this capacity in adult patients with normal lungs and individuals with restrictive pulmonary disease. Restrictive pulmonary disease is characterized by decreases in total lung capacity and all the components that comprise this capacity. Clinically, the most detectable changes are reductions in the tidal volume and vital capacity. IRV = inspiratory reserve volume, TV = tidal volume, ERV = expiratory reserve volume; RV = residual volume, FRC = functional residual capacity.

Adult Respiratory Distress Syndrome

Adult respiratory distress syndrome is characterized by abnormal permeability of pulmonary capillary endothelium, leading to leakage of fluid containing high concentrations of protein into the pulmonary parenchyma and alveoli.[1,2] There are associated decreases in functional residual capacity and lung compliance and increased perfusion of unventilated alveoli, resulting in venous admixture and severe arterial hypoxemia.

ETIOLOGY

Adult respiratory distress syndrome is most often associated with hemorrhage or septic shock. Complement activation that predis-

poses to leukocyte aggregation in the lungs may accompany trauma and sepsis. Likewise, proteinases and lipases released during acute pancreatitis can damage the pulmonary capillary endothelium. Oxygen can injure the alveolar and pulmonary epithelium, emphasizing the need to administer the lowest inspired oxygen concentrations compatible with acceptable arterial oxygenation. Phosgene and oxides of nitrogen in the inhaled smoke from fires may injure the lung structure. Disseminated intravascular coagulation damages pulmonary capillaries, as well as the endothelium of other vascular beds. Pulmonary contusion frequently manifests as adult respiratory distress syndrome. Even when trauma involves only one hemithorax, both lungs may be affected, suggesting that mechanical forces are transmitted bilaterally. Patients who seem to make an uneventful recovery from near drowning may subsequently develop diffuse pulmonary edema with all the features of adult respiratory distress syndrome.[3] This edema appears to be the result of direct osmotic damage to the lungs by hyperosmotic or hypo-osmotic fluid. Finally, chemotherapeutic drugs, particularly bleomycin and busulfan, have been associated with dose-related pulmonary fibrosis and the development of an adult respiratory distress syndrome (see Chapter 30).

MANIFESTATIONS

Classically, patients who are developing adult respiratory distress syndrome manifest progressive tachypnea, and radiographs of the chest show bilateral and diffuse pulmonary infiltrates. This picture on radiographs, which resembles that of pulmonary edema, can progress to complete opacification. Clinically, this pulmonary edema is not associated with evidence of left ventricular dysfunction. Compliance of the lungs becomes progressively reduced, reflecting transudation of intravascular fluid into the lungs. As a result, increased positive airway pressures are necessary to generate given tidal volumes. Pulmonary hypertension may be due in part to obliteration of capillaries by fibrotic changes.

Atelectasis is a prominent feature of adult respiratory distress syndrome. Arterial hypoxemia occurs early in the course of this disease and is often associated with decreases in the arterial partial pressures of carbon dioxide. Thrombocytopenia may be prominent. Superinfections with bacterial and fungal pathogens often ensue. Multiple organ failure may develop.

TREATMENT

Inspired concentrations of oxygen must be progressively increased to maintain acceptable arterial oxygenation (see Chapter 16). One recommendation is to institute mechanical ventilation of the lungs via a tube placed in the trachea whenever greater than 50 percent oxygen is required to maintain acceptable oxygenation. An ominous sign is an increasing arterial partial pressure of carbon dioxide, as this change is associated with patient exhaustion. Likewise, arterial pH is usually normal or even elevated early in the course of this process, only to fall precipitously as terminal stages are reached. In extreme cases, even 100 percent oxygen plus positive end-expiratory pressure is not sufficient to prevent arterial hypoxemia.

Extracorporeal membrane oxygenation has been instituted in desperate situations, in attempts to provide time for the lungs to recover from insults that initiated respiratory failure. The need for systemic heparinization during extracorporeal membrane oxygenation has led to a high incidence of complications. Overall, this therapy has not been shown to increase survival.[4]

Currently, the speculated involvement of the complement cascade, neutrophil aggregation, and lung prostaglandins in pulmonary capillary membrane damage and pulmonary fibrosis provide a basis for new pharmacologic approaches in the treatment of adult respiratory distress syndrome. For example, corticosteroids by inhibiting complement-induced granulocyte aggregation could theoretically be useful in these patients. Indeed, specific therapy to prevent or reverse pathophysiologic sequences that destroy pulmonary architecture rather than further refinements in management of ventilation (positive end-expiratory pressure, high frequency ventilation, extracorporeal membrane oxygenation) will probably be necessary to dramatically improve outcome in patients with adult respiratory distress syndrome.[1,2]

Aspiration Pneumonitis

Aspiration pneumonitis is traditionally thought to be most likely to occur following inhalation of gastric fluid with a pH below 2.5 in a volume that exceeds 0.4 ml·kg^{-1}.[5] This acidic fluid is rapidly distributed into the alveoli, leading to destruction of surfactant-producing cells and damage to the pulmonary capillary endothelium. As a result, atelectasis occurs, and intravascular fluid leaks into the lungs. The clinical picture elicited by inhalation of acidic gastric fluid is similar to the adult respiratory distress syndrome.

MANIFESTATIONS

Arterial hypoxemia is the most consistent manifestation of aspiration pneumonitis. In addition, there may be tachypnea, bronchospasm, and pulmonary vascular vasoconstriction, with associated pulmonary hypertension. Radiographs of the chest may not reveal evidence of aspiration pneumonitis for 6 hours to 12 hours after inhalation of gastric fluid.[6] Such evidence is most often seen in the right lower lobe.

TREATMENT

Assuming a tracheal tube is placed immediately after inhalation of gastric fluid, it is reasonable to inject small volumes of saline (5 ml) into the lungs and aspirate through the tracheal tube. It must be appreciated, however, that gastric fluid is rapidly distributed to peripheral parts of the lungs and that lavage with large volumes of fluid could exaggerate this spread. The pH of gastric fluid should be measured as it reflects the pH of aspirated fluid. Measurement of tracheal aspirate is of doubtful value since inhaled gastric fluid is likely to be rapidly diluted by airway secretions.

The most effective treatment of aspiration pneumonitis is oxygen supplementation of the inhaled gases plus ventilation of the lungs, using positive end-expiratory pressure (see the section Treatment of Respiratory Failure in Ch. 16). Intravenous administration of aminophylline or inhalation of a nebulized mist containing beta-2 adrenergic agonist drugs may be effective in relieving bronchospasm. Although acid-injured lungs may be susceptible to bacterial infections, there is no evidence that antibiotics administered prophylactically decrease the incidence of these infections or alter outcome after aspiration of gastric fluid. Use of corticosteroids for treatment of aspiration pneumonitis is controversial. There is animal evidence that corticosteroids administered immediately after inhalation of acid gastric fluid may be effective in reducing pulmonary damage.[7] Conversely, other data show no beneficial

effects[8,9] or suggest that their use may enhance the development of gram-negative pneumonia.[10] Despite the absence of confirmatory evidence that corticosteroids are beneficial, it is not uncommon for the treatment of aspiration pneumonitis to include the empiric use of pharmacologic doses of methylprednisolone (30 mg·kg^{-1}) or dexamethasone (1 mg·kg^{-1}). Hypoalbuminemia, resulting from extravasation of protein-containing fluids into the lungs, is logically treated with albumin solutions. This approach, however, must be tempered by the possibility that these solutions will also leak across damaged pulmonary capillary endothelium and draw additional intravascular fluid into the lungs (see Chapter 16).

Neurogenic Pulmonary Edema

Neurogenic pulmonary edema begins with a massive outpouring of sympathetic nervous system impulses from the injured central nervous system.[11] This centrally mediated sympathetic nervous system overactivity typically occurs when brain injury is in the area of the hypothalamus. Excessive sympathetic nervous system activity results in intense and generalized peripheral vasoconstriction, leading to shifts of blood volume into the pulmonary circulation. Presumably, increased pulmonary capillary pressures lead to transudation of fluid into the interstitium of the lungs. In addition, pulmonary hypertension and hypervolemia can injure blood vessels of the lung. As a result of this injury, altered pulmonary capillary permeability can persist after normalization of systemic and pulmonary vascular pressures. Digitalis is not indicated in treatment of neurogenic pulmonary edema, since cardiac function is normal, as emphasized by normal pulmonary artery occlusion pressures.

Opioid-Induced Pulmonary Edema

Opioid overdoses, particularly with heroin, can lead to fulminant pulmonary edema.[12] Altered pulmonary capillary permeability is suggested by the protein-rich nature of pulmonary edema fluid. As in patients with neurogenic pulmonary edema, the function of the left ventricle is not impaired, as reflected by normal pulmonary artery occlusion pressures.

High Altitude Pulmonary Edema

Pulmonary edema in the absence of left ventricular failure may occur when individuals overexert before acclimating to high altitudes.[13] Pathogenesis of this pulmonary edema is unknown but may be due to intense hypoxic pulmonary artery vasoconstriction or massive sympathetic nervous system discharge triggered by cerebral hypoxia. Treatment of high altitude pulmonary edema is with oxygen and return to lower altitudes.

CHRONIC INTRINSIC RESTRICTIVE PULMONARY DISEASE

Chronic intrinsic restrictive pulmonary disease is characterized by the presence of pulmonary fibrosis. Anatomic loss of the pulmonary vascular bed due to progression of pulmonary fibrosis can lead to pulmonary hypertension and the development of cor pulmonale. Pneumothorax is common when pulmonary fibrosis is far advanced. Examples of this disease include hypersensitivity pneumonitis, sarcoidosis, eosinophilic granuloma, and alveolar proteinosis.

Hypersensitivity Pneumonitis

Hypersensitivity pneumonitis is characterized by diffuse interstitial granulomatous reactions in the lungs after inhalation of dust that contains fungus, spores, or animal or vegetable

material.[14] Signs and symptoms of hypersensitivity pneumonitis include the onset of dyspnea and cough 4 hours to 6 hours after inhalation of the antigens, followed by leukocytosis and eosinophilia. Arterial hypoxemia can occur despite hyperventilation. Radiographs of the chest show multiple pulmonary infiltrates.

Repeated episodes of hypersensitivity pneumonitis lead to extensive pulmonary fibrosis. Other causes of pulmonary fibrosis include radiation, as administered for treatment of tumors of the chest or mediastinum. In addition, inhalation of substances such as asbestos, diatomaceous earth, and silicone dioxide are retained in the lungs, resulting in scarring and fibrosis.

Sarcoidosis

Sarcoidosis has a predilection for the lungs, leading to extensive pulmonary fibrosis with resulting pulmonary hypertension and cor pulmonale. Diffusion capacity for carbon monoxide across alveolar capillary membranes may be reduced, despite the presence of normal arterial blood gases. Laryngeal sarcoid occurs in 1 percent to 5 percent of patients and may interfere with passage of an adult-sized tracheal tube.[15] The significance of increased activity of angiotensin-converting enzymes present in the pulmonary capillary endothelium of these patients is not known. These enzymes are responsible for inactivating bradykinin and converting angiotensin I to active angiotensin II. Corticosteroids are frequently used to treat sarcoidosis associated with restrictive pulmonary disease.

Eosinophilic Granuloma (Histiocytosis X)

Pulmonary fibrosis accompanies the disease process known as eosinophilic granuloma. Corticosteroids are beneficial if extensive pulmonary fibrotic changes have not already occurred.

Alveolar Proteinosis

Alveolar proteinosis is characterized by filling of alveoli with destroyed type II alveolar cells.[16] This process can occur independently or secondary to administration of chemotherapeutic substances classified as alkylating drugs. Pneumocystis carinii infection is another cause of alveolar proteinosis. Dyspnea and severe arterial hypoxemia are typical clinical manifestations of this disease.

CHRONIC EXTRINSIC RESTRICTIVE PULMONARY DISEASE

Restrictive pulmonary disease in the absence of any abnormalities of the elastic properties of the lungs most often reflects extrinsic disorders that interfere with the expansion of the lungs. Examples of such processes include disorders of the pleura (fibrosis, effusion), thoracic cage (kyphoscoliosis, pectus excavatum), and diaphragm (obesity, ascites, pregnancy). The lungs become compressed and lung volumes are reduced. The work of breathing is increased due to the abnormal mechanical properties of the chest and increased airway resistance due to reduced lung volumes. The thoracic deformity also compresses pulmonary vessels, which increases pulmonary vascular resistance and eventually leads to right ventricular dysfunction. Recurrent pulmonary infections resulting from poor cough dynamics may lead to the development of obstructive components to the pulmonary disease.

PREOPERATIVE PREPARATION

Preoperative preparation of patients with restrictive pulmonary disease includes an assessment of the severity of the disease and treatment of reversible components. A preoperative history of dyspnea that limits activity and can be attributed to restrictive pulmonary disease is an indication for the performance of pulmonary function studies and measurement of arterial blood gases. Reduction of the vital capacity from normal values of about 70 mg·kg^{-1} to below 15 ml·kg^{-1}, or the demonstration of resting elevated arterial partial pressures of carbon dioxide, suggests that these patients are at high risk for developing exaggerated pulmonary dysfunction in the postoperative period. It should be remembered that lack of patient effort, presence of pain, advanced age (vital capacity decreases 3 ml·kg^{-1} to 4 ml·kg^{-1} every 10 years after about 30 years of age), or the presence of obstructive airways disease can also contribute to measurements of reduced vital capacities. Preoperative preparation also includes eradication of acute pulmonary infections, improvement of sputum clearance, treatment of cardiac dysfunction, exercises to improve respiratory muscle strength, and training with respiratory therapy techniques that will be used postoperatively.

MANAGEMENT OF ANESTHESIA

Restrictive pulmonary disease does not influence the choice of drugs used for induction or maintenance of general anesthesia. The need to minimize depression of ventilation that may persist into the postoperative period should be considered when selecting these drugs. Regional anesthesia can be considered for peripheral operations, but it must be appreciated that sensory levels above T-10 can be associated with impairment of respiratory muscle activity necessary for patients with restrictive lung disease to maintain acceptable ventilation. Controlled ventilation of the lungs during the intraoperative period seems prudent, so as to optimize oxygenation and ventilation. High inflation pressures delivered from the ventilator may be necessary to inflate poorly compliant lungs and/or thorax. Mechanical ventilation of the lungs in the postoperative period is often required for those patients with impairment of pulmonary function documented preoperatively. Certainly tracheal tubes should not be removed until patients have met established criteria for extubation (see Chapter 16). It should be appreciated that restrictive pulmonary disease contributes to decreased lung volume, making it difficult to generate an effective cough for removal of secretions from the airway in the postoperative period.

REFERENCES

1. Rinaldo JE, Rogers RM. Adult respiratory-distress syndrome. Changing concepts of lung injury and repair. N Engl J Med 1982;306:900–9
2. Bone RC, Jacobs ER. Advances in pharmacologic treatment of acute lung injury and septic shock. In: Stoelting RK, Barash PG, Gallagher TJ, eds. Advances in Anesthesia. Chicago. Year Book Medical Publishers 1986;4:327–45
3. Orlowski JP. Prognostic factors in drowning and the postsubmersion syndrome. Crit Care Med 1978;6:94
4. Zapol WM, Snider MT, Hill JD, et al. Extracorporeal membrane oxygenation in severe acute respiratory failure. A randomized prospective study. JAMA 1979;242:2193–2201
5. Roberts RB, Shirley MA. Reducing the risk of acid aspiration during cesarean section. Anesth Analg 1974;53:859–68
6. Browne CH, Chew HER, Clarke E, et al. The management of pulmonary aspiration syndrome. Intensive Care Med 1977;3:257–66
7. Dudley WR, Marshall BE. Steroid treatment for acid-aspiration pneumonia. Anesthesiology 1974;40:136–41
8. Downs JB, Chapman RL, Modell JH, Hood CI. An evaluation of steroid therapy in aspiration pneumonitis. Anesthesiology 1974;40:129–35
9. Wynne JW, DeMarco FJ, Hood CI. Physiological effects of corticosteroids in food-stuff aspiration. Arch Surg 1981;116:46–9
10. Wolfe JE, Bone RC, Ruth WE. Effects of corticosteroids in the treatment of patients with gastric aspiration. Am J Med 1977;63:719–22
11. Robin ED, Theodore J. Speculations on neurogenic pulmonary edema (NPE) (editorial). Am Rev Respir Dis 1976;113:405–11
12. Katz S, Aberman A, Frand UI, et al. Heroin pulmonary edema: Evidence for increased pulmonary capillary permeability. Am Rev Respir Dis 1972;106:472–4
13. Straub NC. Pulmonary edema. Physiol Rev 1974;54:678–811
14. Pepys J, Simon G. Asthma, pulmonary eosinophilia, and allergic alveolitis. Med Clin North Am 1973;57:573–91
15. Wills MH, Harris MM. An unusual airway complication with sarcoidosis. Anesthesiology 1987;66:554–5
16. Phillips J, Simon L, Robin ED, et al. Pulmonary alveolar proteinosis: Respiratory medicine rounds of Stanford University Hospital. West J Med 1976;124:29–35

16

Recognition and Management of Respiratory Failure

Respiratory failure is not a single disease entity but instead a combination of pathophysiologic derangements that can arise from a variety of etiologic insults (Table 16-1). Development of respiratory failure can be acute, chronic, or acute superimposed on a chronic disease process. A knowledge of the causes of respiratory failure, as well as the associated pathophysiology, is essential for establishing logical therapy of this disease.[1,2]

DIAGNOSIS

Respiratory failure is invariably associated with arterial hypoxemia due to the mismatch of ventilation to perfusion. Functional residual capacity and lung compliance are decreased, and ventilation of unperfused alveoli is increased. There is often bilateral diffuse opacification of the lungs on radiographs of the chest. Pulmonary artery occlusion pressures are usually less than 15 mmHg, despite the frequent presence of pulmonary edema. Increased pulmonary vascular resistance and pulmonary hypertension are likely to develop when respiratory failure persists.

A guideline for establishing the diagnosis of acute respiratory failure is the presence of arterial partial pressures of oxygen below 50 mmHg, despite supplemental oxygen. This guideline assumes the absence of right-to-left intracardiac shunts. Arterial partial pressures of carbon dioxide in the presence of respiratory failure can be elevated, normal, or decreased, depending on the relationship of alveolar ventilation to the metabolic production of carbon dioxide. Arterial partial pressures of carbon dioxide that exceed 50 mmHg, in the absence of respiratory compensation for metabolic alkalosis, are consistent with the diagnosis of acute respiratory failure.

Acute is distinguished from chronic respiratory failure on the basis of the relationship of the arterial carbon dioxide partial pressures to the pH. For example, acute failure is often associated with abrupt increases in the arterial partial pressures of carbon dioxide and corresponding decreases in the pH. Conversely, in the presence of chronic respiratory failure, the arterial pH is usually between 7.36 and 7.44, despite elevated partial pressures of carbon dioxide. This normal pH reflects compensation by virtue of renal tubular reabsorption of bicarbonate.

It should be apparent that serial measurements of arterial blood gases and pH are necessary to (1) establish the diagnosis of respiratory failure, (2) determine the need for mechanical support of ventilation, (3) assess

235

TABLE 16-1. Etiology of Respiratory
Failure

Primary Pulmonary Dysfunction
  Obstructive pulmonary disease
  Restrictive pulmonary disease
  Pneumonia
  Adult respiratory distress syndrome
  Inhaled toxins-gastric fluid, smoke, phosgene
  Oxygen toxicity
  Fat embolism
  Pulmonary contusion
  Loss of chest wall stability

Cardiovascular Dysfunction
  Hemorrhagic shock
  Sepsis
  Left ventricular cardiac failure
  Fluid overload
  Microembolization
  Massive blood transfusion
  Disseminated intravascular coagulation
  Postcardiopulmonary bypass

Central Nervous System Dysfunction
  Increased intracranial pressure
  Depressant drug overdose
  Central alveolar hypoventilation

Neuromuscular Dysfunction
  Myasthenia gravis
  Spinal cord transection
  Guillain-Barré
  Tetanus
  Muscular dystrophy
  Drug-induced neuromuscular blockade-
    muscle relaxants, antibiotics

Miscellaneous
  Pancreatitis
  Uremia
  Morbid obesity

the effects of therapy, and (4) confirm when patients no longer need mechanical support of ventilation. Respiratory failure can be categorized as arterial hypoxemia plus (1) normocarbia and normal lungs, (2) hypercarbia and normal lungs, and (3) hypercarbia and abnormal lungs.

Normocarbia and Normal Lungs

Respiratory failure characterized by arterial hypoxemia and normal or even decreased arterial partial pressures of carbon dioxide is frequently designated as adult respiratory distress syndrome (see Chapter 15). This form of respiratory failure can occur in the presence or absence of co-existing pulmonary disease. Transudation of intravascular fluid into interstitial spaces of the lungs or alveoli reflects diffuse damage to alveolar capillary membranes characteristic of the adult respiratory distress syndrome. The cause of this damage is unknown; proposed mechanisms include liberation of vasoactive substances, activation of complement pathways, release of prostaglandins, and production of endotoxins.

Hypercarbia and Normal Lungs

Respiratory failure characterized by arterial hypoxemia and hypercarbia, which occurs in patients with previously normal lungs, is due to alveolar hypoventilation secondary to (1) depression of the central nervous system, (2) abnormalities of the neuromuscular junction, or (3) loss of chest integrity. When patients are breathing air, the arterial partial pressures of oxygen are likely to decrease in proportion to the increases in the arterial partial pressures of carbon dioxide. As a guideline, the arterial partial pressures of oxygen will decrease about 1 mmHg for every 1 mmHg increase in the arterial partial pressures of carbon dioxide. Arterial hypoxemia that results from alveolar hypoventilation is readily corrected by increasing the inspired concentrations of oxygen. In contrast to the adult respiratory distress syndrome, this form of respiratory failure is not characterized by an increase in the alveolar-to-arterial difference for oxygen. Mechanical ventilation of the lungs will be necessary to maintain normal arterial partial pressures of carbon dioxide for as long as the causes for alveolar hypoventilation persist.

Hypercarbia and Abnormal Lungs

Respiratory failure characterized by arterial hypoxemia and hypercarbia that occurs in patients with abnormal lungs is most often associated with chronic obstructive airways disease. In these patients, there is a decrease in arterial oxygenation due to a mismatch of ventilation to perfusion. Pulmonary gas exchange can become so inefficient that elimination of carbon dioxide is inadequate despite a normal or even increased minute ventilation.

TREATMENT OF RESPIRATORY FAILURE

Treatment of respiratory failure is directed at supporting pulmonary function until the lungs can recover from the insults that initiated pulmonary dysfunction. Specific therapeutic measures include (1) administration of supplemental oxygen, (2) intubation of the trachea and mechanical support of ventilation of the lungs, (3) positive end-expiratory pressure, (4) maintenance of intravascular fluid volume, (5) facilitation of the removal of secretions from airways, and (6) control of infection.

Administration of Supplemental Oxygen

Administration of supplemental oxygen is used to maintain the arterial partial pressures of oxygen above 60 mmHg. The shape of the oxyhemoglobin dissociation curve is such that saturation of hemoglobin with oxygen, and thus the arterial content of oxygen decreases abruptly when the arterial partial pressures of oxygen decrease below 60 mmHg (see Fig. 25-1). Increasing the arterial partial pressures of oxygen much above 100 mmHg is of little benefit, since saturation of hemoglobin with oxygen is already nearly 100 percent. Ideally, the inspired concentrations of oxygen to achieve acceptable oxygenation should not exceed 50 percent for prolonged periods of time. Administration of more than 50 percent oxygen for greater than 24 hours introduces the risk for developing pulmonary oxygen toxicity. Therefore, use of positive end-expiratory pressure is

often recommended when the arterial partial pressures of oxygen cannot be maintained above 60 mmHg while breathing less than 50 percent oxygen.

Supplemental oxygen can be provided using a nasal cannula, Venturi mask, or nonrebreathing mask. Adequate arterial oxygenation can be achieved in many patients using low flow oxygen (1 L·min^{-1} to 2 L·min^{-1}) delivered through a nasal cannula, or by the use of a Venturi mask, which can supply inspired oxygen concentrations ranging from 24 percent to 40 percent. A Venturi mask uses high flows of oxygen, such that inspired concentrations of oxygen are not influenced by the breathing rate or tidal volume of the patient; with a low flow system, the inspired concentrations of oxygen will vary inversely with the minute ventilation of the patient. A nonrebreathing reservoir mask is capable of delivering inspired concentrations of oxygen that approach 80 percent. Regardless of the methods used, responses to treatment can be determined only by measuring the partial pressures of oxygen in arterial blood.

Intubation of the Trachea and Mechanical Support of Ventilation

Intubation of the trachea and mechanical support of ventilation of the lungs should be considered in the presence of (1) arterial partial pressures of oxygen that remain below 60 mmHg, despite inspired concentrations of oxygen that exceed 50 percent; (2) increasing arterial partial pressures of carbon dioxide associated with reductions in arterial pH; (3) evidence of fatigue of the respiratory muscles; (4) loss of protective upper airway reflexes; and (5) an ineffective cough mechanism. Hypophosphatemia is common in patients with pulmonary infections and may contribute to skeletal muscle weakness and poor contractility of the diaphragm occasionally associated with acute respiratory failure. In experimental models of sepsis, blood flow to the diaphragm increases from a baseline of less than 5 percent of cardiac output to 20 percent or more in spontaneously breathing animals. Mechanical ventilation of the lungs prevents this large capture of blood by muscles of respiration and improves tissue oxygen delivery.[3]

INTUBATION OF THE TRACHEA

Intubation of the trachea can be performed initially by either the oral or nasal route. Tubes placed in the trachea via the nose tend to provide greater stability with fixation and are better tolerated by patients. Oral placement of tracheal tubes permits use of large internal diameter (at least 8 mm) tubes, which facilitates suctioning of secretions from the trachea and passing of a fiberoptic bronchoscope into the trachea.

Tubes selected for placement in the trachea should be equipped with low pressure and large volume cuffs, so as to minimize the likelihood of damage to the underlying tracheal mucosa. These cuffs should be inflated with just enough air to prevent audible leaks of gas during positive pressure ventilation of the lungs. Pressures measured in the cuffs at the volume necessary for a gas-tight seal should not exceed 25 cm H_2O.[4] Although use of highly compliant cuffs has reduced damage produced on the underlying tracheal mucosa, the risk of damage to the vocal cords and larynx from prolonged translaryngeal intubation still remains. Therefore, a tracheotomy is often considered when intubation of the trachea is expected to be required for several days. In addition, a tracheotomy may be preferable to a translaryngeal tube when pulmonary secretions are copious.

MECHANICAL SUPPORT OF VENTILATION

Mechanical support of ventilation of the lungs is most often provided with volume-cycled rather than pressure-cycled ventilators. This preference is based on better maintenance of constant tidal volumes with volume-cycled ventilators during changes in airway resistance and/or lung compliance. Tidal volumes delivered by pressure-cycled ventilators tend to vary inversely with changes in airway resis-

tance and directly with changes in lung compliance. The disadvantage of volume-cycled ventilators is the inability of these devices to compensate for the development of leaks in the delivery system. For example, a leak of gas around the tracheal tube cuff could result in hypoventilation, despite the continued delivery of unchanged inspiratory volumes. Pressure-cycled ventilators continue to deliver constant inspired volumes in the presence of a leak until a preset time is elapsed or a specific airway pressure is achieved.

Initial ventilator settings typically include a breathing rate of 6 breaths·min to 12 breaths·min, tidal volume 10 ml·kg^{-1} to 15 ml·kg^{-1}, and an inspired concentration of oxygen near 50 percent. Use of a slow breathing rate is of greatest benefit in patients with chronic obstructive airways disease who require prolonged periods for exhalation so as to minimize the likelihood of air trapping (see Chapter 14). Large tidal volumes using slow inspiratory flow rates optimize the distribution of ventilation, particularly in the presence of regional differences in airway resistance. Subsequent adjustments in ventilator settings and inspired concentrations of oxygen are based on measurements of arterial blood gases and pH. The goal is to achieve arterial partial pressures of oxygen between 60 mmHg and 100 mmHg, arterial partial pressures of carbon dioxide between 36 mmHg and 44 mmHg, and a pH between 7.36 and 7.44.

High Frequency Positive Pressure Ventilation. High frequency positive pressure ventilation has been introduced as an alternative to the more conventional mode of intermittent positive pressure ventilation.[5,6] Characteristics of high frequency ventilation include (1) ventilatory frequency of 60 breaths·min^{-1} to 100 breaths·min^{-1}, (2) inspiratory-to-expiratory ratio less than 0.3, (3) small tidal volumes that result in low mean positive airway pressures during inspiration, and (4) provision of continuous positive intratracheal and subatmospheric intrapleural pressures throughout the ventilatory cycle. A major advantage ascribed to this form of ventilation is failure of airway resistance and lung compliance to influence the efficacy of ventilation. In addition, maintenance of low mean airway pressures results in minimal effects on cardiac output, and the likelihood of pulmonary barotrauma is reduced. Furthermore, it has been observed that high frequency positive pressure ventilation produces reflex suppression of spontaneous ventilation, allowing mechanical support without the need for sedatives, muscle relaxants, or mechanical hyperventilation of the lungs. Disadvantages of high frequency ventilation include increased expense and complexity of the required equipment.

The mechanism of gas exchange produced by high frequency positive pressure ventilation remains unclear. Nevertheless, such ventilation has been shown to be effective in patients undergoing treatment for acute respiratory failure, laryngoscopy, bronchoscopy, and repair of bronchopleural fistula.[7,8] Not all reports, however, demonstrate decisive advantages of high frequency positive pressure ventilation over more traditional approaches in the management of acute respiratory failure or bronchopleural fistula.[9,10] Maintenance of low mean airway pressures makes high frequency ventilation a consideration for management of patients with increased intracranial pressure who require mechanical support of breathing. Furthermore, patients with circulatory shock and acute respiratory failure maintain higher mean arterial pressures, cardiac output and oxygen delivery during high frequency ventilation than during continuous positive pressure ventilation.[11]

High frequency oscillation is similar to high frequency positive pressure ventilation, except the respiratory frequency is in the range of 15 Hz or 900 oscillations·min^{-1}. The method of ventilation has also been shown to achieve acceptable gas exchange with minimal adverse effects on circulation.[6] In addition, the incidence of pulmonary barotrauma should be low.

Positive End-Expiratory Pressure

Positive end-expiratory pressure is the maintenance of positive airway and intrathoracic pressure during the entire ventilator cycle, with superimposed intermittent inflation of the lungs by cyclic increases in positive pressure. Addition of positive end-expiratory pressure to the ventilator cycle is often recommended if the arterial partial pressures of oxygen cannot be maintained above 60 mmHg, while patients are breathing 50 percent oxygen[1,2] Short-term administration of greater than 50 percent oxygen to maintain adequate arterial oxygenation is acceptable, but it must be recognized that pulmonary oxygen toxicity is a hazard when oxygen concentrations greater than 50 percent are administered for more than 24 hours.[3] It is presumed that positive end-expiratory pressure increases arterial oxygenation, lung compliance, and the functional residual capacity, by expanding previously collapsed but perfused alveoli.[11] As a result, the match of ventilation to perfusion is improved, and the magnitude of right-to-left intrapulmonary shunting of blood is reduced. It should be recognized that positive end-expiratory pressure is unlikely to improve arterial oxygenation when arterial hypoxemia is due to hypoventilation or is associated with a normal or even increased functional residual capacity.

Positive end-expiratory pressure is useful in preventing absorption atelectasis, which is most likely to occur in alveoli that are poorly ventilated but contain gases highly soluble in blood. Examples of gases that predispose to absorption atelectasis are nitrous oxide and oxygen. Conversely, nitrogen is poorly soluble in blood. As a result, nitrogen is more likely than nitrous oxide or oxygen to remain in alveoli and thus reduce the likelihood of atelectasis should ventilation to that area of the lungs be reduced. Nevertheless, the value of using nitrogen to minimize absorption atelectasis remains unproven.

Initially, positive end-expiratory pressure is added in 2.5 cmH$_2$O to 5 cmH$_2$O increments, until the arterial partial pressures of oxygen are greater than 60 mmHg, while patients are breathing less than 50 percent oxygen. The goal is to deliver the amount of positive end-expiratory pressure that maximally improves arterial oxygenation without substantially reducing cardiac output or increasing the risk of pulmonary barotrauma. Optimal levels of positive end-expiratory pressure, as reflected by maximal oxygen transport (arterial oxygen content times cardiac output), are also often associated with the best improvement in static lung compliance (Fig. 16-1).[12] The level of positive end-expiratory pressure that produces maximal oxygen transport without overdistention of alveoli, as reflected by the static lung compliance, has been characterized as "best PEEP".[12] The majority of patients manifest maximal improvement in arterial oxygen transport and lung compliance with levels of positive end-expiratory pressure below 15 cmH₂O.

An important adverse effect of positive end-expiratory pressure is a reduction in the cardiac output, due to interference with venous return and a leftward displacement of the ventricular septum, which restricts filling of the left ventricle.[13] It is conceivable that improvements in arterial oxygenation produced by positive end-expiratory pressure could be offset by reductions in tissue blood flow due to decreases in cardiac output. The potential for positive end-expiratory pressure to reduce

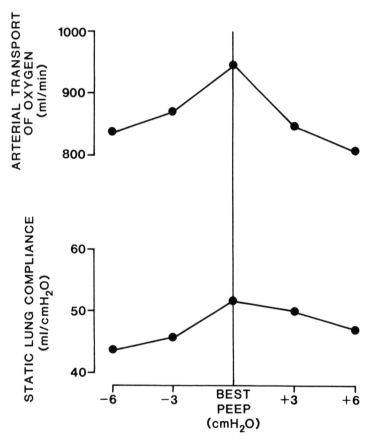

FIG. 16-1. Arterial transport of oxygen (arterial oxygen content times cardiac output) and static lung compliance were measured in 15 patients with acute respiratory failure being treated with continuous mechanical ventilation of the lungs and varying levels of positive end-expiratory pressure. The amount of positive end-expiratory pressure in each patient that resulted in the largest arterial oxygen transport was also associated with the greatest static lung compliance. This amount of positive end-expiratory pressure was defined as "best PEEP." Positive end-expiratory pressure that was 3 cmH₂O or 6 cmH₂O above or below "best PEEP" resulted in lower values for arterial oxygen transport, and the static lung compliance was less. (Data adapted from Suter PM, Fairley HB, Isenberg MD. Optimum end-expiratory airway pressure in patients with acute pulmonary failure. N Engl J Med 1975;292:284–9)

cardiac output is exaggerated in the presence of decreased intravascular fluid volume and/or normal lungs, which permit maximal transmission of increased airway pressures.[14] Replacement of intravascular fluid volume and administration of drugs to increase myocardial contractility can be used to minimize adverse effects of positive end-expiratory pressure on cardiac output. Pulmonary artery catheters are useful for monitoring adequacy of tissue blood flow, as reflected by cardiac output and mixed venous partial pressures of oxygen, particularly when high levels of positive end-expiratory pressure (greater than 15 cmH$_2$O) are used. It must be appreciated that levels of positive end-expiratory pressure that exceed 10 cmH$_2$O can interfere with interpretation of pulmonary artery occlusion pressures as reflections of left atrial pressures. This reflects transmission of intra-alveolar pressures to pulmonary capillaries, which is then measured as pulmonary artery occlusion pressure. Likewise, transmission of positive end-expiratory pressure to pulmonary capillaries will increase resistance to blood flow through the lungs. The resulting increases in pulmonary vascular resistance are associated with elevated pulmonary artery pressures and right ventricular filling pressures.

Another hazard of positive end-expiratory pressure is pulmonary barotrauma. Barotrauma is presumed to reflect overdistention and rupture of alveoli due to excessive levels of positive end-expiratory pressure. Overdistention of alveoli may be reflected by decreased lung compliance. Pneumothorax, pneumomediastinum, and subcutaneous emphysema are examples of pulmonary barotrauma that can be produced by excessive positive end-expiratory pressure. Abrupt deterioration of arterial oxygenation and cardiovascular function during positive end-expiratory pressure should arouse suspicion of a pneumothorax.

Maintenance of Intravascular Fluid Volume

Maintenance of intravascular fluid volume, as well as optimal water content of the lungs, is crucial for management of patients with respiratory failure. For example, excessive accumulation of fluid in the lungs is characteristic of many forms of respiratory failure, particularly the entity designated as adult respiratory distress syndrome. Conversely, respiratory failure associated with chronic obstructive airways disease and chronic restrictive pulmonary disease is not classically accompanied by increased total lung water. Regardless of the etiology of respiratory failure, mechanical ventilation of the lungs, especially in combination with positive end-expiratory pressure, can be associated with fluid retention.[15]

Central venous pressure is not a reliable guide for monitoring intravascular fluid volume in patients with respiratory failure. A more reliable monitor is measurement of the pulmonary artery occlusion pressure; the normal level being 12 mmHg to 15 mmHg. Values above or below this range can reflect excessive or inadequate intravascular fluid volume respectively. It must be remembered that pulmonary artery occlusion pressures can be falsely elevated by positive end-expiratory pressure.

Additional monitors of intravascular fluid volume include measurement of urine output and body weight. Urine outputs of 0.5 ml·kg^{-1}·hr^{-1} to 1 ml·kg^{-1}·hr^{-1} are consistent with an adequate cardiac output and intravascular fluid volume. Normally, daily weight loss of 0.2 kg to 0.4 kg is anticipated in adult patients receiving conventional intravenous fluid therapy. A stable or increasing body weight implies excessive fluid retention.

Adverse alterations in intravascular fluid volume and water content of the lungs are treated with drug-induced diuresis and/or attempts to maximize pulmonary lymph flow.

DRUG-INDUCED DIURESIS

Drug-induced diuresis, using furosemide, is particularly effective in reducing excessive accumulations of fluids in the lungs. Evidence of beneficial effects from diuresis is improvement in arterial oxygenation and resolution of pulmonary infiltrates on radiographs of the chest. Diuresis requires careful titration to avoid excessive reductions in the intravascular fluid volume, which could lead to decreases in cardiac output and development of tissue ischemia.

PULMONARY LYMPH FLOW

The principle factors that favor movement of fluid from the pulmonary vasculature into the interstitium of the lungs are increases in pulmonary vascular pressures and decreases in plasma oncotic pressures. Under normal circumstances, this interstitial fluid is removed via the lung lymphatics. As long as this interstitial fluid is continuously removed, the diffusion distance for respiratory gases remains small and adequate gas exchange is maintained. When the volume of fluid entering the pulmonary interstitium exceeds the volume flow capacity of the lung lymphatics, pulmonary edema ensues and gas exchange deteriorates. Pulmonary lymph flow may be impeded by increases in systemic venous pressures as produced by volume infusions and positive pressure ventilation of the lungs. At the same time, infusion of crystalloid solutions, which reduce plasma oncotic pressures and increase pulmonary arterial pressures, or sepsis associated with production of endotoxin, which damages the pulmonary capillary endothelium, results in greater interstitial movement of fluid. The lungs attempt to maximize pulmonary lymph flow to remove excess edema fluid, but the large infused volume of crystalloid solutions needed to maintain cardiac function may have so elevated systemic venous pressures that pulmonary lymph flow is drastically reduced. In this situation, use of colloid solutions, such as heat-treated plasma protein fractions, might be more effective, since a small total volume could be given, thus avoiding a dilution effect on plasma oncotic pressures while at the same time minimizing increases in systemic venous pressures and pulmonary arterial pressures so as to maximize the efficiency of pulmonary lymph flow.[16] Successful application of these principles requires careful monitoring of systemic venous pressures, pulmonary arterial pressures, and plasma oncotic pressures. Drugs administered to improve cardiac contractility and/or to reduce pulmonary vascular resistance may further reduce fluid movement to the interstitium of the lungs and also improve pulmonary lymph flow.

Facilitation of the Removal of Secretions from the Airways

Optimal removal of secretions from the airways is facilitated by adequate systemic hydration of patients and humidification of inspired gases. In addition, chest physiotherapy is important to enhance the postural drainage of secretions and to stimulate effective coughing. Tracheal suction with a sterile catheter is also useful in stimulating active expiratory efforts and removal of secretions from the airways. Fiberoptic bronchoscopy is useful for removing inspissated secretions that are contributing to atelectasis.

Control of Infection

Control of infection using specific antibiotic therapy based on sputum culture and sensitivity is a valuable adjunct to the management of respiratory failure. Use of prophylactic antibiotics, however, without proven specificity for the infectious organism, is not recommended, since this practice can lead to overgrowth of resistant bacteria or fungi. Not uncommonly, the earliest evidence of infection in patients with respiratory failure is further deterioration of pulmonary function.

MONITORING OF TREATMENT

Monitoring of treatment of respiratory failure depends on evaluation of pulmonary gas exchange and cardiac function. Measurement of (1) arterial and venous blood gases, (2) arterial pH, (3) cardiac output, (4) cardiac filling pressures, (5) intrapulmonary shunt, and (6) static lung compliance are the most informative with respect to the status of respiratory failure and responses to treatment. A pulmonary artery catheter is useful for making many of these measurements.

Oxygen Exchange

Adequacy of oxygen exchange across alveolar capillary membranes is reflected by the arterial partial pressures of oxygen. The efficacy of this exchange is reflected by the difference between the calculated alveolar partial pressures of oxygen and the measured partial pressures of oxygen in arterial blood (Table 16-2).

TABLE 16-2. Calculation of the Alveolar-to-Arterial Difference for Oxygen

$$A\text{-a}DO_2 = P_AO_2 - PaO_2$$

$$P_A = (P_B - P_{H_2O})F_IO_2 - \frac{PaCO_2}{0.8}$$

$A\text{-a}DO_2$	=	alveolar-to-arterial difference for oxygen, mmHg
P_AO_2	=	alveolar partial pressure of oxygen, mmHg
PaO_2	=	arterial partial pressure of oxygen, mmHg
P_B	=	barometric pressure, mmHg
P_{H_2O}	=	partial pressure of water vapor, 47 mmHg at 37 Celsius
F_IO_2	=	inspired concentration of oxygen
$PaCO_2$	=	arterial partial pressure of carbon dioxide, mmHg
0.8	=	respiratory exchange ratio to compensate for the fact that less carbon dioxide is transferred into the alveolus than is oxygen removed from the alveolus.
Example:		Arterial blood gases are PaO_2 100 mmHg ($F_IO_2 = 0.5$) and $PaCO_2$ 40 mmHg. The P_B is 747 mmHg and the P_{H_2O} is 47 mmHg. Calculation of the P_AO_2 and $A\text{-a}DO_2$ is as follows:

$$P_AO_2 = (747 - 47)0.5 - 40/0.8$$

$$P_AO_2 = 350 - 50$$

$$P_AO_2 = 300 \text{ mmHg}$$

$$A\text{-a}DO_2 = 300 - 100$$

$$A\text{-a}DO_2 = 200 \text{ mmHg}$$

TABLE 16-3. Calculation of the Ratio of Arterial to Alveolar Oxygen Partial Pressure

$$a/A = PaO_2/P_AO_2$$

a/A	=	ratio of arterial-to-alveolar partial pressure of oxygen
PaO_2	=	arterial partial pressure of oxygen, mmHg
P_AO_2	=	alveolar partial pressure of oxygen, mmHg (see Table 16-2 for calculation)
Example:		Arterial blood gases are PaO_2 250 mmHg and $PaCO_2$ 40 mmHg breathing 50 percent oxygen. The P_B is 747 mmHg and the P_{H_2O} is 47 mmHg.

$$P_AO_2 = (747 - 47)0.5 - 40/0.8$$

$$P_AO_2 = 350 - 50$$

$$P_AO_2 = 300 \text{ mmHg}$$

$$a/A = 250/300$$

$$a/A = 0.83 \text{ (normal greater than 0.75)}$$

Indeed, calculation of alveolar-to-arterial differences for oxygen, when patients are breathing pure oxygen, provides an estimate of the magnitude of right-to-left intrapulmonary shunting of blood. Conversely, calculation of alveolar-to-arterial differences for oxygen, when patients are breathing air, reflects mismatch of ventilation to perfusion, as well as right-to-left intrapulmonary shunting of blood. A useful clinical guideline is the estimate that each 20 mmHg of alveolar-to-arterial difference for oxygen measured while patients are breathing pure oxygen represents venous admixture equivalent to 1 percent of the cardiac output. This guideline, however, will underestimate the true magnitude of venous admixture when the saturation of hemoglobin with oxygen is less than 100 percent or the cardiac output is elevated. Finally, alveolar-to-arterial differences for oxygen due to diffusion block of oxygen transfer across alveolar capillary membranes have never been proven.

A disadvantage of monitoring the alveolar-to-arterial difference for oxygen is the normal range changes with varying inspired concentrations of oxygen. For this reason, the ratio of alveolar-to-arterial oxygen partial pressures may be useful, as this value is less dependent on inspired oxygen concentrations (Table 16-3).[17] For example, patients with alveolar-to-arterial oxygen partial pressure ratios of 0.5 will have arterial oxygen partial pressures equal to 50 percent of the alveolar oxygen partial pressures regardless of the inspired concentrations of oxygen. Ratios less than 0.75 suggest the lungs are not working well as oxygen exchangers.

Carbon Dioxide Exchange

Adequacy of alveolar ventilation relative to the metabolic production of carbon dioxide is depicted by the arterial partial pressures of carbon dioxide. The efficacy of the transfer of carbon dioxide across alveolar capillary membranes is reflected by the ratio of dead space ventilation to tidal volume (Table 16-4). This ratio depicts areas in the lungs that receive adequate ventilation but inadequate or no pulmonary blood flow. Normally, the dead space-to-tidal volume ratio is less than 0.3 but may increase to 0.6 or greater when there is an increase in the number of alveoli that are ventilated but not perfused. For example, an increased dead space-to-tidal volume ratio occurs in the presence of (1) decreased cardiac output due to anesthetic drugs or reductions in intravascular fluid volume, (2) pulmonary embolism, and (3) respiratory failure.

TABLE 16-4.   Calculation of the Dead Space to Tidal Volume Ratio

$$V_D/V_T = \frac{PaCO_2 - P_ECO_2}{PaCO_2}$$

V_D/V_T = ratio of dead space to tidal volume
$PaCO_2$ = arterial partial pressure of carbon dioxide, mmHg
P_ECO_2 = mixed exhaled partial pressure of carbon dioxide, mmHg

Example: The $PaCO_2$ and P_ECO_2 are 40 mmHg and 30 mmHg respectively during controlled ventilation of the lungs with isoflurane in oxygen. The calculated V_D/V_T ratio is:

$$V_D/V_T = \frac{40 - 30}{40}$$

$$V_D/V_T = 10/40$$

$$V_D/V_T = 0.25$$

Mixed Venous Partial Pressures of Oxygen

Mixed venous partial pressures of oxygen and arterial-to-venous differences for oxygen reflect the cardiac output and extraction of oxygen by tissues. For example, reductions in cardiac output in the presence of unchanged tissue oxygen consumption causes the mixed venous partial pressures of oxygen to decrease and the arterial-to-venous differences for oxygen to increase. These changes reflect the continued extraction of the same amount of oxygen by the tissues from a reduced tissue blood flow. Mixed venous partial pressures of oxygen below 30 mmHg or arterial-to-venous differences for oxygen that exceed 6 ml·dl^{-1} indicate the need to increase cardiac output to insure adequate tissue oxygenation. A properly placed pulmonary artery catheter permits sampling of mixed venous blood via the distal port.

Factors that Influence Accuracy of Blood Gas Measurements

The recommendation that arterial blood gases should be corrected for differences between the patient's body temperature and the temperature of the measuring electrode is based on known temperature-dependent solubility of oxygen and carbon dioxide in blood. For example, placing blood from patients with body temperatures less than 37 degrees Celsius into electrodes maintained at 37 degrees Celsius means that more molecules enter the gas phase to be sensed as partial pressure than would be present in vivo at the lower body temperature of the patient. Nomograms are available to correct blood gases and pH measurements for temperature. Nevertheless, it has been argued that normal partial pressures of carbon dioxide and normal pH measured at electrode temperatures of 37 degrees Celsius reflect an unperturbed acid-base status of patients, regardless of the body temperature that existed at the time the samples were drawn.[18]

If this concept is accepted, it is unnecessary to correct measurements of carbon dioxide partial pressures and pH for temperature. Temperature correction of the partial pressures of oxygen remains necessary to assess oxygenation. Furthermore, calculation of alveolar-to-arterial differences for oxygen requires temperature correction of oxygen and carbon dioxide partial pressures. Nomograms are available to correct blood gas and pH measurements for temperature. When nomograms are not available, a clinically useful guideline for temperature correction is to decrease the arterial partial pressures of oxygen and carbon dioxide 6 percent and 4 percent respectively for every degree Celsius the patient's body temperature is below the temperature of the electrodes, which are usually maintained at 37 degrees Celsius.

Another consideration in the interpretation of arterial blood gases is consumption of oxygen by leukocytes and platelets that could result in an in vitro reduction of oxygen partial pressures. For this reason, blood samples are placed on ice, especially if the time between obtaining the samples and analysis will exceed 20 minutes.[19] Another source of error is introduced by the presence of air bubbles in blood samples. For example, carbon dioxide can pass along partial pressure gradients from the blood into the air bubble resulting in a false-low measurement of the partial pressures of carbon dioxide actually present in patients. Likewise, oxygen can pass to or from the air bubble, depending on the partial pressure of this gas in the blood, resulting in false-low or false-high measurements of the partial pressures of oxygen actually present.

Arterial pH

Arterial pH measurements are necessary to detect acidemia or alkalemia. For example, metabolic acidosis predictably accompanies arterial hypoxemia and inadequate delivery of oxygen to tissues. Furthermore, acidemia due to respiratory or metabolic derangements is associated with cardiac dysrhythmias and increased pulmonary vascular resistance due to constriction of the pulmonary vasculature.

Alkalemia, as reflected by increases in arterial pH, is most often associated with iatrogenic mechanical hyperventilation of the lungs or drug-induced diuresis that leads to loss of chloride and potassium. As with acidemia, the incidence of cardiac dysrhythmias is increased by metabolic or respiratory alkalosis.[20] Presence of alkalemia in patients recovering from respiratory failure can delay or prevent successful weaning from mechanical support of ventilation because of compensatory hypoventilation by patients in attempts to restore total body carbon dioxide stores. The phenomenon known as posthyperventilation hypoxia reflects arterial hypoxemia due to hypoventilation that develops in the absence of supplemental oxygen administration to patients in whom previous mechanical hyperventilation of the lungs has led to depletion of carbon dioxide stores.[21]

Cardiac Ouput

Measurement and maintenance of a normal cardiac output is essential for assuring adequate delivery of oxygen to tissues and evaluating responses to therapeutic interventions during the treatment of respiratory failure. Cardiac output is most frequently measured by thermodilution techniques, using a properly placed pulmonary artery catheter.

Cardiac Filling Pressures

Properly placed pulmonary artery catheters permit measurement of right atrial pressures and pulmonary artery occlusion pressures. Measurement of these cardiac filling pressures, combined with the values for cardiac output, permits construction of right ventricular and left ventricular function curves for use in guiding fluid administration and drug therapy. In addition, measurement of cardiac filling pressures and mean pulmonary artery pressures via the pulmonary artery catheter, plus knowledge of the mean arterial pressure,

TABLE 16-5. Calculation of Pulmonary and Systemic Vascular Resistance

$$PVR = \frac{MPAP - PA_o}{CO} \times 80$$

$$SVR = \frac{MAP - CVP}{CO} \times 80$$

PVR = pulmonary vascular resistance, dynes-sec-cm^{-5}
MPAP = mean pulmonary artery pressure, mmHg
PA$_o$ = pulmonary artery occlusion pressure, mmHg
CO = cardiac output, L·min^{-1}
SVR = systemic vascular resistance, dynes-sec-cm^{-5}
MAP = mean arterial pressure, mmHg
CVP = central venous pressure, mmHg
80 = factor for conversion to dynes-sec-cm^{-5}
Example: The following cardiovascular measurements are obtained via a pulmonary artery catheter and radial artery catheter: MPAP = 15 mmHg, PA$_o$ 8 mmHg, MAP 90 mmHg, CVP = 5 mmHg, and CO 5 L·min^{-1}. Calculated PVR and SVR is:

$$PVR = \frac{15 - 8}{5} \times 80$$

PVR = 112 dynes-sec-cm^{-5}

(normal 50–140 dynes-sec-cm^{-5})

$$SVR = \frac{90 - 5}{5} \times 80$$

SVR = 1360 dynes-sec-cm^{-5}

(normal 900–1500 dynes-sec-cm^{-5})

permits calculation of pulmonary and systemic vascular resistances (Table 16-5).

Intrapulmonary Shunt

Right-to-left intrapulmonary shunting of blood occurs when there is perfusion of alveoli that are not ventilated. The net effect is decreased arterial partial pressures of oxygen, reflecting dilution of oxygen in blood exposed to ventilated alveoli, with blood containing less oxygen coming from unventilated alveoli. Calculation of the shunt fraction provides a reliable assessment of the match of ventilation to perfusion and serves as a useful estimate of responses to therapeutic interventions during treatment of respiratory failure (Tables 16-6, 16-7).

Physiologic shunt normally comprises 2 percent to 5 percent of the cardiac output. This degree of right-to-left intrapulmonary shunting reflects passage of pulmonary arterial blood directly to the left side of the circulation via bronchial and Thebesian veins. It should be appreciated that determination of the shunt fraction while patients are breathing less than 100 percent oxygen reflects the contribution of mismatch of ventilation to perfusion as well as the right-to-left intrapulmonary shunt. Calculation of the shunt fraction from measurements made while patients are breathing pure oxygen eliminates the contribution of mismatch of venti-

TABLE 16-6. Calculation of the Intrapulmonary Shunt Fraction

$$Q_S/Q_T = \frac{CcO_2 - CaO_2}{CcO_2 - CvO_2}$$

Q$_S$ = fraction of pulmonary blood flow not exposed to ventilated alveoli
Q$_T$ = Total pulmonary blood flow
CcO$_2$ = oxygen content in pulmonary capillary blood exposed to a ventilated alveolus, ml·dl^{-1}
CaO$_2$ = oxygen content of arterial blood, ml·dl^{-1}
CvO$_2$ = oxygen content of mixed venous blood, ml·dl^{-1}
Calculation of the oxygen content of arterial blood (same for venous and capillary) is as follows:
CaO$_2$ = (Hb × 1.39)SaO$_2$ + PaO$_2$ × 0.003
Hb = hemoglobin concentration, g·dl^{-1}
1.39 = oxygen bound by hemoglobin, ml·g^{-1}
SaO$_2$ = saturation of hemoglobin with oxygen, percent
PaO$_2$ = arterial partial pressure of oxygen, mmHg
0.003 = solubility coefficient for oxygen in plasma, ml·mmHg^{-1}·dl^{-1}
Calculation of the shunt fraction using the oxygen content of pulmonary capillary blood, mixed venous blood, and arterial blood requires the presence of a pulmonary artery catheter. Furthermore, the number of calculations makes the equation too complex for routine clinical use. An acceptable alternative equation is shown in Table 16-7.

TABLE 16-7. Calculation of the Intrapulmonary Shunt Fraction

$$^*Q_S/Q_T = \frac{\text{A-aDO}_2(0.003)}{(\text{CaO}_2 - \text{CvO}_2) + (\text{A-aDO}_2)(0.003)}$$

Q_S = fraction of pulmonary blood flow not exposed to ventilated alveoli

Q_T = total pulmonary blood flow

A-aDO_2 = alveolar-to-arterial difference for oxygen (see Table 16-2 for calculation)

$\text{CaO}_2 - \text{CvO}_2$ = arterial-to-venous oxygen content difference (assume as 5 ml dl^{-1} or calculate oxygen content as described in Table 16-6)

0.003 = solubility coefficient for oxygen in plasma

Example: The A-aDO_2 in a patient breathing pure oxygen is 200 mmHg. Assuming a $\text{CaO}_2 - \text{CvO}_2$ difference of 5 ml dl^{-1}, the intrapulmonary shunt fraction is calculated as follows:

$$Q_S/Q_T = \frac{\text{A-aDO}_2(0.003)}{(\text{CaO}_2 - \text{CvO}_2) + (\text{A-aDO}_2)(0.003)}$$

$$Q_S/Q_T = \frac{200 \times 0.003}{5 + (200)(0.003)}$$

$$Q_S/Q_T = \frac{0.6}{5.6}$$

$Q_S/Q_T = 0.107$ or 10.7 percent of total pulmonary blood flow

* This equation can be used when patients are breathing pure oxygen and arterial partial pressures of oxygen are greater than 150 mmHg, so as to assure maximum saturation of hemoglobin with oxygen.

lation to perfusion, but the fraction may be falsely elevated because of absorption atelectasis or attenuation of regional hypoxic pulmonary vasoconstriction.

Static Lung Compliance

Static lung compliance is determined by dividing the tidal volume by the difference between the plateau airway pressure at end-inspiration (resulting from a period of no flow for 1 second to 1.5 seconds) and the end-expiratory pressure.[12] This measurement is a useful indicator of lung volumes and of the ideal level of positive end-expiratory pressure for use in the treatment of respiratory failure (see the section Positive End-Expiratory Pressure).

Therefore, measurement of static lung compliance is a practical alternative to measurement of mixed venous partial pressures of oxygen or of cardiac output when attempting to establish "best PEEP."

CESSATION OF MECHANICAL SUPPORT OF VENTILATION

Cessation of mechanical support of ventilation (weaning) can be considered to occur in three stages. The first step is cessation of mechanical inflation of the lungs, followed by removal of the secured airway provided by the tube in the trachea, and then elimination of the need for supplemental oxygen.

Cessation of Mechanical Inflation of the Lungs

Arbitrary guidelines that have been proposed as indicating the feasibility of cessation of mechanical inflation of the lungs include (1) vital capacity greater than 15 ml·kg^{-1}, (2) alveolar-to-arterial differences for oxygen less than 350 mmHg while patients are breathing pure oxygen, (3) arterial partial pressures of oxygen greater than 60 mmHg while patients are breathing less than 50 percent oxygen, (4) maximal inspiratory pressure greater than -20 cmH_2O with airway occlusion, and (5) dead space-to-tidal volume ratio less than 0.6.[22] Ultimately, decisions to attempt cessation of mechanical inflation of the lungs must be individualized, considering not only the status of pulmonary function but also the co-existence of other abnormalities. For example, the level of consciousness, cardiac function, arterial capacity to carry oxygen, intravascular fluid volume, electrolyte balance, and nutritional status must be optimized before attempted cessation of mechanical ventilation of the lungs. Likewise, control of infection is important before this step in the weaning process is initiated.

A T-tube and intermittent mandatory ventilation are the two methods employed for initiating the first stage in the cessation of mechanical support of ventilation.

T-TUBE

T-tube weaning is initiated by connecting the tube in the patient's trachea to a device (T-tube) through which humidified and oxygen-enriched gases are delivered. In addition, 2.5 cmH_2O to 5 cmH_2O of continuous positive airway pressure is often delivered via the T-tube to the airway. Use of continuous positive airway pressure prevents decreases in functional residual capacity associated with cessation of positive pressure ventilation.[23] Indeed, incompetence of the glottic opening produced by the presence of a translaryngeal tracheal tube seems to interfere with the maintenance of a normal functional residual capacity. Initially, patients are allowed to breathe spontaneously for 5 minutes to 10 minutes each hour. Tachycardia, tachypnea (greater than 35 breaths·min^{-1}), or alterations in the level of consciousness during these brief periods of spontaneous ventilation confirm that the weaning attempt has been premature, and mechanical support is immediately reinstituted. When pulmonary function has recovered to the extent that weaning from mechanical ventilation is appropriate, it will be possible to lengthen gradually the periods of spontaneous ventilation.

INTERMITTENT MANDATORY VENTILATION

Intermittent mandatory ventilation permits patients to breathe spontaneously between mechanically delivered tidal volumes, using the same inspired concentrations of oxygen and level of positive end-expiratory pressure provided by mechanical inflation of the lungs.[24] The mechanical tidal volume can be provided as a nonsynchronous mandatory breath delivered at a preset interval or as a synchronized breath initiated by the patient's spontaneous respiratory effort. Cessation of mechanical support of ventilation is initiated by gradually decreasing the number of me-

chanical breaths delivered each minute. Ideally, the rate of intermittent mandatory ventilation is sequentially decreased as long as the arterial partial pressures of carbon dioxide are maintained at levels that result in an arterial pH between 7.36 and 7.44.

An advantage of intermittent mandatory ventilation is gradual rather than abrupt conversion to spontaneous ventilation. In addition, this mode of ventilation is associated with low mean airway pressures, which minimizes interference to venous return and reduces the likelihood of pulmonary barotrauma. The presence of spontaneous breathing during intermittent mandatory ventilation also maintains use of muscles of respiration, which should reduce the likelihood of disuse atrophy. Nevertheless, respiratory muscles continue to be stretched during mechanical ventilation, such that disuse atrophy probably does not occur.

Removal of the Secured Airway

Removal of the secured airway provided by the tube in the trachea should be considered when patients tolerate 2 hours of spontaneous ventilation during T-tube weaning or when they achieve an intermittent mandatory ventilation rate of 1 breath·min^{-1} to 2 breaths·min^{-1} without deterioration of arterial blood gases, central nervous system, or cardiac status. For example, arterial partial pressures of oxygen should be maintained above 60 mmHg when patients are breathing less than 50 percent oxygen. Likewise, arterial partial pressures of carbon dioxide should be less than 50 mmHg or the arterial pH should be above 7.3. It should be remembered that patients with chronic obstructive airways disease may manifest high arterial partial pressures of carbon dioxide but a nearly normal arterial pH because of compensatory increases in plasma concentrations of bicarbonate. Additional important criteria, which must be satisfied before removal of the secured airway, include (1) need for less than 5 cmH_2O positive end-expiratory pressure, (2) ventilatory rate less than 30 breaths·min^{-1}, and (3) vital capacity greater than 15 ml·kg^{-1}. In addition, patients should be alert, with active laryngeal reflexes and the ability to generate an effective cough, so as to clear secretions from the airways.

Elimination of the Need for Supplemental Oxygen

Supplemental oxygen is often needed after removal of the secured airway. This need reflects persistence of areas of mismatch of ventilation to perfusion. Weaning from supplemental oxygen is accomplished by gradual reductions in the inspired concentrations of oxygen, as guided by monitoring of the arterial partial pressures of oxygen. Patients with chronic obstructive airways disease associated with retention of carbon dioxide require careful titration of the inspired concentrations of oxygen. In these patients, inspired concentrations of oxygen are often adjusted to maintain arterial partial pressures of oxygen near 60 mmHg (90 percent saturation). The basis for this recommendation in the past has been that higher arterial partial pressures of oxygen could eliminate the hypoxic drive to ventilation provided by the carotid bodies leading to decreased minute ventilation and accumulation of carbon dioxide. Conversely, increased dead space ventilation, rather than removal of the hypoxic stimulus to ventilation, may be the principal explanation for increased partial pressures of carbon dioxide that occasionally accompany administration of supplemental oxygen to patients with chronic obstructive airways disease.[25]

REFERENCES

1. Bone RC, Jacobs ER. Advances in pharmacologic treatment of acute lung injury and septic shock. In: Stoelting RK, Barash PG, Gallagher TJ, eds. Advances in Anesthesia. Chicago. Year Book Medical Publishers 1986:327–45
2. Hudson LD. Causes of the adult respiratory distress syndrome: Clinical recognition. Clin Chest Med 1982;3:195–212
3. Deneke SM, Fanburg BL. Normobaric oxygen toxicity of the lung. N Engl J Med 1980;303:76–86
4. Bernard AV, Cotrell JE, Sivakumaran C, et al. Adjustment of intracuff pressure to prevent aspiration. Anesthesiology 1979;50:363–6
5. Sjostrand U. High-frequency positive-pressure ventilation (JFPPV): A review. Crit Care Med 1980;8:345–64
6. O'Rourke PP, Crone RK. High-frequency ventilation. A new approach to respiratory support. JAMA 1983;250:2845–7
7. Borg U, Eng Erikson I, Sjostrand U. High-frequency positive-pressure ventilation (HFPPV): A review based upon its use during bronchoscopy and laryngoscopy and microlaryngeal surgery under general anesthesia. Anesth Analg 1980;59:594–603
8. Carlon GC, Ray C, Klain M, McCormick PM. High-frequency positive-pressure ventilation in management of a patient with bronchopleural fistula. Anesthesiology 1980;52:160–2
9. Brichant JF, Rouby JJ, Viars P. Intermittent positive pressure ventilation with either positive end-expiratory pressure or high frequency jet ventilation (HFJV), or HFJV alone in human acute respiratory failure. Anesth Analg 1986;65:1135–42
10. Bishop MJ, Benson MS, Sato P, Pierson DJ. Comparison of high-frequency jet ventilation with conventional mechanical ventilation for bronchopleural fistula. Anesth Analg 1987;66:833–8
11. Fusciardi J, Rouby JJ, Barakat T, DMai H, Godet G, Viars P. Hemodynamic effects of high-frequency jet ventilation in patients with and without circulatory shock. Anesthesiology 1986;65:485–91
12. Suter PM, Fairley HB, Isenberg MD. Optimum end-expiratory airway pressure in patients with acute pulmonary failure. N Engl J Med 1975;292:284–9
13. Jardin F, Farcot J-C, Boisante L, et al. Influence of positive end-expiratory pressure on left ventricular performance. N Engl J Med 1981;304:387–92
14. Trichet B, Falke K, Togut A, Laver MB. The effect of preexisting pulmonary vascular disease on the response to mechanical ventilation with PEEP following open-heart surgery. Anesthesiology 1975;42:56–67
15. Kumar A, Pontoppidan H, Baratz RA, Laver MB. Inappropriate response to increased plasma ADH during mechanical ventilation in acute respiratory failure. Anesthesiology 1974;40:215–21

16. Laine GA, Allen SJ, William JP et al. A new look at pulmonary edema. NIPS 1986;1:150–3

17. Doyle DJ. Arterial/alveolar oxygen tension ratio: A critical appraisal. Can Anaesth Soc J 1986;33:471–4

18. Ream AK, Reitz BA, Silverberg G. Temperature correction of PCO_2 and pH in estimating acid-base status: An example of the emperor's new clothes? Anesthesiology 1982;56:41–4

19. Nanji AA, Whitlow KJ. Is it necessary to transport arterial blood samples on ice for pH and gas analysis. Can Anaesth Soc J 1984;31:568–71

20. Lawson NW, Butler GH, Ray CT. Alkalosis and cardiac arrhythmias. Anesth Analg 1973;52:951–64

21. Sullivan SF, Patterson RW. Posthyperventilation hypoxia: Theoretical considerations in man. Anesthesiology 1968;29:981–6

22. Feeley TW, Hedley-White J. Weaning from controlled ventilation and supplemental oxygen. N Engl J Med 1975;292:903–6

23. Annest SJ, Gottlieb M, Paloski WH, et al. Detrimental effects of removing end-expiratory pressure prior to endotracheal extubation. Ann Surg 1980;191:539–45

24. Downs JB, Kirby RR. Intermittent mandatory ventilation. A new approach to weaning patients from mechanical ventilators. Chest 1973;64:331–5

25. Aubier M, Murciano D, Milic-Emili J, et al. Effects of the administration of oxygen on ventilation and blood gases in patients with chronic obstructive pulmonary disease during acute respiratory failure. Am Rev Resp Dis 1980;122:747–54

17

Acid-Base Disturbances

Maintenance of arterial concentrations of hydrogen ions over a narrow range is necessary to (1) ensure optimal function of enzymes, (2) maintain proper distribution of electrolytes, (3) prevent reductions in myocardial contractility, (4) minimize alterations in systemic and pulmonary vascular resistance, and (5) maintain optimal saturation of hemoglobin with oxygen at prevailing arterial partial pressures of oxygen. Direct effects of alkalemia on cardiac contractility are less striking than those of acidemia. Although acidemia reduces myocardial contractility, little clinical effect is seen until pH falls below 7.2. Since acidemia also induces release of catecholamines, much of the direct depressant effects are mitigated in mild acidemia. When arterial pH is below 7.1, however, cardiac responsiveness to catecholamines decreases and compensatory inotropic effects are diminished. Cardiac dysrhythmias in the presence of alkalemia may be accentuated by hypokalemia. Alkalemia also produces cerebral and coronary artery vasoconstriction and shifts the oxyhemoglobin dissociation curve to the left, thus impairing tissue oxygenation.

Normal hydrogen ion concentrations in arterial blood and extracellular fluid are 36 nM·L^{-1} to 44 nM·L^{-1}. This concentration is traditionally expressed as the pH, which is the negative logarithm of the hydrogen ion concentration. Hydrogen ion concentrations of 36 nM·L^{-1} to 44 nM·L^{-1} correspond to a pH of 7.44 to 7.36, respectively (Table 17-1). Main-

tenance of pH over a narrow range despite continued production of nonvolatile acids during metabolism is accomplished by neutralization of these hydrogen ions with endogenous buffers. Important buffers present in plasma include proteins, bicarbonate, and reduced hemoglobin. In addition, kidneys are important for the excretion of nonvolatile acids.

DIFFERENTIAL DIAGNOSIS OF ACID-BASE DISTURBANCES

Differential diagnosis of acid-base disturbances is based on direct measurements of arterial pH and arterial partial pressures of carbon dioxide, plus derived estimates of plasma concentrations of bicarbonate using a nomogram (Fig. 17-1).[1,2] These measurements are used to categorize acid-base disturbances as (1) respiratory acidosis, (2) respiratory alkalosis, (3) metabolic acidosis, and (4) metabolic alkalosis. Ultimately the distinction between respiratory and metabolic causes of acidemia or alkalemia is based on measurement of the arterial partial pressures of carbon dioxide and estimation of the plasma concentrations of bicarbonate (Figs. 17-2, 17-3 and 17-4, Table 17-2).

Arterial blood is in normal acid-base balance when the (1) hydrogen ion concentration

TABLE 17-1. Relation of Hydrogen Ion Concentrations to pH

Hydrogen Ion Concentrations $(nM \cdot L^{-1})$	pH
80	7.10
63	7.20
50	7.30
44	7.36
42	7.38
40	7.40
38	7.42
36	7.44
32	7.50
25	7.60
20	7.70

is 40 ± 4 nM·L^{-1}, (2) pH is 7.36 to 7.44, (3) partial pressure of carbon dioxide is 40 ± 4 mmHg, and (4) bicarbonate concentration is 24 ± 2 mEq·L^{-1}. Acidemia is present when arterial pH is less than 7.36; alkalemia is present when arterial pH is greater than 7.44. By definition, arterial partial pressures of carbon dioxide greater than 44 mmHg represent hypoventilation; hyperventilation is present when arterial partial pressures of carbon dioxide are less than 36 mmHg. Hypoventilation is synonomous with respiratory acidosis, and hyperventilation is synonomous with respiratory alkalosis. Acidemia and alkalemia not related to alterations in the arterial partial pressures of carbon dioxide are considered to be primary metabolic disturbances.

Interpretation of acid-base disturbances and prediction of compensatory responses require an understanding of the Henderson-Hasselbalch equation (Table 17-3). This equation emphasizes that a normal pH depends upon maintenance of an optimal 20-to-1 ratio of the concentration of bicarbonate to the concentration of carbon dioxide. Acid-base disturbances characterized by changes in plasma concentrations of bicarbonate are predictably accompanied by appropriate compensatory changes in plasma concentrations of carbon dioxide secondary to alterations in alveolar ventilation. If changes in plasma concentrations of bicarbonate and carbon dioxide are proportional, such that a 20-to-1 ratio is maintained, the pH will remain near or within a normal range despite disturbances of acid-base balance (Fig. 17-2). For example, acid-base disturbances due to respiratory acidosis or alkalosis are compensated for by renal-induced changes in plasma concentrations of bicarbonate. Changes in plasma concentrations of bicarbonate will attenuate the impact of chronic alterations in the arterial partial pressures of carbon dioxide on arterial pH. Indeed, this form of renal compensation can return the ratio of the concentration of bicarbonate to the concentration of carbon dioxide to about 20 to 1. As a result, arterial pH in the presence of chronic respiratory acidosis or alkalosis remains relatively normal, despite persistent alterations in the arterial partial pressures of carbon dioxide (Table 17-2). Acid-base disturbances due to metabolic acidosis or alkalosis are compensated for by ventilation-

TABLE 17-2. Direction of Changes During Acute and Chronic Acid-Base Disturbances

	pH	PaCO$_2$	HCO$_3$
Respiratory acidosis			
Acute	Moderate decrease	Marked increase	Slight increase
Chronic	Slight decrease	Marked increase	Moderate increase
Respiratory alkalosis			
Acute	Moderate increase	Marked decrease	Slight decrease
Chronic	Slight increase to no change	Marked decrease	Moderate decrease
Metabolic acidosis			
Acute	Moderate to marked decrease	Slight decrease	Marked decrease
Chronic	Slight decrease	Moderate decrease	Marked decrease
Metabolic alkalosis			
Acute	Marked increase	Moderate increase	Marked increase
Chronic	Marked increase	Moderate increase	Marked increase

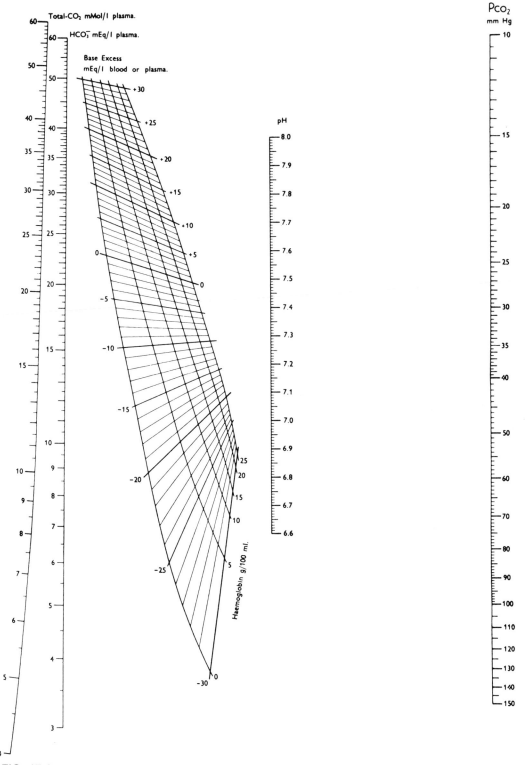

FIG. 17-1. The Siggaard-Andersen alignment nomogram is used to derive the estimated plasma concentration of bicarbonate based on the measured pH and partial pressure of carbon dioxide. For example, a straight line connecting the points between a partial pressure of carbon dioxide equivalent to 40 mmHg and a pH of 7.4 will transect the column representing the plasma concentration of bicarbonate at 24 mEq· L^{-1}. (Siggaard-Andersen O. Blood acid-base alignment nomogram. Scand J Clin Lab Invest 1963;15:211–7)

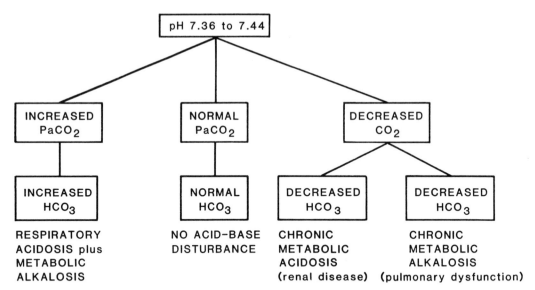

FIG. 17-2. A diagnostic approach to the interpretation of a normal arterial pH based on the arterial partial pressure of carbon dioxide and concentration of bicarbonate. The likely primary acid-base disturbance responsible for the designated changes, as well as the complicating metabolic abnormality, are listed below each column.

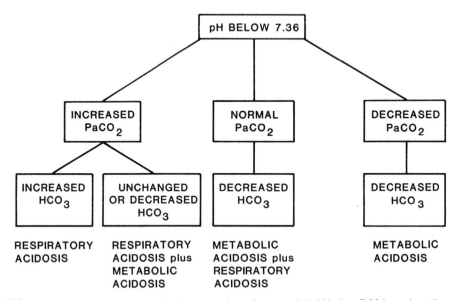

FIG. 17-3. A diagnostic approach to the interpretation of an arterial pH below 7.36 based on the arterial partial pressure of carbon dioxide and concentration of bicarbonate. The likely primary acid-base disturbances responsible for the designated changes, as well as the complicating metabolic or respiratory abnormality, are listed below each column.

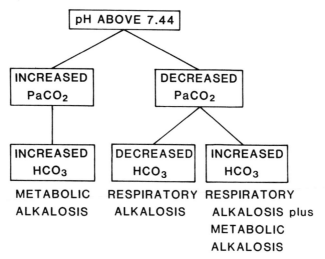

FIG. 17-4. A diagnostic approach to the interpretation of an arterial pH above 7.44 based on the arterial partial pressure of carbon dioxide and concentration of bicarbonate. The likely primary acid-base disturbance responsible for the designated changes, as well as the complicating metabolic abnormality, are listed below each column.

TABLE 17-3. Henderson-Hasselbalch Equation

$$pHa = pK + \log \frac{HCO_3}{0.03 \times PaCO_2}$$

pHa = negative logarithm of the arterial concentration of hydrogen ions
pK = 6.1 at 37 degrees Celsius
HCO_3 = concentration of bicarbonate, $mEq \cdot L^{-1}$
0.03 = solubility coefficient for carbon dioxide in plasma, ml $mmHg^{-1} \cdot dl^{-1}$
$PaCO_2$ = arterial partial pressure of carbon dioxide, mmHg

Substitution of average values for pHa (7.4) and $PaCO_2$ (40 mmHg) results in a calculated bicarbonate (HCO_3) concentration equivalent to 24 $mEq \cdot L^{-1}$. Maintenance of a normal concentration of bicarbonate relative to the concentration of carbon dioxide results in an optimal ratio of about 20 to 1 (24 $mEq \cdot L^{-1}$ divided by 1.2). This optimal ratio of 20 to 1 allows the maintenance of a relatively normal arterial pH (7.36 to 7.44) despite deviations from normal in the concentrations of bicarbonate or the partial pressures of carbon dioxide.

$$CO_2 + H_2O \rightleftharpoons H_2CO_3 \rightleftharpoons HCO_3^- + H^+$$

FIG. 17-5. Hydration of carbon dioxide results in carbonic acid (H_2CO_3), which can subsequently dissociate into bicarbonate and hydrogen ions.

TABLE 17-4. Adjustments for Impact of Ventilation on Plasma Concentrations of Bicarbonate

Changes in Arterial Partial Pressures of Carbon Dioxide	Changes in Bicarbonate Concentrations from 24 mEq·L^{-1}
Acute 10 mmHg increase	Increase 1 mEq·L^{-1}
Acute 10 mmHg decrease	Decrease 2 mEq·L^{-1}
Chronic 10 mmHg increase	Increase 3 mEq·L^{-1}
Chronic 10 mmHg decrease	Decrease 5 mEq·L^{-1}

induced changes in the arterial partial pressures of carbon dioxide (Table 17-2).

Interpretation of nomogram-derived estimates of plasma concentrations of bicarbonate as a reflection of acid-base disturbances due to metabolic processes requires an adjustment for the impact of ventilation. For example, increases in the partial pressures of carbon dioxide will lead to the hydration of carbon dioxide to carbonic acid, with subsequent increases in the plasma concentrations of bicarbonate (Fig. 17-5). Conversely, lowering arterial partial pressures of carbon dioxide will reverse the direction of this reaction, resulting in reductions in the plasma concentrations of bicarbonate. These changes are reasonably linear and permit the use of certain guidelines acceptable for clinical interpretation and management of acid-base disturbances (Table 17-4). For example, using these guidelines, hypoventilation leading to acute increases in the arterial partial pressures of carbon dioxide to 70 mmHg would result in normalized plasma concentrations of bicarbonate equivalent to 27 mEq·L^{-1}, assuming normal values equal to 24 mEq·L^{-1}.

RESPIRATORY ACIDOSIS

Respiratory acidosis occurs as a result of elevated arterial partial pressures of carbon dioxide due to decreased alveolar ventilation, resulting from (1) reduced central nervous system stimulation of ventilation secondary to depressant drugs, (2) disorders of neuromuscular function produced by depressant drugs or diseases, and (3) intrinsic pulmonary disease. Very rarely, respiratory acidosis may result from increased metabolic production of carbon dioxide.

The initial effect of an increase in the arterial partial pressures of carbon dioxide is an increase in the concentration of hydrogen ions, due to hydration of carbon dioxide (Fig. 17-5). Since carbon dioxide readily crosses lipid membranes, such as the blood-brain barrier, reductions in pH produced by hydration of carbon dioxide occur to similar extents in arterial blood and cerebrospinal fluid pH. The response to this reduction in pH is stimulation of ventilation via the carotid bodies and the medullary chemoreceptors located in the ventrolateral surface of the fourth cerebral ventricle.[3] It is estimated that about 85 percent of the ventilatory response to carbon dioxide is mediated by stimulation of the medullary chemoreceptors, with the carotid bodies playing a minor role. With time, cerebrospinal fluid pH is restored to normal by active transport of bicarbonate into cerebrospinal fluid.[3] Restoration of cerebrospinal fluid pH to normal removes the stimulus to ventilation provided by the medullary chemoreceptors. Therefore, the volume of ventilation after restoration of cerebrospinal fluid pH to normal is less than that present during the initial phase of respiratory acidosis.

Absolute reductions in arterial pH in the presence of respiratory acidosis depend on the magnitude of elevation in the arterial carbon dioxide partial pressures and the degree of compensation provided by secondary increases in the plasma concentrations of bicarbonate. It is estimated that the plasma concentrations of bicarbonate increase about 1 mEq·L^{-1} for every 10 mmHg increase in the arterial partial pressures of carbon dioxide above 40 mmHg (Table 17-4). This compensatory increase in the plasma concentrations of bicarbonate occurs within seconds of increases in the arterial partial pressures of carbon dioxide, so as to limit the magnitude of the decreases in arterial pH (Fig. 17-5).

The kidneys are also important for increasing the arterial concentrations of bicarbonate in response to accumulation of carbon dioxide in the plasma. For example, as the arterial partial pressures of carbon dioxide increase, renal tubular cells augment excretion of hydrogen ions, which results in increased reabsorption of bicarbonate into the circulation. In contrast to rapid increases in the arterial concentrations of bicarbonate produced by hydration of carbon dioxide, compensation provided by the kidneys operates slowly, requiring 48 hours to 72 hours for maximal responses to occur. Furthermore, because reabsorbed bicarbonate cannot easily cross lipid cell membranes, the pH of intracellular water is not altered to the same extent as is that of the blood or extracellular fluid. In contrast, because carbon dioxide crosses lipid cell membranes easily, bicarbonate produced by hydration of carbon dioxide has similar buffering effects in all body compartments. Eventually, renal tubular reabsorption of bicarbonate increases the plasma concentrations by about 2 mEq·L^{-1} for every 10 mmHg elevation in the arterial partial pressures of carbon dioxide (Table 17-4). Thus, the total increase in the arterial concentration of bicarbonate produced by hydration of carbon dioxide and renal reabsorption of bicarbonate is about 3 mEq·L^{-1} for every 10 mmHg increase in the arterial partial pressures of carbon dioxide above 40 mmHg (Table 17-4). Addition of bicarbonate to plasma at a time that chloride is being excreted with ammonium results in the characteristic hypochloremia of chronic respiratory acidosis.

Treatment of respiratory acidosis is by correction of the disorder responsible for hypoventilation. Mechanical ventilation of the lungs will be necessary when elevations of the arterial partial pressures of carbon dioxide are marked. It must be remembered that rapid lowering of chronically elevated arterial partial pressures of carbon dioxide by mechanical hyperventilation will reduce body stores of carbon dioxide more rapidly than the kidneys can produce corresponding reductions in the plasma concentrations of bicarbonate. The resulting metabolic alkalosis can result in neuromuscular irritability and excitation of the central nervous system, manifesting as seizures. Therefore, it is mandatory to reduce chronic elevations of the arterial partial pressures of carbon dioxide slowly, so as to permit sufficient time for renal tubular elimination of bicarbonate to occur.

Respiratory Acidosis and Associated Metabolic Acidosis

Respiratory acidosis may be complicated by metabolic acidosis when renal perfusion is decreased to the extent that reabsorption mechanisms via the kidneys are impaired (Fig. 17-3). For example, cardiac output and renal blood flow may be so reduced in patients with chronic obstructive airways disease and cor pulmonale that acidemia develops. When metabolic acidosis accompanies primary respiratory acidosis, the increases in plasma concentrations of bicarbonate are more than 3 mEq·L^{-1} for each 10 mmHg increase in the arterial partial pressures of carbon dioxide.

Respiratory Acidosis and Associated Metabolic Alkalosis

Respiratory acidosis complicated by metabolic alkalosis is suggested by increases in the plasma concentrations of bicarbonate that exceed 3 mEq·L^{-1} for every 10 mmHg increase in the arterial partial pressures of carbon dioxide (Fig. 17-2). Causes of complicating metabolic alkalosis include (1) acute hyperventilation of the lungs in the presence of chronic elevations of the arterial partial pressures of carbon dioxide, (2) decreased plasma concentrations of chloride, and (3) reduced body stores of potassium. For example, reductions in the plasma concentrations of chloride facilitate renal reabsorption of bicarbonate, leading to metabolic alkalosis. Decreased intracellular concentrations of potassium stimulate renal tubules to excrete hydrogen ions, which may produce metabolic alkalosis or aggravate a coexisting alkalosis due to a chloride deficiency. Treatment of metabolic alkalosis associated with respiratory acidosis is with avoidance or mechanical hyperventilation of the lungs and intravenous administration of potassium chloride.

RESPIRATORY ALKALOSIS

Respiratory alkalosis is always due to alveolar hyperventilation (Table 17-5). Reductions in the arterial partial pressures of carbon dioxide decrease the stimulus to breathe normally mediated by the carotid bodies and medullary chemoreceptors. Active transport of bicarbonate out of the central nervous system subsequently restores the pH of cerebrospinal fluid to normal. As a result, activity of the medullary chemoreceptors becomes normal and the volume of ventilation is increased, despite persistence of decreased arterial partial pressures of carbon dioxide. By the same mechanism, hyperventilation to 20 mmHg during anesthesia that lasts 2 hours results in the initiation of spontaneous ventilation at lower arterial partial pressures of carbon dioxide than were present before hyperventilation (Fig. 17-6).[4] This initiation of ventilation reflects a normal cerebrospinal fluid pH, which maintains ventilation via stimulation from the medullary chemoreceptors despite persistent hypocarbia. Likewise, continued hyperventilation, upon returning to sea level from altitude, reflects maintenance of ventilation by medullary chemoreceptors, exposed to a normal cerebrospinal fluid pH.

Three events occur simultaneously during hyperventilation to reduce the plasma concen-

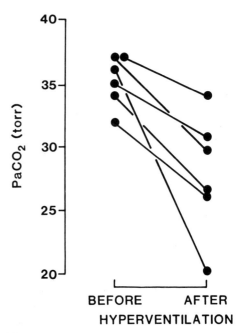

FIG. 17-6. The arterial partial pressure of carbon dioxide ($PaCO_2$) present during spontaneous ventilation before and after hyperventilation of the lungs to a $PaCO_2$ of 20 mmHg for 2 hours was measured in six adult patients. The presence of spontaneous ventilation at a lower $PaCO_2$ after passive hyperventilation of the lungs reflects restoration of cerebrospinal fluid pH to normal despite persistent reductions in arterial partial pressures of carbon dioxide. This is equivalent to resetting the threshold of the medullary chemoreceptors to carbon dioxide. (Data adapted from Edelist G, Osorio A. Postanesthetic initiation of spontaneous ventilation after passive hyperventilation. Anesthesiology 1969;31:22–7)

trations of bicarbonate and thus offset the increases in arterial pH that occur in response to lowering of the arterial partial pressures of carbon dioxide. First, as the arterial pH increases, blood and body buffers react with bicarbonate to produce carbon dioxide. The second mechanism for compensation is generation of lactic acid from glycolysis secondary to stimulation of phosphofructokinase, the rate-limiting enzyme for glycolysis; as the arterial pH increases, so does the activity of this enzyme. Both mechanisms operate rapidly to reduce the plasma concentrations of bicarbonate by about $1\ mEq\cdot L^{-1}$ for every 10 mmHg decrease in the

TABLE 17-5.   Causes of Alveolar Hyperventilation

Iatrogenic—mechanical or self-induced
Decreased barometric pressure
Central nervous system injury
Arterial hypoxemia
Pulmonary vascular disease
Hepatic disease
Sepsis
Elevations of body temperature
Pregnancy
Salicylate overdose

arterial partial pressures of carbon dioxide (Table 17-4). The third compensatory mechanism is increased renal tubular reabsorption of hydrogen ions, which becomes maximal by 48 hours to 72 hours and can reduce the plasma concentrations of bicarbonate by about 3 mEq· L^{-1} for every 10 mmHg reduction in the arterial partial pressures of carbon dioxide. Thus, reduction in the plasma concentrations of bicarbonate produced by these three mechanisms is about 5 mEq·L^{-1} for every 10 mmHg decrease in the arterial partial pressures of carbon dioxide (Table 17-4). This degree of metabolic compensation is sufficient to return arterial pH to normal in patients with chronic reductions in the arterial partial pressures of carbon dioxide (Table 17-2). Chloride is retained to offset declines in plasma concentrations of bicarbonate and maintain electroneutrality. Thus, mild hypokalemia and hyperchloremia characterize respiratory alkalosis.

Treatment of chronic respiratory alkalosis is directed at correcting underlying disorders responsible for hyperventilation. During anesthesia, this is most often accomplished by adjusting the ventilator to decrease alveolar ventilation. In addition, dead space can be added to the breathing circuit to increase rebreathing of exhaled gases that contain carbon dioxide. Carbon dioxide may also be delivered from a metered source to be added to the inspired gases in attempts to reestablish normal partial pressures of carbon dioxide in the arterial blood.

METABOLIC ACIDOSIS

Metabolic acidosis is characterized by decreases in arterial pH due to accumulation of nonvolatile acids, a frequent occurrence during major organ dysfunction (Table 17-6). Plasma bicarbonate concentrations decrease due to buffering of nonvolatile acids in the circulation.

Compensatory responses to metabolic acidosis are initiated in attempts to maintain a normal arterial pH despite reductions in the plasma concentrations of bicarbonate. For ex-

TABLE 17-6. Causes of Metabolic Acidosis

Anaerobic glycolysis due to decreased delivery of oxygenated blood to tissues

Cirrhosis of the liver with decreased removal of lactate

Diabetic ketoacidosis

Impaired excretion of hydrogen ions due to renal dysfunction

ample, there is enhanced excretion of hydrogen ions in the form of ammonium by renal tubular cells. Another compensatory mechanism is increased alveolar ventilation, mediated by hydrogen ion stimulation of the carotid bodies. Subsequent reductions in the arterial partial pressures of carbon dioxide are rapidly reflected as corresponding decreases in the partial pressures of carbon dioxide in the cerebrospinal fluid. As a result, the pH of the cerebrospinal fluid increases, leading to inhibition of the activity of the medullary chemoreceptors and blunting of the increases in ventilation produced by the carotid bodies. With time, the pH of the cerebrospinal fluid normalizes, reflecting active transport of bicarbonate into the central nervous system. Therefore, initial inhibition to ventilation provided by the medullary chemoreceptors is removed, and there are further, although delayed, increases in alveolar ventilation. A third compensatory mechanism is the use of buffers present in bone to neutralize nonvolatile acids present in the circulation. Indeed, chronic metabolic acidosis is commonly associated with loss of bone mass.

Metabolic acidosis will reduce the arterial partial pressures of carbon dioxide about 1 mmHg for every 1 mEq·L^{-1} reduction in the plasma concentrations of bicarbonate. When metabolic acidosis is complicated by respiratory acidosis, the magnitude of reduction in the arterial partial pressures of carbon dioxide is less than 1 mmHg for every 1 mEq·L^{-1} reduction in the plasma concentrations of bicarbonate. Patients with lactic acidosis hyperventilate to a greater degree than patients with other forms of metabolic acidosis such as ketoacidosis. This may reflect the brain's participation in lactic acid production, thereby directly exposing chemoreceptors to acid and obviating

TABLE 17-7. Calculation of the Dose of Sodium Bicarbonate to Treat Metabolic Acidosis

$$\frac{\text{Sodium}}{\text{Bicarbonate}} = \frac{\text{Body}}{\text{Weight}} \times \frac{\text{Plasma}}{\text{Bicarbonate}} \times \frac{\text{Extracellular Fluid}}{\text{Volume as a Fraction of}}$$
$$\text{Concentration} \qquad \text{Body Mass (0.2)}$$

Example: A previously healthy 30-year-old 80-kg man is successfully resuscitated following cardiopulmonary arrest due to an accidental overdose of a volatile anesthetic. Analysis of arterial blood drawn 3 minutes after resuscitation reveals (1) pH 7.20, (2) arterial partial pressure of carbon dioxide 60 mmHg, and (3) plasma bicarbonate concentration 16 mEq·L^{-1}. The normalized bicarbonate concentration corrected for the elevated partial pressure of carbon dioxide would be 26 mEq·L^{-1} (see Table 17-4). Therefore, the difference between the normalized and actual plasma concentration of bicarbonate is 10 mEq·L^{-1}.

The calculated dose of sodium bicarbonate to replace the bicarbonate deficit would be 160 mEq (80 kg × 10 mEq·L^{-1} × 0.2). About one-half of this calculated dose of sodium bicarbonate should be administered intravenously, followed by a repeat measurement of the arterial pH to evaluate the impact of therapy.

the need for transport of hydrogen ions from the periphery. In contrast to lactic acidosis, ketoacids produced by diabetics are only synthesized in the liver and must be transported across the blood-brain barrier before stimulation of ventilation occurs.

Metabolic acidosis is treated by removing the causes for the accumulation of nonvolatile acids in the circulation. Intravenous administration of sodium bicarbonate is indicated if metabolic acidosis is associated with myocardial depression or cardiac dysrhythmias. A commonly used formula to calculate doses of sodium bicarbonate to treat metabolic acidosis is based on deviation of the plasma concentrations of bicarbonate from normal values of 24 mEq·L^{-1}, the percent of body mass that is extracellular fluid (assumed to be 20 percent), and ideal body weight (Table 17-7). A useful approach is to administer about one-half the calculated dose of sodium bicarbonate, followed by repeat measurements of the arterial pH to evaluate the impact of therapy. Acute correction of chronic metabolic acidosis is associated with maintenance of ventilation at higher levels than anticipated, until the pH of cerebrospinal fluid is restored to normal.

METABOLIC ALKALOSIS

Metabolic alkalosis is characterized by loss of nonvolatile acid from extracellular fluid (Table 17-8). For example, vomiting and nasogastric suction result in loss of hydrochloric

acid, with subsequent metabolic alkalosis. Diuretics that inhibit reabsorption of sodium and potassium by proximal renal tubules result in increased excretion of potassium and hydrogen ions, leading to metabolic alkalosis. Another cause of metabolic alkalosis is overzealous intravenous administration of sodium bicarbonate to treat metabolic acidosis. Conversion of lactate present in intravenous fluid solutions to bicarbonate by the liver can also contribute to metabolic alkalosis.

Compensatory responses evoked by metabolic alkalosis include decreased renal tubular excretion of hydrogen ions and alveolar hypoventilation. Increases in the arterial partial pressures of carbon dioxide will initially stimulate medullary chemoreceptors and thus offset the compensatory effect of alveolar hypoventilation. With time, the pH of cerebrospinal fluid is normalized, and the volume of ventilation decreases, despite persistence of compensatory increases of the arterial partial pressures of carbon dioxide. Nevertheless, if the arterial partial pressures of carbon dioxide again increase, cerebrospinal fluid pH will fall,

TABLE 17-8. Causes of Metabolic Alkalosis

Vomiting
Nasogastric suction
Chloride wasting diarrhea
Villous adenoma of the colon
Diuretic therapy
Hyperaldosteronism
Cushing's syndrome
Exogenous corticosteroid administration
Bartter's syndrome
Alkali ingestion

and the same sequence will be repeated. Indeed, respiratory compensation for pure metabolic alkalosis is never complete. As a result, the arterial pH remains elevated in patients with primary metabolic alkalosis (Table 17-2).

Depletion of intravascular fluid volume is often the most important factor in the maintenance of metabolic alkalosis. Indeed, hypovolemia should be considered in postoperative patients who develop metabolic alkalosis. Since loss of potassium often parallels loss of sodium, hypokalemia is frequently present when hypovolemia complicates metabolic alkalosis. Skeletal muscle weakness also accompanies hypokalemia. Urinary chloride excretion is usually less than 10 $mEq \cdot L^{-1}$ in the presence of metabolic alkalosis associated with depletion of intravascular fluid volume.[5]

Treatment of metabolic acidosis is directed at resolution of those events responsible for the acid-base derangement, plus appropriate replacement of electrolytes. On occasion, intravenous infusion of hydrogen ions in the form of ammonium chloride or 0.1 N hydrochloric acid (no greater than 0.2 $mEq \cdot kg^{-1} \cdot hr^{-1}$) is used to facilitate the return of the arterial pH to near normal. Administration of acid requires insertion of a central venous catheter, as peripheral injections can causes sclerosis of veins and hemolysis.

REFERENCES

1. Narins RG, Emmett M. Simple and mixed acid-base disorders: A practical approach. Medicine 1980;59:161–87
2. Siggard-Andersen O. Blood acid base alignment nomogram. Scand J Clin Lab Invest 1963; 15: 211–7
3. Mitchell RA, Singer MM. Respiration and cerebrospinal fluid pH in metabolic acidosis and alkalosis. J Appl Physiol 1965;20:905–11
4. Edelist G, Osorio A. Postanesthetic initiation of spontaneous ventilation after passive hyperventilation. Anesthesiology 1969;31:222–7
5. Sherman RA, Eisinger RP. The use (and misuse) of urinary sodium and chloride measurements. JAMA 1982;247:3121–4

18

Diseases of the Nervous System

Perhaps in no other area of anesthesia is the selection of drugs, technique of ventilation of the lungs, and choice of monitors more important than in the care of patients with diseases involving the central nervous system. In addition, concepts for cerebral protection and resuscitation may assume unique importance in these patients.

INTRACRANIAL TUMORS

Intracranial tumors may be primary or metastatic. Primary tumors occur most often in patients between 40 and 60 years of age. The majority of intracranial tumors that occur in adults are supratentorial. Conversely, most intracranial tumors in children are infratentorial.

Signs and Symptoms

The major mechanism for the production of signs and symptoms by intracranial tumors is increased intracranial pressure. Symptoms of increased intracranial pressure include headache, nausea and vomiting, mental changes, and disturbances of consciousness. During the early stages of intracranial hypertension, it is common for symptoms to be most prominent in the early morning hours. Patients will be awakened by dull headaches followed by spontaneous vomiting. Symptoms will then subside until the next morning. Presumably, increases in the arterial partial pressures of carbon dioxide and the associated cerebral vasodilation that accompanies sleep produce an increase in intracranial contents that exceeds the limits of compensation and intracranial pressure increases (Fig. 18-1). Progressive increases in intracranial pressure eventually result in unexplained fatigue and drowsiness. Papilledema is often accompanied by visual disturbances. Generalized and/or focal seizures that appear in adult years suggest the presence of intracranial tumors. Systemic blood pressure is increased, in an attempt to maintain cerebral perfusion pressure in the presence of intracranial hypertension. As the blood pressure increases, there are corresponding reductions in heart rate, due to reflex activation of the carotid sinus by hypertension. Local tissue destruction by infiltration or compression leads to symptoms determined by the area of the brain involved. For example, mental and behavioral changes are prominent in patients who develop an intracranial tumor in the frontal cortex. Cerebral edema surrounding an expanding intracranial tumor, particularly one with a rapid growth rate, occurs frequently. This edema may contribute to loss of neurologic function, giving the false imppression

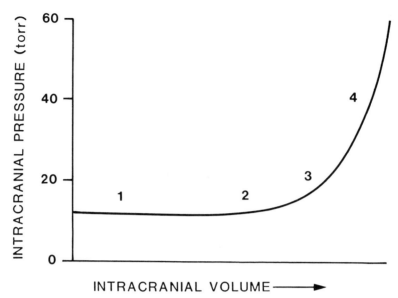

FIG. 18-1. Pressure-volume compliance curves depict the impact of increasing intracranial volume on intracranial pressure. As volume increases from point 1 to point 2 on the curve, the pressure does not increase, since cerebrospinal fluid is shifted from the cranium into the spinal subarachnoid space. Patients with intracranial tumors but between points 1 and 2 on the compliance curve are unlikely to manifest clinical symptoms of increased intracranial pressure. Patients who are on the rising portion of the pressure-volume compliance curve (3) can no longer compensate for increases in volume and pressure begins to increase. Clinical symptoms of elevated intracranial pressure are likely. Additional elevations in volume at this point (3), as produced by increased cerebral blood flow during anesthesia, can precipitate abrupt rises in intracranial pressure (4).

that the tumor is large and highly destructive. The presence of edema around an intracranial tumor is thought to result from increased permeability of tumor capillaries, which allows protein and fluid to penetrate into adjacent normal brain tissues. This abnormal permeability is the basis for isotope uptake observed on the brain scan and for the lucency of tissues on computed tomography.

Intracranial tumors may result in displacement of the brain and compression of neural tissues at distant sites. The most common examples are supratentorial tumors that lead to herniation of the uncus of the temporal lobe through the incisura of the tentorium. This results in compression of the oculomotor nerve at the tentorial notch and causes the homolateral pupil to be dilated and unreactive. Apnea and unconsciousness follow if the midbrain is compressed. Compression of the posterior cerebral artery against the edge of the tentorium

may lead to occipital lobe infarction and contralateral hemianopia. Compression of the cerebral peduncle produces contralateral hemiplegia. A posterior fossa tumor leads to obstruction of the normal flow of cerebrospinal fluid, and resulting increases in intracranial pressure predispose to herniation of the cerebellar tonsils through the foramen magnum, which manifests as a decreased level of consciousness and slow respiratory rate.

Type of Intracranial Tumors

The frequency of intracranial tumors is estimated to be about 5 per 100,000 population.[1] Gliomas constitute the majority of these tumors (Table 18-1).[1] The frequency of metastatic tu-

TABLE 18-1. Types and Incidence of Brain Tumors

Tumor Type	Approximate Incidence (% of Total)
Gliomas	
Glioblastoma	10–12
Astrocytoma	6–10
Medulloblastoma	3–4
Meningioma	13–18
Pituitary adenoma	8–18
Acoustic neuroma	8–9
Metastatic	4

mors is probably much higher than reported, since many of these lesions are never detected.

GLIOBLASTOMAS

Glioblastomas are highly malignant and infiltrative intracranial tumors, which most often arise in a cerebral hemisphere. Areas of necrosis and surrounding cerebral edema give a picture of patchy density on computed tomography. Patients with glioblastomas have a poor prognosis, with an average survival time less than 6 months after the diagnosis.

ASTROCYTOMAS

Astrocytomas begin as slow-growing lesions in cerebral hemispheres, leading to symptoms of increased intracranial pressure. These tumors occur more frequently in children than adults. Treatment is surgical excision, often combined with radiotherapy. Astrocytomas that occur in pediatric patients are unlikely to recur after surgical excision. Conversely, astrocytomas that develop in adults tend to recur.

MEDULLOBLASTOMAS

Medulloblastomas are the most common intracranial tumors occurring in children. These tumors typically arise in the cerebellum. Treatment with combination therapy that includes surgical excision, radiation, and che-

motherapy has improved the survival of patients with these tumors.

MENINGIOMAS

Meningiomas are slow-growing benign intracranial tumors that most often originate from arachnoidal cells. The great vascularity of these tumors accounts for the ease with which they are visualized on isotope brain scans. Meningiomas often infiltrate the skull and provoke osteoblastic activity, which is evident on the radiograph of the skull. These tumors can occur at any age but are most frequently found in middle-aged women. Treatment is surgical removal and the prognosis is good.

ANTERIOR PITUITARY TUMORS

Anterior pituitary tumors account for 8 percent to 18 percent of all intracranial tumors. Nearly 80 percent of anterior pituitary tumors that occur in adults can be classified as chromophobe adenomas. Corresponding tumors in children are designated a craniopharyngiomas. Basophilic and eosinophilic adenomas constitute the remaining categories of anterior pituitary tumors. Classification of pituitary adenomas is based on the staining properties of granules present in the cells of the tumor.

CHROMOPHOBE ADENOMAS

Chromophobe adenomas rarely secrete hormones. Instead, these tumors produce panhypopituitarism by virtue of expansion and compression of normal anterior pituitary tissue. Signs and symptoms of hormone deficiency that accompany panhypopituitarism due to chromophobe adenomas are variable and often unpredictable (see Chapter 23). In addition, suprasellar extension of these adenomas characteristically produces bitemporal hemianopia due to compression of the optic chiasm. Evidence of increased intracranial pressure can occur if the adenoma interferes with drainage of cerebrospinal fluid. Pressure on the floor of the third ventricle or on the hypothalamus due to extension of these tumors can result in decreased levels of consciousness. Finally, chromophobe adenomas of the anterior pituitary may be part of an inherited syndrome, characterized by multiple endocrine neoplasia that also includes abnormalities in the thyroid gland, parathyroid glands, and adrenal cortex (see Chapter 23).

Basophilic Adenomas. Basophilic adenomas frequently produce adrenocorticotrophic hormone and are common causes of hyperadrenocorticism. Signs and symptoms related to visual field defects or increases in intracranial pressure are rare, as these adenomas do not extend beyond the confines of the sella turcica until late in their course.

Eosinophilic Adenomas. Eosinophilic adenomas are likely to secrete growth hormone, resulting in acromegaly (see Chapter 23).

Treatment. Surgical excision by a transfrontal or transphenoidal approach and destruction by radiotherapy are the most frequent treatments used for anterior pituitary tumors. Potential endocrine deficiencies, particularly hypoadrenocorticism, must be recognized when preparing patients for anesthesia and surgery (see Chapter 23).

An alternative primary treatment is with the dopaminergic agonist bromocriptine.[2] Bromocriptine has been found to control hypersecretion of growth hormone and/or prolactin by anterior pituitary tumors. Furthermore, bromocriptine may decrease the size of these tumors, leading to reversal of symptoms due to suprasellar extension of tumor. Therefore, it is conceivable that treatment with bromocriptine will replace surgical excision in selected patients.

ACOUSTIC NEUROMAS

Acoustic neuromas are benign neurofibromas of the 8th cranial nerve. These tumors arise within the internal auditory meatus, where they can produce erosion and widening of the auditory canal. Initial manifestations of acoustic neuromas are progressive unilateral nerve deafness. As tumors grow, they can exert pressure on the cerebellum, resulting in ataxia. The prognosis of patients with this diagnosis is good after successful surgical excision.

METASTATIC INTRACRANIAL TUMORS

Metastatic intracranial tumors are most often from primary sites in the lung and breast. Malignant melanomas, hypernephromas, and intestinal carcinomas are also likely to metastasize to the central nervous system. Metastatic intracranial tumors are the likely diagnosis when diagnostic tests reveal the presence of more than one lesion. Excision of accessible metastatic intracranial tumors can reduce symptoms of increased intracranial pressure and prolong the life of patients. Furthermore, benign primary intracranial tumors can co-exist with carcinomas elsewhere, with the most frequent example being the association of meningiomas and carcinoma of the breast.

Diagnosis

In addition to the classic symptoms and findings on neurologic examination, the presence of intracranial tumors can be substantiated by specific diagnositic evaluations, which include computed tomography, radiography of the skull, angiography, pneumoencephalography, and the electroencephalogram.

COMPUTED TOMOGRAPHY

Computed tomography is the best method for establishing the diagnosis of intracranial tumors. However, it may be difficult to differentiate intracranial tumors from cerebral infarctions on computed tomography.

RADIOGRAPHY OF THE SKULL

Radiography of the skull may reveal enlargement of the sella turcica in the presence of pituitary adenomas, or widening of the internal auditory meatus due to acoustic neuromas. Osteoblastic lesions visible on radiography of the skull suggest the presence of a metastatic process. Osteoblastic activity may be evident in patients with meningiomas.

ANGIOGRAPHY

Angiography is most valuable for documentation of the vascular supply of intracranial tumors, so as to facilitate subsequent surgical excision.

PNEUMOENCEPHALOGRAPHY

Pneumoencephalography is rarely used, as computed tomography is noninvasive and less hazardous. Nevertheless, pneumoencephalography may be necessary to establish the practicality of a transphenoidal approach to parasellar tumors.

ELECTROENCEPHALOGRAM

Electroencephalography is most helpful for the initial diagnosis of intracranial tumors. The value of the electroencephalogram is for determining the epileptogenic nature of intracranial tumors.

MANAGEMENT OF ANESTHESIA FOR REMOVAL OF INTRACRANIAL TUMORS

Management of anesthesia for removal of intracranial tumors mandates a thorough understanding of pressure-volume compliance curves, monitoring of intracranial pressure, methods to decrease intracranial pressure, and

determinants of cerebral blood flow. Indeed, management of these patients in the perioperative period is based on maintenance of intracranial pressure in a normal range, and recognition that autoregulation of cerebral blood flow may be impaired.

Pressure-Volume Compliance Curves

Pressure-volume compliance curves reflect changes produced by expanding intracranial tumors (Fig. 18-1). These curves plot changes in intracranial pressure that accompany alterations in intracranial volume produced by tumors. As tumors gradually enlarge, cerebrospinal fluid in the cranium is shifted into the spinal subarachnoid space, thus preventing an increase in intracranial pressure above its normal value of about 15 mmHg. In addition, increased absorption of cerebrospinal fluid attenuates any increase in pressure that would be produced by expanding tumors. At this stage, there are minimal clinical symptoms suggestive of intracranial tumors. Eventually, a point is reached on pressure-volume compliance curves, where even small increases in intracranial volume produced by expanding tumors result in marked increases in the intracranial pressure. It is at this point on pressure-volume compliance curves that anesthetic drugs and techniques that affect cerebral blood volume can adversely and abruptly increase intracranial pressure.

Marked increases in intracranial pressure can interfere with delivery of adequate blood flow to the brain. For example, cerebral perfusion pressure is determined by the difference between mean arterial pressure and right atrial pressure. When intracranial pressure is greater than right atrial pressure, the cerebral perfusion pressure is determined by the difference between mean arterial pressure and intracranial pressure. Should cerebral perfusion pressure be substantially reduced because of increased intracranial pressure, there are compensatory increases in blood pressure in attempts to restore perfusion pressure and thus maintain cerebral blood flow. Ultimately, this compensatory mechanism fails, and cerebral ischemia occurs.

Monitoring Intracranial Pressure

Intracranial pressure can be continuously monitored by catheters placed through a burr hole into a cerebral ventricle, or by transducers placed on the surface of the brain (Richmond bolt). A normal intracranial pressure wave is pulsatile and varies with cardiac impulses and respiration. The mean pressure should remain below 15 mmHg. The importance of monitoring intracranial pressure in patients with space-occupying intracranial tumors is emphasized by the observation that alterations in intracranial pressure may not be accompanied by changes in the neurologic examination or vital signs. Furthermore, the first evidence of hazardous elevations in intracranial pressure in unresponsive patients may be sudden bilateral pupillary dilation, associated with herniation of the brain stem through the foramen magnum. Delay of treatment to reduce intracranial pressure until these signs appear may be unrewarding, as irreversible brain damage is likely.

PLATEAU WAVES

Abrupt increases in intracranial pressure observed during continuous monitoring are known as plateau waves (Fig. 18-2).[3] Characteristically, intracranial pressure increases from normal or near normal levels to as high as 100 mmHg. During these increases, patients often become overtly symptomatic, and spontaneous hyperventilation can occur. Typically, plateau waves last 10 minutes to 20 minutes, after which intracranial pressure rapidly decreases to levels below that present before the onset of the wave. The mechanism for these sudden increases is unknown. It is thought, however, that abrupt increases in intracranial

blood volume are responsible. This increased blood volume eventually initiates decreases in cerebrospinal fluid volume, leading to subsequent reductions in intracranial pressure.

CAUSES OF PLATEAU WAVES

Events that can be identified as initiating causes for plateau waves include anxiety, painful stimulation, and the induction of anesthesia. Indeed, in normal patients anxiety and painful stimulation can elicit large increases in oxygen uptake and cerebral blood flow. This increase, in the presence of intracranial tumors, can lead to abrupt elevations of intracranial pressure. Therefore, noxious stimuli should be avoided in patients with intracranial tumors, regardless of the level of consciousness. Hence, the liberal use of analgesics to avoid pain even in the unresponsive patient is indicated. Obviously, support of ventilation to avoid hypercarbia secondary to drug-induced depression of ventilation will be necessary when opioids are used. Likewise, establishment of a depth of anesthesia sufficient to block the response to laryngoscopy or noxious surgical stimulation is an important concept.

Methods to Decrease Intracranial Pressure

Methods to decrease intracranial pressure include posture, hyperventilation of the lungs; cerebrospinal fluid drainage; and administration of hyperosmotic drugs, diuretics, corticosteroids, and barbiturates. It is not possible to identify reliably the level of intracranial pressure in an individual patient that can interfere with regional cerebral blood flow. Therefore, a frequent recommendation is to treat sustained elevations of intracranial pressure that exceed 20 mmHg. Treatment may be indicated when intracranial pressure is less than 20 mmHg if the appearance of occasional plateau waves suggests low intracranial compliance.

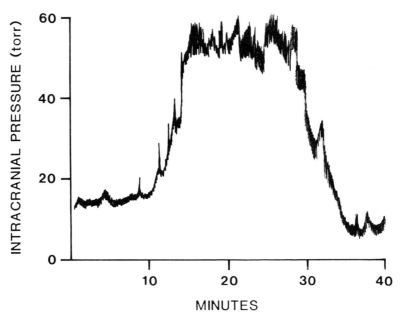

FIG. 18-2. Schematic diagram of a plateau wave. The rise in intracranial pressure typically occurs abruptly, from normal or near normal pressures. Plateau waves persist for 10 minutes to 20 minutes, followed by rapid reductions in pressure, often to levels below those present before the onset of the wave.

POSTURE

Posture is important for assuring optimal venous drainage from the brain. For example, elevation of the head to about 30 degrees will encourage venous outflow from the brain and lower intracranial pressure, if cerebrospinal fluid pathways are patent. It should also be appreciated that extreme flexion or rotation of the head can obstruct the jugular veins and restrict venous outflow from the brain. The head-down position is to be avoided, as this position can markedly increase intracranial pressure.

HYPERVENTILATION

Hyperventilation of the lungs is an effective and rapid method to lower intracranial pressure. In adults, the recommendation is to maintain the arterial partial pressures of carbon dioxide between 25 mmHg and 30 mmHg. A theoretical risk of extreme hyperventilation of the lungs is reduction in cerebral blood flow to the point that cerebral ischemia occurs.

Nevertheless, there is no evidence that cerebral ischemia occurs when the arterial partial pressures of carbon dioxide are above 20 mmHg.[4] Nevertheless, since no additional beneficial therapeutic effect is demonstrable by lowering the arterial partial pressures of carbon dioxide to extremely low levels, it seems reasonable to strive to achieve a level of 25 mmHg to 30 mmHg when treating elevations of intracranial pressure. The duration of the efficacy of hyperventilation of the lungs for reducing intracranial pressure is unknown. In volunteers, however, the effect of hyperventilation wanes with time, and cerebral blood flow returns to normal after about 6 hours.[5]

In children, it may be appropriate to instigate more aggressive hyperventilation of the lungs than recommended for adults, so as to maintain the arterial partial pressures of carbon dioxide between 20 mmHg and 25 mmHg. Presumably, the increased therapeutic benefit of this lower arterial partial pressure of carbon dioxide reflects the relatively high cerebral blood flow that may be present in children, particularly in the presence of acute head injury. Also, in contrast to adults, there is a suggestion that hyperventilation of the lungs in children is associated with sustained reductions in cerebral blood flow beyond 6 hours.

CEREBROSPINAL FLUID DRAINAGE

Cerebrospinal fluid drainage, either from the lateral cerebral ventricles or lumbar subarachnoid space, is an effective method for reducing intracranial volume and pressure. Lumbar drainage in patients with increased intracranial pressure is not recommended, since herniation of the cerebellum through the foramen magnum might occur. Therefore, lumbar drainage is usually reserved for patients undergoing operations on the pituitary gland or surgery for treatment of intracranial aneurysms, when surgical exposure may be difficult.

HYPEROSMOTIC DRUGS

Hyperosmotic drugs, such as mannitol and urea, are important and effective methods for reducing intracranial pressure. These drugs produce transient increases in the osmolarity of plasma, which acts to draw water from tissues, including the brain. The purpose of therapy with hyperosmotic drugs is not to dehydrate the patient, but rather to draw fluid from the brain, along an osmotic gradient. As such, it is an error not to replace some of the intravascular fluid lost via the kidneys (see the section Fluid Therapy). Failure to replace intravascular fluid volume can result in hypotension and jeopardize maintenance of adequate cerebral perfusion pressures. Likewise, urinary loss of electrolytes, particularly potassium, may require careful monitoring and replacement. It is also important to recognize that an intact blood-brain barrier is necessary for mannitol or urea to exert their maximum beneficial effects on brain size. If the blood-brain barrier is disrupted, these drugs may pass into the brain and cause cerebral edema, with an increase in brain size. The brain eventually adapts to sustained elevations in plasma osmolarity, such that chronic use of hyperosmotic drugs is likely to become less effective.

Mannitol. Mannitol is administered intravenously in doses of 0.25 g·kg^{-1} to 1.0 g·kg^{-1} over 15 minutes to 30 minutes. There is little difference in intracranial pressure lowering effects with this dose range, but higher doses may last longer.[6] Smaller doses require less volume for administration, and the risk of serum hyperosmolarity is avoided. Using this dose range of mannitol, it is estimated that 100 ml of water is removed from the brain. After administration, a decrease in intracranial pressure is seen within 30 minutes, and maximum effects occur within 1 hour to 2 hours. Urine output can reach 1 L to 2 L within 1 hour after starting the administration of mannitol. Appropriate infusion of crystalloid and colloid solutions is often necessary to prevent adverse changes in plasma concentrations of electrolytes and intravascular fluid volume due to the brisk diuresis. Conversely, mannitol can initially increase intravascular fluid volume, emphasizing the need to monitor carefully those patients with severe intracranial hypertension or limited cardiac reserve. Mannitol also has direct vascular vasodilating properties that can contribute to increased cerebral blood volume and intracranial pressure. The duration of the hyperosmotic effect of mannitol is about 6 hours. It is important to note that mannitol is not associated with a high incidence of rebound increases in intracranial pressure after this time. Furthermore, the incidence of venous thrombosis after the administration of mannitol is low.

Urea. Urea is administered intravenously in doses of 1 g·kg^{-1} to 1.5 g·kg^{-1} over a 15 minute to 30 minute period. Initial decreases in intracranial pressure begin about 30 minutes after administration. Rebound increases in intracranial pressure occur after 3 hours to 7 hours, and last about 12 hours, before once again beginning to decline slowly. Rebound hypertension reflects penetration of urea molecules into the brain and subsequent passage of water along a concentration gradient when blood urea levels begin to decrease. Another disadvantage of urea is a high incidence of venous thrombosis and the possibility of tissue necrosis, should extravasation of the urea occur.

DIURETICS

Diuretics, particularly furosemide and ethacrynic acid, have been used in attempts to promote reductions in intracranial pressure. Diuretics are particularly useful when there is evidence of increased intravascular fluid volume and pulmonary edema. In this instance, promotion of diuresis and systemic dehydration can improve arterial oxygenation, with concomitant reductions in intracranial pressure.

Furosemide. Furosemide (1 mg·kg^{-1}), administered intravenously to patients with normal intracranial pressure undergoing craniotomy for treatment of intracranial tumors or aneurysms, is more effective in reducing intracranial pressure than is mannitol (1 g·kg^{-1})

(Fig. 18-3).[7] Furosemide does not significantly alter plasma osmolarity or concentrations of potassium. Conversely, mannitol increases plasma osmolarity and plasma concentrations of potassium are decreased. Based on these observations, it has been recommended that furosemide replace mannitol for treatment of patients with increased intracranial pressure, particularly if the blood-brain barrier is altered, or if there is increased water content of the lungs.[7]

CORTICOSTEROIDS

Corticosteroids are effective in lowering increased intracranial pressure due to localized cerebral edema that develops around intracranial tumors. The drugs most frequently

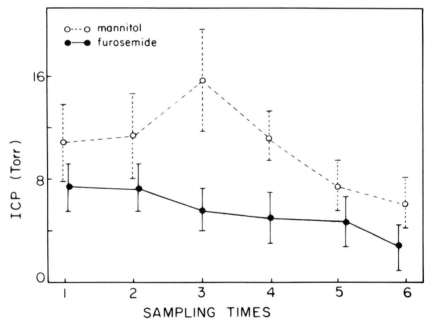

FIG. 18-3. Control of intracranial pressure (mean ± SE) was measured preoperatively (1) and after the induction of anesthesia (2) in 20 adult patients scheduled for removal of intracranial tumors. Mannitol (1 g·kg^{-1}) or furosemide (1 mg·kg^{-1}) was then given in random sequence as a rapid intravenous injection at the time of the skin incision. Intracranial pressure was subsequently measured at the onset of diuresis (3), peak diuresis (4), completion of diuresis (5), and postoperatively (6). Intracranial pressure was increased at the onset of mannitol-induced diuresis (3). In contrast, intracranial pressure was reduced at all measurement times after administration of furosemide. (Cottrell JE, Robustelli A, Post K, Turndorf H. Furosemide- and mannitol-induced changes in intracranial pressure and serum osmolality and electrolytes. Anesthesiology 1977;47:28–30)

used are dexamethasone or methylprednisolone. The mechanism for the beneficial effect of corticosteroids is not known but may involve stabilization of capillary membranes and/or reductions in the production of cerebrospinal fluid. Patients with metastatic intracranial tumors and glioblastomas respond best to corticosteroids. Improvement in neurologic status and disappearance of such signs of increased intracranial pressure as headache or nausea and vomiting frequently occur within 12 hours to 36 hours after initiating treatment with corticosteroids. Furthermore, mortality after removal of supratentorial intracranial tumors in patients treated with dexamethasone before and after surgery is decreased, compared with patients not receiving corticosteroids. Likewise, mortality after acute head injury is decreased in patients treated with corticosteroids. Blood glucose concentrations should be monitored in patients treated with corticosteroids. Finally, the incidence of pulmonary infections or gastrointestinal hemorrhage has not been shown to be increased by short-term use of corticosteroids.

BARBITURATES

Barbiturates administered in high doses are particularly effective in treating increased intracranial pressure that develops after acute head injury, especially when other more traditional methods of treatment have failed (see the section Head Injury).

Determinants of Cerebral Blood Flow

Determinants of cerebral blood flow include the (1) arterial partial pressures of carbon dioxide, (2) arterial partial pressures of oxygen, (3) arterial blood pressure and autoregulation, (4) venous blood pressure, and (5) anesthetic drugs and techniques. Cerebral blood vessels receive innervation from the autonomic nervous system, but the impact on cerebral blood flow is minimal. For example, it is estimated that neurogenic control can alter cerebral blood flow by only 5 percent to 10 percent.[8] Furthermore, stellate ganglion block does not significantly increase cerebral blood flow.

ARTERIAL PARTIAL PRESSURES OF CARBON DIOXIDE

Variations in the arterial partial pressures of carbon dioxide produce corresponding changes in cerebral blood flow (Fig. 18-4). As a guideline, cerebral blood flow (normal = 50 ml·100 g^{-1}·min^{-1}) increases 1 ml·100 g^{-1}·min^{-1} for each 1 mmHg increase in the arterial partial pressures of carbon dioxide above 40 mmHg. A similar reduction in cerebral blood flow occurs during hypocarbia, such that cerebral blood flow is reduced about 50 percent when the arterial partial pressures of carbon dioxide are 20 mmHg. The impact of the arterial partial pressure of carbon dioxode on cerebral blood flow is mediated by pH variations in the cerebrospinal fluid around and inside the walls of arterioles. A decrease in pH causes intense cerebral vasodilation, and an increased pH causes vasoconstriction. Corresponding changes in resistance to blood flow produce predictable effects on cerebral blood flow.

The ability of hypocapnia to lower cerebral blood flow and reduce intracranial pressure is the basis for modern neuroanesthesia. Concern that cerebral hypoxia due to vasoconstriction can occur when the arterial partial pressures of carbon dioxide are lowered below 20 mmHg has not been substantiated.[4] Nevertheless, because there is no evidence of increased therapeutic benefit at extremely low partial pressures, it seems reasonable to recommend maintaining the arterial partial pressures of carbon dioxide between 25 mmHg and 30 mmHg during anesthesia for removal of intracranial tumors.

The long-term value of hypocapnia for reducing intracranial pressure is offset by return of cerebrospinal fluid pH to normal, permitting increases in cerebral blood flow despite persistent reductions in the arterial partial pressures of carbon dioxide.[5] This adaptive change, which reflects active transport of bicarbonate ions into or from the cerebrospinal fluid, requires about 6 hours to return the pH to normal.

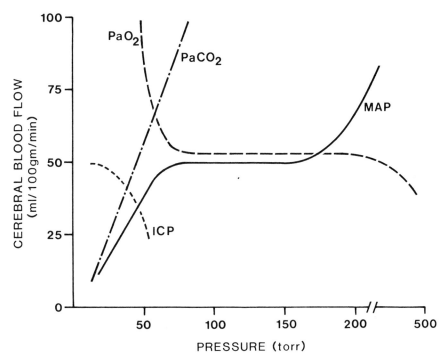

FIG. 18-4. Schematic depiction of the impact of intracranial pressure (ICP), arterial partial pressure of oxygen (PaO_2), arterial partial pressure of carbon dioxide ($PaCO_2$), and mean arterial partial pressure (MAP) on cerebral blood flow.

When adaptation to the effects of carbon dioxide has occurred, it is crucial to avoid arterial hypoxemia and to provide effective sedation and analgesia with appropriate drugs.

The influence of carbon dioxide on local cerebral blood flow may be altered by acidosis, which often surrounds intracranial tumors. For example, acid metabolites from tumors diffuse into adjacent tissues, causing maximal vasodilation and increased blood flow around the tumors. These vessels have lost their responsiveness to carbon dioxide, and vasomotor paralysis is present. Increased blood flow in the area of intracranial tumors has been termed luxury perfusion.[8] When the arterial partial pressures of carbon dioxide are allowed to increase, blood flow will be shunted away from tumors. This reflects vasodilation of normal vessels but no change in vessels already maximally dilated, so that the pressure gradient for blood flow tends to be reversed. This phenomenon has been termed the intracerebral steal

syndrome. Conversely, hypocapnia constricts normal vessels, whereas those manifesting vasomotor paralysis are not altered, leading to a change in pressure gradients that favor flow to acidotic areas surrounding tumors. This response is referred to as the inverse steal or Robin Hood phenomenon. The relative importance of these phenomena is unknown, but it is likely that their occurrence is rare. In the absence of regional cerebral blood flow measurements, it is not known if an individual patient will respond physiologically or paradoxically to alterations in the arterial partial pressures of carbon dioxide. Therefore, the logic of treating focal cerebral ischemia with deliberate hypoventilation or hyperventilation of the lungs is questionable. The prudent approach would be to maintain normal or moderately reduced arterial partial pressures of carbon dioxide when cerebral steal responses are a consideration. If a reduction in intracranial pressure is the goal, the recommendation remains to keep the arterial partial pressures of carbon dioxide between 25 mmHg and 30 mmHg. Inhaled anesthetics do not alter responsiveness of the cerebral circulation to changes in the arterial partial pressures of carbon dioxide.

ARTERIAL PARTIAL PRESSURES OF OXYGEN

Decreases in the arterial partial pressures of oxygen do not produce significant increases in cerebral blood flow until a threshold value of about 50 mmHg is reached (Fig. 18-4).[9] Below this threshold, there is abrupt cerebral vasodilation, and cerebral blood flow increases. Furthermore, the combination of arterial hypoxemia and hypercarbia exerts synergistic effects with an elevation in cerebral blood flow that exceeds the increase that would be produced by either factor alone.

ARTERIAL BLOOD PRESSURE AND AUTOREGULATION

The ability of the brain to maintain cerebral blood flow at a constant level despite changes in mean arterial pressure is known as autoregulation (Fig. 18-4). Autoregulation is an active vascular response, characterized by arterial constriction when the distending blood pressure is increased, and arterial dilation in response to a reduction in the blood pressure. Upper and lower limits of mean arterial pressure with maintenance of autoregulation have been defined. For example, in normotensive patients, the lower limit of mean arterial pressure associated with autoregulation is about 60 mmHg. Below this threshold, cerebral blood flow decreases, and becomes directly related to mean arterial pressure. Indeed, at mean arterial pressures of 40 mmHg to 55 mmHg, symptoms of cerebral ischemia appear, in the form of nausea, dizziness, and slow cerebration. Autoregulation of cerebral blood flow also has an upper limit, above which flow becomes directly proportional to the mean arterial pressure. This upper limit of autoregulation in normotensive patients is a mean arterial

pressure of about 150 mmHg. Above this threshold, cerebral blood flow increases, causing an overdistention of the walls of cerebral blood vessels. As a result, fluid is forced across vessel walls into brain tissue, producing cerebral edema.[10]

Autoregulation of cerebral blood flow is altered in the presence of chronic hypertension. Specifically, the autoregulation curve is displaced to the right, such that higher mean arterial pressures are tolerated before cerebral blood flow becomes pressure dependent. However, adaptation of cerebral vessels to increased blood pressures requires 1 month to 2 months. Indeed, acute hypertension, as seen in children with glomerulonephritis or in patients with toxemia of pregnancy, often produces signs of central nervous system dysfunction at levels of mean arterial pressure tolerated by patients who are chronically hypertensive. Likewise, acute hypertensive episodes associated with stimulation of laryngoscopy or surgery may cause a breakthrough of autoregulation. The lower limit of autoregulation is also shifted upward in chronically hypertensive patients, such that these patients do not tolerate acute blood pressure reductions to the same low levels as do normotensive patients. After gradual reductions in blood pressure occur using antihypertensive therapy, however, the tolerance of the brain to hypotension may improve, as the autoregulation curve shifts back toward its original position.[10]

Autoregulation of cerebral blood flow may be lost or impaired in a variety of conditions, including the presence of intracranial tumors or head trauma and the administration of volatile anesthetics. The loss of autoregulation in blood vessels that surround intracranial tumors reflect acidosis leading to maximum vasodilation, such that blood flow becomes pressure dependent.

In animals, autoregulation of cerebral blood flow in response to changes in blood pressure is retained during administration of 1 MAC isoflurane but not halothane (Fig. 18-5).[11] It is speculated that loss of autoregulation during administration of halothane is responsible for the greater brain swelling seen in animals anesthetized with this drug compared with isoflurane.

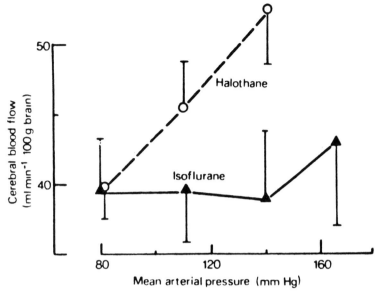

FIG. 18-5. In animals, autoregulation of cerebral blood flow in response to changes in blood pressure is retained during administration of 1 MAC isoflurane but not halothane. (Eger EI. Pharmacology of isoflurane. Br J Anaesth 1984;56:71S–99S)

VENOUS BLOOD PRESSURE

Venous blood pressure is usually low in the supine or standing position, such that mean arterial pressure is the predominant determinant of cerebral perfusion pressure. An increase in cerebral blood flow may increase pressure in cerebral veins, due to the rigid bony orifices that surround the venous exits from the cranium. Furthermore, rigidity of dural layers surrounding intracranial venous sinuses may result in increased venous pressure when cerebral blood flow is increased. An increase in central venous pressure is directly transmitted to intracranial veins. The impact of increased central venous pressure on cerebral perfusion pressure and intracranial pressure must be appreciated when considering the use of positive airway pressure during intracranial surgery or in patients with increased intracranial pressure. Indeed, the use of positive end-expiratory pressure may produce adverse elevations in intracranial pressure and thus decrease cerebral perfusion pressure in patients with intracranial tumors.[6,12] Finally, elevated venous pressure can contribute to increased bleeding during intracranial surgery.

ANESTHETIC DRUGS

Volatile anesthetics administered during normocapnia in concentrations above 0.6 MAC are potent cerebral vasodilators and produce dose-dependent increases in cerebral blood flow (Fig. 18-6).[13] These drug-induced increases in cerebral blood flow are greatest with halothane, intermediate with enflurane, and least for isoflurane and occur despite concomitant reductions in cerebral metabolic oxygen requirements. Ketamine is also a potent cerebral vasodilator. Normally, the tendency for intracranial pressure to increase in response to elevations in cerebral blood flow is prevented by displacement of cerebrospinal fluid from the cranium. In patients with intracranial tu-

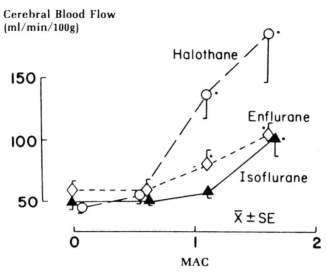

Cerebral Blood Flow (ml/min/100g)

FIG. 18-6. Volatile anesthetics administered during normocapnia in concentrations above 0.6 MAC are potent cerebral vasodilators and produce dose-dependent increases in cerebral blood flow. These drug-induced increases in cerebral blood flow are greatest with halothane, intermediate with enflurane and least for isoflurane. (Eger EI. Isoflurane (Forane). A Compendium and Reference. Anaquest, A Division of BOC, Inc., Madison, WI, 1986;1–160)

mors, however, this compensatory mechanism may fail, such that drug-induced increases in cerebral blood flow produce abrupt elevations of intracranial pressure. In contrast to volatile anesthetics and ketamine, barbiturates and opioids are classified as cerebral vasoconstrictors. Drugs that produce cerebral vasoconstriction predictably reduce cerebral blood flow.

HALOTHANE

Halothane produces dose-related elevations in cerebral blood flow. For example, 0.6 MAC halothane produces minimal changes in cerebral blood flow and intracranial pressure, while 1.1 MAC concentrations of halothane can increase cerebral blood flow nearly three-fold (Fig. 18-6).[13] Introduction of halothane into the inspired gases, simultaneously with the initiation of mechanical hyperventilation of the lungs sufficient to lower the arterial partial pressures of carbon dioxide to about 25 mmHg, does not reliably prevent drug-induced elevations in cerebral blood flow and intracranial pressure in patients with intracranial tu-

mors.[14] Conversely, establishment of hypocarbia for 10 minutes before adding halothane to the inspired gases prevents increases in intracranial pressure. Presumably, prior hypocarbia attenuates or blocks the cerebral vasodilating effects of halothane, which lead to increased cerebral blood flow.

Animals exposed to halothane demonstrate time-dependent decreases in the previously elevated cerebral blood flow, beginning after about 30 minutes and reaching predrug levels after 150 minutes.[15] This normalization of cerebral blood flow reflects concomitant increases in cerebral vascular resistance.

ENFLURANE

Enflurane, like halothane, can cause abrupt increases in the intracranial pressure of patients with intracranial tumors. As with halothane, hypocarbia produced simultaneously with the administration of enflurane does not always protect against an increase in the intracranial pressure. In addition to increased cerebral blood flow, this increased intracranial pressure may reflect the ability of enflurane to increase both the rate of production and resistance to reabsorption of cerebrospinal fluid.[16] Another disadvantage of enflurane is the unique ability of this volatile anesthetic to produce central nervous system seizure activity.[17]

ISOFLURANE

Isoflurane has been shown to increase intracranial pressure when administered to patients with intracranial tumors who are ventilated with this drug at normocarbia.[18] In contrast to halothane, the initiation of hyperventilation of the lungs, simultaneously with the introduction of isoflurane into the inspired gases, prevents the increase in intracranial pressure that occurs at normocarbia. Unlike enflurane, isoflurane does not alter production of cerebrospinal fluid.[19] Furthermore, isoflurane decreases resistance to absorption. Although isoflurane and enflurane are chemical isomers, excitation of the central nervous system produced by enflurane is not seen with isoflurane.[17]

Isoflurane produces reductions in cerebral metabolic oxygen requirements that exceed those produced by an equivalent MAC concentrations of halothane.[20] The greater decrease in cerebral metabolic oxygen requirements produced by isoflurane may explain why cerebral blood flow increases are minimal below 1.1 MAC (Fig. 18-6).[13] For example, decreased cerebral metabolism means that less carbon dioxide is produced, which thus opposes the cerebral vasodilating effects of isoflurane. It is conceivable that isoflurane might produce greater than expected increases in cerebral blood flow when administered to patients with co-existing drug or disease-induced depression of cerebral blood flow.

NITROUS OXIDE

In contrast to volatile anesthetics, nitrous oxide has less of an effect on cerebral blood flow. As a result, nitrous oxide is unlikely to increase intracranial pressure in patients with intracranial tumors who are maintained at normocarbia. Nevertheless, indirect evidence suggests that nitrous oxide is a cerebral vasodilator. This evidence is the reduction in cerebral metabolic rate produced by nitrous oxide, which in the presence of an unchanged cerebral blood flow is equivalent to a relative increase in cerebral blood flow. Agreeing with this reasoning is the observed increase in intracranial pressure in patients with intracranial tumors who breathed 66 percent nitrous oxide.[21,22] Despite this observation, it seems reasonable to consider nitrous oxide much less likely than volatile anesthetics to increase intracranial pressure in patients with intracranial tumors perhaps reflecting restriction of the dose of this drug to less than 1 MAC. Furthermore, nitrous oxide, in contrast to volatile anesthetics, does not interfere with autoregulation of cerebral blood flow. It must be remembered that administration of nitrous oxide to patients who have undergone recent air contrast studies of the cerebral ventricles can result in abrupt increases in intracranial pressure.[23] This reflects the greater solubility of nitrous oxide, as compared with nitrogen, such that nitrous oxide enters the air cavities more rapidly than nitrogen can leave them. Since the cerebral ventricles are relatively noncompliant, the increased gas volume produced by nitrous oxide manifests as an increase in intracranial pressure. A radiograph of the skull to document the presence of any residual air in the cerebral ventricles should be obtained before administering nitrous oxide to any patient who has undergone a recent air contrast study. An arbitrary 48 hour to 72 hour period is not reliable for assuring that complete absorption of air has occurred. This is emphasized by the demonstration on a radiograph of residual air in the cerebral ventricles as long as 5 days after an air contrast study.[24] Nitrous oxide administered during a craniotomy and after closure of the dura may contribute to development of a tension pneumocephalus. Tension pneumocephalus by this mechanism reflects entrance of nitrous oxide into air cavities, which are present in the subdural space.[25]

KETAMINE

Ketamine is a potent cerebral vasodilator capable of increasing cerebral blood flow by more than 60 percent during normocarbia.[26]

This vasodilation is so pronounced that intracranial pressure increases even in the absence of intracranial tumors. The magnitude of the increase is exaggerated in patients with intracranial pathology. Prior administration of thiopental can block the increase.[26] Furthermore, increases in intracranial pressure produced by ketamine can be aborted by the subsequent administration of thiopental. Nevertheless, the effect of thiopental on intracranial pressure in the presence of ketamine is not sufficiently predictable to justify the use of ketamine in patients with intracranial tumors.

Ketamine, like enflurane, has been shown to be a cerebral stimulant capable of producing seizure activity.[27] Conceivably, regional increases in neuronal activity could be responsible for increases in cerebral blood flow unrelated to direct cerebral vasodilating effects of ketamine.

BARBITURATES

Barbiturates such as thiopental are potent cerebral vasoconstrictors, capable of reducing cerebral blood flow with subsequent reductions in previously elevated intracranial pressure. Cerebral vasoconstriction produced by barbiturates and the subsequent impact on cerebral blood flow and intracranial pressure are dose-related. Furthermore, the reduction in cerebral blood flow produced by barbiturates is even greater if hypocarbia is also present. Deep thiopental anesthesia during normocarbia results in about a 50 percent reduction in both cerebral metabolic oxygen consumption and cerebral blood flow.

OPIOIDS

Opioids administered to animals are cerebral vasoconstrictors, resulting in reductions in cerebral blood flow. In humans maintained at normocarbia, fentanyl does not alter cerebral blood flow. During normocarbia, the combination of nitrous oxide and morphine does not significantly alter cerebral blood flow or autoregulation in normal humans. The combination of droperidol and fentanyl causes a reduction in cerebral blood flow and intracranial

pressure in patients with normal cerebrospinal fluid pathways, as well as in individuals with intracranial tumors. Although opioids are typically classified as cerebral vasoconstrictors, it must be appreciated that this effect is readily abolished by vasodilation, as can accompany opioid-induced ventilatory depression.

MUSCLE RELAXANTS

Muscle relaxants that cause the release of histamine could act as cerebral vasodilators, leading to increases in cerebral blood flow and intracranial pressure. For example, d-tubocurarine is thought to increase intracranial pressure via its ability to stimulate the release of histamine.[28] Another disadvantage of d-tubocurarine is its propensity to reduce mean arterial pressure, which may jeopardize the adequacy of cerebral perfusion pressure, particularly in patients with co-existing increases in intracranial pressure.

Intracranial pressure is not altered after administration of atracurium or vecuronium to anesthetized patients undergoing surgery for removal of intracranial tumors.[29,30] These data suggest atracurium may be used for skeletal muscle relaxation during neurosurgical operations, despite its potential to evoke histamine release and cause stimulation of the central nervous system.

Succinylcholine administered to patients with intracranial tumors causes modest and usually transient increases in intracranial pressure (Fig. 18-7).[31] This response could reflect histamine release and/or increased venous pressure due to elevated intra-abdominal and intrathoracic pressures in response to skeletal muscle contractions. Indeed, prevention of succinylcholine-induced skeletal muscle fasciculations by prior administration of a nondepolarizing muscle relaxant prevents increases in intracranial pressure associated with this drug (Fig. 18-7).[31]

Preoperative Evaluation

Preoperative evaluation of patients with intracranial tumors is directed toward estab-

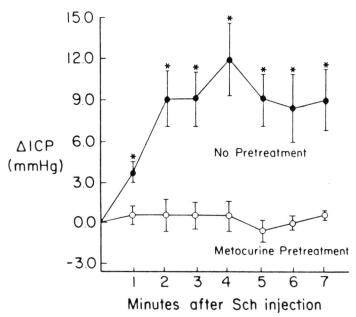

FIG. 18-7. Changes in intracranial pressure (ICP) after administration of succinylcholine 1 mg·kg^{-1} (no pretreatment) or metocurine 0.03 mg·kg^{-1} followed by succinylcholine (metocurine pretreatment) to patients with brain tumors. Mean ± SE. *P < 0.05 compared to baseline prior to injection of succinylcholine. (Stirt JA, Grosslight KR, Bedford RF, Vollmer D. "Defasciculation" with metocurine prevents succinylcholine-induced increases in intracranial pressure. Anesthesiology 1987;67:50–3)

lishing the presence or absence of increased intracranial pressure. Symptoms of increased intracranial pressure include nausea and vomiting, alterations in the level of consciousness, mydriasis and decreased reactivity of the pupils to light, papilledema, bradycardia, hypertension, and disturbances of breathing. Evidence of a midline shift of the brain (greater than 0.5 cm) with computed tomography also suggests the presence of increased intracranial pressure.

Preoperative Medication

Preoperative medication that produces sedation or ventilatory depression should be avoided in patients with intracranial tumors. It must be remembered that patients with intracranial pathology may be extremely sensitive to central nervous system depressant ef-fects of drugs such as opioids. Opioid-induced hypoventilation can lead to increased cerebral blood flow and consequent increases in intracranial pressure. It is difficult to distinguish nausea and vomiting that occurs after administration of preoperative medication from that due to progressive increases in intracranial pressure. Likewise, drug-induced sedation can mask alterations in the level of consciousness that accompany intracranial hypertension. Considering all the potential adverse effects of preoperative medication, it is an inescapable conclusion that pharmacologic premedication should be used sparingly, if at all, in patients with intracranial tumors. Certainly no preoperative depressant drugs should be administered to patients who manifest depressed levels of consciousness. In alert adult patients with intracranial tumors, oral administration of diazepam (5 mg to 10 mg) may provide anxiety relief without introducing hazards of ventilatory depression. The decision to administer anticholinergic drugs or H-2 receptor antagonists is not influenced by the presence or absence of increased intracranial pressure.

Induction of Anesthesia

Induction of anesthesia must be achieved with drugs that produce rapid and reliable anesthesia with minimal effects on cerebral blood flow. This goal is often achieved with the intravenous injection of thiopental (4 mg·kg^{-1} to 6 mg·kg^{-1}), preceded by preoxygenation and voluntary spontaneous hyperventilation. The reduction in cerebral blood flow and increase in the perfusion to metabolism ratio make thiopental a useful induction drug in the presence of increased intracranial pressure. Benzodiazepines and etomidate also reduce cerebral blood flow and, in this regard, would be acceptable drugs for induction of anesthesia. Thiopental is followed by the administration of two to three times the ED95 dose of vecuronium, atracurium, or pancuronium. The use of d-tubocurarine is not recommended because of potential adverse effects of drug-induced histamine release and hypotension on cerebral blood flow. Administration of succinylcholine may be associated with modest and transient increases in intracranial pressure (Fig. 18-7).[31] Mechanical hyperventilation of the lungs is instituted after the administration of muscle relaxants with the goal of reducing the arterial partial pressures of carbon dioxide to between 25 mmHg and 30 mmHg.

Intubation of the trachea by direct laryngoscopy is carried out when intense skeletal muscle paralysis is confirmed by the absence of evoked responses to the peripheral nerve stimulator. Administration of additional doses of thiopental or potent short-acting opioids before initiation of direct laryngoscopy may reduce the pressor response to this painful stimulus. Likewise, intravenous lidocaine 1.5 mg·kg^{-1}, administered about 1 minute before beginning direct laryngoscopy, may be effective in attenuating increased blood pressure and intracranial pressure, which may accompany intubation of the trachea (Fig. 18-8).[32] Laryngotracheal lidocaine does not seem to be as effective as intravenous lidocaine for reducing the magnitude of these responses. It is important to recognize that abrupt increases in blood pressure in the absence of autoregulation in the area of pathology may be accompanied by cerebral edema and undesirable elevations in blood flow and intracranial pressure. Hypotension should also be avoided, as brain ischemia can occur when cerebral perfusion pressure decreases and autoregulation is not intact. Any reaction during placement of the tube in the trachea due to inadequate skeletal muscle relaxation can further increase intracranial pressure, by vitrue of elevations in venous pressure. Likewise, reactions to movement of the tube after it is placed in the trachea must be prevented, emphasizing the need to maintain skeletal muscle paralysis beyond the period of laryngoscopy. An adequate depth of anesthesia as well as complete skeletal muscle paralysis is necessary, since perception of noxious stimulation can abruptly increase cerebral oxygen requirements and cerebral blood flow. After intubation of the trachea, the lungs are ventilated at a rate and tidal volume predicted to maintain the arterial partial pressures of carbon dioxide between 25 mmHg and 30 mmHg. Positive end-expiratory pressure is not recommended, as this could impair cerebral venous drainage and increase intracranial pressure.[6,12]

Maintenance of Anesthesia

Maintenance of anesthesia is often achieved with nitrous oxide plus intravenous supplementation with opioids and/or barbiturates. Fentanyl or similar opioids are attractive selections, as these drugs are unlikely to alter adversely intracranial pressure. Some would question the wisdom of using nitrous oxide in situations where the likelihood of air embolism is great, as with operations performed in the sitting position. Volatile anesthetics are administered with caution because of their potential to increase cerebral blood flow and to interfere with autoregulation. Nevertheless, low concentrations of volatile drugs (less than 0.6 MAC) may be useful for preventing or treating increases in blood pressure related to noxious surgical stimulation. In

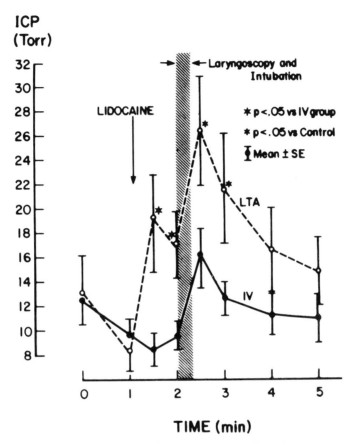

FIG. 18-8. Changes in intracranial pressure (ICP) in response to direct laryngoscopy and intubation of the trachea were measured after the administration of either laryngotracheal (LTA) or intravenous (IV) lidocaine to adult patients undergoing craniotomy for removal of intracranial tumors. An increase in ICP occurred after direct instillation of lidocaine (LTA) into the trachea. Furthermore, LTA lidocaine did not prevent the increase of intracranial pressure in response to intubation of the trachea. In contrast, the initial administration of IV lidocaine did not increase the ICP, and elevations of ICP in response to intubation of the trachea were minimal. (Hamill JF, Bedford RF, Weaver DC, Colohan AR. Lidocaine before endotracheal intubation: Intravenous or laryngotracheal? Anesthesiology 1981;55:578–81)

addition to lowering blood pressure, administration of volatile anesthetics increase the depth of anesthesia and reduce the likelihood that painful stimulation could increase cerebral blood flow. Use of volatile anesthetics requires modest hyperventilation of the lungs to maintain the arterial partial pressures of carbon dioxide between 25 mmHg and 30 mmHg. The minimal effects of isoflurane on cerebral blood flow compared with other volatile anesthetics, plus the acceptability of initiating hyperventilation of the lungs simultaneously with introduction of this drug, make isoflurane a useful volatile anesthetic in patients undergoing intracranial operations.

Peripheral vasodilating drugs, such as trimethaphan, nitroprusside, or nitroglycerin, increase cerebral blood flow and intracranial pressure, despite simultaneous reductions in systemic blood pressure.[33] Therefore, selection of peripheral vasodilators to treat intraoperative hypertension may be questioned in patients with increased intracranial pressure.

Spontaneous movement by patients must

be rigidly avoided during intracranial operations. Such movement can result in disastrous increases in intracranial pressure, excessive bleeding into the operative site, and a brain that bulges into the wound, making surgical exposure difficult. Therefore, in addition to adequate depths of anesthesia, skeletal muscle paralysis is often maintained during intracranial surgery.

Fluid Therapy

Selection of inappropriate fluid solutions or infusion of excessive amounts of crystalloid solutions can adversely influence intracranial pressure in patients with intracranial tumors. Glucose and water solutions are not recommended, since they are rapidly and equally distributed throughout total body water. If the concentrations of glucose in blood decrease more rapidly than brain glucose, brain water becomes relatively hyperosmolar and brain tissues accumulate water, leading to cerebral edema. Furthermore, metabolism of glucose in the brain leaves free water in excess. A hypertonic salt solution, such as 5 percent glucose in lactated Ringer's solution, is an appropriate fluid selection. This solution will initially tend to reduce brain water by increasing the osmolarity of plasma. Regardless of the crystalloid solution selected, it must be remembered that any solution administered in large amounts can increase brain water and elevate intracranial pressure in patients with intracranial tumors. Therefore, the rate of fluid infusion should not exeed 1 $ml \cdot kg^{-1} \cdot hr^{-1}$ to 3 $ml \cdot kg^{-1} \cdot hr^{-1}$ in the perioperative period. Intravascular fluid volume depletion due to blood loss during surgery should be corrected with whole blood or colloid solutions and not with large volumes of balanced salt solutions.

Monitoring

Continuous monitoring of blood pressure via a catheter in a peripheral artery is essential, to detect rapidly, excessive increases or decreases in cerebral perfusion pressure. In addition, ready access to arterial blood for analysis of oxygenation and ventilation is important. A monitor of end-exhaled partial pressure of carbon dioxide is helpful as a continuous indirect reflection of the arterial pressure of carbon dioxide. This monitor is also useful for detecting the occurrence of venous air embolism (see the section Venous Air Embolism). A continuous monitor of intracranial pressure is of obvious value, but this monitor cannot be considered as routine during surgery in every patient with an intracranial tumor. Nasopharyngeal or esophageal temperature should be monitored to detect unexpected alterations in body temperature and to permit appropriate correction of blood gases. A catheter inserted into the bladder is mandatory if diuresis is to be produced during the intraoperative period.

A catheter placed in the right atrium is helpful for guiding the rate of intravenous fluid infusion. Furthermore, this catheter may be important for aspirating air from the heart, should venous air embolism occur (see the section Venous Air Embolism). The position of the catheter can be confirmed by (1) a radiograph of the chest; (2) the configuration of the P waves on the electrocardiogram, with the saline-filled catheter acting as a unipolar lead; or (3) the transduced venous pressure wave form. The impracticality of obtaining a radiograph of the chest in the operating room and the electroshock hazards of recording the electrocardiogram from the catheter are disadvantages to these approaches. Therefore, observation of phasic pressure wave forms recorded from the catheter seems an acceptable criterion for confirming its central venous location. An additional approach is to advance the catheter until right ventricular pressure wave forms are observed and then withdraw the catheter until the pressure trace becomes atrial. In view of reductions in mortality from venous air embolism provided by aspiration of air from right atrial catheters, it would seem prudent to consider placement of a catheter into the right atrium whenever venous air embolism is judged to be a likely occurrence during surgery. An extension of this recommendation would be placement of a pulmonary artery catheter as an alternative.[34]

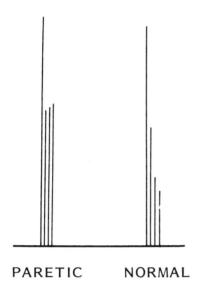

PARETIC   NORMAL

FIG. 18-9. Schematic diagram of a train-of-four ratio recorded from the paretic and normal upper extremities of a patient who had received metocurine. The greater train-of-four ratio recorded from the paretic extremity (0.6), compared to the normal arm (0.3), reflects resistance of the abnormal arm to the effects of nondepolarizing muscle relaxants. (Moorthy SS, Hilgenberg JC. Resistance of nondepolarizing muscle relaxants in paretic upper extremities of patients with residual hemiplegia. Anesth Analg 1980;59:624–7. Reprinted with permission from IARS.)

A peripheral nerve stimulator is essential for monitoring the persistence of skeletal muscle paralysis. Should paresis or paralysis of an upper extremity be associated with intracranial tumors, it is important to appreciate the presence of resistance (e.g., decreased sensitivity) to the effects of nondepolarizing muscle relaxants on the paretic extremity compared with the normal extremity (Fig. 18-9).[35] Therefore, monitoring skeletal muscle paralysis with the leads of the peripheral nerve stimulator placed on the paretic arm may be misleading. For example, evoked responses may be erroneously interpreted as inadequate skeletal muscle paralysis. Likewise, at the conclusion of surgery, the same responses could be assumed to reflect recovery from the effects of the muscle relaxants when substantial neuromuscular blockade persists. Resistance to muscle relaxants may reflect proliferation of ace-

tylcholine responsive extrajunctional cholinergic receptor sites which may occur within 48 hours to 72 hours after denervation (see the section Chronic Spinal Cord Transection).

Monitoring for venous air embolism with a Doppler transducer is indicated in patients undergoing intracranial operations. The transducer is placed to the right of the sternum, between the third and sixth intercostal spaces. Correct positioning is verified by rapid injection of 5 ml to 10 ml of crystalloid solution into the right atrial catheter. Turbulence created by this injection of fluid creates a signal (roaring sound) similar to that caused by air. Amounts of air as small as 0.25 ml can be detected by the transducer. Air is detected as a change in the signal from the transducer because the air-blood interface is a much better acoustical reflector than erythrocytes alone. In addition, audible sounds from the transducer provide early warning of changes in cardiac rate or rhythm.

Monitoring of the electrocardiogram is necessary to detect cardiac dysrhythmias related to the presence of intracranial tumors or for surgical stimulation of vital medullary centers. Indeed, patients with intracranial tumors can manifest abnormalities on the electrocardiogram that are presumed to reflect increased activity of the sympathetic nervous system due to increased intracranial pressure.[36] More important, alterations in cardiac rate or rhythm as sudden respiratory movements may reflect surgical retraction or manipulation of the brain stem or cranial nerves. Indeed, the cardiovascular centers, respiratory control areas and nuclei of the lower cranial nerves lie in close proximity in the brain stem. Manipulation of the brain stem may cause hypertension and bradycardia or hypotension and tachycardia. Cardiac dysrhythmias range from acute sinus dysrhythmias to ventricular premature beats or ventricular tachycardia.

Position

Craniotomy for removal of supratentorial tumors is usually performed with patients supine and the head elevated 10 degrees to 15 degrees to facilitate venous drainage from the brain. Excessive flexion or rotation of the head should be avoided, as these positions can impair jugular vein patency and impede venous outflow.

The sitting position is often used for exploration of the posterior cranial fossa, which may be necessary to resect intracranial tumors, clip aneurysms, decompress cranial nerves, or implant electrodes for cerebellar stimulation. Advantages of the sitting position include excellent surgical exposure and facilitation of venous and cerebrospinal fluid drainage, so as to minimize blood loss and elevations of the intracranial pressure. These advantages are offset by reductions in blood pressure and cardiac output produced by this posture and by the potential hazard of cranial nerve damage and venous air embolism. For these reasons, the lateral or prone position may be selected instead. If the sitting position is used, it is mandatory to maintain a high index of suspicion for venous air embolism (see the section Venous Air Embolism). A serious postoperative complication following posterior fossa craniotomy is apnea due to hematoma formation. Cranial nerve injuries involving innervation to the pharynx and larynx makes these patients vulnerable to aspiration.

Venous Air Embolism

Venous air embolism is a potential hazard whenever the operative site is above the level of the heart, such that the pressure in the veins is subatmospheric. Although this complication is most often associated with neurosurgical procedures, venous air embolism can also occur during operations involving the neck, thorax, abdomen, and pelvis and during open heart procedures, repair of liver and vena caval lacerations, total hip replacement, and vaginal delivery associated with placenta previa. Patients undergoing intracranial surgery are at an increased risk, not only because the operative site is usually above the level of the heart, but also because veins may not collapse due to attachments to bone or dura. Indeed, the cut edge

of bone constituting the skull is a common site for entry of air into veins held open by bone.

PATHOPHYSIOLOGY

The exact mechanism by which venous air embolism leads to cardiovascular collapse is undetermined. Presumably, when air enters the right ventricle, there is interference with blood flow into the pulmonary artery. Pulmonary edema and reflex bronchoconstriction may result from movement of air into the pulmonary circulation. Death is usually secondary to acute cor pulmonale and cardiovascular collapse, plus arterial hypoxemia from obstruction to right ventricular ejection into the pulmonary artery.

Air can probably pass through pulmonary vessels in small amounts to reach the coronary and cerebral circulations; large quantities of air can travel directly to the systemic circulation through a right-to-left intracardiac shunt, as provided by a patent foramen ovale. Indeed, use of the sitting position inherently predisposes neurosurgical patients to paradoxical air embolism since the normal interatrial pressure gradient frequently becomes reversed in this position.[37] When the likelihood of venous air embolism is increased, it is useful, but not mandatory, to place a right atrial catheter before beginning surgery (see the section Monitoring). Death due to paradoxical air embolism results from obstruction of the coronary arteries by air, leading to myocardial ischemia and ventricular fibrillation. Neurologic damage follows air embolism to the brain.

DETECTION

Early detection of venous air embolism is essential to successful treatment of this complication. A Doppler transducer placed over the right heart is the most sensitive indicator of intracardiac air.[38] Indeed, the amount of air detected by the transducer is often not clinically significant. In this regard, the transducer does not provide information as to the volume of air that has entered the venous circulation. Sudden decreases in the end-exhaled partial pressures of carbon dioxide may reflect increased dead space due to continued ventilation of alveoli no longer perfused because of obstruction of their vascular supply by air. Increases in right atrial and pulmonary artery pressure reflect acute cor pulmonale and correlate with abrupt reductions in the end-exhaled partial pressures of carbon dioxide.[34] Although these changes are less sensitive indicators for the presence of air than the Doppler transducer, their occurrence correlates with the size of the venous air embolism.[38] An increase in end-tidal nitrogen concentrations, as during continuous mass spectrometry monitoring, may also reflect venous air embolism. Changes in end-tidal nitrogen concentrations precede decreases in the end-tidal carbon dioxide partial pressures or increases in pulmonary artery pressure.[39]

During controlled ventilation of the lungs, sudden attempts by patients to initiate spontaneous breaths may be the first indication of the occurrence of venous air embolism. Indeed, the slow infusion of air into an animal model consistently produced an alteration in the pattern of breathing characterized by a sudden "gasp".[40] Hypotension, tachycardia, cardiac dysrhythmias, and cyanosis are late signs of venous air embolism. Certainly the detection of the characterisic "mill-wheel" murmur through the esophageal stethoscope is a late sign of catastrophic venous air embolism.

TREATMENT

A change in the signal from the Doppler transducer should alert the surgeons to identify and occlude the site of venous air entry by irrigating the operative site with fluid and by applying occlusive material to all bone edges. Aspiration of air should be attempted through the right atrial catheter. The ideal location of the right atrial catheter tip is controversial, but evidence suggests that a superior vena cava location (junction of the superior vena cava with the right atrium) is preferable as this seems to provide the most rapid aspiration of air.[41] Right atrial multiorifice catheters allow a larger amount of air to be aspirated than single orifice catheters. A pulmonary artery catheter because of its small lumen size and slow speed of blood return is not uniquely useful for aspirating air

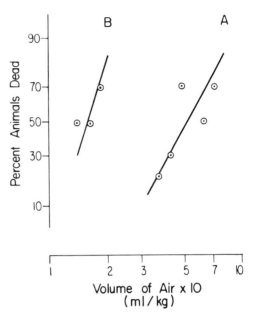

FIG. 18-10. The volume of air injected into a peripheral vein that produced death was measured in animals anesthetized with halothane plus nitrous oxide (**B**), or halothane alone (**A**). The calculated volume of air necessary to produce death in 50 percent of animals was 0.16 ml·kg^{-1} in the presence of nitrous oxide (**B**), and 0.55 ml·kg^{-1} during the administration of halothane without nitrous oxide (**A**). Presumably, the rapid passage of nitrous oxide into air bubbles, with resultant expansion of the air bubbles, was responsible for the increased lethal effect of venous air embolism in the presence of nitrous oxide (**B**). (Munson ES, Merrick HC. Effect of nitrous oxide on venous air embolism. Anesthesiology 1966;27:783–7)

but may provide additional evidence that venous embolism has occurred by virtue of increases in pulmonary artery pressure. Nitrous oxide is immediately discontinued to avoid increasing the size of the venous air bubbles (Fig. 18-10).[42] Indeed, elimination of nitrous oxide from the inspired gases after the detection of venous air embolism results in decreases in pulmonary artery pressures. At the same time that oxygen is substituted for nitrous oxide, it may be helpful to apply positive end-expiratory pressure, so as to increase venous pressure. Despite the logic of this maneuver, the prophylactic use of positive end-expiratory pressure has not been found to be of value in the prevention of venous air embolism. Furthermore, positive end-expiratory pressure could reverse the interatrial pressure gradient and predispose to passage of air across a patent foramen ovale into the left atrium. Extreme hypotension may require support of perfusion pressure with sympathomimetic drugs. Likewise, marked reductions in cardiac output may require infusion of beta-adrenergic agonist drugs such as dopamine or dobutamine. Bronchospasm should be treated initially with aminophylline. If bronchospasm persists, use of beta-2 agonist drug, either by aerosol or intravenously, may be necessary. The traditional admonition to place patients in the lateral position with the right chest uppermost is rarely possible or safe during intracranial operations. It is likely that valuable time, which could be better spent aspirating air and supporting circulation, could be lost attempting to attain this position. Furthermore, appropriate monitoring should allow early detection of venous air embolism, such that significant occlusion of the right ventricular outflow tract with air does not occur.

After the successful treatment of venous air embolism, the surgical procedure can be resumed. However, the decision to reinstitute administration of nitrous oxide must be individualized. If it is decided not to use nitrous oxide, maintenance of an adequate depth of anesthesia will probably require administration of volatile anesthetics. Should nitrous oxide be added again to the inspired gases, it is possible that residual air in the circulation could again produce symptoms. Indeed, increases in pulmonary artery pressures after resumption of breathing nitrous oxide should be viewed as evidence that residual air persists despite apparent successful treatment of venous air embolism.[34] Transfer of patients to hyperbaric chambers in attempts to reduce air bubble size and improve blood flow in the brain is likely to be helpful only if the transfer can be accomplished within 8 hours.

Postoperative Management

Ideally, effects of anesthetics and muscle relaxants are dissipated or pharmacologically reversed at the conclusion of surgery. This fa-cilitates the monitoring of neurologic status and recognition of any adverse effects produced by the surgery. It is important to prevent reactions to the tube in the trachea as patients are allowed to awaken. Intravenous lidocaine (0.5 mg·kg^{-1} to 1.5 mg·kg^{-1}) may be used to attenuate initial responses to the continued presence of the tube in the trachea as the patient awakens. It must be appreciated, however, that this local anesthetic can produce central nervous system depression and reduce activity of protective upper airway reflexes. If patients were alert preoperatively, it may be reasonable to place a nasal airway during anesthesia and remove the tracheal tube at the conclusion of surgery, so as to avoid potentially adverse reactions to the tube. Conversely, if consciousness was depressed preoperatively, it is best to delay extubation of the trachea until it can be confirmed that airway reflexes are present and spontaneous ventilation is sufficient to prevent accumulation of carbon dioxide. Reductions in body temperature (less than 34 degrees Celsius) that occur intraoperatively must be considered as causes for slow postoperative awakening. It may be inappropriate to remove the tracheal tube in the presence of hypothermia, regardless of the preoperative mental status.

CEREBROVASCULAR DISEASE

Cerebrovascular disease can be manifested as (1) transient ischemic attacks, with temporary impairment of cerebral function; (2) minor stroke, where recovery to a normal or near normal state is possible; and (3) major stroke, often resulting in severe and permanent disability or death. Stroke is the third leading cause of death in the United States. Only heart disease and cancer exceed stroke as causes of mortality. The major risk factors for the development of cerebrovascular disease are diabetes mellitus and hypertension. Indeed, effective treatment of hypertension has reduced mortality due to stroke.

Transient Ischemic Attacks

Transient ischemic attacks are temporary and focal episodes of neurologic dysfunction that develop suddenly and last a few minutes to several hours, but never more than 24 hours. Resolution of the episode is rapid, and residual neurologic defects do not occur. The peak age for the development of transient ischemic attacks is during the seventh decade. Such attacks may occur as often as several times daily. Untreated, about one-third of patients will suffer minor or major strokes within 5 years. Among those patients who experience transient ischemic attacks and then develop a stroke, about 20 percent will do so within 1 month, and about 50 percent within 1 year. Overall, the incidence of stroke is about 5 percent in each year after transient ischemic attacks.

Causes of transient ischemic attacks are presumed to be thromboembolism of fibrin-platelet aggregates or atheromatous debris from an atherosclerotic plaque in an extracranial blood vessel. The transient nature of the attack is explained by the rapid fragmentation and dissolution of the microemboli. Disease of the carotid artery or vertebrobasilar arterial system is most often responsible for transient ischemic attacks (Fig. 18-11). It is important to distinguish neurologic dysfunction due to disease of the carotid artery from that due to vertebrobasilar arterial disease, as the prognosis and treatments are different. Radionuclide angiography can also be used to detect carotid artery occlusive disease, and the ability to do a brain scan with this technique is helpful in ruling out intracranial tumors or subdural hematomas.

CAROTID ARTERY DISEASE

The bifurcation of the common carotid artery is a frequent site of atheromatous disease. Disease located in the carotid artery is suggested by complaints of transient ipsilateral monocular visual loss, often associated with a contralateral paresis or sensory disturbance. Transient visual loss (amaurosis fugax) is due to retinal ischemia secondary to the passage of emboli into the ophthalmic artery. Passage of microemboli into the ophthalmic artery is predictable, as this artery is the first branch of the internal carotid artery. Indeed, fundoscopy during the period of blindness can reveal emboli in the retinal arteries.

A neurologic examination performed after transient ischemic attacks is likely to be normal, as changes are usually mild and their evolution complete within a few seconds. Tingling, numbness or clumsiness of an extremity, momentary difficulty in mentation or in verbal expression if the dominant cerebral hemisphere is involved may be described. Disturbance of consciousness is rare.

Auscultation may reveal a bruit over the common carotid artery in the neck. Indeed, asymptomatic cervical bruits occur in 4 percent of the population over 40 years of age, but the risk of myocardial infarction is greater than cerebral vascular accident in these patients.[43] There is no evidence that the incidence of postoperative stroke is increased in these patients who undergo non-neurologic surgery.[44] Absence of a bruit does not rule out the presence of significant stenosis of the carotid artery. For example, a bruit may disappear when the degree of stenosis is so severe that blood flow is minimal. Certainly, the absence of a palpable carotid artery pulse in the neck suggests severe occlusive disease.

The absence of a superficial temporal artery pulse on the same side as the absent carotid artery pulse confirms occlusion of the common carotid artery. In many instances of carotid artery occlusive disease sympathetic nervous system fibers will be involved, and Horner's syndrome will be present.

VERTEBROBASILAR ARTERIAL DISEASE

Vertebrobasilar arterial disease manifests as symptoms referable to ischemia of the posterior portions of the brain, including the occipital lobes and brain stem. Bilateral disturbance of vision results from inadequate blood flow via the posterior cerebral arteries that supply the visual cortex. Visual symptoms range from blurring to total blindness. Diplopia is a common complaint. Attacks of vertigo, ataxia, and nausea and vomiting suggest circulatory disturbances, either in the labyrinth of the inner ear or in the vestibular nuclei of the medulla. Other symptoms of brain stem ischemia include dysarthria, dysphagia, perioral numbness, and weakness or paresthesias of all four limbs.

A sudden loss of postural tone in the legs,

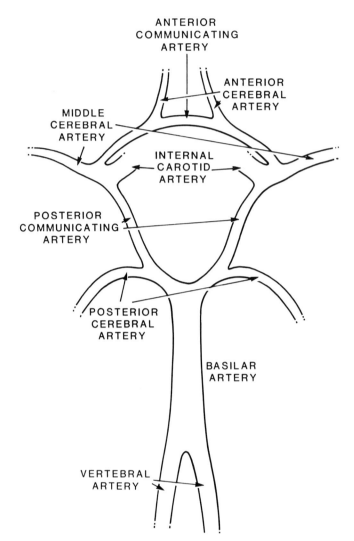

FIG. 18-11. Schematic diagram of the cerebral circulation and circle of Willis. The cerebral blood supply is from two vertebral and two internal carotid arteries. The posterior portion of the brain is supplied by the vertebral arteries, and the anterior portion by the internal carotid arteries. The vertebral arteries arise from the subclavian arteries and join to form the basilar artery, which divides into the posterior cerebral arteries. The internal carotid arteries divide into the middle cerebral arteries and anterior cerebral arteries. The posterior communicating arteries arise from the internal carotid arteries, while the anterior communicating arteries join the anterior cerebral arteries to complete the circle of Willis.

while consciousness is maintained, is characteristic of basilar artery disease. Typically, patients abruptly fall to the ground, often into a kneeling position. Attempts to arise at once serve to distinguish this event from syncope due to third-degree atrioventricular heart block.

Episodes of transient global amnesia are most likely related to vertebrobasilar arterial disease. Characteristically, there is an abrupt onset of memory loss and confusion. During the attack, there is retrograde amnesia, but self-identity is usually preserved. Attacks subside after several minutes to hours, and are ultimately associated with amnesia, permanent only for the period of the ischemic episode. It is presumed that insufficient blood flow to portions of the temporal lobes or thalamus supplied by the posterior cerebral arteries is responsible.

In contrast to patients with carotid artery occlusive disease, patients with vertebrobasilar arterial insufficiency are more likely to describe a relation between symptoms and abrupt changes in posture. Orthostatic hypotension or a low blood pressure for the age of the patient are often present. In addition, vertebral arteries may be compressed by osteoarthritis of the cervical spine and movements of the head, particularly hyperextension. Occasionally, vertebrobasilar arterial insufficiency is associated with a bruit over the subclavian artery, and radiographs of the cervical spine may reveal calcification of the vertebral arteries.

SUBCLAVIAN STEAL SYNDROME

Symptoms of claudication of an exercised arm, accompanied by manifestations of vertebrobasilar arterial insufficiency, constitute the subclavian steal syndrome. For example, occlusion of the subclavian artery or innominate artery, while the major cranial vessels remain patent, can result in reversal of the direction of blood flow in the vertebral artery, leading to symptoms of vertebrobasilar arterial insufficiency. These hemodynamic changes are accentuated during exercise of the arm on the affected side.

Diagnosis of subclavian steal syndrome depends on the presence of a clinical history consistent with vertebrobasilar arterial insufficiency that is associated with exercise-induced claudication of the arm. In addition, physical examination may reveal a bruit over the subclavian artery. There may be a palpable delay in the time of arrival of the radial pulse on the affected side, and a difference in systolic blood pressure of over 20 mmHg in the two arms. Stenosis of the left subclavian artery is responsible for this syndrome in about 70 percent of patients. Subclavian endarterectomy may be curative.

MEDICAL TREATMENT OF TRANSIENT ISCHEMIC ATTACKS

Medical treatment of transient ischemic attacks is preferred in patients with vertebrobasilar arterial disease or multiple vascular lesions. Medical management consists of long-term administration of antiplatelet aggregating drugs or coumarin anticoagulants. Evidence for the effectiveness of oral anticoagulants in protecting against stroke is not well defined as it is for aspirin. Nevertheless, warfarin may be selected for medical management of women who develop transient ischemic attacks, or for men who do not tolerate aspirin. Spontaneous hemorrhage is the major hazard of oral anticoagulant therapy. It must be remembered that drugs commonly used in these patients (phenytoin, barbiturates, salicylates) can affect prothrombin time. Treatment with oral anticoagulants should be continued for 6 months to 12 months after transient ischemic attacks, as this is the period of greatest risk for the development of stroke.

Patients with vertebrobasilar arterial insufficiency who have symptoms associated with low blood pressure or with postural changes may benefit from oral administration of ephedrine. If symptoms are produced by extension or rotation of the head, a cervical collar may be helpful.

SURGICAL TREATMENT OF TRANSIENT ISCHEMIC ATTACKS

Cartoid endarterectomy is the most commonly performed surgical procedure for treatment of patients with histories of transient ischemic attacks. For example, about 75 percent of patients have an obstructive lesion at a surgically accessible site, most commonly at the bifurcation of the common carotid artery. Typically, a carotid endarterectomy is considered for patients with documented occlusive lesions of greater than 80 percent in the carotid artery and histories of transient ischemic attacks or stroke with good neurologic recovery. The presence of an ulcerated atherosclerotic plaque is also an indication for carotid endarterectomy. Approximately 80 percent of patients improve or become asymptomatic after carotid endarterctomy surgery. However, there is no evidence that surgically treated patients have a lower incidence of stroke or longer survival than medically treated patients. Carotid endarterectomy is not likely to be considered in patients with acute strokes or strokes in progress because of the greater than 50 percent incidence of postoperative hemorrhagic infarction. When the vascular occlusion is beyond the anatomic confines of the neck a surgical bypass procedure may be considered (see the section Intracranial Vascular Occlusive Disease).

Management of Anesthesia for Carotid Endarterectomy Surgery

The goal during management of anesthesia for carotid endarterectomy surgery is to maintain cerebral perfusion pressure and cerebral blood flow. The most critical period is the time of surgical occlusion of the common, internal, and external carotid arteries. The vast majority of patients can tolerate this occlusion by using collateral channels provided by the circle of Willis (Fig. 18-11). For example, occlusion of one carotid artery is tolerated because of collateral circulation through the contralateral carotid artery or the vertebral arteries. Other important arterial collaterals are available through the external carotid artery via the ophthalmic artery or occipital artery to the distal internal carotid artery. Nevertheless, in some patients, there may be inadequate cerebral blood flow during the carotid artery occlusion, which is necessary for performance of the endarterectomy.

PREOPERATIVE EVALUATION

In addition to the neurologic evaluation, these patients should be carefully examined for cardiovascular and renal disease. It is predictable that patients with cerebrovascular occlusive disease will also manifest occlusive disease in other arteries. Indeed, coronary artery

disease is a major cause of morbidity and mortality after carotid endarterectomy surgery. The incidence of mortality after this surgery is reduced when patients with angina pectoris are treated with coronary artery bypass grafting before the endarterectomy or when both operations are performed simultaneously.[45] Chronic hypertension is a common finding. It is important to establish the range of normal blood pressure in these patients preoperatively to provide a rational guideline for the range of blood pressure maintenance during surgery. Effects of changes in head position on cerebral function should be ascertained since extreme head rotation, flexion, or extension in patients with co-existing vertebral artery disease could lead to angulation and compression of the artery. Recognition of this response preoperatively allows hazardous head positions (especially hyperextension) to be avoided when patients are unconscious during general anesthesia, particularly during direct laryngoscopy for intubation of the trachea. Palpation of the carotid artery is not recommended, as this maneuver could displace fragments of the occlusive lesion, resulting in cerebral embolism.

CHOICE OF ANESTHESIA

Carotid endarterectomy surgery can be performed with regional or general anesthesia.

Regional Anesthesia. Cervical plexus block produced by injection of local anesthetics (lidocaine or bupivacaine) at the transverse processes of C3–C4 (deep cervical plexus block) followed by infiltration of local anesthetics along the posterior inferior border of the sternocleidomastoid muscle (superficial cervical plexus block) provides the advantage of being able to monitor cerebral function of patients by voice contact when the carotid artery is occluded. Nevertheless, strokes still can occur postoperatively, despite the apparent maintenance of normal cerebral function during regional anesthesia.[46] A disadvantage of regional anesthesia includes a more pronounced cardiovascular response to manipulation in the area of the carotid sinus, as compared with general anesthesia. Furthermore, any cerebral protective effect produced by drugs used for general anesthesia is lost.

General Anesthesia   General anesthesia is acceptably produced by intravenous injection of barbiturates, benzodiazepines, or etomidate followed by administration of nitrous oxide plus volatile drugs or opioids for maintenance of anesthesia. Skeletal muscle paralysis is often produced to allow reduction in the depth of anesthesia in response to hypotension, without introducing the possibility of unwanted patient movement. Although differences among volatile anesthetics as regards neurologic outcome following carotid endarterectomy surgery are not detectable, it seems likely that isoflurane offers some brain protection if volatile anesthetics are selected.[46] For example, critical cerebral blood flow (flow below which the majority of patients develop ipsilateral electroencephalographic signs of ischemia within 3 minutes of clamping the carotid artery) is lower during administration of isoflurane (8 ml·100 g^{-1}·min^{-1} to 10 ml·100 g^{-1}·min^{-1}) than during administration of enflurane or halothane (18 ml·100 g^{-1}·min^{-1} to 20 ml·100 g^{-1}·min^{-1}). Nevertheless, thiopental remains the appropriate drug to select in specific circumstances where pharmacologic brain protection is indicated.

Regardless of the drugs selected for anesthesia, the goal is to maintain arterial blood pressure in a normal range for that patient. Prolonged and excessive reductions in blood pressure may jeopardize cerebral perfusion pressure and the adequacy of cerebral blood flow via collateral channels. When reductions in blood pressure below the normal range for that patient do not respond to decreases in concentrations of anesthetic drugs, it may be necessary to return the blood pressure to a normal level (not above) by continuous infusions of sympathomimetic drugs such as phenylephrine or metaraminol. Despite the universal concern that hypotension can lead to stroke, there is lack of evidence to support this opinion, and some evidence to suggest that reductions in blood pressure are not precipitating factors in the genesis of stroke.[47] The questionable role of hypotension in the production of stroke should not be interpreted as a license to allow blood pressure to remain below normal levels

during anesthesia, particularly during the time of clamping of the carotid artery. On the other hand, it should also be recognized that transient reductions in blood pressure during the intraoperative period cannot be automatically incriminated as the only etiology, when postoperative neurologic deficits manifest.

The hazard of uncontrolled hypertension during surgery is cerebral edema, particularly in diseased areas of the brain with altered ability to autoregulate cerebral blood flow (see the section Management of Anesthesia for Removal of Intracranial Tumors). In addition, efforts to elevate artificially blood pressure above normal values for that patient may contribute to postoperative myocardial infarction in patients with co-existing coronary artery disease. Indeed, the incidence of postoperative myocardial infarction is substantially increased in patients with coronary artery disease in whom intraoperative blood pressure is artificially elevated with sympathomimetic drugs such as metaraminol.[48]

Surgical manipulation in the area of the carotid sinus during mobilization of the carotid artery may be interpreted as stretch by afferent nerve endings in this area, leading to reflex bradycardia and hypotension (see the section Carotid Sinus Syndrome). Conversely, during carotid artery occlusion, decreased pressure within the isolated portion of the artery could initiate sympathetic nervous system activity via the carotid sinus, resulting in tachycardia and hypertension. These intraoperative effects can be modified by intravenous injection of atropine or by local infiltration of the area of the carotid sinus with 3 ml to 5 ml of 1 percent lidocaine, so as to block afferent activity from the baroreceptor.

Present evidence suggests barbiturates may prolong the brain's tolerance to focal ischemia as may be produced by clamping the carotid artery during carotid endarterectomy (see the section Cerebral Protection and Resuscitation). In this regard, it may be reasonable to administer thiopental (4 mg·kg^{-1} to 6 mg·kg^{-1}) immediately before clamping the carotid artery. Nevertheless, there is no specific data to indicate that barbiturates used in this manner reduce morbidity after carotid endarterectomy.[49]

Ventilation of the lungs during carotid endarterectomy surgery is with a tidal volume and respiratory rate that maintains the arterial partial pressures of carbon dioxide near 35 mmHg. Manipulation of the arterial partial pressure of carbon dioxide in attempts to increase cerebral blood flow by vasodilation or to produce the inverse steal phenomenon (see the section Management of Anesthesia for Removal of Intracranial Tumors) is not recommended. Such manipulation can produce paradoxical and unpredictable cerebrovascular responses in individual patients and cannot be relied on to protect the brain.

Monitors during general anesthesia for carotid endarterectomy surgery should include continuous recording of blood pressure via a catheter placed in a peripheral artery. In addition to providing the necessary continuous observation of cerebral perfusion pressure, this monitor provides ready access to arterial blood for analysis of blood gases. Measurement of the end-tidal carbon dioxide partial pressures is useful. In view of the likely presence of coronary artery disease is these patients, it would seem prudent to monitor an appropriate lead of the electrocardiogram for signs of myocardial ischemia.

Monitoring for Adequacy of Cerebral Perfusion During Carotid Endarterectomy Surgery

The goal of monitoring for adequacy of cerebral perfusion is to detect that patient whose cerebral collateral circulation is inadequate to prevent cerebral ischemia during occlusion of the carotid artery. Ideally, this information should identify that patient who requires an intraluminal shunt across the surgically clamped carotid artery. Although some surgeons routinely insert shunts regardless of data obtained from monitors of cerebral perfusion, it must be appreciated that a brief period of carotid occlusion will still be necessary during placement of the shunt. Furthermore, shunts can interfere with surgical exposure and in some instances may induce cerebral emboli-

zation. Neurologic deficits have been shown to occur, even when shunts are routinely used. This may reflect inevitable cerebral ischemia during insertion of shunts, embolization from the carotid artery, or spontaneous distal thrombosis as part of the natural course of the disease.

Methods to monitor adequacy of cerebral perfusion include measurements of jugular venous oxygen saturations, electroencephalogram, regional cerebral blood flow, stump pressures, evoked potentials, and oculoplethysmography.

JUGULAR VENOUS OXYGEN SATURATION

Juglar venous oxygen saturation reflects the relationship between total cerebral blood flow and total cerebral oxygen consumption. Therefore, regional areas of brain ischemia will not be reliably detected in venous blood flowing from the brain.

ELECTROENCEPHALOGRAM

The electroencephalogram, using 16 leads, is a reliable method for diagnosing regional cerebral ischemia. Recording and interpretation, however, are too complex at present to make this a routine monitor. Furthermore, it must be appreciated that the electroencelphalogram will be influenced not only by cerebral ischemia but also by anesthetic drugs, body temperature, and the arterial partial pressures of carbon dioxide. Alternatives to recording the conventional electroencephalogram include compressed and density-modulated spectral array analysis. In addition, a one-channel electroencephalographic filter-processor, known as the cerebral function monitor, is available.

Compressed Spectral Array Analysis. Compressed spectral array analysis provides a three-dimensional pictorial representation of the electroencephalogram, compressed with respect to time. Using this form of display, it is possible to compress the continuous recording of the electroencephalogram for 1 hour onto a single sheet of paper the size of an anesthesia record. This compression allows trends to be easily observed, without the disadvantage of having to scan voluminous amounts of paper recordings (equivalent to 300 pages·hr^{-1}). Despite this advantage, compressed spectral array analysis remains infrequently used because of its complexity and requirement for expensive equipment.

Density-Modulated Spectral Array Analysis. Density-modulated spectral array analysis provides a time-compressed display similar to the compressed spectral array. The advantage of the former is its less complex and less expensive equipment.[50]

Cerebral Function Monitor. The cerebral function monitor provides a compressed recording of the electroencephalogram roughly equivalent to the integrated microvoltage from a single channel.[51] As a result, it may not be sufficiently discriminating for detection of regional cerebral ischemic changes that can occur in the brain during carotid endarterectomy surgery.

REGIONAL CEREBRAL BLOOD FLOW MEASUREMENT

Regional cerebral blood flow measurement by use of isotope-washout techniques, alone or in combination with the electroencephalogram, is an ideal method for monitoring the adequacy of the flow. Regional cerebral blood flows should be maintained above 18 ml·100 g^{-1}·min^{-1}. At present, this technique is too complex for routine operating room use.

STUMP PRESSURE

Stump pressure is the direct measurement of pressures in the internal carotid artery distal to the surgical clamp. Therefore, stump pressures reflect the transmitted pressure via the circle of Willis (Fig. 18-11). Stump pressure is determined by the adequacy of collateral cir-

culation, cerebral perfusion pressure, and cerebral vascular resistance. The latter is increased by barbiturates and hypocarbia; reductions occur in response to volatile drugs and hypercarbia. It must be appreciated that variations in cerebral vascular resistance influence the interpretation of stump pressure and its correlation with cerebral blood flow.[52] For example, an adequate stump pressure during regional anesthesia or anesthetic techniques using nitrous oxide and opioids are probably higher than that required during administration of volatile drugs. This speculation is based on the predictable presence of a higher cerebral vascular resistance in awake patients or patients receiving nitrous oxide plus opioids, as compared with the lower resistance associated with volatile anesthetics. Furthermore, it is likely that administration of barbiturates just before clamping of the carotid artery will elevate stump pressure, by virtue of cerebral vasoconstriction produced by barbiturates. Nevertheless, available data suggest that stump pressures above 60 mmHg provide adequate perfusion of normal areas of the brain during general anesthesia, regardless of the drugs administered (Fig. 18-12).[52] The implication of this observation is that an intraluminal shunt should be used when stump pressures are less than 60 mmHg. Despite its drawbacks, measurement of stump pressure has the advantages of being simple and readily available in most operating rooms.

EVOKED POTENTIALS

Analysis of cortical somatosensory evoked potentials in response to a specific extrinsic stimulus can be used to reflect neuronal function, as well as intactness of sensory or motor pathways. As with the multiple lead electroencephalogram, recording and interpretation of evoked potentials remain complex. Volatile anesthetics produce dose-related and drug-specific depression in the amplitude and an increase in the latency of auditory-evoked, visual-evoked (most sensitive) and somatosensory-evoked potentials.[53] For example, in neurologically intact patients, a monitorable cortical wave form is maintained in the pres-

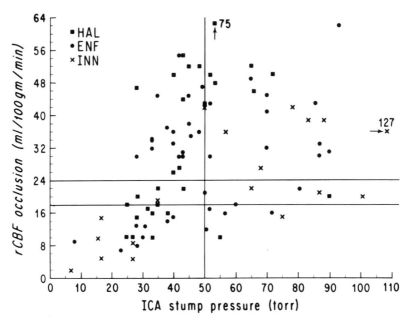

FIG. 18-12. Scattergram of regional cerebral blood flows (rCBF) plotted against internal carotid artery (ICA) stump pressures in patients anesthetized with nitrous oxide plus halothane (HAL), enflurane (ENF), and Innovar (INN). A stump pressure above 60 mmHg was associated with a rCBF greater than 18 ml·100 g^{-1}·min^{-1} in the majority of patients (McKay RD, Sundt TM, Michenfelder JD, et al. Internal carotid artery stump pressure and cerebral blood flow during carotid endarterectomy: Modification by halothane, enflurane, and Innovar. Anesthesiology 1976;45:390–9)

ence of 60 percent nitrous oxide plus 1 MAC halothane, but not isoflurane or enflurane. Nitrous oxide alone may decrease the amplitude of cortical somatosensory evoked potentials.[54] Although less than volatile anesthetics, morphine and fentanyl also produce depressant effects on somatosensory evoked potentials, with low dose continuous infusions of these opioids producing less depression than intermittent injections.[55] Acute hyperventilation of the lungs does not significantly alter amplitude or latency of somatosensory-evoked potentials.[56]

OCULOPLETHYSMOGRAPHY

Oculoplethysmography assesses supraorbital arterial blood flow as a reflection of the adequacy of blood flow through the intraluminal shunt placed at surgery. A delay in the ocular pulse signifies inadequate flow through the shunt and alerts the surgeon to the need for adjusting its position.[57]

Postoperative Problems Following Carotid Endarterectomy Surgery

Postoperative problems after carotid endarterectomy include lability of systemic blood pressure, airway compression due to hematoma formation at the operative site, loss of carotid body function, myocardial infarction, and stroke.[48,58,59]

Hypertension is frequently observed in the immediate postoperative period and is most common in patients with co-existing hypertension.[60] Blood pressure elevation is often greatest 2 hours to 3 hours after surgery and may persist for 24 hours. It is important to lower blood pressure to normal ranges to avoid hazards of cerebral edema and myocardial ischemia. Indeed, the incidence of neurologic deficits is increased threefold in patients who become hypertensive postoperatively.[61] Continuous infusion of nitroprusside is an acceptable treatment to lower blood pressure acutely. When hypertension persists, longer-acting drugs such as labetalol or hydralazine, with or without propranolol, should be considered. The mechanism for hypertension is not known but may reflect increased intravascular fluid volume, altered activity of the carotid sinus, or loss of carotid sinus function due to denervation at the time of surgery. Likewise, hypotension can be explained on the basis of increased afferent nerve activity perceived by a carotid sinus previously shielded by an atheromatous plaque. Treatment of hypotension is with vasopressors such as phenylephrine, infusion of fluids, and infiltration of the carotid sinus with a local anesthetic.

Destruction of the nerve supply to the carotid body, like that to the carotid sinus, is also likely during carotid endarterectomy surgery.[59] Unilateral loss of carotid body function is unlikely to alter the ability of patients to increase ventilation in response to reductions in the arterial partial pressures of oxygen. The ventilatory response to hypoxia, however, is lost in patients who have undergone a bilateral carotid endarterectomy. Should arterial hypoxemia occur, these patients would be less able to compensate with increases in alveolar ventilation, as compared with patients who have intact carotid body function.

Damage to peripheral nerves may occur during exposure of the carotid artery. For example, trauma to the facial nerve may manifest as unilateral perioral weakness, whereas hypoglossal nerve damage results in weakness of the tongue. Persistent hoarseness in the postoperative period may reflect surgical trauma to the recurrent laryngeal nerve.

Postoperative stroke usually occurs as a result of cerebral embolism or hemorrhagic infarction. Angiography is necessary to exclude cerebral thrombosis at the operative site. Morbidity and mortality after carotid endarterectomy are similar whether surgery is performed under regional or general anesthesia.[62]

Intracranial Occlusive Vascular Disease

Occlusive vascular disease involving the internal carotid artery and middle cerebral artery may be treated with microvascular extracranial-intracranial bypass grafting. Typically, the extracranial superficial temporal artery is anastomosed to a cortical branch of the middle cerebral artery. Nevertheless, patients with symptomatic atherosclerotic disease of the internal carotid artery show no evidence that extracranial-intracranial arterial bypass surgery prevents cerebral ischemic events. Vertebrobasilar arterial disease can be treated by anastomosis of the occipital branch of the external carotid artery to the posterior inferior cerebellar artery. Management of anesthesia for these tedious and long surgical procedures includes the same principles as detailed for removal of intracranial tumors (see the section Management of Anesthesia for Removal of Intracranial Tumors).

Minor or Major Stroke

Minor or major stroke is caused by cerebral thrombosis, cerebral embolism, or intracranial hemorrhage.

CEREBRAL THROMBOSIS

Cerebral thrombosis may be manifest as neurologic dysfunction that progresses over several minutes to hours. Dysfunction may be minor and transient or severe and irreversible. Nearly 50 percent of patients who experience a stroke have had one or more previous transient ischemic attacks. Commonly, thrombotic events occur during sleep, presumably reflecting decreased blood pressure and cerebral blood flow that are likely to occur during this time. Symptoms of cerebral thrombosis depend on the cerebral vessel that becomes occluded by thrombus. The middle cerebral artery, or a branch of this artery, is most frequently occluded. When the main trunk is occluded, infarction of a large portion of the cerebral hemisphere will result, producing symptoms of hemiplegia, homonymous hemianopsia, and, if the dominant hemisphere is involved, an expressive and receptive aphasia. Thrombosis of the anterior cerebral artery characteristically produces a more profound degree of impairment in the leg than in the face and arm. Vertebrobasilar arterial thrombosis is suggested by ipsilateral cranial nerve palsy combined with contralateral hemiplegia. Infarction of the medulla produces ipsilateral paralysis of the tongue and contralateral paralysis of the limbs, while the face is spared.

Cerebral thrombosis is most likely to develop in patients who have extensive atherosclerosis associated with essential hypertension or diabetes mellitus. Indeed, treatment of essential hypertension with antihypertensive drugs has greatly reduced the incidence of stroke. Other causes of cerebral thrombosis include (1) hypotension, as can follow a myocardial infarction; (2) inflammatory diseases of blood vessels, as associated with temporal arteritis, polyarteritis nodosa, and systemic lupus erythematosus; and (3) hematologic disorders, including polycythemia, thrombotic thrombocytopenic purpura, and sickle cell anemia. Use of oral contraceptive drugs has been alleged to be associated with an increased incidence of cerebral thrombosis.

Treatment of cerebral thrombosis may include attempts to arrest propagation of the thrombus. Therefore, if the cerebrospinal fluid is clear, these patients may receive heparin initially, followed by chronic anticoagulation with warfarin. Aspirin is an alternative to oral anticoagulants.

CEREBRAL EMBOLISM

Cerebral embolism is most commonly from the heart, in the presence of mitral valve disease plus atrial fibrillation, prosthetic heart valves, or subacute bacterial endocarditis. Occasionally, cerebral embolism represents fat, tumor cells, or air. Unlike cerebral thrombosis, the symptoms of cerebral embolism have an abrupt onset. Headache on the affected side is common. Neurologic deficits will depend on the vessel that is occluded. Emboli are responsible for the majority of ischmeic events that occur in the distribution of the carotid arteries, whereas thrombosis is likely to include vertebrobasilar vessels (Fig. 18-11). Diagnosis of cerebral embolism, although suggested by the abruptness of the onset, is definitive only if strokes occur in patients with valvular heart disease, with or without atrial fibrillation, or if there are emboli elsewhere in the body. Echocardiography may be useful in determining the source of emboli. For example, studies using contrast media with and without a Valsalva maneuver are useful in detecting right-to-left intracardiac shunts that may be associated with paradoxical embolism. Treatment of cerebral embolism in the acute phase is the same as for a cerebral thrombosis. Long-term administration of anticoagulants is helpful in preventing recurrent cerebral embolism.

INTRACRANIAL HEMORRHAGE

Intracranial hemorrhage accounts for about 10 percent of all strokes that occur in the United States.[63] The most common cause is rupture of small arterioles or microaneurysms in association with chronic hypertension, in patients 65 years to 85 years of age. Intracranial aneurysms result from a congenital weakness in the media of cerebral arteries, which can rupture, leading to intracranial hemorrhage at any age, although most often in the fourth through sixth decade. Congenital intracranial aneurysms may be single or multiple. About 50 percent occur in the middle cerebral artery. Approximately 30 percent of congenital aneurysms are present in the region where the anterior communicating artery joins the anterior cerebral arteries. The most important factor predisposing to rupture of congenital intracranial aneurysms is size.[64] Intracranial aneurysms greater than 10 mm in diameter are associated with a high incidence of spontaneous rupture. Hypertension is also thought to predispose to an increased incidence of rupture, but this has not been confirmed. Age, sex, and number and location of intracranial aneurysms do not influence incidence. Mycotic aneurysms are caused by weakening of the arterial wall around a septic embolus from the heart.

Intracranial hemorrhage can also be due to an arteriovenous malformation. Finally, systemic anticoagulation with heparin or warfarin in associated with an increased likelihood of intracranial hemorrhage.

Signs and Symptoms. Signs and symptoms of intracranial hemorrhage reflect the site of hemorrhage and the development of increased intracranial pressure. Rupture of an intracranial aneurysm results in a hematoma that displaces brain structures. For example, with hemorrhage deep in the cerebral hemispheres, there is flaccid hemiplegia, hemianesthesia, and hemianopia. Vomiting and a sudden violent headache are common. Hypertension is often present. Fever and leukocytosis reflect meningeal irritation from blood. Cerebral vasospasm frequently accompanies rupture of congenital intracranial aneurysms. If vasospasm occurs in vessels supplying the hypothalamus, the resulting ischemia may lead to stimulation of the heart through sympathetic nervous system pathways resulting in appearance of Q waves, prolonged Q-T intervals and ST elevation on the electrocardiogram. It is important to recognize that when these abnormalities are seen on the electrocardiogram after subarachnoid hemorrhage they most likely reflect a neurologic mechanism and not myocardial damage.[65] Nimodipine, a calcium entry blocker, reduces the incidence of cerebral vasospasm after subarachnoid hemorrhage.[66] This drug may be useful in preparation of patients undergoing aneurysm repair. Coma and decerebrate rigidity may result from large increases in intracranial pressure. Cerebellar hemorrhage leads to unsteadiness of gait, nuchal rigidity, and peripheral facial weakness. Mortality may exceed 50 percent in the first month following rupture of congenital intracranial aneurysms.[66] Another 30 percent of patients will experience repeat episodes of intracranial hemorrhage during this time period.

In contrast to the rapid onset of neurologic dysfunction associated with hemorrhage due to rupture of intracranial aneurysms, leakage of blood from a low-pressure arteriovenous malformation does not always produce an abrupt onset of symptoms. In fact, many patients experience repeated bouts of intracranial hemorrhage from the arteriovenous malfor-

mation with little permanent neurologic deficit.

Diagnosis. Computed tomography and cerebral angiography are used to establish the diagnosis of intracranial hemorrhage. Hemorrhage appears as a hyperdense area on computed tomography, whereas dysfunction due to transient ischemia will not result in abnormalities. Several hours to days following an ischemic event leading to irreversible damage, lucent areas will be visible on computed tomography. When hemorrhage has been extensive, the cerebrospinal fluid is usually bloody and under increased pressure. Lumbar puncture, if performed, should be accomplished using a small needle because of the risk of herniation after fluid is withdrawn. Xanthochromia develops in the spinal fluid within 4 hours and distinguishes subarachnoid hemorrhage from traumatic taps. The presence of known increased intracranial pressure is an indication not to perform a lumbar puncture.

Treatment. Immediate management of patients with intracranial hemorrhage is directed toward reduction of increased intracranial pressure (see the section Methods to Decrease Intracranial Pressure). The prognosis of massive intracranial hemorrhage is grave, with nearly 80 percent of patients dying during the acute illness. There is considerable controversy regarding the management of patients who have experienced intracranial hemorrhage due to rupture of congenital aneurysms. For example, high doses of aminocaproic acid may be effective in decreasing the incidence of repeat hemorrhage. Others, however, do not find this protective effect. Furthermore, aminocaproic acid may increase the incidence of venous thromboembolism and aggravate vasospasm associated with intracranial hemorrhage. Cerebral vasospasm may be reduced by treatment with the calcium entry blocker, nimodipine.[66] Although early operative intervention after rupture of congenital intracranial aneurysms has been traditionally deemed hazardous, other evidence suggests that prompt surgical treatment is no more dangerous than the natural course of the disease. Likewise, there is no consensus on the management of patients with congenital intracranial aneurysms that have not ruptured. Nevertheless, it is likely that surgical intervention will be planned when the demonstrated diameter of an intact aneurysm exceeds 7 mm.

INITIAL APPEARANCE OF LOCALIZED NEUROLOGIC DYSFUNCTION IN THE POSTOPERATIVE PERIOD

Localized neurologic dysfunction that manifests initially in the immediate postoperative period in a previously normal patient most likely reflects intraoperative cerebral ischemia or hemorrhage. Neurologic dysfunction occurring after cardiopulmonary bypass is most likely due to air emboli, which are especially prone to occur when cardiac chambers are opened to perform surgery (i.e., cardiac valve replacement).[67] Examination of these patients includes (1) review of the history for predisposing causes (transient ischemic attacks, atrial fibrillation); (2) physical examination (neurologic evaluation, auscultation of the heart and major vessels; and (3) review of the intraoperative course. Computed tomography and possibly echocardiography are indicated when new neurologic deficits manifest postoperatively (see the section Minor or Major Stroke). Electroencephalograms are not useful in the initial diagnosis of acute localized neurologic dysfunction. Optimal management of these patients mandates consultation with appropriate specialists as the likelihood of improvements may be dependent on prompt surgical intervention (i.e., evacuation of subdural hematomas). Before surgical intervention in these patients the goals are to maintain cerebral perfusion pressure and to control intracranial pressure.

Anesthesia for Surgical Resection of Congenital Intracranial Aneurysms

The goal during management of anesthesia for resection of congenital intracranial aneurysms is to prevent dangerous elevations in systemic blood pressure and to facilitate surgical exposure and control of the aneurysms by producing controlled hypotension.

PREOPERATIVE EVALUATION

Preoperative evaluation of these patients must assess mental status and estimate intracranial pressure. Sedation before the induction of anesthesia is desirable to reduce apprehension, but it must be titrated to prevent hypoventilation and associated increases in cerebral blood flow. Oral administration of benzodiazepines combined with intramuscular scopolamine, produces desirable anxiety relief and sedation, without introducing significant cardiopulmonary depression. Pretreatment with nimodipine may protect against cerebral vasospasm in these patients.[66]

INDUCTION OF ANESTHESIA

Induction of anesthesia is often achieved with an intravenous injection of barbiturates, benzodiazepines or etomidate followed by muscle relexants to permit easy control of ventilation and to facilitate subsequent intubation of the trachea. The use of succinylcholine is questionable, in view of the report of exaggerated potassium release after administration of this drug to patients undergoing general anesthesia for repair of previously ruptured cerebral aneurysms.[68] It is mandatory to prevent excessive and prolonged elevations in blood pressure that predictably occur in response to direct laryngoscopy and intubation of the trachea. Pressor responses to intubation of the trachea can be minimized by limiting the duration of direct laryngoscopy to less than 15 seconds and by the intravenous administration of lidocaine, 1.5 mg·kg^{-1}, to 2 minutes before beginning laryngoscopy.[69] Intravenous lidocaine can also attenuate increases in intracranial pressure associated with intubation of the trachea (Fig. 18-8).[32] Should blood pressure increase despite these precautions, it may be useful to administer nitroprusside 1 μg·kg^{-1} to 2 μg·kg^{-1} as a rapid intravenous injection.[70]

MAINTENANCE OF ANESTHESIA

Maintenance of anesthesia is acceptably achieved with nitrous oxide plus a volatile anesthetic. Potent volatile drugs are useful for preventing and treating excessive elevations in blood pressure that can occur in response to surgical stimulation. Volatile anesthetics are also likely to reduce the dose of vasodilator drugs necessary for production of controlled hypotension. Furthermore, unchanged cerebral blood flow and decreased cerebral metabolic oxygen requiremeents during administration of isoflurane indicates that global cerebral oxygen supply-demand balance is favorably altered in patients anesthetized with this anesthetic.[71] Management of ventilation, fluid therapy, use of monitors, and treatment of increased intracranial pressure are similar to that described for patients undergoing removal of intracranial tumors (see the section Management of Anesthesia for Removal of Intracranial Tumors).

CONTROLLED HYPOTENSION

Surgical exposure and control of intracranial aneurysms are facilitated by production of controlled hypotension. Continuous intravenous infusion of nitroprusside, using a calibrated pump, is most often used to achieve desired degrees of reductions in blood pressure. In the presence of adequate anesthesia, as provided by volatile anesthetics, the dose of nitroprusside seldom exceeds 3 $\mu g \cdot kg^{-1} \cdot min^{-1}$. Propranolol can be used to slow the heart rate, if reflex tachycardia which accompanies reductions in blood pressure, offsets, the hypotensive effects of nitroprusside. The maximum acceptable infusion rate of nitroprusside is 8 $\mu g \cdot kg^{-1} \cdot min^{-1}$ to 10 $\mu g \cdot kg^{-1} \cdot min^{-1}$, not to exceed 1.5 $mg \cdot kg^{-1}$ for a 1 hour to 3 hour administration, or 0.5 $mg \cdot kg^{-1} \cdot hr^{-1}$ for chronic infusion.[72] If the dose of nitroprusside approaches this infusion rate, it is important to monitor arterial pH at intervals that do not exceed 1 hour. Appearance of metabolic acidosis in patients receiving high doses of nitroprusside suggests the development of cyanide toxicity, and infusion of the drug should be immediately discontinued.

If circulatory collapse is not present, the patient should be treated with sodium thiosulfate 150 $mg \cdot kg^{-1}$, administered rapidly intravenously.[72] Thiosulfate acts as a sulfur donor to convert cyanide to thiocyanate. If cyanide toxicity is severe, with deteriorating hemodynamics and severe acidosis, treatment is the slow intravenous administration of sodium nitrate 5 $mg \cdot kg^{-1}$ to convert hemoglobin to methemoglobin.[73] Methemoglobin acts as an antidote to cyanide toxicity by converting cyanide to cyanmethemoglobin.

Alternative drugs to nitroprusside for producing controlled hypotension are trimethaphan, nitroglycerin, and labetalol. Trimethaphan is both a ganglionic blocker and a peripheral vasodilator. Although trimethaphan provides excellent minute-to-minute control of blood pressure, its use for neuroanesthesia is limited because this drug produces mydriasis, and thus interferes with evaluation of neurologic status. Perhaps more important is the observation in animals that trimethaphan decreases cerebral blood flow more than cerebral metabolic oxygen requirements, thus decreasing brain oxygen reserve during controlled hypotension produced by this drug.[74] Furthermore, tachyphylaxis commonly develops to the blood pressure-lowering effects of trimethaphan. Nitroglycerin acts predominantly on capacitance vessels to decrease blood pressure by reductions in venous return. As such, reductions in blood pressure produced by nitroglycerin may be more dependent on intravascular fluid volume, as compared with nitroprusside. In addition, nitroglycerin is less potent than nitroprusside for reducing blood pressure. For example, equivalent reductions in blood pressure were achieved using 4.7 $\mu g \cdot kg^{-1} \cdot min^{-1}$ of nitroglycerin and 2.5 $\mu g \cdot kg^{-1} \cdot min^{-1}$ of nitroprusside.[75] Labetalol is a mixed alpha- and beta-adrenergic receptor antagonist, which produces prompt reductions in blood pressure when administered intravenously, making it a potentially useful drug for production of controlled hypotension.

It is important to recognize that reductions in the arterial partial pressures of oxygen often accompany production of drug-induced controlled hypotension. Therefore, it is important to monitor arterial oxygenation during drug-induced reductions in blood pressure. Drugs used to produce controlled hypotension also act as cerebral vasodilators. As a result, cerebral blood flow and intracranial pressure can increase, despite reductions in systemic blood pressure. This increase in intracranial pressure has been documented with nitroprusside and can be attenuated by inducing hyperventilation of the lungs before administration of the drug.[33] In view of this effect, it might be prudent to withhold administration of vasodilating drugs until after the dura is opened.

The estimated safe level of controlled hypotension can be calculated on the basis of predicted cerebral blood flow, limits of autoregulation of cerebral blood flow, and arterial partial pressures of carbon dioxide. For example, in normotensive awake individuals, cerebral blood flow is about 50 ml·100 g^{-1}·min^{-1}. Evidence of cerebral ischemia on the electroencephalogram does not occur when cerebral blood flow remains above 25 ml·100 g^{-1}·min^{-1}.[76] Assuming cerebral blood flow decreases linearly below perfusion pressures of 60 mmHg, blood flow to the brain would be reduced to 25 ml·100 g^{-1}·min^{-1} when cerebral perfusion pressures are about 35 mmHg. This cerebral perfusion pressure corresponds to a mean arterial pressure of about 45 mmHg, assuming a central venous pressure of 10 mmHg (cerebral perfusion pressure is mean arterial pressure minus central venous pressure). It must be remembered that cerebral blood flow is also decreased about 1 ml for each mmHg reduction in the arterial partial pressures of carbon dioxide. Therefore, it is important to maintain the arterial partial pressures of carbon dioxide near 35 mmHg during controlled hypotension. Based on these concepts, safe cerebral perfusion pressures during controlled hypotension would be produced by a mean arterial pressures of about 50 mmHg. This mean arterial blood pressure corresponds to a systolic blood pressure of about 60 mmHg to 70 mmHg. It should also be appreciated that patients will safely tolerate mean arterial pressures below 50 mmHg for short periods, as may be needed to place a clip on an intracranial aneurysm.[77] Tolerance to low pefusion pressures is also improved by the zero intracranial pressure present when the dura is open. Conversely, hypotension produced by hemorrhage is not as well tolerated, as are similar decreases

in blood pressure produced by vasodilating drugs. Presumably, development of cerebral ischemia during hemorrhagic hypotension reflects sympathetic nervous system discharge leading to increased cerebral metabolic oxygen requirements. As a result, evidence of cerebral ischemia during hemorrhage is likely to develop at levels of blood pressure and cerebral blood flow that would be considered safe when produced by vasodilating drugs and in the absence of sympathetic nervous system stimulation.

Should controlled hypotension be considered in patients who are hypertensive, it is important to appreciate the likely rightward shift of the curve for autoregulation of cerebral blood flow. The lower limit of 60 mmHg assumed for autoregulation in normotensive patients (mean arterial pressure 90 mmHg) should be adjusted upward an equal amount for each 1 mmHg that the mean arterial pressure exceeds 90 mmHg. Therefore, the lower limit of autoregulation would be 85 mmHg in chronically hypertensive patients, with mean arterial pressures of 115 mmHg. This lower limit of autoregulation value should be used in place of 60 mmHg in calculating the safe level of controlled hypotension.

An alternative to these calculations as a guideline to the safe level of controlled hypotension is to reduce mean arterial pressuress no more than 30 mmHg to 40 mmHg below the normal awake levels. This guideline assumes a central venous pressure of 10 mmHg or less and arterial partial pressures of carbon dioxide near 35 mmHg.

The need to monitor blood pressure accurately requires strict attention to accurate calibration of the transducer used to measure arterial pressure and to proper positioning of the height of the transducer relative to heart level. Accuracy of systolic blood pressures measured from a catheter placed in a peripheral artery of the upper extremity can be confirmed by inflating an encircling cuff placed proximal to the artery until no blood flow is present. The encircling cuff is connected to a mercury manometer. Slow deflation of the occlusive cuff is permitted, until the first sign of pulsatile blood flow is detected from the peripheral artery. The pressure on the mercury manometer when this "reflow" occurs represents true systolic blood pressure. Confirmation by this method is known as the return-to-flow technique. This confirmation is essential, since false-high readings of systolic blood pressure from the intra-arterial catheter could lead to unrecognized and potentially ischemic levels of cerebral perfusion pressure during controlled hypotension. Equally important in confirming the accuracy of blood pressures recorded from the arterial catheter is proper positioning of the arterial pressure transducer. As a guideline, blood pressure decreases about 0.7 mmHg for every centimeter the head is above the level of the heart. Therefore, recording mean arterial pressure from a transducer placed at heart level would not accurately reflect perfusion pressure at the brain, if the head was elevated above the heart level. For example, when the head is elevated 20 cm above heart level, cerebral perfusion pressure will be about 14 mmHg less than the mean arterial pressure present at heart level. If controlled hypotension were produced to a mean arterial pressure of 50 mmHg as recorded from a transducer at heart level, the actual perfusion pressure at the brain would be about 36 mmHg. A useful approach during controlled hypotension is to place the transducer at the same height as the circle of Willis. From a practical standpoint, an arterial pressure transducer placed at the level of the external auditory canal will reflect mean arterial pressure at the circle of Willis.

ACUTE HEAD TRAUMA

Acute head trauma is often associated with other injuries, including cervical spine injury and thoracoabdominal trauma. Initial therapy is establishment of a patent upper airway and control of hemorrhage. Radiographs of the spine and chest are indicated when vital signs have stabilized. Neurologic dysfunction can be monitored according to the Glasgow coma scale (Table 18-2).[78] Use of this scale provides a practical system for following the neurologic status of patients who have sustained head injury. Physical examination should establish the level of consciousness and determine the

TABLE 18-2. Glasgow Coma Scale

Eye Opening	
Spontaneous	4
To speech	3
To pain	2
Nil	1
Best Motor Response	
Obeys	6
Localizes	5
Withdraws (flexion)	4
Abnormal flexion	3
Extensor response	2
Nil	1
Verbal Response	
Oriented	5
Confused conversation	4
Inappropriate words	3
Incomprehensible sounds	2
Nil	1

(Modified from Jennett B, Teasdale G. Aspects of coma after severe head injury. Lancet 1977;1:878–81)

presence of any localizing neurologic signs. The most useful diagnostic procedure is computed tomography. The possibility of an epidural or subdural hematoma should be considered in patients who have incurred head trauma. Likewise, the potential presence of increased intracranial pressure should be considered in the management of anesthesia for patients who require emergency surgery because of acute head trauma.

Epidural Hematoma

Epidural hematoma results from arterial bleeding into the space between the skull and dura due to rupture of meningeal arteries in association with a fracture of the skull. Typically, these patients experience a brief period of unconsciousness, after which there is a rapid progression of headache, lateralizing neurologic signs, and coma. Other patients never regain consciousness after the initial injury. Radiographs of the skull usually reveal a fracture, commonly across the middle meningeal artery groove. Uncal herniation, brain stem compression, and death occur within hours of the injury, unless immediate surgical decompression of the clot, via burr holes, is performed.

Subdural Hematoma

Subdural hematoma results from lacerated or torn bridging veins that bleed into the space between the dura and the arachnoid. The cerebrospinal fluid, which is subarachnoid, remains clear. Symptoms characteristically evolve gradually over several days because the hematoma results from slow venous bleeding. The most common cause is head trauma, which may be considered so minor that the responsible event has been forgotten by the patient. Trivial head injury leading to a subdural hematoma is particularly likely in elderly patients. Occasionally, a subdural hematoma is spontaneous, as in patients being treated with anticoagulants.

Headache is a universal complaint of patients with a subdural hematoma. Drowsiness and obtundation are characteristic findings, but these changes may fluctuate in magnitude from hour to hour. Lateralizing neurologic signs, manifesting as hemiparesis, hemianopsia, and language disturbances, eventually occur. Elderly patients may have an unexplained progressive dementia. Diagnosis of subdural hematoma is confirmed by computed tomography. Conservative medical management has been proposed for patients whose conditions have stablilized.[79] Nevertheless, the most frequent treatment is surgical evacuation of the clot.

DEGENERATIVE DISEASES OF THE NERVOUS SYSTEM

Degenerative diseases of the nervous system may reflect defects in the development of the neural tube, which may not result in symptoms until adulthood. Often, a hereditary pattern is responsible for these disorders. Pathologic processes may be diffuse or involve only neurons that are anatomically and functionally related.

Aqueductal Stenosis

Aqueductal stenosis is caused by congenital narrowing of the cerebral aqueduct that connects the third and fourth ventricles. Obstructive hydrocephalus can develop in infancy, when the narrowing is severe. Lesser degrees of obstruction result in a slowly progressive hydrocephalus, which may not be evident until adulthood. Symptoms of aqueductal stenosis are those of increased intracranial pressure. Seizure disorders are present in about one-third of patients. Computed tomography confirms the presence of obstructive hydrocephalus, but angiography may be necessary to exclude the possibility of posterior fossa tumors. Aqueductal stenosis sufficient to produce signs of hydrocephalus and increased intracranial pressure is treated by ventricular shunting. Management of anesthesia for creation of a ventricular shunt must consider the likely presence of increased intracranial pressure in these patients.

Arnold-Chiari Malformation

The Arnold-Chiari malformation consists of the downward displacement of the tonsillar portion of the cerebellum and caudal portions of the medulla through the foramen magnum into the upper cervical spinal canal. Cerebellar herniation results in the formation of arachnoidal adhesions, which leads to obstruction of the flow of cerebrospinal fluid from the fourth ventricle. This obstruction can lead to hydrocephalus and increased intracranial pressure. In addition, there is progressive entrapment of cranial nerves, and torsion of the brain stem.

SIGNS AND SYMPTOMS

Signs and symptoms of the Arnold-Chiari malformation appear at any age. The most common complaint is that of an occipital headache, often extending into the shoulders and arms, with a corresponding cutaneous dysesthesia. Pain is aggravated by coughing or movements of the head. Visual disturbances, intermittent vertigo, and ataxia are prominent symptoms. Signs of syringomyelia are present in about 50 percent of patients with this disorder.

TREATMENT

Treatment of the Arnold-Chiari malformation is surgical decompression by freeing adhesions and enlarging the foramen magnum. Management of anesthesia must consider the possibility of associated increased intracranial pressure.

Syringomyelia

Syringomyelia is a chronic and slowly progressive degeneration of the spinal cord, leading to cavitation. Presumably, this degeneration reflects an abnormality of embryologic development associated with obstruction to the outflow of cerebrospinal fluid from the fourth ventricle. The pressure of cerebrospinal fluid is directed into the central canal of the spinal cord, which eventually leads to cyst formation.

SIGNS AND SYMPTOMS

Signs and symptoms of syringomyelia usually begin in the third or fourth decades of life. Early complaints are those of dissociated sensory impairment in the upper extremities, reflecting destruction of crossing fibers that convey the sensation of pain and temperature. As the cavitation of the spinal cord progresses, there is destruction of lower motor neurons, with the development of skeletal muscle weakness and wasting, with areflexia. Thoracic scoliosis may result from weakness of paravertebral muscles. Extension of the cavitation process cephalad into the medulla results in syringobulbia, characterized by paralysis of the palate, tongue, vocal cords, and loss of sensation over the face.

TREATMENT

There is no known treatment effective in arresting the progressive degeneration of the spinal cord or medulla. Surgical procedures designed to restore the normal flow of cerebrospinal fluid or to plug the central cavity have not been predictably effective.

MANAGEMENT OF ANESTHESIA

Management of anesthesia in patients with syringomyelia or syringobulbia should consider neurologic deficits associated with this disease. Thoracic scoliosis can contribute to poor matching of ventilation to perfusion. The presence of lower motor neuron disease, leading to skeletal muscle wasting, suggests the possibility that hyperkalemia can develop after the administration of succinylcholine.[80] Likewise, co-existing skeletal muscle weakness could be associated with exaggerated responses to nondepolarizing muscle relaxants. Body temperature should be monitored, as thermal regulation may be impaired. Selection of drugs for induction and maintenance of anesthesia is not influenced by the disease. The possible presence of reduced or absent protective airway reflexes should be remembered when considering removal of the tracheal tube in the postoperative period.

Amyotrophic Lateral Sclerosis

Amyotrophic lateral sclerosis is a degenerative disease of motor cells throughout the central nervous system and spinal cord that most commonly afflicts males between 40 years and 60 years of age. Limitation of the degenerative process to the motor cortex is designated primary lateral sclerosis, and limitation to the brain stem nuclei is known as pseudobulbar palsy. Werdnig-Hoffmann disease resembles amyotrophic lateral sclerosis, except that manifestations of this disease occur in the first 3 years of life. Although the cause of amyotrophic lateral sclerosis is not known, there is occasionally a genetic pattern, and the possibility of a viral etiology has been proposed.

SIGNS AND SYMPTOMS

Signs and symptoms of amyotrophic lateral sclerosis reflect upper and lower motor neuron dysfunction. A frequent initial manifestation is atrophy, weakness, and fasciculations of skeletal muscles, often beginning in the intrinsic muscles of the hand. With time, atrophy and weakness involves most skeletal muscles, including those of the tongue, pharynx, larynx, and chest. Early symptoms of bulbar involvement include fasciculations of the tongue, and dysphagia leading to pulmonary aspiration. For reasons that are not clear, ocular muscles are spared. An inability to control emotional responses is characteristic. Complaints of cramping and aching sensations, particularly in the lower extremities, are common. Carcinoma of the lungs has been associated with amyotrophic lateral sclerosis. Plasma creatine kinase concentrations are normal, distinguishing this disease from chronic polymyositis. There is no treatment, and death is likely within 6 years after the onset of clinical symptoms.

MANAGEMENT OF ANESTHESIA

Patients with lower motor neuron diseases such as amyotrophic lateral sclerosis are vulnerable to hyperkalemia after administration of succinylcholine.[80] Furthermore, these patients may manifest prolonged responses to nondepolarizing muscle relaxants. Indeed, changes of amyotrophic lateral sclerosis, as manifested on the electromyogram, resemble myasthenia gravis. Bulbar involvement with dysfunction of pharyngeal muscles may predispose these patients to pulmonary aspiration. There is no evidence that a specific anesthetic drug or combination of drugs is best for administration to patients with this disease.

Friedreich's Ataxia

Friedreich's ataxia is an autosomal recessive inherited condition, which is characterized by degeneration of the spinocerebellar and pyramidal tracts. Cardiomyopathy is present in 90 percent of cases, and kyphoscoliosis, causing a steady deterioration of pulmonary function, is present in nearly 80 percent of affected individuals. Ataxia is the typical presenting symptom. Dysarthria, nystagmus, skeletal muscle weakness and spasticity, and diabetes mellitus may be present. Friedreich's ataxia is usually fatal by early adulthood often due to cardiac failure.

Management of anesthesia for Friedreich's ataxia is as described for amyotrophic lateral sclerosis. In addition, the potential for exaggerated negative inotropic effects of anesthetic drugs in the presence of cardiomyopathy should be considered. Although experience is limited, response to muscle relaxants seems normal.[81] The likelihood of postoperative respiratory failure may be increased especially in the presence of kyphoscoliosis.

Paralysis Agitans

Paralysis agitans (Parkinson's disease) is a degenerative disease of the central nervous system characterized by loss of dopaminergic fibers present in the basal ganglia of the brain. As a result of the degeneration of these fibers, there is depletion of dopamine in the basal ganglia. Dopamine is presumed to be a neurotransmitter, which acts by inhibiting the rate of firing of neurons that control the extrapyramidal motor system. Depletion of dopamine results in diminished inhibition of the extrapyramidal motor system and an unopposed action of acetylcholine.

Although the cause of paralysis agitans is usually unknown, this disease has been observed to develop after encephalitis, intoxication with carbon monoxide, and chronic ingestion of antipsychotic drugs. Males between 40 years and 60 years of age are most often afflicted.

SIGNS AND SYMPTOMS

Classic signs and symptoms of paralysis agitans are decreased spontaneous movements, rigidity of the extremities, facial immobility, a shifting gait, and a rhythmic resting tremor. These symptoms reflect diminished inhibition of the activity of the extrapyramidal motor system due to depletion of dopamine from the basal ganglia. Skeletal muscle rigidity first appears in proximal limb muscles of the neck. The earliest manifestation can be loss of associated arm swing when walking and absence of head rotation when turning. Facial immobility is characterized by infrequent blinking and a paucity of emotional responses. Tremor is characterized as rhythmic, alternating flexion and extension of the thumb and digits at a rate of four to five movements per second. These movements are often described as a pill-rolling tremor. The tremor is prominent in the resting limb but disappears briefly during the course of a movement, which distinguishes it from an essential or familial tremor. Seborrhea, oily skin, pupillary abnormalities, diaphragmatic spasms, and oculogyric crises are frequent. Dementia and depression are often noted.

TREATMENT

Treatment of paralysis agitans is designed to increase concentrations of dopamine in the basal ganglia or to decrease neuronal effects of acetylcholine. Drugs most often used to achieve these goals are levodopa, anticholinergics, and antihistamines.

Levodopa. Exogenous administration of dopamine will not increase concentrations of this inhibitory neurotransmitter in the basal ganglia, since dopamine cannot cross the blood-brain barrier. However, the immediate precursor of dopamine, levodopa, does cross the barrier and is then converted to dopamine in the central nervous system by a decarboxylase enzyme. Therefore, the oral administration of levodopa (4 g·day^{-1} to 6 g·day^{-1}) can be used to increase central nervous system concentrations of dopamine. It must be appreciated that the decarboxylating enzyme responsible for the conversion of levodopa to dopamine in the central nervous system is also present in the systemic circulation and other tissues. As a result, administration of levodopa results in total body increases in concentrations of dopamine. Furthermore, conversion of levodopa to dopamine in the systemic circulation limits the amount of drug available for transfer to the central nervous system. For this reason, levodopa is often combined with a drug that inhibits activity of decarboxylase enzyme in the systemic circulation. Indeed, the combination of levodopa with such an enzyme inhibitor, carbidopa, often permits a 75 percent reduction in the dose of levodopa, with associated decreases in dose-related adverse side effects of this drug.

Adverse side effects of levodopa manifest on the cardiovascular, gastrointestinal, and central nervous systems. Dopamine resulting from levodopa can increase myocardial contractility and heart rate and predispose to cardiac irritability. Norepinephrine stores in the heart may become depleted by chronic levodopa administration. High dopamine concentrations result in peripheral vasoconstriction; low levels of dopamine are known to increase renal blood flow, glomerular filtration rate, and excretion of sodium. Renin release is also reduced during levodopa therapy. As a result of these renal effects of dopamine, it is likely that intravascular fluid volume will be decreased, and activity of the renin-angiotensin-aldosterone system will be reduced. Therefore, orthostatic hypotension may be a common finding in patients being chronically treated with levodopa. Another mechanism for orthostatic hypotension is decreased production of norepinephrine in sympathetic nervous system nerve endings due to the negative feedback inhibition of high concentrations of dopamine on the synthesis of catecholamines. In addition, dopamine replaces norepinephrine at many sites and, because of its weaker pressor actions, is less able to support blood pressure. Some central nervous system side effects of dopamine contribute to hypotension.

Gastrointestinal side effects of levodopa therapy are reflected by nausea and vomiting, which most likely reflect stimulation of the chemoreceptor trigger zone by dopamine. Central nervous system effects of chronic levodopa therapy most often manifest as psychiatric symptoms, which include agitation, confusion, depression, and overt psychosis. The most serious problem is the appearance of dyskinesis, which develops in about 80 percent of patients after a year or more of treatment with levodopa.

Anticholinergic and Antihistaminic Drugs.   Anticholinergic drugs may be the initial selections for therapy when symptoms of paralysis agitans are mild. Antihistaminic drugs are also useful for the control of mild symptoms of extrapyramidal motor system overactivity, particularly as produced by phenothiazines or butyrophenones.

MANAGEMENT OF ANESTHESIA

Management of anesthesia in patients with paralysis agitans is based on an understanding of the treatment of this disease and of the associated potential adverse drug effects. Levodopa therapy should be continued in the perioperative period, including the usual morning dose on the day of surgery. The elimination half-time of levodopa and the resulting dopamine are short, so that interruption of therapy for more than 6 hours to 12 hours can result in abrupt loss of therapeutic benefits derived from this drug. Indeed, abrupt withdrawal of levodopa can result in skeletal muscle rigidity that interferes with the maintenance of adequate ventilation.[82]

The possibility of orthostatic hypotension, cardiac dysrhythmias, and even hypertension must be kept in mind during administration of anesthesia to patients being treated with levodopa. Selection of drugs to be administered in the preoperative medication and for the production of anesthesia must consider the ability of phenothiazines and butyrophenones to antagonize the effects of dopamine in the basal ganglia. Therefore, droperidol, as present in Innovar, would not be a wise selection in the patient being treated with levodopa. Use of ketamine may be questionable because of the possible provocation of exaggerated sympathetic nervous system responses. Nevertheless, ketamine has been successfully used in a patient being treated with levodopa.[82] Cardiac dysrhythmias may be more likely to occur when halothane is selected, although this speculation has not been documented. The presence of decreased intravascular fluid volume may be manifested as reductions in blood pressure during induction of anesthesia, requiring aggressive administration of crystalloid or colloid solutions. Choice of muscle relaxants does not seem to be influenced by the presence of paralysis agitans. Nevertheless, there is a report of a single patient who developed hyperkalemia after the intravenous administration of succinylcholine.[83] Reinstitution of levodopa therapy in the postoperative period is as important as maintaining treatment up to the time of induction of anesthesia.

Hallervorden-Spatz Disease

Hallervorden-Spatz disease is a rare autosomal recessive disorder of basal ganglia, which follows a slowly progressive course from its onset in late childhood to death in about 10 years. No specific laboratory tests are diagnostic for this condition, and no effective treatment is known. Dementia and dystonia with torticollis, and scoliosis are commonly present. Dystonic posturing is likely to disappear with induction of anesthesia, although skeletal muscle contractures and bony changes may accompany chronic forms of the disease, leading to immobility of the temporomandibular joints and cervical spine, even in the presence of deep general anesthesia or neuromuscular blockade.

Management of anesthesia must consider the possibility of being unable to position optimally the patient for intubation of the trachea after induction of anesthesia.[84] Noxious stimulation, as produced by attempted awake intubation of the trachea, may intensify dystonia. For these reasons, induction of anesthesia may be best achieved by inhalation of anesthetic gases and maintenance of spontaneous ventilation. Administration of succinylcholine is questionable since skeletal muscle wasting and diffuse axonal changes in the brain, which may involve upper motor neurons, could accentuate potassium release after administration of this drug. Any required skeletal muscle relaxation is probably best provided by increased concentrations of volatile anesthetics or nondepolarizing muscle relaxants. Emergence from anesthesia will be predictably accompanied by return of dystonic posturing.

Huntington's Chorea

Huntington's chorea is a premature degenerative disease of the central nervous system characterized by marked atrophy of the caudate nucleus and, to a lesser degree, of the putamen and globus pallidus.[85] Biochemical abnormalities include deficiencies in the basal ganglia of acetylcholine and its synthesizing enzyme choline acetyltransferase and gamma-aminobutyric acid. A selective loss of gamma-aminobutyric acid may reduce inhibition of the dopamine nigrostriatal system. This disease is transmitted as an autosomal dominant trait, but its delayed appearance to 35 years to 40 years of age interferes with effective genetic counseling.

SIGNS AND SYMPTOMS

Signs and symptoms of Huntington's chorea consist of progressive dementia combined with choreoathetosis. Chorea is usually considered the first sign of Huntington's chorea, although behavioral changes (depression, dementia) may precede by several years the onset of involuntary movements. Involvement of pharyngeal muscles makes these patients susceptible to pulmonary aspiration. The disease progresses over several years, and accompanying mental depression makes suicide a prominent cause of death. The duration of Huntington's chorea from onset to the patient's death averages 17 years.

TREATMENT

Treatment of Huntington's chorea is symptomatic and directed at reducing choreiform movements. Haloperidol or chlorpromazine have been used to control chorea and emotional lability associated with this disease. The most useful therapy for control of involuntary movements is with drugs that interfere with the neurotransmitter effects of dopamine. As such, butyrophenones and phenothiazines may be helpful in the management of these patients. Diazepam and lithium have also been tried, with varying success.

MANAGEMENT OF ANESTHESIA

Experience with the management of anesthesia in these patients is too limited to propose specific drugs or techniques. Nitrous oxide combined with opioids plus droperidol would seem like a useful approach in view of the potential antagonism of dopamine by droperidol. Nevertheless, use of nitrous oxide plus volatile anesthetics is also acceptable. Delayed awakening and generalized tonic spasms have been observed after the administration of thiopental to a single patient.[86] The importance of this observation, if any, is not clear. Decreased plasma cholinesterase activity, with prolonged responses to succinylcholine, have been reported.[87] Likewise, it has been suggested that these patients may be sensitive to the effects of nondepolarizing muscle relaxants.[88] Preoperative and postoperative sedation with butyrophenones or phenothiazines may be helpful in controlling choreiform movements. The increased hazards of pulmonary aspiration must be remembered if pharyngeal muscles are involved.

Spasmodic Torticollis

Spasmodic torticollis is thought to result from disturbances of basal ganglia function. The most frequent mode of presentation is spasmodic contraction of nuchal muscles, which may progress to involve limb and girdle muscles. Hypertrophy of the sternocleidomastoid muscle may be present. Spasm may involve muscles of the vertebral column, leading to lordosis and scoliosis and impairment of ventilation. Treatment is not particularly effective, but a bilateral anterior rhizotomy at C-1 and C-3, with a subarachnoid section of the spinal accessory nerve, may be attempted. This operation may result in postoperative paralysis of the diaphragm, manifesting as respiratory distress. There are no known problems related to the selection of anesthetic drugs, but spasm of nuchal muscles may interfere with maintenance of a patent upper airway before institution of skeletal muscle paralysis. Furthermore, awake intubation of the trachea may be necessary, if chronic skeletal muscle spasm has led to fixation of the cervical vertebrae.

Shy-Drager Syndrome

Shy-Drager syndrome is characterized by failure of the autonomic nervous system in association with widespread parenchymatous degeneration in the central nervous system and spinal cord. Although the primary defect is loss of neuronal cells, an element of sympathetic nervous system dysfunction can result from the depletion of norepinephrine from peripheral efferent nerve endings. Idiopathic orthostatic hypotension, rather than the Shy-Drager syndrome, is considered to be present when autonomic nervous system dysfunction occurs in the absence of central nervous system degeneration.

SIGNS AND SYMPTOMS

Signs and symptoms of the Shy-Drager syndrome are related to failure of the autonomic nervous system, as manifested by orthostatic hypotension, urinary retention, bowel dysfunction, diminishhed sweating, and sexual impotence. Postural hypotension is often severe enough to produce syncope. Plasma concentrations of norepinephrine fail to show normal increases after standing or exercise. Sweating may be absent, pupillary reflexes sluggish, and control of breathing abnormal. Further evidence of autonomic nervous system dysfunction is failure of baroreceptor reflexes to produce increases in heart rate or vasoconstriction in response to hypotension. Symptoms of paralysis agitans often develop in these patients.

TREATMENT

There is no specific treatment for this syndrome, and death usually occurs within 8 years of diagnosis. Death is most often due to cerebral ischemia due to prolonged hypotension. Theoretically, orthostatic hypotension might be lessened by treatment with selective alpha-2 adrenergic antagonists, such as yohimbine, which would facilitate continued release of norepinephrine from postganglionic nerve endings. Levodopa is administered to reduce the symptoms of paralysis agitans.

MANAGEMENT OF ANESTHESIA

Management of anesthesia is based on understanding the impact of reduced autonomic nervous system activity on cardiovascular responses to such events as changes in body position, positive airway pressure, and acute blood loss, as well as on the effects produced by the administration of negative inotropic anesthetic drugs. Preoperative evaluation may elicit such signs of autonomic nervous system dysfunction as orthostatic hypotension and absence of beat-to-beat variability in heart rate associated with deep breathing. Despite the obvious vulnerability of these patients to events likely to occur during the perioperative period, clinical experience has been that most tolerate general anesthesia without undue risk.[89] The key to management of these patients is close monitoring of blood pressure, and rapid correction of hypotension by the infusion of crystalloid or colloid solutions. Continuous measurement of arterial blood pressure and cardiac filling pressures is useful for guiding the rate of intravenous fluid infusion. If a vasopressor is needed, it should be appreciated that these patients can exhibit exaggerated responses to drugs that act by provoking the release of norepinephrine. Presumably, this excessive response reflects denervation hypersensitivity. An appropriate selection to treat hypotension pharmacologically would be direct-acting drugs such as phenylephrine. Even doses of phenylephrine should be initially reduced, until the response of each individual patient can be confirmed. The risk of hypotension after administration of spinal or epidural anesthesia detracts from the use of these techniques in affected patients. Excessive reductions in cardiac output, due to myocardial depression from volatile anesthetic drugs, can result in exaggerated hypotension, since such compensatory responses as vasoconstriction or tachycardia are unlikely, in view of absent carotid sinus activity in these patients. Likewise, positive pressure ventilation of the lungs or acute blood loss are not readily compensated for by increases in sympathetic nervous system activity. Bradycardia, which contributes to hypotension, is best treated with atropine. Signs of the depth of anesthesia may be less apparent in these patients because of decreased responses of the sympathetic nervous system to noxious stimulation. Induction of anesthesia with diazepam and fentanyl, plus pancuronium for skeletal muscle paralysis, has been described in these patients, followed by maintenance of anesthesia with low doses of volatile anesthetics, combined with nitrous oxide.[89] Administration of muscle relaxants with minimal to absent effects on circulation would also seem a useful alternative to pancuronium. Thiopental, as used for induction of anesthesia, might provoke exaggerated reductions in blood pressure if the rate of administration is rapid or the intravenous fluid volume decreased. Conversely, the possibility of accentuated blood pressure elevations after administration of ketamine should be considered.

Familial Dysautonomia

Familial dysautonomia (Riley-Day syndrome) is an inherited disorder of central nervous system dysfunction, which manifests as disturbances of autonomic nervous system, sensory, motor, and psychic function (see Chapter 35). Inheritance of this syndrome is as an autosomal recessive trait, with symptoms appearing in infancy or early childhood. Children of Jewish descent are most often affected.

SIGNS AND SYMPTOMS

Sudden alterations in blood pressure, ranging from hypertension to hypotension, are characteristic of familial dysautonomia. Orthostatic hypotension may be prominent in these patients. The presence of hypertension distinguishes this disease from the Shy-Drager syndrome. Hypotension is presumed to reflect absence of normal sympathetic nervous system activity and decreased carotid sinus reflex responses. Indeed, failure of the heart rate to increase in response to reductions in blood pressure is a characteristic finding. Furthermore, there is an absence of increased circulating concentrations of norepinephrine in response to exercise, or on assuming the standing position. Episodes of hypertension are thought to reflect denervation hypersensitivity and an inability to enlist compensatory parasympathetic nervous system responses. Absence of normal sensory perception makes these patients vulnerable to unrecognized trauma or self-mutilation. Infants have difficulty swallowing, and aspiration pneumonia is common. Older children manifest deficient tear formation, excess salivation, emotional lability, retarded growth, and erratic temperature control. Ventilatory responses to carbon dioxide are depressed.

MANAGEMENT OF ANESTHESIA

Management of anesthesia and potential adverse responses are similar to those described for Shy-Drager syndrome. In addition, these patients may have reduced anesthetic requirements based on diminished sensory perception. Stimuli associated with intubation of the trachea may result in exaggerated hypertension. Volatile anesthetics may produce hypotension necessitating administration of sympathomimetics, which in these patients may produce exaggerated responses. Induction and maintenance of anesthesia using opioids with intermittent administration of volatile anesthetics to control blood pressure has been described.[90,91] Use of skeletal muscle relaxants with minimal circulatory effects would seem prudent. Succinylcholine has been administered to these patients, although the risk of increased potassium release in patients with progressive neurologic disease has been described. Regional anesthesia does not seem to be an attractive choice in view of the cardiovascular instability characteristic of this disease. The potential for the development of hyperpyrexia must be considered, in view of the decreased ability of these patients to perspire. Preoperative pulmonary infections are likely because of recurrent pulmonary aspiration. Likewise, vomiting in the postoperative period introduces the risk of aspiration. Indeed, the need to mechanically ventilate the lungs for a period of time postoperatively should be considered.

Congenital Insensitivity to Pain

Congenital insensitivity to pain with anhidrosis (CIPA) is a rare disorder that leads to self-mutilation and defective thermoregulation. Plasma concentrations of catecholamines may be reduced and autonomic nervous system dysfunction may be present. Skeletal muscle weakness and joint laxity are characteristic. Management of anesthesia includes preoperative medication to relieve apprehension in an often mentally retarded patient, monitoring of body temperature and avoidance of joint extension.[92] Use of anticholinergic drugs is questionable considering the presence of anhidrosis, as well as potential autonomic nervous system dysfunction.

Progressive Blindness

Degenerative diseases of the central nervous system limited to the optic nerve and retina include Leber's optic atrophy, retinitis pigmentosa, and the Kearns-Sayer syndrome.

LEBER'S OPTIC ATROPHY

Leber's optic atrophy is characterized by degeneration of the retina and atrophy of the optic nerve, culminating in blindness. Transmission of this disease is as a sex-linked autosomal recessive trait. The defect responsible for optic atrophy is most likely related to an abnormality of cyanide metabolism. Therefore, these patients should not receive nitroprusside.

RETINITIS PIGMENTOSA

Retinitis pigmentosa is a genetically determined disease characterized by degeneration of the retina. Examination of the retina reveals areas of pigmentation, particularly in the peripheral regions. Vision is lost from the periphery of the retina toward the center, until total blindness develops.

KEARNS-SAYER SYNDROME

Kearns-Sayer syndrome is characterized by retinitis pigmentosa associated with progressive external ophthalmoplegia, which typically manifests before 20 years of age. Cardiac conduction abnormalities, ranging from bundle branch block to third-degree atrioventricular heart block, are common in these patients. Third-degree atrioventricular heart block can occur abruptly, leading to death before an artificial cardiac pacemaker can be inserted. Generalized degeneration of the central nervous system has been observed. This finding, plus the often elevated concentration of protein in the cerebrospinal fluid, suggests a viral etiology for this disease.

Although this is an extremely rare syndrome, it is conceivable that one could encounter patients who require surgery for procedures other than the insertion of artificial cardiac pacemakers. Management of anesthesia requires a high index of suspicion and prior preparation to treat third-degree atrioventricular heart block, should this cardiac conduction abnormality occur during the perioperative period (see Chapter 5). This preparation includes the immediate availability of isoproterenol for infusion as a chemical pace-maker so as to maintain an adequate heart rate until external cardiac pacing can be established. Experience is too limited to recommend specific drugs for the induction and maintenance of anesthesia. Apparently, the response to succinylcholine and nondepolarizing muscle relaxants is not altered, suggesting that this disease does not involve the neuromuscular junction.[93]

Alzheimer's Disease

Alzheimer's disease is characterized by progressive dementia, which typically occurs after 60 years of age and may afflict 20 percent of the population who are 80 years of age or older.[94,95] The disease occurs with the same frequency in either sex. In addition to age, risk factors for Alzheimer's disease include its occurrence in a parent or sibling, a history of serious head trauma as associated with boxing, and the presence of trisomy 21. It is estimated that more than 2 million persons in the United States suffer from this disease, which is the principal reason for admission to nursing homes. Alzheimer's disease reduces life expectancy, with total incapacitation usually occurring within 8 years after the diagnosis.

PATHOPHYSIOLOGY

A diagnosis of definite Alzheimer's disease, in addition to clinical findings and laboratory tests to exclude other causes of dementia (neurosyphilis, toxins, vasculitis, metabolic disorders), requires histopathologic evidence obtained via brain biopsy or at autopsy. The principal morphologic changes in the brain include cortical atrophy, loss of neurons, and the presence of neurofibrillary tangles and neuritic plaques.

The most striking morphologic findings in Alzheimer's disease are the abnormal fibrous proteins, which make up the characteristic neurofibrillary tangles. Aluminum and silicon are present in the neuritic plaques of these tangles. There is no evidence, however, that exposure to exogenous aluminum, as may be present in antacids or renal dialysates increases the risk of Alzheimer's disease.

There is a 40 percent to 90 percent decrease in the activity of the biosynthetic enzyme, choline acetyltransferase, in the cerebral cortex and hippocampus of patients with Alzheimer's disease (i.e., a cholinergic deficit).[94] There is a strong correlation between changes in mental status scores and loss of choline acetyltransferase. In this regard, it is noteworthy that the anticholinergic drug, scopolamine, produces confusion and memory loss, which resemble changes seen in the early stages of Alzheimer's disease. If Alzheimer's disease is principally a deficit in cholinergic function, it is likely that drugs could restore the biochemical deficiency. For example, physostigmine, an anticholinesterase drug that slows the hydrolysis of acetylcholine, has been demonstrated to have modest beneficial effects on various aspects of cognitive functioning in occasional patients in the early stages of Alzheimer's disease.[96] Tetrahydroaminoacridine, a centrally active anticholinesterase drug, is sometimes effective when administered orally for long-term palliative treatment.[97] Another drug, which may provide symptomatic relief in some patients, is ergoloid, a combination of three ergot alkaloids.

Alzheimer's disease is not simply a cholinergic deficit, as other neurotransmitters may also be deficient. For example, somatostatin, a peptide neurotransmitter, which may be involved in cortical connectivity, is decreased in the brains of patients with Alzheimer's disease to almost the same extent as choline acetyltransferase. A concomitant reduction in the population of somatostatin receptors contrasts with the relative maintenance of muscarinic receptor density. A deficiency of norepinephrine seems to occur with greater frequency in younger patients with this disease. Neurotransmitters not reduced in patients with Alzheimer's disease include dopamine, gamma-aminobutyric acid, substance P, cholecystokinin and vasoactive intestinal peptide.

SIGNS AND SYMPTOMS

Dementia is characterized by intellectual deterioration in an adult severe enough to interfere with occupational or social performance. Cognitive changes include not only disturbances in memory, but also disturbances in other cognitive areas, such as language use, the ability to learn necessary skills, think abstractly, and make judgments. Initially, retention of new information is impaired followed by global dementia. Social avoidance and anxiety are common. Irritability, agitation, and physical aggression toward family members may develop. Seizures are not likely to occur.

MANAGEMENT OF ANESTHESIA

Management of anesthesia is based on an understanding of the pathophysiology of this disease. The major problem in the perioperative period is dealing with a patient unable to comprehend the environment or to cooperate with those responsible for providing medical care. Sedative drugs, as might be used in preoperative medication, should rarely be administered to these patients, as further mental confusion could result. Certainly, centrally acting anticholinergic drugs should not be included in the preoperative medication, whereas reversal of nondepolarizing neuromuscular blockade might logically include glycopyrrolate rather than atropine. Maintenance of anesthesia can be acceptably achieved with inhaled or injected drugs. A possible advantage of an inhaled drug would be a more predictable return to the level of preoperative mental function after surgery. Possible drug interactions based on co-existing treatment with centrally acting anticholinesterase drugs should be considered.

Creutzfeldt-Jakob Disease

Creutzfeldt-Jakob disease (subacute spongiform encephalopathy) is a rare, noninflammatory disease of the central nervous system caused by a transmissible, slow infectious pathogen known as prions.[98] Prions differ from viruses in lacking RNA or DNA. The incubation period for this disease is prolonged, being measured in months or years. It affects one to two individuals per million population. Lab-

oratory values are not helpful in diagnosis of the disease, although an occasional patient may show evidence of hepatic dysfunction. Alterations in autonomic nervous system function characterized by failure of the heart rate to increase in response to atropine may be present. There is no known treatment.

Creutzfeldt-Jakob disease is potentially iatrogenically transmissible, as emphasized by its occurrence in two patients 2.3 years and 2.5 years after stereotactic electroencephalographic exploration with silver electrodes sterilized in alcohol and formaldehyde but previously implanted in an infected patient.[99] The disease has also been observed in exposed medical personnel. Disposable anesthetic equipment should be used, and other equipment autoclaved for 1 hour at temperatures of at least 121 degrees Celsius or alternatively soaked in a 0.5 percent solution of sodium hypochlorite. Contact with infected tissue and blood is best prevented by use of gloves and gowns. Accidental percutaneous exposure to infected tissue or blood should be followed by thorough cleaning of the wound with iodine or sodium hypochlorite.

Leigh's Syndrome

Leigh's syndrome (subacute necrotizing encephalomyelopathy) is a chronic neurologic disease usually diagnosed before 4 years of age.[100] Symmetric lesions are usually found in the brain stem and lateral walls of the third ventricle, explaining the common clinical features, which include hypotonia, ataxia, breathing difficulties, propensity to aspiration, altered temperature regulation, and occurrence of seizures. The syndrome is progressive and marked by remissions and acute exacerbations, which may develop after surgery.

The most likely enzyme abnormality is a defect in activation of pyruvate dehydrogenase. Indeed, increased blood lactate and pyruvate concentrations are frequently present. In this regard, crystalloid solutions containing lactate are avoided to minimze any iatrogenic contribution to co-existing lactic acidosis. Likewise, iatrogenic respiratory alkalosis due to intraoperative hyperventilation of the lungs could result in inhibition of pyruvate carboxylase and accentuation of lactic acidosis. Selection of drugs for anesthesia may be influenced by the ability of barbiturates and inhaled drugs to interfere with mitochondrial respiration. Nevertheless, experience in management of these patients is too limited to allow specific recommendations for drug selection.

Multiple Sclerosis

Multiple sclerosis is an acquired disease of the central nervous system characterized by random and multiple sites of demyelination of corticospinal tract neurons in the brain and spinal cord.[101,102] Neuropathologic changes consist of loss of the myelin covering the axons in the form of demyelinative plaques. The disease does not affect the peripheral nervous system. Multiple sclerosis is a disease of young adults, with the onset of symptoms before 15 years or after 40 years of age being rare.

ETIOLOGY

The relationship between geographic latitude and the risk of developing multiple sclerosis is striking. For example, the incidence is high (75 to 150 per 100,000 population) in the northern temperate zone in North America and Europe and in the southern portions of New Zealand and Australia. There is a low incidence of this disease near the equator. Studies of migrant populations have disclosed that factors determining susceptibility are acquired before 15 years of age. In addition, the incidence of multiple sclerosis is greater in urban dwellers and among affluent socioeconomic groups. Evidence for the role of genetic factors is demonstrated by the 12-fold to 15-fold increase of the disease among first-degree relatives. In addition, a high percentage of patients share common histocompatibility antigens. For example, 60 percent of patients share the antigen designated as HLA-DW2, whereas only 18 percent of patients without the disease have this antigen. These features of multiple sclerosis lend support to theories of a viral etiology. Conceivably, a viral infection initiates an altered immune reaction against myelin in genetically susceptible individuals. Indeed, several viruses can cause demyelination of the central nervous system in animals, but to date none has been shown to be causative for multiple sclerosis.

SIGNS AND SYMPTOMS

Symptoms of multiple sclerosis reflect sites of demyelination in the central nervous system and spinal cord. For example, disease of the optic nerve causes visual disturbances; involvement of the cerebellum leads to gait disturbances; and lesions of the spinal cord cause limb paresthesias and weakness, as well as urinary incontinence and sexual impotence. Ascending spastic paresis of skeletal muscles is often prominent. Optic neuritis is characterized by diminished visual acuity and defective pupillary reaction to light. Demyelination of pathways in the brain stem that coordinate eye movement cause paresis of the medial rectus muscle on lateral conjugate gaze. Nystagmus is seen in the abducting eye. Intramedullary disease of the cervical cord is suggested by an electrical sensation, which runs down the back into the legs in response to flexion of the neck (Lhermitte's sign). Typically, symptoms develop over the course of a few days, remain stable for a few weeks, and then improve. Since remyelination in the central nervous system probably does not occur, remission of symptoms probably results from correction of transient chemical and physiologic disturbances, which have interfered with nerve conduction in the absence of complete demyelination. There is an increased incidence of seizure disorders in patients with multiple sclerosis.

The course of multiple sclerosis is characterized by exacerbation of symptoms at unpredictable intervals over a period of several years. Residual symptoms eventually persist during remission, leading to severe disability from visual failure, incoordination, spastic weakness, and urinary incontinence. Nevertheless, the disease in some patients remains benign, with infrequent mild episodes of demyelination followed by prolonged, and occasionally permanent, remission. Onset of multiple sclerosis after 35 years of age is most likely to be associated with a slow progression.

DIAGNOSIS

Diagnosis of multiple sclerosis must be made on clinical grounds, as there are no specific laboratory tests.[102,103] Certain laboratory findings, however, support the clinical diagnosis. For example, alterations in color vision may indicate the presence of subclinical optic neuropathy caused by demyelination in the optic nerve. Visual, brain stem-, auditory-, and somatosensory-evoked responses can be used to demonstrate slowing of nerve conduction due to demyelination in specific areas of the central nervous system. Computed tomography may demonstrate demyelinative plaques. Immersion of patients in water at a temperature of 40 degrees Celsius may cause the appearance of new symptoms or the recurrence of previously experienced symptoms.[103] The mechanism by which immersion in hot water provokes symptoms of multiple sclerosis is not known, but it is likely that elevated temperature causes complete blocking of conduction in demyelinated nerves. Indeed, raising the body temperature 0.5 degrees Celsius in animals with experimental demyelination can produce complete conduction blockade. One of the most widely used diagnostic tests for multiple sclerosis is examination of the cerebrospinal fluid. Approximately 70 percent of patients with multiple sclerosis have elevations of immunoglobulin G proteins in the cerebrospinal fluid. This elevation of cerebrospinal fluid protein is not specific for multiple sclerosis, as similar changes occur with infections, connective tissue diseases, encephalopathies, and neurosyphilis. Another test using cerebrospinal fluid is measurement of myelin basic protein by radioimmunoassay. Elevation of this protein indicates destruction of myelin.

TREATMENT

No treatment is curative for multiple sclerosis. Treatment with adrenocorticotrophic hormone or corticosteroids will shorten the du-

ration of an acute attack, but there is no evidence these drugs influence the ultimate progression of the disease. Nonspecific measures include avoidance of excessive fatigue, emotional stress, and marked temperature changes. Stress as produced by surgery is unwise, and elective surgical procedures are rarely performed. Pregnancy seems to introduce no special risk. Drugs used in the the treatment of skeletal muscle spasticity associated with multiple sclerosis include diazepam, dantrolene, and baclofen. Hepatic function should be monitored in patients treated with dantrolene, as this drug can produce liver damage. Painful dyesthesias, toxic seizures, and attacks of paroxysmal dysarthria and ataxia are best treated with carbamazepine. Immunosuppressive therapy has been provided with azathioprine and cyclophosphamide, but data to support the efficacy of this treatment are lacking. Plasmapheresis may produce a beneficial response in some patients.

MANAGEMENT OF ANESTHESIA

Management of anesthesia in patients with multiple sclerosis must consider the impact of surgical stress on the natural progression of the disease. For example, regardless of the anesthetic technique or drugs selected for use during the perioperative period, it is likely that symptoms of multiple sclerosis will be exacerbated during the postoperative period. In this regard, increases in body temperature that follow surgery may be more likely than drugs to be responsible for exacerbation of multiple sclerosis in the postoperative period. Furthermore, the unpredictable cycle of exacerbations and remissions of this disease could lead to the incorrect association of changing manifestations with drugs or events present in the perioperative period. Certainly, the changing neurologic picture in patients with this disease must be appreciated when considering the selection of regional anesthesia. Indeed, spinal anesthesia has been implicated in postoperative exacerbations of multiple sclerosis, whereas exacerbation of the disease after epidural anesthesia or peripheral nerve blocks have not been described.[104] For this reason, epidural anesthesia has been used in parturients with multiple sclerosis.[105] The mechanism by which spinal anesthesia may exacerbate multiple sclerosis is unknown but could reflect local anesthetic neurotoxicity. In this regard, the lack of a protective nerve sheath around the spinal cord and the associated demyelination of multiple sclerosis may render the spinal cord more susceptible to potential neurotoxic effects of local anesthetics. Epidural anesthesia may be less of a risk than spinal anesthesia because concentrations of local anesthetics in the white matter of the spinal cord are three to four times greater after spinal as compared to epidural administration.

General anesthesia is most often chosen, and there are no unique interactions between multiple sclerosis and drugs used to provide anesthesia. There is no evidence to support recommendations for selection of inhaled or injected anesthetic drugs. Selection of muscle relaxants should consider the possibility of exaggerated release of potassium after administration of succinylcholine to these patients. Prolonged responses to muscle relaxants would be consistent with co-existing weakness (myasthenia-like) and decreased skeletal muscle mass. Conversely resistance to the effects of nondepolarizing muscle relaxants has been observed, perhaps reflecting proliferation of extrajunctional cholinergic receptors characteristic of upper motor neuron lesions.[106] Supplementation with corticosteroids may be indicated when these drugs are being used in chronic treatment. Efforts must be made in the perioperative period to recognize and prevent even modest increases in body temperature (greater than 1 degree Celsius), as this change might lead to deterioration of nerve tissue at sites of demyelination. Careful neurologic evaluation in the postoperative period should be performed to detect any new symptoms of multiple sclerosis.

Optic Neuritis

Optic neuritis represents a demyelinating disease of the central nervous system that is limited to the optic nerve. Eventually, about 50 percent of these patients will show evidence of multiple sclerosis. Study of patients with optic neuritis should include examination of the cerebrospinal fluid and determination of histocompatibility antigens.

Transverse Myelitis

Transverse myelitis is inflammation of the spinal cord, which can follow viral infections or radiation. Multiple sclerosis can initially manifest as transverse myelitis. The cause of transverse myelitis, however, is most often unknown. The onset of this disease process is characterized by a rapid ascending weakness of the legs, associated with bladder paralysis and a sensory level in the thoracic region. The entire progression of symptoms can occur over a period of hours, and permanent sequelae are likely. When transverse myelitis is preceded or followed by bilateral optic neuritis, the diagnosis is Devic's disease or neuromyelitis optica.

NEUROPATHIES

Neuropathies may involve cranial or peripheral nerves. Cranial mononeuropathies are represented by idiopathic facial paralysis (Bell's palsy), trigeminal neuralgia (tic douloureux), glossopharyngeal neuralgia, vestibular neuronitis, and cranial neuropathy due to cancer. Peripheral entrapment neuropathies are represented by the carpal tunnel syndrome, ulnar nerve palsy, brachial plexus neuropathy, radial nerve palsy, meralgia paresthetica, and peroneal nerve palsy. Metabolic neuropathy can be due to drugs, alcohol, vitamin B_{12} deficiency, diabetes mellitus, hypothyroidism, uremia, and porphyria. Neuropathy associated with systemic diseases can reflect cancer, sarcoidosis, collagen vascular disease, and acute idiopathic polyneuritis (Guillain-Barré syndrome). Peroneal muscular atrophy (Charcot-

Marie-Tooth disease) and Refsum's disease are examples of hereditary neuropathies.

Idiopathic Facial Paralysis

Idiopathic facial paralysis (Bell's palsy) is characterized by the rapid onset of motor weakness or paralysis of all facial muscles innervated by the facial nerve. Often the onset is first noted on arising in the morning and looking into a mirror. Additional symptoms can include loss of taste sensation over the anterior two-thirds of the tongue, hyperacusis, and diminished salivation and lacrimation. There is no cutaneous sensory loss, emphasizing that the facial nerve is a motor nerve. The cause of idiopathic facial paralysis is presumed to be inflammation and edema of the facial nerve, most often in the facial canal of the temporal bone. A viral-induced inflammatory mechanism (perhaps herpes simplex virus) may be the cause. Indeed, the onset of this neuropathy is often preceded by a viral prodrome.

Spontaneous recovery usually occurs over about 12 weeks. If no recovery occurs in 16 weeks to 20 weeks, the disease is probably not idiopathic facial paralysis. Prednisone, 1 mg·kg^{-1}, daily for 5 days to 10 days depending on the degree of facial nerve paralysis, dramatically relieves pain and reduces the number of patients who experience complete denervation of the facial nerve. The eye should be covered to protect the cornea. Surgical decompression of the facial nerve may be required for persistent or severe cases of idiopathic facial paralysis, or facial paralysis secondary to trauma. Trauma to the facial nerve can reflect stretch injury produced by excessive traction on the angle of the mandible during maintenance of an airway in an unconscious patient.[107] Uveoparotid fever (Heerfordt's syndrome) is a variant of sarcoidosis characterized by bilateral anterior uveitis, parotitis, and mild pyrexia plus the presence of facial nerve paralysis in 50 percent to 70 percent of patients. Facial nerve paralysis associated with uveoparotid fever that appears in the postoperative period may be attributed erroneously to mechanical pressure over the nerve during general anesthesia.[108]

Trigeminal Neuralgia

Trigeminal neuralgia (tic douloureux) is characterized by sudden attacks of brief but intense unilateral facial pain triggered by local sensory stimuli to the affected side of the face.[109] The second and third divisions of the trigeminal nerve are usually involved. Trigeminal neuralgia most often manifests after 50 years of age. Appearance of this neuralgia before 50 should arouse suspicion of multiple sclerosis. Indeed, about 2 percent of patients with multiple sclerosis also experience trigeminal neuralgia. This is consistent with histologic evidence of degeneration or absence of myelin along the trigeminal nerve of patients with trigeminal neuralgia. The etiology of these changes is unknown, but proposed mechanisms include viral infections and vascular compression of the nerve.

TREATMENT

Medical treatment of trigeminal neuralgia is with anticonvulsant drugs such as phenytoin, carbamazepine, and baclofen. The rationale for the use of these drugs is based on the analogy of paroxysmal neuronal discharges in epilepsy and the possibility that similar discharges may produce the sudden attacks of pain characteristic of trigeminal neuralgia. Surgical treatment consists of selective radiofrequency destruction of trigeminal nerve fibers, transection of the sensory root of the trigeminal nerve, and microsurgical decompression of the trigeminal nerve.

MANAGEMENT OF ANESTHESIA

There are no special considerations for the management of anesthesia in patients with trigeminal neuralgia. Patients undergoing surgical therapy of trigeminal neuralgia, however, may experience dramatic and life-threatening increases in blood pressure during radiofrequency destruction of nerve fibers, requiring treatment with nitroprusside.[109] Potential effects of anticonvulsant drug therapy on hepatic microsomal enzyme activity should be remembered when selecting drugs, particularly enflurane or halothane. In addition, carbamazepine can cause altered hepatic function, leukopenia, and thrombocytopenia, emphasizing the importance of evaluating these systems preoperatively in patients receiving this drug.

Glossopharyngeal Neuralgia

Glossopharyngeal neuralgia is characterized by attacks of intense pain in the throat, neck, tongue, and ear. Swallowing, chewing, coughing, or talking can trigger the pain. This neuralgia can also be associated with severe bradycardia and syncope, presumably reflecting activation of the motor nucleus of the vagus nerve. Hypotension, seizures due to cerebral ischemia, and even cardiac arrest can occur in some patients.

DIAGNOSIS

Glossopharyngeal neuralgia is usually idiopathic but has been described in patients with cerebellopontine angle vascular anomalies and tumors, vertebral and carotid artery occlusive disease, arachnoiditis, and extracranial tumors arising in the area of the pharynx, larynx, and tonsils. The presence of glossopharyngeal neuralgia is supported by the occurrence of pain in the distribution of the glossopharyngeal nerve, presence of a site in the oropharynx, which when stimulated reproduces the symptoms, and relief of pain by topical anesthesia of the oropharynx.

In the absence of pain, cardiac symptoms associated with glossopharyngeal neuralgia may be confused with sick sinus syndrome or carotid sinus syndrome (see Chapter 4). Sick sinus syndrome can be ruled out by the absence of characteristic changes on the electrocardiogram. Failure of carotid sinus massage to produce cardiac symptoms rules out the presence of carotid sinus hypersensitivity. Glossopharyngeal nerve block is useful for differentiating glossopharyngeal neuralgia from atypical trigeminal neuralgia. This block does not differentiate glossopharyngeal neuralgia from the carotid sinus syndrome, since afferent pathways of both syndromes are mediated by the glossopharyngeal nerve. Topical anesthesia of the oropharynx blocks receptors in the trigger area responsible for initiating glossopharyngeal neuralgia and thus distinguishes this response from the carotid sinus syndrome.

TREATMENT

Treatment of glossopharyngeal neuralgia associated with cardiac symptoms should be aggressive, as these patients are vulnerable to sudden death. Cardiovascular symptoms are treated with atropine, isoproterenol, and/or an artificial cardiac pacemaker. Pain associated with this syndrome is managed by chronic administration of anticonvulsant drugs, such as phenytoin or carbamazepine. Topical anesthesia of the pharyngeal or oral mucosa, or a glossopharyngeal nerve block, effectively relieves pain, but only for the duration of the effect of the local anesthetic. Prevention of cardiovascular symptoms and provision of predictable pain relief is provided by the intracranial section of the glossopharyngeal nerve and the upper two roots of the vagus nerve. Although permanent pain relief after repeated glossopharyngeal nerve blocks is possible, this neuralgia is sufficiently life-threatening to justify intracranial section of nerves in patients unresponsive to medical therapy.

MANAGEMENT OF ANESTHESIA

Preoperative evaluation is directed at assessing the intravascular fluid volume and cardiac status.[110,111] A significant deficit of intravascular fluid volume may be present, as these patients avoid oral intake and its associated pharyngeal stimulation in attempts to prevent triggering painful attacks. Furthermore, drooling and loss of saliva can contribute to loss of intravascular fluid volume. A preoperative history of syncope or documented bradycardia, concurrent with the presence of neuralgia, introduces the consideration for placement of a prophylactic transvenous artificial cardiac pacemaker before induction of anesthesia.

Continuous monitoring of the electrocardiogram and of arterial blood pressure via a catheter in a peripheral artery is indicated. Topical anesthesia of the oropharynx with lidocaine is useful for preventing bradycardia and hypotension, which occur in response to triggering of this syndrome during direct laryngoscopy and intubation of the trachea. Furthermore, intravenous administration of atropine or glycopyrrolate just before laryngoscopy is recommended.[110]

Cardiovascular changes in response to surgical manipulation and intracranial section of cranial nerve roots should be expected. For example, bradycardia and hypotension are likely during manipulation of the vagus nerve. An anticholinergic drug must be immediately available to treat this vagal-mediated response. Hypertension, tachycardia, and ventricular premature beats can occur after section of the glossopharyngeal nerve and the upper two roots of the vagus nerve. These events may reflect sudden loss of sensory input from the carotid sinus. Hypertension is usually transient but may persist in some patients into the postoperative period. Persistence of hypertension is due to increased sympathetic nervous system activity, as emphasized by prompt reductions in blood pressure produced by alpha-adrenergic blockade with phentolamine or ganglionic blockade with hexamethonium. Hydralazine has also been effective in treating hypertension in the postoperative period. Experience is too limited to permit recommendations for specific anesthetic drugs or muscle relaxants. Thiopental, nitrous oxide, halothane, succinylcholine, and pancuronium have been administered to these patients without adverse or unusual responses.[110] The possibility of the development of vocal cord paralysis after section of the vagus nerve should be considered, if airway obstruction occurs after the tube is removed from the trachea.

Vestibular Neuronitis

Vestibular neuronitis manifests as vertigo, vomiting, and gait disturbances. These symptoms are thought to reflect irritation of the vestibular portion of the 8th cranial nerve. Absence of hearing loss distinguishes vestibular neuronitis from endolymphatic hydrops (Ménière's disease). Vestibular neuronitis is a benign condition, and no specific treatment is necessary.

Cranial Neuropathy in Cancer

Cranial nerve palsies can reflect compression or infiltration by leukemia or lymphomas. Metastatic disease from the breast or lung may invade the trigeminal nerve, causing numbness of the chin or cheek. Similar invasion of the hypoglossal nerve produces atrophy of the tongue.

Carpal Tunnel Syndrome

Carpal tunnel syndrome is the most frequent of the entrapment neuropathies. The median nerve is compressed, and perhaps rendered ischemic, in the confined space between the carpal bones and the flexor retinaculum of the wrist. Resulting symptoms include pain and paresthesias in the thumb, index, and middle fingers, often with nocturnal exacerbations. Neurologic signs include sensory loss in the distribution of the median nerve (Fig. 18-13)[112] and weakness and atrophy of the abductor pollicis brevis in the thenar eminence. Tinel's sign is the provocation of pain by percussion over the median nerve at the wrist.

Carpal tunnel syndrome occurs most often in women 30 years to 50 years of age or in association with pregnancy. There is an increased incidence in patients with acromegaly, hypothyroidism, multiple myeloma, or amyloidosis. Bilateral carpal tunnel syndrome is not uncommon. Diagnosis of this syndrome is by demonstration of a conduction delay in the median nerve at the wrist. Surgical decompression is the recommended treatment, if conservative measures, such as immobilization and local injection of corticosteroids, are not effective.

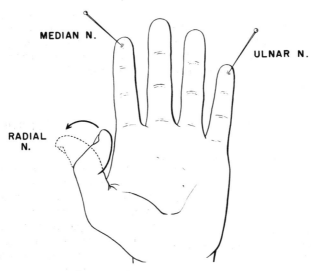

FIG. 18-13. Schematic diagram for the rapid identification of peripheral nerve injuries to the upper extremity. Injury to the musculocutaneous nerve results in loss of biceps function and inability to flex the forearm; injury to the axillary nerve results in loss deltoid function and inability to abduct the arm. (Nicholson MJ, McAlpine FS. Neural injuries associated with surgical positions and operations. In: Martin JT, ed. Positioning in Anesthesia and Surgery. Philadelphia. WB Saunders, 1978;193–224)

Ulnar Nerve Palsy

The ulnar nerve is vulnerable to trauma and external compression at the condylar groove of the elbow. Severe or recurrent injury can lead to local fibrosis and entrapment of the ulnar nerve, manifesting as weakness, atrophy, and sensory loss in the ulnar field of the hand (Fig. 18-13).[112] Nerve conduction studies reveal localized conduction blockade at the elbow. Surgical transposition of the nerve in the antecubital fossa may be necessary.

Brachial Plexus Neuropathy

Localized weakness of one or both arms, developing after a viral-like infection, may signal the onset of brachial plexus neuropathy. Initially, patients describe pain across the shoulder and into the upper arm. Pain subsides over a period of a few days, but weakness or paralysis then becomes manifest. Muscles of the shoulder girdle, particularly the deltoid muscle, are most often affected. Sensory loss is usually not prominent. There is no specific treatment, and complete recovery can be expected, although this may take 1 year to 2 years. Nerve conduction velocity studies confirm the diagnosis and avoid unncessary myelography.

Radial Nerve Palsy

Radial nerve palsy due to compression of the radial nerve manifests as wrist drop and paralysis of the extensor muscles of the fingers (Fig. 18-13).[112]

Meralgia Paresthetica

Entrapment of the lateral femoral cutaneous nerve as it passes under the inguinal ligament can cause burning pain over the anterolateral aspect of the thigh. Hypalgesia and hypesthesia are present in the involved area. Obesity and tight belts can contribute to its development. Relief of pain can be obtained by weight loss, removal of mechanical pressure produced by clothing, and block of the lateral femoral cutaneous nerve with local anesthetics.

Peroneal Nerve Palsy

Peroneal nerve palsy reflects compression of the common peroneal nerve at the level of the head of the fibula. Improper positioning in the lithotomy position or prolonged periods with the legs crossed may be responsible for damage to this nerve. Manifestations are foot drop and sensory loss over the dorsum of the foot (Fig. 18-14).[112]

Fabella Syndrome

Peroneal nerve palsy may be due to compression of the common peroneal nerve by a sesamoid bone (fabella) embedded in the tendinous portion of the gastrocnemius muscle.[113] This bone is present in about 12 percent of patients. A fabella should be considered one of the causes of peroneal nerve palsy, especially after long operations in the supine position in which a leg strap is applied tightly above the knees. Fabella syndrome, in addition to skeletal muscle weakness and sensory changes, is accompanied by local tenderness and pain in the area of the fabella, which is intensified by full extension of the knees.

Drug-Induced Neuropathies

Drugs known to produce a peripheral neuropathy include isoniazid, vincristine, hydralazine, disulfiram, and phenytoin. Discontinuation of the drug is usually followed by spontaneous recovery. Isoniazid-induced peripheral neuropathy can be prevented by pyridoxine therapy. Folic acid deficiency can accompany phenytoin therapy. Finally, heavy metals such as lead, arsenic, and mercury can cause peripheral polyneuropathies.

Alcohol

Polyneuropathy of chronic alcoholism is nearly always associated with a nutritional deficiency. Presumably, a vitamin deficiency is important in the pathogenesis of alcoholic neuropathy. Symptoms characteristically begin in the lower extremities, with pain and numbness in the feet. Weakness and tenderness of the intrinsic muscles of the feet, absent Achilles tendon reflexes, and hypalgesia in a stocking distribution are the early findings. Restoration of a proper diet, abstinence from alcohol, and multivitamin therapy promote a slow but predictable resolution of the neuropathy.

Vitamin B$_{12}$ Deficiency

The earliest neurologic symptoms of vitamin B$_{12}$ deficiency resemble the neuropathy typically seen in patients who use alcohol in excess. Paresthesias in the legs, with a sensory loss in a stocking distribution and absent Achilles tendon reflexes, are characteristic findings. Similar neurologic findings have been reported in dentists who are chronically exposed to nitrous oxide.[114] This is of concern, since nitrous oxide is known to inactivate certain vitamin B$_{12}$-dependent enzymes, which could lead to a deficiency of this essential vitamin (see Chapter 31).[115]

Diabetes Mellitus

The frequency of peripheral neuropathy in patients with diabetes mellitus increases with age of the patients and the duration of the dis-

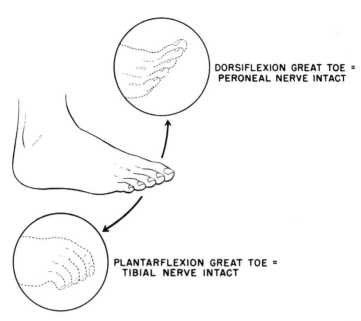

DORSIFLEXION GREAT TOE = PERONEAL NERVE INTACT

PLANTARFLEXION GREAT TOE = TIBIAL NERVE INTACT

FIG. 18-14. Schematic diagram for the rapid identification of peripheral nerve injuries of the lower extremity. Injury to the femoral nerve results in loss of quadriceps function. (Nicholson MJ, McAlpine FS. Neural injuries associated with surgical positions and operations. In: Martin JT, ed. Positioning in Anesthesia and Surgery. Philadelphia. WB Saunders, 1978;193–224)

ease. Strictness of control of blood glucose concentrations does not appear to influence development of neuropathies. Protein concentrations in cerebrospinal fluid are often increased, and nerve conduction studies are slowed. The electromyogram may show evidence of denervation. Sciatic neuropathy in patients with diabetes mellitus is not associated with pain in response to straight leg raising, serving to distinguish this neuropathy from lumbar disc disease. Spontaneous and complete recovery from this peripheral neuropathy usually occurs, but the rate of return of normal nerve function is unpredictable.

Hypothyroidism

A distal sensory neuropathy may be one of the first signs of myxedema. Delayed relax-

ation of tendon reflexes, especially the Achilles tendon reflex, is characteristic.

Uremia

A distal polyneuropathy with sensory and motor components often occurs in the extremities of patients with chronic renal failure. Symptoms tend to be more prominent in the legs than in the arms. Presumably, metabolic abnormalities are responsible for axonal degeneration and segmental demeylination, which accompany this neuropathy. Slowing of nerve conduction has been correlated with elevated plasma concentrations of parathyroid hormone and myoinositol, which is a component of myelin. An improvement in nerve conduction velocity often occurs within a few days after renal transplantation. Hemodialysis does not seem to be equally effective in reversing the polyneuropathy.

Porphyria

The neuropathy associated with porphyria is distinctive in that it is predominantly motor. Cranial nerves and respiratory muscles may be involved by the neuropathic process.

Cancer

Peripheral sensory and/or motor neuropathies occur in patients with a variety of malignancies, especially those involving the lung, ovary, and breast. Polyneuropathy that develops in older patients should always arouse suspicion of undiagnosed cancer. The myasthenic syndrome (Eaton-Lambert syndrome) is characteristically observed in patients with carcinoma of the lung. This syndrome, however, is an abnormality of the neuromuscular junction rather than nerves.

Sarcoidosis

Polyneuropathy is a frequent finding in patients with sarcoidosis. Facial nerve paralysis on one or both sides may result from involvement of this nerve in the parotid gland.

Collagen Vascular Diseases

Collagen vascular diseases are commonly associated with peripheral neuropathies. The most common conditions are systemic lupus erythematosus, polyarteritis nodosa, rheumatoid arthritis, and scleroderma. Detection of multiple mononeuropathies suggests vasculitis of nerve trunks and should stimulate a search for the presence of collagen vascular diseases.

Acute Idiopathic Polyneuritis

Acute idiopathic polyneuritis (Guillain-Barré syndrome) is characterized by the sudden onset of weakness or paralysis that typically manifests in the legs and then spreads cephalad over a few days to involve skeletal muscles of the arms, trunk, and head. Bulbar involvement is most frequently manifested as bilateral facial paralysis. Difficulty in swallowing and impaired respiration due to intercostal muscle paralysis are the most serious symptoms. Because of lower motor neuron involvement, paralysis is flaccid, and corresponding tendon reflexes are diminished. Sensory disturbances occur as paresthesias, which are most prominent in the distal part of the extremities and usually precede the onset of paralysis. Pain often exists in the form of headache, backache, or tenderness of skeletal muscles to deep pressure.

Autonomic nervous system dysfunction is a prominent finding in patients with acute idiopathic polyneuritis. Wide fluctuations in blood pressure, sudden profuse diaphoresis, peripheral vasoconstriction, resting tachycardia, and cardiac conduction abnormalities on the electrocardiogram reflect alterations in the level of autonomic nervous system activity. Orthostatic hypotension may be so severe that elevating the head on a pillow leads to syncope. Sudden death associated with this disease is most likely due to autonomic nervous system dysfunction. A rare but documented complication is increased intracranial pressure.

The disease has been linked to viral infections, vaccinations, and immunosuppressive therapy. Support for a viral etiology is the observation that this syndrome develops after respiratory or gastrointestinal tract infections in about one-half of patients.

DIAGNOSIS

Diagnosis of acute idiopathic polyneuritis is based on the typical clinical findings. The diagnosis is supported by the finding of increased concentrations of protein in the cerebrospinal fluid, although cell counts remain normal. Rises in protein concentrations, which may be delayed for 1 week to 2 weeks after the onset of the clinical symptoms, are presumed to result from inflammation of nerve roots in the subarachnoid space.

TREATMENT

Treatment of acute idiopathic polyneuritis is mainly symptomatic. The major hazards are respiratory insufficiency, autonomic nervous system dysfunction, and thromboembolism. The value of corticosteroids in the treatment of this disease is not documented.

Vital capacity should be monitored; when it is less than 15 ml·kg^{-1}, the need to support ventilation of the lungs must be considered. Measurement of arterial blood gases will help guide the adequacy of ventilation. Pharyngeal muscle weakness, even in the absence of ventilatory failure, may necessitate placement of a cuffed tube in the trachea, so as to protect the lungs from aspiration of secretions and gastric fluid. Autonomic nervous system dysfunction may require treatment of hypertension or hypotension.

Complete spontaneous recovery from acute idiopathic polyneuritis can occur in a few weeks, when segmental demyelination is the predominant pathologic change. Axonal degeneration, however, as shown by electromyography, may result in slow recovery over several months, with some degree of permanent weakness remaining. Mortality from this syndrome is usually less than 5 percent.

MANAGEMENT OF ANESTHESIA

Altered function of the autonomic nervous system and the presence of lower motor neuron lesions are the two important considerations for management of anesthesia in patients with acute idiopathic polyneuritis. Compensatory cardiovascular responses may be absent, resulting in profound hypotension in response to changes in posture, blood loss, or positive airway pressure. Conversely, noxious stimulation, as during direct laryngoscopy, could manifest as exaggerated increases in blood pressure, reflecting the labile activity of the autonomic nervous system in these patients. In view of these unpredictable changes in blood pressure, it would seem prudent to monitor blood pressure continuously via a catheter in a peripheral artery. A possible exaggerated response to indirect-acting vasopressors should be appreciated, when considering treatment of hypotension with drugs rather than intravenous infusion of fluids.

Succinylcholine should not be administered, since the possibility of excessive potassium release exists in the presence of lower motor neuron lesions.[80] Nondepolarizing muscle relaxants with minimal circulatory effects would seem to be better selections than pancuronium. Even if spontaneous respiration is present preoperatively, it is likely that depression from anesthetic drugs will necessitate mechanical ventilation of the lungs during surgery. Certainly, continued support of ventilation is likely to be necessary in the postoperative period.

Peroneal Muscular Atrophy (Charcot-Marie-Tooth Disease)

Peroneal muscular atrophy is a rare degenerative disease of the peripheral nervous system being transmitted as an autosomal dominant trait. The hallmark of the disease is peroneal muscle atrophy. High pedal arches and club feet are common and pes cavus may be present. The onset of this disease is typically in the second decade of life. Later, mild distal sensory impairment develops, and eventually the process spreads to involve the upper extremities. Pregnancy may be associated with exacerbations of this disease. Incapacitation is rare and death usually occurs from other causes. Skeletal muscle atrophy and weakness suggests caution in the use of succinylcholine in these patients. Regional anesthetic techniques are often avoided because of the coexisting neurologic dysfunction.

Refsum's Disease

Refsum's disease is a multisystem disorder manifested by ichthyosis, deafness, retinitis pigmentosa, cardiomyopathy, cerebellar ataxia, and polyneuropathy. The metabolic defect responsible for this disease reflects a failure to oxidize the fatty acid phytic acid, which subsequently accumulates in excessive concentrations. Transmission of Refsum's disease is as an autosomal recessive trait.

Moebius Syndrome

Moebius syndrome is a rare congenital dysplasia of the cranial nerves. The spinal accessory and facial nerves are most often affected, resulting in esotropia or partial facial paralysis. Occasionally, involvement of other cranial nerves manifests as difficulties in mastication, swallowing, and coughing, often leading to aspiration and recurrent pulmonary infections.

SPINAL CORD

Spinal cord transection is the description of damage to the spinal cord that manifests as paralysis of the lower extremities (paraplegia) or all the extremities (quadriplegia). Anatomically, the spinal cord is not divided, but the effect physiologically is the same as if it were. Spinal cord transection above the level of C2–C4 is incompatible with survival, as innervation to the diaphragm is likely to be destroyed. The most common cause of spinal cord transection is trauma. The most frequent nontraumatic cause of spinal cord transection is multiple sclerosis. In addition, infections or vascular and developmental disorders may be responsible for permanent damage to the spinal cord.

Pathophysiology

Spinal cord transection initially produces flaccid paralysis, with total absence of sensation below the level of injury. In addition, there is loss of temperature regulation and spinal cord reflexes below the level of injury. Reductions in systemic blood pressure and bradycardia are common findings. Abnormalities on the electrocardiogram are frequent during the acute phase of spinal cord transection and include ventricular premature beats and ST-T wave changes suggestive of myocardial ischemia. This initial phase, occurring after acute transection of the spinal cord is known as spinal shock and typically lasts 1 week to 3 weeks. During this period, the major cause of morbidity and mortality is impaired alveolar ventilation, combined with inability to protect the airway and to clear bronchial secretions. Aspiration of gastric fluid or contents, pneumonia, and pulmonary embolism are constant threats during spinal shock.

Several weeks after acute transection of the spinal cord, there is gradual return of spinal cord reflexes; and patients enter a chronic stage, characterized by overactivity of the sympathetic nervous system and involuntary skeletal muscle spasms. Sequelae of this chronic stage, which jeopardize the patient's well-being, include impaired alveolar ventilation, cardiovascular instability manifesting as autonomic hyperreflexia, chronic pulmonary and/or genitourinary tract infections, anemia, and altered thermoregulation.

Mental depression and pain are very real problems after spinal cord injury. Root pain is localized at or near the level of the transection. Visceral pain is produced by distention of the bladder or bowel. Phantom body pain can occur in areas of complete sensory loss. As a result of mental depression and/or the presence of pain, these patients may be ingesting drugs, which must be considered when planning management of anesthesia.

Respiratory System

Spontaneous ventilation is impossible if the level of spinal cord transection results in paralysis of the diaphragm. A transection between the level of C2–C4 may result in apnea due to denervation of the diaphragm. When function of the diaphragm is intact, tidal volume is likely to remain adequate. Nevertheless, the ability to cough and clear secretions from the airway is likely to be impaired because of decreased expiratory reserve volume. Indeed, acute transection of the spinal cord at the cervical level is accompanied by marked reductions in vital capacity.[116] Furthermore, arterial hypoxemia is a consistent finding early in the period after cervical spinal cord injury. Tracheobronchial suctioning has been associated with bradycardia and cardiac arrest in these patients, emphasizing the importance of establishing optimal arterial oxygenation before undertaking this maneuver.[117]

Autonomic Hyperreflexia

Autonomic hyperreflexia is a disorder that appears following resolution of spinal shock and in association with return of the spinal cord reflexes.[118] This reflex response can be initiated by cutaneous or visceral stimulation below the level of spinal cord transection. Distention of a hollow viscus, such as the bladder or rectum, is a common stimulus. The incidence of autonomic hyperreflexia depends on the level of spinal cord transection. For example, about 85 percent of patients with spinal cord transections above T-6 will exhibit this reflex; it is unlikely to be associated with transections below T-10. Surgery, however, is a particularly potent stimulus to the development of autonomic hyperreflexia, and even patients with no previous history of this response may be at risk during operative procedures.

PATHOPHYSIOLOGY

Stimulation below the level of spinal cord transection initiates afferent impulses that enter the spinal cord below that level (Fig. 18-15). These impulses elicit reflex sympathetic activity over the splanchnic outflow tract. In neurologically intact individuals, this outflow is modulated by inhibitory impulses from higher centers in the central nervous system. In the presence of spinal cord transection, however, this outflow is isolated from inhibitory impulses, such that generalized vasoconstriction persists below the level of injury. Vasoconstriction results in elevations of blood pressure, which are then perceived by the carotid sinus. Subsequent activation of the carotid sinus results in decreased efferent sympathetic nervous system activity from the central nervous system, which manifests as a predominance of parasympathetic nervous system activity in the periphery. This predominance, however, cannot be produced below the level of spinal cord transection, as this part of the body remains neurologically isolated. Therefore, vasoconstriction persists below the level of spinal cord transection. If the level of spinal cord transection is above the level of splanchnic outflow (T4–T6), vasodilation in the neurologically intact portion of the body is insufficient to offset the effects of vasoconstriction, as reflected by persistent hypertension.

SIGNS AND SYMPTOMS

Hypertension and bradycardia are the hallmarks of autonomic hyperreflexia.[118] Stimulation of the carotid sinus from hypertension manifests as bradycardia and cutaneous vasodilation above the level of spinal cord transection. Hypertension persists, since vasodilation cannot occur below the level of injury. Nasal stuffiness reflects vasodilation. Patients may complain of headache and blurred vision, as manifestations of severe hypertension. Precipitous increases in blood pressure can lead to cerebral, retinal, or subarachnoid hemorrhage and increased operative blood loss. Loss of consciousness and seizures can occur. Cardiac dysrhythmias are also present in the majority of patients. Pulmonary edema reflects acute left ventricular failure, due to increased afterload produced by elevations in blood pressure.

TREATMENT

Treatment of autonomic hyperreflexia can be with ganglionic blocking drugs (trimethaphan, pentolinium), alpha-adrenergic antago-

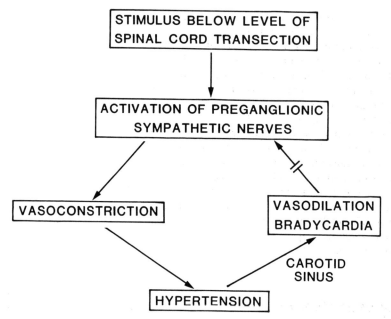

FIG. 18-15. Schematic diagram of the sequence of events associated with the clinical manifestations of autonomic hyperreflexia. Impulses that produce vasodilation cannot reach the neurologically isolated portion of the spinal cord, such that vasoconstriction and hypertension persist.

nists (phentolamine, phenoxybenzamine), direct-acting vasodilators (nitroprusside), and general or regional anesthesia.[118,119] Drugs that lower blood pressure by central actions alone, either on the vasomotor center or on higher centers, are not effective.

Although the most practical approach to lowering blood pressure in awake patients would seem to be with intravenous infusions of nitroprusside, clinical experience with the use of nitroprusside for this purpose has not been reported. Intravenous phentolamine has been recommended, but large doses may be required, emphasizing that the hypertension of autonomic hyperreflexia is not due to increased circulating levels of catecholamines. Institution of epidural anesthesia has been reported to be effective for the treatment of autonomic hyperreflexia provoked by uterine contractions.[120] In this same patient an attempt to control blood pressure with nitroprusside had not been successful. Epidural administration of meperidine has been used during labor to control autonomic hyperreflexia.[121]

Genitourinary Tract System

Renal failure is the leading cause of death in patients with chronic spinal cord transections. Chronic urinary tract infections and immobilization predispose to the development of renal calculi. Amyloidosis of the kidney can manifest as proteinuria, leading to decreases in concentrations of albumin in the plasma.

Musculoskeletal System

Prolonged immobility leads to osteoporosis, skeletal muscle atrophy, and development of decubitus ulcers. Pathologic fractures can occur when moving these patients. Pressure points should be well protected and padded to minimize the likelihood of trauma to the skin and development of decubitus ulcers.

Management of Anesthesia

Management of anesthesia in patients with transections of the spinal cord is largely determined by the duration of the injury.[118] Regardless of the duration of spinal cord transection the institution of preoperative hydration is helpful in preventing hypotension during the induction and maintenance of anesthesia.

ACUTE SPINAL CORD TRANSECTION

Patients with acute transections of the spinal cord may require special precautions in the management of the airway. For example, further damage to the spinal cord could result from extension of the head in the presence of cervical fractures. Topical anesthesia and placement of the tube into the trachea using a fiberoptic laryngoscope is an alternative to rapid sequence induction of anesthesia with intravenous anesthetics and muscle relaxants. Absence of sympathetic nervous system compensatory responses makes these patients particularly likely to develop extreme reductions in blood pressure in response to acute changes in body posture, blood loss, or positive airway pressure. Liberal intravenous infusion of crystalloid solutions may be necessary to fill the vascular space, which has been abruptly increased by vasodilation. Likewise, blood loss should be replaced promptly in these patients. Breathing is best managed by mechanical ventilation of the lungs, as abdominal and intercostal muscle paralysis, combined with general anesthesia, makes maintenance of adequate spontaneous ventilation unlikely. Hypothermia should be guarded against, as these patients tend to become poikilothermic below the level of spinal cord transection. Anesthesia is maintained with drugs that will assure central nervous system sedation and facilitate tolerance of the endotracheal tube. Nitrous oxide combined with volatile or injected drugs is satisfactory for this purpose. Inspired concentrations of oxygen should be adjusted in response to measurement of arterial blood gases; bear in mind that arterial hypoxemia is a frequent finding after acute spinal cord transection.

The need for muscle relaxants will be dictated by the operative site and the level of spinal cord transection. If muscle relaxants are necessary, the sympathomimetic effects of pancuronium make this drug an attractive choice. Succinylcholine is unlikely to provoke an excessive release of potassium in the first few hours after acute spinal cord transection. Nevertheless, it would seem reasonable to avoid use of this drug, except for the rare instances where the rapid onset of short-duration, skeletal-muscle paralysis is mandatory.

CHRONIC SPINAL CORD TRANSECTION

The most important goal during management of anesthesia for patients with chronic transections of the spinal cord is prevention of autonomic hyperreflexia. Surgery is an intense stimulus for its development, emphasizing that patients who have a negative history for this reflex response are vulnerable to its occurrence during operation. General anesthesia, which includes volatile drugs, is effective in preventing this response.[118] Epidural and spinal anesthesia are also effective, but it may be technically difficult to perform these procedures in the spinal cord injury patient. Furthermore, control of the level of anesthesia is not easy to attain. Nevertheless, low spinal anesthesia seems particularly effective in preventing autonomic hyperreflexia.[119] Conversely, epidural anesthesia has been reported to be occasionally ineffective in preventing hypertension during urologic endoscopic procedures in patients with spinal cord injury.[122] Perhaps this could be predicted, as epidural anesthesia may not always provide adequate sacral anesthesia. Block of afferent pathways with topical local anesthetics applied to the urethra, as for cystoscopic procedures, is often not effective in preventing autonomic hyperreflexia, since this anesthesia does not block bladder muscle proprioceptors, which are stimulated by bladder distention. Regardless of the technique selected for anesthesia, it is important to have drugs such as nitroprusside immediately available to treat precipitous hypertension. Nitroprusside administered as rapid intravenous injections of 1 μg·kg^{-1} to 2 μg·kg^{-1} is an effective method for treating sudden hypertension.[70] Persistence of hypertension will require continuous intravenous infusions of nitroprusside. It is also important to appreciate that autonomic hyperreflexia may manifest postoperatively, when effects of the anesthetics begin to dissipate.

Muscle relaxants may be necessary to facilitate intubation of the trachea and to prevent reflex skeletal muscle spasms in response to surgical stimulation. Nondepolarizing muscle relaxants are used for this purpose, since succinylcholine is likely to provoke release of po-

tassium, particularly in patients in whom spinal cord injury is less than 6 months old.[123] Indeed, there is evidence that increased release of potassium after administration of succinylcholine can begin to occur within 4 days of denervation injury (Fig. 18-16).[124] Peak release of potassium after administration of succinylcholine occurs when the injury is about 14 days old. Cardiac arrest due to succinylcholine-induced hyperkalemia, however, has been observed as early as 7 days after spinal cord transection.[124] Furthermore, the magnitude of potassium release does not seem to be dose-

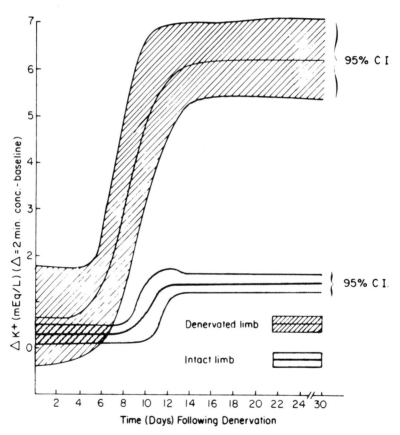

FIG. 18-16. Changes in plasma potassium concentrations (average and 95 percent confidence interval) in venous effluent from denervated and intact limbs were measured 2 minutes following administration of succinylcholine to baboons anesthetized with phencyclidine. Half-peak increases in plasma potassium concentrations occurred 8.4 days after denervation, and maximum increases appeared 14 days after the injury. Increases in plasma potassium concentrations, however, were detectable as early as 4 days after denervation. (John DA, Tobey RE, Homer LD, Rice CL. Onset of succinylcholine-induced hyperkalemia following denervation. Anesthesiology 1976;45:294–9)

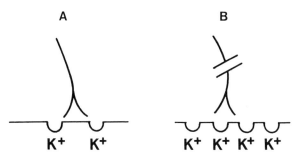

FIG. 18-17. Schematic diagram of the neuromuscular junction before (**A**) and after denervation (**B**). Denervation is associated with a proliferation of extrajunctional cholinergic receptors that participate in the exchange of potassium in response to depolarization induced by acetylcholine. As a result, prolonged depolarization of the neuromuscular junction, as produced by succinylcholine, leads to hyperkalemia.

dependent, as evidenced by the development of hyperkalemia after intravenous administration of 20 mg of succinylcholine to a paraplegic adult patient.[125] It must also be appreciated that prior administration of nonparalyzing doses of nondepolarizing muscle relaxants does not reliably attenuate the release of potassium in response to succinylcholine.

Excess release of potassium presumably reflects proliferation of extrajunctional cholinergic receptors that are responsive to acetylcholine (Fig. 18-17). These receptor sites may develop within 48 hours to 72 hours of denervation and thus provide an increased number of sites for potassium exchange to occur during succinylcholine-induced depolarization.[126] All factors considered, it would seem reasonable to avoid use of succinylcholine in patients with transection of the spinal cord that is more than 24 hours old. The duration of susceptibility to the hyperkalemic effects of succinylcholine is not known, but the risk is probably reduced after 3 months to 6 months. Nevertheless, the presence of resistance to effects of nondepolarizing muscle relaxants in a patient 463 days after burn injury suggests persistence of the same extrajunctional receptors presumed to be responsible for succinylcholine induced hyperkalemia.[127] If this is true, patients could remain at risk for the hyperkalemic effects of succinylcholine far beyond the speculated 3 month to 6 month period after spinal cord transections. In this regard, the advantages attributed to succinylcholine could be equally attained with nondepolarizing muscle relaxants.

CEREBRAL PROTECTION AND RESUSCITATION

Cardiac arrest, stroke, and head injury are the events most likely to require attempts directed towards cerebral protection and resuscitation.

Cardiac Arrest

The early doctrine that 4 minutes to 6 minutes of global cerebral ischemia produced by cardiac arrest results in irreversible brain injury is no longer tenable.[128] Evidence suggests that central nervous system neurons can tolerate 20 minutes to 60 minutes of complete anoxia without always sustaining irreversible injury. Furthermore, events that follow cerebral ischemia may be more likely than the initial insult to produce permanent brain damage. For example, profound cerebral hypoperfusion (cerebral blood flow often less than 10 percent of normal) with areas of no reflow may occur 15 minutes to 90 minutes after resuscitation from circulatory arrest. This massive and progressive increase in cerebral small vessel resistance may reduce blood flow below levels sufficient to maintain neuronal viability. Regardless of the time from cardiac arrest to initiation of cardiopulmonary resuscitation, more than 6 minutes of closed chest massage is associated with increased neurologic morbidity.[128]

Historically, management of patients who fail to awaken after cardiac arrest has included hypothermia, hyperventilation of the lungs, and large doses of corticosteroids. Enthusiasm for hypothermia has waned because of the absence of convincing data that this complex procedure induced after cardiac arrest is beneficial. Nevertheless, recent animal data suggest that even mild reductions of body temperature (1 degree Celsius to 3 degree Celsius) present at the time of arterial hypoxemia may contribute to cerebral protection.[129,130] Certainly, hypothermia is the only method available to depress cellular oxygen requirements below that needed for normal function (e.g., isoelectric electroencephalogram). Hyperventilation of the lungs, in the absence of increased intracranial pressure, has not been shown to improve outcome after cardiac arrest and, like hypothermia, cannot be routinely recommended. Therapy with corticosteroids remains a common intervention, but the value of these drugs is also controversial. Perhaps a low risk-to-benefit ratio has contributed to their continued use. Administration of calcium during and after cardiopulmonary resuscitation may be questionable in view of the possible role of neuronal calcium overloading in small vessel vasoconstriction and postresuscitation cerebral hypoperfusion.[128] In this regard, calcium antagonists may find a role in prevention or attenuation of postresuscitation cerebral hypoperfusion.

BARBITURATES

Use of barbiturates in brain protection after ischemic insults is based on the ability of these drugs to produce dose-related reductions in cerebral metabolic oxygen requirements until maximum reductions of about 50 percent are achieved. This maximum reduction corresponds to an isoelectric electroencephalogram and is evidence that additional doses of barbiturates are not necesssary. This drug-induced reduction in oxygen requirements reflects depression of mentation and not a decrease in oxygen needed to maintain cellular

viability. From this evidence, one can predict that barbiturate protection would occur only if the ischemic insult did not interfere with basal cellular metabolism, as evidenced by the continued presence of electrical activity on the electroencephalogram.[131] During cardiac arrest (e.g., global ischemia), the electroencephalogram becomes flat in 20 seconds to 30 seconds, and subsequent administration of barbiturates would not be expected to improve neurologic outcome. Indeed, administration of thiopental, 30 mg·kg^{-1}, as a single intravenous injection to comatose survivors of cardiac arrest, does not increase survival or improve neurologic outcome.[132] Likewise, controlled animal studies fail to demonstrate improved neurologic outcomes when administration of thiopental precedes or follows global cerebral ischemia.[133,134] In contrast to global ischemia, incomplete ischemia with maintenance of electrical activity on the electroencephalogram is likely to be associated with improved neurologic outcome when barbiturates are administered to produce metabolic suppression. Consistent with this concept is the observation that neuropsychiatric complications after cardiopulmonary bypass, which are presumably due to embolism, clear more rapidly in patients treated prospectively with thiopental (average dose 39.5 mg·kg^{-1}) to maintain electroencephalographic silence.[135] Other patients at risk for incomplete cerebral ischemia who might benefit from prior production of electroencephalographic silence with barbiturates include those scheduled for carotid endarterectomy and thoracic aneurysm resections. In view of these data from patients and animals, it does not seem appropriate to recommend administration of barbiturates to patients who have been resuscitated from cardiac arrests.

POSTANOXIC ENCEPHALOPATHY

Neurologic sequelae after episodes of acute cerebral hypoxia range from mild psychiatric disturbances to irreversible vegetative states. Cortical blindness is a potential complication. Presence of coma after successful cardiopulmonary resuscitation is a grave prognostic sign. In one series, only 20 percent of patients who were comatose after cardiopulmonary resuscitation survived, and nearly one-half of them had permanent neurologic defects.[136]

BRAIN DEATH

The need to define and confirm irreversible brain damage occurring after successful cardiopulmonary resuscitation is apparent. Diagnosis of brain death in the very young is difficult, as it is well documented that the immature brain is resistant to the damaging effects of arterial hypoxemia. In the absence of hypothermia (body temperature above 32 degrees Celsius), plus elimination of a depressant drug overdose as the cause for coma, the criteria for establishment of brain death in adults are as follows:[137]

1. Coma (absent cerebral responsivity) due to known structural or metabolic insults that has persisted for 12 hours. Coma due to overdoses of depressant drugs must be ruled out by history and appropriate laboratory studies.
2. Vital brain stem function absent, as reflected by fixed and unreactive pupils, absent oculocephalic reflexes, no ocular responses to ice water irrigation of the ears, and no spontaneous ventilation, despite normal to elevated arterial partial pressures of carbon dioxide and oxygen. Spinal reflex activity does not preclude the diagnosis of brain death.
3. Cortical function absent, as reflected by an isoelectric electroencephalogram at maximum gain for 60 minutes. Again, this assumes that depressant drug overdoses are not present.
4. Absence of cerebral circulation, or a critical defect of cerebral circulation, as determined by angiography, even in the presence of depressant drug overdoses.

Recording of somatosensory-evoked potentials is useful for monitoring comatose patients and predicting neurologic outcome. Measurement of somatosensory-evoked potentials may also be useful in confirming the presence of brain death.

Stroke

Stroke models in laboratory animals have been shown to benefit from the administration of barbiturates before or after initiation of the stroke.[137] Nevertheless, lesions resulting from the abrupt occlusion of a single cerebral vessel in an otherwise healthy animal cannot be equated to that encountered in often geriatric patients with co-existing cerebrovascular disease. On the basis of current animal data, production of barbiturate coma in stroke patients cannot be recommended. More important is the recognition from animal models that the brain does not immediately infarct after occlusion of a single major vessel; rather, irreversible damage may not occur for as long as 2 hours to 3 hours.

Head Injury

The greatest success in cerebral protection and resuscitation has been in patients who experience head injury. In contrast to patients who suffer cardiac arrest or stroke, these patients are often young, and co-existing cerebrovascular disease is minimal or absent. Routine monitoring of intracranial pressure is essential for guiding management of these patients. Administration of hyperosmotic drugs and corticosteroids, and institution of mechanical hyperventilation of the lungs to produce arterial partial pressures of carbon dioxide between 25 mmHg and 30 mmHg, are standard interventions to reduce intracranial pressure.

BARBITURATES

Administration of barbiturates is recommended when intracranial pressure remains elevated despite traditional therapy. This recommendation is based on the predictable ability of these drugs to reduce intracranial pressure, presumably by decreasing cerebral blood volume secondary to cerebral vascular vasoconstriction. In addition, drug-induced decreases in neuronal metabolism can lead to even further reductions in cerebral blood volume, by decreasing cerebral blood flow in response to metabolic autoregulation.

The goal of barbiturate therapy is to maintain intracranial pressure below 20 mmHg without the occurrence of plateau waves. An effective regimen is the intravenous administration of an initial dose of pentobarbital (3 mg·kg^{-1} to 5 mg·kg^{-1}), followed by a continuous rate of infusion to maintain blood concentrations of the barbiturate between 3 mg·dl^{-1} to 6 mg·dl^{-1} [138,139] An alternative to measuring blood concentrations of pentobarbital every 12 hours to 24 hours is to adjust infusion rates to maintain an isoelectric electroencephalogram, which confirms the presence of maximum drug-induced depression of cerebral metabolic requirements for oxygen. Barbiturates also reduce the dose of mannitol necessary to keep intracranial pressure below 20 mmHg. This reduction in the dose decreases the likelihood of plasma hyperosmolarity and electrolyte disturbances secondary to diuresis. Discontinuation of barbiturate infusion can be considered when intracranial pressure has remained in a normal range for 48 hours.

Hazards of barbiturate therapy, as used to lower intracranial pressure, include hypotension, which can jeopardize the maintenance of an adequate cerebral perfusion pressure. Such hypotension is particularly likely in elderly patients and in the presence of decreased intravascular fluid volume. In patients, doses of thiopental or methohexital sufficient to produce an isoelectric electroencephalogram, produce peripheral vasodilation and myocardial depression.[140,141] In animals, thiopental is more likely than pentobarbital to produce hypotension and ventricular fibrillation when administered in doses sufficient to cause electrical silence in the brain.[142] Inotropic support of cardiac output may be necessary in some patients being treated with barbiturates.

Failure of barbiturates to lower intracranial pressure is a grave prognostic sign. Even when barbiturates are effective, the overall morbidity and mortality in head trauma patients has not been shown to be improved by the use of these drugs, as compared with patients treated aggressively with diuretics, corticosteroids, and hyperventilation.[143]

SEIZURE DISORDERS

Adult onset seizure disorders (epilepsy) are present when manifestations of seizure activity begin after 20 years of age (Table 18-3).[144] Idiopathic seizure disorders usually begin in childhood. The onset of seizures in adult life must arouse suspicion of focal brain disease.

Pathophysiology

Seizure disorders are not a disease, but symptomatic expressions of disorders of neuronal function. Seizures result from excessive discharges of large numbers of neurons, which become depolarized in a synchronized fashion. A focal area of neuronal hyperexcitability in the cerebral cortex may remain localized, if there is a surrounding field in which the neuarons are hyperpolarized and inexcitable. Conversely, hyperactive neurons may impinge on the adjoining cerebral cortex, recruiting more neurons and generating sufficient energy to spread via anatomic connections to the thalmus and brain stem. In such instances, massive synchronous discharges appear and result in generalized seizures. The concept that generalized seizures can result from localized areas in the cerebral cortex is the basis for using the initial symptomatology or aura as a clue to the location of the focal discharge. For example, generalized seizures after an aura of an ill-defined odor indicates focal lesions in the temporal lobe. Electroencephalography is the most important test for both the initial evaluation and the periodic follow-up of seizure disorders. The presence of structural brain disease can be investigated by means of radiographs of the skull, isotope brain scan, or computed tomography.

Treatment

Drugs used to treat adult onset seizures disorders may be used alone or in combination, depending on the type of seizures (Table 18-

TABLE 18-3. Classification of Adult Seizure Disorders

Type	Features	Effective Drugs
Grand mal	Generalized motor seizures with loss of consciousness	Phenytoin Barbiturates
Peti mal	Brief loss of awareness with little or no motor activity	Ethosuximide Trimethadione Valproic acid
Akinetic	Brief loss of consciousness and postural muscle tone	Phenytoin Phenobarbital Clonazepam
Myoclonic	Isolated clonic jerks common in degenerative and metabolic brain disease	Clonazepam Valproic acid
Psychomotor	Impaired consciousness plus bizarre behavior	Primidone Phenytoin Carbamazepine
Focal cortical (Jacksonian)	Focal motor or sensory disturbances	Phenytoin Phenobarbital

3). Most anticonvulsant drugs can be classified as barbiturates, hydantoins, or benzodiazepines (Table 18-4). Valproic acid is a branched-chain carboxylic acid. Concentrations of anticonvulsant drugs in the plasma are useful in guiding therapy and for recognizing toxicity. Although the exact mechanism of action is not known, it seems that anticonvulsant drugs act by reducing the spread of excitation from seizure foci to normal neurons. It is estimated that complete drug-induced control of seizures can be achieved in up to 50 percent of patients plus significant improvement in another 25 percent.

PHENYTOIN

Phenytoin is the primary drug administered for treatment of all types of epilepsy with the exception of petit mal epilepsy. Side effects associated with chronic phenytoin therapy include gastrointestinal irritation, megaloblastic anemia, skin rash, peripheral neuropathy, and gingival hyperplasia. Excessive plasma concentrations of phenytoin manifest as nystagmus, ataxia, and diplopia. Sedation does not accompany treatment with phenytoin. Phenytoin is metabolized in the liver and rarely associated with hepatotoxicity. This drug is not effectively absorbed after intramuscular injection and is therefore administered either orally or intravenously.

PHENOBARBITAL

Phenobarbital is effective in treatment of all forms of epilepsy with the exception of petit mal epilepsy. Sedation is the principal side effect but becomes less with chronic administration and is further mimimized by administration of the drug at night. Skin rash and

TABLE 18-4. Drugs Used for Treatment of Seizure Disorders

Drug	Trade Name	Half-time (Hours)	Therapeutic Blood Level ($\mu g \cdot ml^{-1}$)
Phenobarbital	Luminal	120	20–50
Phenytoin	Dilantin	24	10–20
Primidone	Mysoline	12	7–15
Carbamazepine	Tegretol	12	4–10
Clonazepam	Clonopin	26	
Ethosuximide	Zarontin	55	50–100
Trimethadione	Tridione	14	20–40
Valproic acid	Depakene	12	

megaloblastic anemia may occur. Toxic plasma concentrations of phenobarbital are associated with nystagmus and ataxia. Phenobarbital is a potent stimulus for inducing the activity of hepatic microsomal enzymes, resulting in enhanced metabolism of drugs. Withdrawal symptoms do not accompany abrupt discontinuation of phenobarbital, as used to treat seizure disorders. Phenobarbital is mainly excreted by the kidneys and renal failure can result in unexpectedly high plasma concentrations of the drug. Alkalemia, as produced by mechanical hyperventilation of the lungs or administration of sodium bicarbonate, increases the ionized fraction of phenobarbital, and enhances its renal excretion.

PRIMIDONE

Primidone is a congener of phenobarbital that is effective in the treatment of grand mal epilepsy, focal cortical epilepsy, and psychomotor epilepsy. This drug is partly metabolized to phenobarbital, which is consistent with side effects of sedation, skin rash, and megaloblastic anemia.

CARBAMAZEPINE

Carbamazepine is useful in treatment of psychomotor epilepsy and trigeminal neuralgia. Common side effects include sedation, ataxia, skin rash, and nausea. Rarely, patients develop bone marrow depression, hepatorenal dysfunction, or congestive heart failure.

ETHOSUXIMIDE

Ethosuximide is effective in treatment of petit mal epilepsy. Side effects include sedation, nausea, and headache.

VALPROIC ACID

Valproic acid is effective in treatment of petit mal epilepsy. Platelet aggregation may be altered by this drug and hepatotoxicity can occur. Valproic acid may inhibit activity of hepatic microsomal enzymes.

TRIMETHADIONE

Trimethadione is effective in the treatment of petit mal epilepsy. Side effects include sedation and blurring of vision. Rare adverse responses include hepatic and renal toxicity, anemia, and skeletal muscle weakness.

CLONAZEPAM

Clonazepam is useful in the treatment of petit mal epilepsy, as well as myoclonic seizures in children. Side effects include sedation, ataxia, increased salivary secretions, and skeletal muscle weakness.

Grand Mal Seizures

Grand mal seizures are reflected by generalized and continuous seizure activity, which prevents adequate ventilation; death is inevitable if treatment is not provided. The first priority of treatment is establishment of a patent upper airway and administration of oxygen. Seizure activity is suppressed by intravenous administration of diazepam 2 mg·min^{-1} until seizures stop or to a total of 20 mg.[145] To prevent recurrence of seizure activity as the effect of diazepam wanes, it is recommended that an infusion of phenytoin, 50 mg·min^{-1} to a total of 18 mg·kg^{-1}, be initiated simultaneously with administration of the benzodiazepine. Phenytoin may be a better choice than diazepam for the management of continuous seizure activity associated with head trauma or global cerebral ischemia as drug-induced alterations of consciousness would be undesirable. In extreme situations, general anesthesia using halothane or isoflurane and skeletal muscle relaxants to provide neuromuscular blockade and facilitate ventilation of the lungs will be necessary to control seizure activity. Treatment with only skeletal muscle relaxants is questionable as continuous firing of neurons (greater than 60 minutes) can result in cell damage despite adequate cerebral oxygenation.[145]

Management of Anesthesia

Management of anesthesia in patients with seizure disorders must consider the impact of anesthetic drugs on organ function, coagulation, and responses to anesthetic drugs (see the section Treatment). Known adverse effects of these drugs should be evaluated with appropriate preoperative tests. Co-existing sedation produced by anticonvulsant drugs may have additive effects with anesthetics, whereas drug-induced enzyme induction could alter responses to other drugs or even contribute to organ toxicity associated with administration of halothane or enflurane.

Selection of drugs used for the induction and maintenance of anesthesia should consider the effects of these drugs on central nervous system electrical activity. For example, methohexital may activate epileptic foci and has been recommended as a method to delineate these foci in patients undergoing surgical treatment of epilepsy.[146] Ketamine has been shown to elicit seizure activity in patients with known seizure disorders, as well as in patients with no known central nervous system disease.[147] Nevertheless, some data do not support ketamine-induced seizure activity in normal patients or individuals with known seizure disorders.[148] In fact, sleep may be a more potent stimulus of seizure activity than ketamine in epileptic patients. Furthermore, concurrent use of ketamine with other drugs, such as aminophylline, may result in lowering of seizure thresholds for both drugs.[149] In view of the availability of drugs, such as thiobarbiturates or benzodiazepines, which do not lower seizure thresholds, it would seem reasonable to avoid administration of potentially epileptogenic drugs to patients with epilepsy. In this regard, central nervous system stimulating effects of laudanosine, a metabolite of atracurium, may merit consideration.

Most inhaled anesthetics, including nitrous oxide, have been reported to produce seizure activity.[150] The presence of halogen atoms is an important determinant of convulsant properties of volatile anesthetics, with fluorine being incriminated as epileptogenic. Nevertheless, seizure activity is very rare following halothane and has not been shown to occur in response to the administration of isoflurane.[150] Conversely, enflurane predictably produces spike and wave activity on the electroencephalogram, which can be accompanied by visible skeletal muscle twitching. These changes occur in normal patients, as well as those with known co-existing seizure disorders. The likelihood of seizure activity is greatest when inspired concentrations of enflurane are above 2.5 percent, and hypocarbia (less than 25 mmHg) is present.[151] Seizure activity, however, on the electrocardiogram has been seen in normal children inhaling concentrations of enflurane as low as 1 percent.[150] Auditory stimulation can also elicit seizure activity during the administration of enflurane. Although adverse effects on the brain are not produced by this seizure activity, the wisdom of administering epileptogenic anesthetics to patients with seizure disorders remains doubtful. Conceivably, enflurane could be used to facilitate identification of seizure foci in patients undergoing diagnostic procedures. Halothane or isoflurane would seem good choices when volatile anesthetics that do not produce seizure activity in the central nervous system are desired. Furthermore, opioids or thiobarbiturates, as used for induction of anesthesia, do not predispose to seizure activity. Regardless of the drugs used for anesthesia, it is important to maintain treatment with the preestablished anticonvulsant drugs throughout the perioperative period.

TOURETTE SYNDROME

Tourette syndrome is a complex neuropsychiatric disorder of lifelong duration with onset during childhood.[152] Symptoms begin as attention deficit disorders and progress to spasmodic repetitious movements, which may be confused with seizures. Intelligence is usually above average, but nonspecific abnormalities are present on the electroencephalogram in about one-half of patients. Some patients exhibit coprolalia (profane vocalizations) and echolalia (repetitious speech).

Drugs administered in attempts to provide symptomatic relief of Tourette syndrome include haloperidol, clonidine, and pimozide. Side effects associated with drug therapy include extrapyramidal symptoms (haloperidol), sedation and reduced anesthetic requirements (clonidine), and cardiac dysrhythmias secondary to prolongation of the Q-T interval (pimozide). Sudden unexpected deaths in patients treated with high doses of pimozide (greater than 0.3 mg·kg^{-1}) have been attributed to cardiac dysrhythmias. There are no unique features of this syndrome that influence the selection of anesthetic drugs or muscle relaxants.

HEADACHES

Headaches are one of the most common symptoms described by patients. In most cases, the cause of headaches is benign, and no treatment is required. Occasionally, headaches may be a symptom of central nervous system disease.

Migraine Headaches

Migraine headaches are most frequent in females between 20 years and 35 years of age. A family history of migraine is present in about 50 percent of patients. The incidence of hypertension and coronary artery disease is increased in these patients.

SIGNS AND SYMPTOMS

Signs and symptoms of migraine headaches commonly begin in childhood (abdominal pain, vertigo, severe motion sickness), but headaches may not manifest until later. Classic migraine headaches begin with prodroma characterized by neurologic symptoms suggestive of cerebral ischemia. Visual and sensory disturbances are common, indicating that posterior portions of the cerebral hemispheres are most susceptible to the effects of decreased blood flow. Blurring of vision and tingling paresthesias of the face are frequent. After about 30 minutes, these symptoms wane and are followed by an intense unilateral headache, often associated with nausea and vomiting. In some patients, vomiting relieves the headache. Typically, headaches subside within 6 hours.

TREATMENT

The most frequently used drug for treatment of migraine headaches is ergotamine. Toxic effects of this drug include hypertension. Treatment with serotonin-blocking drugs, such as methysergide, is indicated when ergot preparations are not effective. Chronic administration of methysergide has been associated with pleuropulmonary and/or retroperitoneal fibrosis. Treatment with beta-adrenergic antagonists that are devoid of intrinsic sympathomimetic activity (propranolol or timolol) decreases the frequency, but not the severity, of migraine headaches.[153]

MANAGEMENT OF ANESTHESIA

Management of anesthesia for patients with a history of migraine headaches should consider the possible adverse interactions of anesthetic drugs with ergot preparations. Specifically, administration of vasopressors to patients being treated with these drugs might produce exaggerated increases in blood pressure. There are no known unique hazards of anesthetic drugs when administered to these patients.

Cluster Headaches

Cluster headaches characteristically occur in men between 20 years and 30 years of age. Attacks occur in clusters, followed by long symptom-free intervals. Typically, patients are awakened by unilateral discomfort behind the eye, which rapidly progresses to an intense and deep pain, which may involve the temple or malar regions. Maximum intensity is reached in 20 minutes to 30 minutes, followed by disappearance of the symptoms over the next 1 hour to 2 hours. Treatment is the same as for migraine headaches.

Increased Intracranial Pressure

Headaches can be the initial manifestations of increased intracranial pressure due to intracranial tumors, abscesses, or hematomas. Commonly, headaches occur in early morning, often awakening the patient. Presumably, this timing reflects decreased alveolar ventilation during physiologic sleep, leading to elevations in the arterial partial pressures of carbon dioxide and corresponding increases in cerebral blood flow. Spontaneous vomiting may accompany headaches. Headaches can also be provoked by coughing, which leads to increased intracranial pressure by impeding venous outflow from the brain.

Benign Intracranial Hypertension

Benign intracranial hypertension (pseudotumor cerebri) is defined as a syndrome characterized by (1) elevations of intracranial pressure above 20 cmH2O, (2) normal composition of cerebrospinal fluid, (3) normal level of consciousness, and (4) absence of focal intracranial lesions.[154] Computed tomography reveals normal or even small ventricular systems. Headaches and bilateral visual disturbances typically occur in obese women with menstrual irregularities. In most patients, no identifiable cause for increased intracranial pressure is found. The condition is self-limited and the prognosis is excellent.

Initial treatment of this syndrome is often repeated lumbar puncture and removal of 20 ml to 30 ml of cerebrospinal fluid. Use of large needles is appropriate to facilitate measurement of cerebrospinal fluid pressure. Furthermore, continued leakage of cerebrospinal fluid through the dural puncture site may be therapeutic. Lumbar puncture would not be safe in patients with increased intracranial pressure secondary to space-occupying lesions. In this situation, lumbar puncture could lead to herniation of the cerebellar tonsils and pressure on the medulla oblongata. In patients with benign intracranial hypertension, the presence of uniform swelling of the brain plus the normal position of the cerebellar tonsils prevents herniation and compression of the brain stem. Thus, lumbar puncture in these patients is not only safe but therapeutic, by allowing drainage of cerebrospinal fluid and reduction in intracranial pressure. Patients who do not respond to repeated lumbar drainage of cerebrospinal fluid may benefit from therapy with corticosteroids to reduce cerebral edema or acetazolamide, which reduces the rate of cerebrospinal fluid production. Chronic administration of acetazolamide can result in acidemia, presumably reflecting inhibition of hydrogen ion secretion by renal tubules. Surgical therapy, most often a lumboperitoneal shunt, is indicated only after medical therapy has failed and vision is deteriorating. Management of anesthesia in these patients is as described for patients with intracranial tumors (see the section Management of Anesthesia for Removal of an Intracranial Tumor).

Symptoms of benign intracranial hypertension may be exacerbated during pregnancy. Nevertheless, vaginal delivery is not contraindicated despite elevations of cerebrospinal fluid pressure during uterine contractions. In fact, spinal anesthesia may be beneficial since continued leakage of cerebrospinal fluid is welcomed.[154] When lumboperitoneal shunts are present, a radiograph is helpful to localize the area of entry of the tube into the subarachnoid space before performance of lumbar punctures. Furthermore, there is a theoretical possibility that local anesthetics injected into the subarachnoid space could escape into the peritoneal cavity resulting in inadequate anesthesia. Therefore, general anesthesia may be a more logical choice in the presence of lumboperitoneal shunts.

HERNIATION OF INTERVERTEBRAL DISCS

The intervertebral disc is composed of a compressible nucleus pulposus surrounded by a fibrocartilaginous anulus fibrosis. The disc acts as a shock absorber between vertebral bodies. Trauma or degenerative changes lead to changes in the intervertebral disc. Nerve root compression results when the nucleus pulposus protrudes through the posterolateral aspect of the anulus fibrosus. Occasionally, central protrusion of the disc may occur. If protrusion is into the cervical or thoracic region, there will be signs of spinal cord compression; signs of cauda equina compression occur if protrusion is into the lumbar region. Low back pain is estimated to occur in almost 80 percent of adults at some time.[155] Among chronic conditions, back problems are the most frequent cause of limitation of activity in persons less than 45 years of age.

Cervical Disc Disease

Lateral protrusion of cervical discs usually occurs at the C5–C6 or C6–C7 intervertebral space. Protrusion can be secondary to trauma or occur spontaneously. Pain starting in the neck that radiates to the shoulder and down the outer aspect of the arm into the thumb is characteristic of C5–C6 disc protrusions. The biceps reflex is reduced, and the biceps muscle is weak. Pain in the scapula, triceps region, and the middle and index fingers reflects protrusion at C6–C7 intervertebral spaces. Symptoms are commonly aggravated by coughing. The same symptoms can be due to osteophytes that compress nerve roots in the intervertebral foramina. Initial treatment of cervical disc protrusion is with traction. Surgical decompres-

sion is necessary if symptoms do not abate with conservative treatment.

Lumbar Disc Disease

The most common sites for disc protrusion are the L4–L5 and L5–S1 intervertebral spaces. Both sites produce low back pain, which radiates down the posterior and lateral aspects of the thigh and calf. A history of trauma is usually associated with sudden back pain that signals protrusion. This trauma, however, may be trivial in nature. Pain is aggravated by coughing or stretching of the sciatic nerve, as produced by straight-leg raising. These mechanical signs help distinguish protrusion from peripheral nerve disorders, as may accompany diabetes mellitus, which lack such signs.

Initial treatment of lumbar disc protrusion is with absolute bed rest plus centrally acting muscle relaxants such as diazepam. In patients without neuromotor deficits, clinical outcome is similar with 2 days of bed rest compared with longer periods.[156] An alternative to surgery may be the placement of corticosteroids in the epidural or subarachnoid spaces.[157] Corticosteroids may reduce inflammation and edema of nerve roots that have resulted from compression. Although not documented in patients, placement of large doses of triamcinolone in epidural spaces of dogs results in evidence of reduced responsiveness of the pituitary-adrenal axis for up to 4 weeks.[158] Treatment of disc protrusions with chymopapain injection is associated with risks of life-threatening allergic reactions. Pretreatment with corticosteroids and H-2 receptor antagonists may not reliably prevent chymopapain-evoked allergic reactions.[159]

SLEEP DISORDERS

It is estimated that one in four adults in the United States suffer from insomnia or the belief they obtain too little sleep. Excessive sleepiness is a less frequent complaint, and most of these patients have narcolepsy. Sleep apnea is a rare form of sleep disorder. Even less frequent are the Kleine-Levine syndrome (hypersomnia with excessive eating), and the Pickwickian syndrome (hypersomnia, hypoventilation, and obesity).

Insomnia

Normal sleep consists of two phases, designated rapid eye movement (REM) sleep and non-REM sleep. A cycle of alternating REM and non-REM phases continues fairly regularly throughout the night. Toward morning, the REM periods become longer. Insomniacs who take sedatives on a chronic basis show marked decreases in the amount of REM sleep. Withdrawal of medication is associated with exaggerated increases in REM sleep. This increase probably explains the appearance of insomnia when these patients discontinue medication that was used to facilitate the onset of physiologic sleep.

Narcolepsy

Narcolepsy is characterized by the uncontrollable urge to sleep at inappropriate times. Cataplexy, which is the sudden loss of postural tone leading to collapse, can accompany narcolepsy. Cataplexy almost always follows strong emotional stimuli, such as laughter or fear. Narcolepsy can be confused with psychomotor seizures, as both conditions can be associated with amnesia and automatic behavior. Most patients with narcolepsy demonstrate an abnormal sleep pattern, characterized by a rapid entrance into the REM phase. Treatment with amphetamines is discouraged because of the risk of habituation. An alternative is the administration of methylphenidate. If cataplexy accompanies narcolepsy, the administration of imipramine is recommended.

Sleep Apnea

Sleep apnea (cessation of air flow at the mouth for greater than 10 seconds) can reflect (1) loss of central nervous system drive to maintain ventilation, (2) mechanical upper airway obstruction, or (3) combinations of both.[160] Absence of neural drive to ventilation when voluntary control of breathing is diminished by sleep (Ondine's curve) is characterized by cessation of respiratory movements and airflow and most likely reflects a defect in the function of the medullary ventilatory center. Conversely, obstructive forms of sleep apnea are due to an abnormal relaxation of the posterior pharyngeal muscles, which may also be related to dysfunction of the medullary ventilatory center. Normally, subatmospheric pressure in the airway generated by contraction of the diaphragm is opposed by contraction of pharyngeal muscles. Obstructive sleep apnea occurs when the balance between these two forces is disturbed. There is persistence of respiratory movements, but airflow is absent due to upper airway obstruction. Awakening occurs when the arterial partial pressures of carbon dioxide rise or oxygen falls. A history of intense snoring is often available from families of patients with obstructive sleep apnea. Morning headaches and inappropriate daytime sedation are common. Repeated bouts of acidosis and hypoxia are presumed to be responsible for cardiac dysrhythmias and pulmonary hypertension that occur in these patients. Positive pressure delivered to the upper airway via the nasal passages may be useful in the management of patients with obstructive sleep apnea. Tracheostomy may be required in some patients.

Anesthetic management of patients with sleep apnea must consider a likely exquisite sensitivity to drugs that depress ventilation.[161] Hypoventilation may occur after administration of preoperative medication and long after discontinuation of anesthetic drugs, emphasizing the need for careful monitoring of ventilation. Postoperative pain relief poses an additional risk, and epidural opioids have been recommended so as to minimize systemic effects of these drugs.[161]

ABNORMAL PATTERNS OF VENTILATION

Abnormal patterns of ventilation in awake patients can be categorized as central neurogenic hyperventilation, Cheyne-Stokes respiration, apneustic breathing, respiratory ataxia or Biot's breathing, and posthyperventilation apnea. These patterns are manifestations of central nervous system diseases.

Central Neurogenic Hyperventilation

Central neurogenic hyperventilation is most often due to acute neurologic insults, as associated with a cerebral thrombosis or cerebral embolism. Hyperventilation is spontaneous and may be so severe that the arterial partial pressures of carbon dioxide are reduced to less than 20 mmHg.

Cheyne-Stokes Respiration

Cheyne-Stokes respiration is a pattern of periodic breathing in which hyperpnea alternates with apnea. The rate of ventilation increases in a crescendo fashion, and then declines until apnea is present. This pattern reflects brain damage after arterial hypoxemia or prolonged reductions in cerebral blood flow.

Apneustic Breathing

Apneustic breathing is characterized by prolonged inspiratory plateaus, in which inspiration is maintained for as long as 30 seconds. Occlusion of the basilar artery leading to pontine infarction is a common cause. Brain damage after arterial hypoxemia, hypoglyce-

mia, or meningitis can also result in this pattern.

Respiratory Ataxia

Respiratory ataxia (Biot's breathing) is characterized by a completely random pattern of ventilation in which shallow and deep breaths occur unpredictably, and with variable pauses. Mechanical support of ventilation may be indicated, as apnea is a frequent complication.

Posthyperventilation Apnea

In normal patients, five voluntary deep breaths will lower the arterial partial pressures of carbon dioxide about 10 mmHg. Nevertheless, apnea does not occur reflecting the presence of voluntary drives to ventilation. Conversely, a similar sequence of deep breaths performed by patients with frontal lobe disease results in apnea, until the arterial partial pressures of carbon dioxide return to normal levels.

EPISTAXIS

Arteries that supply the nasal chamber and give rise to epistaxis are terminal branches of the internal carotid artery (ethmoidal arteries) and external carotid artery (sphenopalatine artery). Epistaxis orginating from the anterior nasal chamber (most often from a blood vessel in the mucus membrane of the nasal septum) often stops spontaneously or as the result of conservative measures, such as external application of pressure or cold. Spontaneous bleeding from posterior aspects of the nasal chamber is likely to be arterial and associated with hypertension. In some instances, blood loss may be extensive with accompanying hypotension. Treatment of posterior nasal hemorrhage usually requires sedation and placement of postnasal packs. In an emergency, a Foley catheter serves as an effective postnasal pack. The tip of this catheter should be covered with antibiotic ointment before being inserted into the nostril and the balloon filled with saline rather than air to prevent loss of pressure and gradual collapse.

Any posterior pack that effectively blocks the postnasal space will also block normal pathways for drainage of secretions, thus predisposing patients to acute sinusitis. Obstruction of the Eustachian tube orifice may result in acute otitis media. For these reasons, systemic antibiotics are routinely administered to these patients. Obstruction of the nasal airway may also result in arterial hypoxemia particularly in elderly debilitated patients.

Surgical ligation of bleeding sites, especially from the ethmoidal area, may be required when packing fails to control epistaxis. Angiography is occasionally used to delineate hemorrhage from the ethmoidal or sphenopalatine arteries. The anterior ethmoidal artery is ligated through an incision along the side of the nose. The sphenopalatine artery is approached surgically by opening the maxillary sinus and ligating the artery in the pterygopalatine fissure.

ENDOLYMPHATIC HYDROPS

Endolymphatic hydrops (Ménière's disease) is a disorder of the membranous labyrinth of the inner ear, characterized by the triad of hearing loss, tinnitus, and vertigo. This disease is most common between 30 years and 60 years of age; in the majority of patients, the etiology is unknown. Endolymphatic hydrops should be distinguished from other causes of vertigo, which include acoustic neuroma, vestibular neuronitis, hypoglycemia, and hypothyroidism. The pathognomonic feature of endolymphatic hydrops is distention of the endolymphatic system of the inner ear. Treatment of this disease is surgical, if bed rest and sedation with benzodiazepines are not effective. Surgical therapy is a labyrinthectomy or section of the vestibular nerve, which requires a craniotomy.

MIDDLE EAR COMPLICATIONS RELATED TO THE USE OF NITROUS OXIDE

The middle ear is an air-filled cavity bounded by the tympanic membrane and the inner ear (Fig. 18-18). During the administration of nitrous oxide, middle ear pressures increase. This increase reflects passage of nitrous oxide into the noncompliant confines of the middle ear. Under normal conditions, this pressure buildup in the middle ear is passively vented via the Eustachian tubes into the nasopharynx. Narrowing of the Eustachian tubes by acute inflammation or the presence of scar tissue, as is likely after an adenoidectomy, impairs the ability of the middle ear to vent passively any pressure increase produced by nitrous oxide. Excessive middle ear pressures could jeopardize the integrity of the tympanic membrane. Indeed, tympanic membrane rupture, manifesting as bright red blood in the external auditory canal, has been described during the administration of nitrous oxide, even in the absence of middle ear disease.[162,163] Disruption of previous middle ear reconstructive surgery has also been observed when nitrous oxide is administered at a later date for operative procedures not involving the ear.[164] Manifestations of this disruption are recurrence of hearing loss in the previously diseased ear, upon awakening from anesthesia. Administration of nitrous oxide during tympanoplasty is well known to result in displacement of freshly placed grafts, reflecting the presence of air bubbles containing nitrous oxide in the middle ear. Postoperative nausea and vomiting could also be due to increased middle ear pressures that persist after administration of nitrous oxide.

Absorption of nitrous oxide after discontinuation of the administration of this drug can also exert deleterious effects on the middle ear. For example, rapid reabsorption of nitrous oxide can result in negative pressures in the middle ear and tympanic membrane rupture. Transient hearing impairment after administration of nitrous oxide to previously normal patients most likely reflects negative pressure in the middle ear.[165] Serous otitis can also be a manifestation of this negative pressure.

Potential adverse effects of nitrous oxide

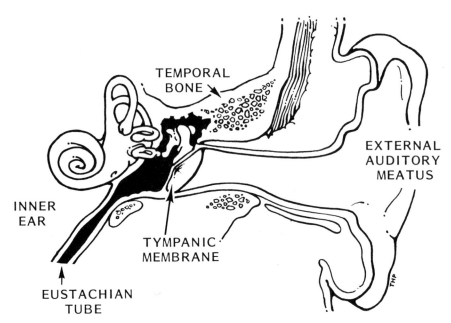

FIG. 18-18. The middle ear is an air-filled cavity bounded by the tympanic membrane and inner ear. Diffusion of nitrous oxide into this cavity can increase middle ear pressures, particularly when passive venting of pressures into the nasopharynx is impaired because of obstruction of the Eustachian tube.

on the middle ear raise questions as to the wisdom of administering this drug to patients with narrowing of the Eustachian tubes due to acute inflammation or scarring. Likewise, a preoperative history of previous middle ear surgery introduces concern. Nevertheless, it is undeniable that many patients with a history of middle ear surgery have received nitrous oxide on subsequent occasions, without detectable detrimental effects on hearing.

lar pressures are 10 mmHg to 20 mmHg, with a value above 25 mmHg considered pathologic.

Glaucoma may be classified as open angle and angle closure. Open angle glaucoma is the most common form, manifesting as a slowly progressive bilateral disorder. It is estimated that 12 percent to 30 percent of blindness in the United States is due to open angle glaucoma. Angle closure glaucoma is less frequent but can be precipitated acutely by mydriasis in susceptible individuals.

GLAUCOMA

Glaucoma is characterized by increased intraocular pressure which, if untreated, leads to blindness, due to interference with blood flow to the retina and compression of the optic disc. Increased intraocular pressure is caused by obstruction to the outflow of aqueous humor from the anterior chamber of the eye into the venous circulation. Normal intraocu-

Treatment

Treatment of glaucoma is with drugs designed to lower intraocular pressure by decreasing resistance to outflow of aqueous humor or by reducing the rate of formation of aqueous humor. Miosis decreases resistance by contracting the ciliary muscle, which stretches the trabecular meshwork in the anterior chamber of the eye. Open angle glaucoma can often be controlled with medical management; angle closure glaucoma will ultimately require surgery.

PARASYMPATHOMIMETICS

Pilocarpine is a short-acting parasympathomimetic drug that produces miosis. Topical administration of this drug three times to four times a day often provides adequate control of intraocular pressure. Carbachol is a parasympathomimetic drug, which can be substituted, if intolerance to pilocarpine develops or if a slightly stronger or longer-acting drug is needed. Echothiophate is a long-acting parasympathomimetic miotic drug. An adverse effect of this drug is inhibition of plasma cholinesterase activity, which persists for about 4 weeks after echothiophate eye drops are discontinued. A potential undesirable effect produced by chronic use of topical miotic drugs is the formation of cataracts.

EPINEPHRINE

Epinephrine, administered topically, reduces intraocular pressure by decreasing the resistance to outflow of aqueous humor from the anterior chamber of the eye into the venous circulation. In addition, epinephrine is likely to reduce the formation of aqueous humor. Epinephrine is variably effective and can produce systemic sympathomimetic symptoms. Furthermore, the use of topical epinephrine is associated with local allergic reactions in about 20 percent of patients.

CARBONIC ANHYDRASE INHIBITORS

Carbonic anhydrase inhibitors, such as acetazolamide, when administered orally, lower intraocular pressure, presumably by reducing formation of aqueous humor.

BETA-ADRENERGIC ANTAGONIST DRUGS

Beta-adrenergic antagonist drugs lower intraocular pressure when given orally or topically. The topical route is preferred because of a lower incidence of systemic side effects. The ability of these drugs to lower intraocular pressure seems to involve decreases in formation of aqueous humor, rather than increases in outflow.

Propranolol lowers intraocular pressure, but its local anesthetic effect when applied topically is undesirable. Timolol is a long-acting, nonselective, beta-adrenergic antagonist drug, without significant local anesthetic effects when applied topically to the cornea. After topical application of a single dose of timolol (one drop of a 0.25 percent solution), intraocular pressure begins to decrease within 20 minutes, and the effect persists even after 24 hours.[166] Timolol does not alter the diameter of the pupil or its reactivity to light. Timolol is absorbed into the systemic circulation after topical application, producing side effects related to blockade of cardiac and noncardiac beta-adrenergic receptors. Indeed, bradycardia and hypotension, which is refractory to atropine treatment, has been observed during anesthesia in patients being treated with topical timolol.[167] In addition, systemic absorption of timolol can result in the appearance of bronchospasm. Lethargy and fatigue are central nervous system effects of topical timolol and other beta-adrenergic antagonist drugs.

Management of Anesthesia

Management of anesthesia for patients with glaucoma includes maintenance of miosis by continuation of parasympathomimetic therapy throughout the perioperative period. For example, topical application of pilocarpine would be appropriate on the morning of surgery. This practice eliminates the likelihood of an attack of acute angle closure glaucoma.

Inclusion of anticholinergic drugs in the preoperative medication is acceptable, since the amount of drug reaching the eye is too little to dilate the pupil.[168] Furthermore, use of anticholinergic drugs in combination with anticholinesterase drugs to reverse nondepolarizing muscle relaxants is acceptable. For example, it is estimated that the intravenous administration of 2 mg of atropine will result in the delivery of only 0.004 mg to the eye. Despite these assurances, it would seem reasonable to limit use of anticholinergic drugs in patients with glaucoma. Indeed, intramuscular scopolamine 0.4 mg produces a significant increase in the diameter of the pupils in healthy subjects and, therefore, may not be an appropriate drug to administer to patients with glaucoma.[169] In contrast, the same dose of atropine does not alter the size of the pupils. Although not evaluated, glycopyrrolate, administered systemically, would predictably also have minimal effects on the diameter of the pupils. Administration of anticholinergic drugs in combination with drugs that produce miosis (opioids, anticholinesterases) may prevent dilating effects on the pupils normally produced by anticholinergic drugs.

Another important goal during administration of anesthesia to patients with glaucoma is prevention of increases in intraocular pressure. Succinylcholine-induced increases in intraocular pressure are maximal 2 minutes to 4 minutes after administration of the muscle relaxant and return to baseline values after about 6 minutes.[168] These increases in intraocular pressure are not reliably obscured by any method, including prevention of skeletal muscle fasciculations by prior administration of nondepolarizing muscle relaxants.[170] Implications of this drug-induced increase in intraocular pressure in patients with glaucoma are not known. Presumably, patients with adequate medical control of glaucoma would not be jeopardized by transient elevations of intraocular pressure produced by succinylcholine. Other events that increase intraocular pressure are hypercarbia and increased central venous pressure. The effect of ketamine on intraocular pressure is unclear, as reports are contradictory.[171] Intraocular pressure is lowered by hypocarbia, decreased central venous pressure as produced by drug-induced osmotic diuresis, opioids, and volatile anesthetic drugs. Fluctuations in arterial pressure and skeletal muscle paralysis produced by the nondepolarizing muscle relaxants exert only minor influences on intraocular pressure, although pancuronium may produce reductions in this pressure.[170]

Interactions of drugs administered during anesthesia with those being used to treat glaucoma must be appreciated. The rare patient being treated with echothiophate is at risk for prolonged paralysis after administration of succinylcholine. If succinylcholine is administered, initial doses should be reduced to 0.1 $mg \cdot kg^{-1}$ and responses observed, using a peripheral nerve stimulator. Bradycardia and exaggerated hypotension have been attributed to beta-adrenergic blockade produced by chronic topical administration of timolol.[172]

Postoperatively, patients with glaucoma should be observed for dilated pupils that are irregular and asymmetric, which can be manifestations of an acute attack of angle closure glaucoma. Patients with such attacks are also likely to complain of pain in and around the eyes, as well as a loss of vision. In contrast, patients with corneal abrasions will complain of pain only in the eyes.

CATARACT EXTRACTION

Patients who require general anesthesia for cataract extraction are likely to be elderly, with co-existing major organ disease. Anesthesia for cataract extraction must assure an immobile patient. Sudden movement or attempts to cough when the eye is open can result in extrusion of vitreous and permanent ocular damage. An adequate depth of anesthesia, with or without skeletal muscle paralysis, is essential. Although succinylcholine increases intraocular pressure, this elevation is transient. Nevertheless, use of intermediate-acting muscle relaxants may serve as useful alternatives. Modest hyperventilation of the lungs to produce hypocarbia and 10 degree to 15 degree head-up tilts to promote venous drainage will likely reduce intraocular pressure during intraocular surgery. It is important to minimize reactions to the endotracheal tube at the conclusion of surgery. Ideally, the tube is removed from the trachea before airway depression from the anesthetic drug has waned. If the tube is left in the trachea as patients awaken, it may be helpful to administer intravenous lidocaine (0.5 $mg \cdot kg^{-1}$ to 1.5 $mg \cdot kg^{-1}$) in attempts to attenuate reflex responses to the presence of the tube.

It is helpful to minimize the incidence of vomiting in the postoperative period. In this regard, use of opioids in the preanesthetic medication is often avoided. Routine aspiration of the stomach at the conclusion of surgery via an orally inserted tube serves not only to remove gastric fluid, but also to decrease gastric distention that could contribute to postoperative nausea and vomiting. A number of antiemetic drugs have been recommended, with questionable efficacy. In a well-controlled study, however, intravenous administration of droperidol, 1.25 mg, 5 minutes before the conclusion of general anesthesia was effective in reducing the incidence of postoperative emesis.[173]

OCULAR TRAUMA

Ocular trauma characterized by penetrating eye injuries requires prompt surgical treatment if the eye is to be salvaged. Management of anesthesia is often complicated by recent ingestion of food by the patient. Therefore, protection of the airway must be balanced against the hazards of producing increases in intraocular pressure and the potential extrusion of intraocular contents. The obvious controversy relates to the use of succinylcholine to facilitate intubation of the trachea. The rapid onset of skeletal muscle paralysis provided by this drug is ideal for prompt placement of a cuffed tube in the trachea. Against the selection of succinylcholine is the predictable increase in intraocular pressure, even when fasciculations are prevented. Despite the controversy associated with the use of succinylcholine, no published case reports describe loss of intraocular contents attributable to this drug. An alternative to succinylcholine is the administration of large doses (0.15 mg·kg^{-1}) of pancuronium, which is alleged to produce rapid onset of skeletal muscle paralysis without the hazard of increased intraocular pressure.[174] The disadvantage of using pancuronium is a prolonged duration of action for what may be a short operation. In this regard, large doses (2–3 × ED$_{95}$) of intermediate-acting muscle relaxants may be useful alternatives. Regardless of the muscle relaxant selection, it is mandatory to confirm the presence of skeletal muscle paralysis by the use of a peripheral nerve stimulator before initiating direct laryngoscopy for intubation of the trachea. Premature placement of the tube in the trachea will provoke movement of the patient and defeat all attempts to minimize hazards of vomiting or elevations in intraocular pressure. Maintenance of anesthesia is acceptably accomplished with inhaled or injected drugs. Timing of the removal of the cuffed tube from the trachea at the end of surgery is determined by the likely presence or absence of gastric contents.

GLOMUS JUGULARE TUMORS

Glomus jugulare tumors (chemodectomas) arise from the glomus body at the dome of the jugular bulb.[175] These tumors are typically slow growing and benign, although they have a propensity for local invasion.

Signs and Symptoms

Symptoms produced by glomus jugulare tumors are related to their vascularity, principally from the external carotid artery and their invasion of surrounding structures. Because of their vascularity, a bruit may be heard over these tumors. Unilateral pulsatile tinnitus is often the patient's initial complaint. Hearing loss results as tumor extension limits mobility of the eardrum or ossicles. Cranial nerve involvement may manifest as dysphagia, recurrent aspiration, upper airway obstruction and difficulty handling secretions. Invasion of the posterior fossa may obstruct the aqueduct of Sylvius and cause hydrocephalus. It is common for glomus jugulare tumors to invade the internal jugular vein and finger-like projections may extend to the right atrium. A mass in the neck occurs when the glomus tumor extends inferiorly and laterally. Occasionally, glomus jugulare tumors secrete norepinephrine and produce symptoms that mimic pheochromocytoma.

Treatment

Surgical excision, often preceded by radiotherapy or embolization to diminish vascularity, is the treatment for glomus jugulare tumors. Preoperative evaluation may include arteriography to evaluate the location and blood supply to the tumor, venography to detect extension into the internal jugular vein, and computed tomography for evidence of intracranial extension. Examination of cranial nerve function is important to evaluate the risk of aspiration. Evidence of increased intracranial pressure is sought when obstructive hydrocephalus is suspected.

Management of Anesthesia

Management of anesthesia is influenced by the potential for massive and rapid blood loss and likely prolonged (often 8 hours or more) operative time. Invasive arterial and venous pressure monitoring is indicated and urine output is followed after placement of a Foley catheter. An internal jugular vein involved by tumor should not be cannulated for placement of right atrial or pulmonary artery catheters. Hypothermia is likely, especially with prolonged surgery, emphasizing the importance of warming inhaled gases and infused fluids. Drugs and techniques to control intracranial pressure may be necessary. Controlled hypotension minimizes blood loss and may facilitate surgical excision of the tumor. Venous air embolism is a hazard, particularly if the internal jugular vein is opened to remove tumor or excision of tumor that has invaded temporal bone results in exposure of veins, which cannot collapse because of bony attachments. In this regard, mechanical ventilation of the lungs may be useful and addition of skeletal muscle paralysis minimizes the likely occurrence of a gasp reflex. Appropriate monitors for detection of venous air embolism are indicated when venous air embolism is considered a hazard (see the section Venous Air Embolism). Sudden unexplained cardiovascular collapse and death during resection of these tumors may reflect occurrence of venous air embolism or tumor emboli. If the surgeon finds it necessary to identify the facial nerve, it may be necessary to avoid profound skeletal muscle paralysis or temporarily pharmacologically antagonize neuromuscular blockade. The choice of anesthetic drugs is not uniquely influenced by the presence of a glomus jugulare tumor, although potential adverse effects of nitrous oxide should be recognized if venous air embolism is likely.

CAROTID SINUS SYNDROME

Carotid sinus syndrome is an uncommon entity caused by exaggeration of normal activity of baroreceptors in response to mechanical stimulation. For example, stimulation of the carotid sinus by external massage, which in normal patients produces slight reductions in heart rate and blood pressure, can produce syncope in affected patients. There is a high incidence of associated vascular disease in these patients. Indeed, carotid sinus syndrome is a known complication of carotid endarterectomy.

Two distinct types of cardiovascular responses may be noted with carotid sinus hypersensitivity. About 80 percent of affected patients manifest a cardioinhibitory reflex mediated by the vagus nerve, which results in profound bradycardia. About 10 percent of patients manifest a vasodepressor reflex mediated by inhibition of sympathetic vasomotor tone with resultant decreases in systemic vascular resistance and profound hypotension. The remaining 10 percent of patients manifest components of both reflexes.

Treatment of carotid sinus syndrome may be with drugs, placement of a permanent demand artificial cardiac pacemaker, or prolonged ablation of the carotid sinus. Anticholinergic drugs and vasopressors are limited by side effects and are rarely effective in patients with vasodepressor or mixed forms of carotid sinus hypersensitivity. Since most patients have the cardioinhibitory type of carotid sinus syndrome, implantation of an artificial cardiac pacemaker is the usual initial treatment. In patients in whom the vasodepressor reflex response is refractory to cardiac pacing, surgical ablation of the carotid sinus may be attempted.

Management of anesthesia is often complicated by hypotension, bradycardia, and cardiac dysrhythmias.[176] Infiltration of lidocaine around the carotid sinus before dissection usually improves hemodynamic stability but may also interfere with determination of the completeness of surgical denervation. Drugs such as atropine, isoproterenol, and epinephrine should be readily available.

NEUROFIBROMATOSIS

Neurofibromatosis is due to an autosomal dominant mutation, which is not limited to racial or ethnic origin (see Chapter 35). Both sexes are affected with equal frequency and severity. Expressivity is variable, but penetrance of the trait is virtually 100 percent. Manifestations are classified as classic (von Recklinghausen's disease), acoustic, and segmental neurofibromatosis. It is estimated that neurofibromatosis affects 80,000 individuals in the United States.

Signs and Symptoms

The diversity of clinical features of neurofibromatosis emphasizes the protean nature of this disease. One feature common to all patients, however, is progression of the disease with time.

CAFÉ AU LAIT SPOTS

Café au lait spots are present in over 99 percent of patients with neurofibromatosis. Six or more spots larger than 1.5 cm in diameter are considered diagnostic. Café au lait spots are usually present at birth and continue to increase in number and sizing during the first decade of life. Café au lait spots vary in size from 1 mm to over 15 cm. Distribution of spots in random, except for disproportionately small numbers on the face. Other than an adverse cosmetic effect, café au lait spots pose no threat to health.

NEUROFIBROMAS

Neurofibromas virtually always involve the skin but they can also occur in deeper peripheral nerves and nerve roots and in or on viscera or blood vessels innervated by the autonomic nervous system. They may be nodular and discrete or diffuse, with extensive interdigitation with surrounding tissues. Although neurofibromas are benign histologically, functional compromise and cosmetic disfigurement may result. Compromise of the airway may occur when neurofibromas develop in the cervical or mediastinal regions. Neurofibromas may be highly vascular. Pregnancy or puberty can lead to increases in the number and size of neurofibromas.

INTRACRANIAL TUMORS

Intracranial tumors occur in 5 percent to 10 percent of patients with neurofibromatosis and account for a major portion of the morbidity and mortality associated with this disease. Computed tomography to rule out the presence of intracranial tumors is indicated when the diagnosis of neurofibromatosis is considered. Histologically, these tumors include astrocytomas, acoustic neuromas, neurilemomas, meningiomas, and neurofibromas. Bilateral presence of acoustic neuromas in a patient with café au lait spots establishes the diagnosis of acoustic neurofibromatosis.

SPINAL CORD TUMORS

Spinal cord tumors in patients with neurofibromas involving the spinal cord presumably derive from sensory or autonomic ganglia, nerve roots, or proximal nerve trunks.

ORTHOPEDIC ABNORMALITIES

Congenital pseudarthrosis is often due to neurofibromatosis. The tibia is involved most often; the radius is the second most frequent site. Ordinarily, only a single site is involved in any one patient. Severity of pseudarthrosis ranges from an asymptomatic radiologic presentation to a need for amputation.

Kyphoscoliosis occurs in about 2 percent of patients with neurofibromatosis. Cervical and thoracic vertebrae are most frequently involved. Paravertebral neurofibromas are often present, but their role, if any, in the development of kyphoscoliosis is not defined. Untreated, this manifestation progresses, leading to cardiorespiratory and neurologic compromise. Short stature is a recognized feature of neurofibromatosis.

CANCER

There is an increased incidence of cancer in patients with neurofibromatosis. Clearly associated cancers include neurofibrosarcomas, malignant schwannomas, Wilms' tumor, rhabdomyosarcoma, and leukemia. Other cancers, including neuroblastomas, medullary thyroid carcinomas, and pancreatic adenocarcinoma, are less clearly associated with neurofibromatosis.

ENDOCRINE DISORDERS

It is a misconception that neurofibromatosis entails diffuse endocrine dysfunction. Associated endocrine disorders, however, include pheochromocytoma, disturbances in reaching puberty, medullary thyroid carcinoma, and hyperparathyroidism. Pheochromocytoma occurs with a frequency of probably less than 1 percent and is virtually unknown in children with neurofibromatosis.

INTELLECTUAL IMPAIRMENT

Intellectual impairment occurs in about 40 percent of patients with neurofibromatosis. Mental retardation is less frequent than is impairment classified as learning disabilities. The intellectual handicap is usually apparent by school age and does not progress with time.

SEIZURES

Major and minor motor seizures are known complications of neurofibromatosis. Seizures may be idiopathic or reflect the presence of intracranial tumors.

CONGENITAL HEART DISEASE

Congenital heart disease, particularly pulmonary stenosis, is said to be relatively frequent among patients with neurofibromatosis. Nevertheless, a true cause and effect relationship has not been established.

Treatment

Treatment of neurofibromatosis is with symptomatic drug therapy (antihistamines for pruritus, anticonvulsants) and appropriately timed surgery. Surgical removal of cutaneous neurofibromas is reserved for those particularly disfiguring or functionally compromising. Progressive kyphoscoliosis is best treated with surgical stabilization. Surgery is indicated for symptoms due to nervous system involvement by neurofibromas or associated endocrine dysfunction.

Management of Anesthesia

Management of anesthesia for patients with neurofibromatosis must consider the multiple clinical features of this disease.[177] Although rare, the possible presence of pheochromocytoma should be considered in the preoperative evaluation. Signs of increased intracranial pressure may reflect the presence of an expanding intracranial tumor. Airway patency may be jeopardized by an expanding neurofibroma. Selection of regional anesthesia must recognize the possible future development of neurofibromas that involve the spinal cord. There are no known unique considerations for the selection of inhaled or injected anesthetic drugs or muscle relaxants in patients with neurofibromatosis.

REFERENCES

1. Cutler RWP. Neurology. In: Rubenstein E, Federman DD, eds. Scientific American Medicine. New York. Scientific American, 1981;11:VI:1–7

2. Spark RF, Baker R, Bienfang DC, Bergland R. Bromocriptine reduces pituitary size and hypersecretion. Requiem for pituitary surgery? JAMA 1982;247:311–6

3. Risberg J, Lundberg N, Ingvar DH. Regional cerebral blood volume during acute transient rises of the intracranial pressure (plateau waves). J Neurosurg 1969;31:303–10

4. Harp JR, Wollman H. Cerebral metabolic effects of hyperventilation and deliberate hypotension. Br J Anaesth 1973;45:256–62

5. Raichle ME, Posner JB, Plum F. Cerebral blood flow during and after hyperventilation. Arch Neurol 1970;23:394–403

6. Marsh ML, Marshall LF, Shapiro HM. Neurosurgical intensive care. Anesthesiology 1977;47:149–63

7. Cottrell JE, Robustelli A, Post K, Turndorf H. Furosemide- and mannitol-induced changes in intracranial pressure and serum osmolality and electrolytes. Anesthesiology 1977;47:28–30

8. Lassen NA, Christensen MS. Physiology of cerebral blood flow. Br J Anaesth 1976;48:719–34

9. Cohen PJ, Alexander SC, Smith TC, et al. Effects of hypoxia and normocarbia on cerebral blood flow and metabolism in man. J Appl Physiol 1967;23:183–9

10. Strandgaard S. Autoregulation of cerebral blood flow in hypertensive patients: The modifying influence of prolonged antihypertensive treatment on the tolerance to acute drug-induced hypotension. Circulation 1976;53:720–7

11. Eger EI. Pharmacology of isoflurane. Br J Anaesth 1984;56:71S–99S

12. Aidinis S, Lafferty J, Shapiro H. Intracranial responses to PEEP. Anesthesiology 1976;45:275–86

13. Eger EI. Isoflurane (Forane). A compendium and reference. Anaquest, A Division of BOC, Inc. Madison, WI, 1986:1–160

14. Adams RW, Gronert GA, Sundt TM, Michenfelder JD. Halothane, hypocapnia, and cerebrospinal fluid pressure in neurosurgery. Anesthesiology 1972;37:510–7

15. Albrecht RF, Miletich DJ, Madala LR. Normalization of cerebral blood flow during prolonged anesthesia. Anesthesiology 1983;58:26–31

16. Artru AA. Effects of halothane, enflurane, isoflurane and fentanyl on resistance to reabsorption of cerebrospinal fluid. Anesth Analg 1984;63:180–5

17. Eger EI, Stevens WC, Cromwell TH. The electroencephalogram in man anesthetized with Forane. Anesthesiology 1971;35:504–8

18. Adams RW, Cucchiara RF, Gronert GA, et al. Isoflurane and cerebrospinal fluid pressure in neurosurgical patients. Anesthesiology 1981;54:97–9

19. Artru AA. Isoflurane does not increase the rate of CSF production in the dog. Anesthesiology 1984;60:193–7

20. Todd MM, Drummond JC. A comparison of the cerebrovascular and metabolic effects of halothane and isoflurane in the cat. Anesthesiology 1984;60:276–80

21. Henriksen HT, Jorgensen PB. The effect of nitrous oxide on intracranial pressure in patients with intracranial disorders. Br J Anaesth 1973;45:486–92

22. Phirman JR, Shapiro HM. Modification of nitrous oxide-induced intracranial hypertension by prior induction of anesthesia. Anesthesiology 1977;46:150–1

23. Saidman LJ, Eger EI. Change in cerebrospinal fluid pressure during pneumoencephalography under nitrous oxide anesthesia. Anesthesiology 1965;26:67–72

24. Artru A, Sohn YJ, Eger EI. Increased intracranial pressure from nitrous oxide five days after pneumoencephalography. Anesthesiology 1978;49:136–7

25. Artur AA. Nitrous oxide plays a direct role in the development of tension pneumocephalus intraoperatively. Anesthesiology 1982;57:59–61

26. Wyte SR, Shapiro HM, Turner P, Harris AB. Ketamine-induced intracranial hypertension. Anesthesiology 1972;36:174–6

27. Winters WD. Epilepsy or anesthesia with ketamine. Anesthesiology 1972;36:309–12

28. Takkanen L, Laitinen L, Johansson G. Effects of d-tubocurarine on intracranial pressure and thalamic electrical impedance. Anesthesiology 1974;40:247–51

29. Rosa G, Orfei P, Sanfilippo M, et al. The effects of atracurium besylate (Tracrium) on intracra-

nial pressure and cerebral perfusion pressure. Anesth Analg 1986;65:381–4

30. Rosa G, Sanfilippo M, Vilardi V, et al. Effects of vecuronium bromide on intracranial pressure and cerebral perfusion pressure. Br J Anaesth 1986;58:437–40

31. Stirt JA, Grosslight KR, Bedford FR, Vollmer D. "Defasciculation" with metocurine prevents succinylcholine-induced increases in intracranial pressure. Anesthesiology 1987;67:50–3

32. Hamill JF, Bedford RF, Weaver, DC, Colohan AR. Lidocaine before endotracheal intubation: Intravenous or laryngotracheal? Anesthesiology 1981;55:578–81

33. Turner JM, Powell D, Gibson RM, McDowall DG. Intracranial pressure changes in neurosurgical patients during hypotension induced with sodium nitroprusside or trimethaphan. Br J Anaesth 1977;49:419–25

34. Marshall WK, Bedford RF. Use of a pulmonary-artery catheter for detection and treatment of venous air embolism: A prospective study in man. Anesthesiology 1980;52:131–4

35. Moorthy SS, Hilgenberg JC. Resistance to nondepolarizing muscle relaxants in paretic upper extremities of patients with residual hemiplegia. Anesth Analg 1980;59:624–7

36. Jachuck SJ, Ramani PS, Clark F, Kalbag RM. Electrocardiographic abnormalities associated with raised intracranial pressure. Br Med J 1975;1:242–4

37. Perkins-Pearson NAK, Marshall WK, Bedford RF. Atrial pressures in the seated position. Implications for paradoxical air embolism. Anesthesiology 1982;57:493–7

38. English JB, Westenshow D, Hodges MR, Stanley TH. Comparison of venous air embolism monitoring methods in supine dogs. Anesthesiology 1978;48:425–9

39. Matjaski J, Petrozza P, Mackenzie CF. Sensitivity of end-tidal nitrogen in venous air embolism detection in dogs. Anesthesiology 1985;63:418–25

40. Adornato DC, Gildenberg PL, Ferrario CM, et al. Pathophysiology of intravenous air embolism in dogs. Anesthesiology 1978;49:120–7

41. Bunegin L, Albin MS, Helsel PE, et al. Positioning the right atrial catheter: A model for reappraisal. Anesthesiology 1981;55:343–8

42. Munson ES, Merrick HC. Effect of nitrous oxide on venous air embolism. Anesthesiology 1966;27:783–7

43. Ropper AH, Wechsler LR, Wilson LS. Carotid bruit and the risk of stroke in elective surgery. N Engl J Med 1982;307:1388–90

44. Chambers BR, Norris JW. Outcome in patients with asymptomatic neck bruits. N Engl J Med 1986;315:860–5

45. Ennix CL, Lawrie GM, Morris GC, et al. Improved results of carotid endarterectomy in patients with symptomatic coronary disease: An analysis of 1546 consecutive cardiac operations. Stroke 1979;10:122–5

46. Michenfelder JD, Sundt TM, Fode N, Sharbrough FW. Isoflurane when compared to enflurane and halothane decreases the frequency of cerebral ischemia during carotid endarterectomy. Anesthesiology 1987;67:336–40

47. Torvik A, Skullerud K. How often are brain infarcts caused by hypotensive episodes? Stroke 1976;7:255–7

48. Riles TS, Kopelman I, Imparato AM. Myocardial infarction following carotid endarterectomy: A review of 683 operations. Surgery 1979;85:249–52

49. Keats AS. Anesthesia for carotid endarterectomy. Cleve Clin Q 1981;48:68–71

50. Fleming RA, Smith NT. An inexpensive device for analyzing and monitoring the electroencephalogram. Anesthesiology 1979;50:456–60

51. Cucchiara RF, Sharbrough FW, Messick JM, Tinker JH. An electroencephalographic filter-processor as an indicator of cerebral ischemia during carotid endarterectomy. Anesthesiology 1979;51:77–9

52. McKay RD, Sundt TM, Michenfelder JD, et al. Internal carotid artery stump pressure and cerebral blood flow during carotid endarterectomy: Modification by halothane, enflurane and Innovar. Anesthesiology 1976;45:390–9

53. Peterson DI, Drummond JC, Todd MM. Effects of halothane, enflurane, isoflurane, and nitrous oxide on somatosensory evoked potentials in humans. Anesthesiology 1986;65:35–40

54. McPherson RW, Mahla M, Johnson R, Traystman RJ. Effects of enflurane, isoflurane, and nitrous oxide on somatosensory evoked potentials during fentanyl anesthesia. Anesthesiology 1985;62:626–33

55. Pathak KS, Brown RH, Cascorbi HF, Nash CL. Effects of fentanyl and morphine on intraoperative somatosensory cortical-evoked potentials. Anesth Analg 1984;63:833–7

56. Schubert A, Drummond JC. The effect of acute hypocapnia on human median nerve somatosensory evoked responses. Anesth Analg 1986;65:240–4

57. Pearce HJ, Kowell J, Tubb DW, Brown HJ. Continuous oculoplethysmographic monitoring during carotid endarterectomy. Am J Surg 1979;138:733–5

58. Liapis CD, Satiani B, Florence CL, Evans WE.

Motor speech malfunction following carotid endarterectomy. Surgery 1981;89:56−9

59. Wade JG, Larson CP, Hickey RF, et al. Effect of carotid endarterectomy on carotid chemoreceptor and baroreceptor function in man. N Engl J Med 1970;282:823−9

60. Asiddao CB, Donegan JH, Whitesell RC, Kalbfleisch JH. Factors associated with perioperative complications during carotid endarterectomy. Anesth Analg 1982;61:631−7

61. Towne JB, Bernhard VM. The relationship of postoperative hypertension to complications following carotid endarterectomy. Surgery 1980;88:575−80

62. Anderson CA, Rich NM, Collins GJ, et al. Carotid endarterectomy: Regional versus general anesthesia. Ann Surg 1980;46:323−7

63. EC/IC Bypass Study Group. Failure of extracranial-intracranial arterial bypass to reduce the risk of ischemic stroke: Results of an international ramdomized trial. N Engl J Med 1985;313:1191−1200

64. Wiebers DO, Whisnant JP, O'Fallon WM. The natural history of unruptured intracranial aneurysms. N Engl J Med 1981;304:696−8

65. White JC, Parker SD, Rogers MC. Preanesthetic evaluation of a patient with pathologic Q waves following subarachnoid hemorrhage. Anesthesiology 1985;62:351−4

66. Allen GS, Ahn HS, Preziosi TJ et al. Cerebral arterial spasm-a controlled trial of nimodipine in patients with subarachnoid hemorrhage. N Engl J Med 1983;308:619−24

67. Slogoff S, Gergis KZ, Keats AS. Etiologic factors in neuropsychiatric complications associated with cardiopulmonary bypass. Anesth Analg 1982;61:903−11

68. Iwatsuki N, Kuroda N, Amaha K, Iwatsuki K. Succinylcholine-induced hyperkalemia in patients with ruptured central aneurysms. Anesthesiology 1980;53:64−7

69. Stoelting RK. Circulatory changes during direct laryngoscopy and tracheal intubation: Influence of duration of laryngoscopy with or without prior lidocaine. Anesthesiology 1977;47:381−3

70. Stoelting RK. Attenuation of blood pressure response to laryngoscopy and tracheal intubation with sodium nitroprusside. Anesth Analg 1979;58:116−9

71. Newman B, Gelb AW, Lam AM. The effect of isoflurane-induced hypotension on cerebral blood flow and cerebral metabolic rate for oxygen in humans. Anesthesiology 1986;58:1−10

72. Michenfelder JD, Tinker JH. Cyanide toxicity and thiosulfate protection during chronic administration of sodium nitroprusside in the dog:

Correlation with a human case. Anesthesiology 1977;47:441−8

73. Tinker JH, Michenfelder JD. Sodium nitroprusside: Pharmacology, toxicology, and therapeutics. Anesthesiology 1976;45:340−54

74. Sivarajan M, Amory DW, McKenzie SM. Regional blood flows during induced hypotension produced by nitroprusside or trimethaphan in the Rhesus monkey. Anesth Analg 1985;64:759−66

75. Fahmy NR. Nitroglycerin as a hypotensive drug during general anesthesia. Anesthesiology 1978;49:17−20

76. Sundt TM, Sharbrough FW, Anderson RE, Michenfelder JD. Cerebral blood flow measurements and electroencephalograms during carotid endarterectomy. J Neurosurg 1974;41:310−20

77. Eckenhoff JE, Enderby GEH, Larson A, et al. Human cerebral circulation during deliberate hypotension and head-up tilt. J Appl Physiol 1963;18:1130−7

78. Jennett B, Teasdale G. Aspects of coma after severe head injury. Lancet 1977;1:878−81

79. Seelig JM, Becker DP, Miller JD, et al. Traumatic acute subdural hematoma. N Engl J Med 1981;304:1511−8

80. Rosenbaum KJ, Neigh JL, Strobel GE. Sensitivity to nondepolarizing muscle relaxants in amyotrophic lateral sclerosis: Report of two cases. Anesthesiology 1971;35:638−41

81. Bird TM, Strunin L. Hypotensive anesthesia for a patient with Freidreich's ataxia and cardiomyopathy. Anesthesiology 1984;60:377−80

82. Hetherington A, Rosenblatt RM. Ketamine and paralysis agitans (letter). Anesthesiology 1980;52:527

83. Gravelee GP. Succinylcholine-induced hyperkalemia in a patient with Parkinson's disease. Anesth Analg 1980;59:444−6

84. Roy RC, McLain S, Wise A, Shaffner LD. Anesthetic management of a patient eith Hallervorden-Spatz disease. Anesthesiology 1983;58:382−4

85. Martin JB, Gusella JF. Huntington's disease. Pathogenesis and management. N Engl J Med 1986;315:1267−76

86. Davies DD. Abnormal response to anesthesia in a case of Huntington's chorea. Br J Anaesth 1966;38:490−1

87. Propert DN. Pseudocholinesterase activity and phenotypes in mentally ill patients. Br J Psychiatry 1979;134:477−81

88. Lamont AMS. Brief report: Anaesthesia and Huntington's chorea. Anaesth Intensive Care 1979;7:189−90

89. Malan MD, Crago RR. Anaesthetic considera-

tions in idiopathic orthostatic hypotension and the Shy-Drager syndrome. Can Anaesth Soc J 1979;26:322–7

90. Beilin B, Maayan CH, Vatashsky E, et al. Fentanyl anesthesia in familial dysautonomia. Anesth Analg 1985;64:72–6

91. Stirt JA, Frantz RA, Gunz EF, Conolly ME. Anesthesia, catecholamines, and hemodynamics in autonomic dysfunction. Anesth Analg 1982;61:701–4

92. Mitaka C, Tsunoda Y, Hikawa Y, et al. Anesthetic management of congenital insensitivity to pain with anhydrosis. Anesthesiology 1985;63:328–9

93. D'Ambra MN, Dedrick D, Savarese JJ. Kearns-Sayer syndrome and pancuronium-succinylcholine-induced neuromuscular blockade. Anesthesiology 1979;51:343–5

94. Katzman R. Alzheimer's disease. N Engl J Med 1986;314:964–73

95. Dementia. Council on Scientific Affairs. JAMA 1986;256:2234–8

96. Hollander E, Mohs RC, Davis KL. Cholinergic approaches to the treatment of Alzheimer's disease. Br Med Bull 1986;42:97–100

97. Summers WK, Majovski LV, Marsh GM, et al. Oral tetrahydroaminoacridine in long-term treatment of senile dementia, Alzheimer type. N Engl J Med 1986;315:1241–5

98. Bockman JM, Kingsburg DT, McKinley MP, et al. Creutzfeldt-Jakob disease prion proteins in human brains. N Engl J Med 1985;312:73–8

99. MacMurdo SD, Jakymec AJ, Bleyaert AL. Precautions in the anesthetic management of a patient with Creutzfeldt-Jacob disease. Anesthesiology 1984;60:590–3

100. Ward DS. Anesthesia for a child with Leigh's syndrome. Anesthesiology 1981;55:90–1

101. McFarlin DE, McFarland HF. Multiple sclerosis. N Engl J Med 1982;307:1183–8; 1246–51

102. Hart RG, Sherman DG. The diagnosis of multiple sclerosis. JAMA 1982;498–503

103. Malhotra AS, Goren H. The hot bath test in the diagnosis of multiple sclerosis. JAMA 1981;246:1113–4

104. Crawford JS, James FM, Nolte H, et al. Regional anesthesia for patients with chronic neurological disease and similar conditions. Anaesthesia 1981;36:821–8

105. Warren TM, Datta S, Ostheimer GW. Lumbar epidural anesthesia in a patient with multiple sclerosis. Anesth Analg 1982;61;1022–3

106. Brett RS, Schmidt JH, Gage JS, et al. Measurement of acetylcholine receptor concentration in skeletal muscle from a patient with multiple sclerosis and resistance to atracurium. Anesthesiology 1987;66:837–9

107. Nightingale PJ, Longreen A. Iatrogenic facial nerve paresis. Anesthesiology 1982;37:322–3

108. Vaghadia H. Facial paresis after general anesthesia. Report of an unusual case: Heerfordt's syndrome. Anesthesiology 1986;64:513–4

109. Sweet WH. The treatment of trigeminal neuralgia (tic douloureux). N Engl J Med 1986;315:174–7

110. Rao NL, Drupin BR. Glossopharyngeal neuralgia with syncope-anesthetic considerations. Anesthesiology 1981;54:426–8

111. Thompson GE, Robb JV. Glossopharyngeal neuralgia-implications for the anesthesiologist. Anesthesiology 1972;37:660–1

112. Nicholson MJ, McAlpine FS. Neural injuries associated with surgical positions and operations. In: Martin JT, ed. Positioning in anesthesia and surgery. Philadelphia. WB Saunders, 1978;193–224

113. Kubota Y, Toyoda Y, Kubota H, et al. Common peroneal nerve palsy associated with the fabella syndrome. Anesthesiology 1986;65:552–3

114. Layzer RB, Fishman RA, Schafer JA. Neuropathy following abuse of nitrous oxide. Neurology 1978;28:504–6

115. Koblin DD, Watson JE, Deady JE, et al. Inactivation of methionine synthetase by nitrous oxide in mice. Anesthesiology 1981;54:318–24

116. Ledsome JR, Sharp JM. Pulmonary function in acute cervical cord injury. Am Rev Respir Dis 1981;124:41–4

117. Frankel HL, Mathias CJ, Spalding JMK. Mechanisms of cardiac arrest in tetraplegic patients. Lancet 1975;2:1183–5

118. Schonwald G, Fish KJ, Perkash I. Cardiovascular complications during anesthesia in chronic spinal cord injured patients. Anesthesiology 1981;55:550–8

119. Lambert DH, Deane RS, Mazuzan JE. Anesthesia and the control of blood pressure in patients with spinal cord injury. Anesth Analg 1982;61:344–8

120. Ravindran RS, Cummins DF, Smith IE. Experience with the use of nitroprusside and subsequent epidural analgesia in a pregnant quadriplegic patient. Anesth Analg 1981;60:1–3

121. Baraka A. Epidural meperidine for control of autonomic hyperreflexia in a paraplegic parturient. Anesthesiology 1985;62:688–90

122. Broecker BH, Hranowsky N, Hackler RH. Low spinal anesthesia for the prevention of autonomic dysreflexia in the spinal cord injury patient. J Urol 1979;122:366–8

123. Gronert GA, Theye RA. Pathophysiology of hyperkalemia induced by succinylcholine. Anesthesiology 1975;43:89–99

124. John DA, Tobey RE, Homer LD, Rice CL. Onset

of succinylcholine-induced hyperkalemia following denervation. Anesthesiology 1976; 45:294–9

125. Tobey RE. Paraplegia, succinylcholine, and cardiac arrest. Anesthesiology 1970;32:359–64

126. Shayevitz JR, Matteo RS. Decreased sensitivity to metocurine in patients with upper motorneuron disease. Anesth Analg 1985;64:767–72

127. Martyn JAJ, Matteo RS, Szyfelbein SK, Kaplan RF. Unprecedented resistance to neuromuscular blocking effects of metocurine with persistence and complete recovery in a burned patient. Anesth Analg 1982;61:614–7

128. White BC, Weigenstein JG, Winegar CD. Brain ischemic anoxia. Mechanisms of injury. JAMA 1984;251:1586–90

129. Berntman L, Welsh FA, Harp JR. Cerebral protective effect of low-grade hypothermia. Anesthesiology 1981;55:495–8

130. Artru AA, Michenfelder JD. Influence of hypothermia or hyperthermia alone or in combination with pentobarbital or phenytoin on survival time in hypoxic mice. Anesth Analg 1981;60:867–70

131. Michenfelder JD. A valid demonstration of barbiturate-induced brain protection in man-at last. Anesthesiology 1986;64:140–2

132. Brain Resuscitation Clinical Trial I Study Group. Randomized clinical study of thiopental loading in comatose survivors of cardiac arrest. N Engl J Med 1986;314:397–403

133. Todd MM, Chadwick HS, Shapiro HM, et al. The neurologic effects of thiopental therapy following experimental cardiac arrest in cats. Anesthesiology 1982;57:76–86

134. Gisvold SE, Safar P, Hendrick HHL, et al. Thiopental treatment after global brain ischemia in pigtailed monkeys. Anesthesiology 1984;60:88–96

135. Nussmeier NA, Arlund C, Slogoff S. Neuropsychiatric complications after cardiopulmonary bypass: Cerebral protection by a barbiturate. Anesthesiology 1986;64:165–70

136. Bell JA, Hodgson HJF. Coma after cardiac arrest. Brain 1974;97:361–72

137. Plum F, Posner JB. The diagnosis of stupor and coma. Philadelphia. FA Davis, 1972:286

138. Smith AL. Barbiturate protection in cerebral hypoxia. Anesthesiology 1977;47:285–93

139. Rockoff MA, Marshall LF, Shapiro HM. High dose barbiturate therapy in humans: A clinical review of 60 patients. Ann Neurol 1979;6:194–9

140. Todd MM, Drummond JC, Sang H. The hemodynamic consequences of high-dose methohexital anesthesia in humans. Anesthesiology 1984;61:495–501

141. Todd MM, Drummond JC, Sang H. The hemodynamic consequences of high-dose thiopental anesthesia. Anesth Analg 1985;64:681–7

142. Roesch C, Haselby KA, Paradise RP, et al. Comparison of cardiovascular effects of thiopental and pentobarbital at equivalent levels of CNS depression. Anesth Analg 1983;62:749–53

143. Ward JD, Becker DP, Miller DJ, et al. Failure of prophylactic barbiturate coma in the treatment of severe head trauma. J Neurosurg 1985;62:383–8

144. Delgado-Escueta AV, Treiman DM, Walsh GO. The treatable epilepsies. N Engl J Med 1983;308:1508–14, 1576–84

145. Delgado-Escueta AV, Wasterlain C, Treiman DM, Porter RJ. Current concepts in neurology. Management of status epilepticus. N Engl J Med 1982;306:1337–40

146. Ford EW, Morrell F, Whisler WW. Methohexital anesthesia in the surgical treatment of uncontrollable epilepsy. Anesth Analg 1982;61:997–1001

147. Ferrer-Allado T, Brechner VL, Dymond A, et al. Ketamine-induced electroconvulsive phenomena in the human limbic and thalamic regions. Anesthesiology 1973;38:333–44

148. Celesia GG, Chen R-C, Bamforth BJ. Effects of ketamine in epilepsy. Neurology 1975;25:169–72

149. Hirshman CA, Krieger W, Littlejohn G, et al. Ketamine-aminophylline-induced decrease in seizure threshold. Anesthesiology 1982;56:464–7

150. Steen PA, Michenfelder JD. Neurotoxicity of anesthetics. Anesthesiology 1979;50:437–53

151. Lebowitz MH, Blitt CB, Dillion JB. Enflurane-induced central nervous system excitation and its relation to carbon dioxide tension. Anesth Analg 1972;51:355–63

152. Morrison JE, Lockhart CH. Tourette syndrome: Anesthetic implications. Anesth Analg 1986;65:200–2

153. Stellar S, Ahrens SP, Meibohm AR, Reines SA. Migraine prevention with timolol. A double-blind crossover study. JAMA 1984;252:2576–80

154. Abouleish E, Ali V, Tang RA. Benign intracranial hypertension and anesthesia for cesarean section. Anesthesiology 1985;63:705–7

155. Deyo RA. Conservative therapy for low back pain. Distinguishing useful from useless therapy. JAMA 1983;250:1057–60

156. Deyo RA, Diehl AK, Rosenthal M. How many days of bed rest for acute low back pain? N Engl J Med 1986;315:1064–70

157. Abram SE. Subarachnoid corticosteroid injection following inadequate response to epi-

dural steroids for sciatica. Anesth Analg 1978;57:313–5

158. Gorski DW, Rao TLK, Glisson SN, et al. Epidural triamcinolone and adrenal response to hypoglycemic stress in dogs. Anesthesiology 1982;57:364–66

159. Bruno LA, Smith DS, Bloom MJ. Sudden hypotension with a test dose of chymopapain. Anesth Analg 1984;63:533–6

160. Bradley TD, Phillipson EA. Pathogenesis and pathophysiology of the obstructive sleep apnea syndrome. Med Clin North Am 1985;69:1169–85

161. Pellecchia DJ, Bretz KA, Barnette RE. Postoperative pain control by means of epidural narcotics in a patient with abstructive sleep apnea. Anesth Analg 1987;66:280–2

162. Owens WD, Gustave F, Sclaroff A. Tympanic membrane rupture with nitrous oxide anesthesia. Anesth Analg 1978;57:283–6

163. White PF. Spontaneous rupture of the tympanic membrane occurring in the absence of middle ear disease. Anesthesiology 1983;59:368–9

164. Man A, Segal S, Ezra S. Ear injury caused by elevated intratympanic pressure during general anesthesia. Acta Anaesth Sand 1980;24:224–6

165. Perreault L, Normandin N, Plamondon L, et al. Tympanic membrane rupture after anesthesia with nitrous oxide. Anesthesiology 1982;57:325–6

166. Kosman ME. Timolol in the treatment of open angle glaucoma. JAMA 1979;241:2301–3

167. Mishra P, Calvey TN, Williams NE, Murray GR. Intraoperative bradycardia and hypotension associated with timolol and pilocarpine eye drops. Br J Anaesth 1983;55:897–9

168. Cunningham AJ. Intraocular pressure-physiol-

ogy and implications for anaesthetic management. Can Anaesth Soc J 1986;33:195–208

169. Garde JF, Aston R, Endler GC, Sison OS. Racial mydriatic response to belladonna premedication. Anesth Analg 1978;57:572–6

170. Meyers EF, Krupin T, Johnson M, Zink H. Failure of nondepolarizing neuromuscular blockers to inhibit succinylcholine-induced increase intraocular pressure, a controlled study. Anesthesiology 1978;48:149–51

171. Ausinsch B, Rayburn RL, Munson ES, Levy NS. Ketamine and intraocular pressure in children. Anesth Analg 1976;55:773–5

172. Mishra P, Calvey TN, Williams NE, Murray GR. Intraoperative bradycardia and hypotension associated with timolol and pilocarpine eye drops. Br J Anaesth 1983;55:897–9

173. Kortilla K, Kauste A, Auvinen J. Comparison of domperidone, droperidol, and metoclopramide in the prevention and treatment of nausea and vomiting after balanced general anesthesia. Anesth Analg 1979;58:396–400

174. Brown EM, Krishnaprasad S, Similer BG. Pancuronium for rapid induction technique for tracheal intubation. Can Anaesth Soc J 1972;26:489–91

175. Ghani GA, Sung Y-F, Per-Lee JH. Glomus jugulare tumors-origin, pathology, and anesthetic considerations. Anesth Analg 1983;62:686–91

176. Brown CQ, Watson CB. Carotid sinus syndrome. Intraoperative management facilitated by temporary transvenous demand pacing. Anesthesiology 1982;56:151–3

177. Krishna G. Neurofibromatosis renal hypertension, and cardiac dysrhythmias. Anesth Analg 1975;54:542–5

19

Diseases of the Liver and Biliary Tract

Rational management of anesthesia in the presence of liver disease requires an understanding of the physiologic functions of the liver. In addition, the impact of anesthesia and surgery on hepatic blood flow has important implications for the management of anesthesia. Liver function tests are essential for detecting unsuspected co-existing liver disease. Furthermore, these tests are helpful in establishing the diagnosis when postoperative liver dysfunction occurs. It is also important to understand the pathophysiology of disease processes that involve the liver (hepatitis, cirrhosis) and the biliary tract.

PHYSIOLOGIC FUNCTIONS OF THE LIVER

Physiologic functions of hepatocytes, the principal cells of the liver, include glucose homeostasis, fat metabolism, protein synthesis, drug and hormone metabolism and bilirubin formation and excretion (Table 19-1). Hepatic sinuses are lined by Kupffer cells, which are capable of phagocytizing bacteria in portal venous blood. This is important since portal venous blood drains the gastrointestinal tract and almost always contains bacteria from the colon.

Glucose Homeostasis

The liver is responsible for the formation, storage, and release of glucose (Fig. 19-1). Glucose enters hepatocytes, where it is stored as glycogen (glycogenesis). Breakdown of glycogen (glycogenolysis) releases glucose back into the systemic circulation, to maintain normal blood glucose concentrations, especially during periods of fasting, as before elective surgery or during sustained exercise. In addition, the liver is the major site of gluconeogenesis. For example, lactate, glycerol, and amino acids are converted to glucose by gluconeogenesis. The combination of glycogenolysis and conversion of fat and proteins to glucose by gluconeogenesis is the mechanism by which the liver maintains glucose homeostasis.

Blood glucose levels are also regulated by hormones, including insulin, glucagon, and epinephrine. Insulin stimulates glycogen synthesis but inhibits gluconeogenesis. Glucagon and epinephrine exert opposite metabolic effects.

It must be remembered that the liver can store only about 75 g of glycogen. This amount of glycogen can be depleted by 24 hours to 48 hours of starvation. Glucose homeostasis depends primarily on gluconeogenesis when glycogen stores are depleted. Anesthesia may inhibit gluconeogenesis, as evidenced by dose-related decreases in the formation of glucose

355

TABLE 19-1.   Physiologic Functions of the Liver

Glucose homeostasis

Fat metabolism

Protein synthesis
   Drug binding
   Coagulation
   Hydrolysis of ester linkages

Drug and hormone metabolism

Bilirubin formation and excretion

from lactate produced by halothane.[1] External sources of glucose during the perioperative period become important when glycogen stores are depleted due to poor preoperative nutrition, and when gluconeogenesis is inhibited by anesthesia.

Fat Metabolism

Lipids reach the liver as chylomicrons, which are subsequently converted to glycerol and fatty acids. In the fasted state, fatty acids may be converted to ketone bodies. Ketone bodies are capable of providing a large proportion of the energy consumption of the body, thus reducing the need for gluconeogenesis. Insulin inhibits oxidation of fatty acids to ketone bodies, whereas glucagon has opposite effects.

In the absence of fasting, fatty acids are esterified in the liver with glycerol to form triglycerides. Triglycerides are important for the synthesis of lipoproteins and cholesterol. Catabolism of cholesterol to bile acids and the subsequent conjugation with bile acids is essential for absorption of fat from the gastrointestinal tract. Fatty liver infiltration as may ac-

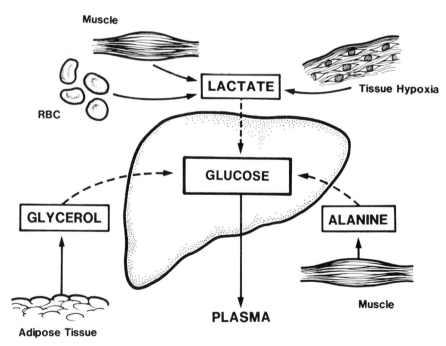

FIG. 19-1.   The liver is responsible for the formation and release of glucose into the systemic circulation. Lactate from skeletal muscles and erythrocytes, glycerol from adipose tissues, and amino acids (alanine) from skeletal muscles enter the liver and are converted to glucose by gluconeogenesis. Tissue hypoxia, when present, is also a source of lactate. Metabolic acidosis can occur when severe hepatic dysfunction interferes with ability of the liver to clear lactate from the systemic circulation. Glucose is stored in the liver as glycogen. Glycogenolysis provides glucose for release into plasma to maintain normal blood glucose concentrations.

company a variety of diseases (obesity, malnutrition, diabetes mellitus, Reye's syndrome) usually reflects excess accumulation of triglycerides in the liver.

Protein Synthesis

Hepatocytes contain components responsible for protein synthesis (rough endoplasmic reticulum), as well as microsomal enzymes (smooth endoplasmic reticulum) necessary for inactivation of drugs. Gamma globulins (immunoglobulins) are important proteins synthesized outside the liver in the reticuloendothelial system; all proteins except gamma globulins and antihemophiliac factor (factor VIII) are produced in the rough endoplasmic reticulum of the liver. Approximately 10 g to 15 g of albumin is produced daily. This level of albumin production maintains plasma albumin concentrations in the range of 3.5 $g \cdot dl^{-1}$ to 5.5 $g \cdot dl^{-1}$. This plasma concentration, plus albumin's high molecular weight (about 69,000), accounts for the fact that albumin provides about 80 percent of the colloid oncotic (osmotic) pressure of plasma.

Liver disease can be associated with altered plasma concentrations of albumin and gamma globulin. For example, severe liver disease is associated with decreased production of albumin. Conversely, gamma globulin concentrations are often increased in the presence of liver disease. This may represent a response to bacteria, which are normally removed from the circulation in the liver by the phagocytic action of Kupffer cells.

Protein synthesis is important in drug binding, coagulation, and hydrolysis of drugs with ester linkages.

DRUG BINDING

Albumin has a large number of reactive groups and therefore can reversibly combine with most drugs likely to be present in the circulation. When liver disease leads to decreased albumin production, fewer protein sites will be available for drug binding. As a result, un-

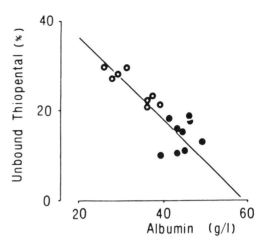

FIG. 19-2. Free (unbound) plasma concentrations of thiopental parallel albumin concentrations in patients with cirrhosis (clear symbols) and those with normal hepatic function (solid symbols). Reduced plasma concentrations of albumin in patients with cirrhosis result in higher free plasma concentrations of thiopental. (Pandele G, Chaux F, Salvadori C, et al. Thiopental pharmacokinetics in patients with cirrhosis. Anesthesiology 1983;59:123–6)

bound pharmacologically active fractions of drugs, such as thiopental, increase and unexpected drug sensitivities can occur (Fig. 19-2).[2] Increased drug sensitivities due to decreased protein binding are most likely to occur when plasma albumin levels are less than 2.5 $g \cdot dl^{-1}$. Acute hepatic dysfunction is not likely to be associated with hypoalbuminemia since the elimination half-time for albumin from the plasma is 14 days to 21 days.

COAGULATION

Hepatocytes are responsible for the synthesis of most clotting factors, including prothrombin; fibrinogen; and factors V, VII, IX, and X. Antihemophiliac factor is the only important procoagulant not synthesized in the liver. Decreased prothrombin production may reflect severe hepatocellular disease or impaired vitamin K absorption due to biliary obstruction and absence of bile salts. Parenteral vitamin K restores prothrombin production when decreases are due to biliary obstruction but may not be effective if hepatocellular disease is severe. Liver disease associated with splenomegaly can alter the normal coagulation mechanism via platelet trapping in the spleen. Another factor predisposing to a bleeding diathesis is failure of a diseased liver to clear plasma activators of the fibrinolytic system. Failure to clear these substances can lead to an enhancement of fibrinolysis.

Clotting abnormalities must be suspected in patients with liver disease. Adequacy of clotting factor levels is evaluated by measuring the prothrombin time, partial thromboplastin time, and bleeding time. Liver function must be dramatically depressed before impaired coagulation manifests, since many of the coagulation factors require only 20 percent to 30 percent of their normal concentrations to prevent bleeding. Nevertheless, plasma half-times of hepatic-produced clotting factors, including prothrombin and fibrinogen, are relatively

brief (hours), and acute liver dysfunction is likely to be associated with clotting abnormalities.

HYDROLYSIS OF ESTER LINKAGES

Plasma cholinesterase (pseudocholinesterase) is a protein produced in the liver, which is responsible for hydrolysis of drugs with ester linkages, such as succinylcholine and certain local anesthetics. Severe liver disease may decrease cholinesterase production to the extent that the duration of apnea after the administration of succinylcholine is prolonged (Fig. 19-3).[3] Prolonged effects of succinylcholine (greater than 30 minutes), however, are unlikely from liver disease alone, and atypical cholinesterase enzyme must be suspected. It should be realized that the plasma half-time for cholinesterase is about 14 days. Therefore,

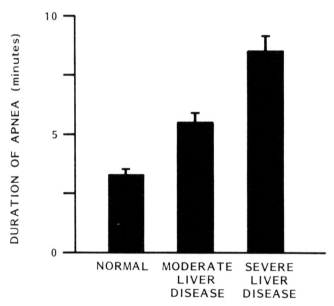

FIG. 19-3. Duration of apnea (Mean ± SE) after the intravenous administration of succinylcholine (0.6 mg·kg^{-1}) is prolonged in the presence of moderate and severe liver disease. In the same study, moderate liver disease was also associated with a twofold decrease in plasma cholinesterase activity, compared with nearly a fourfold decrease in patients with severe liver disease. (Data adapted from Foldes FF, Swerdlow M, Lipschitz E, et al. Comparison of the respiratory effects of suxamethonium and suxethonium in man. Anesthesiology 1956;17:559–68)

acute liver failure is unlikely to be associated with a slowed rate of succinylcholine hydrolysis.

Drug Metabolism

Conversion of lipid soluble drugs to more water soluble and less active substances is under the control of microsomal enzymes present in smooth endoplasmic reticulum of hepatocytes. Availability of drugs to hepatocytes is influenced by hepatic blood flow and the fraction of drug, which is bound to plasma proteins. Clearance of drugs from the plasma that have high hepatic extraction ratios (lidocaine, propranolol) is greatly influenced by hepatic blood flow, whereas drugs with low hepatic ratios are more influenced by changes in microsomal enzyme activity and protein binding.

Chronic liver disease may interfere with metabolism of drugs by virtue of reduced numbers of enzyme-containing hepatocytes and/or decreased hepatic blood flow, which typically accompany cirrhosis of the liver. Indeed, prolonged elimination half-times for diazepam,[4] lidocaine,[5] meperidine,[6] morphine,[7] and alfentanil[8] have been demonstrated in patients with cirrhosis of the liver. This emphasizes

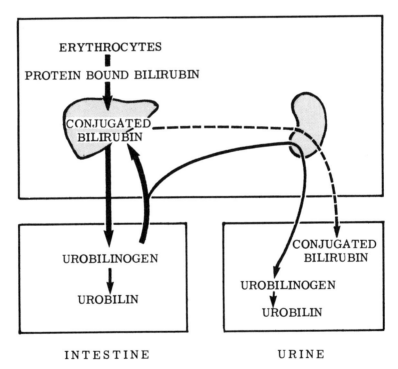

FIG. 19-4. Protein-bound bilirubin derived from destroyed erythrocytes is poorly soluble in water and thus does not appear in the urine. Bilirubin is made water soluble by conjugation in the liver with glucuronic acid. Conjugated bilirubin is excreted into the biliary canaliculi and transported to the small intestine. Bilirubin is converted to urobilinogen and urobilin by bacteria in the gastrointestinal tract. A small amount of urobilinogen is reabsorbed into the systemic circulation from the gastrointestinal tract for recirculation through the liver (enterohepatic circulation) or renal excretion. Understanding the formation and elimination of bilirubin is important for the interpretation of plasma and urine measurements of this substance, and for categorization of liver dysfunction as prehepatic, intrahepatic, or posthepatic.

that repeated injections of these drugs are more likely to produce cumulative effects in patients with severe liver disease. Conversely, cirrhosis of the liver does not substantially alter elimination half-times of thiopental[2] or fentanyl[9] compared with normal patients.

It is conceivable that accelerated drug metabolism and resulting resistance to pharmacologic effects of drugs may accompany cirrhosis of the liver. This may reflect production of additional microsomal enzymes (enzyme induction) as reduced numbers of hepatocytes are exposed to drugs for metabolism.

Volatile anesthetics may interfere with clearance of drugs from plasma by virtue of reductions in hepatic blood flow and/or inhibition of drug metabolizing enzymes. Despite reductions in hepatic blood flow, decreases in drug clearance during administration of halothane seem to be principally due to inhibition of hepatic microsomal enzymes.[10]

Bilirubin Formation and Excretion

Bilirubin, 250 mg·day^{-1} to 350 mg·day^{-1} is produced from the breakdown of heme-containing compounds (hemoglobin, myoglobin) in the reticuloendothelial system (Fig. 19-4). This bilirubin enters the circulation where it is firmly bound to albumin for transport to the liver. Protein-bound bilirubin (unconjugated) is not water soluble, and urinary excretion is minimal. Conjugation of bilirubin with glucuronic acid in the liver renders bilirubin water soluble. This conjugation is under the control of the enzyme glucuronyltransferase, which is susceptible to enzyme induction. A small amount of conjugated bilirubin enters the circulation and undergoes renal excretion. The remaining conjugated bilirubin is excreted into the biliary canniculi and eventually into the small intestine, where it is converted to urobilinogen and urobilin by action of bacteria. Some urobilinogen may be reabsorbed back into the circulation, where it is either recirculated through the liver (enterohepatic circulation) or excreted by the kidneys.

HEPATIC BLOOD FLOW

The liver is the only major organ that receives a dual afferent blood supply (Fig. 19-5). Total hepatic blood flow is about 1,450 ml·min^{-1} (e.g., 25 percent to 30 percent of the cardiac output) with 1,100 ml provided by the portal vein (e.g., about 75 percent of the total) and the remainder by the hepatic artery. On a weight basis, hepatic blood flow is about 100 ml·100 g^{-1}·min^{-1}. The highly saturated arterial blood supplies about two-thirds of the oxygen used by the liver. Therefore, oxygen delivery to the liver may be marginal, since the majority of blood flow is with desaturated hemoglobin delivered via the portal vein. Indeed, cells adjacent to hepatic venules are particularly susceptible to hypoxia. The resulting cell damage is designated as centrilobular necrosis. Furthermore, any reduction in the arterial oxygen partial pressures greatly reduces oxygen delivery to the liver.

Hepatic artery blood flow maintains nutrition of connective tissues and walls of bile ducts. For this reason, interruption of hepatic artery blood flow can be fatal because of ensuing necrosis of vital liver structures. Blood from the hepatic artery, after it supplies the structural elements of the liver, empties into hepatic sinuses to mix with portal venous blood. This combination of hepatic arterial and portal venous blood provides oxygen and nutrients to hepatocytes.

Determinants of Hepatic Blood Flow

Hepatic blood flow is determined by perfusion pressure (mean arterial or portal vein pressure minus hepatic vein pressure) and splanchnic vascular resistance. Mean portal venous pressure is about 10 mmHg; the hepatic venous pressure averages 5 mmHg. Splanchnic vessels are innervated by sympathetic vasoconstrictor nerve fibers (T$_3$–T$_{11}$) traveling with splanchnic nerves. Splanchnic nerve stimulation, as produced by arterial hypoxemia, hy-

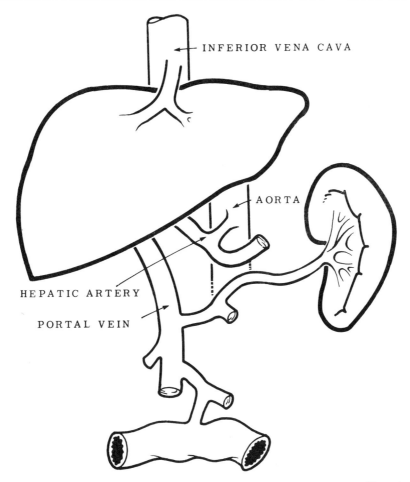

FIG. 19-5. The liver receives a dual afferent blood supply, with about 75 percent of hepatic blood flow provided by the low pressure portal vein. The remainder of hepatic blood flow is derived from the hepatic artery. Autoregulation of hepatic blood flow is controversial. If autoregulation does occur, however, it seems to influence only that blood flow delivered by the hepatic artery. The two afferent blood supplies to the liver join at the hepatic sinusoids, and venous effluent enters the hepatic veins and subsequently the inferior vena cava. Total hepatic blood flow is determined by the perfusion pressure across the liver (mean portal vein or arterial pressure minus hepatic vein pressure) and splanchnic vascular resistance. Cirrhosis of the liver increases resistance to flow through the portal vein and decreases hepatic blood flow.

percarbia, or endogenous or exogenous catecholamines, results in hepatic artery and portal vein vasoconstriction, with concomitant reductions in blood flow through these vessels. The hepatic circulation is also supplied with beta-adrenergic receptors. Indeed, beta-adrenergic blockade is associated with reductions in hepatic blood flow. Positive pressure ventilation of the lungs with high inspiratory pressures or congestive heart failure also result in decreases in hepatic blood flow, presumably by increasing central venous pressure (hepatic vein pressure) and thus decreasing hepatic perfusion pressure. Whether autoregulation of hepatic blood flow occurs is controversial. In a dog model, autoregulation of hepatic blood flow occurs during the fed metabolically active state but not during fasting.[11]

Impact of Anesthetic Drugs on Hepatic Blood Flow

Inhaled anesthetics, as well as regional anesthesia, reduce hepatic blood flow 20 percent to 30 percent in the absence of surgical stimulation.[12,13] These changes reflect drug or technique-induced effects on perfusion pressure and/or splanchnic vascular resistance. For example, reductions in hepatic blood flow associated with volatile anesthetics, as well as regional anesthesia (T_5 sensory level) are most likely due to decreased perfusion pressure.[14] Isoflurane administered to animals is less likely to decrease hepatic blood flow than is halothane.[14] Nitrous oxide plus d-tubocurarine and controlled ventilation of lungs decreases hepatic blood flow by reducing perfusion pressure and increasing splanchnic vascular resistance.[13] Reductions in arterial carbon dioxide partial pressures produced by deliberate hyperventilation of the lungs leads to decreased sympathetic nervous system activity. As a re-

sult, splanchnic vascular resistance is reduced, and hepatic blood flow tends to improve during nitrous oxide and muscle relaxant anesthesia.[13] Halothane unmasks direct relaxant effects of carbon dioxide on vascular smooth muscle, so that hypercarbia leads to decreased splanchnic vascular resistance.[12]

Another important determinant of hepatic blood flow is surgical stimulation. During halothane anesthesia, the magnitude of reduction in hepatic blood flow during surgical stimulation is greater during cholecystectomies than during operations (herniorrhaphies) distant from the liver (Fig. 19-6).[15]

Ideally, reductions in hepatic blood flow would be accompanied by similar reductions in liver oxygen consumption. However, during anesthesia, hepatic blood flow decreases more than splanchnic oxygen consumption.[16] Conceivably, this could result in anaerobic metabolism reflected by excess lactate production. Nevertheless, increased splanchnic lactate production has not been observed during anesthesia.[12] Therefore, it seems unlikely that re-

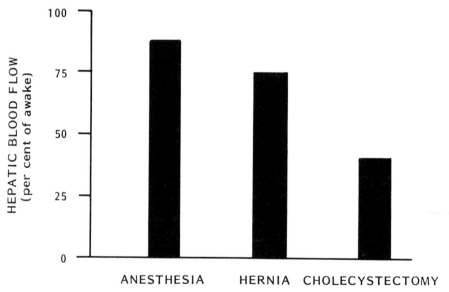

FIG. 19-6. Hepatic blood flow, as a percent of the awake value, is reduced during nitrous-oxide-halothane anesthesia. Surgical stimulation (hernia or cholecystectomy) further reduces flow, with the greatest reductions occurring during cholecystectomy. These data suggest that the nearness of the operative site to the liver and not the drugs used for anesthesia is the most important factor in decreasing hepatic blood flow. (Data adapted from Gelman SI. Disturbances in hepatic blood flow during anesthesia and surgery. Arch Surg 1976;111:881–3)

ductions in hepatic blood flow produced by anesthetic drugs or techniques jeopardize viability of hepatocytes. It must be recognized, however, that these measurements are all from patients without known liver disease. It is conceivable that underlying liver disease would make hepatocytes more vulnerable to adverse effects produced by reductions in hepatic blood flow.

Selective hepatic artery constriction has been observed in patients without liver disease during halothane anesthesia.[17] The mechanism and clinical significance of this hepatic artery constriction are unknown.

LIVER FUNCTION TESTS

The ability to interpret liver function tests is useful for appreciating the presence of liver disease preoperatively and to facilitate the differential diagnosis of postoperative liver dysfunction. It is important to remember that liver function tests are rarely specific. Furthermore, in view of the enormous reserve of the liver,

considerable hepatic damage must be present before liver function tests are altered. Indeed, cirrhosis may produce little alteration in liver function, and only when some additional insult (operation) produces further deterioration does the underlying liver disease become obvious.

Halothane, but not isoflurane or enflurane, is associated with transient elevations of bromosulfophthalein retention following prolonged administration (8.8 MAC hours to 11.6 MAC hours) in the absence of surgical stimulation (Fig. 19-7).[18,19] Likewise, clearance of antipyrine from the plasma was delayed in patients exposed to halothane but not enflurane or meperidine.[20] Transient elevations of liver transaminase enzymes occur after prolonged administration of enflurane but not halothane or isoflurane (Fig. 19-8).[18,19] These changes following prolonged administration of halothane and enflurane are statistically significant but not clinically important. In the presence of surgical stimulation, bromosulfophthalein retention and elevations of liver transaminase enzymes transiently follow even the administration of isoflurane, suggesting that changes in hepatic blood flow evoked by pain-

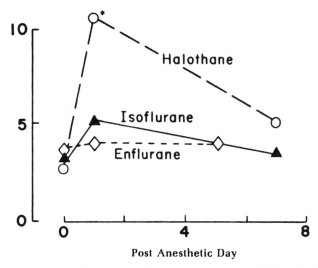

FIG. 19-7. Halothane, but not isoflurane or enflurane, is associated with transient elevations of bromsulphalein (BSP) retention after prolonged administration (8.8 MAC hours to 11.6 MAC hours) to volunteers in the absence of surgical stimulation. (Eger EI. Isoflurane (Forane). A compendium and reference. Anaquest, A Division of BOC, Inc. Madison, WI, 1986:1–160)

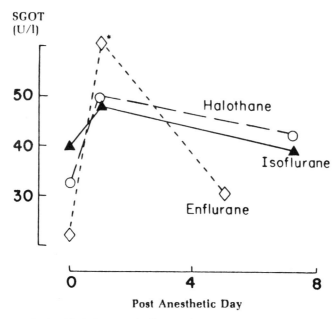

FIG. 19-8. Enflurane, but not halothane or isoflurane, is associated with transient elevations of plasma concentrations of glutamic oxalic transaminase (SGOT) after prolonged administration (8.8 MAC hours to 11.6 MAC hours) to volunteers in the absence of surgical stimulation. (Eger El. Isoflurane (Forane). A compendium and reference. Anaquest, A Division of BOC, Inc. Madison, WI, 1986:1–160)

ful stimulation can adversely alter hepatic function independent of volatile anesthetics.

Postoperatively, the magnitude of liver dysfunction as reflected by liver function tests is exaggerated by operations near the liver (Fig. 19-9).[21] The specific anesthetic drug does not influence the magnitude of postoperative liver dysfunction as reflected by liver function tests (Fig. 19-9).[21] Despite the logic that postoperative liver dysfunction is likely to be greater in the presence of co-existing liver disease, there is evidence that halothane anesthesia does not exacerbate hepatic dysfunction in cirrhotic rats (Fig. 19-10).[22]

Liver function tests may reveal different responses in hepatic function after repeated anesthesia and operation. For example, in one study the maximum plasma transaminase changes occurring after a second anesthetic with halothane within 7 days were ten times greater than those seen after the first administration of halothane.[23] Other studies, however, have not confirmed an exaggerated derangement of liver function tests after repeated administration of halothane.[24,25]

Liver function tests include measurement of plasma concentrations of bilirubin, transaminase enzymes, alkaline phosphatase, and albumin and determination of bromsulphalein excretion.

Bilirubin

Interpretation of plasma bilirubin measurements (normal plasma concentrations 0.3 mg·dl^{-1} to 1.1 mg·dl^{-1}) depends on understanding the formation and elimination of the various bilirubin fractions (Fig. 19-4). Protein-bound (indirect-reacting or unconjugated) bilirubin (normal plasma concentrations 0.2 mg·dl^{-1} to 0.7 mg·dl^{-1}) cannot be excreted by the kidneys, whereas conjugated (direct-reacting) bilirubin (normal plasma concentrations 0.1 mg·dl^{-1} to 0.4 mg·dl^{-1}) may appear in the urine. Overt jaundice is present when plasma bilirubin concentrations exceed 3 mg·dl^{-1}.

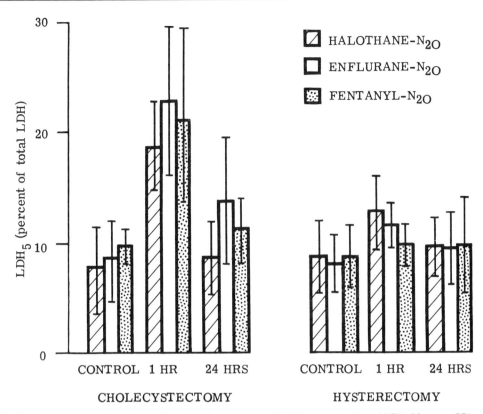

FIG. 19-9. Isoenzyme fractions of lactic dehydrogenase (LDH5 percent of total LDH, Mean ± SD) were measured before, and 1 hour and 24 hours after, elective cholecystectomy or hysterectomy. Anesthesia was with 60 percent inspired nitrous oxide plus halothane, enflurane, or fentanyl. Each anesthetic group included 10 patients. Normal LDH5 is 5 percent to 16 percent of the total LDH. LDH5 did not change after hysterectomy. In contrast, LDH5 values 1 hour after cholecystectomy were increased above control ($P<0.05$) and above corresponding values ($P<0.05$) in those patients undergoing hysterectomy. LDH5 values 24 hours after cholecystectomy were not different from control or corresponding measurements after hysterectomy. These data suggest that the site of operation and not the drugs used for anesthesia is responsible for postoperative elevations of LDH5. (Viegas OJ, Stoelting RK. LDH5 changes after choleystectomy or hysterectomy in patients receiving halothane, enflurane, or fentanyl. Anesthesiology 1979;51:556–8)

Increases in plasma concentrations of un- conjugated bilirubin are likely to accompany hemolysis of erythrocytes. Hemolysis is fur- ther suggested by decreases in the hematocrit or increases in the reticulocyte count. In- creases in plasma concentrations of conjugated bilirubin reflect impaired ability to secrete bili- rubin into the biliary tract (i.e., cholestasis) due either to hepatocellular disease or bile obstruction as produced by tumor or stones. Often, there is no correlation between plasma levels of bilirubin and severity of liver dis- ease.

Transaminase Enzymes

Hepatocytes contain large amounts of transaminase enzymes, so that acute hepato- cellular damage, as may occur in response to arterial hypoxemia, drugs, or viruses, will cause these enzymes to spill into the circula- tion. Other tissues including heart, lungs, and skeletal muscles also contain transaminase en- zymes. Therefore, measurement of plasma transaminase concentrations may not be spe- cific for liver damage. Indeed, postoperative

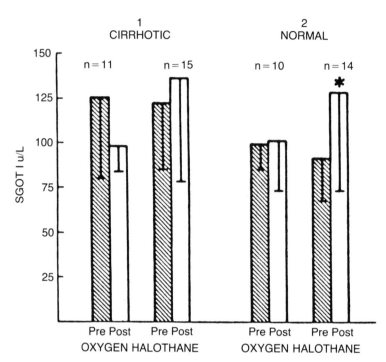

FIG. 19-10.   Cirrhotic or normal rats were exposed to pure oxygen or 1.8 percent halothane in oxygen for 3 hours. Compared with pretreatment values (Pre) measurements of plasma glutamic oxalacetic transaminase concentrations (Post) after treatment were elevated (P<0.05) only in normal rats receiving halothane. (Maze M, Smith CM, Baden JM. Halothane anesthesia does not exacerbate hepatic dysfunction in cirrhotic rats. Anesthesiology 1985;62:1–5)

increases in plasma transaminase concentrations may reflect skeletal muscle damage from intramuscular injections given preoperatively or damage to skeletal muscles during surgery. Nevertheless, marked elevations of plasma transaminase concentrations (three times normal or greater) in the postoperative period should suggest acute hepatocellular damage. The magnitude of plasma transaminase enzyme elevations typically parallel the severity of hepatocellular damage. Acute biliary tract obstruction as due to cholelithiasis may also cause elevations of plasma transaminase concentrations. Initially, elevated transaminase concentrations decline as hepatocellular recovery occurs or on rare occasions as a reflection of continued hepatocellular damage such

that too few hepatocytes remain to serve as a source of enzymes.

Commonly measured transaminase enzymes are glutamic oxaloacetic transaminase (aspartate aminotransferase, SGOT), glutamic pyruvic transaminase (alanine aminotransferase, SGPT), and lactic dehydrogenase (LDH). Normal plasma concentrations of these enzymes depend on the specific method of analysis used by an individual laboratory.

GLUTAMIC OXALACETIC TRANSAMINASE

This enzyme is present not only in large quantities in hepatocytes but also in the heart, kidneys, and skeletal muscles. Therefore, extrahepatic sources must always be considered when plasma concentrations of this enzyme are elevated in the postoperative period. It is important to remember that this enzyme can be elevated in the asymptomatic prodromal phase of viral hepatitis.

GLUTAMIC PYRUVIC TRANSAMINASE

This enzyme is considered more specific for liver than the oxaloacetic transaminase enzyme. Nevertheless, extrahepatic changes still exert an important influence on the interpretation of levels.

LACTIC DEHYDROGENASE

This enzyme is widely distributed in the body, being found primarily in the liver, erythrocytes, heart, and skeletal muscles. Measurement of plasma lactic dehydrogenase is a relatively insensitive index of hepatocellular damage. Greater sensitivity is provided by measuring the isoenzyme-5 fraction of lactic dehydrogenase, felt to be specific for hepatocytes.[21]

Alkaline Phosphatase

Alkaline phosphatase enzyme is present in bile duct cells, such that even slight degrees of biliary obstruction are manifested by elevations (three times normal or greater) of plasma concentrations of this enzyme. Therefore, this test helps differentiate between hepatic dysfunction due to biliary obstruction and that due to hepatocellular damage. Despite the predominant presence of this enzyme in bile duct cells, it is well recognized that elevations of plasma alkaline phosphatase concentrations can also accompany hepatocellular disease. As with transaminase enzymes, there are also extrahepatic stores of alkaline phosphatase, particularly in bone.

Albumin

The liver is the sole site of synthesis of albumin, and hepatocellular damage predictably results in decreased plasma concentrations (normal concentrations 3.5 $g \cdot dl^{-1}$ to 5.5 $g \cdot dl^{-1}$). Plasma albumin concentrations less than 2.5 $g \cdot dl^{-1}$ may signify significant liver disease. In addition, excessive protein loss as associated with the nephrotic syndrome, protein-losing enteropathies, thermal injuries or exfoliative dermatitis may result in hypoalbuminemia, even in the absence of decreased synthesis due to liver disease. Loss of albumin into ascitic fluid is another cause of reduced plasma albumin concentrations due to excessive loss with or without decreased protein synthesis by the liver.

Half-times for albumin in the plasma, are 14 days to 21 days, emphasizing that acute liver dysfunction will not be reflected by decreased plasma albumin levels. Altered responses to drugs due to decreased protein binding are most likely to occur when plasma albumin concentrations are less than 2.5 $g \cdot dl^{-1}$. Albumin-to-globulin ratios have little significance as a measure of hepatic function, since immunoglobulin production does not take place in the liver.

DIFFERENTIAL DIAGNOSIS OF POSTOPERATIVE HEPATIC DYSFUNCTION

When postoperative hepatic dysfunction occurs, a predetermined approach, including serial liver function tests and a search for extrahepatic causes of hepatic dysfunction, facilitates the differential diagnosis.

Liver Function Tests

Causes of hepatic dysfunction, most often manifesting as jaundice, can be categorized as prehepatic, intrahepatic or hepatocellular, and posthepatic or cholestatic based on repeated measurements of the plasma concentrations of bilirubin, transaminase enzymes, and alkaline phosphatase (Table 19-2).

PREHEPATIC DYSFUNCTION

Prehepatic dysfunction, as follows hemolysis, hematoma resorption, or bilirubin overload from stored whole blood, is characterized by (1) increased plasma bilirubin concentrations, predominantly the unconjugated fraction; (2) normal plasma transaminase concentrations; and (3) normal plasma alkaline phosphatase concentrations.

INTRAHEPATIC DYSFUNCTION

Intrahepatic dysfunction, as due to viral hepatitis, drug toxicity, sepsis, arterial hypoxemia, or cirrhosis, is characterized by (1) increased plasma bilirubin concentrations, predominantly conjugated; (2) markedly increased plasma transaminase concentrations; and (3) normal to slightly elevated plasma alkaline phosphatase concentrations.

POSTHEPATIC DYSFUNCTION

Posthepatic dysfunction as may accompany a retained common duct stone is characterized by (1) increased plasma bilirubin concentrations, predominantly conjugated; (2)

normal to slightly elevated plasma transaminase concentrations; and (3) markedly elevated plasma alkaline phosphatase concentrations. The urine will also contain large amounts of conjugated bilirubin but little or no urobilinogen.

There are two exceptions to the generalization that measurement of alkaline phosphatase and transaminase concentrations can serve to distinguish between posthepatic and intrahepatic dysfunction. First, in contrast to chronic biliary tract injury, acute injury to the biliary tract, such as that caused by a stone entering the common duct postoperatively, may not always evoke an immediate rise in plasma alkaline phosphatase concentrations. Second, biliary tract obstruction associated with infection may be associated with striking elevations in plasma transaminase concentrations.

Extrahepatic Causes of Hepatic Dysfunction

Causes of postoperative hepatic dysfunction are difficult to confirm because few pathognomonic features are unique to specific etiologies. Furthermore, liver function often returns to normal without specific treatment. In this regard, the following steps should be taken in search of extrahepatic causes of hepatic dysfunction before assuming, without supporting

TABLE 19-2. Liver Function Tests and Differential Diagnosis

Hepatic Dysfunction	Bilirubin	Transaminase Enzymes	Alkaline Phosphatase	Causes
Prehepatic	Unconjugated (indirect)	Normal	Normal	Hemolysis Hematoma resorption Bilirubin overload from whole blood
Intrahepatic (hepatocellular)	Conjugated (direct)	Elevated	Normal to slightly elevated (less than twice normal)	Viral Drugs Sepsis Hypoxemia Cirrhosis
Posthepatic (cholestatic)	Conjugated	Normal to slightly elevated	Elevated (more than twice normal)	Stones Sepsis

evidence, that anesthetic drugs are the responsible hepatotoxins.

1. Review all drugs administered, as every drug, regardless of how innocuous it may seem, must be considered as a potential cause of hepatocyte damage. Administration of catecholamines or sympathomimetics may evoke splanchnic vasoconstriction sufficient to interfere with an adequate hepatic blood flow.
2. Check for sources of sepsis. The development of jaundice is common in patients with severe infection.
3. Evaluate bilirubin load. A 500 ml transfusion of fresh whole blood contains 250 mg of bilirubin. This bilirubin load increases as the age of transfused blood increases. Patients with normal hepatic function can receive large amounts of blood without appreciable increases in bilirubin concentrations. This response can be different in patients with co-existing hepatic disease.
4. Rule out occult hematomas. Resorption of large hematomas may produce hyperbilirubinemia for several days. Furthermore, patients with Gilbert's syndrome have limited ability to conjugate bilirubin, and even small increases in bilirubin load may lead to jaundice (see the section Gilbert's Syndrome).
5. Rule out hemolysis. Reductions in the hematocrit or increases in the reticulocyte count may reflect hemolysis of erythrocytes.
6. Review perioperative records. Evidence of hypotension, arterial hypoxemia, hypoventilation, and hypovolemia must be considered as possible etiologic factors in postoperative hepatic dysfunction.
7. Consider extrahepatic abnormalities. Extrahepatic causes of hepatic dysfunction include congestive heart failure, respiratory failure, pulmonary embolism, and renal insufficiency.
8. A phenomenon designated benign postoperative intrahepatic cholestasis has been described in association with extensive and prolonged surgery, especially if complicated by hypotension, arterial hypoxemia and massive blood transfusion.[26] Jaundice, in association with conjugated hyperbilirubinemia, is usually apparent 1 day to 2 days postoperatively and may persist for 2 weeks to 4 weeks. Liver function tests other than plasma bilirubin concentrations may be normal or mildly deranged. Patients who experience these responses are often elderly.

ACUTE HEPATITIS

Acute hepatitis is an inflammatory disease of hepatocytes, which is most often due to viral infections or ingestion of toxic drugs. Rarely, acute hepatitis, characterized by fatty infiltration of the liver, is associated with pregnancy. Other causes of acute hepatitis include sepsis and congestive heart failure.

Viral Hepatitis

Causative organisms responsible for viral hepatitis include (1) type A virus; (2) type B virus; (3) non-A, non-B virus; (4) Epstein-Barr virus (EBV); and (5) cytomegalovirus (see Chapter 12). Many cases of viral hepatitis are unrecognized because they remain subclinical or anicteric. It is likely that a number of patients undergo elective operations while in asymptomatic prodromal phases of viral hepatitis.[27]

The onset of viral hepatitis can be gradual or sudden. The most characteristic early symptoms, occurring in 90 percent or more of patients, include dark urine, fatigue, and anorexia. Nausea, fever, and abdominal discomfort occur in over 50 percent of patients. Concentrations of plasma transaminase enzymes are elevated 7 days to 14 days before the onset of jaundice and begin to decline shortly after jaundice is noticeable. Plasma bilirubin concentrations do not usually exceed 20 mg·dl^{-1} unless liver disease is severe or hemolysis is also present. Mild anemia and lymphocytosis are common. Severe and potentially fatal hepatitis is suggested by plasma albumin concentration below 2.5 g·dl^{-1} or markedly prolonged prothrombin times. Failure of vitamin K to improve prothrombin synthesis emphasizes the severity of the underlying hepatocellular disease. Nevertheless, in most patients, the clinical course of viral hepatitis is uneventful, and recovery of liver function is complete. Characteristic features of hepatitis due to type A, B, and non-A, non-B virus are summarized in Table 19-3.

TYPE A VIRUS

Hepatitis due to type A virus is also referred to as infectious or short incubation hepatitis. This form of hepatitis is highly infectious; cross-infection within families is common. Transmission of the virus is believed to be by the fecal-oral route or by ingestion of food contaminated with sewage. Viremia occurs 1 day to 25 days before the onset of symptoms, but transmission by plasma or blood products rarely occurs. The incubation period for type A hepatitis is short, ranging from 2 weeks to 6 weeks.

The period of potential infectivity of patients harboring type A virus is 2 weeks to 3 weeks before and after the onset of clinical symptoms. This corresponds to the maximum duration of virus excretion in the feces. During this time, strict attention to stool isolation and appropriate hand washing by all personnel in attendance is mandatory.

Antibodies of the immunoglobulin M or G class appear during early acute illness and persist in most patients for 3 months to 4 months. The presence of this protein in plasma of patients with acute hepatitis is considered diagnostic of recent infections with type A virus.[28] Patients with hepatitis A antibodies are probably immune to the disease on reexposure. Indeed, nearly one-half the adult population of the United States has high plasma concentrations of antibodies against type A virus. Pooled gamma globulin (0.02 ml·kg^{-1}) greatly reduces the severity of type A hepatitis when given during the incubation period. Furthermore, pooled gamma globulin will provide protection against the disease for about 6 months. Prognosis in patients who develop type A hepatitis is good, with symptoms disappearing and plasma transaminase concentrations decreasing in 3 weeks to 4 weeks. Chronic liver disease does not develop and a chronic carrier state does not occur.

TYPE B VIRUS

Hepatitis due to type B virus is also referred to as serum or post-transfusion hepatitis and is probably the most common type of viral hepatitis. Transmission is usually via parenteral routes such as blood transfusion or percutaneous inoculation. Nevertheless, it has become increasingly apparent that nonparenteral

TABLE 19-3.   Characteristic Features of Viral Hepatitis

Features	Type A (Infectious Hepatitis)	Type B (Serum Hepatitis)	Non-A, Non-B
Causative agent	27 nm RNA	42 nm DNA; core and surface components	Similar to Type B
Transmission	Fecal-oral	Parenteral Oral-oral	Parenteral Oral-oral
Incubation period	2–6 weeks	4–24 weeks	2–20 weeks
Period of infectivity	2–3 weeks in late prodromal phase and early clinical stages	During HB$_s$Ag positivity	Unknown
Prophylaxis	Hygiene Immune serum globulin	Hygiene Hepatitis B immune globulin Vaccine	Hygiene ?Immune serum globulin
Massive hepatic necrosis	Rare	Uncommon	Uncommon
Carrier state	No	Yes	Yes
Chronic hepatitis	No	Yes	Yes

routes (oral-to-oral and sexual) can also be responsible. The incubation period for type B hepatitis is from 4 weeks to 24 weeks.

Electron microscopic and immunologic techniques have led to the identification of several viral particles associated with type B hepatitis. Of these materials, the Dane particle may be synonymous with type B virus.[29] The Dane particle consists of the hepatitis B surface antigen (HB_sAg) and a core particle designated as the hepatitis B core antigen (HB_cAg) and E antigen (HB_eAg). Antibodies (anti-HB_s, anti-HB_c) may develop against these antigens.

Monitoring plasma titers of these antigens as well as their antibodies may be helpful in (1) following the course of hepatitis, (2) determining immunity, (3) assessing the state of infectivity of patients, and (4) facilitating the screening of blood. For example, HB_sAg is detectable by radioimmunoassay in the plasma of nearly all patients with hepatitis B several weeks before the onset of symptoms. About 25 percent of infected adults develop clinical hepatitis.[30] Titers of HB_sAg are usually decreasing by the time of onset of clinical symptoms and are negligible by 6 weeks. Therefore, the presence of HB_sAg in plasma indicates the potential for infectivity. Antibodies to HB_sAg (anti-HB_s) appear in about 90 percent of patients during convalescence, and remain elevated as long as HB_sAg persists in plasma. The incidence of anti-HB_s antibodies in the general population is about 10 percent, indicating that hepatitis B is self-limited in most patients. Anti-HB_c antibodies become detectable soon after the onset of symptoms and persist for months to years, serving as a marker for prior or chronic hepatitis B infections. HB_eAg are found only in the nuclei of hepatocytes, and antibodies to this antigen (anti-HB_e) can serve as markers of previous infections. Furthermore, the presence of HB_eAg may reflect the patient's potential for infectivity and/or development of chronic disease states.

Persistence of HB_sAg for longer than 6 months in the absence of antibodies indicates that the patient is a chronic carrier and potentially infective to others. Approximately 1 in every 200 adults in the United States is classified as a chronic carrier on this basis. These patients do not appear to be susceptible to reactivation of the virus when subjected to anesthesia and operation. Furthermore, HB_sAg is rarely present in plasma of patients with unexplained jaundice in the postoperative period. An unknown percentage of chronic carriers of HB_sAg develop chronic active hepatitis, which often progresses to cirrhosis of the liver with esophageal varices and ascites. Primary hepatocellular carcinoma is also 220 times more likely to develop in chronic carriers.

PROPHYLAXIS

Prevention of hepatitis B infection is desirable, considering the potential risks associated with this infection. Those who administer anesthesia because of their exposure to blood or other body fluids, such as oral secretions, deserve special consideration in prophylaxis and prevention. Indeed, personnel who administer anesthesia are about five times more likely to show serologic evidence of prior or current hepatitis B infection than the general population.[30,31] Avoiding exposure to infected patients is not reliable prophylaxis, considering infective patients who are asymptomatic and unrecognized. Furthermore, hepatitis B virus can survive on contaminated surfaces at room temperature for as long as 6 months. In this regard, heating to 60 degrees for 4 hours, heat or steam sterilization or 2 percent glutaraldehyde destroy the hepatitis virus. Immunization with hepatitis B vaccine is a highly effective means (protective antibody response in over 90 percent of vaccinated individuals) of protecting personnel at risk. Procedures used to prepare the inactivated hepatitis B vaccine will inactivate all known viruses, including those responsible for acquired immunodeficiency syndrome.[32] Postoperative prophylaxis with hepatitis B immune globulin is recommended for prophylaxis of personnel exposed to patients known to be infective for hepatitis.

Several types of patients may present for anesthesia and operation with a high likelihood for harboring HB_sAg. These include patients on hemodialysis, immunosuppressed patients, drug addicts, and male homosexuals. Proper management of potentially infective patients in the perioperative period includes the wearing of gloves by all those involved in caring for these patients, the use of disposable equipment, and clear labeling of blood specimens as possibly coming from patients with hepatitis.

NON-A, NON-B VIRUS

Hepatitis due to non-A, non-B virus is also referred to as hepatitis C and probably includes several as yet undetected viruses. The route of transmission seems to be by inoculation, and the incubation period is 2 weeks to 20 weeks. Over 80 percent of hepatitis due to blood transfusion is felt to be due to these viruses. It is not known if immunity develops to this type of hepatitis, but pooled gamma globulin reduces the incidence of the clinical disease. Chronic liver disease is not an uncommon complication and a chronic carrier state is frequent. Mortality rate for this type of hepatitis has not been defined, but it may be similar to that for hepatitis B. This form of hepatitis is a diagnosis of exclusion since serologic markers are not available.

Drug-Induced Hepatitis

Several classes of drugs, including but not limited to antibiotics, antihypertensives, anticonvulsants, analgesics, tranquilizers, and anesthetics, are occasionally associated with hepatic dysfunction that may be indistinguishable histologically from viral hepatitis. These are most often idiosyncratic drug reactions, which are unpredictable and not dose-dependent. Clinical signs of liver dysfunction usually occur 2 weeks to 6 weeks after starting drug therapy but can be seen as early as the first day or as late as 6 months. Treatment is early recognition of alterations in liver function and discontinuation of the responsible drug.

ANESTHETIC DRUGS

All anesthetic drugs studied in the hypoxic rat model that includes enzyme induction may produce centrilobular necrosis, but the incidence is greatest with halothane, followed in order by fentanyl and nitrous oxide.[33] In this same model, thiopental, enflurane, and isoflurane produce minimal and similar hepatic changes. The combination of nitrous oxide with halothane accentuates hepatic injury produced by halothane in the hypoxic rat model.[34] In patients, there is no evidence that enflurane or isoflurane are hepatotoxic.[35,36] Based on the estimated use of enflurane and isoflurane, the alleged incidence of anesthetic dysfunction produced by these anesthetics, as indicated by the number of published reports, is less than the spontaneous attack rate of viral hepatitis.[37]

Small changes in inhaled hypoxic concentrations of oxygen may influence the likelihood of centrilobular necrosis after administration of inhaled or injected anesthetic drugs. For example, hepatic damage occurs in the hypoxic rat model after administration of all studied anesthetic drugs when inhaled concentrations of oxygen are 10 percent (Fig. 19-11).[38] Conversely, hepatic damage occurs after administration of halothane, but not enflurane or isoflurane, when inhaled concentrations of oxygen are 12 percent or 14 percent. Furthermore, hypoxia in the absence of anesthetic drugs can produce hepatic damage in the rat model.[39] In this regard, it seems likely that hepatic damage that occurs after administration of anesthesia could be related to changes associated with the administration of any anesthetic drug and not unique effects of any specific drug. Specifically, any anesthetic drug could contribute to inadequate hepatocyte oxygenation by depression of hepatic blood flow and/or alveolar ventilation. Consistent with the rat model, hepatocyte hypoxia could be greater with halothane than isoflurane because of greater reductions in hepatic blood flow produced by halothane.[14] Furthermore, anesthetic drugs could alter regional distribution of hepatic blood flow or interfere with the ability of hepatocytes to use oxygen. Further evidence for the role of hepatocyte hypoxia in the production of hepatic damage is the observation that reductions in body temperature to 32 degrees Celsius prevent centrilobular necrosis in the hypoxic rat model after administration of enflurane and isoflurane but not halothane.[38] The protective effect of hypothermia presum-

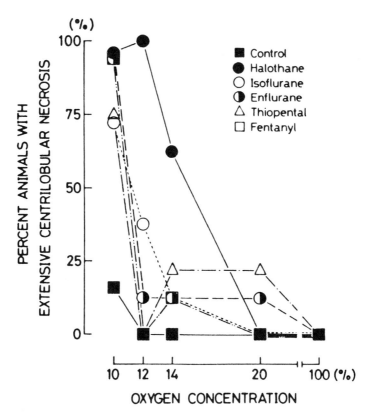

FIG. 19-11. The percent of rats having extensive hepatic necrosis 24 hours after exposure to different anesthetic drugs for 2 hours at the oxygen concentration indicated. Nearly all animals receiving anesthetic drugs manifested hepatic necrosis while breathing 10 percent oxygen. When inhaled, oxygen concentrations were increased above 12 percent halothane was the only anesthetic associated with hepatic necrosis in more than 50 percent of animals. (Shingu K, Eger EI, Johnson BH, et al. Effect of oxygen concentration on anesthetic-induced hepatic injury in rats. Anesth Analg 1983;62:146–50. Reprinted with permission from IARS.)

ably reflects decreased hepatic oxygen requirements. Co-existing hepatic disease, such as cirrhosis, may be associated with marginal hepatocyte oxygenation, which would be further jeopardized by effects of anesthetic drugs on hepatic blood flow and/or alveolar ventilation. Despite the theoretical adverse effects of co-existing liver disease, it has been demonstrated that postanesthetic hepatic dysfunction is minimal and similar in cirrhotic and noncirrhotic rats (Fig. 19-10).[22]

Halothane-Associated Hepatic Dysfunction. Halothane-associated hepatic dysfunction is a diagnosis of exclusion based on elim-

ination of other possible causes as likely explanations (see the section Extrahepatic Causes of Hepatic Dysfunction). Undoubtedly, halothane has been wrongly incriminated in many patients when a more detailed investigation (laboratory tests, electron microscopy) would have exonerated the anesthetic. Severe and occasionally fatal liver damage is extremely rare, being estimated to occur between 1 in 22,000 and 1 in 35,000 administrations of halothane.[40,41] This incidence is considerably lower than the incidence of unexpected liver disease in asymptomatic adult patients scheduled for elective surgery. For example, unsuspected liver dysfunction is present in about 1 in every 700 adults scheduled for elective surgery and about 1 in every 2,000 to 2,500 of these patients subsequently develop jaundice even without imposition of anesthesia and surgery.[42,43] Postoperative non-A, non-B hepatitis may occur in more than 3 percent of patients undergoing surgical procedures not requiring blood transfusions.[44] Nevertheless, most cases of alleged halothane-associated hepatic dysfunction have occurred in middle-aged obese women, especially with repeat administration of halothane within 4 weeks of a previous halothane anesthetic. Typically, hepatic dysfunction manifests as elevated body temperature and increased plasma concentrations of transaminase enzymes in the first 7 days postoperatively or sooner if a repeated halothane anesthetic is involved. Eosinophilia may be present and jaundice may or may not occur. The increased incidence of hepatic dysfunction associated with repeat administration of halothane at short intervals may reflect additive hepatic damage, which was produced but not clinically apparent with the first exposure. Conceivably, sufficient time between halothane exposures should allow regeneration of hepatocytes. This speculation has led to attempts to recommend safe intervals between halothane exposures. Any recommendation as to safe intervals, however, is empiric. In view of alternatives to halothane (enflurane, isoflurane, opioids), it would seem logical to avoid repeating halothane anesthesia. Certainly halothane should not be administered to patients who have experienced postoperative hepatic dysfunction for unknown reasons after previous operations that included administration of halothane. Pediatric patients seem to be uniquely resistant to the development of halothane-associated hepatic dysfunction, even with repeated short interval exposures, although alleged cases have been described.[45]

The mechanism responsible for halothane-associated hepatic dysfunction is unknown, but theories invoke toxic reactive intermediary metabolites or a cell-damaging, immune-mediated hypersensitivity response (e.g., an allergic reaction). With respect to toxic metabolites, it is speculated that products of reductive metabolism can bind irreversibly (covalently) to intracellular constituents of hepatocytes and cause their destruction. Halothane is the only volatile anesthetic drug that undergoes reductive metabolism in the presence of low oxygen partial pressures with the possible production of highly reactive intermediary metabolites. Fluoride is a final metabolite when reductive metabolism of halothane occurs. The fact that anesthetic drugs that do not undergo reductive metabolism can cause hepatic necrosis in the hypoxic rat model has cast doubt on the role of toxic intermediary metabolites in the production of liver injury.

An allergic response as a mechanism for halothane-associated hepatic dysfunction is suggested by eosinophilia and accelerated liver dysfunction after repeat exposures to halothane. Conversely, it is difficult to accept the likelihood of antibody production evoked by a small nonprotein molecule such as halothane. Nevertheless, reductive metabolites of halothane that bind covalently to liver cells could act as haptens. Support for such responses is the observation that plasma from some patients recovering from halothane-associated hepatic dysfunction contains antibodies that bind to surfaces of specially prepared hepatocytes that have been exposed to halothane.[46] A possible genetic role is suggested by variations in the susceptibility of the liver to toxic metabolites of halothane in different strains of rats, as well as the occurrence of hepatitis after administration of halothane anesthesia to three pairs of closely related women (mother-daughter, sisters, first cousins) with a common ethnic origin (Mexican-Indian or Mexican-Spanish).[47] A familial or constitutional susceptibility factor is suggested by demonstration of damage to lymphocytes from patients with suspected halothane-associated hepatic dysfunction when exposed to electrophilic metabolites.[48] Genetic factors could be important in determining the likelihood that susceptible patients will form antibodies or use reductive pathways of metabolism for halothane.

There is speculation that two types of halothane-associated hepatic dysfunction could exist.[37] The more common reaction could involve quantitative enhancement of reductive metabolism of halothane by factors including obesity, decreased hepatic blood flow as a result of the anesthetic drugs and retractors, plus the unpredictable impact of genetic characteristics and various enzyme inducing drugs. The net result is a purely biochemical insult to the liver produced by reductive metabolites of halothane. Onset of detectable liver dysfunction is within 1 day to 3 days postoperatively but usually remains mild and does not progress to life-threatening hepatic necrosis. A repeat halothane anesthetic at a short interval to these patients might produce sufficient additional liver damage to convert subclinical hepatic dysfunction to overt hepatic dysfunction. Conversely, sufficient time between halothane exposures might allow recovery from hepatocyte damage and repeat halothane anesthetics are not followed by symptomatic hepatic dysfunction. The second type of speculated reaction is rare but more severe, being able to progress to fatal hepatic necrosis. As with the first type of reaction, the basic event is metabolism, but instead of producing direct damage to hepatocytes, these metabolites conjugate with liver macromolecules and the resulting complexes act as haptens. This reaction is slower to develop than the first, perhaps requiring 6 days to 14 days to become clinically manifest, and can be detected by the presence of circulating antibodies. Clearly, a repeat halothane anesthetic to these patients, regardless of the time interval between administrations, will be followed by symptomatic hepatic dysfunction. Further investigations are needed to support the validity of these proposed forms of halothane-associated hepatic dysfunction.[37]

CHRONIC HEPATITIS

Chronic hepatitis is an unresolving disease caused by a virus, drugs, inborn errors of metabolism, or unknown factors. Indeed, a specific cause for chronic hepatitis can be found in only 10 percent to 20 percent of patients, and most of these will be associated with type B virus. Drugs known to cause chronic hepatitis include alpha-methyldopa and dantrolene, isoniazid, nitrofurantoin, acetaminophen, aspirin, and alcohol. In the majority of patients, the disease begins insidiously, so that the time of onset is uncertain.

Chronic hepatitis is categorized as chronic active hepatitis or chronic persistent hepatitis,

based on clinical features (Table 19-4) and interpretation of a liver biopsy.[49] Factors that determine the specific type of chronic hepatitis that develops are unknown.

Chronic Active Hepatitis

Chronic active hepatitis is the most serious form of chronic hepatitis, ultimately resulting in cirrhosis and hepatic failure. There is widespread inflammation and destruction of hepatocytes. Plasma bilirubin, transaminases, and gamma globulin levels are elevated. Reduction in plasma albumin concentrations and prolongation of the prothrombin time are suggestive of severe hepatic dysfunction.

Patients with chronic active hepatitis who are negative for the HB_sAg are often treated with corticosteroids with or without azathioprine. This therapy is associated with improvement in liver function tests, a reduction in clinical symptoms and improved survival. Treatment is commonly required for 3 years to 5 years. Over one-half of patients treated with corticosteroids for longer than 18 months develop severe complications, including diabetes mellitus, hypertension, and osteoporosis with vertebral collapse. In contrast, treatment of HB_sAg-positive chronic active hepatitis has been reported to have an overall harmful effect, and the use of corticosteroids in these patients is controversial.[50]

Chronic Persistent Hepatitis

Chronic persistent hepatitis is a benign nonprogressive inflammatory disease largely confined to portal areas. Despite its benign course, plasma transaminase abnormalities may persist for years. Plasma transaminase concentrations may also cycle between normal and elevated levels. Plasma bilirubin concentrations do not exceed $3 \text{ mg} \cdot dl^{-1}$, gamma globulin is normal to slightly elevated, and albumin concentrations and prothrombin time are normal (Table 19-4).[49] Nutritional support,

TABLE 19-4.   Differentiating Features in Chronic Hepatitis

Features	Chronic Active Hepatitis	Chronic Persistent Hepatitis
Jaundice	Common	Rare
Transaminases	Markedly elevated	Mildly elevated
Bilirubin	Elevated	Normal
Gamma globulin	Elevated	Normal
Prothrombin time	Prolonged	Normal
Albumin	Decreased	Normal
HB$_s$Ag (incidence)	10%–20%	10%–20%

(Data from Boyer JL. Chronic hepatitis: A perspective on classification and determinants of prognosis. Gastroenterology 1976:76:1161–71)

avoidance of potential hepatotoxins, and continued observation of these patients is the accepted treatment.

ACUTE HEPATIC FAILURE

Fulminant hepatic failure, regardless of the etiology, is associated with a poor prognosis. Plasma transaminase enzyme concentrations often rise to high levels that parallel the extent of hepatic injury. Enzyme concentrations, however, do not correlate with prognosis. If massive necrosis continues, enzyme levels may decrease due to lack of remaining hepatocytes to serve as sources for these enzymes. Hepatic encephalopathy manifests as personality changes, motor abnormalities (asterixis), and alterations in the level of consciousness. Cerebral edema and increased intracranial pressure often accompany hepatic encephalopathy and are the most likely causes of death.

Hyperventilation is a constant feature of early hepatic failure and most likely reflects stimulation of ventilation by ammonia. Ammonia is produced in the gastrointestinal tract by bacterial-induced deamination of amino acids and other nitrogenous substances. Ammonia is then delivered by the portal vein circulation to the liver where it is converted to urea. When hepatic failure is present, this highly toxic substance accumulates not only because of hepatocyte damage, but also because of the development of shunts between portal and systemic circulations.

Hypoglycemia is frequent and most likely reflects (1) insufficient degradation of insulin by the liver, (2) glycogen depletion, or (3) impaired glucose formation by gluconeogenesis. Normally, the liver removes about two-thirds of the insulin delivered to it in the portal vein, thus limiting the amount of insulin that reaches the systemic circulation. In addition, failure of the liver to remove lactic acid from the circulation for conversion to glucose by gluconeogenesis is consistent with the development of metabolic acidosis in patients with acute hepatic failure.

Cardiac output tends to be elevated, reflecting low peripheral vascular resistance and increased arteriovenous shunting. Renal failure with associated electrolyte disturbances is common. These patients have an increased susceptibility to infection, probably because of impaired polymorphonuclear leukocyte function. Over one-half of these patients develop a bleeding diathesis. Thrombocytopenia is likely, and accumulation of fibrin degradation products can reflect the presence of disseminated intravascular coagulation or the inability of the diseased liver to clear these substances from the circulation. Anemia, often from bleeding esophageal varices and/or poor nutrition, may be prominent. Intrapulmonary shunting is increased, resulting in a tendency to develop arterial hypoxemia.

Treatment

Treatment of acute hepatic failure is often supportive, including correction of coagulation abnormalities and electrolyte derangements, treatment of bacterial infections, and use of neomycin and/or lactulose to decrease plasma ammonia concentrations. Avoidance of factors that may aggravate encephalopathy (gastrointestinal hemorrhage, dietary protein, hypokalemia, sepsis, surgery) is important. Orthotopic liver transplantation may be considered in selected patients (see the section Orthotopic Liver Transplantation).

Management of Anesthesia

Only surgery designed to correct life-threatening situations should be considered in patients with acute hepatic failure. Preoperatively, correction of coagulation abnormalities with fresh frozen plasma should be considered. Certainly depressant or sedative drugs are not indicated. Nitrous oxide may be sufficient to provide analgesia and total amnesia. Use of volatile anesthetics must be questioned in view of possible adverse effects on a damaged liver, and barbiturates and opioids may produce prolonged effects in the absence of normal rates of hepatic metabolism. Muscle relaxants are appropriate for providing operative exposure and facilitating the management of ventilation. Choice of muscle relaxants must consider the impact of decreased hepatic function and often associated renal dysfunction on clearance of these drugs from the plasma. Since the plasma half-time of cholinesterase is 14 days, it is unlikely that acute liver failure will be associated with prolonged responses to succinylcholine.

Provision of exogenous glucose is important, and, in long operations, plasma glucose measurements to confirm the absence of hypoglycemia are prudent. Blood should be warmed and administered at as slow a rate as is practical to minimize the likelihood of citrate intoxication. Careful monitoring of arterial blood gases, pH, and electrolyte status is indicated, as these patients are vulnerable to developing arterial hypoxemia, metabolic acidosis, and decreased plasma potassium, calcium, and magnesium concentrations. Hypotension and its potential adverse effects on hepatic blood flow and hepatocyte oxygenation must be appreciated. Urine output should

be maintained with intravenous fluid infusions and, if necessary, by administration of mannitol. Invasive monitoring, including arterial and pulmonary artery catheters, is helpful in guiding perioperative management. These patients are vulnerable to infections, emphasizing the importance of aseptic techniques during insertion of intravascular catheters.

ORTHOTOPIC LIVER TRANSPLANTATION

Orthotopic liver transplantation is the only curative therapy for patients in hepatic failure. Hepatoma, biliary tract tumors, and genetically determined metabolic disturbances may also be treated with liver transplantation. Preoperative disturbances include encephalopathy, hypokalemia, hypocalcemia, renal failure, intrapulmonary shunting, anemia, thrombocytopenia, and disseminated intravascular coagulation. The urgent nature of the operation often limits the time available to optimize these disturbances before proceeding with surgery.

Management of Anesthesia

Management of anesthesia for liver transplantation includes invasive monitoring of arterial pressure and cardiac filling pressures.[51] The radial artery is preferred over infradiaphragmatic sites because the abdominal aorta is occasionally cross-clamped during hepatic arterial anastomosis. Clamping of the inferior vena cava dictates placement of venous access catheters above the diaphragm. Massive blood and fluid requirements require the presence of several venous catheters. Most patients have delayed gastric emptying times from ascites-induced increased intra-abdominal pressures, emphasizing the importance of gaining rapid protection of the airway with a cuffed tracheal tube. Ketamine is a useful drug for induction of anesthesia, especially if co-existing hypovolemia is present. Prolongation of the action of succinylcholine (1 mg·kg^{-1} to 2 mg·kg^{-1}) administered to facilitate intubation of the trachea is not a clinical problem because of the duration of surgery and the hemodilutional effect of multiple blood volume exchanges. Atracurium, which lacks significant dependence on hepatic or renal function, is a useful alternative to succinylcholine when rapid onset of skeletal muscle paralysis is not considered essential.

Maintenance of anesthesia is often with isoflurane with or without opioids. Large doses of opioids are not recommended in view of the role of the liver in the clearance of these drugs. Nitrous oxide is not administered because of possible bowel distention and the risk of air embolization at the time of revascularization of the liver, reflecting air previously trapped in the liver. Hepatic and renal routes of elimination must be considered in selection of muscle relaxants during maintenance of anesthesia.

The preeminent problem during liver transplantation is massive blood loss, requiring use of cell-saver devices. Calcium administration is often required to treat citrate-induced hypocalcemia and myocardial depression. Citrate-induced hypocalcemia is particularly likely in the absence of functioning hepatocytes plus hypothermia that often accompanies this operation. Indeed, hypothermia almost always occurs despite warming of infused fluids and inhaled gases. Venoveno bypass (femoral vein to axillary vein), used to decompress portal veins, contributes to hypothermia. Thrombocytopenia invariably occurs.

Circulatory changes during liver transplantation may include decreased venous return when the inferior vena cava is clamped requiring use of inotropes or sympathomimetics. Venoveno bypass or partial cardiopulmonary bypass may be an alternative for minimizing blood loss and reducing circulatory changes produced by clamping the inferior vena cava. Hypotension also may accompany unclamping of the inferior vena cava, perhaps reflecting washout of negative inotropic or vasodilating factors from the liver, which occurs even with the use of venoveno bypass. Metabolic acidosis during surgery is predictable and

combined with electrolyte disturbances and hypothermia may lead to cardiac dysrhythmias. Life-threatening hyperkalemia may accompany unclamping of previously clamped vessels. Hypoglycemia and hyperglycemia have been observed during liver transplantation. Maintenance of urine output is important and oliguria may reflect co-existing renal dysfunction or hypovolemia. Postoperatively, metabolism of the citrate complex leads to metabolic alkalosis and elevation of total plasma calcium concentrations while ionized calcium levels remain normal or depressed. It is common to support ventilation of the lungs via a tracheal tube for 24 hours to 48 hours after surgery.

CIRRHOSIS OF THE LIVER

Cirrhosis of the liver is a chronic disease process, which destroys the hepatic parenchyma and subsequently replaces it with collagen. This eventually results in disorganization of lobular architecture and interference with normal physiologic functions of the liver. Alcohol is the most frequent cause of cirrhosis in the United States. Other causes include drugs or toxins, viral infections (hepatitis), congestive heart failure, primary biliary cirrhosis, hemochromatosis, and Wilson's disease.

Regardless of the etiology of cirrhosis, the net effects on liver function are similar. Specifically, reductions in the number of hepatocytes leads to an impairment of all the physiologic functions of the liver (see the section Physiologic Functions of the Liver). The second important change produced is a reduction in hepatic blood flow due to increased intrahepatic resistance to flow through the portal vein (i.e., portal hypertension) reflecting the fibrotic process associated with cirrhosis. As a result of this increased resistance, the proportion of hepatic blood flow delivered via the portal vein is decreased, and the contribution to total hepatic blood flow from the hepatic artery is increased. Therefore, decreases in systemic perfusion pressure or arterial oxygenation are more likely to jeopardize the adequacy of hepatic blood flow and delivery of oxygen to the liver in patients with cirrhosis, as compared to normal patients. Despite these predictable changes, liver function tests are usually normal or only slightly deranged. Often, it is only when additional insults, such as anesthesia and surgery, are imposed that cirrhosis becomes manifest as changes in liver function tests.

Alcoholic Cirrhosis (Laennec's Cirrhosis)

Cirrhosis due to alcohol ingestion occurs in about 10 percent of those who consume the equivalent of 80 g of alcohol daily for 10 years to 15 years. It is estimated that alcoholism afflicts about 10 million persons in the United States. Alcoholic cirrhosis typically progresses through the stages of acute alcoholic hepatitis and portal vein hypertension.

ACUTE ALCOHOLIC HEPATITIS

Acute alcoholic hepatitis is characterized by jaundice in association with elevations of the plasma transaminase enzyme concentrations. Ascites occurs in nearly one-half of patients. If hepatic destruction is severe, plasma albumin concentrations may be reduced below 3 g·dl^{-1} and the prothrombin time prolonged.

PORTAL VEIN HYPERTENSION

Typically, portal vein hypertension does not develop until several years after the first attack of alcoholic hepatitis. Patients develop anorexia and lose skeletal muscle mass, particularly in the face, neck, and forearms. The most striking finding on physical examination is the presence of hepatomegaly, with or without splenomegaly and ascites. Ascites is due to decreased oncotic pressure secondary to low plasma albumin concentrations (usually less than 2.5 g·dl^{-1}), elevated resistance to blood flow through the portal vein system, and in-

creased secretion of antidiuretic hormone. Despite the loss of skeletal muscle mass, body weight is often maintained due to accumulation of ascitic fluid. Palmar erythema; spider angiomas over the face, upper back, and arms; and subcutaneous bleeding with minor trauma (capillary fragility related to vitamin C and prothrombin deficiency) are prominent.

Laboratory changes in the presence of portal hypertension include a hematocrit between 30 percent and 35 percent, most likely due to chronic gastrointestinal bleeding, hemolysis, or folic acid deficiency. Hyponatremia is probably related to increased secretion of antidiuretic hormone. Blood urea nitrogen concentrations are often below 10 mg·dl^{-1}, which most likely reflects the absence of dietary protein intake. Elevation of blood urea nitrogen concentrations to above 20 mg·dl^{-1} in patients with alcoholic cirrhosis suggests deteriorating renal function. Plasma bilirubin, transaminases, and alkaline phosphatase concentrations are likely to be mildly to moderately elevated.

EXTRAHEPATIC COMPLICATIONS OF ALCOHOLIC CIRRHOSIS

Several important extrahepatic complications are associated with alcoholic cirrhosis that has progressed to portal vein hypertension:[52] (1) circulatory changes, (2) arterial hypoxemia, (3) renal failure, (4) gallstones, (5) duodenal ulcer, (6) esophageal varices, (7) hepatic encephalopathy, and (8) spontaneous bacterial peritonitis.

Circulation. A hyperdynamic circulation characterized by an increased cardiac output is often present in patients with cirrhosis. This increased cardiac output has been attributed to increased intravascular fluid volume, decreased viscosity of blood secondary to anemia, and arteriovenous communications particularly in the lungs. Conversely, cardiomyopathy manifesting as congestive heart failure can occur in patients with alcoholic cirrhosis. Megaloblastic anemia is frequent and is probably due to antagonism of folate by alcohol, rather than dietary deficiencies.

Arterial Hypoxemia.   Despite the fact that hyperventilation is often present, many patients with alcoholic cirrhosis manifest arterial hypoxemia. One possible explanation is impaired movement of the diaphragm due to the accumulation of ascitic fluid. In addition, right-to-left intrapulmonary shunts may develop in the presence of portal vein hypertension, leading to arterial hypoxemia. Arterial hypoxemia may reflect pneumonia, a frequent occurrence in alcoholic patients. The vulnerability to developing pneumonia may reflect the ability of alcohol to inhibit phagocytic activity normally present in the lungs. As a result, bacteria inhaled into the respiratory tract are more likely to produce pneumonia. Indeed, the majority of lung abscesses are found in chronic alcoholic patients. Finally, regurgitation of gastric contents is made more likely by alcohol-induced reductions in lower esophageal sphincter tone.

Renal Failure.   Cirrhosis is associated with reductions in renal blood flow and glomerular filtration rate, which precedes overt renal dysfunction by several months. Increased activity of the renin-angiotensin-aldosterone system may be responsible for decreased renal blood flow in these patients. Abrupt oliguria in association with cirrhosis (hepatorenal syndrome) has a mortality of over 60 percent.

Hypoglycemia.   Hypoglycemia is a constant threat in alcoholic patients. This may reflect glycogen depletion due to malnourishment plus alcohol-induced glycogenolysis and interference with gluconeogenesis. The liver is responsible for clearing lactic acid from the circulation and subsequently converting lactate to glucose by gluconeogenesis. Severe liver disease may impair this function, contributing not only to hypoglycemia but also to the development of metabolic acidosis.

Gallstones.   The incidence of gallstones is increased in patients with cirrhosis. This response most likely reflects an increased bilirubin load, related to chronic hemolytic anemia due to splenomegaly. Gallstones can increase morbidity and mortality in patients

with cirrhosis if they precipitate acute cholecystitis or pancreatitis. Furthermore, the presence of gallstones complicates the differential diagnosis should jaundice occur.

Duodenal Ulcer.   Peptic ulcer disease is twice as common in patients with cirrhosis, as compared with the general population. Bleeding from peptic ulcers contributes to anemia and presents an increased ammonia load to the gastrointestinal tract, which may aggravate hepatic encephalopathy. Furthermore, hemorrhage from duodenal ulcers is difficult to distinguish from bleeding due to esophageal varices.

Gastroesophageal Varices.   Gastroesophageal varices are massively dilated submucosal veins, allowing the passage of splanchnic venous blood from the high pressure portal system to the low pressure azygous and hemiazygous thoracic veins. Esophageal varices are thin-walled submucosal veins beneath the squamous epithelium of the esophagus. It is important to recognize that not all patients with cirrhosis of the liver develop esophageal varices and not all patients with varices will bleed from their varices.[53] However, when it does occur variceal hemorrhage is usually from the distal esophagus or proximal stomach and often is hemodynamically significant.

Treatment of active variceal bleeding is with whole blood to maintain the hematocrit near 30 percent. In patients with coagulopathy due to hypoprothrombinemia and/or thrombocytopenia, fresh frozen plasma and/or platelets are necessary. In those patients with vigorous hemorrhage, especially in patients with hepatic encephalopathy, intubaton of the trachea may be performed to prevent pulmonary aspiration and facilitate endoscopic evaluation of the bleeding site. Once the acutely hemorrhaging patient has been resuscitated, a variety of approaches are available for control of bleeding and prevention of its recurrence. Balloon tamponade controls variceal hemorrhage in 40 percent to 80 percent of patients with endoscopically documented variceal hemorrhage.[53] This therapy is best preceded by intubation of the trachea. Endoscopic variceal sclerotherapy under general anesthesia may be useful for control of acute variceal hemorrhage. The value of intravenous vasopressin is controversial (see Chapter 20). There seems to be no advantage of selective intra-arterial vasopressin infusion. Portasystemic shunts remain the mainstay of surgical treatment for portal hypertension. The distal splenorenal (Warren) shunt is the most commonly performed elective surgical therapy for management of portal hypertension, but hepatic encephalopathy remains a risk.

Hepatic Encephalopathy. Development of hepatic encephalopathy is associated with a high mortality. Mental obtundation, asterixis, and fetor hepaticus are thought to occur because nitrogenous waste products, specifically ammonia, have direct access to the systemic circulation due to portasystemic shunting. Asterixis is the flapping motion of the hands caused by intermittent loss of extensor muscle tone. This finding is the hallmark of hepatic encephalopathy. Treatment of encephalopathy is the elimination of exogenous sources of ammonia by restriction of dietary protein intake and control of gastrointestinal bleeding. Oral neomycin is poorly absorbed from the gastrointestinal tract and, by decreasing the bacterial population, will reduce the amount of urea converted to ammonia by bacterial ureases. Lactulose is effective in decreasing concentrations of ammonia, by virtue of its ability to reduce the pH of the gastrointestinal tract. For example, lactulose-induced acidosis favors the conversion of ammonia to poorly soluble and thus poorly absorbed ammonium.

Impaired Immune Defense. Alcohol ingestion broadly suppresses immune defense mechanisms, rendering alcoholic patients vulnerable to bacterial and viral infections, tuberculosis, and development of cancer.[54] Spontaneous bacterial peritonitis develops in nearly 10 percent of patients with alcoholic liver disease and ascites. These responses emphasize that the individual using alcohol in excess, either episodically or on a regular basis, should be viewed as being immunosuppressed.

Care of the Chronic Alcoholic Patient in the Perioperative Period

Chronic consumption of alcohol results in the development of tolerance, physical dependence, and multisystem organ dysfunction. A knowledge of the pathophysiologic changes produced by chronic alcohol abuse is important for the management of these patients in the perioperative period.

MINOR ALCOHOL WITHDRAWAL SYNDROME

Abrupt discontinuation of alcohol ingestion is followed by compensatory neuronal excitability and catecholamine release. Minor withdrawal symptoms occur in the majority of alcoholic patients within 6 hours to 8 hours after abstinence. Symptoms include tremulousness, insomnia, and irritability. Autonomic nervous system imbalance may be reflected by hypertension, tachycardia, and cardiac dysrhythmias. These features of minor alcohol withdrawal syndrome usually wane or disappear within 48 hours without specific therapy.

SEVERE ALCOHOL WITHDRAWAL SYNDROME (DELERIUM TREMENS)

A severe alcohol withdrawal syndrome following acute cessation of alcohol ingestion occurs in about 5 percent of alcoholic patients. This syndrome represents a medical emergency, as mortality may approach 15 percent. Compared with the mild alcohol withdrawal syndrome, the onset of the severe alcohol withdrawal syndrome is delayed, being most likely to appear 48 hours to 72 hours after cessation of drinking.[52]

Signs and Symptoms. Manifestations of a severe alcohol withdrawal syndrome include tremulousness, disorientation, and hallucinations. There is increased activity of the sympathetic nervous system, with catecholamine release leading to diaphoresis, hyperpyrexia, tachycardia, and hypertension. Indeed, chronic alcohol abuse leads to the development of additional beta-adrenergic receptors such that biologic responses to catecholamines are exaggerated during alcohol withdrawal.[55] In some patients, grand mal seizures may be the first indication of the alcohol withdrawal syndrome. When seizures occur, hypoglycemia must be ruled out as a possible cause. Biochemically, the most likely findings during severe alcohol withdrawal syndrome are hypomagnesemia, hypokalemia, and respiratory alkalosis. This triad of changes increases the likelihood of cardiac dysrhythmias.

Treatment.   Treatment of a severe alcohol withdrawal syndrome consists of prompt sedation, vitamin replacement (especially thiamine), and correction of fluid and electrolyte disorders. Oral or intravenous diazepam is frequently used for sedation. A recommended regimen is diazepam, 10 mg intravenously, followed by 5 mg every 5 minutes until the patient becomes calm but remains awake.[56] The dose of diazepam required to achieve this state ranges from 45 mg to 90 mg. Propranolol may be effective in suppressing manifestations of sympathetic nervous system hyperactivity. Replacement of magnesium and potassium is important to minimize the development of serious cardiac dysrhythmias. Lidocaine is usually effective when cardiac dysrhythmias occur.

WERNICKE-KORSAKOFF SYNDROME

Symptoms of this syndrome include ataxia due to loss of neurons in the cerebellum (Wernicke's encephalopathy) and loss of memory (Korsakoff's psychosis). The majority of these patients show signs of polyneuropathy. Postural hypotension, ocular palsies, and nystagmus are prominent. Treatment is with thiamine. This symptom complex is not a withdrawal syndrome, but its occurrence establishes that the patient is or has been physically dependent on alcohol.

MANAGEMENT OF ANESTHESIA IN THE SOBER ALCOHOLIC PATIENT

It is estimated that 5 percent to 10 percent of all patients with cirrhosis of the liver undergo surgery in the last 2 years of life. Postoperative morbidity is increased, especially with respect to poor wound healing, bleeding, infection and deterioration of hepatic function including encephalopathy. Preoperative criteria may correlate with the surgical risk and postoperative outcome of patients with cirrhosis of the liver undergoing major surgery (Table 19-5).[57]

Management of anesthesia in the sober patient with alcoholic liver disease is based on an understanding of pathophysiologic changes associated with chronic liver disease (see the section Extrahepatic Complications of Alcoholic Cirrhosis). The optimal anesthetic drug choice or technique in the presence of liver disease is not known. It is important to remember, however, that a constant feature of chronic liver disease is decreased hepatic blood flow due to increased resistance to flow through the portal vein.

Surgical stimulation can even further reduce perfusion of the liver (Fig. 19-6).[15] In view of the decreased flow, it follows that hepatic blood flow and hepatocyte oxygenation are more dependent on hepatic artery flow than in normal patients. Furthermore, postoperative liver dysfunction is likely to be exaggerated in patients with chronic liver disease, regardless of the drug or drugs administered for anesthesia.

Thus, it would seem prudent to select drugs for production of anesthesia that do not increase splanchnic vascular resistance and, at the same time, undergo minimal metabolism. In this regard, nitrous oxide, enflurane, and isoflurane are attractive choices. Among the volatile anesthetics, isoflurane may be associated with the best maintenance of hepatic blood flow and hepatocyte oxygenation. There is no evidence, however, that halothane, when administered to animals or patients with cirrhosis, causes adverse effects on liver function (Fig. 19-10).[22] Nevertheless, it should be recognized that events likely to favor reductive metabolism of halothane (enzyme induction

TABLE 19-5. Prediction of Surgical Risk Based on Properative Evaluation

	Minimal	Modest	Marked
Bilirubin (mg·dl^{-1})	<2	2–3	>3
Albumin (g·dl^{-1})	>3.5	3–3.5	<3
Prothrombin time (seconds prolonged)	1–4	4–6	6
Encephalopathy	None	Moderate	Severe
Nutrition	Excellent	Good	Poor
Ascites	None	Moderate	Marked

(Data from Strunin I. Preoperative assessment of the patient with liver dysfunction. Br J Anaesth 1978;50:25–34)

from alcohol and malnutrition plus hepatocyte hypoxia from decreased hepatic blood flow) are predictably present in patients with cirrhosis. Opioids or benzodiazepines are valuable adjuncts to nitrous oxide with or without volatile anesthetics, but it must be appreciated that cumulative drug effects are likely if liver disease is severe enough to slow metabolism.

Response to Anesthetic Drugs. Tolerance of alcoholic patients to alcohol is paralleled by similar resistance (cross-tolerance) to other central nervous system depressant drugs, such as barbiturates and volatile anesthetics. Indeed, there is evidence that chronic alcohol abuse increases anesthetic requirements (MAC) for halothane[58] and isoflurane (Fig. 19-12).[59] The most likely explanation is cellular tolerance. Furthermore, increased phospholipid content has been observed in brain tissues of known alcoholic patients.[58] This increased lipid content parallels increased solubility of halothane in the central nervous system. An increased anesthetic requirement in mice selectively bred for their susceptibility to alcohol, however, was not associated with a different phospholipid, fatty acid, or cholesterol composition of synaptic nerve membranes.[60] Alcohol is also a potent enzyme-inducing drug. It is likely that alcohol accelerates its own metabolism, as well as that of other drugs. Nevertheless, an accelerated rate of metabolism would seem unlikely to exert a major impact on anesthetic requirements for inhaled anesthetics that undergo minimal degradation. Furthermore, metabolism would alter the amount of inhaled anesthetic needed to achieve a given brain partial pressure but would not alter the partial pressure required to produce anesthesia.

In contrast to resistance to depressant drugs, co-existing, alcohol-produced cardiomyopathy could make these patients unusually sensitive to cardiac depressant effects of volatile drugs. Likewise, decreased protein binding of drugs in the presence of reduced plasma albumin concentrations due to liver disease would theoretically increase the pharmacologic effects of a barbiturate such as thiopental.[2] Profound hypotension during anesthesia has been observed in chronic alcoholic patients who are receiving disulfiram.[61] This hypotension may reflect depletion of sympathetic nervous system neurotransmitters, as disulfiram inhibits the enzyme (dopamine beta oxidase) necessary for the conversion of dopamine to norepinephrine.

Muscle Relaxants. The role of the liver in the clearance of muscle relaxants must be considered when selecting these drugs for administration to patients with cirrhosis of the liver. Succinylcholine is acceptable, although severe liver disease may reduce plasma cholinesterase activity to prolong modestly the duration of action of this drug. The increased volume of distribution that accompanies cirrhosis may result in the need for greater initial doses of nondepolarizing muscle relaxants to produce given plasma concentrations of drugs, but the resulting neuromuscular blockade may be prolonged if these drugs depend on hepatic metabolism. Indeed, elimination half-times of pancuronium are prolonged, and the clearance is decreased in patients with cirrhosis compared with normal patients.[62] Metocurine and d-tubocurarine do not depend on hepatic me-

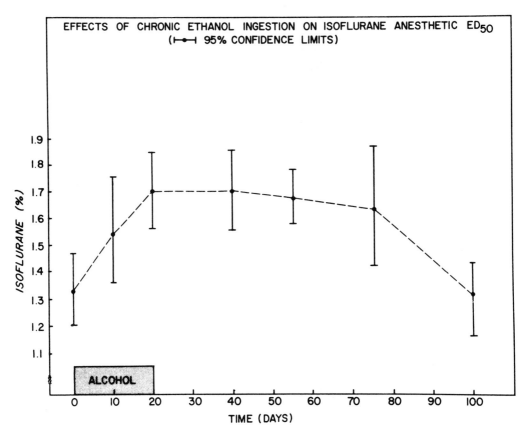

FIG. 19-12. The effect of chronic alcohol (ethanol) ingestion on isoflurane anesthetic ED50 was determined during 20 days of continuous exposure to alcohol and for 80 days after discontinuing the alcohol. Isoflurane values on days 20, 40, 55, and 75 were significantly elevated ($P<0.05$) above the control value. Therefore, tolerance by these alcoholic mice persisted through 55 days after discontinuing alcohol. These mice had lost their anesthetic tolerance 100 days after discontinuing alcohol. (Johnston RE, Kulp RA, Smith TC. Effects of acute and chronic ethanol administration on isoflurane requirement in mice. Anesth Analg 1975;54:277–81. Reprinted with permission from IARS.)

tabolism. Hepatic dysfunction does not alter elimination half-times of atracurium.[63] Elimination half-times of vecuronium in the presence of hepatic dysfunction are not increased until the dose exceeds 0.1 mg·kg.[63] This prolonged elimination half-time with large doses of vecuronium is consistent with dependence of this drug on hepatic clearance mechanisms.

Altered protein binding of muscle relaxants has previously been speculated to account for resistance to the effects of muscle relaxants, especially d-tubocurarine, occasionally observed in patients with cirrhosis. Nevertheless, the extent and importance of protein binding

of nondepolarizing muscle relaxants to either albumin or gamma globulin is not clearly defined. Furthermore, protein binding of d-tubocurarine is not altered by hepatic disease.[64] All factors considered, intermediate-acting muscle relaxants, especially atracurium, would be attractive selections to produce skeletal muscle paralysis in patients with severe liver disease.

Monitoring. Monitoring of intraoperative arterial blood gases, pH, and urine output, plus provision of exogenous glucose, are important principles. Arterial hypoxemia may be exaggerated intraoperatively if drugs used for anesthesia produce vasodilation of co-existing portasystemic and intrapulmonary shunts.[65] Intravenous infusion of glucose during the perioperative period is important, not only to prevent hypoglycemia, but also to reduce the likelihood of deposition of potentially harmful lipid soluble metabolic products of volatile anesthetics in hepatocytes. Repeated blood glucose determinations would be helpful in long surgical procedures. Intraoperative maintenance of urine output, particularly in patients with co-existing jaundice, is important for reducing the chances of postoperative renal failure. Mannitol may be necessary to establish diuresis.

The need for invasive intraoperative monitoring is determined by the extent and urgency of the surgery. Management of anesthesia for surgical creation of portacaval shunts includes monitoring of intra-arterial and cardiac filling pressures. Institution of neomycin or lactulose therapy in the preoperative period will decrease the ammonia load and help prevent hepatic encephalopathy. Use of fresh blood is recommended, both to reduce the ammonia load and to provide coagulation factors. A practical point is the avoidance of unnecessary esophageal instrumentation in patients with known esophageal varices.

MANAGEMENT OF ANESTHESIA IN THE INTOXICATED ALCOHOLIC PATIENT

In contrast to the chronic but sober alcoholic, the acutely intoxicated patient requires less anesthetic, since there is an additive depressant effect between alcohol and anesthetics. The acutely intoxicated patient also withstands stress and blood loss poorly. Furthermore, alcohol tends to reduce tolerance of the brain to hypoxia. Surgical bleeding may reflect alcohol-induced interference with platelet aggregation. Intoxicated patients may be more vulnerable to regurgitation of gastric contents, as alcohol slows gastric emptying and reduces tone of the lower esophageal sphincter.

Alcohol, even in moderate doses, causes increased circulating catecholamines, most likely reflecting inhibition of neurotransmitter uptake back into presynaptic nerve endings. The influence of this phenomena, if any, on the development of intraoperative cardiac ventricular dysrhythmias or on susceptibility to exogenous epinephrine is unknown.

Primary Biliary Cirrhosis

Primary biliary cirrhosis is a chronic, progressive and often fatal cholestatic liver disease characterized by destruction of intrahepatic bile ducts, portal inflammation and scarring and the eventual development of cirrhosis and liver failure.[66] Over 90 percent of patients are women between 30 years and 65 years of age. Liver function tests reveal a cholestatic pattern in which plasma alkaline phosphatase concentrations are elevated to at least three times normal. Elevated plasma concentrations of cholesterol and lipids reflect marked reductions in secretion of bile. Antimitochondrial antibody tests are positive in 95 percent of patients. Jaundice may not develop until 5 years to 10 years after onset of generalized pruritus. Bile duct patency is evaluated with ultrasonography or computed tomography. Scleroderma, Sjögren's syndrome, arthropathy, osteoporosis, and hypothyroidism are associated with this disease.

Treatment of primary biliary cirrhosis is symptomatic and includes relief of pruritus by lowering bile acids with cholestyramine and replacing fat soluble vitamins. Drugs that have been tried without consistent efficacy include penicillamine, colchicine, chlorambucil and cyclosporine.[66] Hepatocyte function is often maintained for many years. Therefore, portal vein hypertension and esophageal varices can usually be treated by a surgical portasystemic shunt, without a serious risk of postshunt encephalopathy. Liver transplantation is a consideration for those in whom liver failure or recurrent bleeding from esophageal varices develops.

Hemochromatosis

Hemochromatosis develops when excessive amounts of iron are deposited in hepatocytes, leading to scarring and cirrhosis. The disease predominates in men, and symptoms are unlikely before 40 years of age. The cause is unknown, although some patients are excessive users of alcohol. Portal vein hypertension is less common than with alcoholic cirrhosis.

Laboratory tests reveal increased plasma iron concentrations. Mild elevations of plasma transaminase and alkaline phosphatase concentrations are common. Reductions in plasma albumin concentrations below 3 g·dl^{-1} or prolongation of the prothrombin time do not occur until late in the disease process. When symptoms of hepatic dysfunction are present, 50 percent of patients will also have symptoms of diabetes mellitus, and 15 percent will have symptoms of congestive heart failure or manifest cardiac dysrhythmias. Repeated phlebotomy (1 unit every week) depletes iron stores (each unit of whole blood contains 200 mg to 250 mg of iron) and is an effective treatment to halt the cirrhotic process and improve pancreatic and cardiac function.

Wilson's Disease

Wilson's disease (hepatolenticular degeneration) is an inherited defect of copper transport and storage, which results in excess tissue levels of copper, with resulting symptoms of neurologic and/or hepatic dysfunction. Jaundice, bleeding from esophageal varices, and moderate elevations of plasma transaminase concentrations reflect hepatic dysfunction. Laboratory tests reveal the absence of ceruloplasmin, a copper-binding globulin. Treatment is with penicillamine, which binds copper and thus promotes its renal excretion. Treatment with penicillamine can be associated with leukopenia, thrombocytopenia, and occasionally a nephrotic syndrome.

IDIOPATHIC HYPERBILIRUBINEMIA

Hyperbilirubinemia may occur in the absence of hemolysis or overt hepatobiliary disease. Unconjugated hyperbilirubinemia will be present if there are defects before conjugation steps in hepatocytes (Fig. 19-4). These conjugation steps render bilirubin water soluble and are under the control of the hepatic enzyme, glucuronyl transferase. If the defect in transport occurs after conjugation, conjugated bilirubin will reenter the circulation to produce a conjugated hyperbilirubinemia (Fig. 19-4).

Gilbert's Syndrome

The most common example of idiopathic hyperbilirubinemia (present in varying degrees in 5 percent to 10 percent of the population) is Gilbert's syndrome, which is inherited as an autosomal dominant trait with variable penetrance. The primary defect is decreased bilirubin uptake by hepatocytes, resulting in elevation of plasma concentrations of unconjugated bilirubin. Plasma bilirubin concentrations seldom exceed 5 mg·dl^{-1}.

Crigler-Najjar Syndrome

The Crigler-Najjar syndrome is a rare form of severe unconjugated hyperbilirubinemia, due to reduced or absent hepatic glucuronyl transferase enzyme. Children with no enzyme activity are jaundiced at birth and develop kernicterus, with plasma bilirubin levels near 30 mg·dl^{-1}. These children seldom survive to adulthood. When some enzyme activity is present, plasma bilirubin concentrations average 15 mg·dl^{-1}, and jaundice is less severe. In these less severely afflicted patients, chronic phenobarbital therapy may reduce jaundice by stimulating glucuronyl transferase enzyme activity.

Dubin-Johnson Syndrome

This syndrome is due to a reduced ability to transport organic ions from hepatocytes into the biliary system, resulting in conjugated hyperbilirubinemia. Inheritance of this syndrome is autosomal recessive.

DISEASES OF THE BILIARY TRACT

It is estimated that 15 million adults in the United States have biliary tract disease, manifested by the presence of gallstones. Gallstones are reported to be present in 10 percent of men and 20 percent of women between 55 years and 65 years of age. Causes of gallstone formation are most likely related to abnormalities in the physiochemical aspects of the various components of bile. Bile is normally composed of cholesterol, bile salts, and phospholipids. Cholesterol is insoluble in water and will precipitate, unless it is maintained in solution by the action of bile salts. Therefore, if bile salts are abnormal or their concentrations are inadequate, hydrophobic cholesterol molecules will precipitate, providing the nidus for the formation of gallstones. Indeed, approximately 90 percent of gallstones are radiolucent, being composed primarily of cholesterol. The remaining gallstones are usually radiopaque and are typically composed of calcium biluribinate.

Diseases of the biliary tract may present as acute cholecystitis, or chronic cholelithiasis and cholecystitis. If chronic cholecystitis has not developed, bile salts such as chenodeoxycholic acid can be administered orally in attempts to lower cholesterol levels in bile and thus favor dissolution of gallstones.[67]

Acute Cholecystitis

Acute cholecystitis is almost always due to obstruction of the cystic duct by gallstones. The cardinal symptom of acute cholecystitis is the abrupt onset of severe pain (colic) in the mid epigastrium, which extends into the right upper abdomen. This pain is typically accentuated by inspiration (Murphy's sign). Local-

ized tenderness potentially indicates perforation with peritonitis. Ileus may be present. Body temperature is usually elevated to between 38 degrees Celsius to 39 degrees Celsius. There is frequently a mild leukocytosis. Plasma bilirubin, alkaline phosphatase, and amylase concentrations are often elevated. Jaundice is present when the cystic duct is completely obstructed by gallstones. Myocardial infarction is distinguished from acute cholecystitis on the basis of the electrocardiogram and measurement of plasma transaminase enzyme concentrations specific for cardiac muscle.

Initial management of patients with acute cholecystitis consists of gastric suction and intravenous fluid and volume replacement, especially if vomiting has been prominent. Despite the fact that opioids can cause spasm of the choledochoduodenal sphincter, it is often necessary to administer these drugs to relieve the intense pain produced by acute cholecystitis. Presence of free air in the abdomen or of peritonitis suggests perforation of the gallbladder and necessitates emergency laparotomy.

Chronic Cholelithiasis and Cholecystitis

Patients who experience repeated attacks of acute cholecystitis eventually develop fibrotic gallbladders, which are not capable of contracting to expel bile. Laboratory tests are usually normal, but elevated plasma bilirubin or alkaline phosphatase concentrations suggest the presence of choledocholithiasis (common bile duct stones) or chronic cholangitis.

CHOLEDOCHOLITHIASIS

Lodgment of gallstones in the common bile duct occurs in about 15 percent of patients who develop chronic choledocholithiasis. Acute common bile duct obstruction is associated with the abrupt onset of intense right upper quadrant pain, shaking chills, and fever. Plasma alkaline phosphatase concentrations are markedly elevated to at least three times normal, bilirubin is 5 mg·dl^{-1} to 10 mg·dl^{-1}, and jaundice is present. Plasma transaminase values are variably elevated. All these changes occur within 48 hours to 96 hours after the onset of abdominal pain. Clinical presentation and liver function tests distinguish acute obstruction of the common bile duct from viral hepatitis, myocardial infarction, ureterolithiasis, and pancreatitis. Treatment is surgical exploration of the common bile duct and removal of the impacted stone or stones.

CHRONIC CHOLANGITIS

Chronic cholangitis is inflammation of the hepatic biliary tree, which develops in response to obstruction of the biliary tract. This response is most often due to chronic and recurrent choledocholithiasis. Fatigue, intermittent chills and fever, and weight loss are common complaints. Plasma alkaline phosphatase concentrations are persistently elevated to at least three times normal.

Management of Anesthesia

Management of anesthesia for cholecystectomy and/or common bile duct exploration is influenced by effects of drugs used for anesthesia on intraluminal pressures in the biliary tract. Specifically, opioids are known to cause spasm of the choledochoduodenal sphincter (Oddi's sphincter). Fentanyl, morphine, and meperidine have been reported to produce sustained choledochal hypertension (Fig. 19-13).[68–70]

Implications of opioid-induced biliary tract hypertension relate to the interpretation of operative cholangiography and measurements of biliary pressure. For example, routine operative cholangiography has been advocated for all cholecystectomies. This recommendation is based on an incidence of unsuspected common duct stones, which may be as high as 4 percent. In addition, biliary manometry is often performed to evaluate the need for a sphincteroplasty. Opioid-induced spasm of the choledochoduodenal sphincter could elevate intrabiliary pressures and at the same time impair passage of contrast medium into the duodenum, erroneously suggesting the need for a sphincteroplasty or the presence of common duct stones. Opioid-induced spasm of the choledochoduodenal sphincter may appear radiologically as a constriction at the distal end of the common bile duct and be misinterpreted as common bile duct stones. In view of these potential adverse effects, it may be prudent to avoid administration of opioids in the management of anesthesia for patients undergoing biliary tract surgery. Nevertheless, opioids have been used in many instances without adverse effects. This emphasizes that not all patients respond to opioids with choledochoduodenal sphincter spasm. Indeed, some feel the incidence of opioid-induced sphincter spasm during cholecystectomy is so low (3 percent or less) that the possibility of this response should not influence the use of opioids during anesthesia.[71] In addition, tachyphylaxis to the spasmogenic effects of opioids on the biliary system may occur. It should also be remembered that intraoperative manipulation of the biliary duct system with probes and use of cold or irritating solutions (radiopaque dyes) may produce spasm of the choledochoduodenal sphincter, which is independent of drugs used to produce anesthesia.

Alternatives to opioids for maintenance of anesthesia during cholecystectomies would include use of volatile anesthetics. The possible presence of liver disease is often a concern when selecting volatile anesthetics for these patients. Nevertheless, there is no evidence that hepatic dysfunction after cholecystectomy is different in patients anesthetized with nitrous oxide plus fentanyl, halothane, or enflurane (Fig. 9-9).[21]

An alternative to avoiding the use of opioids entirely in patients undergoing biliary tract operations is the intraoperative reversal of opioid effects should the cholangiogram or biliary pressures be abnormal. Opioid-induced choledochoduodenal sphincter spasm can be reversed with naloxone (Fig. 19-13).[69,70] Naloxone, however, is not a practical approach, as this drug reverses analgesia and necessitates introduction of other drugs such as volatile anesthetics to insure adequate anesthesia. A more attractive approach is the intravenous administration of 1 mg to 2 mg of glucagon, which has been shown to reverse opioid-induced

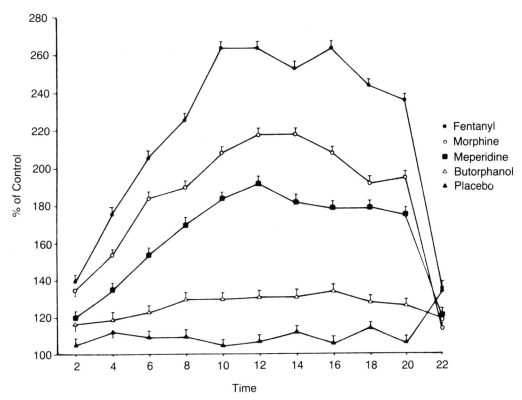

FIG. 19-13. In patients anesthetized with nitrous oxide-enflurane, the intravenous administration (over 60 seconds) of fentanyl (1.5 μg·kg^{-1}), morphine (0.15 mg·kg^{-1}), and meperidine (1 mg·kg^{-1}) resulted in increased pressures in the common bile duct (% of control). Changes in common bile duct pressures after intravenous administration of butorphanol (0.03 mg·kg^{-1}) were modest. Intravenous administration of naloxone (5 μg·kg^{-1}) 20 minutes after injection of the opioids resulted in prompt decreases in common bile duct pressures. Mean ± SD. (Radnay PA, Duncalf D, Navakovic M, Lesser ML. Common bile duct pressure changes after fentanyl, morphine, meperidine, butorphanol, and naloxone. Anesth Analg 1984;63:441–4. Reprinted with permission from IARS.)

spasm of the choledochoduodenal sphincter.[72] Hypersensitivity is a rare but potential problem with glucagon. Hyperglycemia is predictable and glucagon administered to awake patients often evokes nausea. Furthermore, glucagon should not be administered to patients with a known or suspected insulinoma or pheochromocytoma.

Emergency surgery for acute cholecystitis or common bile duct obstruction associated with vomiting may necessitate volume and electrolyte replacement. Many of these patients will have ileus and should be considered at increased risk for pulmonary aspiration of gastric contents. Delayed elimination of pancuronium has been observed in patients with obstruction of the common bile duct.[73]

REFERENCES

1. Biebuyck JF. Effects of anaesthetic agents on metabolic pathways: Fuel utilization and supply during anaesthesia. Br J Anaesth 1973;45:263–8
2. Pandele G, Chaux F, Salvadori C, et al. Thiopental pharmacokinetics in patients with cirrhosis. Anesthesiology 1983;59:123–6

3. Foldes FF, Swerdlow M, Lipschitz E, et al. Comparison of the respiratory effects of suxamethonium and suxethonium in man. Anesthesiology 1956;17:559–68

4. Klotz U, Avant GR, Hoyumpa A, et al. The effects of age and liver disease on the disposition and elimination of diazepam in adult man. J Clin Invest 1975;55:347–59

5. Thomson PD, Rowland M, Melmon KL. The influence of heart failure, liver disease, and renal failure on the disposition of lidocaine in man. Am Heart J 1971;83:417–21

6. Klotz U, McHorse TS, Wilkerson GR, et al. The effect of cirrhosis on elimination of meperidine in man. Clin Pharmacol Ther 1974;16:667–75

7. Mazoit J-X, Sandouk P, Zetlaoui P, Scherrmann J-M. Pharmacokinetics of unchanged morphine in normal and cirrhotic subjects. Anesth Analg 1987;66:293–8

8. Ferrier C, Marty J, Bouffard Y, et al. Alfentanil pharmacokinetics in patients with cirrhosis. Anesthesiology 1985;62:480–4

9. Haberer JP, Schoeffler P, Couderc E, Duvaldestin P. Fentanyl pharmacokinetics in anaesthetized patients with cirrhosis. Br J Anaesth 1982;54:1267–72

10. Reilly CS, Wood AJJ, Koshakji RP, Wood M. The effect of halothane on drug disposition in intrinsic drug metabolizing capacity and hepatic blood flow. Anesthesiology 1985;63:70–6

11. Norris CP, Barnes GE, Smith EE. Autoregulation of superior mesenteric blood flow in fasted and fed dogs. Am J Phyysiol 1979;237:H1174

12. Kennedy WF, Everett GB, Cobb LA, Allen GA. Simultaneous systemic and hepatic hemodynamic measurements during high spinal anesthesia in normal man. Anesth Analg 1970;49:1016–24

13. Cooperman LH, Warden JC, Price HL. Splanchnic circulation during nitrous oxide anesthesia and hypocarbia in normal man. Anesthesiology 1968;29:254–8

14. Gelman S, Fowler KC, Smith LR. Liver circulation and function during isoflurane and halothane anesthesia. Anesthesiology 1984;61:726–30

15. Gelman SI. Disturbances in hepatic blood flow during anesthesia and surgery. Arch Surg 1976;111:881–3

16. Cooperman LH. Effects of anesthetics on the splanchnic circulation. Br J Anaesth 1972;44:967–70

17. Benumof JL, Bookstein JJ, Saidman LJ, Harris R. Diminished hepatic arterial flow during halothane administration. Anesthesiology 1976:45:545–51

18. Eger EI. Isoflurane (Forane). A Compendium and Reference. Anaquest, A Division of BOC, Inc. Madison, WI, 1986:1–160

19. Eger EI, Calverley RK, Smith NT. Changes in blood chemistries following prolonged enflurane anesthesia. Anesth Analg 1976;55:547–9

20. Cousins MJ, Gourlay GK, Knights KM, et al. A randomized prospective controlled study of metabolism and hepatotoxicity of halothane in humans. Anesth Analg 1987;66:299–308

21. Viegas OJ, Stoelting RK. LDH_5 changes after cholecystectomy or hysterectomy in patients receiving halothane, enflurane, or fentanyl. Anesthesiology 1979;51:556–8

22. Maze M, Smith CM, Baden JM. Halothane anesthesia does not exacerbate hepatic dysfunction in cirrhotic rats. Anesthesiology 1985;62:1–5

23. Brohunt J. Liver reaction after halothane and diethyl ether anesthesia. Acta Anaesthesiol Scand 1967;11:201–20

24. Wright R, Eade OE, Chisholm OM, et al. Controlled prospective study of the effect on liver function of multiple exposures to halothane. Lancet 1975;1:817–20

25. Trowell J, Peto R, Crampton-Smith A. Controlled trial of repeated halothane anaesthetics in patients with carcinoma of the uterine cervix treated with radium. Lancet 1975;1:821–3

26. LaMont JT, Isselbacher KJ. Postoperative jaundice. N Engl J Med 1973;288:305–7

27. Dykes MHM, Gilbert JP, McPeek B. Halothane in the United States. An appraisal of the literature on halothane hepatitis and the American reaction to it. Br J Anaesth 1972;44:925–34

28. Syndman DR, Dienstag JL, Stedt B, et al. Use of IgM-hepatitis A antibody testing. Investigating a common-source, food-borne outbreak. JAMA 1981;245:827–30

29. Dane DS, Cameron CH, Briggs M. Virus-like particles in serum of patients with australia-antigen-associated hepatitis. Lancet 1970;1:695–8

30. Oxman MN. Hepatitis B vaccination of high-risk hospital personnel. Anesthesiology 1984;60:1–3

31. Berry AJ, Isaacson IJ, Hunt D, Kane M. The prevalence of hepatitis B viral markers in anesthesia personnel. Anesthesiology 1984;60:6–9

32. Francis DP, Feorino PM, Mcdougal S, et al. The safety of the hepatitis B vaccine. Inactivation of the AIDS virus during routine vaccine manufacture. JAMA 1986;256:869–72

33. Fassoulaki A, Eger EI, Johnson BH, et al. Nitrous oxide, too, is hepatotoxic in rats. Anesth Analg 1984;63:1076–80

34. Ross JAS, Monk SJ, Duffy SW. Effect of nitrous oxide on halothane-induced hepatotoxicity in

hypoxic, enzyme induced rats. Br J Anaesth 1984;56:527–33

35. Eger EI, Smuckler EA, Ferrell LD, et al. Is enflurane hepatotoxic? Anesth Analg 1986;65:21–30

36. Stoelting RK, Blitt CD, Cohen PJ, Merin RG. Hepatic dysfunction after isoflurane anesthesia. Anesth Analg 1987;66:147–53

37. Brown BR, Gandolfi AJ. Adverse effects of volatile anaesthetics. Br J Anaesth 1987;59:14–23

38. Shingu K, Eger EI, Johnson BH, et al. Effect of oxygen concentration, hyperthermia, and choice of vendor on anesthetic-induced hepatic injury in rats. Anesth Analg 1983;62:146–50

39. Shingu K, Eger EI, Johnson BH. Hypoxia per se can produce hepatic damage without death in rats. Anesth Analg 1982;61:820–3

40. Summary of the national halothane study. JAMA 1966;197:775–88

41. Mushin WW, Rosen M, Jones EV. Post-halothane jaundice in relation to previous administration of halothane. Br Med J 1971;3:18–22

42. Schemel WH. Unexpected hepatic dysfunction found by multiple laboratory screening. Anesth Analg 1976;55:810–2

43. Wataneeyawech M, Kelly KA. Hepatic diseases unsuspected before surgery. NY State J Med 1975;75:1278–81

44. Dienstag JL, Non-A, non-B hepatitis. I. Recognition, epidemiology, and clinical features. Gastroenterology 1983;85:439–62

45. Lewis RB, Blair M. Halothane hepatitis in a young child. Br J Anaesth 1982;54:349–52

46. Vergani D, Tsantoulas D, Eddleston ALWF, et al. Sensitization to halothane-altered liver components in severe hepatic necrosis after halothane anesthesia. Lancet 1978;2:801–3

47. Hoft RH, Bunker JP, Goodman HI, Gregory PB. Halothane hepatitis in three pairs of closely related women. N Engl J Med 1981;304:1023–4

48. Farrell B, Prendergast D, Murray M. Halothane hepatitis: Detection of a constitutional susceptibility factor. N Engl J Med 1985;313:1310–4

49. Boyer JL. Chronic hepatitis: A perspective on classification and determinants of prognosis. Gastroenterology 1976;70:1161–71

50. Lam KC, Lai CL, Ng RP, et al. Deleterious effect of prednisolone in HB_sAg-positive chronic active hepatitis. N Engl J Med 1981;304:380–6

51. Borland LM, Cook DR. Anesthesia for organ transplantation. In: Stoelting RK, Barash PG, Gallagher TJ, eds. Advances in Anesthesia. Chicago: Year Book Medical Publishers 1986:1–36

52. Eckardt MJ, Harford TC, Kaelber CT, et al. Health hazards associated with alcohol consumption. Anesthesiology 1981;56:648–66

53. Cello JP, Crass RA, Grendell JH, Trunkey DD. Management of the patient with hemorrhaging esophageal varices. JAMA 1986;256:1480–4

54. MacGregor RR. Alcohol and immune defense. JAMA 1986;256:1474–9

55. Banerjee SP, Sharma VK, Khanna JM. Alterations in beta-adrenergic receptor binding during ethanol withdrawal. Nature 1976;276:407–9

56. Thompson WL, Johnson AD, Maddrey WL, et al. Diazepam and paraldehyde for treatment of severe delerium tremens: A controlled trial. Ann Intern Med 1975;82:175–80

57. Strunin L. Preoperative assessment of the patient with liver dysfunction. Br J Anaesth 1978;50:25–34

58. Han YH. Why do chronic alcoholics require more anesthesia? Anesthesiology 1969;30:341–2

59. Johnston RE, Kulp RA, Smith TC. Effects of acute and chronic ethanol administration on isoflurane requirement in mice. Anesth Analg 1975;54:277–81

60. Koblin DD, Deady JE. Anaesthetic requirement in mice selectively bred for differences in ethanol sensitivity. Br J Anaesth 1981;53:5–10

61. Diaz JH, Hill GE. Hypotension with anesthesia in disulfiram-treated patients (letter). Anesthesiology 1979;51:366–8

62. Duvaldestin P, Agoston S, Henzel D, et al. Pancuronium pharmacokinetics in patients with liver cirrhosis. Br J Anaesth 1978;50:1131–6

63. Bell CF, Hunter JM, Jones RS, Utting JE. Use of atracurium and vecuronium in patients with oesophageal varices. Br J Anaesth 1985;57:160–8

64. Martyn JAJ, Matteo RS, Greenblatt DJ, Lebowitz PW, Savarese JJ. Pharmacokinetics of d-tubocurarine in patients with thermal injury. Anesth Analg 1982;61:241–6

65. Kaplan JA, Bitner RL, Dripps RD. Hypoxia, hyperdynamic circulation, and the hazards of general anesthesia in patients with hepatic cirrhosis. Anesthesiology 1971;35:427–31

66. Kaplan MM. Primary biliary cirrhosis. N Engl J Med 1987;316:521–7

67. Thistle JL, Hofmann AF, Ott BJ, Stephens DH. Chemotherapy for gallstone dissolution. I. Efficacy and safety. JAMA 1978;239:1041–6

68. Murphy P, Saleman J, Roseman DL. Narcotic anesthetic drugs. Arch Surg 1980;115:710–1

69. Radnay PA, Duncalf D, Novakovic M, Lesser ML. Common bile duct pressure changes after fentanyl, morphine, meperidine, butorphanol, and naloxone. Anesth Analg 1984;63:441–4

70. McCammon RL, Viegas OJ, Stoelting RK, Dryden GE. Naloxone reversal of choledochoduodenal sphincter spasm associated with narcotic administration. Anesthesiology 1978;48:437

71. Jones RM, Detmer M, Hill AB, Bjoraker DE. Incidence of choledochoduodenal sphincter spasm during fentanyl-supplemented anesthesia. Anesth Analg 1981;60:638–40

72. Jones RM, Fiddian-Green R, Knight PR. Narcotic-induced choledochoduodenal sphincter spasm reversed by glucagon. Anesth Analg 1980;59:946–7

73. Westra P, Vermeer GA, deLange AR, et al. Hepatic and renal disposition of pancuronium and gallamine in patients with extrahepatic cholestasis. Br J Anaesth 1981;53:331–8

20

The Gastrointestinal System

The principal function of the gastrointestinal tract is to provide the body with a continual supply of water, nutrients, and electrolytes. Each part of the gastrointestinal tract is adapted for specific functions, such as a conduit for passage of food in the esophagus, storage of food in the stomach, and digestion and absorption in the small intestine and proximal colon.

DISORDERS OF THE ESOPHAGUS

Important disorders involving the esophagus are (1) diffuse esophageal spasm, (2) chronic peptic esophagitis, (3) hiatal hernia, (4) carcinoma of the esophagus, (5) achalasia, and (6) esophageal diverticulum. Dysphagia is the classic symptom present at some stage in all disorders of the esophagus. A barium contrast examination of the esophagus should be performed in patients complaining of dysphagia.

Diffuse Esophageal Spasm

Diffuse esophageal spasm occurs most frequently in geriatric patients. Alterations in autonomic nervous system innervation are presumed to be responsible. Contraction of esophageal muscle can produce high intraluminal pressures with referred pain to the chest. Dysphagia is characteristically intermittent. Failure of food or liquid to traverse the esophagus in association with pain may occur on one occasion but not at other times, despite ingestion of similar foods. Treatment is symptomatic and often unsatisfactory. Some patients respond temporarily to nitroglycerin or long-acting nitrates.[1]

Chronic Peptic Esophagitis

The diagnostic feature of chronic peptic esophagitis is retrosternal discomfort (heartburn), which is relieved by antacids. Often, there is regurgitation of small amounts of acidic gastric contents into the pharynx. This regurgitation can occur during sleep, leading to pulmonary aspiration and the development of pneumonia. The underlying defect leading to esophagitis seems to be decreases in the resting tone of the lower esophageal sphincter.

LOWER ESOPHAGEAL SPHINCTER

The lower esophageal sphincter is a specialized structure, physiologically different from the body of the esophagus. The impor-

393

tance of this sphincter relates to its prevention of reflux of acidic gastric contents into the esophagus. When tone of this sphincter is decreased, barrier pressure (lower esophageal sphincter pressure minus gastric pressure) is reduced, and gastric fluid can reflux into the esophagus. Gastroesophageal reflux is likely to occur when barrier pressure is less than 13 cmH_2O.[2] Even more important is the fact that this reflux may be the forerunner of pulmonary aspiration.

Decreased Tone of the Lower Esophageal Sphincter. History of esophagitis in the preoperative period should alert one to the increased likelihood of esophageal reflux, especially if lower esophageal sphincter tone is further reduced by drugs used during the perioperative period. Indeed, anticholinergic drugs (atropine, scopolamine, glycopyrrolate), as used for preoperative medication, have been documented to reduce tone of the lower esophageal sphincter, leading to reductions in barrier pressures (Fig. 20-1).[3]

Theoretically, anticholinergic drugs used as part of the preoperative medication could increase the incidence of silent regurgitation and the likelihood of pulmonary aspiration during general anesthesia. Although this potentially adverse effect of anticholinergic drugs has not been documented, it has been reported that silent regurgitation of gastric contents occurs in 25 percent to 70 percent of patients receiving a general anesthetic.[4] Other drugs known to decrease lower esophageal sphincter tone include nicotine (cigarettes) and alcohol. Scleroderma and dermatomyositis may also involve the esophagus, resulting in decreases of lower esophageal sphincter tone, which leads to reflux esophagitis.

Increased Tone of the Lower Esophageal Sphincter. Increased tone of the lower esophageal sphincter might be a useful method for preventing gastroesophageal reflux. Intravenous administration of metoclopramide (10 mg)[5] and domperidone (0.15 $mg \cdot kg^{-1}$)[6] (Fig. 20-2) have been shown to increase barrier pressures by increasing resting lower esophageal sphincter tone. Furthermore, these drugs prevent reductions in lower esophageal sphincter tone produced by atropine.[5,7] Conceivably, metoclopramide or domperidone could be used

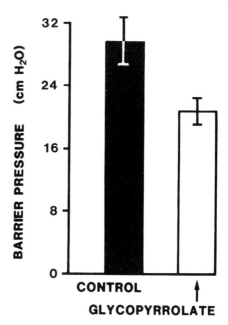

FIG. 20-1. Barrier pressure (lower esophageal sphincter pressure minus gastric pressure, Mean ± SE) was calculated before (control) and after intravenous administration of glycopyrrolate (0.3 mg) to eight healthy volunteers. Glycopyrrolate significantly reduced ($P < 0.05$) mean barrier pressure. (Data adapted from Brock-Utne JG, Rubin J, Welman S, et al. The effect of glycopyrrolate (Robinul) on the lower esophageal sphincter. Can Anaesth Soc J 1978;25:144–6)

as part of the preoperative medication, particularly in patients with known gastroesophageal reflux, to reduce the incidence of silent regurgitation during anesthesia. Succinylcholine increases lower esophageal sphincter tone, but barrier pressures are unchanged, since fasciculations are associated with increases in gastric pressure.[8]

MANAGEMENT OF ANESTHESIA.

Preoperative evaluation of patients with chronic peptic esophagitis should include careful physical examination plus radiographs of the chest to rule out the co-existence of pneumonia due to inhalation of gastric contents. The decision to include anticholinergic drugs in the preoperative medication must be weighed against the known ability of this class

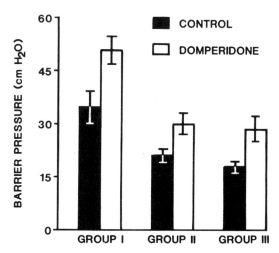

FIG. 20-2. Barrier pressure (lower esophageal sphincter pressure minus gastric pressure, Mean ± SE) was calculated before (control) and after intravenous administration of domperidone (0.2 mg·kg^{-1}) to nonpregnant patients (group I), pregnant patients with no symptoms of esophagitis (group II), and pregnant patients with a history suggestive of esophageal reflux (group III). Control barrier pressure was significantly greater ($P < 0.05$) in group I patients as compared with pregnant patients. Domperidone significantly increased ($P < 0.05$) barrier pressure in all patient groups. (Data adapted from Brock-Utne JG, Downing JW, Dimopoulos GE, et al. Effect of domperidone on lower esophageal sphincter tone in later pregnancy. Anesthesiology 1980;52:321–3)

of drugs to reduce tone of the lower esophageal sphincter.[3] Combining anticholinergic drugs with metoclopramide or domperidone will negate effects of anticholinergic drugs on the lower esophageal sphincter.[5,7] Consideration should be given to the preoperative use of antacids or H-2 antagonists, so as to increase the pH of the gastric fluid before the induction of anesthesia. Most important, protection of the airways during anesthesia by placement of a cuffed tube in the trachea is indicated.

Hiatal Hernia

Hiatal hernia is a protrusion of a portion of the stomach through the hiatus of the diaphragm and into the thoracic cavity. Esophagitis and hiatal hernia may co-exist, although each can also occur independently. Antacid therapy or administration of H-2-receptor antagonists is the initial treatment of patients with hiatal hernia who have symptoms of reflux esophagitis. Patients resistant to medical treatment may benefit from surgical restoration

of the gastroesophageal junction and fundal plication (Nissen procedure).[9] Management of anesthesia is as described for surgery in patients with chronic peptic esophagitis.

Carcinoma of the Esophagus

Carcinoma of the esophagus causes only subtle dysphagia early in its course; the disease is usually far advanced when the diagnosis is confirmed. A significant number of these patients abuse alcohol and/or smoke heavily. Therefore, the likelihood of underlying liver disease, chronic obstructive airways disease, and cross-tolerance with depressant drugs must be considered in the management of anesthesia for these patients. Furthermore, severe weight loss often parallels reductions in intravascular fluid volume, which manifests as hypotension during induction and/or maintenance of anesthesia.

Achalasia

Achalasia is a syndrome characterized by co-existence of aperistalsis and hypertonia of the lower esophageal sphincter leading to marked dilation of the esophagus. These changes are usually associated with a decreased number of neurons in the myenteric plexus of the esophageal muscle layers. Therapy may include dilation and/or myotomy of the lower esophageal sphincter and, in some cases, partial surgical resection of the esophagus.

Esophageal Diverticulum

The most important esophageal diverticulum, Zenker's diverticulum, develops in the upper esophagus. Regurgitation of previously ingested food from the diverticulum occurs frequently and predisposes patients to pulmonary aspiration. Therefore, these patients are at risk during the perioperative period, even in the absence of oral intake. Surgical excision of the diverticulum is often performed in two stages, with an initial mobilization of the pouch, followed by complete excision after granulation tissue has formed.

PEPTIC ULCER DISEASE

Anatomically and functionally, the stomach is divided into the cardia, body, and antrum (Fig. 20-3). The cardia joins the esophagus and contains mucus-secreting cells. The body of the stomach contains parietal cells, which secrete hydrogen ions and intrinsic factor, and the chief cells, which secrete pepsinogen. The antrum contains G cells, which synthesize and secrete a hormone known as gastrin.

The stomach is innervated by the vagus nerve. Therefore, increased vagal activity stimulates parietal cells to secrete hydrogen ions and the G cells to release gastrin. Gastrin enters the circulation and reaches the parietal cells,

further stimulating these cells to secrete hydrogen ions. Thus, gastrin serves as the regulatory hormone of acid secretion. Hydrogen ion secretion is also stimulated by ingestion of food and histamine-mediated activation of H-2 receptors.

The daily production of gastric fluid is about 2000 ml. Hydrogen ions when undiluted produce a pH below 1.[10] This acidic fluid is diluted and buffered by swallowed saliva. The average pH of gastric fluid was 4.7 in volunteers who had fasted for 18 hours to 24 hours, and 81 percent of these subjects had pH values above 3.5.[11] Gastric fluid does not accumulate in the stomach during fasting or physiologic sleep. It is possible, however, that stress and emotional upset, as likely in the preoperative period, may increase production of gastric hydrogen ions and fluid.[12]

Duodenal Ulcer Disease

Development of a chronic ulcer in the duodenum just beyond the pylorus constitutes peptic ulcer disease of the duodenum (Fig. 20-3). Because the clinical syndrome and response to treatment are similar for ulcers occurring in the distal antrum of the stomach and the pylorus, these are also considered to be duodenal. The highest incidence of chronic duodenal ulceration is found in men between 45 years to 65 years of age and in women older than 55 years. Causes of duodenal ulceration are not known, but both hydrochloric acid and pepsin are required for the development of ulcers. Patients with duodenal ulcer disease may have an increased number of parietal cells and accentuated gastrin release in response to ingestion of food. Emotional stress has been implicated in the development of a peptic ulcer, but no distinct personality types have emerged as predisposing factors. Aspirin, on a regular basis, is a gastric irritant and probably predisposes individuals to duodenal ulcer development. The incidence of duodenal ulcer disease seems to be increased in patients with chronic obstructive airways disease, rheumatoid arthritis, cirrhosis of the liver, and hyperparathyroidism.

The typical complaint of duodenal ulcer-

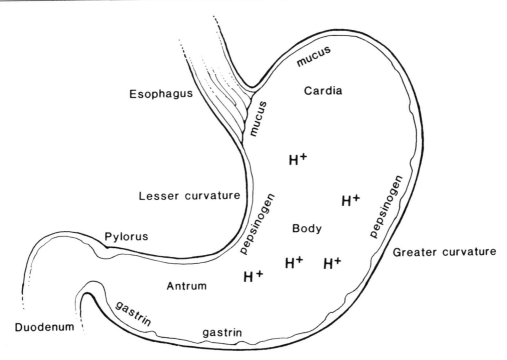

FIG. 20-3. The three major anatomic areas of the stomach are the cardia, body, and antrum. The body comprises nearly 90 percent of the stomach. Mucus-secreting cells are present in the area designated as the cardia. Parietal cells, which secrete hydrogen ions and intrinsic factor, as well as chief cells that secrete pepsinogen, are located in the body. The antrum contains G cells, which secrete gastrin. Ulceration that occurs in the distal antrum, in the pylorus, and in the duodenum immediately beyond the antrum is considered as peptic ulcer disease of the duodenum. Most gastric ulcers develop in the lesser curvature of the stomach.

ation is a deep pain in the midepigastrum, which is relieved after ingestion of food or antacids. Plasma electrolyte concentrations and liver function tests are almost always normal. Acute and chronic bleeding from ulcers may produce an iron deficiency anemia.

COMPLICATIONS

The most serious complications of duodenal ulcer disease are (1) bleeding, (2) intestinal obstruction due to edema or fibrosis in the region of the ulcer, and (3) perforation into the peritoneal cavity or pancreatic bed. Severely ill patients may be at increased risk for developing peptic ulcer disease and gastrointestinal bleeding. Hourly administration of antacids to maintain gastric fluid pH above 3.5 has been used to decrease the incidence of

bleeding. H-2-receptor antagonists may be effective alternatives to antacids. Diagnosis of intestinal obstruction depends on demonstration of retained gastric fluid volumes greater than 300 ml, 30 minutes after oral ingestion of 750 ml of saline. Surgery is necessary when intestinal obstruction does not respond to nasogastric suction. Duodenal ulcer perforation produces sudden and severe epigastric pain, which requires laparotomy and sealing of the perforation. Occasionally, acute pancreatitis results from posterior ulcers that penetrate into the pancreatic bed.

TREATMENT

Liquid antacids are the mainstay of duodenal ulcer therapy. Important potential complications of antacid therapy are (1) acid rebound, (2) milk-alkali syndrome, (3) phosphorus depletion, and (4) diarrhea. Acid rebound is the marked increase in gastric hydrogen ion secretion that takes place after neutralization of gastric contents. This complication occurs only after administration of antacids containing calcium carbonate. The milk-alkali syndrome is hypercalcemia, increased plasma creatinine concentrations, and systemic alkalosis, associated with excessive ingestion of milk plus a calcium carbonate antacid. Hypercalcemia associated with malignant tumors, renal insufficiency, or hyperparathyroidism may mimic the milk-alkali syndrome. Phosphorus depletion can occur in patients who ingest large doses of aluminum salts because these antacids bind phosphate ions in the intestinal tract and prevent their absorption. Individuals with phosphorus depletion may experience anorexia, skeletal muscle weakness, and malaise. Diarrhea due to antacid therapy reflects the fact that magnesium is poorly absorbed and water is retained in the small intestine by osmosis.

An alternative to initial therapy of peptic ulcer disease with antacids is treatment with an H-2 receptor antagonists such as cimetidine. Cimetidine relieves the pain of duodenal ulcer in about 70 percent of patients within 4 weeks.[9] The rate of healing of duodenal ulcers can be evaluated most accurately by endoscopy. Intractable peptic ulcer disease is treated by proximal gastric vagotomy with partial gastrectomy.[9] Delayed gastric emptying is a potential complication of vagotomy. Anemia is common after peptic ulcer surgery. Osteomalacia develops in 15 percent to 30 percent of patients after partial gastrectomy. In otherwise asymptomatic patients, elevated plasma alkaline phosphatase concentrations may be reflections of previously unsuspected bone disorders.

Anticholinergic drug therapy for duodenal ulcer disease is based on the fact that these drugs competitively inhibit the actions of acetylcholine, which stimulates acid-secreting cells in the stomach. Effectiveness of anticholinergic drug therapy is limited by dose-related adverse side effects, such as blurring of vision and urinary retention.

Gastrin Secreting Tumors (Gastrinomas)

Gastrinomas secrete gastrin, which, when released into the circulation, stimulates parietal cells in the body of the stomach to produce massive amounts of hydrochloric acid. When gastrinomas are associated with persistent pain, multiple ulcers, and diarrhea, they are designated the Zollinger-Ellison syndrome. Treatment is initially with H-2-receptor antagonists in attempts to control hyperacidity before surgical resection of the gastrinoma is attempted. If the preoperative response to H-2-receptor antagonists is favorable and a resectable tumor is present, no further surgery is necessary.[9] Total gastrectomy is necessary when medical control of hyperactivity is not optimal or when primary tumors cannot be excised. Gastrinomas are often malignant with metastases. Adenomas of the pituitary, parathyroid, pancreas, or adrenal glands occur in about 20 percent of patients with gastrinomas.

Management of anesthesia must consider gastric hypersecretion and the likelihood of large gastric fluid volumes at the time of induction of anesthesia. Esophageal reflux is common in these patients despite the ability of gastrin to increase lower esophageal sphincter tone. Depletion of intravascular fluid volume and electrolyte imbalance (hypokalemia and metabolic alkalosis) may accompany profuse watery diarrhea. Hypoproteinemia could alter pharmacokinetics of injected drugs, and cimetidine could influence the rate of hepatic breakdown of some drugs, reflecting inhibition of cytochrome P-450 oxidative pathways. Hyperparathyroidism with hypercalcemia, hyperthyroidism, acromegaly, and excess corticosteroid secretion are associated endocrine abnormalities that could influence management of anesthesia in these patients.

Gastric Ulcer Disease

Most gastric ulcers occur on the lesser curvature of the stomach (Fig. 20-3) and are associated with normal gastric hydrogen ion secretion or even hypochlorhydria. Weight loss is common due to the associated pain and anorexia. Malignancy must be considered, especially if gastric acid secretion is absent. Surgical excision of the ulcer is indicated if complete healing has not occurred after 12 weeks of medical therapy with antacids. Surgical procedures involving partial gastric resection are associated with the risk of the dumping syndrome characterized by nausea, vomiting, diarrhea, tachycardia, postural hypotension, and diaphoresis following food intake.

IRRITABLE BOWEL SYNDROME (SPASTIC OR MUCOUS COLITIS)

Patients with irritable bowel syndrome complain of generalized abdominal discomfort, often confined to the left lower quadrant. There may be constipation but more commonly the frequency of stools is increased, and the feces are often covered with mucus. Many patients have associated symptoms of vasomotor instability, including tachycardia, hyperventilation, fatigue, diaphoresis, and headaches. Air trapped in the splenic flexure may produce pain in the left shoulder, which radiates down the left arm. This latter symptom is the reason for the occasional designation of this disease as the splenic flexure syndrome.

Despite the frequent occurrence of irritable bowel syndrome, there is no known etiologic agent or structural or biochemical defect. The syndrome appears to be an intense intraabdominal response to emotional tension.

INFLAMMATORY BOWEL DISEASE

Ulcerative colitis and granulomatous ileocolitis (Crohn's disease) are inflammatory bowel diseases. The prognosis and treatment of each disease differs.

Ulcerative Colitis

Ulcerative colitis is an inflammatory disease of the rectum and distal colon, which in severe cases may involve the entire colon. The cause is unknown, and remissions and exacerbations are common. The disease is more common among women and individuals of Jewish extraction. Symptomatic ulcerative colitis usually occurs between 25 years and 45 years of age. The majority of patients have mild disease, characterized by intermittent diarrhea and occasional cramping abdominal pain. Fatigue, low grade fever, and weight loss occur during exacerbations.

Associated complications of ulcerative colitis are colonic and extracolonic (Table 20-1). Toxic megacolon is a form of fulminant ulcerative colitis manifested by the sudden onset of high fever (40 degrees Celsius), tachycardia, dehydration, and marked dilation of the colon. Intestinal perforation is associated with marked rebound pain, except when high doses of corticosteroids mask the symptoms. Extracolonic complications of ulcerative colitis include erythema nodosum, inflammation of the iris and conjunctiva, migratory arthritis, ankylosing spondylitis, and hepatic dysfunction. Liver dysfunction may manifest as fatty infiltration, pericholangitis, or cirrhosis. Carci-

TABLE 20-1. Complications Associated with Ulcerative Colitis

Complications	Incidence (%)
Colonic	
Toxic megacolon	1–3
Intestinal perforation	3
Carcinoma of colon	2.5–5
Hemorrhage	4
Stricture of colon	10
Extracolonic	
Erythema nodosum	3
Iritis	5–10
Ankylosing arthritis	5–10
Fatty infiltration of liver	40
Pericholangitis	30–50
Cirrhosis of liver	3

(Data from Gray GM. Inflammatory bowel disease. In: Rubenstein E, Federman DD, eds. Scientific American Medicine. New York. Scientific American. 1980;4IV:1–17)

noma of the colon is ten times more likely in affected patients leading some to recommend frequent colonoscopies (every 1 year to 3 years) with multiple mucosal biopsies in hopes of detecting dysplastic changes that antedate the development of cancer. Nevertheless, there is no evidence that surveillance colonoscopy is useful.[13]

Patients with mild ulcerative colitis are best managed with antidiarrheal drugs and sulfa drugs such as sulfasalazine. Patients with severe disease require hospitalization to facilitate restoration of extracellular fluid volume and electrolytes. Intravenous administration of corticosteroids or adrenocorticotropic hormone is indicated in these patients. A proctocolectomy may be necessary if there is no response to therapy.

Granulomatous Ileocolitis (Crohn's Disease)

Granulomatous ileocolitis manifests as chronic inflammation of all layers of the bowel. The peak incidence of this disease is between the age of 20 years and 40 years. The cause is unknown. About one-half of patients have both ileal and colonic involvement; the remainder are equally divided among those with only small intestine disease (regional ileitis) or with disease confined to the colon.

Granulomatous ileocolitis, in contrast to ulcerative colitis, is chronic and slowly progressive, seldom leads to cancer, and has a low mortality rate. Another difference is that surgery may not be curative; in fact, surgery is often followed by recurrence of this disease. Extracolonic complications are similar in prevalance to those observed in patients with ulcerative colitis (Table 20-1). Mild anemia is common, and reduced plasma albumin concentrations reflect protein loss through diseased bowel mucosa. Intra-abdominal fistulas or perirectal abscesses occur in nearly 50 percent of patients. A high percentage of patients with granulomatous ileocolitis have renal stones and gallstones.

Treatment of granulomatous ileocolitis is similar to that of ulcerative colitis. Corticosteroids produce a prompt remission but must be continued chronically to maintain asymptomatic states. Enteral or parenteral nutrition is indicated when weight loss and malnutrition are prominent.

Pseudomembranous Enterocolitis

The etiology of pseudomembranous enterocolitis is unknown. Commonly associated events include antibiotic therapy (especially clindamycin and lincomycin), bowel obstruction, uremia, congestive heart failure, and intestinal ischemia. Clinical manifestations include fever, watery diarrhea, dehydration, hypotension, cardiac dysrhythmias, skeletal muscle weakness, intestinal ileus, and metabolic acidosis.

Management of Anesthesia

Surgical treatment of inflammatory bowel disease most often involves resection of varying lengths and portions of the gastrointestinal tract. Management of anesthesia requires preoperative evaluation of intravascular fluid volume and electrolyte status, and assessment of both colonic and extracolonic complications (Table 20-1) that may be associated with the inflammatory bowel process. For example, anemia due to chronic gastrointestinal hemorrhage may introduce the need for preoperative transfusion of whole blood or erythrocytes. Arthritis may influence management of the upper airway. Underlying liver disease should be considered in selection of drugs used to maintain anesthesia and provide skeletal muscle relaxation. The need to provide additional corticosteroids in the perioperative period is introduced when these drugs have been used as part of medical therapy. Adverse effects associated with enteral or parenteral nutrition must also be remembered if hyperalimentation has been used preoperatively (see Chapter 24).

Traction on abdominal mesentery in association with surgical mobilization and resection of portions of the gastrointestinal tract may cause afferent sympathetic nervous system stimulation that results in vasodilation of the splanchnic vasculature.[14] This vasodilation may manifest as reductions in blood pressure, although compensatory increases in cardiac output often mask this response. Alterations in heart rate and central venous pressure in response to traction on abdominal mesentery are not predictable.

Reversal of nondepolarizing muscle relaxants with anticholinesterase drugs will increase intraluminal pressures in the gastrointestinal tract (Fig. 20-4).[15] Inclusion of atropine or glycopyrrolate does not modify this effect on the gastrointestinal tract. It has been suggested, but not proven, that these drug-induced increases in intraluminal pressure increase the risk of colon suture line dehiscence.[16,17] Until definitive data are available, it is reasonable to consider carefully the advantages of pharmacologic reversal of neuromuscular blockade relative to the potential adverse effects on new suture lines in the colon.

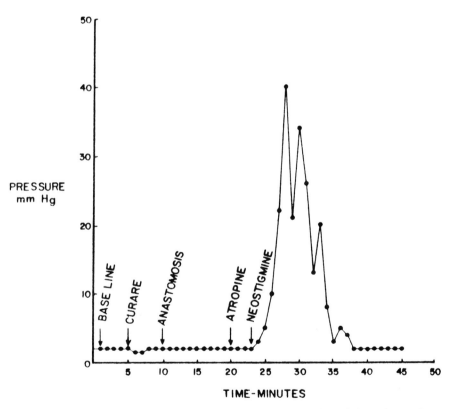

FIG. 20-4. Intraluminal colonic pressures were measured after division of the colon and a standard two-layer anastomosis. Data are from a single dog. Anesthesia was with intravenous pentobarbital and skeletal muscle paralysis was produced with d-tubocurarine (curare, 0.2 mg·kg^{-1}). Antagonism of neuromuscular blockade was with the rapid intravenous administration of atropine (0.012 mg·kg^{-1}) followed by neostigmine (0.035 mg·kg^{-1}). Intracolonic pressures were transiently increased after administration of neostigmine. Nevertheless, there was no evidence that this muscarinic-induced elevation of intracolonic pressures caused disruption of the freshly completed bowel anastomosis. (Yellin YE, Newman J, Donovan AJ. Neostigmine-induced hyperperistalsis. Effects of security on colonic anastomoses. Arch Surg 1973;106:779–81. Copyright 1973, American Medical Association.)

CARCINOID TUMORS

Carcinoid tumors arise from enterochromaffin tissues and are typically found in the gastrointestinal tract. Indeed, carcinoid tumors are the most common neoplasms of the small intestine, with the highest incidence being in the appendix, where these tumors can mimic acute appendicitis. On occasion, carcinoid tumors arise in the bronchi, where they are histologically indistinguishable from undifferentiated small cell carcinomas. Rarely, carcinoid tumors arise from the ovaries. The estimated incidence of carcinoid tumors is 8 per 100,000 persons. Diagnosis of carcinoid tumor is supported by elevated urinary excretion of 5-hydroxyindoleacetic acid, which is the degradation produce of serotonin.

Carcinoid Syndrome

Carcinoid syndrome is present when vasoactive substances released from the cells of carcinoid tumors results in clinical symptoms.[18] These substances include serotonin, prostaglandins, histamine, and kallikreins. Kallikreins are important because they activate a plasma factor (kininogen), which subsequently produces a group of polypeptides (kinins), which includes bradykinin. Normally, release of vasoactive substances produces minimal if any symptoms, as the liver is able to inactivate effectively these substances before they reach the systemic circulation. Manifestations of the carcinoid syndrome occur when output of vasoactive substances overwhelms the ability of the liver to inactivate these substances. Hepatic metastases are usually present when manifestations of carcinoid syndrome develop. Indeed, presence of carcinoid tumors in the liver may permit direct access to the circulation of vasoactive substances produced by these metastatic cells. Nevertheless, only about 5 percent of patients with carcinoid tumors develop the carcinoid syndrome.[19]

Carcinoid tumors in the bronchi or ovaries may produce symptoms of the carcinoid syndrome earlier than similar tumors located in

TABLE 20-2. Manifestations of the Carcinoid Syndrome

Bronchoconstriction—asthma
Tricuspid regurgitation and/or pulmonary stenosis
Premature atrial beats and supraventricular tachydysrhythmias
Episodic cutaneous flushing or cyanosis
Venous telangiectasia
Chronic abdominal pain and diarrhea
Hepatomegaly
Hyperglycemia
Decreased plasma albumin concentrations

the jejenum or ileum because pulmonary or ovarian tumors do not drain into the portal venous system. As a result, vasoactive substances are not inactivated in the liver. Carcinoid tumors in the appendix have never been reported to produce the carcinoid syndrome.

Vasoactive substances released by carcinoid tumors produce changes in the respiratory tract, heart, skin, and gastrointestinal tract (Table 20-2). These changes may be life-threatening and constitute the carcinoid syndrome.

RESPIRATORY TRACT

Bronchoconstriction in patients with known carcinoid tumors reflects release of vasoactive substances capable of producing constriction of airway smooth muscle. Conventional therapy for bronchospasm is not helpful. Indeed, catecholamines are known to provoke release of serotonin and kallikreins from tumor cells. Corticosteroids, although effective as prophylactic measures by stabilizing lysosomal membranes and preventing the generation of kinins, are probably ineffective once vasoactive substances have been liberated.

CARDIOVASCULAR SYSTEM

Tricuspid regurgitation or pulmonary stenosis represent the type of right-sided valvular heart lesions, which may result from valve cusp distortion produced by metastases from carcinoid tumors. Valves on the left side of the heart are spared, which may reflect the ability of pulmonary parenchymal cells to inactivate vasoactive substances. Patients with the carcinoid syndrome have a high incidence of premature atrial beats and supraventricular tachydysrhythmias.

SKIN

Episodic cutaneous flushing initially involves the face and neck and with increasing intensity and duration may spread to involve the trunk and upper extremities. During cutaneous flushing, arterial blood pressure is usually reduced, and cardiac output is likely to be elevated. Bradykinin is a potent vasodilator and seems the most likely cause of cutaneous flushing. Venous telangiectasia, when present, is most prominent on the nose, upper lip, and butterfly area of the face. Cyanosis of the face and upper body may also be present.

GASTROINTESTINAL TRACT

Chronic intermittent abdominal pain and diarrhea are manifestations of the carcinoid syndrome. Diarrhea is most likely due to elaboration of serotonin by carcinoid tumor cells and is often effectively controlled with the antiserotonin drug methysergide. Flushing attacks associated with gastric carcinoids are mediated by histamine and can be prevented by combinations of H-1 and H-2-receptor antagonists. Hepatomegaly often reflects extensive hepatic metastases from carcinoid tumors.

MISCELLANEOUS FINDINGS

Mild hyperglycemia and decreased plasma albumin levels may be present in patients with carcinoid tumors. Hyperglycemia most likely reflects the ability of serotonin to mimic metabolic effects of epinephrine and to stimulate glycogenolysis and gluconeogenesis. Decreased concentrations of plasma albumin may reflect diversion of tryptophan from production of protein to synthesis of serotonin. Normally, less than 2 percent of dietary tryptophan is used for synthesis of serotonin, but in patients with carcinoid tumors, up to 60 percent of this amino acid can be used by the tumor cells.[19]

Management of Anesthesia

Carcinoid tumors and their manifestations have important implications for the management of anesthesia.[20] Patients with the carcinoid syndrome may present in the operating room for primary resection of the carcinoid tumor or removal of hepatic metastases. On occasion, these patients may require replacement of a heart valve. Preoperative preparation of these patients with drugs that block effects of vasoactive substances secreted by carcinoid tumor cells would seem logical. For example, effects of histamine may be attenuated by combinations of diphenhydramine and cimetidine, so as to block both H-1 and H-2 receptors. Cyproheptadine (Periactin) has both antiserotonin and antihistamine activity and in animals effectively blocks histamine- and serotonin-induced bronchoconstriction.[21] The usual adult dose of this drug is 4 mg orally three to four times daily. The most prominent side effect is drowsiness. Ketanserin is a competitive serotonin receptor antagonist, which has been administered to these patients to attenuate and treat vasoconstricting, bronchoconstricting, or platelet-aggregating effects of serotonin.[22] This drug appears to be particularly useful in treatment of hypertensive episodes that occur in patients with carcinoid tumors. Long-acting analogs of somatostatin may be effective in controlling flushing and diarrhea. In one report, a life-threatening carcinoid crisis was promptly reversed by the intravenous administration of a somatostatin analog.[23] Somatostatin is a releasing factor secreted by the hypothalamus, which inhibits subsequent release of endogenous peptides including serotonin. Aminocaproic acid has been advocated as an antibradykinin drug, but its efficacy has not been proven, and its use may introduce such serious complications as systemic clotting.[20] Administration of morphine to these patients is not recommended, since this opioid may stimulate release of serotonin and histamine. Droperidol may have mild antiserotonin activity, but this desirable effect is often offset with undesirable responses that include prolonged sedation or dysphoria. Adequate preoperative hydration to minimize intraoperative hypotension is important.

No specific anesthetic drugs or techniques have been proven superior in patients with carcinoid tumors.[13] Since hypotension may stimulate release of vasoactive substances from tumor cells, it is important to consider potential adverse effects of deep anesthesia or effects of peripheral sympathetic nervous system blockade as produced by regional anesthetic techniques. Catecholamines are known to activate kallikreins. This would theoretically detract from the use of ketamine or sympathomimetic drugs that elevate blood pressure by stimulating release of endogenous norepinephrine. Drugs known to be associated with histamine release (d-tubocurarine, metocurine, atracurium, succinylcholine, morphine) must be used cautiously. Increased central nervous system serotonin levels are associated with sedation, suggesting that anesthetic requirements might be decreased in these patients.

Intraoperative complications that have been observed in these patients include hypotension, bronchospasm, and occasionally hypertension and tachycardia, particularly during manipulation of the tumors.[22] Tachycardia and hypertension are most likely due to serotonin release and are managed by increasing the depth of anesthesia or a administration of vasodilators or a specific antiserotonin drug such as ketanserin. There is no satisfactory anesthetic regimen for the prevention or treatment of bronchospasm. In one case report, bronchospasm was unresponsive to all forms of therapy, including inhalation of halothane and intravenous administration of ketamine.[24] All factors considered, general anesthesia with nitrous oxide and short-acting opioids, plus muscle relaxants that produce minimal circulatory effects, is a logical approach.

DISEASES OF THE PANCREAS

Acute Pancreatitis

Conditions that predispose to acute pancreatitis include excessive ingestion of alcohol, gallstones, hypercalcemia, blunt abdominal trauma, and posterior penetrating peptic ulcer disease. The hallmark of acute pancreatitis is elevated plasma amylase concentrations. Patients are acutely ill, with excruciating pain in the epigastrium and a moderately elevated body temperature. Breathing may be painful if there are associated pleural effusions, and respiratory failure may occur. White blood cell counts are elevated. Bilirubin and alkaline phosphatase concentrations may be increased due to compression of the common bile duct by the edematous head of the pancreas or a stone in the common bile duct. Intestinal ileus is common. Hypotension and hypovolemia are related to exudation of plasma into the pancreatic area. Acute renal failure may occur if hypotension is prolonged. Hypocalcemia may develop, and patients should be observed for signs of tetany. Severe hemorrhagic pancreatitis may result in diabetic coma. Treatment of acute pancreatitis is with nasogastric suction plus fluid and electrolyte repletion with or without peritoneal dialysis. Pancreatectomy is best reserved for fulminant pancreatitis that is unresponsive to other treatments. Hypoglycemia is a life-threatening risk after this surgery.[9]

Chronic Pancreatitis

Chronic pancreatitis characteristically presents in emaciated men who are a chronic alcoholics. Predisposing conditions in addition to alcoholism include severe biliary tract disease and blunt trauma, which may have occurred many years earlier. Plasma amylase concentrations are often normal during recurrent episodes of chronic pancreatitis. Jaundice occurs in about 10 percent of patients. Maldigestion of fat and protein supervenes when about 80 percent of the pancreas is destroyed. Mild diabetes mellitus is common. Fatty liver infiltration is particularly likely when chronic alcohol abuse is also present.

Pancreatic Neoplasms

Hallmarks of pancreatic duct cell adenocarcinoma are persistent epigastric pain, anorexia, and weight loss. Appearance of jaundice usually indicates the disease is incurable. Complications of pancreatic neoplasms include gastrointestinal bleeding and diabetes mellitus.

GASTROINTESTINAL BLEEDING

Gastrointestinal bleeding is responsible for about 2 percent of all adult hospital admissions in the United States. About 10 percent to 20 percent of these patients undergo surgery for control of bleeding. In almost one-half of patients the cause of bleeding is not determined. Specific sites of bleeding are suggested by the history. For example, epigastric pain that precedes passage of black stools by 1 week to 2 weeks suggests peptic ulcer disease. Weight loss, anorexia, and chronic anemia may reflect gastric carcinoma. Lower abdominal pain, fever, and bloody diarrhea are common in the presence of diverticulitis. Passage of bright red blood via a nasogastric tube suggests a Mallory-Weiss tear at the esophagogastric junction, hemorrhagic esophagitis, or bleeding esophageal varices.

Immediate attention should be given to assessing the degree of hypovolemia produced by gastrointestinal bleeding. Heart rate increases of 10 beats·min^{-1} to 20 beats·min^{-1} and decreases in systolic blood pressure of 10 mmHg to 20 mmHg, which occur when patients sit upright from a reclining position, suggest that significant blood loss has occurred. Hematocrits may be normal despite significant blood loss, reflecting hemoconcentration. Blood urea nitrogen concentrations may exceed 40 mg·dl^{-1} when gastrointestinal bleeding is severe, reflecting the absorbed nitrogen load secondary to blood in the small intestine. Plasma creatinine concentrations in this situation are usually normal. Prolonged hypotension secondary to massive gastrointestinal bleeding may produce centrilobular liver necrosis, as evidenced by massive elevations of plasma transaminase enzyme concentrations. In addition, prolonged hypotension from hemorrhage is associated with mesenteric insufficiency, acute renal failure, and myocardial ischemia.

Most acute gastrointestinal bleeding is self-limited, such that 80 percent to 90 percent of patients treated with conservative medical management cease bleeding within 24 hours to 48 hours. Demonstration of a bleeding arterial site by angiography may be treated by intravenous or selective intra-arterial infusions of vasopressin. Localized vasoconstriction resulting from vasopressin will control bleeding in over one-half of patients. A risk of vasopressin infusions is selective coronary artery vasoconstriction. Direct intravascular injection of sclerosants into esophageal varices (sclerotherapy) controls bleeding in over 90 percent of patients.[9] Portacaval shunts may be indicated for emergency control of bleeding from esophageal varices, although mortality is often great. Prophylaxis against stress-related bleeding from the gastrointestinal tract may be provided by maintaining gastric fluid pH above 3.5 by administration of antacids or H-2-receptor antagonists.

DISEASES PRODUCING MALABSORPTION

Malabsorption classically refers to altered food absorption due to disease or resection of the small intestine. In addition, deficiencies of pancreatobiliary secretions may produce severe nutritional deficiencies. Quantitative analysis of fecal fat excretion (steatorrhea) is the most sensitive diagnostic test for detecting malabsorption or maldigestion. Malabsorption caused by small intestine diseases differs from malabsorption caused by deficiencies of pancreatobiliary secretions (Table 20-3). For example, weight loss, vitamin deficiencies, and anemia due to folic acid deficiencies are more likely with small intestine diseases than with pancreatobiliary diseases. Plasma albumin levels below 2.5 g·dl^{-1}, reflecting protein loss through damaged gastrointestinal mucosa, are common with diseases of the small intestine. Hypocalcemia and hypomagnesemia may result in tetany and mental confusion in patients with small intestine diseases. The hallmark of pancreatobiliary diseases is marked steatorrhea.

TABLE 20-3. Differential Features of Malabsorption

Features	Small Intestine Disease	Deficiency of Pancreatobiliary Secretions
Weight loss	Marked	Mild
Vitamin deficiency (A,B,E,K,B$_{12}$)	Common	Rare
Anemia	Common (usually megaloblastic)	Rare (unless associated with alcoholism)
Hypoalbuminemia	Common	Rare
Hypomagnesemia	Common	Rare
Xylose absorption	Decreased	Normal
Steatorrhea	Moderate (less than 35 g day^{-1})	Marked (40–80 g day^{-1})

(Data from Gray GM. Diseases producing malabsorption and maldigestion. In: Rubenstein E, Federman DD, eds. Scientific American Medicine. New York. Scientific American, 1980;4 XI:1–15)

Diseases of the Small Intestine Causing Malabsorption

DIABETES MELLITUS

A significant number of patients with diabetes mellitus develop autonomic nervous system neuropathy that causes decreased activity of the small intestine. Malabsorption occurs in nearly one-fourth of these patients and is most likely related to bacterial overgrowth. Watery diarrhea is prominent, and fecal fat excretion is increased. Broad spectrum antibiotics may be effective in treatment of this disorder.

CELIAC SPRUE

Celiac sprue is characterized by weight loss despite an adequate appetite. Megaloblastic anemia is common. Women of short stature (mean height 150 cm) are most often affected. Treatment is removal of gluten from the diet.

TROPICAL SPRUE

Individuals living in tropical regions, including Puerto Rico, may develop small intestine lesions that result in severe malabsorption, with weight loss and marked megaloblastic

anemia. The etiology is most likely an infectious agent, which remains unidentified. Both anemia and malabsorption are responsive to folic acid therapy.

SMALL INTESTINE RESECTION

Extensive jejunal resection results in only mild malabsorption because of compensation by the ileum. In contrast, resection of 75 percent or more of the ileum results in severe malnutrition, diarrhea, electrolyte imbalances, and vitamin B$_{12}$ insufficiency. There is often an increased incidence of cholelithiasis and nephrolithiasis. These complications of extensive small bowel resection are similar to those that follow jejunoileal bypass surgery for treatment of morbid obesity. In addition, fatty liver infiltration is a common complication associated with intestinal bypass surgery. Gastric bypass surgery, in which a fundic pouch is created by transection or stapling of the stomach so as to provide early satiety, seems the preferred surgical method to treat morbid obesity.

ISCHEMIC DISEASE

Atherosclerosis of blood vessels supplying the small intestine results in inadequate blood flow, which is manifested as abdominal pain 15 minutes to 2 hours after a meal. Malabsorption is usually not severe, but weight loss may occur, since patients avoid eating to escape postprandial discomfort. Most of these patients also have associated vascular disease at such other sites as the brain and heart.

RADIATION ENTERITIS

Treatment of intra-abdominal malignant processes, particularly lymphomas, with radiation may produce enteritis and malabsorption. Corticosteroids may be necessary in management of chronic radiation enteritis.

Diseases of the Pancreatobiliary System Causing Maldigestion

CHRONIC PANCREATITIS

Chronic alcoholism that leads to chronic pancreatitis is the most common cause of pancreatic exocrine insufficiency. A significant percentage of these patients also have diabetes mellitus.

BILE SALT DEFICIENCY

Bile salt deficiency may occur as a result of bacterial overgrowth, regional enteritis, or extensive ileal resection. Resulting malabsorption is usually mild and rarely nutritionally significant, although bile salts are necessary for absorption of fat-soluble vitamins.

POSTGASTRECTOMY STEATORRHEA

Destruction of the pyloric sphincter may allow nutrients to precede pancreatic secretions in transit through the small intestine, producing maldigestion syndromes.

DIVERTICULOSIS AND DIVERTICULITIS

Colonic diverticulosis is characterized by multiple outpouchings of the colonic mucosa, most often located in the sigmoid colon. Colonic diverticula are seen on barium enema examinations in over 30 percent of patients more than 60 years of age. The pathogenesis of diverticulosis has not been clearly established. Despite the frequency of diverticulosis, serious complications such as bleeding or diverticular inflammation are rare. Less than 2 percent of patients experience bleeding, but when it does occur, the degree of hemorrhage is often massive.[25] The majority of patients cease bleeding spontaneously. Inflammation develops most often in narrow-necked diverticula located in the sigmoid colon. Left lower quadrant abdominal pain with fever and chills is characteristic. Surgical therapy is indicated when favorable responses to medical management (nasogastric suction, intravenous fluids, and antibiotics) do not occur within 24 hours to 48 hours. After acute attacks have subsided, elective surgery may be indicated if frequent and recurrent attacks of diverticulitis have occurred or if there is evidence of fistula formation or low-grade intestinal obstruction.

REFERENCES

1. Orlando RC, Bozmski EM. Clinical and manometric effects of nitroglycerin in diffuse esophageal spasm. N Engl J Med 1973;289:23–5
2. Haddad JK. Relation of gastroesophageal reflux to yield sphincter pressures. Gastroenterology 1970;58:175–84
3. Brock-Utne JG, Welman RS, Dimopoulos GE, et al. The effect of glycopyrrolate (Robinul) on the lower esophageal sphincter. Can Anaesth Soc J 1978;25:144–6
4. Blitt CD, Gutman HL, Cohen DD, et al. Silent regurgitation and aspiration with general anesthesia. Anesth Analg 1970;49:707–13
5. Brock-Utne JG, Rubin J, Downing JW, et al. The administration of metoclopramide with atropine (a drug interaction effect on the gastroesophageal sphincter in man). Anaesthesia 1976;31:1186–90

6. Brock-Utne JG, Downing JW, Dimopoulos GE, et al. Effect of domperidone on lower esophageal sphincter tone in late pregnancy. Anesthesiology 1980;52:321–3

7. Brock-Utne JG. Domperidone antagonizes the relaxant effect of atropine on the lower esophageal sphincter. Anesth Analg 1980;59:921–4

8. Smith G, Dalling R, Williams TIR. Gastrooesophageal pressure gradient changes produced by induction of anaesthesia and suxamethonium. Br J Anaesth 1978;50:1137–42

9. Welch CE, Malt RA. Abdominal surgery. N Engl J Med 1983;308:624–33; 685–95; 753–60

10. Hollander F. Composition and mechanism of formation of gastric acid secretion. Science 1949;110:57–63

11. Kuna S. The pH of gastric juice in the normal resting stomach. Arch Int Pharmacodyn Ther 1964;151:79–97

12. Mahl GF, Karpe R. Emotions and hydrochloric acid secretion during psychoanalytic hours. Psychosom Med 1953;15:312–26

13. Collins RH, Feldman M, Fordtran JS. Colon cancer, dysplasia, and surveillance in patients with ulcerative colitis. A critical review. N Engl J Med 1987;316:1654–8

14. Seltzer JL, Ritter DE, Starsnic MA, Marr AT. The hemodynamic response to traction on the abdominal mesentery. Anesthesiology 1985;63:96–9

15. Yellin AE, Newman J, Conovan AJ. Neostigmine-induced hyperperistalsis. Effects on security of colonic anastomoses. Arch Surg 1973;106:779–81

16. Aitkenhead AR. Anaesthesia and bowel surgery. Br J Anaesth 1984;56:95–101

17. Hunter AR. Colorectal surgery for cancer: The anaesthetist's contribution? Br J Anaesth 1986;58:825–6

18. Oates JA. The carcionoid syndrome. N Engl J Med 1986;315:702–4

19. Weidner FA, Ziter FMH. Carcinoid tumors of the gastrointestinal tract. JAMA 1981;245:1153–5

20. Mason RA, Steans PA. Carcinoid syndrome: Its relevance to the anaesthetist. Anaesthesia 1976;31:228–42

21. Stone CA, Wenger HC, Ludden CT, et al. Antiserotonin-antihistamine properties of cyproheptadine. J Pharmacol Exp Ther 1961;131:73–84

22. Casthely PA, Tablons M, Griepp RB, et al. Ketanserin in the preoperative and intraoperative management of a patient with carcinoid tumor undergoing tricuspid valve replacement. Anesth Analg 1986;65:809–11

23. Marsh HM, Martin JK, Kvols LK, et al. Carcinoid crisis during anesthesia: Successful treatment with a somatostatin analogue. Anesthesiology 1987;66:89–91

24. Miller R, Boulukos PA, Warner RRP. Failure of halothane and ketamine to alleviate carcinoid syndrome-induced bronchospasm during anesthesia. Anesth Analg 1980;59:621–3

25. Heald RJ, Ray IE. Bleeding in diverticular disease of the colon. Proc R Soc Med 1972;65:779–82

21

Renal Disease

The kidneys are essential for maintaining an ideal total body water content, as well as ensuring that the solute composition of this water is optimal. Co-existing renal disease can predispose patients to perioperative morbidity and mortality. Furthermore, the possibility of impaired renal function during the intraoperative and postoperative period should be considered in otherwise healthy patients undergoing major operations.

Management of patients in the perioperative period with respect to renal function requires an understanding of the (1) functional anatomy of the kidneys, (2) glomerular filtration rate, (3) renal blood flow, (4) endocrine functions of the kidneys, (5) tests used for evaluation of renal function, (6) effects of anesthetics on renal function, (7) changes characteristic of chronic renal disease, (8) management of anesthesia for patients with chronic renal disease, (9) differential diagnosis of perioperative oliguria, and (10) knowledge of disease processes involving the kidneys. Management of anesthesia for renal transplantation and transurethral resection of the prostate also introduces unique considerations.

FUNCTIONAL ANATOMY OF THE KIDNEY

The functional unit of the kidney is the nephron (Fig. 21-1). Each kidney contains approximately 1.2 million nephrons; this number does not increase after birth. The two components of nephrons are the glomerulus and the renal tubule.

Glomerulus

The glomerulus is a network of capillaries originating from an afferent arteriole. These capillaries are surrounded by the dilated blind end of the nephron, known as Bowman's capsule. Each tuft of capillaries arises from a single afferent arteriole and is drained by an efferent arteriole. Therefore, glomerular capillaries are unique because they are the only capillaries anatomically interposed between two sets of arterioles. As a consequence of this anatomic arrangement, the hydrostatic pressure inside these capillaries can be varied by changing the tone of either the afferent or efferent arterioles.

Renal Tubule

The renal tubule consists of the proximal convoluted tubule, the loop of Henle, and the distal convoluted tubule. Distal ends of several distal convoluted tubules join to form collecting tubules, which subsequently drain into the renal pelvis.

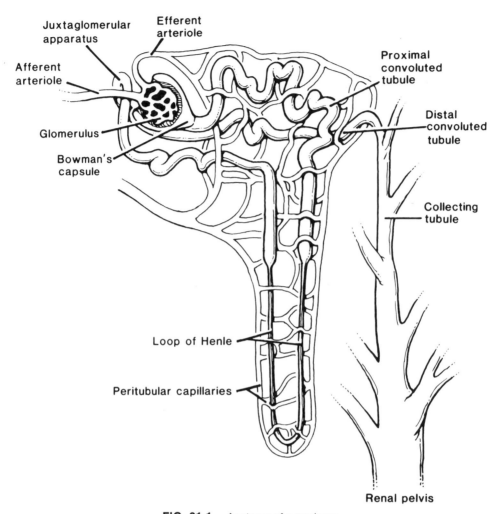

FIG. 21-1.   Anatomy of a nephron.

PROXIMAL CONVOLUTED TUBULE

The proximal convoluted tubule is a direct continuation of Bowman's capsule. About 65 percent of the total filtered sodium, chloride, and water is reabsorbed from proximal convoluted tubules back into peritubular capillaries. Reabsorption of sodium into peritubular capillaries is against a concentration gradient and, therefore, requires the expenditure of energy. Furthermore, reabsorption of sodium is obligatory in that it is not related to the need of the body for sodium or water. Conversely,

reabsorption of chloride and water back into peritubular capillaries at proximal convoluted tubules is passive.

Glucose is actively reabsorbed from proximal convoluted tubules back into peritubular capillaries against a concentration gradient. However, there is a maximum rate of transfer for glucose back into peritubular capillaries (e.g., threshold). When blood glucose concentrations exceed about 180 mg·dl^{-1}, the reabsorption threshold is exceeded and glucose appears in the urine.

Most of the filtered potassium is reabsorbed back into peritubular capillaries from proximal convoluted tubules. Potassium is also secreted by distal convoluted tubules into peritubular capillaries.

Phosphate reabsorption at proximal convoluted tubules is under the control of the parathyroid glands. Increased circulating levels of parathormone reduce reabsorption back into peritubular capillaries such that phosphate excretion in the urine is enhanced. Conversely, reabsorption of calcium back into peritubular capillaries from proximal convoluted tubules is enhanced by parathormone.

LOOP OF HENLE

The loop of Henle is a continuation of the straight portions of proximal convoluted tubules. The depth that the loops of Henle extend into the medulla varies according to the location of the glomerulus from which they are derived. About 85 percent of the loops of Henle are derived from nephrons with glomeruli in the outer two-thirds of the renal cortex. Therefore, these loops extend only a short distance into the renal medulla before turning back into the cortex. The remaining loops of Henle are derived from juxtamedullary glomeruli and penetrate deeply into the renal medulla.

About 25 percent of total filtered sodium is reabsorbed from loops of Henle, particularly the ascending limbs, via an active process. In contrast to sodium, less water is reabsorbed from loops of Henle so that fluid passing along these loops becomes hypotonic relative to plasma. Eventual formation of concentrated urine involves (1) creation of a hypertonic medullary interstitium and (2) equilibration of fluid in the renal tubules with the hypertonic fluid in the medullary interstitium. It is principally the loops of Henle that are responsible for formation of hypertonic fluid in the medullary interstitium via the countercurrent multiplier system.

DISTAL CONVOLUTED TUBULE AND COLLECTING TUBULE

Distal convoluted tubules can reabsorb sodium, chloride, and water principally under the influence of aldosterone. Furthermore, secretion of potassium and hydrogen ions and ammonia occurs at distal convoluted tubules.

The osmolarity of the filtrate present in distal convoluted tubules and collecting tubules is under the control of antidiuretic hormone. Antidiuretic hormone is released from the posterior pituitary in response to increased plasma osmolarity, as can follow hemorrhage or dehydration. This hormone increases permeability of distal convoluted tubules and collecting tubules to water. As a result, water is reabsorbed back into peritubular capillaries, and a small volume of highly concentrated urine enters the renal pelvis. Conversely, an excess of total body water and subsequent decrease in plasma osmolarity inhibits release of antidiuretic hormone and leads to excretion of high volumes of urine with low osmolarity.

Secretion of hydrogen ions by renal tubular cells of distal convoluted tubules facilitates the elimination of acid metabolites, which result from normal dietary intake. The capacity of this system is limited because the lowest urine pH that the kidneys can achieve by hydrogen ion secretion is 4.5. These same renal tubular cells, however, can also secrete ammonia, which combines with hydrogen ions to form ammonium. This permits the further secretion of hydrogen ions into the urine. The source of hydrogen ions secreted by renal tubular cells is not known but most likely results from the dissociation of carbonic acid. As a result, inhibition of carbonic anhydrase enzyme impairs the ability of renal tubular cells to secrete hydrogen ions and to acidify urine.

In the presence of systemic acidosis, hydrogen ions are secreted into distal convoluted tubules in preference to potassium by renal tubular cells. Conversely, systemic alkalosis favors the elimination of potassium and retention of hydrogen ions. The secretion of potassium or hydrogen ions into distal convoluted tubules also depends on the exchange of these ions with sodium. For example, aldosterone and corticosteroids enhance the reabsorption of sodium into distal convoluted tubules, which facilitates the secretion of hydrogen ions and potassium. Clinically, the end result of excessive aldosterone or corticosteroid production can be hypokalemic metabolic alkalosis and secretion of an acid urine. Conversely, in the absence of adrenal cortical function (Addison's disease), there is increased sodium loss into the urine, and plasma potassium concentrations increase while arterial pH decreases.

Decreased ability of the kidneys to eliminate hydrogen ions leads to metabolic acidosis. Indeed, metabolic acidosis is a predictable feature of renal failure. Metabolic acidosis due to specific renal tubular defects in the absence of glomerular insufficiency is known as renal tubular acidosis. Patients with renal tubular acidosis are characterized by an inappropriately elevated urinary pH (5.5 or greater) despite the presence of hyperchloremic acidosis.

GLOMERULAR FILTRATION RATE

Hydrostatic pressure in the glomerular capillaries is about 50 mmHg. This pressure acts to force water and low molecular weight substances through glomerular capillaries into Bowman's space. Outward filtration forces produced by hydrostatic pressures are opposed primarily by the plasma oncotic pressure. Oncotic pressure in glomerular capillaries increases from 25 mmHg at the afferent arterioles to 35 mmHg in the efferent arterioles. This increased oncotic pressure is due to the filtration of plasma crystalloids but not protein. The net pressure for glomerular filtration will thus be greater at the afferent ends. Despite relatively low filtration pressures, the glomerular capillaries are able to filter about 125 ml·min^{-1} or near 200 L·day^{-1}. About 90 percent of the fluid resulting from glomerular filtration is reabsorbed during its passage along renal tubules and returned to the circulation via peritubular capillaries.

Knowledge of factors that influence the glomerular filtration rate is helpful in predicting the impact of pathologic changes on renal function. For example, decreased systemic arterial pressure decreases hydrostatic pressure in the glomerular capillaries, and outward filtration is predictably reduced. Hemorrhage or dehydration can increase oncotic pressure of plasma, which leads to decreased filtration

pressures. Likewise, ureteral obstruction can increase hydrostatic pressure in Bowman's capsule and thus oppose glomerular filtration.

RENAL BLOOD FLOW

The kidneys represent about 0.5 percent of the total body weight but receive 20 percent to 25 percent of the resting cardiac output. About two-thirds of the total renal blood flow is to the renal cortex. Renal blood flow remains constant at mean arterial pressures ranging from 60 mmHg to 160 mmHg. This ability to maintain renal blood flow is known as autoregulation. Autoregulation is achieved by adjustment of the afferent arteriolar tone and subsequent resistance imparted to blood flow. By virtue of maintaining renal blood flow, the glomerular capillary hydrostatic pressure and the glomerular filtration rate remain unchanged despite alterations in perfusion pressure.

It is important to appreciate that changes in renal blood flow are pressure dependent outside the range of mean arterial pressures associated with autoregulation. Renal blood flow is also influenced by the autonomic nervous system and the renin-angiotensin system. Sympathetic nervous system stimulation produces renal vascular vasoconstriction, with marked reductions in renal blood flow and glomerular filtration rate. This response occurs despite maintenance of perfusion pressures in ranges associated with autoregulation. Furthermore, any reduction in renal blood flow will initiate renin release, which, along with catecholamine release, can further reduce total blood flow, as well as alter distribution of blood flow in the kidneys. Prostaglandins may produce vasodilation and offset, to some extent, renal artery vasoconstriction, which results from the release of renin.

ENDOCRINE FUNCTION OF THE KIDNEYS

In addition to serving as target organs for various hormones, the kidneys are involved in both the metabolism and secretion of regulatory substances. For example, insulin is inactivated by the kidneys.[1] This may explain why glucose tolerance improves in diabetic patients in the presence of renal failure.

Renin is a proteolytic enzyme secreted into the circulation by specialized smooth muscle cells of afferent arterioles and modified segments of distal convoluted tubules known as the macula densa. Together, these specialized areas are designated the juxtaglomerular apparatus (Fig. 21-1). This apparatus secretes renin in response to (1) beta-adrenergic stimulation, (2) decreased perfusion pressure in afferent arterioles, and (3) reductions in the sodium load delivered to distal convoluted tubules. Beta-adrenergic antagonist drugs such as propranolol, may be effective in decreasing the release of renin.

Renin acts in the plasma on alpha-2-globulins synthesized in the liver (angiotensinogen) to form angiotensin I. Angiotensin I is then split by converting enzyme in the lungs to form angiotensin II. Renal effects of angiotensin II include renal artery vasoconstriction with subsequent decreases in renal blood flow and glomerular filtration rate and inhibition of renal tubular reabsorption of sodium. Furthermore, angiotensin II is an important stimulus for the release of aldosterone from the adrenal cortex.

Prostaglandins are produced in the renal medulla and appear to modulate the effect of other hormones. They are released in response to such stimuli as increased sympathetic nervous system activity or elevated levels of circulating angiotensin II. Prostaglandins designated as PGE_2 and PGI_2 are vasodilators and function to attenuate vasoconstriction in the renal vasculature produced by increased sympathetic nervous system activity and angiotensin II. In contrast, PGF_2 is a potent vasoconstrictor that enhances effects of sympathetic nervous system activity. Prostaglandins also seem to be important for optimal effects of antidiuretic hormone on collecting ducts.

TESTS USED FOR EVALUATION OF RENAL FUNCTION

Baseline renal function is defined by standard laboratory tests that evaluate glomerular filtration rate and renal tubular function (Table

TABLE 21-1. Tests Used for Evaluation of Rena Function (Normal Values)

Glomerular Filtration Rate	Renal Tubular Function
Blood urea nitrogen (10–20 mg·dl^{-1})	Urine specific gravity (1.003–1.030)
Plasma creatinine (0.7–1.5 mg·dl^{-1})	Urine osmolarity (38–1400 mOsm·L^{-1})
Creatinine clearance (110–150 ml·min^{-1})	Urine sodium (130–260 mEq·day^{-1})

(Data from Conn HF, ed. Current Therapy. Philadelphia. W.B. Saunders 1980;916–25)

21-1). It must be emphasized that many of these tests are not sensitive measurements and that significant renal disease can be present despite normal laboratory values. Indeed, at least half of normal renal function may be lost before tests of glomerular filtration rate become abnormal. Furthermore, clinical evidence of renal failure becomes evident only after more than 75 percent of nephrons are nonfunctional. Trends are more useful than single determinations in evaluating renal function. Furthermore, most renal diseases interfere with glomerular filtration rate as well as renal tubular function. This is predictable, since renal tubular cells are dependent on glomerular filtration for delivery of water and solutes for selective renal tubular secretion and reabsorption.

Blood Urea Nitrogen

In normal patients ingesting an average diet, blood urea nitrogen concentrations vary inversely with the glomerular filtration rate. Nevertheless, blood urea nitrogen concentrations are not sensitive indices of glomerular filtration rate because urea clearance also depends on the production rate and tubular reabsorption rate of urea. As a result, blood urea nitrogen concentrations can be abnormal despite a normal glomerular filtration rate. For example, the production rate of urea is increased by high protein diets or gastrointestinal bleeding (hemoglobin is digested as is blood in ingested meat). Other causes for increased blood urea nitrogen concentrations despite a normal glomerular filtration rate include increased catabolism during febrile illnesses and enhanced renal tubular reabsorption of urea due to slow movement of fluid through renal tubules. Slow renal tubular flow allows more time for the action of the antidiuretic hormone. Indeed, increased blood urea nitrogen levels observed during dehydration or fluid deprivation most likely reflect increased urea reabsorption back into peritubular capillaries. When slow movement of fluid through renal tubules is responsible for elevation of blood urea nitrogen concentrations, the plasma creatinine remains normal.

Blood urea nitrogen levels can remain normal in the presence of a low protein diet (starvation, hemodialysis patients) despite marked reductions in glomerular filtration rate. Conversely, low levels of blood urea nitrogen can reflect an excess of total body water content. Nevertheless, despite these extraneous influences, blood urea nitrogen concentrations above 50 mg·dl^{-1} almost always reflect a decreased glomerular filtration rate.

Plasma Creatinine

Plasma creatinine concentrations are specific indicators of glomerular filtration rate. In contrast to blood urea nitrogen concentrations, plasma creatinine levels are not influenced by protein metabolism or the rate of fluid flow through renal tubules. Furthermore, production of creatinine is constant when skeletal muscle mass is unchanging, and there is no renal tubular reabsorption of creatinine after it is filtered. A minor problem is that some creatinine is secreted by the renal tubules back into peritubular capillaries. In general, 50 percent increases in plasma creatinine concentrations reflect similar decreases in the glomerular filtration rate. A small increase in plasma creatinine concentrations, as compared with a previous admission to the hospital, can represent marked deteriorations in renal function.

It must be appreciated that acute reductions in the glomerular filtration rate are not immediately reflected by measurement of plasma creatinine concentrations, as it takes 24 hours to 72 hours for equilibration to occur, especially if there is concurrent rapid infusion of fluids. In patients who are not hypercatabolic, plasma creatinine concentrations will not rise more rapidly than 1 mg·dl^{-1} to 2 mg·dl^{-1} each day. Even at the maximal rate of rise in the absence of concurrent dilution, at least 8 hours are required for plasma creatinine concentrations to increase from normal levels to that suggestive of acute renal failure. Even with the total absence of renal function, plasma creatinine concentrations plateau, apparently as a result of nonrenal (gastrointestinal tract) excretion or inhibition of production of creatinine.[2]

It is important to appreciate the impact of skeletal muscle mass on plasma creatinine concentrations. For example, normal plasma creatinine values are higher in muscular men than in women. Conversely, plasma creatinine concentrations can remain within normal limits in geriatric patients, even though the glomerular filtration rate decreases progressively by 1 percent·yr^{-1} to 2 percent·yr^{-1} between 25 years and 65 years of age.[3] Maintenance of normal plasma creatinine values in geriatric patients reflects decreased creatinine production due to reduced skeletal muscle mass that accompanies aging. Indeed, mild elevations in plasma creatinine concentrations in geriatric patients should suggest significant renal disease. Likewise, in patients with chronic renal failure, measured plasma creatinine concentrations may not accurately reflect the glomerular filtration rate because of decreased creatinine production in the presence of reduced skeletal muscle mass.

Creatinine Clearance

Creatinine clearance is the most reliable measurement for accurate assessment of the glomerular filtration rate. This test measures the ability of glomeruli to excrete creatinine into the urine for given plasma creatinine concentrations. Creatinine clearance does not depend on corrections for age or the presence of a steady state. The major disadvantage of this test is the need for accurate urine collections.

Mild renal dysfunction is present when creatinine clearance values are 50 ml·min⁻¹ to 80 ml·min⁻¹. Moderate renal dysfunction is present when values are below 25 ml·min⁻¹; the doses of drugs that depend on renal excretion, such as long-acting nondepolarizing muscle relaxants, should be reduced; and electrolyte and water replacement must be carefully monitored. Patients with creatinine clearance values below 10 ml·min⁻¹ can be considered anephric and will require hemodialysis for water and electrolyte homeostasis.

Urine Concentrating Ability

Diagnosis of renal tubular dysfunction is established by demonstrating that the kidneys do not produce appropriately concentrated urine in the presence of an adequate physiologic stimulus for the release of antidiuretic hormone. In the absence of diuretic therapy or glycosuria, a urinary-specific gravity above 1.018 after an overnight fast makes impaired ability of renal tubules to reabsorb water and concentrate urine an unlikely diagnosis.[4] Conversely, if urine osmolarity does not rise significantly above the osmolarity of plasma (at least 300 mOsm·L⁻¹) after standard periods of water deprivation, an impaired ability of renal tubules to concentrate urine is likely.

Exogenous antidiuretic hormone (vasopressin) may be administered after confirmation that urine osmolarity does not increase significantly in response to a physiologic stimulus, such as overnight fasting. Caution should be exercised in administering vasopressin to patients with suspected coronary artery disease, as this drug can produce coronary artery vasoconstriction. If urine osmolarity increases in response to exogenous administration of vasopressin, the diagnosis of diabetes insipidus is established. If administration of vasopressin does not increase the osmolarity of urine, it is reasonable to conclude that renal tubules are unable to reabsorb water because of an unresponsiveness to antidiuretic hormone. This unresponsiveness is known as nephrogenic diabetes insipidus. Fluoride nephrotoxicity, after administration of anesthesia with drugs such as methoxyflurane[5] and, rarely, enflurane,[6] is an example of nephrogenic diabetes insipidus. Other causes include lithium, amphotericin B, osmotic diuretics, hypercalcemia, hypokalemia, and chronic pyelonephritis.

Sodium Excretion

Decreased ability to conserve sodium occurs with diseases that primarily involve the renal tubules (pyelonephritis, polycsytic kidney disease) and with the diuretic phase of acute renal failure. Adrenal insufficiency and hypoaldosteronism are also associated with sodium wasting. Indeed, urinary excretion of greater than 40 mEq·L⁻¹ of sodium suggests a decreased ability of renal tubules to reabsorb sodium. It is likely that signs of hypovolemia (postural hypotension, tachycardia, decreased central venous pressure) will be present when there is excessive renal tubular excretion of sodium.

EFFECTS OF ANESTHETICS ON RENAL FUNCTION

Anesthetic drugs can alter renal function indirectly by their effects on the systemic circulation, sympathetic nervous system, and endocrine function. In rare instances, drugs used for anesthesia produce direct nephrotoxicity. This may manifest as decreased intrinsic clearance of drugs or be delayed due to toxic metabolites. Although confirmatory data are not available, it is not unlikely that depressant effects of anesthetics on function of diseased kidneys are greater than those which occur in the absence of kidney disease.

Systemic Circulation

Drugs used to produce anesthesia may alter renal function by decreasing renal perfusion pressure and·or increasing renal vascular resistance. Regardless of the mechanism, the net effect is a decrease in the renal blood flow, glomerular filtration rate, and urine output during anesthesia.

Inhaled anesthetic drugs most likely depress renal function by producing decreases in cardiac output and systemic blood pressure. Nitrous oxide plus equivalent concentrations of halothane, enflurane, and isoflurane produce similar reductions in renal blood flow and glomerular filtration rate.[7–9] During administration of halothane, these reductions in renal blood flow and glomerular filtration rate are attenuated by preoperative hydration and administration of low concentrations of volatile anesthetics so as to maintain blood pressure near normal levels (Table 21-2).[10] Although similar data are not available for enflurane or isoflurane, it seems likely that preoperative hydration and maintenance of blood pressure would produce similar effects.

Alterations in autoregulation of renal blood flow due to effects produced by volatile anesthetics could exaggerate changes in renal function, which occur in response to circulatory effects produced by anesthetics. In an isolated and perfused dog kidney autoregulation of renal blood flow is not altered by halothane, with or without thiopental or nitrous oxide (Fig. 21-2).[11] Conversely, halothane does interfere with autoregulation of renal blood flow in a sheep model.[12] The impact, if any, of other anesthetics on autoregulation of renal blood flow has not been evaluated.

Changes in renal function during barbiturate opioid-nitrous oxide anesthesia are similar to those observed during administration of low concentrations of volatile anesthetics. Droperidol-fentanyl[13] or high doses of morphine

$(2 \text{ mg} \cdot \text{kg}^{-1})$[14] produce no significant changes in renal blood flow or glomerular filtration rate. However, the addition of nitrous oxide to droperidol-fentanyl or morphine results in renal function changes similar to those observed during administration of volatile anesthetics.[14,15] This response most likely reflects reductions in cardiac output produced by the addition of nitrous oxide to the other drugs being administered.

Sympathetic Nervous System

The renal vasculature is richly innervated by the sympathetic nervous system. Conceivably, drugs that stimulate the sympathetic nervous system could increase renal vascular resistance, leading to reductions in renal blood flow and glomerular filtration rate. Indeed, renal blood flow and glomerular filtration rate have been observed to decrease during ketamine anesthesia, despite increases in cardiac output and mean arterial pressure.[16] Conversely, drugs that inhibit sympathetic nervous system activity might reduce renal vascular resistance. Support for this mechanism is the observation that low concentrations of halothane partially restore renal blood flow when administered to animals with hemorrhagic shock.[17] This response most likely reflects a decrease in renal vascular resistance.

Sympathetic nervous system blockade secondary to regional anesthesia results in minimal changes in renal blood flow and glomer-

TABLE 21-2. Impact of Inspired Concentrations of Halothane and Preoperative Hydration on Renal Function

Inspired Halothane Concentration (%)	Preoperative Hydration	% Decrease from Control	
		Renal Blood Flow	Glomerular Filtration Rate
0.5–1.0	No	61	48
	Yes	12	8
1.2–3.0	No	69	58
	Yes	47	40

(Data from Barry KG, Mazze RI, Schwartz FD. Prevention of surgical oliguria and renal hemodynamic suppression by sustained hydration. N Engl J Med 1964;270:1371–7)

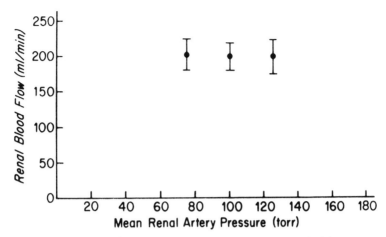

FIG. 21-2. Renal blood flow in dogs (Mean ± SE) was similar at mean arterial pressures of 75 mmHg, 100 mmHg, and 125 mmHg, in the presence of 0.9 percent end-exhaled halothane. These observations suggest that autoregulation of renal blood flow is not altered by halothane anesthesia. (Bastron RD, Perkins FM, Payne JL. Autoregulation of renal blood flow during halothane anesthesia. Anesthesiology 1977;46:142–4)

ular filtration rate[18,19] because baseline renal hemodynamics are minimally influenced by sympathetic nervous system activity. When alterations in renal hemodynamics occur during regional anesthesia, the most likely explanation is a decrease in the systemic arterial pressure.

Endocrine Function

Anesthetic drugs can influence hemodynamics and function by producing changes in antidiuretic hormone release or in the activity of the renin-angiotensin system.

ANTIDIURETIC HORMONE

Decreased urinary output during anesthesia suggests the release of antidiuretic hormone. Plasma antidiuretic hormone levels, however, do not change during halothane or morphine (1 mg·kg^{-1} to 2 mg·kg^{-1}) anesthesia (Fig. 21-3).[20] Painful stimulation in association with the onset of surgery, however, results in significant increases in circulating levels of an-

tidiuretic hormone. Hydration before induction of anesthesia attenuates rises in plasma antidiuretic hormone levels produced by surgical stimulation.

Positive pressure ventilation of the lungs, as well as positive end-expiratory pressure, may be associated with fluid retention. The short-term antidiuretic effect of positive end-expiratory pressure is mainly due to hemodynamic impairment of renal function characterized by reductions in cardiac output and renal blood flow.[21] Associated increases in plasma renin activity, plasma aldosterone, and antidiuretic hormone concentrations may participate in fluid retention during more prolonged uses of positive end-expiratory pressure.

RENIN-ANGIOTENSIN

Suggestions that anesthetics increase renin release have not been confirmed in animals during halothane, enflurane, or morphine-nitrous oxide anesthesia.[22,23] Renin levels, however, have been shown to increase during halothane or enflurane anesthesia when sodium depletion is present.[24] This suggests that preoperative hydration is important in de-

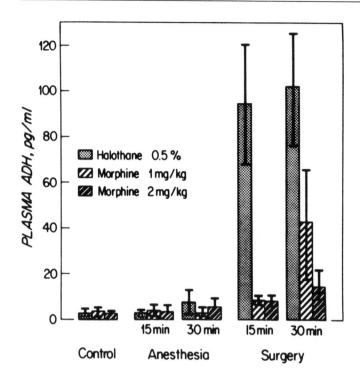

FIG. 21-3. Plasma antidiuretic hormone (ADH) levels (Mean ± SE) in adult patients were not altered from control measurements during anesthesia with nitrous oxide (50 percent) plus halothane or morphine. Thiopental (2 mg·kg^{-1}) was also administered to patients who subsequently received halothane. Surgical stimulation increased plasma ADH concentration, with the greatest elevation occurring in those patients receiving halothane. (Philbin DM, Coggins CH. Plasma antidiuretic hormone levels in cardiac surgical patients during morphine and halothane anesthesia. Anesthesiology 1978;49:95–8)

termining the intraoperative release of renin. Increases in circulating renin levels produced by surgical stimulation are indeed attenuated by hydration.

Direct Nephrotoxicity

In a sense, all anesthetics are direct nephrotoxins, as they produce generalized depression of measurable renal function. This depression of renal function, however, is transient and usually clinically insignificant. Nevertheless, halothane, but not spinal anesthesia (sensory level T4), interferes with renal clearance of drugs, such as cefotoxin, suggesting halothane-induced impairment of energy requiring transfer processes in the kidney.[12] These changes persisted as long as 24 hours after administration of halothane.

Delayed nephrotoxicity secondary to fluoride resulting from metabolism of volatile anesthetics may also occur (Table 21-3).[5,8,9,25] For example, methoxyflurane produces a dose-related nephrotoxicity related to its metabolism to fluoride.[5] Typically, this renal failure is characterized by an inability to concentrate urine. Polyuria leads to dehydration, with hypernatremia and increased plasma osmolarity. Detectable renal dysfunction is likely after ad-

TABLE 21-3. Plasma Fluoride Concentrations in Nonobese Adults[5,8,9,25]

	Dose (MAC hours)	Maximum Plasma Fluoride (μM·L^{-1})	Time of Maximum Increase (Hours Postanesthesia)
Methoxyflurane	2.5	61	24
Enflurane	2.5	22	4
Isoflurane	4.5	4.4	6
Halothane	4.5	No change	

ministration of a dose of methoxyflurane that results in plasma fluoride levels that exceed 50 μM·L^{-1}. Because of this nephrotoxicity potential, methoxyflurane is not recommended for anesthesia in the presence of co-existing renal disease or for operations associated with a high incidence of postoperative renal dysfunction, such as resection of abdominal aortic aneurysms. In the absence of increased risks for developing renal dysfunction, the dose of methoxyflurane should not exceed 2 hours using a 1 MAC concentration.

Conceivably, fluoride nephrotoxicity could result from administration of other volatile anesthetics. Nevertheless, defluorination of halothane[25] and isoflurane[9] is insufficient

to lead to plasma fluoride levels capable of producing nephrotoxicity (Table 21-3). In contrast, metabolism of enflurane to fluoride, although much less than with methoxyflurane, is potentially great enough to produce nephrotoxicity, particularly after prolonged administration.[8] Indeed, the administration of enflurane for prolonged periods (1 MAC for 9.6 hours) can result in decreased urine concentrating ability during a time when plasma fluoride levels average 15 μM·L^{-1} (Fig. 21-4).[26] Urine concentrating ability is not changed after similar exposures to halothane. This suggests that potentially nephrotoxic levels of plasma fluoride may be much less than the speculated level of 50 μM·L^{-1}. In contrast, shorter anes-

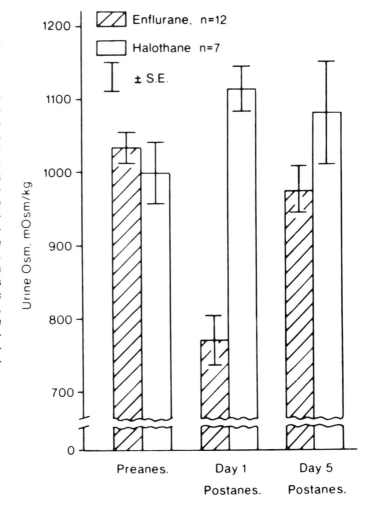

FIG. 21-4. The ability to concentrate urine (maximum urine osmolarity) in response to exogenous vasopressin was measured in volunteers without renal disease before (preanes) and 1 day and 5 days after anesthesia (postanes) with enflurane (9.6 MAC hours) or halothane (13.7 MAC hours). MAC hours were determined by multiplying the end-exhaled concentration of the volatile anesthetic, as a fraction of MAC, times the duration of exposure in hours. The ability to concentrate urine in response to vasopressin was decreased on day 1 after enflurane but not halothane anesthesia. By day 5 after anesthesia, mean values for enflurane patients had returned to preanesthetic levels. (Mazze RI, Calverley RK, Smith NT. Inorganic fluoride nephrotoxicity: Prolonged enflurane and halothane anesthesia in volunteers. Anesthesiology 1977;46:265–71)

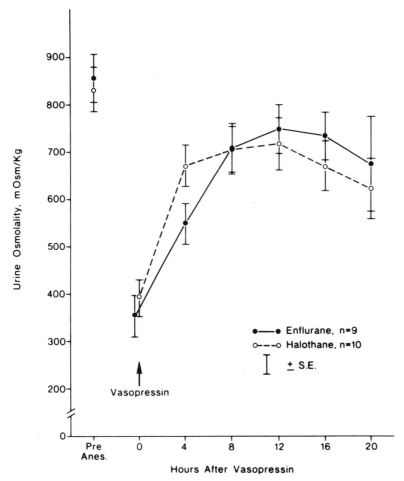

FIG. 21-5. The ability to concentrate urine after administration of exogenous vasopressin was similar in surgical patients without renal disease after anesthesia with enflurane (2.7 MAC hours) or halothane (4.9 MAC hours). See Fig. 21-4 for definition of MAC hours. (Cousins MJ, Greenstein LR, Hitt BA, Mazze RI. Metabolism and renal effects of enflurane in man. Anesthesiology 1976;44:44–53)

thetic exposures (1 MAC for 2.7 hours) reveal no difference between enflurane or halothane with respect to urine concentrating ability or intraoperative changes in renal blood flow, glomerular filtration rate, or urine output (Fig. 21-5).[8]

Use of enflurane in patients vulnerable for developing postoperative renal dysfunction may be questioned. This concern is based on the realization that excretion of fluoride depends on the glomerular filtration rate. Therefore, it is likely that patients with decreased glomerular filtration rates will maintain elevated circulating levels of fluoride for longer periods of time than normal patients. Nephrotoxicity depends on the duration of the exposure of renal tubules to fluoride, as well as on the levels of plasma fluoride. Therefore, it is possible that patients with decreased glomerular filtration rates are at an increased risk in the presence of plasma fluoride concentrations usually considered nontoxic (i.e., below 50 $\mu M \cdot L^{-1}$). Indeed, postoperative renal dysfunction has been reported after administration of enflurane to a patient with co-existing renal disease.[6] Nevertheless, a large series of patients with chronic renal disease (plasma creatinine concentrations 1.5 mg·dl^{-1} to 3.0 mg·dl^{-1}), undergoing elective operations with halothane or enflurane, manifested evidence of improved renal function postoperatively (Fig. 21-6).[27] Furthermore, peak plasma fluoride concentrations (19 μmol·L^{-1}), as well as the rate of disappearance of fluoride from the circulation in these patients, was similar to that in patients without renal disease. Presumably, storage of fluoride in bone offsets the effect of reduced glomerular filtration rate on fluoride clearance from the plasma and thus prevents sustained exposure of renal tubules to this potential nephrotoxin. Based on these observations, it is not possible to justify recommendations to avoid routinely administration of enflurane for nonrenal surgery to patients with co-existing renal dysfunction. It is undeniable, however, that the differential diagnosis of postoperative renal dysfunction may be unnecessarily complicated if enflurane, rather than equally acceptable alternative drugs, are administered to patients with co-existing renal disease or is administered to patients undergoing operations associated with a high incidence of postoperative renal dysfunction. In this regard, minimal metabolism of isoflurane and halothane to fluoride suggests that renal dysfunction is unlikely from nephrotoxic metabolites after administration of these drugs.

Obese patients have been shown to have higher plasma fluoride concentrations after administration of methoxyflurane or enflurane, as compared with nonobese patients.[28,29] Nevertheless, the incidence of renal dysfunction has not been reported to increase after administration of these drugs to obese patients. Likewise, enzyme induction produced by administration of phenobarbital does not significantly increase defluorination of enflurane. Isoniazid administration does increase defluorination of enflurane. Plasma fluoride concentrations during and after enflurane anesthesia may also be influenced by the pH of the urine (Fig. 21-7).[30] For example, mean maximal plasma concentrations of fluoride are 26.4 μM·L^{-1} in patients with a urinary pH of 5.08. Conversely, mean maximal plasma concentrations of fluoride are 13.5 μM·L^{-1} when the urinary pH is 8.16. These data suggest that it is possible to influence the renal excretion of fluoride after enflurane anesthesia by manipulation of the urinary pH.

CHANGES CHARACTERISTIC OF CHRONIC RENAL FAILURE

Chronic renal failure is characterized by a progressive decrease in the number of functioning nephrons, leading to an irreversible re-

FIG. 21-6. Plasma creatinine concentrations in patients with chronic renal disease declined similar amounts after elective operations with general anesthesia produced by enflurane or halothane. Mean ± SE. (Data adapted from Mazze RI, Sivenpiper TS, Stevenson J. Renal effects of enflurane and halothane in patients with abnormal renal function. Anesthesiology 1984;60:161–3)

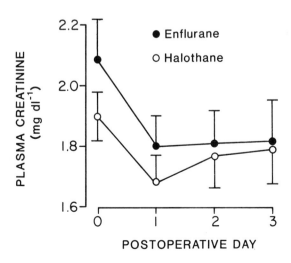

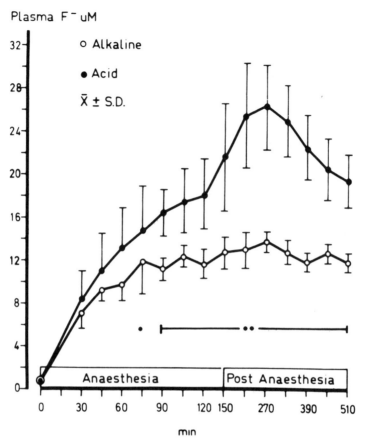

FIG. 21-7. Plasma fluoride (F⁻) concentrations were measured during and after administration of enflurane to adult patients. Acetazolamide was administered to one group of patients to produce an acidic urine (pH 5.08), while the second group received ammonium chloride to alkalinize the urine (pH 8.16). F⁻ concentrations increased rapidly in patients with a low urine pH. Conversely, in patients with an alkaline urine, F⁻ levels increased less and remained nearly constant after 75 minutes of anesthesia. Maximal F⁻ concentrations occurred 2 hours after the conclusion of anesthesia in both groups and were 26.4 ± 7.9 $\mu M \cdot L^{-1}$ and 13.5 ± 2.4 $\mu M \cdot L^{-1}$ in the acidic-urine and alkaline-urine groups respectively. *P < 0.05 and **P < 0.01-alkaline compared to acid urine groups. (Jarnberg P-O, Ekstrand J, Irestedt L. Renal fluoride excretion and plasma fluoride levels during and after enflurane anesthesia are dependent on urinary pH. Anesthesiology 1981;54:48–52)

duction in glomerular filtration rate. The end result of chronic renal disease is renal failure, requiring hemodialysis or renal transplantation. Common diseases leading to chronic renal failure are chronic glomerulonephritis, tubulointerstitial diseases, diabetic nephropathy, and polycystic kidney disease. Rational management of anesthesia in these patients requires an understanding of those changes characteristic of chronic renal failure (Table 21-4).

Chronic Anemia

Normochromic, normocytic anemia occurs in almost all patients with chronic renal failure who have plasma creatinine concentrations greater than 3.5 mg·dl⁻¹. The degree of anemia often parallels the degree of chronic renal dysfunction but remains relatively constant after end-stage renal failure has occurred.

TABLE 21-4. Changes Characteristic of Chronic Renal Failure

Chronic Anemia
    Increased cardiac output
    Oxyhemoglobin dissociation curve shifted to the right

Coagulopathies
    Platelet dysfunction
    Systemic heparinization

Altered Hydration and Electrolyte Balance
    Unpredictable intravascular fluid volume
    Hyperkalemia
    Hypermagnesemia
    Hypocalcemia

Metabolic Acidosis

Systemic Hypertension
    Congestive heart failure
    Attenuated sympathetic nervous system activity due to therapy with antihypertensive drugs

Increased Susceptibility to Infection
    Decreased activity of phagocytes
    Immunosuppressant drugs—corticosteroids

Hemoglobin concentrations in the range of 5 $g \cdot dl^{-1}$ to 8 $g \cdot dl^{-1}$ are hallmarks of chronic renal failure. Decreased production of erythropoietin in the presence of elevated blood urea nitrogen levels is the most likely explanation for the decreased manufacture of erythrocytes. Furthermore, survival time for erythrocytes is shortened about 50 percent in the presence of chronic uremia, reflecting erythrocyte membrane fragility. In addition, a hemorrhagic tendency manifested by menorrhagia or chronic gastrointestinal bleeding may contribute to anemia in these patients (see the section Coagulopathies). This anemia is well tolerated because of its slow onset. Indeed, preoperative transfusions are not routinely indicated. When transfusions are required, the use of erythrocytes, rather than whole blood, minimizes the risks of fluid overload.

The greatest hazard of anemia is decreased oxygen-carrying capacity, which can result in tissue hypoxia. Indeed, transfusion of erythrocytes may be effective treatment of angina pectoris in patients with chronic renal disease. This decreased oxygen-carrying capacity is compensated for by increased tissue blood flow due to decreased blood viscosity. In addition, release of oxygen from hemoglobin to tissues is facilitated by a shift of the oxyhemoglobin dissociation curve to the right, due to metabolic acidosis and an increased concentrations of 2,3-diphosphyglycerate.

The importance of increased tissue blood flow in offsetting the effects of anemia emphasizes the need to minimize decreases in cardiac output produced by anesthetic drugs and positive pressure ventilation of the lungs. These goals are achieved by the administration of low concentrations of volatile anesthetics or use of opioids and use of a slow breathing rate, so as to insure sufficient time between each mechanical breath for venous return to occur.

Coagulopathies

Coagulopathies must be suspected in patients with chronic renal failure. The most likely coagulation defect is decreased platelet adhesiveness. Although the mechanism is not known, the accumulation of metabolic acids may interfere with factor VIII activity and subsequent platelet aggregation. Bleeding time is a useful test to evaluate the status of coagulation in patients with chronic renal failure and uremia, as prothrombin time and partial thromboplastin time are not predictably altered. Patients with plasma creatinine concentrations below 6 $mg \cdot dl^{-1}$ generally exhibit normal platelet function. Hemodialysis is the most effective treatment for platelet dysfunction in these patients.

In addition to platelet abnormalities, patients needing hemodialysis may require systemic or regional heparinization to maintain patency of vascular shunts. Persistence of prolongation of prothrombin time and plasma thromboplastin time after hemodialysis is more likely after systemic heparinization. The problem can be further compounded if co-existing liver disease has interfered with production of procoagulants. Thus, the possibility of impaired coagulation must be remembered in patients with chronic renal failure, particularly when considering regional anesthetic techniques.

Hydration and Electrolyte Balance

Disturbances in hydration and electrolyte balance (hyperkalemia, hypermagnesemia, hypocalcemia) frequently occur in patients with chronic renal failure. Estimates of blood volume status may be made by comparing body weight before and after hemodialysis, consideration of vital signs (blood pressure with position changes, heart rate) and measurement of atrial filling pressures. Regardless of blood volume status, these patients often respond to induction of anesthesia as if they are hypovolemic. The likelihood of hypotension during induction of anesthesia may be increased if sympathetic nervous system function is attenuated by antihypertensive drugs or uremia. Attenuated sympathetic nervous system activity impairs compensatory peripheral vasoconstriction, so that small decreases in blood volume, institution of positive pressure ventilation of the lungs, abrupt changes in body position, or drug-induced myocardial depression can result in exaggerated reductions in blood pressure.

The most serious electrolyte abnormality in patients with chronic renal failure is hyperkalemia (see Chapter 27). Hazards of hyperkalemia are cardiac conduction abnormalities and dysrhythmias. Because of the potential dangers of hyperkalemia, it is a common recommendation not to perform elective surgery unless plasma potassium concentrations are less than 5.5 $mEq \cdot L^{-1}$. Even when hemodialysis has been performed in the previous 6 hours to 8 hours, it is important to measure plasma potassium concentrations before induction of anesthesia, as unexpected hyperkalemia can occur rapidly. If surgery cannot be delayed, plasma potassium concentrations can be lowered acutely by deliberate hyperventilation of the lungs and·or glucose-insulin infusions. Sodium bicarbonate is indicated if metabolic acidosis accompanies hyperkalemia. Intravenous administration of calcium is effective in restoring normal cardiac conduction in the presence of hyperkalemia.

Increased plasma magnesium levels may accompany chronic renal failure, especially when the glomerular filtration rate declines below 10 $ml \cdot min^{-1}$. Magnesium-containing antacids may accentuate hypermagnesemia in these patients. Hypermagnesemia results in central nervous system depression and can lead to hypotension, depression of ventilation, and coma. Potentiation of depolarizing and nondepolarizing muscle relaxants may accompany increased plasma concentrations of magnesium.[31]

The association of hypocalcemia with chronic renal failure reflects the presence of hyperphosphatemia and decreased intestinal absorption of calcium secondary to decreased activity of vitamin D. Decreased vitamin D activity emphasizes the fact that the kidneys are responsible for the final step in the conversion of this vitamin to its highly active metabolite, 1,25-dihydroxycholecalciferol. Chronic hypocalcemia in these patients stimulates the parathyroid glands with resulting bone decalcification, development of osteodystrophic abnormalities, and vulnerability to pathologic fractures as during positioning for anesthesia and surgery.

Plasma sodium concentrations are usually normal in patients with chronic renal disease because the osmoreceptor mechanism is functioning, so that thirst prevents hypernatremia. Dementia is most likely due to aluminum toxicity, either from aluminum in the dialysate fluid or aluminum salts in antacids administered to prevent hyperphosphatemia.[32]

Metabolic Acidosis

The kidneys normally excrete 40 mEq to 60 mEq of hydrogen ions every day. Chronic renal disease interferes with this excretion and metabolic acidosis can result. Associated changes often include decreases in plasma bicarbonate concentrations and arterial partial pressures of carbon dioxide. Hemodialysis is effective in restoring the arterial pH to nearly normal values. In patients requiring emergency surgery, intravenous administration of sodium bicarbonate may be necessary to correct severe acidosis (pH less than 7.15).

Systemic Hypertension

Hypertension is a frequent complication of chronic renal disease. Sustained hypertension can lead to cardiomegaly and congestive heart failure. Cardiac failure can be aggravated by the arteriovenous fistula used for hemodialysis. Preoperative hypertension is most often due to fluid overload and is amenable to treatment by hemodialysis. When hypertension does not respond to hemodialysis, use of antihypertensive drugs is necessary. Associated changes often include decreases in plasma bicarbonate concentrations and arterial partial pressures of carbon dioxide.

Management of hypertension in the perioperative period can be with vasodilators such as hydralazine or nitroprusside. Cyanide from the breakdown of nitroprusside is unlikely to cause toxicity in these patients. Indeed, animal data have demonstrated resistance to the development of cyanide toxicity in the absence of renal function.[33] The most likely explanation for this resistance is decreased renal excretion of thiosulfate. Thiosulfate serves as an endogenous sulfur donor and facilitates conversion of cyanide to thiocyanate.

In addition to hypertension, patients with chronic renal failure are prone to the development of coronary artery disease. Painless pericarditis with associated pericardial effusions may result in unexpected interference with venous return in the perioperative period.

Infection

The most serious problem facing patients with chronic renal failure is infection. Indeed, the most common cause of death in patients with renal failure is sepsis, often originating from a pulmonary infection. Susceptibility to infection can be partially explained by the use of immunosuppressive drugs, including corticosteroids. Strict attention to asepsis is important when placing vascular cannulae and endotracheal tubes in these patients.

A high incidence of viral hepatitis in patients with chronic renal disease most likely reflects frequent use of blood products, as well as effects of immunosuppression. Approximately one-third of patients with chronic renal failure who become infected with hepatitis virus become chronic carriers.

Central and Peripheral Venous System Abnormalities

Abnormalities of central and peripheral nervous system function may accompany chronic renal failure. Tiredness, insomnia, irritability, and mental depression are common. Seizures may accompany uremia or reflect cerebral edema from acute hypertension. Uremia-induced peripheral neuropathies include painful paresthesias of the extremities, skeletal muscle weakness, and occasional sensory defects. The median and common peroneal nerves are most commonly affected. Autonomic nervous system dysfunction commonly accompanies uremia and may contribute to attenuated compensatory responses to sudden changes in blood volume or positive pressure ventilation of the lungs, especially if patients are also being treated with antihypertensive drugs.

Gastrointestinal and Endocrine Dysfunction

Gastric fluid volume and acidity are likely to be increased in patients with chronic renal failure. These changes combined with delayed gastric emptying associated with uremia may place these patients at increased risk for regurgitation and pulmonary aspiration.

Diabetes mellitus is commonly present in patients with chronic renal failure. Overproduction of parathyroid hormone and subsequent osteodystrophy reflects attempts of the parathyroid glands to correct hypocalcemia (see the section Hydration and Electrolyte Balance).

MANAGEMENT OF ANESTHESIA FOR PATIENTS WITH CHRONIC RENAL FAILURE

Preoperative Preparation

Preoperative preparation of patients with chronic renal failure includes consideration of concomitant drug therapy and evaluation of recent laboratory measurements (especially plasma potassium concentrations).[34] Insulin and corticosteroid replacement regimens may require alteration. Signs of digitalis toxicity should be sought in treated patients, emphasizing the role of renal clearance of this and other drugs. Antihypertensive drug therapy is usually continued. Preoperative medication must be individualized, remembering that these patients may have increased gastric fluid volumes and at the same time exhibit unexpected sensitivity to central nervous system depressants.

Induction of Anesthesia

Induction of anesthesia and intubation of the trachea can be safely accomplished with intravenous drugs including barbiturates, benzodiazepines, or etomidate plus succinylcholine. An alternative to succinylcholine would be intermediate-acting muscle relaxants, especially atracurium (see the section Muscle Relaxants). None of these anesthetic induction drugs or muscle relaxants depend significantly on renal excretion for clearance from plasma. Logic would suggest slow injections of intravenous anesthetic drugs such as barbiturates to minimize drug-induced reductions in blood pressure. Exaggerated pharmacologic effects produced by barbiturates could also reflect reduced protein binding of drugs, resulting in more unbound drug to act at receptor sites. Indeed, the amount of pharmacologically active (not protein bound) thiopental in plasma is increased in patients with chronic renal failure.[35] Furthermore, the blood-brain barrier may not be intact in the presence of uremia. This could also increase the incidence of excessive drug effects, particularly as reflected by central nervous system depression. Furthermore, autonomic nervous system dysfunction may interfere with compensatory responses resulting in exaggerated drug-induced changes in blood pressure.

Potassium release after administration of succinylcholine is not exaggerated in patients with chronic renal failure.[36] Caution is necessary, however, when preoperative plasma potassium concentrations are in high normal ranges, since this combined with maximum drug-induced potassium release (0.5 mEq·L^{-1} to 1.0 mEq·L^{-1} could result in dangerous hyperkalemia. Furthermore, use of small doses of nondepolarizing muscle relaxants before administration of succinylcholine (pretreatment) does not reliably prevent potassium release after injection of succinylcholine.[37] Prolonged responses to succinylcholine have been attributed to decreased cholinesterase activity due to cholinesterase enzyme absorption onto the hemodialysis membrane. This does not occur, however, with currently used hemodialysis membranes, and responses to succinylcholine are not altered.[38]

Maintenance of Anesthesia

In patients with chronic renal disease but who are not dependent on hemodialysis, or in patients vulnerable to renal dysfunction because of advanced age, co-existing obstructive jaundice, sepsis, diabetes mellitus, or the need for major abdominal vascular surgery, the maintenance of anesthesia is often achieved with nitrous oxide combined with isoflurane, halothane, or short-acting opioids. Enflurane may be avoided due to concerns for potential adverse effects of fluoride on the diseased kidneys (see the section Direct Nephrotoxicity).

Potent volatile anesthetics are useful in controlling intraoperative hypertension and reducing doses of muscle relaxants needed for adequate surgical relaxation. The high incidence of associated liver disease in patients with chronic renal disease, however, should be considered when selecting these drugs, particularly halothane. Furthermore, excessive depression of cardiac output is a potential hazard of volatile anesthetics. Reductions in tissue blood flow must be minimized in the presence of anemia to avoid jeopardizing tissue oxygen delivery. Opioids decrease the likelihood of cardiovascular depression and avoid the concern of liver toxicity. Nevertheless, opioids are not reliably effective in controlling intraoperative blood pressure elevations. Furthermore, prolonged central nervous system and respiratory depression from small doses of opioids has been described in anephric patients.[39] Conceivably, pharmacologically active metabolites of opioids accumulate in the circulation and cerebrospinal fluid when renal function is absent.

Maintenance of anesthesia in patients requiring chronic hemodialysis is often achieved with nitrous oxide combined with isoflurane or enflurane. Isoflurane or enflurane provides sufficient potency to reduce excessive increases in blood pressure due to surgical stimulation. These drugs also decrease the dose of nondepolarizing muscle relaxants needed to produce skeletal muscle relaxation. Furthermore, use of isoflurane or enflurane in the presence of co-existing liver disease is less controversial than the use of halothane. Excessive plasma fluoride elevations do not occur in anephric patients receiving enflurane, since storage of fluoride in bone is able to offset the lack of its renal excretion.[40]

Regional Anesthesia

Brachial plexus block is useful for placement of vascular shunts necessary for chronic hemodialysis. In addition to providing analgesia, this form of regional anesthesia also abolishes vasospasm and provides optimal surgical conditions by producing maximal vascular vasodilation. Duration of brachial plexus block produced by local anesthetics may be shortened by nearly 40 percent in patients with chronic renal failure.[41] It is thought that elevated tissue blood flow (that is, increased cardiac output) results in a more rapid clearance of local anesthetics from active sites leading to shorter durations of block. This shortened duration of action supports the use of bupivacaine, especially if prolonged surgery is expected. Adequacy of coagulation should be confirmed and the presence of uremic neuropathies excluded before regional anesthesia is performed in these patients. Co-existing metabolic acidosis may decrease the seizure threshold for local anesthetics.

Muscle Relaxants

Renal disease slows the rate of decline in plasma concentrations of long-acting nondepolarizing muscle relaxants (Fig. 21-8).[42–44] Prolonged responses are predictable if usual doses of these drugs are administered to these patients. Alternatively, the intermediate-acting muscle relaxant, atracurium, and to a lesser extent vecuronium, are independent of renal mechanisms for their clearance from plasma. Indeed, the duration of neuromuscular blockade is not altered when large doses of atracurium or vecuronium are administered to anephric patients (Fig. 21-9).[45] Excretion of laudanosine, the principal metabolite of atracurium, however, is prolonged in the presence of renal failure.[46] Laudanosine lacks effects at the neuromuscular junction but at high plasma concentrations may produce stimulation of the central nervous system. Patients with renal failure show a higher plasma concentration of vecuronium at 25 percent and 75 percent recovery compared to patients with normal renal function,[47] which suggests an apparent tolerance to the drug. This tolerance is consistent with a slower onset of action of vecuronium in patients with renal failure. A similar but less prominent degree of tolerance may also occur after administration of atracurium to patients in renal failure.[45] Atracurium, and to a somewhat lesser extent vecuronium, would seem to

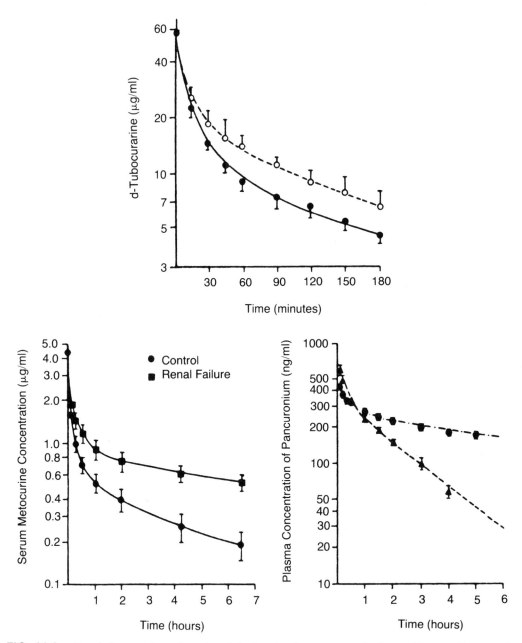

FIG. 21-8. Renal disease slows the rate of decline in plasma concentrations of long-acting muscle relaxants with the greatest impact being on pancuronium. (Data adapted from Brotherton WP, Matteo RS. Pharmacokinetics and pharmacodynamics of metocurine in humans with and without renal failure. Anesthesiology 1981;55:273–6; McLeod K, Watson MJ, Rawlings MD. Pharmacokinetics of pancuronium in patients with normal and impaired renal function. Br J Anaesth 1976;48:341–5; Miller RD, Matteo R, Benet LZ, Sohn YJ. Influence of renal failure on the pharmacokinetics of d-tubocurarine in man. J Pharmcol Exp Ther 1977;202:1–7)

FIG. 21-9. Time to recovery of twitch response to 10 percent of control (T-10) after rapid intravenous administration of atracurium (0.5 mg·kg^{-1}) or vecuronium (0.1 mg·kg^{-1}) to normal or anephric patients during nitrous oxide-fentanyl-thiopental anesthesia. Absence of renal function does not prolong the duration of action of either drug, although variability in response was greatest in anephric patients receiving vecuronium. Mean ± SD. (Hunter JM, Jones RS, Utting JE. Comparison of vecuronium, atracurium and tubocurarine in normal patients and in patients with no renal function. Br J Anaesth 1984;56:941–50)

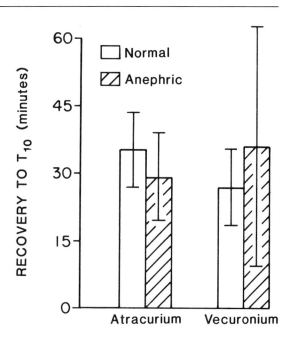

be the most useful nondepolarizing muscle relaxants for administration to patients with severe renal disease.

Renal excretion accounts for about 50 percent of the elimination of neostigmine and about 75 percent of the elimination of edrophonium and pyridostigmine. As a result, elimination half-times of these drugs are greatly prolonged by renal failure (Fig. 21-10).[48] Therefore, recurarization is unlikely because plasma clearance of anticholinesterase drugs will be delayed as long, if not longer, than the nondepolarizing muscle relaxants. When skeletal muscle weakness persists or recurs postoperatively, other causes of recurarization such as inadequate initial antagonism of neuromuscular blockade, respiratory acidosis, electrolyte derangements, or drug-induced effects, as from antibiotics, must be considered.

Ventilation

Management of ventilation of the lungs during anesthesia should be designed to maintain normocapnia and minimize effects of pos-

itive intrathoracic pressure on cardiac output. Hypoventilation with resulting respiratory acidosis is undesirable, as decreases in arterial pH can result in transfer of potassium from cells into the circulation, so as to accentuate hyperkalemia. Conversely, respiratory alkalosis from hyperventilation of the lungs shifts the oxyhemoglobin dissociation curve to the left and reduces tissue oxygen availability. This change is particularly undesirable in patients with anemia. Changes in cardiac output produced by positive pressure ventilation of the lungs can be minimized by using a slow breathing rate, to allow sufficient time for venous return during pauses between mechanical breaths.

Fluid Management

Patients with renal failure but not requiring hemodialysis, as well as those patients without renal disease undergoing operations associated with a high incidence of postoperative renal failure, may benefit from preoperative hydration with 10 ml·kg^{-1} to 20 ml·kg^{-1} of intravenous balanced salt solutions. Lactated Ringer's solution (4 mEq·L^{-1} of potas-

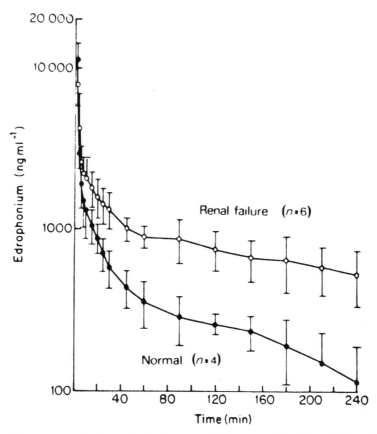

FIG. 21-10. Plasma concentrations of edrophonium decline more slowly in patients with renal failure than in normal patients. Delayed clearance of edrophonium (and other anticholinesterase drugs) parallels delayed clearance of nondepolarizing muscle relaxants (see Fig. 21-8). (Morris RB, Cronnelly R, Miller RD, et al. Pharmacokinetics of edrophonium in anephric and renal transplant patients. Br J Anaesth 1981;53:1311–3)

sium) or other potassium-containing fluids should not be administered to anuric patients. Preservation of renal function intraoperatively depends on minimizing cardiovascular depression, avoiding events that produce renal vasoconstriction and maintaining an adequate intravascular fluid volume. Urine output should be maintained between 0.5 ml·kg^{-1}·hr^{-1} to 1 ml·kg^{-1}·hr^{-1} in the operative and immediate postoperative period. This is best achieved by intravenous fluid replacement with balanced salt solutions, 3 ml·kg^{-1}·hr^{-1} to 5 ml·kg^{-1}·hr^{-1}. In general, when urine output is less than 0.5 ml·kg^{-1}·hr^{-1}, glomerular filtration rate can be assumed to be reduced. A small dose of furosemide (5 mg intravenously) will often increase urine output if oliguria is due to antidiuretic hormone release, but not if it is due to hypovolemia and reduced renal blood flow. Rapid infusion of balanced salt solutions (500 ml) should increase urine output if hypovolemia is present. Stimulation of urine output with an osmotic (mannitol) or tubular (furosemide) diuretic in the absence of adequate intravascular fluid volume replacement is discouraged. Indeed, the most likely reason for oliguria is an inadequate circulating fluid volume, which can only be further compromised by a drug-induced diuresis.

If fluid replacement is not effective in restoring urine output, a diagnosis of congestive heart failure should be considered. Dopamine is a useful drug for treating oliguria due to congestive heart failure. In addition, mechanical obstruction of the urinary catheter or pooling of urine in the dome of the bladder due to a head-down position should be considered in the differential diagnosis of oliguria.

Patients dependent on hemodialysis require special attention with regard to perioperative fluid management. Absence of renal function narrows the margin of safety between insufficient and excessive fluid administration to these patients. Noninvasive operations require replacement of only insensible water losses with 5 percent dextrose in water (5 ml·kg^{-1} to 10 ml·kg^{-1}). The small amount of urine output can be replaced with 0.45 percent sodium chloride. Thoracic or abdominal surgery can be associated with loss of significant intravascular fluid volume to interstitial spaces. This loss is often replaced with balanced salt solutions or 5 percent albumin solutions (Plasmanate). Infusion of erythrocytes may be considered when oxygen carrying capacity must be increased or blood loss replaced.

Monitoring

Minor surgical procedures can be monitored by noninvasive methods. Permanent vascular shunts should be protected and their patency monitored with a Doppler sensor to confirm continued patency during the operative procedure.

Continuous monitoring of intra-arterial blood pressure is helpful when major operative procedures are being performed. A femoral or dorsalis pedis artery is often used, since patients may require availability of arteries in the upper extremity for placement of vascular shunts. Intravenous fluid replacement is guided by central venous pressure measurements and urine output. A pulmonary artery catheter can be useful if interpretation of central venous measurements is questionable, as in the presence of co-existing chronic obstructive airways disease or left ventricular dysfunction. Furthermore, measurement of thermodilution cardiac outputs and calculation of systemic vascular resistance can be helpful in guiding doses of anesthetic drugs and recognizing the need for inotropic drugs, such as dopamine. Because of their immunosuppressed state, strict asepsis is mandatory for placement of intravascular catheters, such as those for measurement of blood pressure or pulmonary artery occlusion pressure.

Postoperative Management

Diagnosis of recurarization should be considered in anephric patients who manifest signs of respiratory insufficiency in the postoperative period (see the section Muscle Relaxants). A weak hand grip or unsustained head lift followed by improvement after intravenous administration of 5 mg to 10 mg of edrophonium confirms the diagnosis.

Hypertension is a frequent problem in the postoperative period. Hemodialysis is the best treatment if fluid excess is the cause. Vasodilator drugs, such as nitroprusside, hydralazine, or labetalol, are effective until the excess fluid can be removed by hemodialysis.

Caution must be exercised in the use of opioids for postoperative analgesia, in view of reports describing exaggerated central nervous system and ventilatory depression after even small doses of opioids.[39] Naloxone should be immediately available to treat this ventilatory depression should it occur. Continuous monitoring of the electrocardiogram is necessary to detect cardiac abnormalities related to hyperkalemia. Continuation of supplemental oxygen in the postoperative period seems prudent, especially in anemic patients.

DIFFERENTIAL DIAGNOSIS OF PERIOPERATIVE OLIGURIA

Causes of perioperative oliguria (urine output less than 0.5 ml·kg^{-1}·hr^{-1}) can be categorized as prerenal, renal, and postrenal (Table 21-5). Postrenal obstruction is uncommon and is diagnosed by zero urine output.

TABLE 21-5. Causes of Postoperative Oliguria

Prerenal (Decreased Renal Blood Flow)
  Hypovolemia
  Decreased renal blood flow due to low cardiac output

Renal (Acute Tubular Necrosis)
  Renal ischemia due to prerenal causes
  Nephrotoxic drugs
  Release of hemoglobin or myoglobin

Postrenal
  Bilateral ureteral obstruction
  Extravasation due to rupture of bladder

Thus, the usual differential diagnosis is between prerenal or renal causes (Table 21-6).

Oliguria due to prerenal causes is characterized by the kidneys' attempt to conserve sodium and to restore intravascular fluid volume. As a result, urinary sodium excretion is often less than 40 $mEq·L^{-1}$, and the urine is concentrated to greater than 400 $mOsm·L^{-1}$. Excretion of sodium-poor and highly concentrated urine confirms that renal tubular function is intact.

Oliguria due to renal causes is characterized by reduced blood flow to the renal cortex and a markedly decreased glomerular filtration rate. Indeed, a speculated mechanism for acute tubular necrosis is renal cortical vasoconstriction (acute vasomotor nephropathy), leading to ischemia of this area of the kidneys. Inability of the renal tubules to reabsorb sodium is evidenced by urinary sodium excretion in excess of 40 $mEq·L^{-1}$. Likewise, urine osmolarity is less than 400 $mOsm·L^{-1}$, reflecting washout of osmotically active particles from the renal medulla, due in part to redistribution of renal blood flow from the cortex to medullary areas of the kidneys. Oliguria that progresses to acute renal failure in surgical patients produces at least 50 percent mortality.[49] Indeed, nearly 50 percent of the acute hemodialysis instituted in the United States is due to perioperative renal failure. The most common cause of acute renal failure is prolonged renal hypoperfusion, due most often to hypovolemia. Untreated, this renal hypoperfusion leads to reduced urine output, reflecting reductions in glomerular filtration rate and renal tubule function. The key strategy in reducing the likelihood of oliguria progressing to acute renal failure is limiting the duration and magnitude of renal hypoperfusion. Indeed, renal blood flow, and in particular renal cortical blood flow, is significantly reduced early in acute renal failure regardless of the etiology. Persistence of renal hypoperfusion for only 30 minutes to 60 minutes may be sufficient to lead to acute renal failure. In this regard, undue reliance on laboratory tests (urinary electrolytes, urine osmolarity, derived indices such as renal failure index, or fractional excretion of sodium) to differentiate prerenal from renal causes of oliguria may delay institution of appropriate therapy.[50] None of these tests or derived indices are sufficiently sensitive or specific to predict whether patients have developed or will develop acute renal failure or who will or will not respond to therapy. Often, the most useful information in the perioperative management of potential acute renal failure is measurement of urine output. All these tests and measurements may be misleading in patients who have recently been treated with diuretics.

Treatment of Oliguria

Aggressive and early treatment of perioperative oliguria is most important for those patients at increased risk for developing acute renal failure. At-risk patients include (1) geriatric patients, (2) patients with sepsis, (3) those with co-existing renal and·or cardiac dysfunction, (4) patients with co-existing jaundice, and (5) those undergoing surgical procedures often associated with postoperative renal dysfunction (abdominal aneurysm resection, cardiac surgery, emergency surgery for trauma).

TABLE 21-6. Differential Diagnosis of Perioperative Oliguria

	Prerenal	Renal
Urinary sodium ($mEq·L^{-1}$)	Below 40	Above 40
Urine osmolarity ($mOsm·L^{-1}$)	Above 400	250–300
Ratio of urine to plasma osmolarity	Above 1.8	Below 1.1

Occurrence of transient oliguria during elective operations in young patients without co-existing renal disease does not require the same aggressive treatment as does oliguria in geriatric patients with co-existing renal disease (Fig. 21-11) (Prough DS, Bowman Gray School of Medicine, Personal communication).

Oliguria in patients considered at risk for development of acute renal failure is initially treated with rapid infusion of 500 ml of balanced salt solutions. Administration of diuretics at this point could produce further detri-

mental effects on renal blood flow if drug-induced diuresis accentuates co-existing hypovolemia. Brisk diuresis in response to a fluid challenge suggests hypovolemia as the cause of oliguria. When this fluid challenge does not produce a therapeutic response, additional fluids may be infused with or without monitoring of atrial filling pressures depending on whether patients are at risk for developing cardiac dysfunction. When patients are at risk for development of cardiac dysfunction and pulmonary artery occlusion pressures are normal

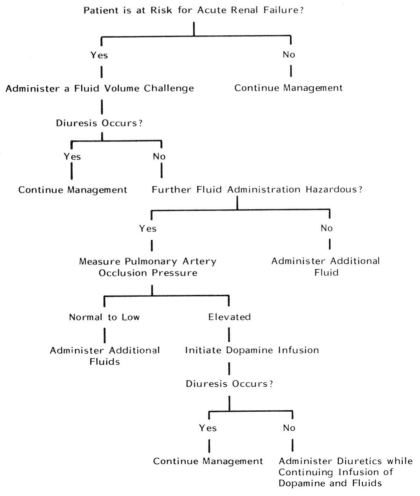

FIG. 21-11. Treatment of perioperative oliguria. (Data adapted from Prough DS, Bowman Gray School of Medicine, personal communication.)

or below normal, treatment with additional intravenous fluids is acceptable. In the presence of elevated pulmonary artery occlusion pressures, the possibility of oliguria and decreased renal blood flow due to low cardiac output should be considered. In this situation, infusion of dopamine, 1 $\mu g \cdot kg^{-1} \cdot min^{-1}$ to 5 $\mu g \cdot kg^{-1} \cdot min^{-1}$ is useful therapy. Failure of dopamine to improve urine output may be an indication to administer diuretics such as mannitol, 0.5 $g \cdot kg^{-1}$ to 1 $g \cdot kg^{-1}$ with or without furosemide 1 $mg \cdot kg^{-1}$ to 3 $mg \cdot kg^{-1}$. Combinations of low-dose dopamine (1 $\mu g \cdot kg^{-1} \cdot min^{-1}$ to 3 $\mu g \cdot kg^{-1} \cdot min^{-1}$) and high-dose furosemide (5 $mg \cdot kg^{-1}$ to 15 $mg \cdot kg^{-1}$) may facilitate conversion of oliguric to nonoliguric renal failure.[52] Although easier to treat with respect to fluid and electrolyte replacement, there is no evidence that conversion of oliguric to nonoliguric renal failure reduces mortality.[53]

DISEASE PROCESSES INVOLVING THE KIDNEY

A number of pathologic processes can as primary diseases involve the kidneys. Likewise, renal abnormalities can occur in association with dysfunction of other organ systems. A knowledge of associated pathology and characteristics of the renal disease is important for planning management of these patients in the perioperative period.

Glomerulonephritis

Acute glomerulonephritis is usually due to deposition of antigen-antibody complexes in the glomeruli. The source of antigens may be exogenous (poststreptococcal infection) or endogenous (collagen diseases). Glomerulonephritis can manifest as acute nephritic syndrome, nephrotic syndrome, or interstitial nephritis. Chronic renal failure can be the end result of glomerulonephritis. Indeed, glomerulonephritis is the most common cause of end-stage renal failure in adults.

ACUTE NEPHRITIC SYNDROME

Acute nephritic syndrome usually occurs in children, and is characterized by a sudden onset of hematuria with red blood cell casts. Proteinuria and hypertension are often present. The pathologic picture is that of cellular proliferation in the glomeruli.

Poststreptococcal glomerulonephritis is the classic entity associated with the acute nephritic syndrome. Renal dysfunction becomes clinically apparent 1 week to 3 weeks after an infection with group A beta-hemolytic streptococci. The disease in children is usually self-limited, and there is no evidence that treatment with corticosteroids or immunosuppressive drugs is beneficial.

Goodpasture's Syndrome. Goodpasture's syndrome is a combination of glomerulonephritis and pulmonary hemorrhage, which occurs most frequently in young males. Antibodies account for the renal lesions and apparently also react with similar antigens in the lungs, producing alveolitis that results in pulmonary hemorrhage. Typically, hemoptysis precedes clinical evidence of renal disease by several months. The prognosis is poor, with most patients progressing to renal failure within 1 year of the diagnosis. There is no known effective drug therapy.

NEPHROTIC SYNDROME

Nephrotic syndrome has a diverse etiology (Table 21-7) but is consistently characterized by increased glomerular permeability to plasma proteins. The classic symptom complex is massive proteinuria, hypoalbuminemia, and hypercholesterolemia. The marked reduction in albumin concentration and the decreased oncotic pressure lead to transfer of fluid from plasma to interstitial fluid spaces, resulting in edema, ascites, pleural effusions, and hypovolemia. Accumulation of fluid in interstitial spaces increases hydrostatic pressure outside of capillaries. This change counters re-

TABLE 21-7. Etiology of the Nephrotic Syndrome

Immunologic-systemic lupus erythematosus
Infections—bacterial, viral
Neoplastic—lung, Hodgkin's disease
Amyloidosis
Diabetes mellitus
Drugs—trimethadione, probenecid
Morbid obesity
Toxemia of pregnancy

duced plasma oncotic pressure and protects against further loss of plasma volume.

Renal biopsy is the standard diagnostic approach. Corticosteroids, usually prednisone, are frequently effective in abolishing proteinuria. Therapy with corticosteroids may be required for several weeks before a persistent remission is established. Cancer chemotherapeutic drugs, such as cyclophosphamide, may also be effective in the management of the nephrotic syndrome.

INTERSTITIAL NEPHRITIS

Interstitial nephritis has been observed as an allergic reaction to a number of drugs, including sulfonamides, allopurinol, phenytoin, and diuretics. Patients exhibit reduced ability to concentrate urine, proteinuria, and hypertension. Glomerular abnormalities on renal biopsy are often minimal. Instead, the renal biopsy shows infiltration of the renal interstitium by inflammatory cells. Corticosteroid therapy may be beneficial.

Polycystic Renal Disease

Polycystic renal disease is inherited as an autosomal dominant trait. The disease typically progresses slowly, until renal failure occurs in middle age. Mild hypertension and proteinuria are common. Decreased urine concentrating ability develops early in the course of the disease. Cysts may also be present in the liver and in the central nervous system, as intracranial aneurysms. Hemodialysis or renal transplantation will eventually be necessary in most patients.

Medullary Sponge Kidney Disease

Medullary sponge kidney disease is characterized by cystic dilation of one or more collecting ducts. It does not lead to reduced nephron function but rather to the development of renal calculi. Nephrolithiasis is the usual method of presentation. Infection is the most common complication.

Fanconi's Syndrome

Fanconi's syndrome results from inherited or acquired disturbances of proximal renal tubular function, causing hyperaminoaciduria, glycosuria, and hyperphosphaturia. There is renal loss of substances normally conserved by proximal renal tubules, including potassium, bicarbonate, and water. Symptoms of Fanconi's syndrome reflect the abnormality of the renal tubules and include polyuria, polydipsia, metabolic acidosis due to loss of bicarbonate, and skeletal muscle weakness related to hypokalemia. Dwarfism with osteomalacia, reflecting loss of phosphate, is prominent in these patients. Indeed, presentation as vitamin D-resistant rickets is frequent. Management of anesthesia must appreciate fluid and electrolyte disorders characteristic of this syndrome and recognize that left ventricular cardiac failure secondary to uremia is often present in the final stages.[54]

Bartter's Syndrome

Bartter's syndrome is characterized by renal juxtaglomerular apparatus hyperplasia, with elevated plasma concentrations of renin, angiotensin II, and aldosterone, Hypokalemic, hypochloremic metabolic alkalosis develops, and there is decreased vascular reactivity to vasopressor actions of angiotensin II and norepinephrine. Despite these changes, patients with Bartter's syndrome are characteristically normotensive. A cardinal feature of this syndrome is overproduction of prostaglandins.

TREATMENT

Treatment of Bartter's syndrome consists of oral supplements to replace sodium and potassium losses. Administration of spironolactone, an aldosterone antagonist, acts to preserve total body potassium. Propranolol has been used to decrease release of renin from the kidneys. Inhibition of prostaglandin synthesis is accomplished with drugs, such as aspirin or indomethacin. Blocking the conversion of angiotensin I to angiotensin II with captopril may be helpful. Surgical removal of the adrenal glands in an effort to control hyperaldosteronism has not proved to be effective.

MANAGEMENT OF ANESTHESIA

Management of anesthesia for patients with Bartter's syndrome is influenced by the status of renal function and the intravascular fluid volume.[55,56] For example, selection of enflurane may not be wise if there is evidence of renal dysfunction preoperatively. Patients treated with spironolactone and propranolol may be hypovolemic but may fail to manifest chronotropic responses because of beta-adrenergic blockade. A brisk diuresis with associated loss of potassium may occur in the perioperative period, requiring careful monitoring of acid-base and electrolyte status. Because of the tendency toward hypokalemic metabolic alkalosis, it is important to avoid hyperventilation of the lungs. It is conceivable, although undocumented, that diminished reactivity of blood vessels to catecholamines could be associated with exaggerated reductions in blood pressure produced by anesthetic drugs. Medications used to treat these patients should be continued throughout the perioperative period, even if it is necessary to administer oral medications via a nasogastric tube.

Amyloidosis

Diffuse amyloid deposition in glomeruli is followed by proteinuria and progressive renal failure. Hypertension occurs in about 50 percent of patients. Diagnosis is confirmed by renal biopsy.

Renal Hypertension

Renal disease is the most frequent cause of secondary hypertension. Accelerated or malignant hypertension is likely to be associated with renal disease. Furthermore, appearance of blood pressure elevations in young patients suggests the diagnosis of renal rather than essential hypertension. Hypertension due to renal dysfunction reflects either parenchymal disease of the kidneys or renal vascular disease.

Chronic pyelonephritis and glomerulonephritis are parenchymal diseases often associated with hypertension, particularly in younger patients. Less common forms of renal parenchymal disease that can cause hypertension include diabetic nephropathy, cystic disease of the kidneys, and renal amyloidosis. Renal vascular disease is characterized by atherosclerosis and accounts for only a small percentage of patients with hypertension. Sudden onset, however, of marked elevations in blood pressure or the presence of hypertension before the age of 30 years should arouse suspicion of renovascular disease. A bruit may be audible on auscultation of the abdomen over the areas of the kidneys. This type of hypertension does not respond well to antihypertensive drugs.

The mechanism for the production of hypertension in the presence of renal disease is not established. Stimulation of the renin-angiotensin-aldosterone system is a possible but unproven mechanism. Alternatively, the kidneys may function to some extent as antihypertensive organs, possibly producing substances with vasodepressor activity. Regardless of the mechanism, treatment of hypertension due to renal parenchymal disease is usually with antihypertensive drugs, including beta-adrenergic antagonist drugs, which inhibit release of renin from the kidneys. Treatment of hypertension due to renal vascular disease is with renal artery endarterectomy or nephrectomy.

Uric Acid Deposition

Acute uric acid nephropathy is distinct from gout and occurs when uric acid crystals are precipitated in the renal collecting tubules or ureters, producing acute oliguric renal failure. This precipitation occurs when the uric acid concentrations reach a saturation point in acidic urine. This is particularly likely to occur when uric acid production is greatly increased, as in patients with myeloproliferative disorders being treated with cancer chemotherapeutic drugs. These patients are particularly vulnerable to uric acid nephropathy if they have good renal function and urine concentrating ability and then become dehydrated or develop acidosis because of reduced caloric intake.

Liver Disease

Renal failure associated with liver disease is designated the hepatorenal syndrome. Renal failure may reflect vigorous attempts to reduce ascites, that lead to excessive reductions in intravascular fluid volume. Patients with hepatocellular or obstructive jaundice have also been observed to develop renal failure. Renal failure in these patients may be due to circulating bacterial endotoxins.

Nephrolithiasis

The majority of renal stones are composed of calcium oxalate (Table 21-8). These stones typically occur in the presence of hypercalciuria or hyperoxaluria. Causes of hypercalcemia and hypercalciuria are primary hyperparathyroidism, vitamin D intoxication, malignancies, and sarcoidosis. Small bowel bypass is associated with hyperoxaluria.

Alterations in the pH of the urine or the presence of metabolic disturbances can result in the formation of renal stones with a composition that differs from the typical calcium oxalate variety (Table 21-8). For example, urinary tract infections and renal tubular acidosis

TABLE 21-8. Composition and Characteristics of Renal Stones

Type of Stone	Incidence (% of Total)	Radiographic Appearance	Etiology
Calcium oxalate	80	Opaque	Hypercalciuria Hyperoxaluria Idiopathic
Magnesium ammonium phosphate	10	Opaque	Persistent alkaline urine (usually due to chronic bacterial infection)
Calcium phosphate	1	Opaque	Persistent alkaline urine (renal tubular acidosis, carbonic anhydrase inhibitors, antibiotics)
Uric acid	5–10	Lucent	Gout
Cystine	1	Opaque	Cystinuria
Xanthine	Rare	Lucent	Xanthine oxidase deficiency

produce persistent elevations of urinary pH and can lead to formation of magnesium ammonium phosphate stones and calcium phosphate stones. Allopurinol may be used to reduce rates of uric acid excretion in hyperuricemic patients. Manipulation of urine pH may also be effective in prevention of certain types of renal stones. Indeed, precipitation of uric acid and subsequent stone formation can be minimized by keeping urine pH above 6.0 with sodium bicarbonate. Conversely, a high urine pH may encourage calcium stone formation. A urine pH less than 6.0, by virtue of ammonium chloride therapy, will increase solubility for magnesium ammonium phosphate and calcium phosphate stones.

EXTRACORPOREAL SHOCK WAVE LITHOTRIPSY

Extracorporeal shock wave lithotripsy is a noninvasive treatment of renal stones that produces destruction of stones by shock waves. As an alternative to percutaneous nephrolithotomy, this approach has the advantages of low morbidity and shorter hospital stay. These are important attributes as the incidence of kidney stones is estimated as 1.5 per thousand.

Patients undergoing lithotripsy are strapped in a semireclining position into a hydraulically operated chairlike support system and then submerged in water from the clavicles down in a large immersion tub. Shock waves (up to 2,000 per treatment) are transmitted through water and focused precisely on the target stone using biplanar fluroscopy. To minimize the risk of initiating cardiac dysrhythmias, shock waves are triggered by the R-wave of the electrocardiogram and delivered to the kidney during the myocardial refractory period. Cardiac dysrhythmias may still occur but are usually self-limited and rarely require treatment with drugs such as lidocaine. Patients with artificial cardiac pacemakers are at risk for experiencing dysfunction of the pacemaker during this form of therapy. The impact of the shock waves at the flank entry site is painful and necessitates anesthesia. Immobilization is also important, as any movement may displace the stone from the predetermined focus site for the shock waves leading to unnecessary trauma

to adjacent tissues, as well as incomplete dissolution of the stone. Even spontaneous or mechanical ventilation of the lungs with associated movement of the diaphragm causes stones to move 30 mm to 32 mm along a vertical axis.[57] In this regard high-frequency positive pressure ventilation allows the stone to remain virtually stationary. Nevertheless, high-frequency positive pressure ventilation may not always provide adequate ventilation in patients undergoing this procedure.[58] Furthermore, expiratory flow limitations during high-frequency positive pressure ventilation may predispose to bronchospasm in vulnerable patients, especially those with co-existing obstructive airways disease. The ability to entrain volatile anesthetics into the anesthetic circuit during high frequency positive pressure ventilation facilitates production of adequate anesthesia.[57] General anesthesia using conventional methods of ventilation and regional anesthesia including epidural and intercostal nerve blocks with local infiltration have been used to provide analgesia during lithotripsy.[59,60] The head-up position during anesthesia can be associated with peripheral pooling of blood. This effect, however, is usually offset by immersion in water, which increases hydrostatic pressures on the abdomen and thorax so that blood pressure is maintained. In patients with limited cardiac reserve displacement of blood into the central circulation by virtue of increases in hydrostatic pressure may result in acute congestive heart failure. Likewise, hydrostatic forces on the thorax result in decreases in chest wall compliance and functional residual capacity. These changes may produce or aggravate ventilation to perfusion mismatches.

The water in the immersion tub must be kept warm to avoid hypothermia. Catheter insertion sites must be protected from immersion. Noise and vibrations associated with this therapy may make auditory monitoring of heart and breath sounds impractical.

Patients who are not candidates for extracorporeal shock wave lithotripsy include those with abdominal aortic aneurysms, spinal cord tumors, or orthopedic implants in the lumbar region. Parturients, obese patients, and patients with known coagulopathies also are not likely candidates.

MANAGEMENT OF ANESTHESIA FOR RENAL TRANSPLANTATION

Management of anesthesia for patients receiving kidney transplants invokes the same principles as detailed for chronic renal failure patients (see the section Management of Anesthesia for Patients with Chronic Renal Disease). This includes hemodialysis before surgery to optimize coagulation and hydration and to improve electrolyte and acid-base balance. Many of these patients are diabetics emphasizing the need to monitor blood glucose concentrations in the perioperative period. In addition, strict asepsis must be adhered to during placement of intravascular catheters and intubation of the trachea.

Regional and general anesthesia have been successfully used during renal transplantation.[61,62] Advantages of regional anesthesia include elimination of the need for intubation of the trachea in immunosuppressed patients, as well as the need for muscle relaxants. These advantages are negated, however, if regional anesthetics must be supplemented with injected or inhaled drugs. Furthermore, blockade of the peripheral sympathetic nervous system, as produced by regional anesthetics, can make control of blood pressure difficult, especially considering the unpredictable intravascular fluid volume status of these patients. Use of regional anesthesia, particularly epidural techniques, is controversial in the presence of abnormal coagulation. For these reasons, general anesthesia is often the preferred approach for management of patients undergoing renal transplantation.

When general anesthesia is selected, a useful approach is administration of nitrous oxide combined with volatile drugs or short-acting opioids. Plasma creatinine concentrations, urine volume, and urine specific gravity after renal transplantation are not different when nitrous oxide plus enflurane, halothane, or fentanyl are used.[63] Nevertheless, use of volatile drugs has some potential disadvantage. For example, administration of enflurane is questionable, since elimination of fluoride depends on glomerular filtration rate, which is often decreased in the early period after renal trans-

plantation. In addition, the likely presence of liver disease in patients undergoing chronic hemodialysis, and the frequent occurrence of hepatic dysfunction after renal transplantation must be remembered when considering the use of halothane. Furthermore, reductions in cardiac output due to negative inotropic effects of volatile drugs must be minimized to avoid jeopardizing the adequacy of tissue oxygen delivery, especially if anemia is present. All factors considered, skeletal muscle relaxing effects of isoflurane, plus its minimal metabolism, make this volatile anesthetic an attractive choice. Disadvantages of opioids used during anesthesia for renal transplantation are their lack of skeletal muscle relaxant effects and the fact that excessive elevations in blood pressure cannot be reliably prevented or treated with these drugs.

Choice of muscle relaxants must consider the unpredictable nature of renal function after renal transplantation. In this regard, pancuronium is more dependent on renal excretion than is d-tubocurarine. Furthermore, the newly transplanted kidney appears able to excrete d-tubocurarine at rates similar to the rates of excretion achieved by two normal kidneys.[44] All factors considered, use of intermediate-acting muscle relaxants, especially atracurium, is attractive for patients undergoing renal transplantation due to the fact these drugs have minimal to absent dependence on renal function for clearance from the plasma. Pharmacokinetics of anticholinesterase drugs as used to antagonize nondepolarizing neuromuscular blockade are unchanged within 1 hour after renal transplantation.[48,64] Regardless of the muscle relaxant chosen, the dose should be carefully titrated and patients closely observed in the early postoperative period for recurrence of skeletal muscle weakness.

Fluid management includes intravenous replacement of intravascular fluid volume lost due to surgical trauma. In addition, intravenous fluids are necessary to optimize intravascular fluid volume and thus maintain renal blood flow to the newly transplanted kidney. Potassium-containing intravenous fluid solutions should be used with caution in these patients. The anuric patient typically requires about 8 ml·kg^{-1} daily to replace insensible water loss. Humidification of inspired gases during surgery reduces this maintenance fluid requirement. Replacement of this insensible water loss, as well as fluid translocated due to surgical trauma, is often with 5 percent glucose solutions with 0.45 percent sodium chloride to minimize sodium load until renal function is established after renal transplantation. Tissue oxygen delivery can be improved by administering erythrocytes. In the absence of cardiopulmonary disease, monitoring central venous pressure is a useful guide to the optimal rate of intravenous fluid infusion. Optimal hydration during the intraoperative period improves early function of the transplanted kidney.[65]

Diuretics are often administered to facilitate urine formation by the newly transplanted kidney. In this regard, an osmotic diuretic such as mannitol will facilitate urine output and reduce excess tissue and intravascular fluid. Unlike loop diuretics (furosemide or ethacrynic acid), mannitol does not depend on renal tubular concentrating mechanisms to produce diuresis.

Cardiac arrest has been described after completion of the renal artery anastomosis to the transplanted kidney.[66] This event occurred with the release of the occlusion clamp and most likely reflected sudden hyperkalemia, due to establishment of blood flow to the transplanted kidney and washout of potassium-containing solutions used to preserve the kidney before transplantation.[67] In addition, if clamping of the external iliac artery is necessary during the renal artery anastomosis, potassium can be released into the circulation from the ischemic limb after removal of the clamp. In addition, unclamping may be followed by hypotension due to the abrupt addition of up to 300 ml to the intravascular fluid space plus release of vasodilating chemicals from previously ischemic tissues. Ideally, this hypotension, when it does occur, is treated with intravenous infusion of fluids.

Acute immunologic rejection of the newly transplanted kidney can occur. This rejection manifests in the vasculature of the transplanted kidney and can be so rapid that inadequate circulation is evident almost immediately after the blood supply to the kidney is established. When rejection occurs this rapidly, it most likely reflects previous sensitization to specific donor antigens, as present in previously transfused blood products. Nevertheless, for unclear reasons, recipients of blood transfusions have a much higher rate of organ survival than recipients who have not received transfusions.[68] Delayed signs of rejection of the transplanted kidney include hyperthermia, deterioration of urine output, and disseminated intravascular coagulation. Prompt removal of the rejected organ is necessary when bleeding due to disseminated intravascular coagulation occurs.

BENIGN PROSTATIC HYPERTROPHY

Benign prostatic hypertrophy reflects glandular and leiomyomatous hyperplasia of the submucosal glands and smooth muscle of the prostatic urethra that typically occurs after 50 years of age. This growth is stimulated by testicular hormones. Initially, patients complain of frequency, nocturia and feeling of incomplete emptying. Obstruction to urine flow may result in urinary retention and renal failure. Definitive therapy is transurethral resection of the prostate (TURP). Because patients are often elderly, they are likely to have coexisting medical diseases, especially cardiopulmonary disorders. The surgical procedure itself is associated with absorption of nonelectrolyte irrigating fluids used to distend the bladder and wash away blood and prostatic tissue. Absorption of this fluid can produce circulatory overload, hyponatremia, and decreases in plasma osmolarity.[69] Two commonly used isomolar irrigating solutions are Cytol (sorbital plus mannitol) and glycine. The amount of irrigating fluid absorbed is determined by the number of venous sinuses opened during the surgical resection, the hydrostatic pressure of the irrigating fluid (determined by the height of the fluid container above the patient), and the duration of the resection (ideally limited to less than 60 minutes).

It is estimated that 10 ml to 30 ml of irrigating fluid are absorbed for every minute of operating time, although volumes exceeding

6000 ml have been absorbed in 75 minutes to 120 minutes, of resection. This absorbed fluid produces hyponatremia, and patients with co-existing cardiac disease are also vulnerable to developing pulmonary edema from acute increases in intravascular fluid volume. Central nervous system changes due to cerebral edema include irritability, confusion, and seizures, especially if plasma sodium concentrations acutely decline below 100 mEq·L^{-1}. Cardiac dysrhythmias and conduction abnormalities may also accompany hyponatremia. Ammonia resulting from metabolism of glycine, which is commonly used as an irrigating fluid, may contribute to central nervous system depression after TURP.[70] Glycine may also act as an inhibitory neurotransmitter in the retina and transient blindness after TURP has been attributed to intravascular absorption of this irrigating fluid.[71]

Management of Anesthesia

Spinal anesthesia has been recommended for TURP since awake patients may demonstrate early signs of excessive intravascular absorption of irrigating fluid or accidental urinary bladder perforation (referred subdiaphragmatic pain). A T-10 sensory level is necessary when regional anesthetics are selected for TURP. General anesthesia may mask these signs but, nevertheless, may be a more desirable approach in patients who cannot co-operate or who require support of ventilation of the lungs. Assessment of blood loss during TURP is difficult because dilution of blood by irrigating fluids and the usual hemodynamic responses of blood loss (e.g., tachycardia and hypotension) are unreliable. Blood transfusion intraoperatively is guided by the preoperative hematocrit, duration and difficulty of the resection, and clinical assessment of the patient's condition. Bleeding is about 15 ml·g^{-1} of resected tissue. Intraoperative monitoring of hematocrit, plasma sodium concentrations and·or osmolarity may be useful in detecting excessive hemodilution due to intravascular absorption of irrigating fluids. Central venous pressure elevations are likely to accompany these changes. Although increases in blood pressure are likely to accompany hypervolemia, hypotension may also occur. Plasma sodium concentrations below 120 mEq·L^{-1} signal excessive hemodilution. Administration of diuretics, and on rare occasions hypertonic saline, may be required to treat hyponatremia.

REFERENCES

1. Stein JH. Hormones and the kidney. The kidney in health and disease. Hosp Pract 1979;14:91–105

2. Mitch WE, Walser M. A proposed mechanism for reduced creatinine excretion in severe chronic renal failure. Nephron 1978;21:248–54

3. Epstein M. Effects of aging in the kidney. Fed Proc 1979;38:168–71

4. Curtis JR, Donovan BA. Assessment of renal concentrating ability. Br Med J 1979;1:304–5

5. Cousins MJ, Mazze RI. Methoxyflurane nephrotoxicity—a study of dose response in man. JAMA 1973;225:1611–6

6. Loehning RW, Mazze RI. Possible nephrotoxicity from enflurane in a patient with severe renal disease. Anesthesiology 1974;40:203–5

7. Mazze RI, Schwartz RD, Slocum HC, Barry KG. Renal function during anesthesia and surgery—the effects of halothane anesthesia. Anesthesiology 1963;24:279–84

8. Cousins MJ, Greenstein LR, Hitt BA, Mazze RI. Metabolism and renal effects of enflurane in man. Anesthesiology 1976;44:44–53

9. Mazze RI, Cousins MJ, Barr GA. Renal effects and metabolism of isoflurane in man. Anesthesiology 1974;40:536–42

10. Barry KG, Mazze RI, Schwartz FD. Prevention of surgical oliguria and renal hemodynamic suppression by sustained hydration. N Engl J Med 1964;270:1371–7

11. Bastron RD, Perkins FM, Pyne JL. Autoregulation of renal blood flow during halothane anesthesia. Anesthesiology 1977;46:142–4

12. Runciman WB, Mather LE, Ilsley AH, et al. A sheep preparation for studying interactions between blood flow and drug disposition. Br J Anaesth 1984;56:1247–58

13. Gorman HM, Craythorne NB. The effects of a new neurolept analgesic agent (Innovar) on renal function in man. Acta Anaesthesiol Scand (Supply) 1966;24:111–8

14. Stanley TH, Gray NH, Bidwai AV, Lordon R. The

effects of high dose morphine and morphine plus nitrous oxide on urinary output in man. Can Anaesth Soc J 1974;21:379–83

15. Jarnberg P-O, Santesson J, Eklund J. Renal function during neurolept anaesthesia. Acta Anaesthesiol Scand 1978;22:167–72

16. Hirasawa H, Yonezawa T. The effects of ketamine and Innovar on the renal cortical and medullary blood flow of the dog. Anaesthesist 1975;24:349–53

17. Macdonald AG. The effect of halothane on renal cortical blood flow on normotensive hypotensive dogs. Br J Anaesth 1969;41:644–54

18. Kennedy WF, Sawyer TK, Gerbershagen HU, et al. Simultaneous systemic cardiovascular and renal hemodynamic measurements during high spinal anesthesia on normal man. Acta Anaesthesiol Scand 1979;37:163–71

19. Kennedy WF, Sawyer TK, Gerbershagen HU, et al. Systemic cardiovascular and renal hemodynamic alterations during peridural anesthesia in normal man. Anesthesiology 1969;31:414–21

20. Philbin DM, Coggins CH. Plasma antidiuretic hormone levels in cardiac surgical patients during morphine and halothane anesthesia. Anesthesiology 1978;49:95–8

21. Annat G, Viale JP, Xuan BB, et al. Effect of PEEP ventilation on renal function, plasma renin, aldosterone, neurophysins and urinary ADH, and prostaglandins. Anesthesiology 1983;58:136–41

22. Bailey D, Miller ED, Kaplan JA, Rogers PW. The renin-angiotensin-aldosterone system during cardiac surgery with morphine-nitrous oxide anesthesia. Anesthesiology 1975;42:538–44

23. Miller ED, Gianfagra W, Ackerly JA, Peach MJ. Converting enzyme activity and pressure responses to angiotensin I and II in the rat awake and during anesthesia. Anesthesiology 1979;50:88–92

24. Miller ED, Ackerly JA, Peach MJ. Blood pressure support during general anesthesia in a renin-dependent state in the rat. Anesthesiology 1978;48:404–8

25. Creasser C, Stoelting RK. Serum inorganic fluoride concentrations during and after halothane, fluroxene and methoxyflurane anesthesia in man. Anesthesiology 1973;39:537–40

26. Mazze RI, Calverley RK, Smith NT. Inorganic fluoride nephrotoxicity: Prolonged enflurane and halothane anesthesia in volunteers. Anesthesiology 1977;46:265–71

27. Mazze RI, Sievenpiper TS, Stevenson J. Renal effects of enflurane and halothane in patients with abnormal renal function. Anesthesiology 1984;60:161–3

28. Young SR, Stoelting RK, Peterson C, Madura JA. Anesthetic biotransformation and renal function

in obese patients during and after methoxyflurane or halothane anesthesia. Anesthesiology 1975;42:451–57

29. Bentley JB, Vaughn RW, Miller MS, et al. Serum inorganic levels in obese patients during enflurane anesthesia. Anesth Analg 1979;58:409–12

30. Jarnberg P-O, Ekstrand J, Irestedt L. Renal fluoride excretion and plasma fluoride levels during and after enflurane anesthesia are dependent on urinary pH. Anesthesiology 1981;54:48–52

31. Ghoneim MM, Long JP. The interaction between magnesium and other neuromuscular blocking agents. Anesthesiology 1970;32:23–7

32. McDermott JR, Smith AI, Ward MK, et al. Brain-aluminum concentrations in dialysis encephalopathy. Lancet 1978;1:901–3

33. Tinker JH, Michenfelder JD. Increased resistance to nitroprusside-induced cyanide toxicity in anuric dogs. Anesthesiology 1980;52:40–7

34. Weir PH, Chung FF. Anaesthesia for patients with chronic renal disease. Can Anaesth Soc J 1984;31:468–80

35. Ghoneim MM, Pandya H. Plasma protein binding of thiopental in patients with impaired renal or hepatic function. Anesthesiology 1975;42:545–8

36. Powell DR, Miller RD. The effect of repeated doses of succinylcholine on serum potassium in patients with renal failure. Anesth Analg 1975;54:746–8

37. Gronert GA, Lambert EH, Theye RA. The response of denervated skeletal muscle to succinylcholine. Anesthesiology 1973;39:13–22

38. Ryan DW. Preoperative serum cholinesterase concentration in chronic renal failure. Br J Anaesth 1977;49:945–9

39. Don HF, Dieppa RA, Taylor P. Narcotic analgesics in anuric patients. Anesthesiology 1975;42:745–7

40. Carter R, Heerdt M, Acchiardo S. Fluoride kinetics after enflurane anesthesia in healthy and anephric patients and in patients with poor renal function. Clin Pharmacol Ther 1977;20:565–70

41. Bromage PR, Gertel M. Brachial plexus anesthesia in chronic renal failure. Anesthesiology 1972;36:488–93

42. Brotherton WP, Matteo RS. Pharmacokinetics and pharmacodynamics of metocurine in humans with and without renal failure. Anesthesiology 1981;55:273–6

43. McLeod K, Watson MJ, Rawlings MD. Pharmacokinetics of pancuronium in patients with normal and impaired renal function. Br J Anaesth 1976;48:341–5

44. Miller RD, Matteo R, Benet LZ, Sohn YJ. Influence of renal failure on the pharmacokinetics of d-tubocurarine in man. J Pharmacol Exp Ther 1977;202:1–7

45. Hunter JM, Jones RS, Utting JE. Comparison of vecuronium, atracurium and tubocurarine in normal patients and in patients with no renal function. Br J Anaesth 1984;56:941–50

46. Fahey MR, Rupp SM, Canfell C, et al. Effect of renal function on laudanosine excretion in man. Br J Anaesth 1985;57:1049–51

47. Bencini AF, Scaf AHJ, Sohn YJ, et al. Disposition and urinary excretion of vecuronium bromide in anesthetized patients with normal renal function or renal failure. Anesth Analg 1986;65:245–51

48. Morris RB, Cronnelly R, Miller RD, et al. Pharmacokinetics of edrophonium in anephric and renal transplant patients. Br J Anaesth 1981;53:1311–3

49. Tilney NL, Lazarus JM. Acute renal failure in surgical patients. Surg Clin North Am 1983;63:357–77

50. Oken DE. On the differential diagnosis of acute renal failure. Am J Med 1981;71:916–20

51. Linder A. Synergism of dopamine and furosemide in oliguric acute renal failure. Nephron 1983;33:121–6

52. Krasna MJ, Scott GE, Scholz PM, et al. Postoperative enhancement of urinary output in patients with acute renal failure using continuous furosemide therapy. Chest 1986;89:294–5

53. Brown CB, Ogg CS, Cameron JS. High dose furosemide in acute renal failure. Clin Nephrol 1981;15:90–6

54. Joel M, Rosales JK. Fanconi syndrome and anesthesia. Anesthesiology 1981;55:455–6

55. Abston PA, Priano LL. Bartter's syndrome: Anesthetic implications based on pathophysiology and treatment. Anesth Analg 1981;60:764–6

56. Nishikawa T, Dohi S. Baroreflex function in a patient with Bartter's syndrome. Can Anaesth Soc J 1985;32:646–50

57. Perel A, Hoffman B, Podeh D, Davidson DJT. High frequency positive pressure ventilation during general anesthesia for extracorporeal shock wave lithotripsy. Anesth Analg 1986;65:1231–4

58. Berger JJ, Boysen PG, Gravenstein JS, et al. Failure of high frequency jet ventilation to ventilate patients adequately during extracorporeal shock-wave lithotripsy. Anesth Analg 1987;66:262–3

59. Duvall JO, Griffith DP. Epidural anesthesia for extracorporeal shock wave lithotripsy. Anesth Analg 1985;64:544–6

60. Malhotra V, Long CW, Meister MJ. Intercostal blocks with local infiltration anesthesia for extracorporeal shock wave lithotripsy. Anesth Analg 1987;66:85–8

61. Linke CL, Merin RG. A regional anesthetic approach for renal transplantation. Anesth Analg 1976;55:69–73

62. Borland LM, Cook DR. Anesthesia for organ transplantation. In: Stoelting RK, Barash PG, Gallagher TJ, eds. Advances in Anesthesia. Chicago. Year Book Medical Publishers 1986:1–36

63. Goldman E, Goldman MC, Sherrill D, Aldrete JA. Enflurane and renal function after transplantation. Anesthesiology 1979;51:S24

64. Cronnelly R, Stanski DR, Miller RD, Sheiner LB. Pyridostigmine kinetics with and without renal function. Clin Pharmacol Ther 1980;28:78–81

65. Carlier M, Squifflet JP. Maximal hydration during anesthesia increases pulmonary artery pressure and improves function of human renal transplants. Transplantation 1982;34:701–4

66. Hirschman CA, Edelstein G. Intraoperative hyperkalemia and cardiac arrests during renal transplantation in an insulin-dependent diabetic patient. Anesthesiology 1979;51:161–2

67. Hirschman CA, Leon D, Edelstein G, et al. Risk of hyperkalemia in recipients of kidneys preserved with an intracellular electrolyte solution. Anesth Analg 1980;59:283–6

68. Opelz G, Terasaki PI. Improvement of kidney-graft survival with increased numbers of blood transfusion. N Engl J Med 1978;299:799–803

69. Wong KC, Wen-Shin L. Anesthesia for urologic surgery. In: Stoelting RK, Barash PG, Gallagher TJ, eds. Advances in Anesthesia. Chicago. Year Book Medical Publishers 1986;4:349–92

70. Roesch RP, Stoelting RK, Lingeman JE, et al. Ammonia toxicity resulting from glycine absorption during a transurethral resection of the prostate. Anesthesiology 1983;58:577–9

71. Ovassapian A, Joshi CW, Brunner EA. Visual disturbance: An unusual symptom of transurethral prostatic resection reaction. Anesthesiology 1982;57:332–4

22

Water and Electrolyte Disturbances

Alterations of water and electrolyte content and distribution can produce multiple organ system dysfunction in the perioperative period. For example, impairment of central nervous system, cardiac, and neuromuscular function are likely in the presence of water and electrolyte (sodium, potassium, calcium, magnesium) disorders. Furthermore, those disorders often accompany events associated with the perioperative period (Table 22-1). Management of patients with water and electrolyte disorders requires an understanding of the distribution of water and electrolytes and the electrophysiology of cells.

portant for the viability of cells. Indeed, water is the medium in which all metabolic reactions occur. Furthermore, all nutrients and solutes of the body are dissolved or suspended in water.

Total body water content is categorized as intracellular or extracellular fluid, according to the location of water relative to cell membranes (Fig. 22-2). Intracellular fluid represents about 55 percent of the total body water content; the remaining water is distributed as extracellular fluid. Extracellular fluid is further divided into interstitial and intravascular (plasma) fluid on the basis of the location of water relative to capillary membranes. Calcu-

DISTRIBUTION OF BODY WATER

Total body water content is greatest at birth, representing about 70 percent of the body weight in kilograms (Fig. 22-1). With increasing age, total body water content decreases, constituting about 60 percent of the body weight of an average adult man and 50 percent of the body weight of an adult woman. This difference is due to the greater fat content of women. Since fat is essentially anhydrous, it contributes to body weight without a proportionate increase in the volume of total body water. Constant total body water content is im-

TABLE 22-1. Etiology of Water and Electrolyte Disturbances

Disease States
  Endocrinopathies
  Nephropathies
  Gastroenteropathies

Drug Therapy
  Diuretics
  Corticosteroids

Nasogastric Suction

Surgical Interventions
  Transurethral resection of prostate
  Translocation of fluid due to tissue trauma
  Resection of portions of the gastrointestinal tract

Management of Anesthesia
  Intravenous fluid administration
  Hyperventilation

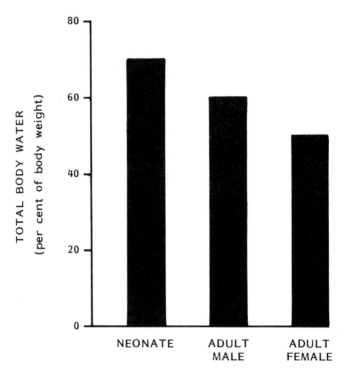

FIG. 22-1. Total body water represents about 70 percent of the body weight (kg) of neonates, 60 percent of adult men, and 50 percent of adult women. Anhydrous fat contributes a disproportionate amount to the body weight of adult women, explaining the decreased amount of body water relative to body weight.

lation of water content of these fluid spaces is summarized in Table 22-2.

The body's main priority is to maintain intravascular fluid volume. Acute reductions in this volume, as occur with fluid deprivation

TABLE 22-2. Calculation of Total Body Water Content and Distribution in an Average 70 kg Adult

	Male (L)	Female (L)
Total body water	42	35
	(70 × 0.6)*	(70 × 0.5)*
Total intracellular water	23	19
	(42 × 0.55)†	(35 × 0.55)†
Total extracellular water	19	16
	(42 × 0.45)	(35 × 0.45)

* Total body water content constitutes 60 percent of the body weight (kg) of an adult man and 50 percent of the body weight of an adult woman.

† Intracellular water represents about 55 percent of the total body water content.

in the preoperative period, blood loss, or surgical trauma that results in tissue edema ("third-space loss"), elicit the release of antidiuretic hormone and renin (Fig. 22-3). Both of these substances subsequently result in responses at renal tubules that lead to restoration of intravascular fluid volume. Furthermore, interstitial fluid is in dynamic equilibrium with intravascular fluid, serving as an available reservoir from which water and electrolytes can be mobilized into the circulation. Conversely, interstitial fluid spaces can accept water and electrolytes if these substances are present in excess amounts in intravascular fluid spaces. Peripheral edema is a manifestation of excess amounts of water in interstitial fluid spaces.

Water moves freely across cell and capillary membranes. Therefore, water content of these fluid compartments is dependent on osmotic, hydrostatic, and oncotic pressures.

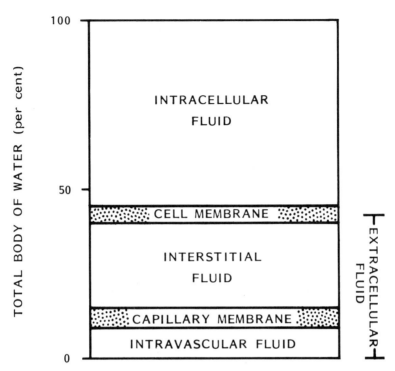

FIG. 22-2. Total body water is designated as intracellular or extracellular fluid, depending on the location of water relative to cell membranes. Water in the extracellular compartment is further subdivided as interstitial or intravascular (plasma) fluid, depending on its location relative to capillary membranes. About 55 percent of total body water is intracellular, 37 percent interstitial, and the remaining 8 percent intravascular.

Osmotic Pressure

The pressure necessary to prevent movement of solvent (water) to another fluid space is designated the osmotic pressure. The amount of osmotic pressure exerted by a solute is dependent on the number of molecules or ions (osmoles) present in the solvent. Osmolarity denotes the concentration of solute (osmoles) present in 1 L of water. Sodium is the most important cation for determining plasma osmolarity. Indeed, plasma osmolarity can be predicted clinically by doubling the plasma sodium concentration (Table 22-3). Low plasma osmolarity (below 285 mOsm·L^{-1}) means a high concentration of water; a high osmolarity (above 295 mOsm·L^{-1}) means a low concentration.

If solutes are present in different concentrations on the two sides of permeable membranes, the solutes and water will move across membranes in response to their individual concentration gradients. The result is equality of all concentrations in the two solutions. If the membranes are permeable to water but not solutes (i.e., semipermeable membranes), then only water will move until its concentration is equal on the two sides.

Intravenous solutions administered to patients are considered isotonic, hypotonic, or hypertonic according to their effective osmotic pressures relative to plasma. Normal saline and 5 percent glucose in water has an osmolarity similar to body fluids. Therefore, these fluids are classified as isotonic solutions. It is important to understand, however, that metabolism and cellular uptake of glucose present in 5 percent glucose in water results in hypotonic solutions. The resulting free water can distrib-

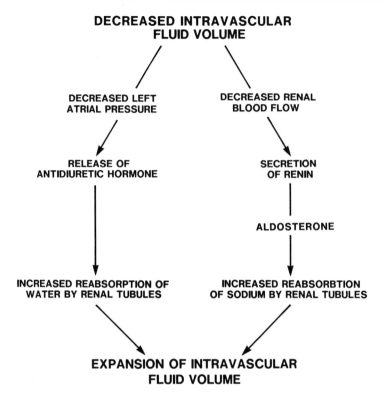

FIG. 22-3.   Acute reductions in intravascular fluid volume elicit changes mediated by antidiuretic hormone and the renin-angiotensin-aldosterone system. These changes lead to increased reabsorption of water and sodium by renal tubules. The net effect of increased water and sodium reabsorption by renal tubules is an expansion of intravascular fluid volume.

ute itself among all fluid compartments with less than 10 percent remaining intravascular. Lactated Ringer's solution, containing 5 percent glucose, is initially hypertonic (about 527 mOsm·L^{-1}), but the hypertonicity diminishes as glucose is metabolized and taken up by cells.

Hydrostatic Pressure and Oncotic Pressure

Movement of water across cell membranes is not influenced by hydrostatic pressure, since transmembrane pressures are low. Conversely, the pressure produced by the heart results in a hydrostatic pressure gradient of approximately 20 mmHg across capillary membranes. If this pressure gradient is not counterbalanced, it tends to force intravascular water into the interstitial fluid compartment. Indeed, were it not for large protein molecules (principally albumin), which cannot freely cross capillary membranes, there would be continuous loss of intravascular fluid volume. The concentrations of these proteins are just sufficient to balance the hydrostatic pressure difference of about 20 mmHg that exists between the intravascular and interstitial fluid compartments. This osmotic effect produced by proteins maintains the circulating plasma volume and is called the colloid osmotic or oncotic pressure. An important way to increase circulating plasma volume is to infuse albumin, which draws water from the interstitial into the intravascular fluid space.

TABLE 22-3. Calculation of Plasma Osmolarity

Plasma osmolarity

$$= 2(\text{Plasma Sodium Concentration}) + \frac{\text{BUN}}{2.8}$$

$$+ \frac{\text{Glucose}}{18}$$

Normal plasma osmolarity is 285 mOsm·L^{-1} to 295 mOsm·L^{-1}. In the presence of normal blood urea nitrogen (BUN, 10 mg·dl^{-1} to 20 mg·dl^{-1}) and blood glucose (60 mg·dl^{-1} to 100 mg·dl^{-1}) levels, plasma osmolarity can be predicted as twice the plasma sodium concentration. As the BUN and·or blood glucose concentrations increase, a greater impact is exerted by these substances on plasma osmolarity.

DISTRIBUTION OF ELECTROLYTES

The distribution and concentration of electrolytes differ greatly among the fluid compartments for body water (Table 22-4). The major cation in intravascular fluid is sodium, plus small amounts of potassium, calcium, and magnesium. In contrast, the major cation in intracellular fluid is potassium. The net effect is a concentration of total cation that is essentially equal throughout body water. These positive charges are balanced by anions such as chloride, bicarbonate, phosphate, and the negative charged sites on proteins.

Sodium is unique in that changes in the concentrations of this ion in extracellular fluid are usually due to changes in the volume of solvent (water) and not changes in total body content of sodium. Therefore, changes in plasma sodium concentrations must be interpreted with respect to total body water content. Indeed, acute changes in plasma sodium concentrations usually reflect alterations in total body water content and not sodium content.

Plasma potassium concentrations are easily measured, but only about 2 percent (80 mEq) of total body potassium content is present in extracellular fluid. Skeletal muscles are the major storage site of potassium.

ELECTROPHYSIOLOGY OF CELLS

Electrophysiology of excitable cells is dependent on intracellular and extracellular concentrations of sodium, potassium, and calcium. An essential characteristic of excitable cells is their ability to maintain concentration gradients for sodium and potassium across their membranes. As a result of this unequal distribution of ions (excess potassium inside and sodium outside cells), there is an electrochemical difference across cell membranes, with the interior of cells being negative relative to the exterior (Fig. 22-4). At rest, the interior of cells is about -90 mV with respect to the outside of cells. The negative electrical potential of cell interiors is designated as the resting membrane potential. Arrival of an appropriate stimulus (electrical, chemical, mechanical) results in altered permeability of cell membranes, such that sodium enters and potassium

TABLE 22-4. Composition (Approximate) of Extracellular and Intracellular Fluids (mEq·L^{-1})

Substance	Extracellular		Intracellular
	Intravascular	Interstitial	
Sodium	140	145	10
Potassium	5	4	150
Calcium	5	2.5	<1
Magnesium	2	1.5	40
Chloride	103	115	4
Bicarbonate	28	30	10

Total anion concentration also consists of phosphates, sulfates, organic acids, and negatively charged sites on proteins.

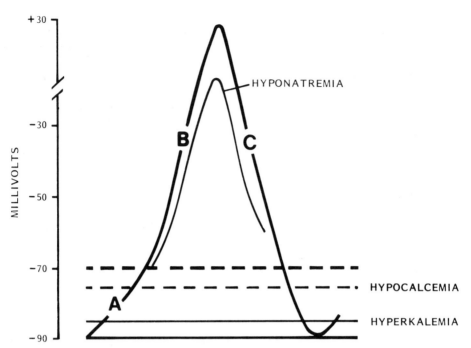

FIG. 22-4. This schematic diagram depicts the electrophysiology of an automatic (pacemaker) cell. The resting membrane potential (−) is normally minus 90 mV. Continuous movement of sodium and potassium across cell membranes results in spontaneous depolarization (A) until the threshold potential (− −) is reached at about − 70 mV. When the threshold potential is reached, there are sudden increases in permeability of cell membranes to sodium, and rapid depolarization (B) leads to the production of an action potential. After propagation of the action potential, permeability of cell membranes is restored, sodium is pumped out of the cells, and repolarization occurs (C). Disturbances of electrolyte concentrations alter the electrophysiology of cells. For example, hyponatremia decreases the amplitude of the action potential. Hyperkalemia results in a less negative resting membrane potential. Hypocalcemia results in a more negative threshold potential.

leaves the cells. The net effect of this change is a decrease in the electrical potential difference (that is, the resting membrane potential becomes less negative) across cell membranes. When the difference across cell membranes is about − 70 mV, there is a sudden additional influx of sodium that produces a reversal of the electrical charge across cell membranes. The result is the production of an action potential. After this maximum depolarization, the permeability of cell membranes is restored and repolarization ensues. Automatic cardiac pacemaker cells differ from contractile cells in that the resting membrane potential is not stable but undergoes spontaneous depolarization until the threshold potential is reached (Fig. 4-3).

Electrophysiology of cells and the resulting action potentials are altered by changes in the concentrations of electrolytes (Fig. 22-4). For example, sodium is necessary for cellular depolarization and generation of an action potential. Indeed, the amplitude of the action potential is decreased in the presence of hyponatremia. Potassium gradients across cell membranes are the most important determinants of resting membrane potentials. An increase in extracellular concentrations of potassium results in less negative resting membrane potentials that are closer to threshold potentials. Conversely, reductions in the extracellular concentrations of potassium make resting membrane potentials more negative. Excitability of cells is partly related to the distance between the resting membrane potential and the threshold potential. Since hyperkalemia brings the resting membrane potential closer to the threshold potential, a smaller impulse is required to elicit an action potential. Therefore, the excitability of cells is considered to be increased. Effects of potassium on the rate of spontaneous depolarization and conduction velocity of neural impulses must also be considered when predicting effects of changes in the concentration of this electrolyte on the excitability of cells. For example, reductions in plasma potassium concentrations increase the rate of spontaneous depolarization, while high concentrations of extracellular potassium slow conduction velocity of neural impulses. All factors considered, it is difficult to predict reliably the effects of changes in plasma concentrations of potassium on the excitability of cells. Calcium is also necessary for the maintenance of threshold potentials.

TOTAL BODY WATER EXCESS

The hallmark of excess total body water content is hyponatremia (plasma sodium concentrations below 135 mEq·L^{-1}) in the presence of a normal or increased intravascular fluid volume. Because the kidneys have an extraordinary ability to excrete increased amounts of water, patients with excess body water are also likely to have impaired renal function. The ability of the kidneys to excrete water is impaired, for example, in patients with excess body water associated with congestive heart failure, nephrosis, and cirrhosis of the liver. Peripheral edema is a manifestation of excess body water that accompanies these disease processes.

Excess body water can also be due to inappropriate secretion of antidiuretic hormone, but edema does not occur (see the section Inappropriate Secreton of Antidiuretic Hormone). Intravascular absorption of large volumes of water, as during transurethral resection of the prostate, can result in iatrogenic water intoxication. Regardless of the etiology, an excess of body water results in reductions of plasma sodium concentrations and decreases in plasma osmolarity.

Signs and Symptoms

Signs and symptoms of total body water excess depend on absolute plasma sodium concentrations and the rate of its decline. When water retention is sufficient to reduce plasma sodium concentrations below 120 mEq·L^{-1}, it is likely that central nervous system signs ranging from confusion to drowsiness will manifest. Further declines to less than 110 mEq·L^{-1} can produce seizures and coma. These central nervous system abnormalities most likely reflect cerebral edema and increased intracranial pressure. Cardiac dysrhythmias, including ventricular fibrillation, can occur when plasma sodium concentrations decreases below 100 mEq·L^{-1}.

Treatment

Emergency treatment of excess body water is to reduce the water content of the brain by administering hypertonic saline or mannitol. As a rough guide, 1 ml of 5 percent saline will increase sodium concentrations of a liter of body water by 1 mEq. For example, to increase plasma sodium concentrations from 130 mEq·L^{-1} to 140 mEq·L^{-1} in a 70 kg adult male (predicted total body water content 42 liters) would require about 420 ml of 5 percent saline (1 ml × 10 mEq × 42 liters). The rate of sodium administration varies from 30 minutes to several hours, depending on the urgency of the situation and should stop once seizures cease or cardiac dysrhythmias are corrected. In contrast to saline, mannitol not only removes water from cells but also results in an osmotic diuresis. Both saline and mannitol will initially expand the extracellular fluid volume.

Management of Anesthesia

Management of anesthesia must consider the likely presence of renal, cardiac, or liver disease as an etiology for excess body water. Decreased excitability of cells due to low plasma sodium concentrations (Fig. 22-4) could result in poor cardiac contractility and increased sensitivity to nondepolarizing muscle relaxants. This former possibility should be considered when hypotension occurs, particularly during administration of anesthetics with known negative inotropic effects. Likewise, the dose of muscle relaxants should be titrated, observing responses evoked by peripheral nerve stimulators.

TABLE 22-5. Factors Associated with Inappropriate Secretion of Antidiuretic Hormone

Postoperative Period

Positive Pressure Ventilation of the Lungs

Endocrine Disorders
  Adrenal cortical insufficiency
  Anterior pituitary damage

Carcinoma of Lung

Central Nervous System Dysfunction
  Infection
  Hemorrhage
  Trauma

Drugs
  Chlorpropamide
  Opioids
  Diuretics
  Antimetabolites

INAPPROPRIATE SECRETION OF ANTIDIURETIC HORMONE

Inappropriate secretion of antidiuretic hormone results in water retention, low output of a highly concentrated urine, and dilutinal hyponatremia.[1] In addition, urinary excretion of sodium is increased, which further lowers plasma sodium concentrations. Despite this excess sodium loss, hypovolemia does not occur, since the concomitant retention of water has expanded the intravascular fluid volume. Secretion of antidiuretic hormone is considered to be inappropriate, since there is no physiologic stimulus present to stimulate elaboration of this hormone.

Inappropriate secretion of antidiuretic hormone has been described after a number of events (Table 22-5). The possible occurence of this response in the postoperative period should be appreciated.[2] For example, a consistent metabolic response to surgery is the release of antidiuretic hormone for up to 96 hours postoperatively.[3] Indeed, acute hyponatremia is the most common acute biochemical change found after surgery. The most likely mechanism for this hyponatremia is acute expansion of intravascular fluid volume secondary to hormone-induced reabsorption of water by renal tubules. This excess hormone release

(aldosterone also) may be an exaggerated response to decreases in intravascular fluid volume that often occurs during invasive operations (Fig. 22-3). Abrupt reductions in the plasma concentrations of sodium (especially below 110 $mEq\cdot L^{-1}$) can lead to cerebral edema and seizures. Indeed, intravenous administration of sodium deficient solutions to oliguric postoperative patients has led to hyponatremia, seizures, and permanent brain damage.[4]

Inappropriately elevated urinary sodium concentrations and osmolarity in the presence of hyponatremia and decreased plasma osmolarity (less than 280 $mOsmol\cdot L^{-1}$) is virtually diagnostic of inappropriate antidiuretic hormone secretion. Treatment is initially with reductions in water intake to 500 $ml\cdot day^{-1}$. Establishment of a negative water balance leads to a spontaneous decreases in the release of antidiuretic hormone and often is the only treatment necessary in postoperative patients in whom the abnormality of antidiuretic hormone secretion is transient. Demeclocycline may be administered to antagonize the effects of antidiuretic hormone on renal tubules. Restriction of fluid intake and administration of demeclocycline, however, are not immediately effective for management of patients manifesting acute neurologic symptoms due to hyponatremia. In these patients, intravenous infu-

sion of hypertonic saline solutions sufficient to elevate plasma concentrations of sodium 0.5 $mEq \cdot L^{-1} \cdot hr^{-1}$ is a useful guideline. Overly rapid correction of symptomatic hyponatremia has been associated with a fatal neurologic disorder known as central pontine myelinolysis.[5]

IATROGENIC WATER INTOXICATION

The most likely cause of iatrogenic water intoxication is intravascular absorption of large volumes of nonelectrolyte solutions used for irrigation during transurethral resection of the prostate (see Chapter 21). The volume of water absorbed during this procedure has been estimated to be 10 ml to 30 ml for every minute of resection time.[6] Dilution of plasma sodium concentrations due to absorption of nonelectrolyte solutions can occur precipitously, leading to grand mal seizures, particularly if plasma sodium concentrations decrease to below 120 $mEq \cdot L^{-1}$.[7] Visual disturbances may accompany cerebral edema. Other evidence of water intoxication is arterial hypertension, bradycardia, increased central venous pressure, mental agitation, and pulmonary edema. In addition, plasma osmolarity and hematocrit are predictably decreased when excess nonelectrolyte solutions have been absorbed.

A high index of suspicion is important in early detection and recognition of iatrogenic water intoxication. Treatment of water intoxication is with saline, guided by repeated measurements of the plasma sodium concentrations. Congestive heart failure may require administration of diuretics (furosemide) and digitalis.

TOTAL BODY WATER DEFICITS

The hallmark of total body water deficits are plasma sodium concentrations above 145 $mEq \cdot L^{-1}$. Pure water deficits are rare, as most conditions leading to water loss are also ac-companied by loss of electrolytes. Causes of pure water loss include deficiencies or absence of antidiuretic hormone (diabetes insipidus) or resistance of renal tubules to the effects of this hormone. For example, pure water loss due to renal tubular unresponsiveness to antidiuretic hormone can accompany hypercalcemia, hypokalemia, and chronic nephritis. Pure water deficits can also occur in elderly or confused patients who do not respond to the sensation of thirst. Prolonged mechanical ventilation of the lungs with unhumidified gases can also lead to substantial water loss.

Signs and Symptoms

Clinical manifestations of deficits of total body water reflect loss of water from all fluid compartments. For example, mucous membranes are dry and skin turgor is reduced. When dehydration is severe, blood pressure, venous pressure, and urine output are reduced, and heart rate is increased. Postural hypotension is often present. Peripheral cyanosis reflects a sluggish peripheral circulation, with marked desaturation of the venous blood. Central nervous system dysfunction (drowsiness, coma) can occur. Because intracellular and extracellular fluid volumes are both reduced, the hematocrit will probably not rise significantly. Blood urea nitrogen and serum creatinine concentrations will increase, as hypovolemia produces decreases in blood pressure and cardiac output that lead to reductions in renal blood flow and glomerular filtration rate. If the kidneys are responding normally, the urine concentrating system will be functioning at its maximum level resulting in a urine with a high osmolarity (above 800 $mOsm \cdot L^{-1}$) and specific gravity (above 1.030). Peripheral edema is absent, emphasizing that reductions in total body water content are responsible for increased plasma sodium concentrations.

Treatment

Treatment of deficits of body water consists of administering free water based on measured reductions in body weight or, more commonly, the magnitude of elevation of plasma sodium concentrations. An acceptable approach is administration of 5 percent dextrose in water, with the volume and rate of administration guided by changes in blood pressure, central venous pressure, urine output, and repeated determinations of plasma sodium concentrations. It should be appreciated that the brain does not necessarily shrink to the same extent that total body water diminishes, particularly if dehydration is gradual. Thus, if correction of the body water deficit is rapid, the brain can take up excessive water, leading to the development of cerebral edema.

Management of Anesthesia

Induction and maintenance of anesthesia in the presence of decreased intravascular fluid volume due to a total body water deficits are likely to be accompanied by reductions in blood pressure. Specifically, peripheral vasodilation produced by opioids, volatile drugs, or d-tubocurarine can unmask hypovolemia. Ketamine is less likely to reduce blood pressure when intravascular fluid volume is reduced. Positive pressure ventilation of the lungs and blood loss are likely to produce exaggerated blood pressure reductions in these patients.

A contracted intravascular fluid volume also results in decreased volume of distribution for drugs such as nondepolarizing muscle relaxants, which are primarily limited in their distribution to extracellular fluid. Conceivably, these patients could have an increased sensitivity to muscle relaxants. Likewise, effects of barbiturates might be exaggerated. Measurements of cardiac filling pressures and urine output are helpful in guiding the volume and rate of intravenous fluid administration.

SODIUM EXCESS

Total body excess of sodium is reflected by plasma sodium concentrations that exceed 145 mEq·L^{-1}. The kidneys closely regulate total body sodium content, such that excess accumulation of sodium is almost impossible unless there is altered renal function. For example, impairment of sodium excretion by the kidneys often occurs in patients with congestive heart failure, nephrotic syndrome, and cirrhosis of the liver with ascites. Increased reabsorption of sodium by renal tubules is a classic response to excess aldosterone secretion by the adrenal cortex. Indeed, in patients with primary aldosteronism, hypernatremia predominates, with little evidence of expansion of the interstitial fluid volume. It must be remembered, however, that the most common cause of hypernatremia is not an excess of total body sodium, but rather a decrease in the total body content of water.

Signs and Symptoms

Peripheral edema is the hallmark of increased total body sodium content. Interstitial fluid spaces, however, can be expanded by as much as 5 liters in normal adults before edema is detectable. Other features of total body sodium excess include ascites, pleural effusion, and an expanded intravascular fluid volume that manifests as hypertension.

Treatment

Treatment of excess total body sodium is facilitation of excretion of sodium via the kidneys. This is accomplished by the administration of diuretics that prevent reabsorption of sodium by the renal tubules.

Management of Anesthesia

Other than the recognition of an increased intravascular fluid volume, there are no specific recommendations regarding management of anesthesia. Although the volume of distri-

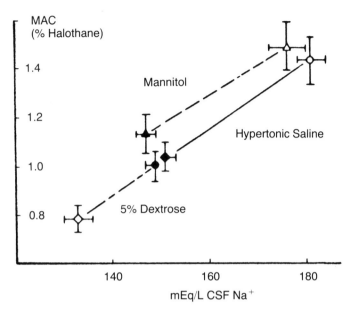

FIG. 22-5. In animals, anesthetic requirements for halothane (MAC) parallel changes in sodium concentrations and osmolarity of cerebrospinal fluid (CSF) produced by infusion of mannitol, hepertonic saline or 5 percent dextrose. (Tanifuji Y, Eger EI. Brain sodium, potassium and osmolality: Effects on anesthetic requirement. Anesth Analg 1978;57:404–10 Reprinted with permission from IARS.)

bution for parenteral drugs is increased, clinical responses produced by these drugs do not seem to be predictably altered. In animals, abrupt increases in sodium concentrations of cerebrospinal fluid and accompanying hyperosmolarity are associated with elevations in anesthetic requirements for halothane (Fig. 22-5).[8]

SODIUM DEFICIT

Reductions in total body sodium content are reflected by decreases in plasma sodium concentrations below 135 mEq·L^{-1}. Excessive loss of sodium can result from vomiting, diarrhea, diaphoresis, third-degree burns, and administration of thiazide diuretics. As with total body sodium excess, it is important to remember that the most common cause of hyponatremia is not a deficiency of total body sodium but rather an excess of total body water.

Signs and Symptoms

Total body sodium deficit is evidenced by decreased intravascular fluid volume and cardiac output. Conversely, hyponatremia due to excess of total body water is associated with an increased intravascular fluid volume. Manifestations of reduced intravascular fluid volume include decreased blood pressure, venous pressure, and glomerular filtration rate, plus an increased heart rate. Hematocrit is typically increased, reflecting reductions in intravascular fluid volume without concomitant loss of erythrocytes.

Reductions of interstitial fluid volume in association with deficits of total body sodium concentrations are reflected by decreases in skin turgor. Because the amount of underlying fat can also affect skin elasticity, a useful site to look for decreased skin turgor is the forehead. Loss of skin elasticity in the extremities cannot be distinguished from poor skin turgor accompanying the aging process.

TABLE 22-6. Calculation of Total Body
Sodium Deficit

Sodium Deficit = 140 − Plasma Sodium

× Total Body Water (weight in kg × 0.6)

Example: The predicted sodium deficit in an 80 kg
male with a plasma sodium concentration of 120
mEq·L^{-1} would be calculated as:

$$= (140 - 120) \times (80 \times 0.6)$$
$$= 20 \qquad \times 48$$
$$= 960 \text{ mEq}$$

Failure of sodium pump mechanisms (sick
cell syndrome) results in passage of sodium
into cells. As a result, other ions leave cells,
and hyponatremia is not associated with the
expected decrease in plasma osmolarity.

Treatment

Treatment of total body sodium deficits is
made difficult by the fact that there is usually
an accompanying loss of body water. An approximation of sodium deficits, however, can
be calculated from plasma sodium concentrations and the predicted total body water content (Table 22-6). Despite substantial calculated deficits of total body sodium, use of
hypertonic saline is usually reserved for symptomatic hyponatremia, which is most likely to
be present when plasma sodium concentrations are below 110 mEq·L^{-1} (see the section
Inappropriate Secretion of Antidiuretic Hormone).

Management of Anesthesia

Considerations for management of anesthesia in the presence of total body deficits of
sodium are similar to those outlined for patients with total body water deficits. In animals, abrupt decreases in sodium concentrations of cerebrospinal fluid and associated

decreases in osmolarity are associated with decreases in anesthetic requirements for halothane (Fig. 22-5).[8]

HYPERKALEMIA

Hyperkalemia (plasma potassium concentrations above 5.5 mEq·L^{-1} can be due to increased total body potassium content or to alterations in distribution of potassium between
intracellular and extracellular sites (Table 22-
7).

Increased Total Body Potassium Content

Increased total body potassium content occurs when the kidneys are unable to excrete
sufficient cation to maintain plasma potassium
concentrations below 5.5 mEq·L^{-1}. Acute oliguric renal failure is the classic cause of hyperkalemia. In contrast, patients with chronic
renal disease do not usually develop hyperkalemia until glomerular filtration rates decrease to less than 15 ml·min^{-1}.[9] Patients with
severe renal disease, but not requiring hemodialysis, may be vulnerable to hyperkalemia if
they are challenged with potassium loads. This
potential hazard must be considered when
penicillin (1.7 mEq of potassium for every 1
million units of penicillin) or banked whole

TABLE 22-7. Causes of Hyperkalemia

Increased Total Body Potassium Content
    Acute oliguric renal failure
    Chronic renal disease
    Decreased aldosterone secretion
        Adrenal cortex disease
        Aldosterone-antagonist diuretics

Altered Distribution of Potassium Between
    Intracellular and Extracellular Sites
    Succinylcholine
    Respiratory or metabolic acidosis
    Lysis of cells due to chemotherapy
    Iatrogenic (exogenous) bolus administration
    Diabetes mellitus

blood (1 mEq of potassium·L^{-1}·day^{-1} of storage) is administered to patients with chronic renal disease. Hypoaldosteronism favors potassium retention such that hyperkalemia can result. Likewise, diuretics such as spironolactone and triamterene, which act as aldosterone antagonists, can interfere with renal elimination of potassium.

Altered Distribution of Potassium

Altered distribution of potassium between intracellular and extracellular sites can result in hyperkalemia, even in the absence of changes in total body content of potassium. For example, release of intracellular potassium and subsequent hyperkalemia after succinyl-choline administration to patients with burns, spinal cord transection, or muscle trauma is well recognized.[10–12] Respiratory or metabolic acidosis favors passage of potassium from intracellular to extracellular locations. Specifically, a 0.1 unit decrease in arterial pH, as produced by a 10 mmHg increase of the carbon dioxide partial pressures, can increase plasma potassium concentrations about 0.5 mEq·L^{-1} (Fig. 22-6).[13] Increased plasma potassium concentrations can result from tumor lysis and release of intracellular constituents, including potassium. This response is most likely to occur in patients receiving cancer chemotherapeutic drugs for treatment of leukemia or lymphoma. Iatrogenic hyperkalemia has been attributed to poor mixing of potassium chloride added to plastic fluid containers, resulting in intravenous delivery of the added potassium chloride to patients as a bolus.[14] The likelihood of inadequate mixing is minimal when potassium chloride is added with plastic containers

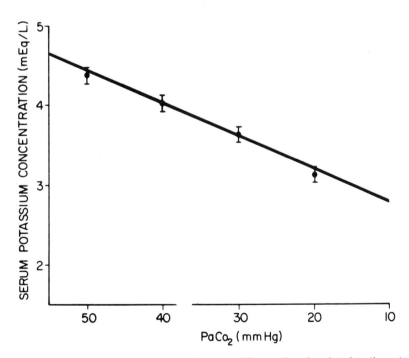

FIG. 22-6. Plasma potassium concentrations (Mean ± SE) are directly related to the arterial carbon dioxide partial pressures ($PaCO_2$). A 10 mmHg change in $PaCO_2$ results in corresponding changes in plasma potassium concentrations of about 0.5 mEq·L^{-1}. (Edwards R, Winnie AP, Ramamurthy S. Acute hypocapneic hypokalemia: An iatrogenic anesthetic complication. Anesth Analg 1977;56:786–92 Reprinted with permission from IARS.)

held in the inverted position with the injection port uppermost. Increased plasma potassium concentrations in patients with diabetes mellitus reflect impaired glucose transfer into cells due to the absence of insulin.[15]

Signs and Symptoms

Adverse effects of hyperkalemia are likely to accompany acute increases in plasma potassium concentrations. In contrast, chronic hyperkalemia is more likely to be associated with normalization of gradients between extracellular and intracellular concentrations of potassium and return of the resting membrane potentials of excitable cells to near normal. Indeed, the fact that patients with chronic elevations of potassium are often asymptomatic supports the greater importance of appropriate potassium gradients across cell membranes rather than the absolute plasma concentrations of potassium.

The most detrimental effect of hyperkalemia is on the cardiac conduction system. Characteristic changes on the electrocardiogram are prolonged P-R intervals with ultimate loss of P waves, broadening of QRS complexes, ST segment elevation, and peaking of T-waves (Fig. 22-7).[16] These changes may be difficult to distinguish from idioventricular rhythm or acute myocardial infarctions. Peaking of T-waves, although diagnostic, occurs in less than 25 percent of patients with hyperkalemia. Appearance of abnormalities on the electrocardiogram depends on the absolute levels of plasma potassium, as well as on the rapidity with which plasma potassium concentrations have increased. For example, cardiac conduction abnormalities are frequently present when plasma potassium concentrations exceed 6.5 mEq·L^{-1}. Nevertheless, these changes can manifest at even lower plasma potassium concentrations if the increase has been acute. Peaked T-waves and ventricular dysrhythmias seem to be most likely when plasma potassium concentrations approach 7 mEq·L^{-1}. Although ventricular fibrillation can occur, the more likely event in the presence of hyperkalemia is cardiac standstill in diastole.

Hyperkalemia is often accompanied by skeletal muscle weakness. The mechanism for this effect is not clear.

Treatment

Treatment of acute hyperkalemia is designed to move potassium from plasma into cells and to antagonize effects of potassium on the heart (Table 22-8). If plasma potassium concentrations are less than 6.5 mEq·L^{-1} and there are no indications of cardiac toxicity on the electrocardiogram, the treatment of hyperkalemia may be conservative, being directed at correction of the underlying problem. The most rapidly acting therapeutic approach for reversal of the cardiac manifestations of hyperkalemia is intravenous administration of calcium. Potassium can be shifted into cells by production of systemic alkalosis (hyperventilation of the lungs or intravenous administration of sodium bicarbonate) or by intravenous injection of glucose combined with regular insulin (2 g glucose for every unit of regular insulin). A common approach is the intravenous infusion of 25 g of glucose combined with 10 units to 15 units of regular insulin. Insulin is given to ensure that glucose enters cells and carries potassium with it. All these treatments represent temporizing measures (e.g., an alteration in the distribution of potassium) until elimination of excess potassium from the body can be accomplished. This latter goal can require use of potassium binding resins (Kayexalate) used as enemas, or institution of peritoneal or hemodialysis.

Management of Anesthesia

Ideally, plasma potassium concentrations should be below 5.5 mEq·L^{-1} before subjecting patients to elective operations that require an anesthetic. If this is not possible, it is important to adjust anesthetic techniques so as to recognize adverse effects of hyperkalemia intraoperatively and to minimize the likelihood of

TABLE 22-8.   Treatment of Hyperkalemia

Treatment	Mechanism	Onset	Duration
Calcium	Direct antagonism	Rapid	15–30 minutes
Sodium bicarbonate	Direct antagonism	15–30 minutes	3–6 hours
	Redistribution		
Glucose and insulin	Redistribution	15–30 minutes	3–6 hours
Kayexelate	Decreased total body content	1–3 hours	
Peritoneal dialysis	Decreased total body content	1–3 hours	
Hemodialysis	Decreased total body content	Rapid	

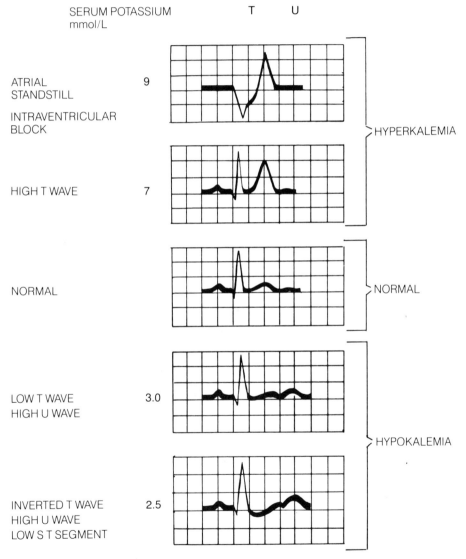

FIG. 22-7.   Schematic representation of typical changes on the electrocardiogram produced by deviations of plasma potassium concentrations from normal levels. Plasma potassium concentrations are the same whether expressed as $mMol \cdot L^{-1}$ or $mEq \cdot L^{-1}$. (Goudsouzian NG, Karamanian A. The electrocardiogram. In: Physiology for the Anesthesiologist. New York. Appleton-Century-Crofts 1977:37.)

additional increases in plasma potassium concentrations. Specifically, it is important to monitor the electrocardiogram continuously to detect adverse cardiac effects produced by hyperkalemia. Ventilation of the lungs must be managed in a way that assures the absence of carbon dioxide accumulation, which would lead to respiratory acidosis and transfer of potassium from intracellular to extracellular sites. Metabolic acidosis due to unrecognized arterial hypoxemia or excessive depths of anesthesia would also contribute to an extracellular distribution of potassium. Mild hyperventilation of the lungs during the intraoperative period would seem logical, since a 10 mmHg decrease in arterial carbon dioxide partial pressures reduces plasma potassium concentrations about 0.5 mEq·L^{-1} (Fig. 22-6).[13] These goals are facilitated by measuring arterial blood gases and pH.

Responses to muscle relaxants must also be considered when hyperkalemia is present. Plasma potassium concentrations increase about 0.3 mEq·L^{-1} to 0.5 mEq·L^{-1}, after administration of 1 mg·kg^{-1} to 2 mg·kg^{-1} of succinylcholine.[17] The implications of a 0.5 mEq·L^{-1} increase must be considered when coexisting plasma potassium concentrations are elevated. Since there is no effective way to prevent release of potassium after administration of succinylcholine, it may be prudent to avoid administration of this drug to patients with elevated plasma potassium concentrations, though institution of hyperventilation before the injection of succinylcholine might provide some degree of protection. Responses to nondepolarizing muscle relaxants in the presence of hyperkalemia are unclear. Presence of skeletal muscle weakness preoperatively would suggest the possibility of decreased muscle re-

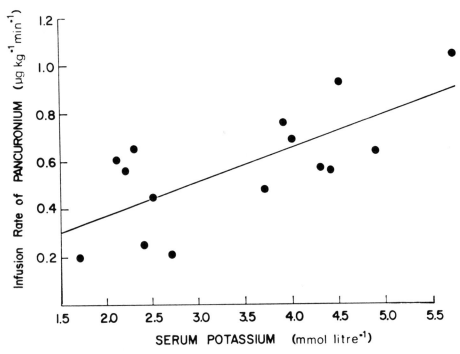

FIG. 22-8. The relationship between the infusion rate of pancuronium necessary to maintain 90 percent depression of twitch tension and plasma potassium concentrations is depicted. Each dot represents data from a single cat. Reductions in plasma potassium concentrations from 4.0 mEq·L^{-1} to 2.0 mEq·L^{-1} reduces by about 50 percent the infusion rate of pancuronium necessary to maintain an unchanging twitch depression. (Miller RD, Roderick LL. Diuretic-induced hypokalemia, pancuronium neuromuscular blockade and its antagonism by neostigmine. Br J Anaesth 1978;50:541–4)

laxant requirements intraoperatively. Evidence from an animal study suggests that dose requirements for pancuronium are directly related to plasma potassium concentrations (Fig. 22-8).[18] A useful approach would seem to be titration of muscle relaxants until desired effects are obtained, as evidenced by monitoring with a peripheral nerve stimulator.

Perioperative intravenous fluids must be selected with the realization that most solutions contain potassium. Lactated Ringer's solution contains 4 mEq·L^{-1}, Normosol-R 5 mEq·L^{-1} and Normosol-M 13 mEq·L^{-1} of potassium. Drugs such as calcium and glucose-insulin must be readily available to treat intraoperative manifestations of hyperkalemia. Unlike alterations in plasma concentrations of sodium, hyperkalemia is not associated with alterations in requirements for volatile anesthetics.[8]

HYPOKALEMIA

Hypokalemia (plasma potassium concentrations below 3.5 mEq·L^{-1} can be due to a decreased total body potassium content or alterations in distribution of potassium between intracellular and extracellular sites (Table 22-9). Chronic hypokalemia is likely to be associated with decreased total body content of potassium, as well as reductions in plasma concentrations of this ion. In contrast, acute hypokalemia is usually due to intracellular translocation of potassium, without a change in total body content.

Clinically, the only practical means of assessing hypokalemia is by measuring plasma concentrations of potassium. Nevertheless, it is important to remember that 98 percent of total body potassium is intracellular and thus not measured by plasma determinations (Table 22-4). Furthermore, as extracellular potassium is lost, intracellular potassium crosses cell membranes along a concentration gradient in an attempt to restore extracellular fluid concentrations and thus maintain the normal ratio of intracellular to extracellular potassium. Indeed, enormous potassium deficits can be present with only a small decrease in plasma

TABLE 22-9. Causes of Hypokalemia

Decreased Total Body Potassium Content
　Gastrointestinal loss
　　Vomiting—diarrhea
　　Nasogastric suction
　　Villous adenoma of the colon
　Renal loss
　　Osmotic-tubular diuretics
　　Hyperglycemia
　　Excess aldosterone secretion
　　Excess endogenous or exogenous cortisol
　　Surgical trauma
　Decreased oral intake

Altered Distribution of Potassium Between
　Intracellular and Extracellular Sites
　Respiratory or metabolic alkalosis
　Glucose-insulin
　Familial periodic paralysis
　Beta-2 agonist stimulation

potassium concentrations. For example, it is estimated that chronic reductions of 1 mEq·L^{-1} in plasma potassium concentrations can reflect total body deficits of 600 mEq to 800 mEq of potassium.

Decreased Total Body Potassium Content

Deficits of total body potassium are most often due to increased chronic loss of this ion via the gastrointestinal tract or the kidneys. Gastrointestinal losses of potassium responsible for hypokalemia include vomiting, diarrhea, laxative abuse, nasogastric suction, and villous adenomas of the colon. Renal losses of potassium occur in response to osmotic and tubular diuretics, hyperglycemia, and excess secretion of aldosterone or cortisol. Trauma as produced by surgery results in loss of potassium (50 mEq·day^{-1} for the first 2 days postoperatively) via the kidneys. Inadequate oral intake of potassium is an uncommon cause of hypokalemia unless the patient's only source of nutrition is potassium-free parenteral fluids.

Differentiating hypokalemia due to gastrointestinal versus renal losses is facilitated by measuring concentrations of potassium in the urine. If the gastrointestinal tract is the source of loss, the kidneys will respond by reducing urinary excretion of potassium to less than 10 mEq·L⁻¹. Conversely, if the kidneys are the source, urine potassium content is likely to exceed 40 mEq·L⁻¹.

Altered Distribution of Potassium

Hypokalemia without changes in total body potassium content occurs when potassium is acutely shifted from the extracellular fluid into cells to replace hydrogen ions, which have left cells to offset increases in arterial pH. For example, plasma potassium concentrations decrease approximately 0.5 mEq·L⁻¹ for every 10 mmHg reduction in the arterial carbon dioxide partial pressure (Fig. 22-6).[13] Hyperventilation of the lungs during anesthesia is the most frequent cause of acute hypokalemia due to changes in the distribution of potassium between cells and extracellular fluid. Another cause of acute hypokalemia due to this mechanism is glucose-insulin infusions that drive potassium into cells without altering the total body content of potassium. The hypokalemic form of familial periodic paralysis is also characterized by abrupt intracellular shifts of potassium from the intravascular fluid space (see Chapter 28).

The sympathetic nervous system modulates distribution of potassium between intracellular and extracellular sites. For example, beta-2 agonist stimulation, as produced by epinephrine, causes reductions in plasma concentrations of potassium reflecting catecholamine-induced intracellular redistribution of potassium (Fig. 22-9).[19] Hypokalemia by this mechanism is a hazard of treating premature labor with beta-2 agonists such as terbutaline and ritodrine.[20]

Signs and Symptoms

Hypokalemia produces adverse effects, which are manifested as changes at the heart, neuromuscular junction, gastrointestinal tract,

and kidneys. It is important to appreciate that responses due to hypokalemia can be different if reductions in potassium concentrations are acute rather than chronic.

HEART

Acute hypokalemia, as produced by hyperventilation of the lungs, is unlikely to produce significant alterations in cardiac contractility or conduction.[21] In contrast, intracellular depletion of potassium, as is likely with chronic hypokalemia, is associated with poor myocardial contractility.[22] Furthermore, abrupt additional decreases in plasma potassium concentrations in the presence of co-existing chronic hypokalemia are more likely to produce cardiac conduction and rhythm abnormalities than is the same degree of hypokalemia produced acutely but in the absence of co-existing total body potassium depletion. It is speculated that sudden decreases in plasma potassium concentrations exert more profound effects on electrochemical gradients for potassium in chronically hypokalemic patients. Orthostatic hypotension in the presence of hypokalemia may reflect autonomic nervous system dysfunction.

Changes on the electrocardiogram produced by hypokalemia characteristically reflect impaired cardiac conduction (Fig. 22-7).[16] The P-R intervals and Q-T intervals are prolonged, ST segments are depressed, T waves are flat, and prominent U waves are present. There is increased automaticity of the atria and ventricles, reflecting the more rapid rate of spontaneous depolarization, which occurs in the presence of hypokalemia (Fig. 22-4). Ventricular fibrillation is a common terminal dysrhythmia in the presence of hypokalemia.

NEUROMUSCULAR JUNCTION

Hypokalemia is associated with skeletal muscle weakness, which is most prominent in the legs and rarely affects muscles innervated by cranial nerves.[23] Induced in cats by the chronic administration of a potassium-losing diuretic, hypokalemia is also associated with increased sensitivity to the effects of pancu-

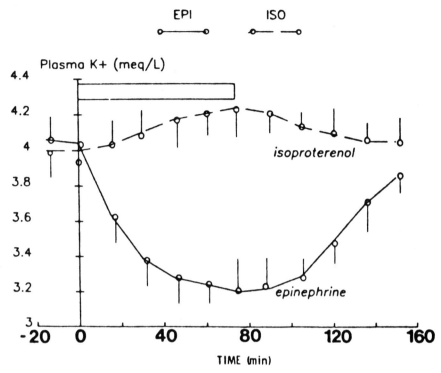

FIG. 22-9. Beta-2 agonist effects of epinephrine (EPI) are responsible for intracellular movement of potassium and associated declines in plasma concentrations of potassium. Plasma potassium concentrations return slowly to control levels after discontinuation of epinephrine infusions. (Brown MJ, Brown DC, Murphy MB. Hypokalemia from beta-2 receptor stimulation by circulating epinephrine. N Engl J Med 1983;309:1414–9)

ronium (Fig. 22-8).[18] In addition, more neostigmine is needed to antagonize neuromuscular blockade produced by pancuronium in the presence of hypokalemia.[18] Nevertheless, the clinical importance of changes in response to muscle relaxants and their antagonists produced by hypokalemia is probably minimal. Indeed, neuromuscular blockade was always antagonized in the presence of hypokalemia.[18]

GASTROINTESTINAL TRACT AND KIDNEYS

Effects of hypokalemia on gastrointestinal and renal function are manifested as ileus and polyuria. Polyuria probably reflects the association of hypokalemia with impaired urine-concentrating ability. Decreased plasma potassium concentrations are associated with de-

creased glomerular filtration rate and renal blood flow.

Treatment

Treatment of hypokalemia depends on whether decreased plasma potassium concentrations are associated with normal or decreased total body potassium content. When total body potassium content is normal, as with acute hypokalemia, treatment begins with correction of the underlying cause, such as excessive intraoperative hyperventilation of the lungs.

Chronic hypokalemia associated with decreased total body potassium content is treated with supplemental potassium chloride. Chloride is important, since hypochloremic metabolic alkalosis is frequently associated with hypokalemia. Despite the common practice of administering supplemental potassium chloride, there is evidence that such therapy may be ineffective and unnecessary.[24,25] For example, about 50 percent of patients with diruetic-induced hypokalemia fail to attain normal plasma concentrations of potassium despite potassium supplementation. Indeed, in many treated patients, most of the ingested supplemental potassium is excreted in the urine despite persistence of hypokalemia. Even in the presence of hypokalemia, measurements of intracellular potassium concentrations are often normal.[26]

It must be appreciated that chronic hypokalemia is often associated with total body potassium deficits exceeding 500 mEq or even 1000 mEq. This emphasizes that potassium content cannot be totally corrected in the 12 hours to 24 hours preceding elective surgery. Nevertheless, intravenous infusions of potassium chloride ($0.2 \text{ mEq·kg}^{-1}\text{·hr}^{-1}$) in the few hours preceding surgery have been suggested to be beneficial even in severely depleted patients.[21] The explanation is not clear, but it is possible that even small amounts of potassium are helpful in normalizing the electrophysiology of cells. Continuous monitoring of the electrocardiogram during intravenous administration of potassium is essential. Repeat plasma potassium measurements every 12 hours to 24 hours should be used to guide continued replacement and rates of infusion. When digitalis toxicity is suspected, potassium chloride can be administered as 0.5 mEq to 1 mEq intravenous boluses every 3 minutes to 5 minutes until the electrocardiogram reverts to normal. A practical point is to administer the potassium in glucose-free solutions; hyperglycemia would favor potassium entrance into cells, which could further exaggerate the degree of hypokalemia.

Management of Anesthesia

Advisability of proceeding with elective surgery in the presence of chronic plasma potassium concentrations below 3.5 mEq·L^{-1} is controversial.[27] It is suggested that chronically hypokalemic patients are at increased risk for developing cardiac dysrhythmias intraoperatively, particularly if plasma potassium concentrations are less than 3 mEq·L^{-1}. Nevertheless, it is impossible to confirm or defend arbitrary plasma potassium concentrations acceptable for elective surgery. Ultimately, the decision to proceed depends on several factors, including the acuteness or chronicity of the potassium changes and the magnitude of the proposed operation. Indeed, the incidence of intraoperative cardiac dysrhythmias is not increased in asymptomatic patients with chronic hypokalemia (2.6 mEq·L^{-1} to 3.5 mEq·L^{-1}) undergoing elective operations.[28]

Administration of anesthesia in the presence of moderate but chronic hypokalemia mandates that those events known to produce hypokalemia be avoided. It must be emphasized that adverse effects of hypokalemia are most likely when acute reductions in plasma potassium concentrations are superimposed on co-existing chronic hypokalemia.

It would seem logical to repeat plasma potassium measurements and obtain an electrocardiogram for evaluation of cardiac rhythm before the induction of anesthesia. During surgery, intravenous fluids should be selected to avoid glucose loads, as hyperglycemia could contribute to hypokalemia. Addition of 10 mEq to 20 mEq of potassium chloride to every liter of intravenous fluid maintenance can be considered but must be weighed against the hazards of too rapid administration should infusion rates be inadvertently increased during the intraoperative period. Use of exogenous epinephrine should be discouraged as beta-2 agonist stimulation may shift potassium intracellularly and exaggerate co-existing hypokalemia (Fig. 22-9).[19] Furthermore, the potassium depleted heart may be vulnerable to arrhythmogenic effects of catecholamines, as well as digitalis and calcium. Hyperventilation of the lungs must be rigorously avoided. Measurement of arterial blood gases and pH is helpful in confirming the proper management of ventilation.

The potential for prolonged responses to nondepolarizing muscle relaxants must be anticipated. A prudent approach is to reduce the initial dose by 30 percent to 50 percent. Administration of subsequent doses should be based on responses shown by a peripheral nerve stimulator. Nevertheless, chronic hypokalemia is likely to be associated with a normal ratio of intracellular to extracellular potassium, so that responses to muscle relaxants may not be altered.

No specific anesthetic drugs or techniques seem superior for administration to patients with hypokalemia. Nevertheless, it should be recalled that chronic hypokalemia has been associated with reduced myocardial contractility and postural hypotension. Therefore, patients with chronic hypokalemia might be unusually sensitive to cardiac depressant effects of volatile anesthetics. Likewise, exaggerated blood pressure reductions in response to positive pressure ventilation of the lungs or blood loss are likely in the presence of reduced sympathetic nervous system activity. Association of chronic hypokalemia with polyuria must also be remembered in choosing anesthetic drugs that are metabolized to fluoride.

It is mandatory to monitor continuously the electrocardiogram in the intraoperative and postoperative period. Appearance of abnormalities on the electrocardiogram related to hypokalemia requires prompt treatment with intravenous infusions of potassium chloride, including consideration of the administration of 0.5 mEq to 1.0 mEq bolus injections until the electrocardiogram reverts to normal.

CALCIUM

Calcium is essential for nerve and muscle excitability and muscle contractility. Total plasma calcium concentrations are maintained between 4.5 $mEq \cdot L^{-1}$ and 5.5 $mEq \cdot L^{-1}$ by the actions of parathyroid hormone. Physiologically active forms of calcium, however, are the ionized fractions, which normally represents about 45 percent of the total plasma concentration. Therefore, normal plasma ionized calcium concentrations are 2.0 $mEq \cdot L^{-1}$ to 2.5 $mEq \cdot L^{-1}$.

Symptoms due to altered concentrations of calcium reflect changes in plasma levels of ionized calcium. This emphasizes the need to evaluate disturbances in calcium homeostasis by measurement of ionized calcium concentrations. It must be remembered that concentrations of ionized calcium are dependent on the arterial pH; for example, acidosis increases the concentration and alkalosis decreases it.

Plasma albumin concentrations must be considered in interpreting plasma calcium measurements. For example, plasma albumin binds nonionized calcium. When plasma albumin concentrations are decreased, there will be less calcium bound to protein. As a result, nonionized calcium is free to return to storage sites such as bone. Therefore, total plasma calcium concentrations can be reduced in the presence of hypoalbuminemia, but symptoms of hypocalcemia do not occur unless ionized calcium concentrations are also reduced. Likewise, elevated plasma albumin concentrations are associated with increased total calcium concentrations, but the ionized fractions can be normal.

Hypercalcemia

The most common causes of hypercalcemia (total plasma calcium concentrations above 5.5 $mEq \cdot L^{-1}$) are hyperparathyroidism and neoplastic disorders with bone metastases.[29] Less common causes include pulmonary granulomatous diseases (sarcoidosis), vitamin D intoxication, and immobilization.

SIGNS AND SYMPTOMS

Hypercalcemia produces changes that manifest on the central nervous system, gastrointestinal tract, kidneys, and heart. Early signs and symptoms include sedation and vomiting. Persistently elevated plasma calcium concentrations (7 $mEq \cdot L^{-1}$ to 8 $mEq \cdot L^{-1}$) can interfere with urine-concentrating ability, and polyuria results. In addition, increased plasma calcium concentrations can contribute to formation of renal calculi. Oliguric renal failure can occur in advanced cases of hypercalcemia. When plasma calcium concentrations exceed 8 $mEq \cdot L^{-1}$, cardiac conduction disturbances, characterized on the electrocardiogram as prolonged P-R intervals, wide QRS complexes, and shortened Q-T intervals occur.

TREATMENT

The cornerstone of treatment of hypercalcemia is hydration with normal saline. Hydration lowers plasma calcium concentrations by dilution, and sodium acts to inhibit the renal reabsorption of calcium. Diuresis produced with furosemide minimizes the risk of overhydration and further facilitates renal elimination of calcium. Ambulation is an important aspect of the treatment, as this reduces calcium release from bone associated with immobilization.

Elevated plasma calcium concentrations secondary to myeloproliferative disorders can be lowered by the administration of the cancer chemotherapeutic drug, mithramycin. This drug, however, acts slowly, and is not helpful in the acute management of patients with hypercalcemia.

MANAGEMENT OF ANESTHESIA

The cardinal principle for management of anesthesia in the presence of hypercalcemia is maintenance of hydration and urine output with intravenous fluids containing sodium. Continuous monitoring of the electrocardiogram is useful to warn of adverse effects on cardiac conduction produced by excessive increases in plasma calcium concentrations. Choice of anesthetic drugs should consider impaired urine-concentrating ability associated with polyuria, which, in the postoperative period, could be confused with anesthetic-induced fluoride nephrotoxicity. Theoretically, hyperventilation of the lungs would be undesirable, as respiratory alkalosis lowers plasma potassium concentrations and would leave actions of calcium unopposed. Nevertheless, by lowering ionized fractions of calcium, alkalosis could also be beneficial. The response to nondepolarizing muscle relaxants is not well defined, but the preoperative existence of skeletal muscle weakness would suggest decreased dose requirements for these drugs.

Hypocalcemia

The most common cause of hypocalcemia (plasma calcium concentrations below 4.5 $mEq \cdot L^{-1}$) is reduced plasma albumin concentrations. Critically ill patients with low plasma albumin concentrations characteristically have low plasma calcium levels but plasma ionized calcium measurements may be normal.[30] Conversely, normal total plasma calcium concentrations in the presence of hypoalbuminemia may indicate increased concentrations of ionized calcium. Other causes of hypocalcemia are acute pancreatitis, hypoparathyroidism, especially after thyroid surgery, decreased plasma magnesium concentrations (malnutrition, sepsis, aminoglycoside administration), vitamin D deficiencies, and renal failure. Radiographic contrast media contains calcium chelators (edetate and citrate) and may acutely lower plasma calcium concentrations. Hyperventilation of the lungs may result in reductions in plasma ionized concentrations of calcium due to alkalosis-induced increases in calcium binding to proteins. Patients given sodium bicarbonate for control of metabolic acidosis can also develop acute ionized hypocalcemia by this mechanism. Increases in plasma free fatty acid concentrations, as associated with total parenteral nutrition, may lower plasma ionized calcium concentrations while not altering total calcium concentrations.[30] Hypocalcemia and hyperphosphatemia due to use of hypertonic phosphate enemas (Fleet enema) has been associated with cardiac arrest during induction of anesthesia.[31]

SIGNS AND SYMPTOMS

Manifestations of hypocalcemia are on the central nervous system, heart, and neuromuscular junction. Numbness and circumoral paresthesias can progress to confusion and occasionally seizures. Abrupt reductions in the ionized portion of total plasma calcium concentrations are associated with hypotension and increased left ventricular filling pressures.[32,33] The Q-T intervals on the electrocardiogram can be prolonged, but this is not a consistent observation, therefore, Q-T intervals are not clinically reliable as guides to the presence of hypocalcemia. Impaired neuromuscular function in the presence of hypocalcemia probably reflects decreased presynaptic release of acetylcholine. Indeed, many patients with chronic hypocalcemia complain of skeletal muscle weakness and fatigue. Rapid decreases in plasma calcium concentrations as can follow a total parathyroidectomy, can produce skeletal muscle spasm, manifested by laryngospasm. Skeletal muscle spasm is most likely to occur when plasma calcium concentrations abruptly decrease below 3.5 $mEq \cdot L^{-1}$.

TREATMENT

Initial management of hypocalcemia is correction of any co-existing respiratory or metabolic alkalosis. Intravenous infusions of calcium should be considered when there are symptoms of hypocalcemia (hypotension, tetany), or when plasma calcium concentrations decrease below 3.5 $mEq \cdot L^{-1}$. Treatment is initially with intravenous administration of 10 percent calcium chloride (1.36 $mEq \cdot ml^{-1}$) or calcium gluconate (0.45 $mEq \cdot ml^{-1}$). Equal elemental calcium doses of calcium chloride (2.5 $mg \cdot kg^{-1}$) or calcium gluconate (7.5 $mg \cdot kg^{-1}$) are equivalent in their ability to increase plasma ionized calcium concentrations.[34] Calcium should be administered until plasma concentrations approach 4 $mEq \cdot ml^{-1}$ or the electrocardiogram returns to a normal pattern.

MANAGEMENT OF ANESTHESIA

Management of anesthesia is designed to prevent further decreases in plasma calcium concentrations and to recognize and treat adverse effects of hypocalcemia, particularly on the heart. During surgery and anesthesia, it is important to appreciate that respiratory or metabolic alkalosis can rapidly decrease plasma ionized calcium concentrations. This can occur during hyperventilation of the lungs or after intravenous administration of sodium bicarbonate for treatment of metabolic acidosis.

Administration of whole blood containing citrate preservative usually does not reduce plasma calcium concentrations because calcium is rapidly mobilized from body stores. Ionized calcium concentrations, however, can be decreased with rapid infusions of blood (500 ml every 5 minutes to 10 minutes) or when metabolism or elimination of citrate is limited by hypothermia, cirrhosis of the liver, or renal dysfunction.[35] Although there is no evidence that co-existing hypocalcemia predisposes patients to citrate intoxication, it would seem prudent to maintain a high index of suspicion when whole blood is administered.

Continuous monitoring of the electrocardiogram to facilitate recognition of changes characteristic of hypocalcemia is important in the perioperative period. Intraoperative hypotension may reflect exaggerated cardiac depression produced by anesthetic drugs in the presence of decreased plasma ionized calcium concentrations. Arterial blood gases, pH, and plasma calcium measurements (particularly plasma ionized calcium concentrations if available) are valuable in guiding intraoperative management. The importance of plasma albumin concentrations must be remembered and administration of protein in the intravenous maintenance and replacement fluids considered. Administration of colloid solutions is particularly important if there is, due to surgical trauma, loss of intravascular fluid into tissues.

Responses to nondepolarizing muscle relaxants could be potentiated by hypocalcemia. Nevertheless, clinical experience is too limited to confirm this speculation. Theoretically, coagulation abnormalities could also accompany extreme reductions in plasma concentrations of calcium. Postoperatively, it should be appreciated that sudden reductions in plasma calcium concentrations can produce skeletal muscle spasm, including laryngospasm.

MAGNESIUM

Total body magnesium stores are about 2000 mEq. The majority of this magnesium is distributed to intracellular spaces (Table 22-4). Excretion of magnesium is by the gastrointestinal tract and kidneys. In its absence in the diet, the kidneys are able to conserve magnesium, excreting less than 1 mEq·day^{-1}. The most important physiologic effect of magnesium is regulation of presynaptic release of acetylcholine from nerve endings.

Hypermagnesemia

Hypermagnesemia is present when plasma magnesium concentrations exceed 2.5 mEq·L^{-1}. The most common causes of hypermagnesemia are iatrogenic, including administration of magnesium sulfate to treat toxemia of pregnancy and excessive individual use of antacids or laxatives. Patients with chronic renal dysfunction are at increased risks for developing hypermagnesemia, since magnesium elimination is dependent on glomerular filtration rate. Indeed, plasma magnesium levels predictably increase when exogenous magnesium is administered to patients with glomerular filtration rates below 30 ml·min^{-1}.

SIGNS AND SYMPTOMS

Important manifestations of hypermagnesemia are on the central nervous system, heart, and neuromuscular junction. Central nervous system depression is manifested as hyporeflexia plus sedation, which may progress to coma. Cardiac depression may be prominent. Skeletal muscle weakness, presumably reflecting reduced acetylcholine release secondary to increased magnesium levels, can be so severe as to impair ventilation. Indeed, the most common cause of death from hypermagnesemia is cardiac and·or respiratory arrest.

TREATMENT

Signs and symptoms of hypermagnesemia can be temporarily reversed with the intravenous administration of calcium. Magnesium elimination can be facilitated by fluid loading and diuresis produced by diuretics. Definitive therapy for persistent and life-threatening hypermagnesemia requires either peritoneal dialysis or hemodialysis.

MANAGEMENT OF ANESTHESIA

Acidosis and dehydration must be prevented intraoperatively, as these events lead to increased plasma magnesium concentrations. Therefore, ventilation of the lungs should be managed to ensure the absence of respiratory acidosis due to hypoventilation. Arterial blood gas and pH determinations are valuable in guiding management of ventilation of the lungs and insuring the absence of systemic acidosis. Intravenous fluid maintenance and replacement should be adjusted to maintain urine output. Stimulation of urine output with a diuretic, such as furosemide, may be necessary.

Hypermagnesemia potentiates the action of nondepolarizing and depolarizing muscle relaxants (Fig. 22-10).[36] This emphasizes the importance of decreasing initial doses of muscle relaxants. Subsequent doses are based on responses observed with a peripheral nerve stimulator.

It is conceivable that cardiac depression produced by anesthetic drugs could be exaggerated in the presence of hypermagnesemia. Furthermore, high magnesium levels produce peripheral vasodilation, which might be accentuated further by drugs used during anesthesia. These speculations remain undocumented, but it would seem prudent to titrate the doses of anesthetic drugs, maintaining a high index of suspicion for magnesium-anesthetic drug interactions should hypotension occur.

Hypomagnesemia

Plasma magnesium concentrations below 1.5 mEq·L^{-1} are associated with chronic alcoholism, malabsorption syndromes, hyperalimentation therapy without added magnesium, and protracted vomiting or diarrhea.

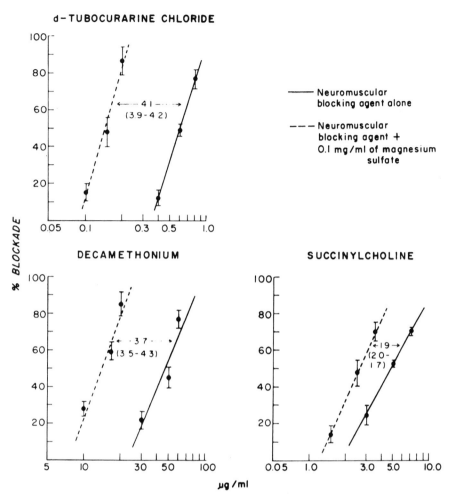

FIG. 22-10. Dose-response curves (Mean ± SE) for production of neuromuscular blockade with or without magnesium sulfate, using the rat phrenic nerve-diaphragm preparation. Displacement of the dose response curve to the left reflects increased sensitivity to neuromuscular blocking effects of the muscle relaxant in the presence of magnesium. (Ghoneim MM, Long JP. The interaction between magnesium and other neuromuscular blocking agents. Anesthesiology 1970;32:23–7)

SIGNS AND SYMPTOMS

Signs and symptoms of hypomagnesemia are similar to those observed in patients with hypocalcemia. Indeed, both hypomagnesemia and hypocalcemia frequently present as combined electrolyte disorders. Predictable manifestations of hypomagnesemia include central nervous system irritability reflected by hyperreflexia and seizures, skeletal muscle spasm, and cardiac irritability. Hypomagnesemia can potentiate digitalis-induced cardiac dysrhythmias.

TREATMENT

Treatment with magnesium sulfate 1 g, administered intravenously for 15 minutes to 20 minutes, is indicated when seizure activity or skeletal muscle spasm is present. Blood pressure, heart rate, and patellar reflexes should be monitored. Depression or disappearance of patellar reflexes is an indication to stop magnesium replacement.

MANAGEMENT OF ANESTHESIA

The importance of hypomagnesemia to the management of anesthesia is primarily related to associated disturbances such as alcoholism, malnutrition, and hypovolemia. Conceivably, decreased plasma magnesium concentrations could interfere with the response to muscle relaxants, but this possibility has not been studied.

REFERENCES

1. Bartter FC, Schwartz WB. The syndrome of inappropriate secretion of antidiuretic hormone. Am J Med 1967;42:790–806
2. Hemmer M, Viquerat CE, Suter PM, Valotton MB. Urinary antidiuretic hormone excretion during mechanical ventilation and weaning in man. Anesthesiology 1980;52:395–400
3. Chung H-M, Kluge R, Schrier RW, Anderson RJ. Postoperative hyponatremia: A prospective study. Arch Intern Med 1986;146:333–6
4. Arieff AI. Hyponatremia, convulsions, respiratory arrest, and permanent brain damage after elective surgery in healthy women. N Engl J Med 1986;314:1529–35
5. Sterns RH, Riggs JE, Schochet SS. Osmotic demyelination syndrome following correction of hyponatremia. N Engl J Med 1986;314:1535–42
6. Hagstrom RS. Studies on fluid absorption during transurethral prostatic resection. J Urol 1955;73:852–9
7. Hurlbert BJ, Wingard DW. Water intoxication after 15 minutes of transurethral resection of the prostate. Anesthesiology 1979;50:355–6
8. Tanifuji Y, Eger EI. Brain sodium, potassium, and osmolality: Effects on anesthetic requirement. Anesth Analg 1978;57:404–10
9. Gonick HC, Kleeman CR, Rubini ME, Maxwell MH. Functional impairment in chronic renal disease. III. Studies of potassium excretion. Am J Med Sci 1971;261:281–90
10. Tolmie JD, Toyee TH, Mitchell GD. Succinylcholine: Danger in the burned patient. Anesthesiology 1967;28:467–70
11. Mazze RI, Escue HM, Houston JB. Hyperkalemia and cardiovascular collapse following administration of succinylcholine to the traumatized patient. Anesthesiology 1969;31:540–7
12. Tobey RE, Jacobson PM, Kahle CT, et al. The serum potassium response to muscle relaxants in neural injury. Anesthesiology 1972;37:332–7
13. Edwards R, Winnie AP, Ramamurthy S. Acute hypocapneic hypokalemia: An iatrogenic anesthetic complication. Anesth Analg 1977;56:786–92
14. Williams RP. Potassium overdosage: A potential hazard of non-rigid parenteral fluid containers. Br Med J 1973;1:714–5
15. Viberti GC. Glucose-induced hyperkalemia: A hazard for diabetics? Lancet 1978;1:690–1
16. Goudsouzian NG, Karamanian A. The electrocardiogram. In: Physiology for the Anesthesiologist. New York. Appleton-Century-Crofts 1977:19–38
17. Stoelting RK, Peterson C. Adverse effects of increased succinylcholine dose following d-tubocurarine pretreatment. Anesth Analg 1975;54:282–8
18. Miller RD, Roderick LL. Diuretic-induced hypokalemia, pancuronium neuromuscular blockade and its antagonism by neostigmine. Br J Anaesth 1978;541–4
19. Brown MJ, Brown DC, Murphy MB. Hypokalemia from beta$_2$-receptor stimulation by circulating epinephrine. N Engl J Med 1983;309:1414–9
20. Hurlbert BJ, Edelman JD, David K. Serum potassium levels during and after terbutaline. Anesth Analg 1981;60:723–5
21. Wong KC, Wetstone D, Martin WE, et al. Hypokalemia during anesthesia: The effects of d-tubocurarine, gallamine, succinylcholine, thiopental, and halothane with or without respiratory alkalosis. Anesth Analg 1973;52:522–8
22. Abbrecht PH. Cardiovascular effects of chronic potassium deficiency in the dog. Am J Physiol 1972;223:555–9
23. Hill GE, Wong KC, Shaw CL, Blatnick RA. Acute and chronic changes in intra- and extracellular potassium and responses to neuromuscular blocking agents. Anesth Analg 1978;57:417–21
24. Papademetriou V, Burris J, Kukich S, Freis ED. Effectiveness of potassium chloride or triamterene in thiazide hypokalemia. Arch Intern Med 1985;145:1986–90
25. Papademetrious V, Fletcher R, Khatri IM, Freis ED. Diuretic-induced hypokalemia in uncomplicated systemic hypertension: Effect of plasma potassium correction on cardiac arrhythmias. Am J Cardiol 1983;52:1017–22
26. Tyson I, Genna S, Jones RL, et al. Studies of po-

tassium depletion using direct measurements of total-body potassium. J Nucl Med 1970;11:426–34

27. Harrington JT, Isner JM, Kassirer JP. Our national obsession with potassium. Am J Med 1982;73:155–9

28. Vitez TS, Soper LE, Wong KC, Soper P. Chronic hypokalemia and intraoperative dysrhythmias. Anesthesiology 1985;63:130–3

29. Mundy GR, Ibbotson KJ, D'Souza SM, et al. The hypercalcemia of cancer. Clinical implications and pathogenic mechanisms. N Engl J Med 1984;310:1718–26

30. Zaloga GP, Chernow B. Hypocalcemia in critical illness. JAMA 1986;256:1924–9

31. Reedy JC, Zwiren GT. Enema-induced hypocalcemia and hyperphosphatemia leading to cardiac arrest during induction of anesthesia in an outpatient surgery center. Anesthesiology 1983;59:578–9

32. Denlinger JK, Nahrwold ML. Cardiac failure associated with hypocalcemia. Anesth Analg 1976;55:34–6

33. Scheidegger D, Drop LJ. The relationship between duration of Q-T interval and plasma ionized calcium concentration: Experiments with acute, steady-state (Ca^{++}) changes in the dog. Anesthesiology 1979;51:143–8

34. Cote CJ, Drop LJ, Danniels AL, Hoaglin DC. Calcium chloride versus calcium gluconate: Comparison of ionization and cardiovascular effects in children and dogs. Anesthesiology 1987;66:465–70

35. Denlinger JK, Nahrwold ML, Gibbs PS, Lecky JP. Hypocalcemia during rapid blood transfusion in anesthetized man. Br J Anaesth 1976;48:995–1000

36. Ghoneim MM, Long JP. The interaction between magnesium and other neuromuscular blocking agents. Anesthesiology 1970;32:23–7

23

Endocrine Disease

Endocrine diseases are characterized by the overproduction or underproduction of single or multiple hormones. Alterations in the physiologic responses to stress and/or changes in homeostatic mechanisms reflect the impact of excessive or deficient amounts of these hormones. Endocrine gland disorders may be the primary reason for surgery or may co-exist in patients requiring operations unrelated to endocrine gland dysfunction. An understanding of the pathophysiology of endocrine gland function is essential for the management of patients in the perioperative period who manifest dysfunction of an endocrine gland.

THYROID GLAND

Thyroid gland dysfunction reflects the overproduction or underproduction of triiodothyronine and/or thyroxine (tetraiodothyronine). These two physiologically active thyroid gland hormones act on cells via the adenylate cyclase system to produce changes in the speed of biochemical reactions, total body oxygen consumption, and energy (heat) production.[1] Symptoms of hyperthyroidism or hypothyroidism reflect the effects of these hormones. Although the exact mechanism by which thyroid gland hormones work is not known, one theory proposes that these sub-

stances activate the enzyme system or systems responsible for maintaining intracellular to extracellular gradients of sodium and potassium.[1] In addition to physiologically active thyroid hormones, the thyroid gland also releases calcitonin (thyrocalcitonin) in response to elevated plasma calcium concentrations. The effect of calcitonin on plasma calcium concentrations is opposite to the effects produced by parathormone (see the section Parathyroid Glands). For example, release of calcitonin lowers plasma calcium concentrations by reducing the passage of calcium from bone into the circulation. Excess secretion of calcitonin can occur in the presence of medullary carcinoma of the thyroid gland. Nevertheless, hypocalcemia does not occur despite excess concentrations of calcitonin in the circulation.

Rational management of the patient with thyroid gland dysfunction requires an appreciation of the synthesis and secretion of thyroid hormones, and the tests of thyroid gland function.

Synthesis and Secretion of Thyroid Hormones

Synthesis and secretion of triiodothyronine and thyroxine occur by a series of reactions, which can be divided into four phases desig-

473

nated as (1) iodide trapping, (2) oxidation and iodination, (3) hormone storage, and (4) proteolysis and release (Fig. 23-1). These reactions are regulated by thyroid stimulating hormone released from the anterior pituitary. Secretion and release of thyroid stimulating hormone are in turn regulated by a negative feedback mechanism involving the circulating level of thyroid hormones and thyrotropin-releasing hormone. Thyrotropin-releasing hormone is secreted by the hypothalamus and transported to the anterior pituitary by the hypophyseal-portal venous system. Therefore, thyroid gland dysfunction can reflect disease processes involving the hypothalamus, the anterior pituitary, or the thyroid gland itself.

IODIDE TRAPPING

Synthesis of thyroid hormones is the only in vivo process that uses iodine. Iodine is absorbed from the gastrointestinal tract and appears in the plasma as inorganic iodide. The ability of thyroid gland epithelial cells to concentrate iodide above concentrations present in plasma is referred to as iodide trapping. The differential concentration gradient of iodide between the thyroid gland and plasma is normally 20 to 1, but may reach a ratio of 500 to 1 in the presence of hyperthyroidism. The passage of iodide into the thyroid gland is accelerated by thyroid stimulating hormone and depressed by increased circulating plasma concentrations of iodide. Iodide trapping is inhibited by inorganic ions such as thiocyanate and perchlorate, accounting for the antithyroid action of these compounds.

OXIDATION AND IODINATION

After entering the thyroid gland, inorganic iodide is oxidized and subsequently incorporated into tyrosine residues to form monoiodotyrosine and diiodotyrosine. Once iodide is bound in these organic compounds, it is no longer diffusible. Oxidation and iodination are accelerated by thyroid stimulating hormone and inhibited by propylthiouracil and methimazole.

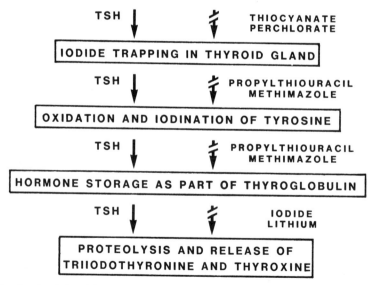

FIG. 23-1. Synthesis of thyroid gland hormone occurs in four steps, which are regulated by thyroid stimulating hormone (TSH). Iodide trapping by thyroid gland cells is inhibited by thiocyanate and perchlorate. Propylthiouracil and methiamazole inhibit formation and storage of active thyroid gland hormones. Iodide and lithium inhibit release of triiodothyronine and thyroxine from the thyroid gland into the circulation.

HORMONE STORAGE

Precursors of thyroid gland hormones are stored in the thyroid gland until coupling of monoiodotyrosine and diiodotyrosine forms triiodothyronine or thyroxine. The thyroid gland is unique among endocrine glands in its ability to store large amounts of hormone. For example, it is estimated that the iodine reserve in the thyroid gland is sufficient for about 100 days.

PROTEOLYSIS AND RELEASE

The proteolytic action of thyroid stimulating hormone is responsible for release of physiologically active thyroid gland hormones into the circulation. Thyroxine constitutes 95 percent of the hormones released; the remainder is triiodythyronine. These hormones are released in combination with three carrier proteins, thyroxine binding globulin, prealbumin, and albumin. Triiodothyronine is less firmly bound to protein than thyroxine, and as a result, has a more rapid onset of effect and a shorter duration of action. For example, the half-time for triiodothyronine is about 12 hours, compared with about 144 hours for thyroxine. Furthermore, triiodothyronine is three times to five times more potent than thyroxine. Triiodothyronine is also produced by the deiodination of thyroxine in the circulation and peripheral tissues, especially the liver and kidneys. The proteolytic step necessary for the release of active hormone from the thyroid gland is stimulated by thyroid stimulating hormone and inhibited by elevated intrathyroidal concentrations of iodide and lithium.

Tests of Thyroid Gland Function

Tests of thyroid gland function are necessary for the detection of hyperthyroidism or hypothyroidism and for the evaluation of an asymptomatic goiter (Table 23-1).[2]

TOTAL PLASMA THYROXINE

Total plasma thyroxine concentrations are the standard screening tests for evaluation of thyroid gland function. For example, this concentration will be elevated in about 90 percent of patients with hyperthyroidism. Conversely, about 85 percent of patients who are hypothyroid will have low concentrations. It must be appreciated that alterations in plasma concentrations of thyroxine binding globulin can alter total serum thyroxine concentrations in the absence of thyroid gland dysfunction. Therefore, events that increase or decrease plasma concentrations of thyroxine binding globulin must be considered when interpreting abnormal measurements of the total serum thyroxine concentration (Table 23-2).

RESIN TRIIODOTHYRONINE UPTAKE

Resin triiodothyronine uptake is an indirect measurement of the unbound plasma concentrations of thyroxine. Therefore, this test clarifies whether abnormalities in total plasma thyroxine concentrations are due to dysfunction of the thyroid gland or reflect alterations in plasma concentrations of thyroxine binding globulin.

FREE THYROXINE

The percent of free thyroxine can be measured by equilibrium dialysis. This value multiplied by the total plasma thyroxine concentration is equivalent to the amount of free thyroxine in the plasma. Measurement of free thyroxine is useful when malnutrition in a hyperthyroid patient results in low levels of thyroxine binding globulin. In such patients, total plasma thyroxine concentration may be normal, while free thyroxine is elevated. As with resin triiodothyronine uptake, this test is independent of plasma concentrations of thyroxine binding globulin.

PLASMA TRIIODOTHYRONINE

Plasma triiodothyronine concentrations are used to detect hyperthyrodism in patients who manifest increased plasma concentrations

TABLE 23-1. Tests of Thyroid Gland Function

Tests	Primary Diagnostic Indication	Normal Value
Total plasma thyroxine	Screening test for thyroid gland function	4.4–9.9 μg·dl^{-1}
Resin triiodothyronine	Distinguish between thyroid gland dysfunction and altered thyroxine binding globulin concentrations	30%–40%
Free thyroxine	Distinguish between thyroid gland dysfunction and altered thyroxine binding globulin concentrations	1–2.1 ng·dl^{-1}
Total plasma triiodothyronine	Detect hyperthyroidism	150–250 ng·ml^{-1}
Radioactive iodine uptake	Deter hyperthyroidism or hypothyroidism	10%–25% at 24 hours
Thyroid stimulating hormone	Detect hypothyroidism	up to 7 units·ml^{-1}
Thyroid scan	Distinguish between benign and malignant disease of the thyroid gland	
Ultrasonography	Distinguish between cystic and solid nodules in the thyroid gland	
Antibodies to thyroid tissue	Hashimoto's thyroiditis	

of triiodothyronine that precede changes in plasma concentrations of thyroxine. Indeed, in some patients, triiodothyronine may be the only thyroid gland hormone produced in excess.

Measurement of plasma triiodothyronine concentrations is not a sensitive test for decreased thyroid gland function. For example, plasma triiodothyronine concentrations may be normal in about 50 percent of hypothyroid patients. This unexpected finding reflects the tendency of hypothyroid patients to produce relatively more triiodothyronine than thyroxine as the thyroid gland fails. Conversely, plasma triiodothyronine concentrations can be low in euthyroid patients with renal failure, cirrhosis of the liver, or malnutrition, as these conditions inhibit peripheral deiodination of thyroxine to triiodothyronine.

RADIOACTIVE IODINE UPTAKE

Radioactive iodine uptake measures the percent of a tracer dose that enters the thyroid gland in a given time period. Radioactive iodine uptake is directly proportional to activity of the thyroid gland. Nevertheless, an overactive thyroid gland does not always cause a high iodine uptake, which detracts from the reliability of this test.

THYROID STIMULATING HORMONE

Measurement of thyroid stimulating hormone activity is the most sensitive screening test for the detection of hypothyroidism. For example, activity of thyroid stimulating hormone may be elevated before the appearance of clinical symptoms of hypothyroidism or the detection of reduced total plasma thyroxine concentrations. This early elevation reflects the extreme sensitivity of the hypothalmic-pituitary axis to even slight decreases in circulating concentrations of physiologically active thyroid gland hormones. Conversely, hypothyroidism due to dysfunction of the hypothala-

TABLE 23-2. Events that Influence Plasma Concentrations of Thyroxine Binding Globulin

Events	Thyroxine Binding Globulin Concentrations
Pregnancy	Increased
Oral contraceptives	Increased
Infectious hepatitis	Increased
Nephrosis	Decreased
Hypoproteinemia (malnourishment)	Decreased
Acromegaly	Decreased

mus and/or pituitary gland will be suggested by a reduced level of thyroid stimulating hormone in the presence of decreased total plasma thyroxine concentrations.

THYROID SCAN

Ability of the thyroid gland to concentrate a labeled substance is determined by radionuclide scanning. Thyroid scan is useful in differentiating between benign and malignant disease of the thyroid gland. Functioning thyroid tissue ("hot") is rarely malignant; nonfunctioning tissue ("cold") may be malignant or benign.

ULTRASONOGRAPHY

Ultrasonography permits reliable discrimination between cystic and solid nodules, which are present in the thyroid gland. A cystic thyroid gland nodule is rarely malignant; a solitary nonfunctioning solid thyroid gland nodule may be malignant 10 percent to 30 percent of the time, and thus requires definitive diagnosis involving surgery.[10]

ANTIBODIES TO THYROID TISSUE

Detection of circulating antibodies to thyroid gland tissue suggests the presence of Hashimoto's thyroiditis. Hyperthyroidism can also be associated with increased circulating levels of antibodies to thyroid gland tissue.

Hyperthyroidism

Hyperthyroidism results from excess secretion (five times to fifteen times normal) of triiodothyronine and/or thyroxine by the thyroid gland. Typically, hyperthyroidism occurs between the ages of 20 years and 40 years, and is about four times more frequent in women than men. The most common manifestation of hyperthyroidism is diffuse toxic goiter (Graves'

disease). The majority of patients with this disorder demonstrate the presence of long-acting thyroid stimulator (LATS) in the plasma, which mimics the effects of thyroid stimulating hormone, producing effects lasting as long as 12 hours in contrast to about 1 hour for thyroid stimulating hormone. Hyperthyroidism during pregnancy occurs in about 0.2 percent of parturients and is most often due to diffuse toxic goiter.[4] It is likely that diffuse toxic goiter is an autoimmune disease, reflecting the presence of an immunoglobulin antibody. Immune suppression could decrease the intensity of diffuse toxic goiter due to an autoimmune response, with exacerbation occurring in the postpartum period upon removal of the immunosuppression. Other variants of hyperthyroidism include toxic adenoma (Plummer's disease), toxic multinodular goiter, and Jod-Basedow's disease. Diagnosis of hyperthyroidism is based on clinical signs and symptoms, plus confirmation of excessive thyroid gland function demonstrated by appropriate tests (see the section Tests of Thyroid Gland Function). Diagnosis of hyperthyroidism during pregnancy is difficult since estrogen-induced increases in thyroxine binding globulin results in elevations of plasma thyroxine concentrations.

SIGNS AND SYMPTOMS

Signs and symptoms of hyperthyroidism reflect the impact of excess amounts of thyroid gland hormones on the speed of biochemical reactions, total body oxygen consumption, and energy (heat) production. For example, thyroid gland hormones cause the uncoupling of oxidative phosphorylation, such that energy cannot be stored and heat production increases. There is weight loss, despite a high caloric intake. Fatigue, emotional lability, diaphoresis, and heat intolerance are characteristic. Exophthalmus is due to an infiltrative process involving the retrobulbar fat and eylids. Retrobulbar edema can be so severe that the optic nerve is compressed, with resultant blindness. A dermopathy characterized by elevated and pruritic skin, especially over the tibia, can develop in patients with diffuse toxic goiter.

A hyperdynamic circulation, characterized by tachycardia, cardiac tachydysrhythmias, and increased cardiac output, suggests excessive activity of the sympathetic nervous system, as well as compensatory attempts to eliminate excess heat. Plasma concentrations of catecholamines are not elevated, suggesting that excess sympathetic nervous system activity reflects the ability of thyroid gland hormones to sensitize adrenergic receptors to exogenous and endogenous catecholamines. Nevertheless, there is no direct evidence that cardiovascular responsiveness to exogenous catecholamines is altered by increased or decreased activity of the thyroid gland.[1] More intriguing is the observation that persistent excessive release of thyroid gland hormones results in an increase in the number of beta-adrenergic receptors.[5] Adrenal cortex hyperplasia in the presence of hyperthyroidism reflects an increased production and use of cortisol. Finally, skeletal muscle weakness is frequently present in patients with excessive activity of the thyroid gland.

TREATMENT

Treatment of hyperthyroidism is with antithyroid drugs, beta-adrenergic blockade, subtotal thyroidectomy, or radioactive iodine.[6] Regardless of the treatment selected, the goal of therapy is to render the patient euthyroid.

Antithyroid Drugs.   Propylthiouracil and methimazole are thiourea derivatives that inhibit oxidation of inorganic iodide. These drugs will render most patients euthyroid in several weeks. A rare but significant complication from treatment with these drugs is agranulocytosis. Intraoperative bleeding due to drug-induced thrombocytopenia or hypoprothrombinemia has been reported in patients being treated with propylthiouracil.[7,8] Continuation of antithyroid drugs beyond the time when a euthyroid condition is produced often results in hypothyroidism. Only about 30 percent of patients, however, remain euthyroid after these drugs are discontinued.[6]

Oral iodide, as Lugol's solution or as a tablet, is effective in reducing vascularity of hyperplastic thyroid glands before surgery. Potassium iodide administered orally or sodium iodide by the intravenous route is also effective in reducing activity of the thyroid gland by preventing the release of active hormones.

Beta-adrenergic Blockade.   Beta-adrenergic blockade with drugs such as propranolol is effective in attenuating manifestations of excessive sympathetic nervous system activity characteristic of hyperthyroidism. For example, propranolol is effective in reducing heart rate and cardiac output in patients with hyperthyroidism. It should be appreciated that propranolol alone does not interfere with synthesis and release of active hormones from the thyroid gland. The combination of oral propranolol (80 mg every 8 hours) and potassium iodide (60 mg every 8 hours), however, is effective in attenuating cardiovascular manifestations of hyperthyroidism, and reducing circulating plasma concentrations of triiodothyronine and thyroxine.[9] Therefore, this combination has been proposed as a useful preoperative preparation for patients with hyperthyroidism.[9] The efficacy of propranolol is attributed to beta-adrenergic blockade and to the ability of this drug to interfere with the deiodination of thyroxine to triiodothyronine in the peripheral circulation and tissues.[10] Nadolol, which has a longer duration of action than propranolol, is effective in controlling sympathetic nervous system manifestations of hyperthyroidism with a single daily oral dose of 160 mg.[11] Furthermore, plasma concentrations of nadolol are maintained at therapeutic concentrations in the 24 hour perioperative period.

Subtotal Thyroidectomy.   Subtotal thyroidectomy is an alternative to prolonged pharmacologic treatment of hyperthyroidism. For reasons not clear, extensive but incomplete removal of the thyroid gland induces remission in the majority of patients with diffuse toxic goiter. Before surgery, patients should be rendered euthyroid with drugs. The combined use of propranolol and potassium iodide for about 10 days is effective for achieving this goal.[9] Alternatively, treatment for 6 weeks to 8 weeks with specific antithyroid drugs, plus an oral iodide solution for 7 days to 10 days before surgery, will produce a euthyroid state and reduce vascularity of the thyroid gland.

Early complications occurring after a subtotal thyroidectomy include manifestations of damage to the laryngeal nerves, tracheal compression, and hypoparathyroidism.[12,13] It should be remembered that the entire sensory and motor supply to the larynx is from two superior and two recurrent laryngeal nerves. The superior nerves provide the motor supply to the cricothyroid muscles and sensation above the level of the vocal cords. The recurrent nerves supply motor innervation to all the muscles of the larynx except the cricothyroid muscles, plus sensation below the level of the vocal cords. In view of the possibility of damage to these nerves, it would seem prudent to evaluate vocal cord movement at the conclusion of surgery. This can be accomplished by indirect or direct laryngoscopy and by asking the patient to phonate by saying "e". Superior laryngeal nerve paralysis is manifest as hoarseness in a patient with a wrinkled appearing vocal cord. Loss of sensation above the vocal cords makes the patient with superior laryngeal nerve damage susceptible to inhalation of secretions present in the pharynx. The most common nerve injury occurring after thyroid gland surgery is damage to the abductor fibers of the recurrent laryngeal nerve. This type of damage, when unilateral, is characterized by hoarseness and a paralyzed vocal cord, which assumes an intermediate position. Bilateral recurrent nerve injury results in aphonia and paralyzed vocal cords, which can flap together producing airway obstruction during inspiration. Selective injury of the adductor fibers of the recurrent laryngeal nerve leaves the abductor fibers unopposed, and pulmonary aspiration is a hazard. Conversely, selective injury of the abductor fibers leaves the adductor fibers unopposed, and airway obstruction can occur. Symptoms attributed to laryngeal nerve injury may actually be due to laryngeal edema. Laryngeal edema is more commonly due to surgical trauma than to difficult intubation of the trachea.

Airway obstruction occurring after a subtotal thyroidectomy can also be due to compression of the trachea. Compression of the trachea can be a manifestation of a hematoma at the operative site or of tracheomalacia due to weakening of the tracheal rings by chronic pressure from a goiter. Indeed, airway obstruction occurring after removal of the tube from the trachea, despite normal vocal cord function, should suggest the diagnosis of tracheomalacia.

Hypoparathyroidism leading to hypocalcemia, after an operation on the thyroid gland, reflects inadvertent surgical removal of the parathyroid glands. This rarely occurs after a subtotal thyroidectomy but is estimated to be the cause of permanent hypoparathyroidism in about 1 percent of patients who undergo total thyroidectomy. Hypocalcemia may also reflect increased uptake of calcium by bone following an abrupt reduction in the circulating levels of thyroid gland hormones produced by surgical removal of the gland. Signs and symptoms of hypocalcemia commonly develop 24 hours to 72 hours postoperatively but may manifest as early as 1 hour to 3 hours after surgery. Laryngeal muscles are the most sensitive to hypocalcemia, and inspiratory stridor progressing to laryngospasm may be the first suggestion that surgically induced hypoparathyroidism is present. Immediate treatment is with intravenous infusion of calcium until laryngeal stridor ceases.

Radioactive Iodine.　Radioactive iodine induces a euthyroid state by destroying thyroid cell function after its entrance into the gland. This form of therapy is not recommended for the pregnant patient because of potential radiation-induced damage to the fetus.

MANAGEMENT OF ANESTHESIA

Elective surgery should never be considered until patients have been rendered euthyroid and the hyperkinetic circulation has been controlled by drug-induced beta-adrenergic blockade, as evidenced by resting heart rates less than 85 beats·min^{-1}. Anesthesia in euthyroid patients does not pose an increased risk. Patients who cannot be rendered euthyroid before surgery may develop adverse responses related to excessive release of thyroid gland hormones during the perioperative period.

Preoperative Medication.　Preoperative medication is both psychological and pharmacologic. Sedation is ideally produced by the oral administration of a barbiturate or benzo-diazepine. Use of an anticholinergic drug is not recommended, since these drugs can interfere with the normal heat regulating mechanism and contribute to increases in heart rate.

Induction of Anesthesia. Induction of anesthesia is ideally accomplished with the in-travenous administration of thiopental. Thio-pental is an attractive selection because its thi-ourea structure lends antithyroid activity to the drug. Nevertheless, it is unlikely that a signif-icant antithyroid effect is produced by this dose. Ketamine is not a good selection because it can stimulate the sympathetic nervous sys-tem. Indeed, tachycardia and hypertension have been reported after administration of ke-tamine to euthyroid patients taking thyroid gland replacement medication.[14] Administra-tion of succinylcholine or nondepolarizing muscle relaxants that lack effects on the car-diovascular system are indicated to facilitate intubation of the trachea.

Maintenance of Anesthesia. Goals dur-ing maintenance of anesthesia for hyperthyroid patients are to avoid administration of drugs that stimulate the sympathetic nervous system and to provide sufficient anesthetic depression to prevent exaggerated responses to surgical stimulation.[15] The possibility of organ toxicity due to altered or accelerated drug metabolism in the presence of hyperthyroidism must also be considered when selecting drugs for main-tenance of anesthesia. Indeed, exposure of triiodothyronine-treated rats to halothane, en-flurane, or isoflurane results in evidence of he-patic centrilobular necrosis in 92, 24, and 28 percent of animals respectively.[16] An undoc-umented but potential concern with enflurane would be nephrotoxicity from increased pro-duction of fluoride due to accelerated metab-olism of the drug. Despite animal evidence of hepatic necrosis after exposure to all volatile anesthetics, the ability of isoflurane to offset adverse sympathetic nervous system responses to surgical stimulation and not sensitize the myocardium to catecholamines makes this an attractive selection to combine with nitrous oxide for maintenance of anesthesia for hy-perthyroid patients. Furthermore, liver func-tion tests are not altered postoperatively in pre-

viously hyperthyroid patients who are rendered euthyroid before surgery and anes-thesia that includes administration of halo-thane or enflurane.[17] Nitrous oxide combined with short-acting opioids is an alternative to use of volatile drugs but has the disadvantage of not providing inhibition of sympathetic ner-vous system activity.

A clinical impression is that hyperthy-roidism leads to increased anesthetic require-ments. Nevertheless, controlled animal studies have not demonstrated a clinically significant change in anesthetic requirements for halo-thane (Fig. 23-2).[18] The discrepancy between clinical impression and objective data is pre-sumed to reflect the increased cardiac output characteristic of hyperthyroidism. Increased cardiac output accelerates uptake of inhaled anesthetics, resulting in the need to raise the inspired concentration of the anesthetic so as to achieve a brain partial pressure similar to that achieved with a lower inspired concen-tration in the euthyroid patient. It should be appreciated that accelerated metabolism of the anesthetic drug does not alter the partial pres-sure of the drug needed in the brain to produce the desired pharmacologic effect. Another fac-tor that should be considered when evaluating anesthetic requirements in the presence of al-tered thyroid gland function is body temper-ature.[19] For example, elevations in body tem-perature due to hyperthyroidism would be expected to increase anesthetic requirements about 5 percent for each degree the temperature rises above 37 degrees Celsius.

Selection of muscle relaxants must con-sider the impact of these drugs on the sym-pathetic nervous system. For example, pan-curonium would not be a logical choice, in view of the ability of this drug to increase heart rate and in some instances to stimulate the sympathetic nervous system. Likewise, hista-mine release after administration of d-tubo-curarine and to a lesser extent after metocurine would be undesirable. Such drugs as vecuron-ium or atracurium, which minimally affect the cardiovascular system, are logical selections in the presence of hyperthyroidism. Conceivably, prolonged responses could occur when tradi-tional doses of muscle relaxants are adminis-tered to patients with co-existing skeletal mus-cle weakness. Furthermore, the incidence of

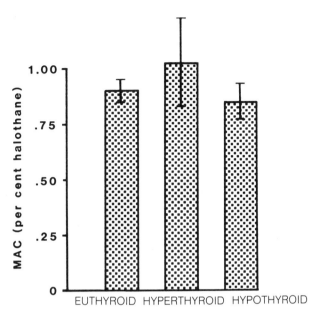

FIG. 23-2. The minimum alveolar concentration of halothane (MAC, Mean ± SD) was determined in euthyroid, hyperthyroid, and hypothyroid dogs. MAC in the presence of hyperthyroidism or hypothyroidism was not significantly altered from values measured in euthyroid dogs. MAC in the presence of hyperthyroidism, however, was greater than values in hypothyroid dogs ($P<0.05$). (Data adapted from Babad AA, Eger EI. The effects of hyperthyroidism and hypothyroidism on halothane and oxygen requirements in dogs. Anesthesiology 1968;29:1087–93).

myasthenia gravis is alleged to be increased in hyperthyroid patients. Therefore, it would seem prudent to reduce the initial dose of muscle relaxants, and closely monitor the effects produced at the neuromuscular junction, using a peripheral nerve stimulator. Reversal of nondepolarizing neuromuscular blockade with anticholinesterase drugs combined with anticholinergic drugs introduces the concern for drug-induced tachycardia. Although experience is too limited to make recommendations, it seems unwarranted to avoid pharmacologic reversal of muscle relaxants in these patients. Perhaps glycopyrrolate, which has less chronotropic effect than atropine, would be an appropriate anticholinergic drug selection.

Treatment of hypotension with sympathomimetic drugs must consider the possibility of exaggerated responsiveness of hyperthyroid patients to catecholamines. Therefore, reduced doses of direct-acting vasopressors such as phenylephrine may be a more logical selection than ephedrine, which acts in part by provoking release of catecholamines.

Monitoring during maintenance of anesthesia in hyperthyroid patients is directed at early recognition of increased activity of the thyroid gland, suggesting the onset of thyroid storm. Constant monitoring of body temperature is particularly important, and means to lower body temperature, including a cooling mattress and cold solutions for intravenous infusion, must be available. The electrocardiogram may reveal tachycardia and/or cardiac dysrhythmias, indicating the need for the intraoperative administration of propranolol or lidocaine. Finally, patients with exophthalmus are susceptible to corneal ulceration and drying, emphasizing the need to protect the eyes during the perioperative period.

Maintenance of beta-adrenergic blockade during the perioperative period is essential in the patient with hyperthyroidism. In this regard, continuous intravenous infusion of propranolol (3 mg·hr^{-1}) to adult patients is associated with the maintenance of therapeutic plasma concentrations of this drug.[20] Conceivably, this form of therapy would protect hyperthyroid patients from sympathetic nervous system stimulation in the perioperative period.

Regional Anesthesia. Regional anesthesia, with its associated blockade of the sympathetic nervous system, is an attractive selection for hyperthyroid patients. Advantages of regional anesthetic techniques are somewhat offset by the possible need to treat associated hypotension. It must be remembered that these patients may manifest exaggerated responses to sympathomimetic drugs. A reduced dose of phenylephrine would be the logical drug selection to treat reductions in blood pressure. Epinephrine should not be added to local anesthetic solutions, as systemic absorption of this catecholamine could produce exaggerated circulatory responses. Finally, awake hyperthyroid patients, despite adequate anesthesia, may require sedation with intravenous drugs, such as midazolam or diazepam, to avoid excessive anxiety and associated activation of the sympathetic nervous system.

THYROID STORM (THYROTOXICOSIS)

Thyroid storm is a severe exacerbation of hyperthyroidism due to sudden excessive release of thyroid gland hormones into the circulation. Hyperthermia, tachycardia, congestive heart failure, dehydration, and shock are likely. Indeed, thyroid storm can mimic the onset of malignant hyperthermia.[21] Hyperglycemia is likely, reflecting thyroid hormone induced impairment of insulin secretion and increased glycogenolysis. Thyroid storm associated with surgery can occur intraoperatively but is more likely to manifest in the first 6 hours to 18 hours after surgery and is nearly always abrupt in onset. Treatment of thyroid storm is both supportive and specific. Intravenous infusion of cold crystalloid solutions containing glucose is indicated. In addition, aggressive infusion of crystalloid solutions is necessary to replace fluid loss that accompanies hyperthermia. A digitalis preparation may be necessary to treat cardiac dysfunction, although high-output congestive heart failure is likely to be refractory to this form of treatment. Drugs used to treat specific manifestations of

TABLE 23-3. Pharmacologic Treatment of Thyroid Storm

Drug	Dosage
Sodium iodide	500–1000 mg IV every 8 hours
Cortisol	100–200 mg IV every 8 hours
Propranolol	1–2 mg IV or a dose sufficient to slow the heart rate to less than 90 beats·min^{-1}
Propylthiouracil	200–400 mg orally every 8 hours

excessive thyroid gland activity include sodium iodide, cortisol, propranolol, and propylthiouracil (Table 23-3). Sodium iodide is effective for acutely reducing the release of physiologically active hormones from the thyroid gland (Fig. 23-1). Increased metabolism and use of corticosteroids during thyroid storm can result in acute primary adrenal insufficiency, requiring exogenous administration of cortisol. Propranolol is necessary to alleviate peripheral effects of thyroid gland hormones on the cardiovascular system. Propylthiouracil is necessary to reduce the synthesis of new thyroid gland hormones, particularly that which can occur from the administration of sodium iodide. Aspirin may displace thyroxine from carrier proteins and should not be used to lower body temperature.

Hypothyroidism

Hypothyroidism is the generic term for exposure of the body to subnormal amounts of physiologically active thyroid gland hormones. Decreased function of the thyroid gland may be secondary to dysfunction of the hypothalamus or anterior pituitary, or primary, due to destruction of the thyroid gland (Table 23-4). The diagnosis of hypothyroidism is based on signs and symptoms, plus confirmation of decreased thyroid gland function demonstrated by appropriate tests (see the section Tests of Thyroid Gland Function). Subclinical hypothyroidism manifested solely by elevated plasma concentrations of thyroid stimulating hormone is present in about 5 percent of the population with a prevalence of

TABLE 23-4. Etiology of Hypothyroidism

Type	Etiology
Secondary Hypothyroidism	
Hypothalamic dysfunction	Deficiency of thyrotropin releasing hormone
Anterior pituitary dysfunction	Deficiency of thyroid stimulating hormone
Primary Hypothyroidism	
Thyroid gland destruction	Previous subtotal thyroidectomy
	Previous I^{131} therapy
	Irradiation of the neck
	Chronic inflammation
Thyroid Gland Hormone Deficiency	Dietary iodine deficiency
	Excess iodide (inhibits release)
	Antithyroid drugs

13.2 percent in healthy geriatric patients[22] (see Chapter 36). Chronic thyroiditis (Hashimoto's thyroiditis) is assumed to be the cause of thyroid dysfunction in most of these patients. Other causes for impaired thyroid function include surgical or medical treatment of hyperthyroidism.

SIGNS AND SYMPTOMS

Signs and symptoms of hypothyroidism depend on the age of onset of thyroid gland dysfunction. For example, deficiency of thyroid gland hormones in the neonatal period can result in cretinism, with mental retardation and reduced physical development. The development of hypothyroidism in adulthood is insidious and may go unrecognized for years because of the gradual onset of the thyroid gland dysfunction.

The only physical findings whose presence has a high statistical correlation with hypothyroidism are delayed ankle reflexes, a husky voice, and the presence of dry skin. Characteristically, there is a generalized reduction in metabolic activity. Lethary is prominent, and intolerance to cold is present. Bradycardia and decreased stroke volume are responsible for up to a 40 percent reduction in cardiac output. Decreased cardiac output combined with increased systemic vascular resistance and decreased blood volume results in prolongation of circulation time and narrowing of the pulse pressure. Peripheral vasoconstriction is characteristic leading to cool and dry skin. Presumably, vasoconstriction is an attempt to minimize loss of body heat. Many of the cardiac manifestations of hypothyroidism (cardiomegaly, pleural effusion, ascites, peripheral edema) mimic congestive heart failure. Overt congestive heart failure, however, is unlikely and if present may indicate co-existing heart disease or an unrecognized myocardial infarction. There is often atrophy of the adrenal cortex and an associated decrease in the production of cortisol. Theoretically, unrecognized hypoadrenocorticism in these patients could lead to cardiovascular collapse during anesthesia and surgery.

Myxedema Coma. Myxedema coma is characterized by congestive heart failure, hypoventilation, spontaneous hypothermia, and a depressed level of consciousness. Hypothermia is presumed to reflect a diminished calorigenic response to catecholamines. Hypoventilation may reflect myxedematous infiltration of the muscles of respiration. In addition, there is a decrease in total production of corticosteroids, which may be associated with atrophy of the adrenal cortex. Finally, inappropriate secretion of antidiuretic hormone by hypothyroid patients can result in hyponatremia due to an impaired ability of the renal tubules to excrete free water.

Subacute Thyroiditis. Subacute thyroiditis is characterized by a viral-like illness associated with a diffusely enlarged and tender thyroid gland. Transient hypothyroidism, which lasts for 2 months to 6 months, occurs in about 25 percent of these patients.

Chronic Thyroiditis (Hashimoto's Thyroiditis). Chronic thyroiditis is an autoimmune disease characterized by progressive destruction of the thyroid gland, culminating in hypothyroidism. An adult with diffuse enlargement of the thyroid gland should have antibody measurements to determine the presence of this disease. Indeed, chronic thyroiditis is the most frequent cause of hypothyroidism in adult patients. Chronic thyroiditis may be associated with other autoimmune processes, including pernicious anemia, myasthenia gravis, primary adrenal insufficiency, and premature ovarian failure. Indeed, the presence of any of these diseases should also direct attention to the function of the thyroid gland.

TREATMENT

Treatment of hypothyroidism is with exogenous replacement of thyroid gland hormones. Thyroid gland hormone concentrations in the circulation must be restored slowly because of the dangers of precipitating angina pectoris, cardiac dysrhythmias, or congestive heart failure. Thyroxine requires up to 10 days to exert a physiologic effect and therefore is not effective for emergency treatment of hypothyroidism. Conversely, intravenous triiodothyrine exerts a physiologic effect within 6 hours and reaches a peak effect within 48 hours to 72 hours. Exogenous administration of cortisol will be necessary if there is evidence of primary adrenal insufficiency. Digitalis preparations to treat congestive heart failure must be used sparingly, as the hypothyroid heart cannot easily perform increased myocardial contractile work.

Chronic treatment of hypothyroidism is with oral levothyroxine or desiccated thyroid, which produces physiologic responses indistinguishable from effects seen with endogenous secretion of the thyroid hormones. Adequacy of therapy and the existence of a euthyroid state are confirmed by normal plasma concentrations of thyroid stimulating hormone. Cardiomyopathy associated with hypothyroidism is reversible with thyroid gland hormone replacement.

Treatment of hypothyroid patients with coronary artery disease poses special problems. For example, attempts to render these patients euthyroid with thyroid hormone replacement may produce myocardial ischemia. In these patients, coronary revascularization surgery is often accomplished first followed by postoperative thyroid hormone replacement.[23]

MANAGEMENT OF ANESTHESIA

Elective surgery should not be performed until patients have been rendered euthyroid. Nevertheless, many cases of hypothyroidism

are unrecognized because of the insidious onset of the disease. The possibility of hypothyroidism must be considered in any patient with a history of a previous subtotal thyroidectomy or of therapy with radioactive iodine. When surgery cannot be delayed in known hypothyroid patients, the important anesthetic considerations include (1) exquisite sensitivity to depressant drugs, (2) hypodynamic cardiovascular system characterized by decreased cardiac output due to reductions in heart rate and stroke volume, (3) slowed metabolism of drugs particularly opioids, (4) unresponsive baroreceptor reflexes, (5) decreased intravascular fluid volume, (6) impaired ventilatory response to arterial hypoxemia and/or elevation of the partial pressures of carbon dioxide, (7) delayed gastric emptying time, (8) impaired clearance of free water resulting in hyponatremia, (9) hypothermia, (10) anemia, (11) hypoglycemia, and (12) primary adrenal insufficiency.[1] There is no direct evidence of a reduced responsiveness of these patients to exogenous catecholamines.[1] Furthermore, reduced circulating concentrations of thyroid hormones may be associated with a reversible conversion of beta-adrenergic receptors to alpha-adrenergic receptors. Indeed, hypothyroidism is associated with reductions in the number of beta-adrenergic receptors.[5]

Preoperative Medication. Preoperative medication for hypothyroid patients should be limited to a preoperative visit and psychological support. Supplemental cortisol may be indicated, since surgical stress could unmask decreased adrenal cortex function that often accompanies hypothyroidism (see the section Corticosteroid Therapy Before Surgery). Opioids can produce ventilatory depression. Sedative drugs or anticholinergic drugs can be administered intravenously on arrival in the operating room, if such therapy is deemed essential.

Induction of Anesthesia. Induction of anesthesia can be accomplished with the slow intravenous administration of ketamine. Barbiturates or benzodiazepines are not the first choices, as it seems these drugs would be more likely than ketamine to produce abrupt reductions in blood pressure. Even ketamine, in the absence of an active sympathetic nervous system, might produce unexpected cardiovascular depression. In some hypothyroid patients, the inhalation of nitrous oxide may be sufficient to produce unresponsiveness. Intubation of the trachea is facilitated by succinylcholine or an appropriate dose of nondepolarizing muscle relaxants.

Maintenance of Anesthesia. Maintenance of anesthesia for hypothyroid patients is best achieved by inhalation of nitrous oxide, plus supplementation, if necessary, with minimal doses of short-acting opioids, benzodiazepines or ketamine.[24] Volatile anesthetics are not recommended because of the exquisite sensitivity of hypothyroid patients to drug-induced myocardial depression. In addition, vasodilation produced by even low concentrations of volatile drugs in the presence of hypovolemia and/or attenuated baroreceptor reflex responses may result in abrupt decreases in blood pressure, suggesting increased sensitivity to the drug. Nevertheless, it should be appreciated that hypothyroidism does not appear to significantly reduce the dose of volatile drugs needed to prevent skeletal muscle responses to a noxious stimulus (Fig. 23-2).[18] Failure of alterations in thyroid activity to change anesthetic requirements may reflect maintenance of a cerebral metabolic requirements for oxygen, which is independent of thyroid activity.[1] The clinical impression that anesthetic requirements are reduced most likely reflects reductions in cardiac output that accelerate establishment of an anesthetizing partial pressure manifesting as a rapid induction of anesthesia. Furthermore, reductions in body temperature below 37 degrees Celsius would be expected to reduce anesthetic requirements for volatile drugs[25], as well as slow hepatic metabolism and renal elimination of injected drugs.

Maintaining skeletal muscle paralysis to provide surgical working conditions, while at the same time minimizing doses of anesthetic drugs, is an appropriate goal for management of hypothyroid patients. Furthermore, controlled ventilation of the lungs is recommended because of the tendency for hypothyroid patients to hypoventilate. Reduced production of carbon dioxide associated with decreased metabolic rates makes hypothyroid patients vulnerable to excessive reductions in the arterial partial pressures of carbon dioxide during controlled ventilation of the lungs. Since cerebral metabolic requirements for oxygen are not likely to be altered in these patients, it is important to avoid excessive hyperventilation of the lungs and associated reductions in cerebral blood flow. Because of its mild sympathomimetic effects, pancuronium may be a useful drug for production of skeletal muscle paralysis in hypothyroid patients. Intermediate acting muscle relaxants would also be acceptable and less likely than pancuronium to produce prolonged neuromuscular blockade. Indeed reduced skeletal muscle activity associated with hypothyroidism suggests the possibility of prolonged responses should traditional doses of muscle relaxants be administered to these patients. The likelihood of reductions in blood pressure after administration of d-tubocurarine detracts from the use of this drug. Finally, reversal of nondepolarizing neuromuscular blockade with anticholinesterase drugs combined with an anticholinergic drug poses no known hazards in hypothyroid patients.

Monitoring of patients with hypothyroidism is directed toward early recognition of congestive heart failure and detection of the onset of hypothermia. Continuous recording of blood pressure via a catheter placed in a peripheral artery, as well as measurement of cardiac filling pressures, is indicated for invasive operations. Measurement of central venous pressure is helpful for guiding the rate of intravenous fluid infusion. In addition to glucose, solutions used for intravenous fluid replacement should contain sodium to minimize the development of hyponatremia due to impaired clearance of free water. Hypotension that requires treatment with infusion of fluids or administration of sympathomimetic drugs introduces the risk of producing congestive heart failure. For example, administration of alpha-adrenergic agonist drugs such as phenylephrine can adversely increase systemic vascular resistance in the presence of a heart that cannot increase its myocardial contractility. In contrast, drugs with beta-adrenergic agonist activity may result in cardiac dysrhythmias. A useful drug to treat hypotension would seem to be small doses of ephedrine (2.5 mg to 5 mg), administered during careful monitoring of cardiac filling pressures and continuous observation of the electrocardiogram. The possibility of acute primary adrenal insufficiency should be remembered when hypotension persists despite treatment with infusion of fluids and/or sympathomimetic drugs. Maintenance of body temperature is facilitated by increasing the temperature of the operating room and warming inhaled gases. In addition, passage of intravenous fluid solutions through a blood warmer would seem prudent.

Recovery from sedative effects of anesthetic drugs may be delayed in hypothyroid patients, resulting in the need for prolonged observation in the postoperative period. Indeed, prolonged postoperative lethargy and inability to wean from mechanical support of ventilation may reflect previously unrecognized hypothyroidism.[26] Removal of tracheal tubes should not be considered until patients are responding and body temperature is near 37 degrees Celsius. It must be appreciated that these patients are extremely vulnerable to ventilatory depressant effects produced by opioids. Therefore, postoperative analgesia, if necessary, should be provided with minimal doses of an opioid or a nonopioid analgesic.

Regional Anesthesia. Regional anesthesia is a useful approach for management of anesthesia in the presence of hypothyroidism. Although supporting evidence is not available, it would seem likely that doses of local anesthetics necessary for peripheral nerve blocks might be reduced. Furthermore, metabolism of amide local anesthetics absorbed into the systemic circulation is likely to be slowed. Conceivably, this could predispose hypothyroid patients to the development of systemic toxicity from local anesthetics.

Carcinoma of the Thyroid Gland

A solitary and nonfunctioning ("cold") nodule in the thyroid gland (see the section Tests of Thyroid Gland Function) will be malignant in 10 percent to 30 percent of patients, with the greatest incidence occurring in patients less than 20 years of age. A history of irradiation delivered to the neck, particularly in childhood, plus a thyroid nodule should arouse suspicion as to the presence of a thyroid gland carcinoma. Production of large amounts of calcitonin by a medullary thyroid gland carcinoma is characteristic. Nevertheless, hypocalcemia does not occur, despite increased secretion of calcitonin. Diagnosis of carcinoma of the thyroid gland can be made only by an open surgical biopsy. The combination of medullary thyroid gland carcinoma and pheochromocytoma is an autosomal dominant disorder known as multiple endocrine neoplasia type II (see the section Multiple Endocrine Neoplasia).

PARATHYROID GLANDS

The four parathyroid glands are located behind each of the two upper and lower poles of the thyroid gland. These glands produce a polypeptide hormone known as parathormone. Parathormone is released into the circulation by a negative feedback mechanism dependent on plasma concentrations of calcium. For example, low plasma calcium concentrations stimulate release of parathormone; an increased concentration suppresses both the synthesis and release of this hormone. Release of parathormone is also influenced by plasma phosphorus concentrations. This reflects the ability of increased phosphorus concentrations to lower plasma concentrations of calcium and thus stimulate the release of parathormone. Finally, reductions in plasma magnesium concentrations can impair release of parathormone, as well as peripheral responses to this hormone.

Parathormone maintains plasma calcium concentrations in a normal range (4.5 mEq·L^{-1} to 5.5 mEq·L^{-1}) by promoting movement of calcium into the blood across three interfaces, represented by the gastrointestinal tract, kidneys, and bone. Gastrointestinal absorption of calcium is enhanced by parathormone-induced synthesis of an active form of vitamin

D. Calcium release from bone is enhanced by parathormone-induced stimulation of osteoclastic activity. The effect of parathormone on the kidney, which leads to calcium entrance into the circulation, is via activation of an enzyme necessary for the synthesis of vitamin D, which in turn leads to increased tubular reabsorption of calcium and enhanced renal tubular clearance of phosphorus.

Hyperparathyroidism

Hyperparathyroidism is present when secretion of parathormone is increased. Plasma calcium concentrations may be elevated, normal, or decreased. Hyperparathyroidism is classified as primary, secondary, or ectopic (pseudohyperparathyroidism).

PRIMARY HYPERPARATHYRODISM

Primary hyperparathyroidism results from excessive secretion of parathormone due to benign parathyroid adenomas, carcinoma of a parathyroid gland, or hyperplasia of the parathyroid glands. A benign parathyroid adenoma is responsible for primary hyperparathyroidism in about 90 percent of patients; carcinoma of a parathyroid gland is responsible in less than 5 percent. Hyperplasia usually involves all four parathyroid glands, although not all the glands may be enlarged to the same degree. Finally, primary hyperparathyroidism can exist in association with other endocrine gland disorders (see the section Multiple Endocrine Neoplasia).

Signs and Symptoms. A broad spectrum of signs and symptoms, for which hypercalcemia is responsible, accompanies primary hyperparathyroidism (Table 23-5). Mild generalized weakness is the most frequent complaint. Renal stones, with or without renal insufficiency, must arouse suspicion of hyperparathyroidism. Polyuria and polydipsia reflect hypercalcemia. Hypertension is a frequent finding. The electrocardiogram may

TABLE 23-5. Manifestations of Hypercalcemia Due to Hyperparathyroidism

Type	Manifestation
Renal	Polydipsia and polyuria
	Renal stones
	Decreased glomerular filtration rate
Cardiac	Hypertension
	Short Q-T interval
	Prolonged P-R interval
Gastrointestinal	Abdominal pain
	Vomiting
	Weight loss
	Peptic ulcer
	Pancreatitis
Skeletal	Bone pain and tenderness
	Skeletal demineralization
	Pathologic fractures
	Collapse of vertebral bodies
Nervous system	Somnolence
	Psychosis
	Decreased pain sensation
Neuromuscular	Skeletal muscle weakness
Articular	Periarticular calcifications
	Gout
Ocular	Calcifications (band keratopathy)
	Conjunctivitis
Hematopoietic	Anemia

reveal short Q-T intervals, while P-R intervals are often prolonged. Cardiac rhythm is usually normal. Peptic ulcer disease is frequent and may reflect potentiation of gastric acid secretion by calcium. Acute and chronic pancreatitis is associated with primary hyperparathyroidism. Even in the absence of peptic ulcer disease or pancreatitis, abdominal pain that often accompanies hypercalcemia can mimic that of an acute surgical abdomen. The classic skeletal consequence of primary hyperparathyroidism is osteitis fibrosa cystica, which reflects accelerated osteoclastic activity. Radiographic evidence of skeletal involvement includes generalized osteopenia, subcortical bone resorption in the phalanges and distal ends of the clavicles, and the appearance of bone cysts. Bone pain and tenderness and pathologic fractures may be present. There may be deficits of memory and cerebration, with or without personality changes or mood disturbances, including hallucinations. Loss of sensation for pain and vibration can occur. Neuromuscular involvement is characterized by skeletal muscle weakness and hypotonia so severe that myasthenia gravis may be suspected. Loss of strength and skeletal muscle mass is most notable in the proximal musculature of the lower extremity. Anemia, even in the absence of renal dysfunction, is a consequence of primary hyperparathyroidism.

Diagnosis. Elevated plasma concentrations of calcium (above 5.5 mEq·L^{-1}) are the most valuable diagnostic indicators of primary hyperparathyroidism. Marked elevations (above 7.5 mEq·L^{-1}) are more likely to occur in patients with carcinoma of a parathyroid gland than in those with benign adenomas or parathyroid gland hyperplasia. Plasma chloride concentrations are usually greater than 102 mEq·L^{-1}. These plasma chloride elevations reflect the influence of parathormone on renal excretion of bicarbonate, producing a mild metabolic acidosis. Plasma phosphorus concentrations are usually low, reflecting increased renal excretion of phosphorus. As the disease progresses, elevations of plasma creatinine concentrations may reflect associated renal dysfunction. Urinary excretion of cyclic adenosine monophosphate is increased in patients with primary hyperparathyroidism. Conversely, hypercalcemia due to causes unrelated to dysfunction of the parathyroid glands is not associated with changes in the urinary excretion of cyclic adenosine monophosphate. Measurement of plasma parathormone concentrations is not always sufficiently reliable to confirm the diagnosis of primary hyperparathyroidism.

Treatment. Lowering of plasma calcium concentrations is initially accomplished by establishing diuresis in response to the administration of intravenous or oral fluids plus furosemide. Emergency treatment of hypercalcemia is usually necessary when plasma calcium concentrations exceed 7.5 mEq·L^{-1}. Rapid lowering of plasma calcium concentrations is best accomplished by the intravenous administration of mithramycin (25 μg·kg^{-1}). Mithramycin inhibits parathormone-induced osteoclastic activity, leading to reductions in plasma calcium concentrations within 12 hours to 36 hours that last 3 days to 5 days. Toxic effects of mithramycin include thrombocytopenia and damage to the liver and/or

kidneys. Hemodialysis can be used to lower plasma calcium concentrations if mithramycin is contraindicated. Calcitonin is also effective for rapidly lowering plasma calcium concentrations, but the effects of this hormone are transient. Rarely, hypercalcemia cannot be medically managed, and emergency parathyroidectomy is required.

Definitive treatment of primary hyperparathyroidism is surgical removal of the parathyroid adenoma or malignant parathyroid gland. Hyperplasia of all four parathyroid glands is treated by excision of all parathyroid tissue except for one-half of one gland. Successful parathyroidectomy is reflected by reductions in the urinary excretion of cyclic adenosine monophosphate and normalization of plasma calcium concentrations within 3 days to 4 days. It should be remembered that postoperative hypoparathyroidism can follow parathyroidectomy for treatment of hyperplasia of the parathyroid glands, particularly in patients with co-existing osteitis fibrosa cystica. Furthermore, even adequate amounts of remaining parathyroid gland may not be able to resume promptly normal parathyroid function. The resultant hypoparathyroidism typically begins to resolve in 7 days to 10 days. Hypomagnesemia may occur postoperatively as a result of unbalanced uptake of magnesium into bone and prior magnesium depletion. Manifestations of hypocalcemia are aggravated and its treatment rendered refractory in the presence of hypomagnesemia. Acute arthritis, including gout and pseudogout, occur with increased frequency in patients with hyperparathyroidism and may be precipitated by parathyroid surgery. Hyperchloremic metabolic acidosis, in association with deterioration of renal function, may occur transiently after parathyroidectomy.

Management of Anesthesia. Management of anesthesia for patients with elevated plasma concentrations of calcium should emphasize the importance of maintaining hydration and urine output (see Chapter 22). Knowledge of the manifestations of hypercalcemia is also important in the perioperative management of these patients (Table 23-5). There is no evidence that specific anesthetic drugs or techniques are indicated. However, the possibility of co-existing renal dysfunction should be remembered when considering the selection of enflurane. The existence of somnolence before the induction of anesthesia introduces the possibility that intraoperative anesthetic requirements will be reduced. Ketamine would be a questionable selection in patients with personality disturbances related to hypercalcemia. Monitoring of the electrocardiogram for evidence of adverse effects of hypercalcemia on the heart is important. Nevertheless, there is evidence that Q-T intervals may not be reliable indices of changes in plasma calcium concentrations during anesthesia.[27] The response of muscle relaxants could be altered in these patients. For example, skeletal muscle weakness associated with hypercalcemia suggests the possibility of decreased muscle relaxant requirements. Conversely, elevated plasma concentrations of calcium might be expected to antagonize effects of nondepolarizing muscle relaxants. Indeed, there is a report of sensitivity to succinylcholine and resistance to atracurium in a patient with hyperparathyroidism.[28] In view of unpredictable responses to these drugs, a prudent approach would seem to be reductions in the initial doses of muscle relaxants and observation of responses produced at the neuromuscular junction by using a peripheral nerve stimulator. Finally, careful positioning of these patients during surgery is necessary, because of the likely presence of osteoporosis and associated vulnerability to pathologic fractures.

SECONDARY HYPERPARATHYROIDISM

Secondary hyperparathyroidism represents an appropriate compensatory increase in the secretion of parathormone in response to disease processes that produce hypocalcemia, hyperphosphatemia, or hypomagnesemia. Renal disease is a common cause. For example, renal disease impairs the elimination of phosphorus, and reduces the hydroxylation of vitamin D. As a result, plasma calcium concentrations are decreased, leading to hyperplasia of the parathyroid glands and increased secretion of parathormone. Malabsorptive diseases of the gastrointestinal tract also result in hy-

pocalcemia and subsequent secondary hyperparathyroidism. Treatment is directed at control of the underlying disease. In contrast to patients with primary hyperparathyroidism, plasma calcium concentrations remain low to normal in these patients.

On occasion, transient hypercalcemia may follow successful renal transplantation. This response reflects the inability of previously hyperactive parathyroid glands to adapt suddenly to normal renal handling of calcium, phosphorus, and vitamin D. The parathyroid glands will usually return to normal size and function with time. In some instances, however, parathyroidectomy may be necessary.

ECTOPIC HYPERPARATHYROIDISM (PSEUDOHYPERPARATHYROIDISM)

Ectopic hyperparathyroidism is due to the production of parathormone, or a substance with similar endocrine effects, by tissues other than the parathyroid glands. Carcinoma of the lung, breast, pancreas, or kidney and lymphoproliferative diseases are most likely to supply ectopic sites for secretion of this hormone, leading to hypercalcemia.

Ectopic hyperparathyroidism is distinguished from primary hyperparathyroidism by a more frequent presence of anemia, serum chloride concentrations less than 102 mEq· L^{-1}, and increased plasma alkaline phosphatase concentrations. A role for prostaglandins in the production of hypercalcemia in these patients is suggested by the calcium lowering effects produced by indomethacin, which is an inhibitor of prostaglandin synthesis.

Hypoparathyroidism

Hypoparathyroidism is present when secretion of parathormone is deficient or peripheral tissues are resistant to the effects of this hormone (Table 23-6). Absence of parathormone secretion is almost always iatrogenic, reflecting inadvertent removal of the parathyroid glands, as during thyroidectomy. Idiopathic

TABLE 23-6. Etiology of Hypoparathyroidism

Decreased to Absent Parathormone
Inadvertent removal of parathyroid glands during thyroidectomy
Parathyroidectomy to treat hyperplasia of parathyroid glands
Idiopathic

Resistance of Peripheral Tissues to the Effects of Parathormone
Pseudohypoparathyroidism
Hypomagnesemia
Chronic renal failure
Gastrointestinal malabsorption
Anticonvulsant drugs

Unknown Mechanism
Acute pancreatitis

parathormone deficiency can be an isolated finding or can occur in association with dysfunction of other endocrine glands, especially the thyroid and adrenal glands. Pseudohypoparathyroidism is an inherited disorder in which release of parathormone is intact, but the kidneys are unable to respond to released hormone. Patients are characterized by mental retardation, obesity, short stature, short metacarpals and metatarsals, and calcification of the basal ganglia. Pseudo-pseudohypoparathyroidism is characterized by the above findings, but plasma calcium concentrations are normal. Parathormone secretion or activity may also be inadequate in the presence of reduced plasma magnesium concentrations, chronic renal failure, gastrointestinal malabsorption, and therapy with anticonvulsant drugs. Indeed, chronic treatment with phenytoin has been implicated as a cause of vitamin D deficiency. Finally, acute pancreatitis, by an unknown mechanism, can result in hypocalcemia.

SIGNS AND SYMPTOMS

Signs and symptoms of hypoparathyroidism reflect the presence of hypocalcemia (see the section Hypocalcemia in Chapter 22). Clinical manifestations of hypocalcemia depend on the rapidity of the reduction in plasma calcium concentrations.

Acute Hypocalcemia. An acute onset of hypocalcemia, as can occur after inadvertent

removal of the parathyroid glands during a thyroidectomy, is likely to manifest as perioral paresthesias, restlessness, and neuromuscular irritability. Such irritability is confirmed by a positive Chvostek's or Trousseau's sign. A positive Chvostek's sign is facial muscle twitching produced by manual tapping over the area of the facial nerve at the angle of the mandible. It must be appreciated, however, that Chvostek's sign is present in 10 percent to 15 percent of patients in the absence of hypocalcemia. A positive Trousseau's sign is carpopedal spasm produced by 3 minutes of limb ischemia, using a tourniquet. Inspiratory stridor reflects neuromuscular irritability of the intrinsic laryngeal musculature.

Chronic Hypocalcemia. Gradual reductions in plasma calcium concentrations are associated with complaints of fatigue and skeletal muscle cramps. Chronic renal failure is probably the most common cause of hypocalcemia. Skeletal muscle spasms that manifest in malnourished patients, particularly alcoholic patients, most likely reflect hypocalcemia due to reduced plasma concentrations of magnesium. Hypocalcemia is associated with prolonged Q-T intervals on the electrocardiogram, and QRS complexes and P-R intervals remain normal. Cardiac rhythm usually remains normal, despite changes on the electrocardiogram. Petit mal or grand mal seizures can be exaggerated by hypocalcemia. Neurologic changes include lethargy, cerebration deficits, and personality changes reminiscent of hyperparathyroidism. Finally, chronic hypocalcemia is associated with the formation of cataracts, calcification involving the subcutaneous tissues and basal ganglia, and thickening of the skull.

DIAGNOSIS

Reduced plasma calcium concentrations (below 4.5 mEq·L^{-1}) are the most valuable diagnostic indicators of hypoparathyroidism. Urinary excretion of calcium and phosphorus is diminished. Low plasma concentrations of parathormone are reflected by low urinary excretion of cyclic adenosine monophosphate.

Hyperphosphatemia is characteristic of pseudohypoparathyroidism.

TREATMENT

Treatment of acute hypocalcemia is with intravenous infusion of calcium until signs of neuromuscular irritability disappear. Chronic hypoparathyroidism is treated by administration of oral calcium and vitamin D, since a practical exogenous parathormone hormone replacement is not available. An alternative is administration of thiazide diuretics. Thiazide diuretics cause sodium depletion without proportional calcium excretion, which tends to increase plasma calcium concentrations.

MANAGEMENT OF ANESTHESIA

Management of anesthesia for patients with hypoparathyroidism is determined by the impact of perioperative events on plasma calcium concentrations (see the section Hypocalcemia in Chapter 22).

DiGeorge Syndrome

DiGeorge syndrome is characterized by hypoplasia or aplasia of the parathyroid glands and thymus gland, resulting in secondary hypocalcemia and propensity to develop sepsis due to defects in cellular immunity.[29] Associated anomalies are often vascular, including right aortic arch, persistent truncus arteriosus, and tetralogy of Fallot. Micrognathia may interfere with adequate exposure of the glottic opening during direct laryngoscopy. Iatrogenic hyperventilation and associated respiratory alkalosis as may occur during anesthesia could accentuate co-existing hypocalcemia. Responses to neuromuscular blocking drugs could be altered in the presence of hypocalcemia. Hemodynamic instability may manifest if hypoparathyroid patients are made acutely hypocalcemic. Ability to measure plasma concentrations of calcium, particularly the ionized fractions, is helpful in the perioperative management of these patients.

ADRENAL CORTEX

The adrenal cortex is responsible for the synthesis of three groups of hormones, classified as glucocorticoids, mineralocorticoids, and androgens. Cholesterol, which is derived from acetate, is the building block for the steroid nucleus necessary for the synthesis of all the hormones produced by the adrenal cortex (Fig. 23-3). The adrenal cortex is divided into three functional zones; the zona fasciculata, zona glomerulosa, and zona reticularis. The zona fasciculata produces glucocorticoids; the zona glomerulosa, mineralocorticoids; and the zona reticularis, androgens.

Cortisol is the most important glucocorticoid secreted by the adrenal cortex. Indeed, endogenous and synthetic corticosteroids are compared to cortisol with respect to glucocorticoid potency (anti-inflammatory effects) and mineralocorticoid potency (salt-retaining effects) (Table 23-7). Prednisolone and prednisone are hydroxylated synthetic derivatives of cortisol and cortisone respectively. Assuming a daily endogenous cortisol production of 20 mg, an equivalent glucocorticoid effect would be produced by 5 mg of prednisolone or prednisone. Methylation of prednisolone to produce methylprednisolone or dexamethasone results in increased glucocorticoid potency and reductions in mineralocorticoid activity (Table 23-7). Therefore, pharmacologic doses of methylprednisolone or dexamethasone can be administered to produce desirable glucocorticoid effects without producing changes characteristic of mineralocorticoid activity.

Glucocorticoids

The principal endogenous glucocorticoid is cortisol. Cortisone is a glucocorticoid, which is secreted in small amounts. Synthesis and release of cortisol is regulated by adrenocor-

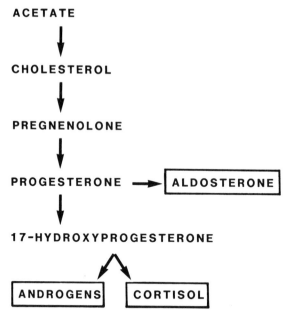

FIG. 23-3.   Schematic diagram of the steps leading to the synthesis of the primary hormones (androgens, cortisol, and aldosterone) secreted by the adrenal cortex.

ticotrophic hormone (ACTH), which is produced in the anterior pituitary. ACTH release is determined by corticotropin-releasing factor from the hypothalamus and a negative feedback mechanism regulated by plasma concentrations of cortisol. In addition, hypoglycemia and stress, as produced by trauma, can stimulate release of ACTH and thus increase plasma concentrations of cortisol.

Daily endogenous production of cortisol is about 20 mg. Most of the circulating cortisol is inactive, as it is bound to an alpha globulin designated as transcortin or cortisol-binding globulin. Resting plasma concentrations of cor-

TABLE 23-7.   Endogenous and Synthetic Corticosteroids

	Glucocorticoid Potency* (Anti-Inflammatory Effects)	Mineralocorticoid Potency* (Salt-Retaining Effects)	Equivalent Oral or IV Dose* (mg)
Cortisol	1	1	20†
Cortisone	0.8	0.8	25
Prednisolone	4	0.8	5
Prednisone	4	0.8	5
Methylprednisolone	5	0	4
Betamethasone	25	0	0.75
Dexamethasone	25	0	0.75
Triamcinolone	5	0	4
Corticosterone	0.35	15	
Fludrocortisone	10	125	
Aldosterone		3000	

* Potencies and equivalent doses are as compared with cortisol.
† Assumed daily endogenous cortisol production.

tisol are 10 $\mu g \cdot dl^{-1}$ to 25 $\mu g \cdot dl^{-1}$ in the morning, and 2 $\mu g \cdot dl^{-1}$ to 10 $\mu g \cdot dl^{-1}$ at midnight. This diurnal variation reflects varying release of ACTH from the anterior pituitary. Cortisol is inactivated in the liver, and metabolites appear in the urine as 17-hydroxysteroids.

Cortisol is the only hormone produced by the adrenal cortex that is essential for life. Physiologic effects of cortisol are diverse. Maintenance of blood pressure by cortisol reflects the importance of this hormone for facilitating conversion of norepinephrine to epinephrine in the adrenal medulla. Cortisol promotes breakdown of proteins and subsequent formation of glucose from the liberated amino acids by gluconeogenesis. Peripheral use of glucose by cells is inhibited by cortisol. Indeed, hyperglycemia in response to cortisol administration reflects gluconeogenesis and decreased peripheral use of glucose. Retention of sodium and excretion of potassium are facilitated by cortisol. In addition, this hormone promotes excretion of water, by increasing glomerular filtration rate and by diminishing reabsorption of water by renal tubules. Finally, cortisol also has well-known anti-inflammatory effects, particularly when plasma concentrations are markedly elevated. Anti-inflammatory effects of glucocorticoids reflect the ability of these substances to (1) stabilize cell membranes, and thus prevent release of lysosomal enzymes; (2) reduce the permeability of capillary membranes, which prevents leakage of proteins into inflamed tissues; and (3) inhibit formation of bradykinin.

Mineralocorticoids

The principal endogenous mineralocorticoid is aldosterone. Corticosterone and desoxycorticosterone are secreted in small amounts. Secretion and synthesis of aldosterone by the adrenal cortex are regulated by the renin-angiotensin system and plasma concentrations of potassium. For example, renin release from the juxtaglomerular cells of the kidneys, in response to hypotension, hyponatremia, or hypovolemia, results in conversion of angiotensinogen to angiotensin I. Angiotensin I is converted to angiotensin II, which acts as a potent stimulus for release of aldosterone from the adrenal cortex. In addition, aldosterone secretion is stimulated by increased plasma potassium concentrations, whereas hypokalemia suppresses its release. Aldosterone regulates extracellular fluid volume by promoting reabsorption of sodium by renal tubules. In addition, aldosterone promotes renal tubular excretion of potassium. Normal daily secretion of aldosterone is 50 μg to 250 μg, resulting in a plasma aldosterone concentration of 1 $ng \cdot dl^{-1}$ to 5 $ng \cdot dl^{-1}$.

Androgens

Testosterone and estradiol are manufactured in only trace amounts by the adrenal cortex. However, these hormones can be produced elsewhere in the body, from androgens synthesized initially in the adrenal cortex. Release of androgens by the adrenal cortex is regulated by ACTH. Androgens are inactivated in the liver, and metabolites appear in the urine as 17-ketosteroids.

Hyperadrenocorticism (Cushing's Disease)

Hyperadrenocorticism can result from excess production of ACTH, excess production of cortisol, and exogenous administration of corticosteroids. Excess production of ACTH by the anterior pituitary is the etiology of hyperadrenocorticism in about two-thirds of patients. The usual cause of excess ACTH production is an anterior pituitary tumor (basophilic adenoma), although excess production of corticotropin-releasing factor in the hypothalamus could also be the mechanism. Hyperadrenocorticism can also result from ectopic production of ACTH by malignant tumors, especially carcinoma of the lung, kidney, and pancreas. Excess production of cortisol by malignant tumors of the adrenal cortex is the etiology in about one-third of patients. Occasionally benign adrenal cortex adenomas result in excess secretion of cortisol.

SIGNS AND SYMPTOMS

Hyperadrenocorticism manifests as hypertension, hypokalemia, hypernatremia, hyperglycemia, increased intravascular fluid volume, and skeletal muscle weakness. Osteoporosis reflects cortisol-induced loss of proteins from bone. Shortening of the thoracic spine may reflect vertebral body collapse from osteoporosis. Obesity, plethoric and round facies, and accumulation of fat between the scapulae are characteristic. Hirsutism is present when hyperadrenocorticism is due to excess secretion of ACTH, reflecting the ability of this hormone to stimulate the release of androgens as well as cortisol. Menstrual irregularities are common. Thromboembolism from hypercoagulability is a hazard. Finally, the incidence of bacterial and fungal infection is increased in patients with hyperadrenocorticism.

DIAGNOSIS

Diagnosis of hyperadrenocorticism is based on a demonstration of increased plasma and urine concentrations of cortisol. Dexamethasone will suppress plasma concentrations of cortisol in normal patients, but not in those with hyperadrenocorticism.

Elevated plasma concentrations of ACTH suggest a pituitary gland tumor or an ectopic hormone-producing tumor as a cause of hyperadrenocorticism. Extremely high plasma concentrations of ACTH are evidence for an ectopic rather than pituitary gland source of excess production. Furthermore, in contrast to the gradual onset of symptoms seen with excess pituitary gland production of ACTH, the clinical presentation in patients with ectopic production of this hormone is that of acute hyperadrenocorticism dominated by mineralocorticoid rather than glucocorticoid effects.

Carcinoma of the adrenal cortex, which produces excess cortisol, is also likely to secrete excess androgens, so that urinary concentrations of 17-ketosteroids are elevated.

Conversely, a benign adenoma in the adrenal cortex usually results in excess production of only cortisol.

TREATMENT

Traditional treatment of hyperadrenocorticism is surgical. For example, transphenoidal microadenectomy is indicated when hyperadrenocorticism is due to excess secretion of ACTH by a pituitary gland tumor. Adrenalectomy is performed for management of patients with carcinoma of the adrenal cortex or a benign adrenal cortex adenoma. Irradiation directed to the pituitary gland or medical treatment with cyproheptadine may be effective in some patients with hyperadrenocorticism due to a pituitary gland tumor.

MANAGEMENT OF ANESTHESIA

Management of anesthesia for patients with hyperadrenocorticism must consider the physiologic effects of excess cortisol secretion.[30] Preoperative evaluation of cardiovascular function, blood pressure, electrolyte balance, acid-base status, and the plasma concentration of glucose are indicated. The extent of osteoporosis must be considered in terms of subsequent positioning for the operative procedure.

Choice of drugs for preoperative medication or production of anesthesia is not influenced by the presence of hyperadrenocorticism. Surgical stimulation will predictably increase release of cortisol from the adrenal cortex. It seems unlikely that this stress-induced release would produce different effects in these patients, as compared with normal patients. Furthermore, attempts to reduce adrenal cortex activity with opioids, barbiturates, or volatile anesthetics are probably futile, since any drug-induced inhibition will likely be overridden by surgical stimulation. Even regional anesthesia may not be effective in predictably preventing increased cortisol secretion during surgery. Muscle relaxant doses should be reduced initially, in view of skeletal muscle weakness, which frequently accompanies hyperadrenocorticism. Furthermore, the presence of hypokalemia could influence the response to muscle relaxants. Mechanical ventilation of the lungs during surgery is recommended, as skeletal muscle weakness, with or without co-existing hypokalemia, may reduce strength in the muscles of respiration. Regional anesthesia is acceptable, but the likely presence of osteoporosis, with possible vertebral body collapse, must be appreciated.

Continuous intravenous infusion of cortisol at a rate equivalent to 100 mg·day^{-1} should be started intraoperatively if the surgery is for a hypophysectomy or bilateral adrenalectomy. Postoperatively, chronic maintenance therapy with corticosteroids will be necessary in these patients.

Hypoadrenocorticism

Hypoadrenocorticism may develop as a result of (1) destruction of the adrenal cortex by granulomatous disease, cancer, or hemorrhage; (2) deficiency of ACTH; and (3) prolonged administration of exogenous corticosteroids, which suppresses the pituitary-adrenal axis. Destruction of the adrenal cortex produces findings classified as primary adrenal insufficiency or Addison's disease. Manifestations of primary adrenal insufficiency are related to the absence of cortisol and aldosterone. Hypoadrenocorticism due to deficiency of ACTH reflects dysfunction of the anterior pituitary leading to panhypopituitarism. In contrast to primary adrenal insufficiency, aldosterone secretion remains normal.

SIGNS AND SYMPTOMS

Primary adrenal insufficiency due to destruction of the adrenal cortex manifests as skeletal muscle weakness, weight loss, and hypotension. Hyperpigmentation is caused by excessive secretion of melanocyte stimulating hormone by the anterior pituitary. Any stress, such as accidental or surgical trauma, can result in circulatory collapse, with hyponatremia, hyperkalemia, hypoglycemia, and hemoconcentration. Elevations in blood urea

nitrogen concentrations reflect reductions in the intravascular fluid volume and decreased renal blood flow due to low cardiac output. The clinical picture may be indistinguishable from shock due to loss of intravascular fluid volume. Hypoadrenocorticism due to dysfunction of the anterior pituitary and deficiency of ACTH is less likely than primary adrenal insufficiency to be associated with severe derangements in plasma concentrations of electrolytes or loss of intravascular fluid volume, since aldosterone secretion is maintained. Panhypopituitarism, however, may be associated with symptoms due to the absence of growth hormone, thyroid stimulating hormone, and gonadotropins, as well as manifestations of deficient secretion of ACTH (see the section Anterior Pituitary).

DIAGNOSIS

Low plasma or urine concentrations of corticosteroids derived from the adrenal cortex suggest the diagnosis of hypoadrenocorticism. Plasma concentrations of ACTH are elevated in the presence of primary adrenal insufficiency and reduced when hypoadrenocorticism is due to dysfunction of the anterior pituitary or inhibition of the pituitary-adrenal axis.

TREATMENT

Treatment of hypoadrenocorticism associated with circulatory collapse is with intravenous cortisol, 100 mg followed by 50 mg every 4 hours to 6 hours during the first 48 hours after the crisis. Intravenous infusion of glucose in saline, colloid solutions, and in some cases whole blood should be administered to restore intravascular fluid volume. Replacement therapy for chronic hypoadrenocorticism is with oral cortisone, 15 mg to 20 mg in the morning and 10 mg to 15 mg in the afternoon. In addition, patients should receive an appropriate corticosteroid to provide mineralocorticoid effects. This effect is monitored by observing patients for weight gain, development of hypertension, or appearance of hypokalemia.

CORTICOSTEROID THERAPY BEFORE SURGERY

Corticosteroid supplementation should be increased whenever patients being treated for chronic hypoadrenocorticism undergo surgical procedures. This recommendation is based on the concern that these patients are susceptible to cardiovascular collapse, since they cannot release additional endogenous cortisol in response to the stress of surgery. More controversial is management of the patients who may manifest suppression of the pituitary-adrenal axis due to current or previous administration of corticosteroids for treatment of diseases such as asthma or rheumatoid arthritis, which are unrelated to pathology in the anterior pituitary or adrenal cortex. The dose of corticosteroid or duration of therapy with a corticosteroid that will produce suppression of the pituitary-adrenal axis is not known. Furthermore, recovery of normal pituitary-adrenal axis function may require as long as 12 months after discontinuation of therapy. In addition, documentation of normal plasma concentrations of cortisol in the preoperative period does not confirm an intact pituitary-adrenal axis or the ability of the adrenal cortex to release cortisol in response to surgical stress. Performance of stimulation tests with infusion of ACTH in the preoperative period is informative but not practical for routine evaluation. Therefore, the clinical approach is often to administer empirically supplemental corticosteroids in the perioperative period when surgery is planned in patients who are being treated with corticosteroids or who have been treated for more than 1 month in the past 6 months to 12 months. Nevertheless, it should be appreciated that cause and effect relationships between intraoperative hypotension and acute hypoadrenocorticism in patients previously treated with corticosteroids have never been documented. [30,31]

In view of possible adverse influences of corticosteroids (retardation of healing, increased susceptibility to infection, gastrointestinal hemorrhage) attempts have been made to rationalize corticosteroid supplementation for surgical patients considered to be at risk of developing adrenocortical insufficiency and to define an appropriate but minimal dose schedule. [30] A rational regimen for corticosteroid supplementation in the perioperative period uses intravenous administration of cortisol. [32,33] For example, administration of intravenous cortisol, 25 mg, at the time of induction of anesthesia, followed by continuous intravenous infusions of cortisol, 100 mg, during the next 24 hours, maintains plasma concentrations of cortisol above normal during major surgery in patients receiving chronic treatment with corticosteroids and manifesting subnormal responses to preoperative infusions of ACTH (Fig. 23-4). [32] These data provide a rational and physiologic approach to low-dose supplementation with corticosteroids in the perioperative period. Empiric use of this regimen should provide adequate plasma concentrations of cortisol in patients considered to be at risk for the presence of a suppressed pituitary-adrenal axis and in whom major surgery is necessary. It is likely that patients undergoing minor operations will need minimal (25 mg intravenously) to no additional corticosteroid coverage during the perioperative period. Even patients treated with corticosteroids and manifesting diminished adrenocortical responses may withstand major surgery without corticosteroid supplementation, emphasizing the need for further information of the role of adrenocortical responses in relation to plasma concentrations of corticosteroids and greater precision in identification of patients who would benefit from supplementation in the perioperative period.

In addition to low-dose intravenous cortisol supplementation, patients receiving daily maintenance doses of a corticosteroid should also receive this dose with the preoperative medication on the day of surgery. The maintenance dose schedule should be continued on the first day after surgery. No objective evidence supports increasing the maintenance dose of corticosteroids preoperatively. [32] Likewise, no evidence supports regimens in the postoperative period that use increased maintenance doses followed by gradual reductions over several days until the original preoperative doses are reached. In those instances when postoperative events could exaggerate needs for exogenous corticosteroid supplementation, the continuous infusion of cortisol 100 mg every 12 hours to 24 hours should be sufficient. Indeed, endogenous cortisol production during stress introduced by major surgery or ex-

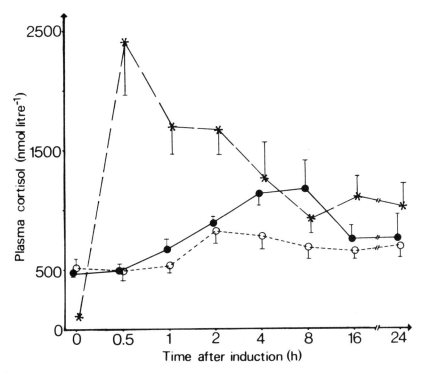

FIG. 23-4. Plasma cortisol concentrations (Mean ± SE) were measured before and after induction of anesthesia for elective surgery in three groups of patients. Control patients (Group I ●—●) had never been treated with corticosteroids. Group II (O—O) consisted of patients receiving long-term corticosteroid treatment who manifested normal increases in plasma concentrations of cortisol in response to preoperative administration of adrenocorticotrophic hormone. These patients, as well as the control patients, did not receive exogenous corticosteroids during the perioperative period. Group III (*– –*) consisted of patients receiving long-term corticosteroid treatment who manifested subnormal changes in plasma concentrations of cortisol in response to preoperative administration of adrenocorticotrophic hormone. These patients received low-dose cortisol substitution during the perioperative period, consisting of intravenous cortisol 25 mg after induction of anesthesia, plus continuous, intravenous infusions of cortisol 100 mg during the next 24 hours. Time courses for changes in the plasma concentrations of cortisol were similar in groups I and II, except at 4 hours and 8 hours after induction of anesthesia when plasma concentrations were greater in group I patients (P < 0.05). Control plasma concentrations of cortisol were significantly lower in group III, compared with the other two groups (P < 0.001). After intravenous administration of cortisol, plasma concentrations increased markedly, and remained significantly above the values present in groups I and II for the next 2 hours (P < 0.01). Thereafter, mean values for the plasma concentrations were similar to those present in the other two groups. (Symreng T, Karlberg BE, Kagedal B, Schildt B. Physiological cortisol substitution of long-term steroid treated patients undergoing major surgery. Br J Anaesth 1981;53:949-53 Copyright © Macmillan Magazines Ltd.)

tensive burns has been reported to range from only 72 mg·day^{-1} to 150 mg·day^{-1}.[34]

MANAGEMENT OF ANESTHESIA

Management of anesthesia for patients with known hypoadrenocorticism introduces no unique problems, other than provision of exogenous corticosteroids, and a high index of suspicion for primary adrenal insufficiency, should intraoperative hypotension occur. Despite frequent suggestions that unexplained intraoperative hypotension and even death reflect unsuspected hypoadrenocorticism, there is no evidence that primary adrenal insufficiency is a likely etiology for these responses.[31] Selection of drugs used for anesthesia is not influenced by the presence of treated hypoadrenocorticism. Plasma cortisol concentrations predictably increase during surgery, but this response is related to the surgical stimulus rather than the anesthetic drugs being administered.

Emergency surgery in the presence of untreated hypoadrenocorticism should be rare. If surgery becomes necessary, however, the perioperative management must include administration of supplemental corticosteroids and intravenous infusion of fluids. Minimal doses of anesthetic drugs should be administered, since these patients are exquisitely sensitive to drug-induced myocardial depression. Invasive monitoring of arterial blood pressure and cardiac filling pressures is indicated. Plasma concentrations of glucose and electrolytes should be measured frequently during the perioperative period. In view of skeletal muscle weakness, initial doses of muscle relaxants should be reduced and responses produced monitored, using a peripheral nerve stimulator.

Hyperaldosteronism

Hyperaldosteronism results from sustained excess secretion of aldosterone from the adrenal cortex.[29] Causes of excess secretion include a functional tumor or tumors, adrenal cortex hyperplasia, and excess production of renin by the kidneys. Primary aldosteronism (Conn's syndrome) is present when excess secretion of aldosterone from a functional tumor occurs independently of a physiologic stimulus. Secondary aldosteronism is present when increased renin secretion is responsible for the excess secretion of aldosterone. Increased secretion of renin is a common finding in patients with renovascular hypertension.

SIGNS AND SYMPTOMS

Signs and symptoms of hyperaldosteronism reflect physiologic effects of aldosterone. For example, increased sodium retention leads to volume-dependent blood pressure elevations. Hypertension is characterized by diastolic blood pressures that range between 100 mmHg to 125 mmHg. Peripheral edema is rare, despite retention of sodium. Aldosterone promotes renal excretion of potassium, resulting in hypokalemic metabolic alkalosis. Skeletal muscle weakness is presumed to reflect the presence of hypokalemia. An impairment of glucose tolerance occurs in about 50 percent of patients. Finally, hypokalemic nephropathy can result in polyuria and an inability to optimally concentrate urine.[35]

DIAGNOSIS

Hyperaldosteronism should be considered in patients with hypertension and plasma potassium concentrations below 3.5 $mEq \cdot L^{-1}$. Confirmation of the diagnosis is by demonstration of increased plasma concentrations of aldosterone and elevated urinary potassium excretion. Typically, urinary potassium excretion in the presence of hyperaldosteronism exceeds 30 $mEq \cdot L^{-1}$, despite co-existing hypokalemia. Measurement of plasma renin activity allows classification of the disease as primary (low renin activity) or secondary (elevated renin activity). The impact of drug therapy on plasma renin activity should be considered when interpreting laboratory measurements of this substance (Table 23-8). Selective adrenal gland venography and scanning studies are helpful for distinguishing hyperaldosteronism due to functional tumors from that produced by adrenal cortex hyperplasia.

TREATMENT

Initial treatment of hyperaldosteronism is with potassium supplementation and administration of competitive aldosterone antago-

TABLE 23-8. Drugs That Alter Plasma Renin Activity

Increased Activity	Decreased Activity
Thiazide diuretics	Propranolol
Nitroprusside	Alpha-methyldopa
Hydralazine	Clonidine
Chlorpromazine	
Thyroxine	

nists such as spironolactone. Hypokalemic skeletal muscle paralysis requires treatment with intravenous potassium and spironolactone. Hypertension may require management with antihypertensive drugs. Accentuation of hypokalemia from drug-induced diuresis is minimized by using potassium-sparing diuretics such as triamterene.

Definitive treatment for aldosterone-secreting tumors is surgical excision. Bilateral adrenalectomy may be necessary if there are multiple aldosterone-secreting tumors. Hyperaldosteronism due to adrenal cortex hyperplasia is managed with the administration of spironolactone.

MANAGEMENT OF ANESTHESIA

Management of anesthesia for treatment of hyperaldosteronism is facilitated by preoperative correction of hypokalemia and treatment of hypertension. Persistence of hypokalemia may modify responses to nondepolarizing muscle relaxants. Furthermore, it must be appreciated that intraoperative hyperventilation can decrease plasma potassium concentrations. Inhaled or injected drugs are acceptable for maintenance of anesthesia. Use of enflurane may be questionable, however, if hypokalemic nephropathy and polyuria exist preoperatively. Measurement of cardiac filling pressures via a right atrial or pulmonary artery catheter is important during surgery to evaluate adequately intravascular fluid volume, as well as responses to intravenous infusion of fluids. Indeed, aggressive preoperative preparation can convert excess intravascular fluid volume status of these patients to unexpected hypovolemia, which manifests as hypotension in response to vasodilating anesthetic drugs, positive pressure ventilation of the lungs, position change, or sudden blood loss. Existence of orthostatic hypotension detected during the preoperative evaluation is a clue to the presence of unexpected hypovolemia in these patients. Acid-base status and plasma electrolyte concentrations should be measured frequently in the perioperative period. Finally, supplementation with exogenous cortisol is probably not necessary for surgical excision of a solitary adenoma in the adrenal cortex; bilateral mo-

bilization of the adrenal glands to excise multiple functional tumors, however, may introduce the need for exogenous administration of cortisol. Continuous intravenous infusions of cortisol 100 mg every 24 hours may be initiated empirically if transient hypoadrenocorticism due to surgical manipulation is a consideration.

ADRENAL MEDULLA

The adrenal medulla is a specialized part of the sympathetic nervous system, capable of synthesizing norepinephrine and epinephrine (Fig. 23-5). The major portion of norepinephrine synthesized in the adrenal medulla is methylated to epinephrine by the action of the enzyme known as phenylethanolamine N-methyltransferase. Distribution of this enzyme is limited almost exclusively to the adrenal medulla, emphasizing the importance of this gland in the production of epinephrine. Indeed, catecholamine output from the adrenal gland is about 75 percent epinephrine and 25 percent norepinephrine.

Activity of phenylethanolamine N-methyltransferase, and thus the production of epinephrine is stimulated by cortisol, which flows through the adrenal medulla from the adrenal cortex. Thus cortisol ultimately regulates production of epinephrine. The half-time of norepinephrine and epinephrine in the circulation is less than 1 minute. This short half-time of catecholamines is due to their enzymatic breakdown by monoamine oxidase and catechol-O-methyltransferase (Fig. 23-5). The major end-products of norepinephrine and epinephrine metabolism are metanephrines and vanillylmandelic acid (3-methoxy, 4-hydroxymandelic acid, VMA) (Fig. 23-5). These metabolites and unchanged catecholamines appear in the urine (Table 23-9). Vanillylmandelic acid comprises about 80 percent of the urinary metabolites of catecholamines; metanephrines account for about 15 percent. Less than 1 percent of the originally released norepinephrine or epinephrine are excreted unchanged in the urine.

The only important disease process asso-

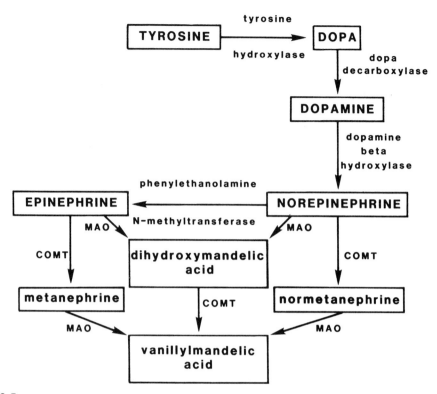

FIG. 23-5. Synthesis of endogenous catecholamines (dopamine, norepinephrine, and epinephrine) involves a series of enzyme controlled steps, beginning with active transport of tyrosine from the circulation into postganglionic sympathetic nerve endings. The rate-limiting enzyme step is conversion of tyrosine to DOPA by tyrosine hydroxylase. Inhibition of tyrosine hydroxylase by drugs or increased plasma concentrations of norepinephrine results in decreased to absent synthesis of catecholamines. Metabolism of norepinephrine and epinephrine to normetanephrine, metanephrine, and vanillylmandelic acid is controlled by the enzymes monoamine oxidase (MAO) and catechol-O-methyltransferase (COMT).

ciated with the adrenal adrenal medulla is pheochromocytoma. Adrenal medulla insufficiency is not known to occur.

Epinephrine

By virtue of its ability to stimulate both alpha-adrenergic and beta-adrenergic receptors, epinephrine has important effects on the cardiovascular system, respiratory system, and metabolism (Table 23-10). For example, epinephrine stimulates beta-adrenergic receptors in the heart to provoke increases in heart rate

and myocardial contractility. Cardiac output is predictably elevated by epinephrine. Increased velocity of impulse transmission through the cardiac conduction system is consistent with the well-known cardiac dysrhythmic effects of epinephrine. Typically, blood pressure is increased by epinephrine, reflecting its cardiac effects, as well as alpha-adrenergic mediated vasoconstriction in the vessels of the kidney and skin. Low doses of epinephrine, however, can reduce blood pressure due to preferential stimulation of beta-adrenergic receptors, particularly in skeletal muscle, resulting in vasodilation. Nevertheless, even low doses of epinephrine are likely to produce predominant alpha-adrenergic effects on the renal vascula-

TABLE 23-9. Urinary Excretion of Catecholamines and Catecholamine Metabolites

	Daily Urinary Excretion	
	Normal	Pheochromo-cytoma
Total metanephrines	0.1–1.6 mg	2.5–4 mg
Vanillylmandelic acid	1–8 mg	10–250 mg
Norepinephrine	<100 μg	
Epinephrine	<1- μg	
Total catecholamines	4–126 μg	200–4,000 μg

ture. Beta-adrenergic effects of epinephrine on bronchial smooth muscle are manifested as bronchodilation.

Metabolic effects of epinephrine include promotion of hepatic glycogenolysis and inhibition of hepatic gluconeogenesis. Alpha-adrenergic stimulation produced by epinephrine inhibits release of insulin. The net effect of these metabolic changes is hyperglycemia. In addition, production of fatty acids is increased by epinephrine.

Norepinephrine

Norepinephrine exerts effects on the cardiovascular system and metabolism by virtue of its stimulation of alpha-adrenergic receptors (Table 23-10). Beta-adrenergic stimulation pro-

duced by norepinephrine on the heart is masked by the predominant alpha-adrenergic stimulation produced on the peripheral vasculature. For example, norepinephrine produces marked increases in blood pressure, reflecting alpha-adrenergic mediated peripheral vasoconstriction in most vascular beds. Hypertension stimulates the carotid sinus, resulting in reflex bradycardia. Heart rate slowing contributes to the unchanged or decreased cardiac output that accompanies hypertension produced by norepinephrine. Indeed, prevention of vasoconstriction by prior administration of an alpha-adrenergic antagonist unmasks beta-adrenergic effects of norepinephrine on the heart, such that cardiac output is likely to increase. Any doubt that norepinephrine has beta-adrenergic effects on the heart should be dispelled when it is recalled that norepinephrine is the neurotransmitter released by postganglionic sympathetic nerve endings. Effects of norepinephrine on conduction velocity of cardiac impulses and propensity to produce cardiac dysrhythmias are similar to the effects produced by epinephrine; metabolic effects of norepinephrine are less than those produced by epinephrine.

Pheochromocytoma

Pheochromocytoma is a catecholamine-secreting tumor, which originates in the adrenal medulla or in chromaffin tissue along the par-

TABLE 23-10. Comparative Effects of Epinephrine and Norepinephrine

Parameter	Epinephrine	Norepinephrine
Heart rate	Minimal increase	Moderate decrease
Stroke volume	Moderate increase	Minimal decrease
Cardiac output	Marked increase	No change to minimal or moderate decrease
Cardiac dysrhythmias	Marked increase	Marked increase
Systolic blood pressure	Marked increase	Marked increase
Diastolic blood pressure	No change to minimal decrease	Moderate increase
Mean arterial pressure	Minimal increase	Moderate increase
Systemic vascular resistance	Minimal decrease	Moderate to marked increase
Renal blood flow	Moderate to marked decrease	Moderate to marked decrease
Skin blood flow	Moderate decrease	Moderate decrease
Muscle blood flow	Marked increase	No change to minimal decrease
Airway resistance	Marked decrease	No change
Blood glucose concentration	Marked increase	No change to minimal increase

avertebral sympathetic chain, extending from the pelvis to the base of the skull.[36] Sympathetic ganglia in the wall of the urinary bladder may be a site for pheochromocytoma. Nevertheless, over 95 percent of pheochromocytomas are found in the abdominal cavity, and about 90 percent originate in the adrenal medulla. About 10 percent of these tumors involve both adrenal glands, and functional tumors in multiple sites are found in nearly 20 percent of patients, especially children. Less than 10 percent of pheochromocytomas are malignant. Pheochromocytomas typically occur in patients 30 years to 50 years of age, but about one-third of reported cases have been in children, 70 percent of whom are males.

MULTIPLE ENDOCRINE NEOPLASIA

Pheochromocytoma is usually an isolated finding, but these tumors can occur in conjunction with other functional endocrine tumors. For example, familial pheochromocytoma may occur in association with medullary thyroid carcinoma or parathyroid adenoma and is designated multiple endocrine neoplasia type II(a) or Sipple's syndrome. Multiple endocrine neoplasia type II(b) is pheochromocytoma in association with medullary thyroid carcinoma, mucosal neuromas and marfanoid habitus. Neurofibromatosis occurs in about 5 percent of patients with pheochromocytoma, but the incidence of the reverse combination is less than 1 percent.[37] There is also an increased incidence of pheochromocytoma in patients with von Hippel-Lindau disease, tuberous sclerosis, and Sturge-Weber syndrome.

SIGNS AND SYMPTOMS

The hallmark of pheochromocytoma is paroxysmal hypertension associated with diaphoresis, headache, tremulousness, and palpitations. The triad of diaphoresis, tachycardia, and headaches in hypertensive patients is highly suggestive of pheochromocytoma. Conversely, absence of this triad virtually rules out the presence of a pheochrom-

ocytoma. Likewise, flushing is so rare that its presence casts doubt on the diagnosis of pheochromocytoma. Nausea and vomiting, personality changes, and visual disturbances may accompany symptoms of pheochromocytoma. Symptoms may last from several minutes to hours and are often followed by fatigue. Weight loss is frequently present. Orthostatic hypotension is a common finding and reflects decreases in intravascular fluid volume associated with sustained hypertension. Indeed, about 50 percent of patients develop persistent elevations in blood pressure, with intermittent exacerbations. Hyperglycemia reflects a predominance of alpha effects (inhibition of insulin release, glycogenolysis) over beta effects (insulin release) produced by the catecholamines secreted by these tumors. Cholelithiasis is observed frequently. Persistent elevations of plasma concentrations of catecholamines can result in necrosis of cardiac muscle and development of a cardiomyopathy. Death resulting from pheochromocytoma is usually due to congestive heart failure, myocardial infarction, or intracerebral hemorrhage. Although less than 0.1 percent of patients with hypertension have a pheochromocytoma, nearly 50 percent of the deaths in patients with unsuspected pheochromocytoma occur during anesthesia and surgery or parturition.

DIAGNOSIS

Definitive diagnosis of pheochromocytoma requires biochemical confirmation of excessive catecholamine production. The most widely used screening procedures are measurements of urinary excretion of catecholamines or metabolites of catecholamines such as metanephrines or vanillylmandelic acid (Table 23-9). Results of urinary determinations of these indices of catecholamines production, however, can be erratic. Indeed, the incidence of false-negative results can be as high as 50 percent.[38] In contrast, measurement of the total plasma concentrations of catecholamines reliably reflects the presence or absence of pheochromocytoma in nearly every patient (Fig. 23-6).[38] Furthermore, plasma concentrations of catecholamines do not correlate with resting

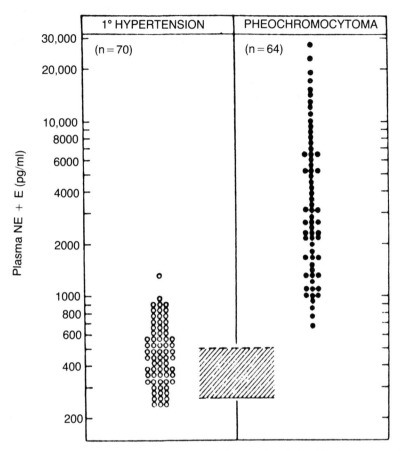

FIG. 23-6. Plasma concentrations of norepinephrine (NE) and epinephrine (E) were measured in patients with essential hypertension and patients with pheochromocytoma. The cross-hatched area represents the Mean ± 2 SD of values in a control group of normotensive patients. Measurement of total plasma concentrations of catecholamines reliably reflects the presence or absence of pheochromocytoma in nearly every patient. (Bravo EL, Gifford RW. Pheochromocytoma: Diagnosis, localization and management. N Engl J Med 1984;311:1298–1303)

mean arterial pressure in patients with pheochromocytoma.[38] Therefore, this measurement serves as a valuable diagnostic approach even in the presence of normotension. Normotension, despite elevated plasma concentrations of catecholamines, presumably reflects decreases in the number or the sensitivity of peripheral adrenergic receptors, in response to high circulating concentrations of the neurotransmitter.

A current recommendation is to measure total plasma concentrations of catecholamines as part of the initial laboratory examination of each patient with hypertension. A value of 1,000 pg·ml^{-1} or less is considered to rule out pheochromocytoma.[38] Values between 1,000 pg·ml^{-1} and 2,000 pg·ml^{-1} are considered equivocal; total plasma concentrations of catecholamines above 2,000 pg·ml^{-1} are considered diagnostic for pheochromocytoma. A glucagon-provocative test may be performed on patients in whom the diagnosis is equivocal. A positive glucagon test is an increase in blood pressure of at least 20/15 mmHg above the response to a cold pressor test and a clear increase (at least threefold) in the simultaneously measured plasma concentrations of catecholamines. A hazard of the glucagon test is excessive increases in blood pressure.

Performance of a suppression test with clonidine has been proposed when the diagnosis of pheochromocytoma, on the basis of plasma catecholamine concentrations (1,000 pg·ml^{-1} to 2,000 pg·ml^{-1}), is equivocal.[38] For example, a single oral dose of clonidine (0.3 mg) reduces plasma concentrations of catecholamines below 500 pg·ml^{-1} only in hypertensive patients who do not have a pheochromocytoma (Fig. 23-7).[38] This reflects the ability of clonidine to suppress increases in plasma catecholamine concentrations that result from the neurogenic release but not from the diffusion of excess catecholamines from a pheochromocytoma into the circulation. Beta-an-

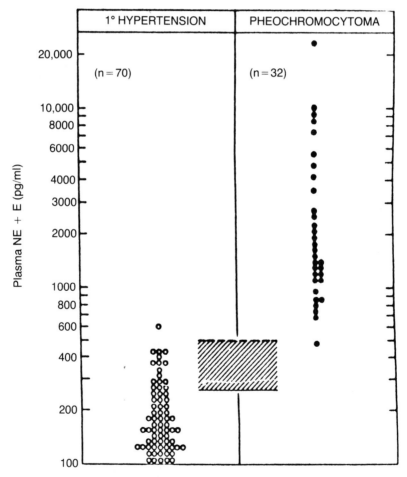

FIG. 23-7. A single oral dose of clonidine (0.3 mg) reduces plasma concentrations of norepinephrine (NE) and epinephrine (E) below 500 pg·ml^{-1} in nearly every patient with essential hypertension. Clonidine does not reduce reliably plasma concentrations of catecholamines in patients with pheochromocytoma. The cross-hatched area represents the Mean ± 2 SD of values in a control group of normotensive patients. (Bravo EL, Gifford RW. Pheochromocytoma: Diagnosis, localization and management. N Engl J Med 1984;311:1298-1303)

tagonist drugs can prevent the catecholamine-lowering effects of clonidine by interfering with hepatic clearance of catecholamines. The dose of clonidine used for the suppression test lowers systolic blood pressure 20 percent to 25 percent in patients with and without a pheochromocytoma. Hypotension may be exaggerated when clonidine is administered in the presence of other antihypertensive drugs or hypovolemia and bradycardia may be accentuated when the drug is given to patients being treated with beta-adrenergic antagonists.

TREATMENT

Treatment of pheochromocytoma is surgical excision of the catecholamine secreting tumor or tumors. Before surgical excision is attempted, however, it is mandatory to treat these patients with drugs such as phenoxybenzamine or prazosin to produce alpha-adrenergic blockade.[36] Prazosin may be preferable, as it is a relatively selective postsynaptic alpha-1 receptor antagonist in contrast to phenoxybenzamine, which acts at alpha-1 and alpha-2 receptors. By sparing alpha-2 receptors, prazosin allows released norepinephrine to exert a negative feedback effect on continued catecholamine release. Alpha-adrenergic blockade prevents vasoconstriction in response to catecholamines, leading to reductions in blood pressure. Return to normotension facilitates increases in intravascular fluid volume. Indeed, decreases in hematocrit are often early indications that intravascular fluid volume has been restored toward normal in response to drug-induced reductions in blood pressure. Normalization of intravascular fluid volume and blood pressure with alpha-adrenergic blockade before surgery also reduces risks of intraoperative hypertension during manipulation of the tumor. Finally, alpha-adrenergic blockade will facilitate release of insulin and reduce the likelihood of hyperglycemia in patients with a pheochromocytoma.

Persistence of tachycardia and/or cardiac dysrhythmias despite the presence of alpha-adrenergic blockade is an indication for administration of drugs such as propranolol to produce beta-adrenergic blockade. It is emphasized that beta-adrenergic blockade should not be instituted in the absence of alpha-adrenergic blockade.[36] This recommendation is based on the theoretical concern that a heart depressed by beta-adrenergic blockade could not maintain an adequate cardiac output should unopposed alpha-mediated vasoconstriction from the release of catecholamines result in abrupt increases in systemic vascular resistance. Labetalol, which produces alpha- and beta-adrenergic blockade, has also been used in the preoperative preparation of these patients.[36]

Inhibition of catecholamine synthesis by blocking enzymes responsible for hydroxylation of tyrosine (Fig. 23-5) would be an attractive treatment for the management of patients with a pheochromocytoma. Alpha-methyltyrosine is a drug that interferes with hydroxylation of tyrosine and thus reduces synthesis of catecholamines. Despite the theoretical value of this drug, its superiority over other drugs for the management of patients with catecholamine-secreting tumors remains undocumented.

Preoperative preparation of patients with a pheochromocytoma also includes attempts to localize the anatomic position of the tumor. Noninvasive techniques include intravenous pyelography with tomography, abdominal ultrasound, and computed tomography. Computed tomography is a particularly valuable technique for localizing a pheochromocytoma greater than 1 cm in diameter and should be the initial localizing procedure.[38] Arteriography can also be used to localize the tumor, but the risk of a hypertensive response during the study is great, even in the presence of alpha-adrenergic blockade.

MANAGEMENT OF ANESTHESIA

Management of anesthesia for patients requiring excision of a pheochromocytoma is based on administration of drugs that do not stimulate the sympathetic nervous system, plus the use of invasive monitoring techniques to facilitate early and appropriate intervention when catecholamine-induced changes in cardiovascular function occur.[36,40–42]

Continuation of alpha-adrenergic antagonist drugs until the day of surgery is controversial. Conceivably, maintenance of alpha-adrenergic blockade could interfere with localization of catecholamine secreting tumors by preventing hypertensive responses during surgical manipulation. In addition, alpha-adrenergic blockade could contribute to refractory hypotension after vascular isolation of the tumor. For these reasons, discontinuation of drug therapy 24 hours to 48 hours before surgery has been proposed.[36] Nevertheless, clinical experience does not support this recommendation, and continuation of alpha-adrenergic antagonist drugs until the day of surgery is appropriate. Likewise, patients who are being treated with beta-adrenergic antagonist drugs should be maintained on them until the induction of anesthesia.

Preoperative Medication. Preoperative medication is indicated to reduce the likelihood of apprehension-induced activation of the sympathetic nervous system. Administration of an oral benzodiazepine plus intramuscular morphine and scopolamine is ideal for producing reliable sedation. Scopolamine is unlikely to produce adverse heart rate changes and is essential for producing a sedative effect.

Induction of Anesthesia. Placement of a catheter in a peripheral artery to provide continuous monitoring of blood pressure is useful before proceeding with induction of anesthesia. In the presence of adequate preoperative medication and local anesthesia, this invasive monitor can be placed without the risk of stimulating the sympathetic nervous system.

Induction of anesthesia is ideally accomplished with the intravenous administration of short-acting barbiturates or benzodiazepines. After the onset of unconsciousness, the depth of anesthesia should be increased by ventilation of the lungs with nitrous oxide plus enflurane or isoflurane.[41,42] Selection of enflurane or isoflurane is based on the ability of these drugs to reduce sympathetic nervous system activity and on their failure to sensitize the heart to dysrhythmic effects of catecholamines. Halothane is not recommended because of the likelihood of cardiac dysrhythmias in the presence of increased plasma concentrations of catecholamines. Mechanical ventilation of the lungs is facilitated by the production of skel-

etal muscle paralysis with nondepolarizing muscle relaxants such as vecuronium or atracurium, which produce minimal cardiovascular effects. The use of succinylcholine has been questioned, since histamine release or compression of an abdominal tumor by drug-induced contractions of skeletal muscles could provoke the release of catecholamines. Nevertheless, clinical experience has not supported predictable adverse effects of this drug when administered to patients with a pheochromocytoma. Certainly, histamine-releasing effects of d-tubocurarine and to a lesser extent metocurine and the vagolytic effects of pancuronium or gallamine would make these drugs unlikely selections. Furthermore, pancuronium may produce stimulation of the sympathetic nervous system and hypertension in patients with pheochromocytoma.[43]

Direct laryngoscopy for intubation of the trachea is considered only after the establishment, with inhaled drugs, of an adequate depth of anesthesia. An adequate depth of anesthesia is essential to minimize increases in blood pressure associated with intubation of the trachea. It is helpful to administer intravenous lidocaine 1 mg·kg^{-1} to 2 mg·kg^{-1} about 1 minute before initiating laryngoscopy, as this drug may attenuate blood pressure responses to intubation of the trachea and reduce the likelihood of cardiac dysrhythmias.[44] In addition, intravenous administration of fentanyl 100 μg to 200 μg or sufentanil 10 μg to 20 μg just before starting direct laryngoscopy may attenuate pressor responses. Equivalent doses of alfentanil may also be administered for this purpose. Nitroprusside or phentolamine should be immediately available ʿor intravenous administration should persistent hypertension accompany intubation of the trachea. Nitroprusside 1 μg·kg^{-1} to 2 μg·kg^{-1} administered intravenously, is effective for treating acute increases in blood pressure.

Maintenance of Anesthesia. Maintenance of anesthesia is ideally accomplished with nitrous oxide plus enflurane or isoflurane.[36,42,43] Delivered concentrations of volatile anesthetic drugs should be adjusted in response to changes in blood pressure. Maintenance of anesthesia with nitrous oxide and an opioid is not ideal, as these drugs do not suppress activity of the sympathetic nervous system, and hypertensive responses are likely. In addition, the ability to reduce the depth of anesthesia should persistent hypotension occur is not easily achieved when injected drugs are used for maintenance of anesthesia. An unconfirmed but theoretical disadvantage of opioids, particularly morphine, would be histamine-induced release of catecholamines. The use of Innovar is questionable, since droperidol has been reported to provoke hypertension in the presence of pheochromocytoma.[45,46] Droperidol may interfere with uptake of norepinephrine back into the postganglionic sympathetic nerve endings or stimulate release of catecholamines directly from the tumor.[46]

A continuous intravenous infusion of nitroprusside or phentolamine will be necessary should hypertension persist despite maximum concentrations (about 1.5 MAC to 2.0 MAC) of volatile anesthetic drugs. Disadvantages of a continuous infusion of phentolamine include development of tachyphylaxis and a longer duration of action than nitroprusside should it become necessary to discontinue infusion because of decreases in blood pressure. Trimethaphan is not recommended because of the frequent occurrence of tachyphylaxis and the possibility of drug-induced release of histamine.

Reductions in blood pressure may accompany decreases in plasma concentrations of catecholamines that occur as the veins draining the pheochromocytoma are surgically ligated. This reduction in blood pressure is treated by decreases in the inhaled concentrations of the volatile drugs and rapid infusion of crystalloid and/or colloid solutions. Persistent hypotension may require continuous intravenous infusions of norepinephrine until the peripheral vasculature can adapt to decreased levels of alpha-adrenergic stimulation.

A pulmonary artery catheter is useful for monitoring the status of intravascular fluid volume in these patients, especially if there is a history of congestive heart failure.[42] Furthermore, ability to measure cardiac output by thermodilution is helpful in evaluating cardiac function and the need for intervention with inotropic or vasodilator drugs. A central venous catheter is an alternative to placement of a pulmonary artery catheter, but left ventricular dysfunction may not be appreciated from this measurement. Furthermore, the capability to measure cardiac output by thermodilution is not possible in the absence of a pulmonary artery catheter.

Monitoring of arterial blood gases, arterial pH, plasma electrolytes, blood glucose concentrations, urine output, electrocardiogram, and body temperature is important during the perioperative period. Mechanical ventilation of the lungs is guided by the arterial partial pressures of carbon dioxide; the inspired concentration of oxygen is determined by the arterial partial pressures of oxygen. Hyperglycemia is typical before excision of the pheochromocytoma; hypoglycemia may occur when plasma catecholamine concentrations decrease after removal of the tumor.[47] Maintenance of a normal blood pressure is important for reducing the incidence of cardiac dysrhythmias. A continuous infusion of lidocaine is appropriate if ventricular cardiac dysrhythmias persist despite maintenance of normal blood pressure. Incremental intravenous injections of beta-adrenergic antagonist drugs, such as propranolol, are indicated for the management of excessive increases in heart rate. Propranolol should be used cautiously in the presence of catecholamine-induced cardiomyopathy, as even minimal beta-adrenergic blockade can accentuate left ventricular dysfunction.

Administration of nondepolarizing muscle relaxants is guided by the response to a peripheral nerve stimulator. Muscle relaxants with insignificant effects on the cardiovascular system are the best selections. Although experience is limited, no evidence suggests that reversal of nondepolarizing neuromuscular blockade with anticholinesterase drugs plus anticholinergic drugs need be avoided after excision of a pheochromocytoma.

Postoperative management of these patients includes continuation of invasive monitoring until the presence of cardiovascular stability is assured. Removal of the tube from the trachea is likely to be possible shortly after surgery, as these patients tend to be young, and co-existing pulmonary disease is unlikely. Failure of the blood pressure to return to normal within 24 hours to 48 hours after excision of a pheochromocytoma is highly suggestive that a catecholamine secreting tumor is still present.[38] Despite the return of blood pressure to normal levels, plasma concentrations of catecholamines often do not return to baseline until 7 days to 10 days after surgery.[38]

Regional Anesthesia. Regional anesthesia for excision of a pheochromocytoma has the attractive features of blocking the sympathetic nervous system and not sensitizing the heart to dysrhythmogenic effects of catecholamines. Nevertheless, postsynaptic alpha-adrenergic receptors can still respond to direct effects of sudden increases in circulating concentrations of catecholamines. A specific disadvantage of a regional anesthetic technique is the absence of sympathetic nervous system activity should hypotension accompany ligation of the veins draining the pheochromocytoma. Furthermore, the volume of spontaneous ventilation may be inadequate during the high abdominal exploration that is often necessary. Finally, selection of a regional technique is practical only if the surgical procedure is performed in a supine position.

TESTIS AND OVARY

The principal hormone secreted by the testes is testosterone. In the adult, testosterone is responsible for spermatogenesis. Dihydrotesterone, a metabolite of testosterone, is responsible for external virilization. Progesterone and estrogen are the principal hormones secreted by the ovaries.

Testicular dysfunction is reflected by Klinefelter's syndrome. Ovarian dysfunction includes physiologic menopause, gonadal dysgenesis syndrome, and polycystic ovary syndrome.

Klinefelter's Syndrome

Klinefelter's syndrome is due to a chromosomal defect characterized by the presence of two X and one Y chromosomes. Manifesta-tions of this syndrome are absent spermatogenesis and small testes. Plasma concentrations of testosterone are reduced. Diagnosis of Klinefelter's syndrome is confirmed by demonstration of clumps of chromatin (Barr bodies) in the nucleus of cells with two X chromosomes. Cells for examination are typically obtained from the oral mucosa. Management of anesthesia is not influenced by the presence of this syndrome.

Physiologic Menopause

A natural decline in ovarian function occurs at an average age of 48 years. Manifestations of the menopause, including vascular symptoms described as hot flashes, are presumed to reflect deficiency of estrogens. A consequence of prolonged estrogen deficiency is osteoporosis. Risk of coronary artery disease is not increased by the occurrence of physiologic menopause.[48] Exogenous administration of estrogen beyond the onset of physiologic menopause may be associated with an increased incidence of endometrial carcinoma of the uterus.

Gonadal Dysgenesis Syndrome (Turner's Syndrome)

Gonadal dysgenesis syndrome is due to the absence of a second X chromosome. Manifestations of this syndrome include primary amenorrhea, immaturity of the genitalia, and short stature. Additional associated features, which may influence the management of anesthesia, include hypertension, short webbed neck, high palate, micrognathia, the occasional presence of coarctation of the aorta and pectus excavatum, and an absent kidney.[49]

Polycystic Ovary Syndrome (Stein-Leventhal Syndrome)

Polycystic ovary syndrome is characterized by increased production of androgens and associated findings of primary amenorrhea, hirsutism, and muscularity. Height is usually normal, and congenital defects are unlikely. Long-term anovulation, as occurs in these patients, may be associated with an increased incidence of endometrial carcinoma of the uterus. Wedge resection of the ovary has been used to improve fertility of these patients. Drug-induced stimulation of ovulation is also effective in management of patients who wish to become pregnant.

PITUITARY GLAND

The pituitary gland (hypophysis) is located in the sella turcica at the base of the brain. The two components of the pituitary gland are the anterior pituitary (adenohypophysis) and posterior pituitary (neurohypophysis). The hypothalamus controls the function of the pituitary gland by virtue of vascular connections between the hypothalamus and anterior pituitary and nerve fibers between the hypothalamus and posterior pituitary.

Anterior Pituitary

The anterior pituitary secretes luteinizing hormone, follicle stimulating hormone, growth hormone, thyroid stimulating hormone, ACTH, prolactin, and melanocyte stimulating hormone. Luteinizing hormone induces ovulation and stimulates the testes to produce androgens. Follicle stimulating hormone stimulates the development of the ovaries or the maturation of the testes. Luteinizing and follicle stimulating hormones are also referred to as gonadotropins or sex hormones. Growth hormone stimulates skeletal development, increases protein synthesis, and decreases the rate of carbohydrate metabolism. Thyroid stimulating hormone regulates the synthesis and release of active thyroid gland hormones. ACTH regulates the release of cortisol and androgens from the adrenal cortex. Prolactin is necessary for lactation; melanocyte stimulating hormone is necessary for formation of mel-

anin pigments. Endorphins are also present in high concentrations in the anterior pituitary gland. It is of interest that endorphins and ACTH are derived from a common molecule.

The hypothalamus secretes hormones, which subsequently regulate the release of hormones from the anterior pituitary. For example, thyrotropin-releasing hormone and corticotrophin-releasing factor are produced in the hypothalamus, and transported via the hypophyseal-portal venous system to the anterior pituitary, where they regulate the release of thyroid stimulating hormone and ACTH, respectively. Secretion of dopamine by the hypothalamus is the factor likely to be responsible for inhibition of prolactin secretion by the anterior pituitary. Indeed, depletion of dopamine by drugs, such as alpha-methyldopa, or blockade of dopaminergic receptors with phenothiazines or butyrophenones results in excessive plasma concentrations of prolactin. Conversely, bromocriptine, a dopaminergic agonist drug, is effective in controlling excess secretion of prolactin by the anterior pituitary. Luteinizing hormone-releasing factor from the hypothalamus is responsible for the release of luteinizing and follicle stimulating hormones from the anterior pituitary. Somatostatin is thought to be a growth hormone release inhibiting factor. The hypothalamus, in turn, is subject to regulation by hormones released from the anterior pituitary, as well as by other areas in the central nervous system. It should be appreciated that there is no neural connection between the hypothalamus and the anterior pituitary.

HYPERSECRETION OF ANTERIOR PITUITARY HORMONES

Hypersecretion of anterior pituitary hormones is not a common cause of disease, with the exception of hyperadrenocorticism. Hypersecretion of ACTH is the most common cause of spontaneous hyperadrenocorticism (Cushing's disease). A basophilic adenoma of the anterior pituitary gland is often the source of excessive ACTH. Excessive secretion of thyroid stimulating hormone is a rare cause of hyperthyroidism. An adenoma of the anterior pituitary is associated with excessive secretion of growth hormone, leading to giantism if the epiphyses have not closed, or acromegaly if the tumor develops in an adult. Excess prolactin production leading to galactorrhea is the most frequent hormonal abnormality associated with an anterior pituitary tumor.

Acromegaly. Acromegaly is due to excess secretion of growth hormone from an eosinophilic adenoma of the anterior pituitary. A diagnosis of acromegaly is likely if an intravenous infusion of glucose fails to lower plasma concentrations of growth hormone. Manifestations of acromegaly reflect parasellar extension of the anterior pituitary adenoma and peripheral effects produced by presence of excess growth hormone (Table 23-11).

An enlarged sella turcica is seen on a radiograph of the skull in nearly every patient. Headache and papilledema reflect increased intracranial pressure due to expansion of the anterior pituitary adenoma. Likewise, visual disturbances are due to compression of the optic chiasm by the expanding anterior pituitary tumor.

Excess growth hormone leads to a general overgrowth of skeletal, soft, and connective tissues. Facial features are coarse, and the hands and feet become enlarged. The mandible increases in thickness and length. A major problem is the overgrowth of soft tissues of the upper airway, characterized by excessive enlargement of the tongue and epiglottis.[50-52]

TABLE 23-11. Manifestations of Acromegaly

Parasellar
  Enlarged sella turcica
  Headache
  Visual field defects
  Rhinorrhea

Excess Growth Hormone
  Skeletal overgrowth (prognathism)
  Soft tissue overgrowth (lips, tongue, epiglottis, vocal cords)
  Connective tissue overgrowth (recurrent laryngeal nerve paralysis)
  Peripheral neuropathy (carpal tunnel syndrome)
  Visceromegaly
  Glucose intolerance
  Osteoarthritis
  Osteoporosis
  Hyperhidrosis
  Skeletal muscle weakness

Polypoid masses reflect overgrowth of pharyngeal tissue. These changes make patients susceptible to upper airway obstruction. Hoarseness and abnormal movement of the vocal cords can reflect thickening of the vocal cords or paralysis of a recurrent laryngeal nerve due to stretching by overgrowth of cartilaginous structures. In addition, involvement of the cricoarytenoid joints can result in alterations in the voice due to impaired movement of the vocal cords. Stridor or a history of dyspnea is also suggestive of involvement of the larynx by acromegaly. Finally, the subglottic diameter of the trachea can be reduced in these patients.[51]

Development of peripheral neuropathy is common due to trapping of nerves by skeletal, connective, and soft tissue overgrowth. Flow through the ulnar artery may be compromised in patients with symptoms of carpal tunnel syndrome. Even in the absence of symptoms of carpal tunnel syndrome about one-half of patients with acromegaly have inadequate collateral blood flow via the ulnar artery in at least one hand.[53]

Hypertension leading to congestive heart failure is more common in patients with acromegaly. The incidence of coronary artery disease seems to be increased. Lung volumes are enlarged, and the mismatch of ventilation to perfusion is likely to be increased. Glucose intolerance and, on occasion, diabetes mellitus requiring treatment with insulin reflect effects of growth hormone on carbohydrate metabolism. A thyroid goiter may be present. Osteoarthritis and osteoporosis are common. The skin becomes thick and oily. Skeletal muscle weakness and complaints of fatigue are frequent.

MANAGEMENT OF ANESTHESIA

Management of anesthesia for patients with acromegaly is complicated by the changes induced by excess secretion of growth hormone. Particularly important are changes in the upper airway.[50-53] Distorted facial anatomy may interfere with the placement of a face mask. Enlargement of the tongue and epiglottis predispose to upper airway obstruction and make difficult visualization of the vocal cords by direct laryngoscopy. The lips to vocal cord distance is increased by overgrowth of the mandible. The glottic opening may be narrowed due to enlargement of the vocal cords, which, combined with subglottic narrowing, may necessitate use of smaller internal diameter tracheal tubes than would have been predicted on the basis of the age or size of the patient. Nasal turbinate enlargement may preclude passage of nasopharyngeal or nasotracheal airways. The preoperative history of dyspnea on exertion or the presence of hoarseness and/or stridor suggests involvement of the larynx by acromegaly. In this instance, indirect laryngoscopy may be indicated to quantitate the extent of vocal cord dysfunction. When difficulty placing a tube in the trachea is anticipated, it is prudent to perform an intubation with the patient awake, preferably using a fiberoptic laryngoscope. Anticipation of the need to use a small internal diameter tracheal tube and minimization of the mechanical trauma to the upper airway and vocal cords are crucial, as additional edema can lead to airway obstruction after the tube is removed from the trachea. In placing a catheter in the radial artery, one must consider the possibility of inadequate collateral circulation at the wrist.[53] Monitoring of plasma glucose concentrations is important if diabetes mellitus accompanies acromegaly. Doses of nondepolarizing muscle relaxants should be guided by the use of a peripheral nerve stimulator, particularly if skeletal muscle weakness exists before the induction of anesthesia. Acromegaly does not influence the selection of drugs for the maintenance of anesthesia.

Galactorrhea. Galactorrhea is the manifestation of excess secretion of prolactin by the anterior pituitary. The most frequent cause is an anterior pituitary tumor. Indeed, plasma concentrations of prolactin should be measured in any patient who experiences the onset of secondary amenorrhea or who manifests evidence of an enlarged sella turcica on radiography of the skull. Plasma concentrations of prolactin that exceed 300 ng·ml^{-1} are suggestive of an anterior pituitary tumor.

HYPOSECRETION OF ANTERIOR PITUITARY HORMONES

Hyposecretion of anterior pituitary hormones usually reflects panhypopituitarism due to compression of the pituitary gland by expansion of a tumor classified as a chromophobe adenoma in adults or a craniopharyngioma in children. Panhypopituitarism (Sheehan's syndrome) that occurs after postpartum hemorrhagic shock is due to vasospasm that leads to necrosis of the anterior pituitary. Head injury or radiation therapy delivered to structures near the anterior pituitary can result in panhypopituitarism. Panhypopituitarism may also be due to surgical hypophysectomy to (1) remove an anterior pituitary tumor, (2) treat diabetic retinopathy, (3) manage severe exophthalmus due to hyperthyroidism, or (4) encourage regression of hormone-dependent cancers. Chemical hypophysectomy, accomplished by injection of absolute alcohol into the sella turcica, using a transphenoidal approach and stereotaxis control, may be performed in attempts to reduce pain associated with metastatic carcinoma.[54]

Gland Dysfunction. The onset and magnitude of individual endocrine gland dysfunction is variable. Signs and symptoms due to deficiency of luteinizing and/or follicle stimulating hormones are early manifestations of anterior pituitary dysfunction. For example, impotence in the male or appearance of secondary amenorrhea may be the first evidence of panhypopituitarism. Deficiency of growth hormone in childhood results in dwarfism; a deficiency of this hormone in adults does not produce symptoms. Hypoadrenocorticism occurs 4 days to 14 days after a surgical hypophysectomy; hypothyroidism is unlikely to manifest before 4 weeks. Treatment of panhypopituitarism is with specific hormone replacement, which may include gonadotropins, cortisol, and thyroxine. Administration of a corticosteroid with mineralocorticoid effects is usually not necessary, since release of aldosterone is maintained in the absence of adrenocorticotrophic hormone.

Posterior Pituitary

The posterior pituitary is composed of terminal endings of neurons that originate in the hypothalamus. Antidiuretic hormone (vasopressin) and oxytocin are the hormones synthesized in the supraoptic and paraventricular nuclei of the hypothalamus and subsequently transported along the hypothalamic neuronal axons for storage in the posterior pituitary. Stimulus for the release of these hormones arises in the hypothalamus.

Primary functions of antidiuretic hormone are regulation of plasma osmolarity and maintenance of extracellular fluid volume. Indeed, the most important physiologic stimulus for release of antidiuretic hormone is activation of osmoreceptors in the hypothalamus. For example, an increase in plasma osmolarity of only 1 percent (normal plasma osmolarity 285 $mOsm \cdot L^{-1}$ to 295 $mOsm \cdot L^{-1}$) stimulates osmoreceptors and causes the release of antidiuretic hormone. Antidiuretic hormone facilitates reabsorption of water by the renal tubules, leading to reductions in plasma osmolarity and increases in osmolarity of the urine. Conservation of free water as a result of the release of antidiuretic hormone also manifests as decreases in urine output. Reductions in intravascular fluid volume, painful stimulation due to accidental trauma or surgery, positive airway pressure, and positive end-expiratory pressure are additional factors that lead to release of antidiuretic hormone and a conservation of free water.[55] It is of interest that reductions in intravascular fluid volume result in release of antidiuretic hormone at a lower plasma osmolarity than would ordinarily stimulate hormone release. In animals, administration of morphine results in the release of antidiuretic hormone. Conversely, the administration of morphine to patients in the absence of surgical stimulation does not alter the plasma concentration of antidiuretic hormone.[55] The physiologic role of oxytocin is to stimulate contraction of the pregnant uterus and to promote milk secretion and ejection by the mammary glands.

Disorders of posterior pituitary function manifest as diabetes insipidus or inappropriate antidiuretic hormone secretion.

DIABETES INSIPIDUS

Diabetes insipidus reflects the absence of antidiuretic hormone release due to destruction of the posterior pituitary or the failure of renal tubules to respond to antidiuretic hormone. Destruction of the posterior pituitary can occur as a result of intracranial trauma, hypophysectomy, or neoplastic invasion of the gland. Diabetes insipidus due to intracranial trauma typically does not become apparent until several days after the injury, and spontaneous recovery usually occurs within 24 hours. Diabetes insipidus, which develops during or immediately after pituitary gland surgery, is generally due to reversible trauma of the posterior pituitary and, therefore, is transient.

Signs and Symptoms. Classic manifestations of diabetes insipidus are polydipsia and a high output of poorly concentrated urine, despite an increased serum osmolarity. Diuresis may be so severe that hypernatremia and hypovolemia become life-threatening. Initial treatment of diabetes insipidus is intravenous infusion of electrolyte solutions if oral intake cannot offset polyuria.

Treatment. Intramuscular hormone replacement is effective in patients with diabetes insipidus due to absence of antidiuretic hormone release but not in the management of diabetes insipidus due to renal tubular unresponsiveness to antidiuretic hormone. Chlorpropamide, an oral hypoglycemic drug that increases sensitivity of renal tubules to endogenous antidiuretic hormone may be all the treatment required when diabetes insipidus is mild, as in patients with incomplete destruction of the posterior pituitary. A rare but potential adverse effect of chlorpropamide is hypoglycemia.

Management of Anesthesia. Management of anesthesia for patients with diabetes insipidus should include monitoring of urine output and serum electrolyte concentrations during the perioperative period.

INAPPROPRIATE ANTIDIURETIC HORMONE SECRETION

Inappropriate antidiuretic hormone secretion can occur in the presence of diverse pathologic processes, including intracranial tumors, hypothyroidism, porphyria, and carcinoma of the lung, particularly undifferentiated small cell carcinoma. Inappropriate secretion of antidiuretic hormone is also alleged to occur in virtually all patients after surgery. An inappropriately elevated urinary sodium concentration and osmolality in the presence of hyponatremia and decreased plasma osmolarity is virtually diagnostic of inappropriate antidiuretic hormone secretion. Hyponatremia is due to dilution, reflecting an expansion of intravascular fluid volume secondary to hormone-induced reabsorption of water by the renal tubules. Abrupt reductions in the plasma concentrations of sodium (especially below 110 $mEq·L^{-1}$) can lead to cerebral edema and seizures. Indeed, intravenous administration of sodium deficient solutions to otherwise healthy but oliguric patients has led to hyponatremia, seizures, and permanent brain damage (see Chapter 22).[56]

Treatment of excess secretion of antidiuretic hormone is with restriction of fluid intake to 500 $ml·day^{-1}$, antagonism of the effects of antidiuretic hormone on the renal tubules by the administration of demeclocycline, and intravenous infusion of sodium chloride 120 $mEq·day^{-1}$ to 360 $mEq·day^{-1}$. Often, restriction of fluid intake is sufficient treatment for inappropriate antidiuretic hormone secretion not associated with symptoms secondary to hyponatremia. Restriction of fluid intake and administration of demeclocycline, however, are not immediately effective for the management of patients manifesting acute neurologic symptoms due to hyponatremia. In these patients, intravenous infusion of hypertonic saline sufficient to elevate plasma concentrations of sodium 0.5 $mEq·L^{-1}·hr^{-1}$ are recommended. Overly rapid correction of chronic hyponatremia has been associated with a fatal neurologic disorder known as central pontine myelinolysis (see Chapter 22).[57]

REFERENCES

1. Murkin JM. Anesthesia and hypothyroidism: A review of thyroxine physiology, pharmacology, and anesthetic implications. Anesth Analg 1982;61:371–83

2. Wellby ML. Laboratory diagnosis of thyroid disorders. Adv Clin Chem 1976;18:103–72
3. Becker SP, Skolinik EM, O'Neill JV. The nodular thyroid. Otolaryngol Clin North Am 1980;13:53–8
4. Burrow GN. The management of thyrotoxicosis in pregnancy. N Engl J Med 1985;313:562–8
5. Maze M. Clinical implications of membrane receptor function in anesthesia. Anesthesiology 1981;55:160–71
6. Waldstein SS. The assessment and management of hyperthyroidism. Otolaryngol Clin North Am 1980;13:13–27
7. Gotta AW, Sullivan CA, Seaman J, Jean-Gilles B. Prolonged intraoperative bleeding caused by propylthiouracil-induced hypoprothrombinemia. Anesthesiology 1972;37:562–3
8. Ikeda S, Schweiss JF. Excessive blood loss during operation in the patient treated with propylthiouracil. Can Anaesth Soc J 1982;29:477–80
9. Feek CM, Sawers JS, Irvine WJ, et al. Combination of potassium iodide and propranolol in preparation of patients with Graves' disease for thyroid surgery. N Engl J Med 1980;302:883–5
10. Verhoeeven RP, Visser TJ, Doctor R, et al. Plasma thyroxine, 3,3', 5'-triiodothyronine during beta-adrenergic blockade in hyperthyroidism. J Clin Endocrinol Metab 1977;44:1002–5
11. Hamilton WFD, Forrest AL, Gunn A, et al. Beta-adrenoreceptor blockade and anesthesia for thyroidectomy. Anaesthesia 1984;39:335–42
12. Caldarelli DD, Holinger LD. Complications and sequelae of thyroid surgery. Otolaryngol Clin North Am 1980;13:85–97
13. Waldstein SS. Medical complications of thyroid surgery. Otolaryngol Clin North Am 1980;13:99–107
14. Kaplan JA, Cooperman LH. Alarming reactions to ketamine in patients taking thyroid medication-treatment with propranolol. Anesthesiology 1971;35:229–30
15. Stehling LC. Anesthetic management of the patient with hyperthyroidism. Anesthesiology 1974;41:585–95
16. Berman ML, Kuhnert L, Phythyon JM, Holaday DA. Isoflurane and enflurane-induced hepatic necrosis in triiodythyronine-pretreated rats. Anesthesiology 1983;58:1–5
17. Seino H, Dohi S, Aiyoshi Y, et al. Postoperative hepatic dysfunction after halothane or enflurane anesthesia in patients with hyperthyroidism. Anesthesiology 1986;64:122–5
18. Babad AA, Eger EI. The effects of hyperthyroidism and hypothyroidism on halothane and oxygen requirements in dogs. Anesthesiology 1968;29:1087–93

19. Steffey EP, Eger EI. Hyperthermia and halothane MAC in the dog. Anesthesiology 1974;41:392–6

20. Smulyan H, Weinberg SE, Howanitz PJ. Continuous propranolol infusion following abdominal surgery. JAMA 1982;247:2539–42

21. Cooper DS. Subclinical hypothyroidism. JAMA 1987;258:246–7

22. Peters KR, Nance P, Wingard DW. Malignant hyperthyroidism or malignant hyperthermia? Anesth Analg 1981;60:613–5

23. Drucker DJ, Burrow GN. Cardiovascular surgery in the hypothyroid patient. Arch Intern Med 1985;145:1585–7

24. Kim JM, Hackman L. Anesthesia for untreated hypothyroidism: Report of three cases. Anesth Analg 1977;56:299–302

25. Regan MJ, Eger EI. The effect of hypothermia in dogs on anesthetizing and apenic doses of inhalation agents. Anesthesiology 1967;28:689–99

26. Levelle JP, Jopling MW, Sklar GS. Perioperative hypothyroidism: An unusual postanesthetic diagnosis. Anesthesiology 1985;63:195–7

27. Drop LJ, Cullen DJ. Comparative effects of calcium chloride and calcium gluceptate. Br J Anaesth 1980;52:501–5

28. Al-Mohaya S, Naguib M, Abdelatif M, Farag H. Abnormal responses to muscle relaxants in a patient with primary hyperparathyroidism. Anesthesiology 1986;65:554–6

29. Flashburg MH, Dunbar BS, August G, Watson D. Anesthesia for surgery in an infant with DiGeorge syndrome. Anesthesiology 1983;58:479–80

30. Weatherill D, Spence AA. Anaesthesia and disorders of the adrenal cortex. Br J Anaesth 1984;56:741–7

31. Knudsen L, Christiansen LA, Lorentzen JE. Hypotension during and after operation in glucocorticoid-treated patients. Br J Anaesth 1981;53:295–301

32. Symreng T, Karlberg BE, Kagedal B. Schildt B. Physiological cortisol substitution of long-term steroid-treated patients undergoing major surgery. Br J Anaesth 1981;53:949–53

33. Kehlet H. A rational approach to dosage and preparation of parenteral glucocorticoid substitution therapy during surgical procedures. Acta Anaesthesiol Scand 1975;19:260–4

34. Hume DM, Bell CC, Bartter FC. Direct measurement of adrenal secretion during operative trauma and convalescence. Surgery 1962;52:174–87

35. Gangat Y, Triner L, Baer L, Puchner P. Primary aldosteronism with uncommon complications. Anesthesiology 1976;45:542–4

36. Hull CJ. Phaechromocytoma. Diagnosis, preoperative preparation and anaesthetic management. Br J Anaesth 1986;58:1453–8

37. Thomas JL, Bernardino ME. Pheochromocytoma in multiple endocrine adenomatosis. JAMA 1981;245:1467–9

38. Bravo EL, Gifford RW. Pheochromocytoma: Diagnosis, localization and management. N Engl J Med 1984;311:1298–1303

39. Rouby JJ, Gory G, Gaveau T, et al. Dangerous rise in pulmonary wedge pressure following aortography in a patient with pheochromocytoma. Anesth Analg 1980;59:154–6

40. Suzukawa M, Michaels IAL, Ruzbarsky J, et al. Use of isoflurane during resection of pheochromocytoma. Anesth Analg 1983;62:100–3

41. Janeczki GF, Ivankovich AD, Glisson SN, et al. Enflurane anesthesia for surgical removal for pheochromocytoma. Anesth Analg 1977;56:62–7

42. Mihm FG. Pulmonary artery pressure monitoring in patients with pheochromocytoma. Anesth Analg 1983;62:1129–33

43. Jones RB, Hill AB. Severe hypertension associated with pancuronium in a patient with a pheochromocytoma. Can Anaesth Soc J 1981;28:394–6

44. El-Naggar M, Suerte E, Rosenthal E. Sodium nitroprusside and lidocaine in the anesthetic management of pheochromocytoma. Can Anaesth Soc J 1977;24:353–9

45. Sumikawa K, Amakata Y. The pressor effect of droperidol on a patient with pheochromocytoma. Anesthesiology 1977;46:359–61

46. Bitter DA. Innovar-induced hypertensive crises in patients with pheochromocytoma. Anesthesiology 1979;50:366–9

47. Martin R, St-Pierre B, Mliner O-R. Phaeochromocytoma and postoperative hypoglycemia. Can Anaesth Soc J 1979;26:260–2

48. Colditz GA, Willette WC, Stampfer MJ, et al. Menopause and the risk of coronary heart disease in women. N Engl J Med 1987;316:1105–10

49. Divekar VM, Kothari MD, Kamdar BM. Anaesthesia in Turner's syndrome. Can Anesth Soc J 1983;30:417–8

50. Kitahata LM. Airway difficulties associated with anaesthesia in acromegaly. Br J Anaesth 1971;43:1187–90

51. Hassan SZ, Matz G, Lawrence AM, Collins PA. Laryngeal stenosis in acromegaly. Anesth Analg 1976;55:57–60

52. Southwick JP, Katz J. Unusual airway difficulty in the acromegalic patient—indications for tracheostomy. Anesthesiology 1979;51:72–3

53. Compkin TV. Radial artery cannulation, potential hazard in patients with acromegaly. Anaesthesia 1980;35:1008–9

54. Katz J, Levin A. Treatment of diffuse metastatic cancer pain by instillation of alcohol into the sella turcica. Anesthesiology 1977;46:115–21

55. Philbin DM, Coggins CH. Plasma antidiuretic hormone levels in cardiac surgical patients during morphine and halothane anesthesia. Anesthesiology 1978;49:95–8

56. Arieff AI. Hyponatremia, convulsions, respiratory arrest, and permanent brain damage after elective surgery in healthy women. N Engl J Med 1986;314:1529–35

57. Sterns RH, Riggs JE, Schochet SS. Osmotic demyelination syndrome following correction of hyponatremia. N Engl J Med 1986;314:1535–42

24

Metabolism and Nutrition

Disorders of metabolism with implications for management of anesthesia range from the common occurrence of diabetes mellitus to the rare patient with porphyria (Table 24-1). The etiology of these disorders is often related to the absence of a specific enzyme. Nutritional disorders may reflect excess caloric intake leading to morbid obesity or voluntary starvation, as in patients with anorexia nervosa, leading to malnutrition (Table 24-2). Enteral and parenteral nutrition have emerged as life-saving therapy in the management of critically ill and malnourished patients. Finally, the trauma of surgery results in predictable endocrine and metabolic responses. These potentially adverse responses can be influenced by the management of anesthesia.

DIABETES MELLITUS

Diabetes mellitus is a chronic systemic disease due to a relative or absolute lack of insulin. Classically, diabetes is manifest as hyperglycemia, glycosuria, and degeneration of small blood vessels.

Classification

Diabetes can be classified as juvenile-onset (also known as insulin-dependent, ketoacidosis-prone, type I, or labile diabetes) or maturity-onset (also known as noninsulin-dependent, nonketoacidosis-prone, type II, or stable diabetes) (Table 24-3). Juvenile-onset diabetes is a distinct disorder from maturity-onset diabetes.[1] Appearance of juvenile-onset diabetes is typically before 16 years of age, and these children usually require exogenous insulin to prevent ketoacidosis. Diabetics who do not need exogenous insulin to prevent ketoacidosis usually develop the disease in adulthood (after 35 years of age) and are said to

---

TABLE 24-1. Disorders of Metabolism

Diabetes mellitus
Nonketotic hyperosmolar hyperglycemic coma
Hypoglycemia
Porphyria
Gout
Pseudogout
Hyperlipidemia
Disorders of carbohydrate metabolism
Disorders of amino acid metabolism
Mucopolysaccharidoses
Gangliosidoses

TABLE 24-2.   Disorders of Nutrition

Morbid obesity
Obesity-hypoventilation syndrome
Malnutrition
Anorexia nervosa
Disorders related to vitamin imbalance

manifest maturity-onset diabetes. Although many maturity-onset diabetics are receiving exogenous insulin, they are usually not ketoacidosis prone. Maturity-onset diabetics comprise over 90 percent of all diabetics and are often obese.

Etiology

The mode of transmission of diabetes mellitus is not defined. Although there is a strong familial tendency for diabetes, the mode of inheritance is controversial.[2] For example, both autosomal dominant and recessive modes of genetic transmission have been implicated in the development of maturity-onset diabetes. Infections caused by mumps, coxsackie B virus, rubella, and cytomegalovirus have been proposed as etiologic agents. Round cell infiltration of the pancreatic islet cells in maturity-onset diabetes and the seasonal variation in juvenile-onset diabetes lend support to an environmental trigger such as a virus. Indeed, in juvenile-onset diabetes, it has been proposed that a viral infection initiates an autoimmune response in which beta cells of the pancreas are destroyed.[2] The demonstration of antibodies to pancreatic islet cells and the association

of diabetes with adrenal and thyroid diseases also suggest an autoimmune mechanism. An estimated 15 percent of maturity-onset diabetics have islet cell antibodies and usually become insulin dependent within 4 years.[2] Early immunotherapy with drugs such as cyclosporine may be beneficial in management of juvenile-onset diabetics.[3]

Obesity seems to play a prominent role in the appearance of maturity-onset diabetes. This is most likely related to a resistance to endogenous insulin, which develops in association with an increase in total body fat stores.[4] Typically, obese nondiabetics require two times to five times the normal amount of endogenous insulin to meet energy requirements. Therefore, in overweight patients with anatomically and/or functionally deficient beta cells, diabetes is unmasked or accentuated by obesity.

Insulin

Insulin in a polypeptide anabolic hormone secreted by the beta cells of the pancreas. Normal daily insulin secretion is equivalent to about 50 units. The important physiologic and metabolic effects of insulin include (1) facilitation of glucose transfer across cell membranes into cells, (2) enhancement of glycogen formation, (3) inhibition of lipolysis and gluconeogenesis, (4) transportation of glucose into adipose tissue for conversion to and storage as fatty acids, and (5) facilitation of the passage of potassium into cells with glucose.

Fasting causes insulin levels to decline. As

TABLE 24-3.   Classification of Diabetes Mellitus

	Juvenile-Onset	Maturity-Onset
Age of onset (years)	Before 16	After 35
Onset	Abrupt	Gradual
Manifestations	Polyphagia	May be asymptomatic
	Polydipsia	
	Polyuria	
Require exogenous insulin	Yes	Not always
Ketoacidosis prone	Yes	No
Blood glucose concentrations	Wide fluctuations	Less marked fluctuations
Nutrition	Thin	Often obese
Vascular complications	Infrequent	Frequent

a result, catabolic hormones use tissue stores to maintain blood glucose concentrations and provide energy for metabolic needs. For example, cortisol causes breakdown of peripheral protein stores. Resistance to the effects of insulin occurs during surgery, most likely reflecting increased plasma concentrations of cortisol and catecholamines. The peak effect of these hormones typically occurs 12 hours to 24 hours postoperatively. Insulin resistance is particularly intense during and after hypothermic cardiopulmonary bypass predisposing these patients to difficulties in control during the perioperative period.[5]

Diagnosis

Diabetes is diagnosed by performing a glucose tolerance test. In this test, blood glucose levels are measured every 30 minutes, after the administration of an oral glucose load. If the amount of insulin released by pancreatic beta cells is deficient or if the release of insulin is slow, blood glucose levels remain high for a prolonged period of time, resulting in an abnormal or diabetic glucose tolerance curve (Table 24-4).

Treatment

Treatment of diabetes includes diet and the use of oral hypoglycemic drugs or the administration of exogenous insulin. Transplan-

TABLE 24-5. Oral Hypoglycemic Drugs

Drug	Generic Name	Trade Name
Sulfonylureas	Tolbutamide	Orinase
	Chlorpropamide	Diabinese
	Acetohexamide	Dymelor
	Tolazamide	Tolinase
	Glyburide	DiaBeta
	Glipizide	Glucotrol
Biguanides	Phenformin	DBI
		Metrol

tation of pancreatic tissue remains an infrequently performed procedure.

ORAL HYPOGLYCEMIC DRUGS

Oral hypoglycemic drugs are used when blood glucose control cannot be attained with diet alone in maturity-onset diabetics. These drugs are classified as sulfonylureas and biguanides (Table 24-5).

Sulfonylureas are presumed to act by stimulating the release of insulin from beta cells of the pancreas. A potential adverse effect is prolonged hypoglycemia. Hypoglycemia is even more likely to occur in patients with impaired renal function. These drugs are also alleged to enhance the effects of thiazide diuretics, barbiturates, and anticoagulants.[6] The popularity of oral hypoglycemic drugs has diminished since the suggestion that sudden death may be more frequent in patients receiving tolbutamide or the biguanide preparation, phenformin.[7] The use of phenformin is further restricted by the propensity of this drug to produce lactic acidosis.

EXOGENOUS INSULIN

There are several types of commercially available preparations of insulin (Table 24-6). The most popular preparation is the single-peak Lente insulin. This form of insulin is the least allergenic of the intermediate-acting insulin preparations. Lente insulin is most frequently employed as the 100 $U \cdot ml^{-1}$ strength (U-100). Insulin-dependent diabetics usually require a combination insulin regimen consisting of regular and Lente insulin before

TABLE 24-4. Glucose Tolerance Test

Time of Sampling after Glucose Load (Minutes)	Blood Glucose Concentrations ($mg \cdot dl^{-1}$)	
	Nondiabetic	Diabetic
Control	Below 100	Above 110
30	Below 160	Above 160
60	Below 160	Above 160
90	Below 140	Above 140
120	100–110	Above 120

TABLE 24-6.   Commercially Available
Preparations of Insulin

Type	Onset (Hours)	Peak Effect (Hours)	Duration (Hours)
Short-acting			
Crystalline	1	2–4	6–8
Semilente	1.5	5–7	12–18
Intermediate			
NPH	1–2	10–20	20–24
Lente	1–2	14–18	20–24
Prolonged			
Protamine	6–8	16–24	24–36
Ultralente	6–8	22–26	24–36

breakfast and a second injection of Lente insulin in the evening. This approach simulates the normal physiologic pattern in which endogenous insulin levels rise rapidly after meals. Rebound hyperglycemia usually occurs after an episode of hypoglycemia (Somogyi effect), emphasizing that the detection of early morning glycosuria may actually reflect a prior episode of hypoglycemia. Obviously, the dose of insulin in this situation should be decreased rather than increased to avoid a repetition of the hypoglycemia that initiated the rebound effect.

Patients treated with protamine containing insulin preparations such as NPH or protamine zinc insulin are 50 times more likely to experience life-threatening allergic responses when protamine is administered intravenously to antagonize the effects of heparin.[8] Presumably, low-dose antigenic stimulation from the insulin preparation evokes the production of antibodies to protamine.[9]

PANCREAS TRANSPLANTATION

Pancreas transplantation (whole grafts, segmental grafts, or processed islet cells) may become a more common treatment for patients with insulin-dependent diabetes mellitus who have labile plasma blood glucose concentrations and who manifest progressive microangiopathy.[10] Vascular thrombosis (splenic artery is usually anastomosed to the donated pancreas after a splenectomy) and exocrine spillage are major problems associated with

pancreas transplantation. When islet cells are transplanted, they are infused into either the liver or the spleen. Management of anesthesia for pancreas transplantation requires frequent monitoring for hypoglycemia or hyperglycemia and consideration of the impact of immunosuppressant drugs.[10]

Complications of Diabetes Mellitus

The most serious acute metabolic complication of diabetes is ketoacidosis. Other complications associated with the progression of diabetes include neuropathies, atherosclerosis, microangiopathy, and an increased incidence of infection. Morbidity and mortality are increased in diabetics undergoing surgery, most often reflecting cardiovascular complications; delayed wound healing, especially when metabolic control is poor; and postoperative wound infections. Gram-negative organisms are a common cause of wound infections.

KETOACIDOSIS

Metabolic acidosis in the presence of hyperglycemia (usually greater than 300 mg·dl^{-1}), plus the history of diabetes, is sufficient to establish the diagnosis of ketoacidosis. The stress of trauma or infection (urinary, biliary, respiratory tract) is often responsible for resistance to insulin, which leads to the development of ketoacidosis. Inhibition of premature labor in insulin-dependent diabetics by administration of a beta-2 agonist may abruptly precipitate ketoacidosis even with prior subcutaneous injections of insulin.[11]

That even small amounts of insulin will suppress the breakdown of adipose tissue by lipases is evidence that an absolute deficiency of circulating insulin is the causative factor in the development of ketoacidosis. In the absence of insulin, fatty acids are converted in the liver to acetoacetic acid, acetone, and beta-hydroxybutyrate, leading to ketoacidosis.

Ketoacids have a low renal threshold, and

about one-half the acid load is excreted in combination with sodium. The resulting hyponatremia accentuates ketoacidosis. Myocardial contractility and peripheral vascular tone are also diminished by ketoacidosis. Furthermore, in the presence of ketoacidosis, potassium leaves the cells, such that the plasma potassium concentrations are likely to be elevated despite the presence of a total body potassium deficit. Indeed, moderate hyperkalemia usually occurs with ketoacidosis. Compensatory responses to ketoacidosis are chloride loss via the kidneys and hyperventilation.

Hyperglycemia associated with ketoacidosis also produces adverse effects. For example, hyperglycemia increases plasma osmolarity, so that water is transferred from cells to the extracellular fluid, producing intracellular dehydration. Furthermore, glucose permeates biologic membranes relatively poorly; when blood glucose concentrations exceed about 180 mg·dl^{-1}, there is glycosuria and a concomitant osmotic diuresis. This diuresis further accentuates hyperosmolarity and is associated with loss of electrolytes, particularly potassium, and decreases in intravascular fluid volume. Hypovolemia may result in circulatory collapse. Despite severe hypotension, there is usually some urine output because of the osmotic effects of glucose.

Definitive treatment of ketoacidosis is the intravenous administration of insulin. In the presence of hypotension and ketoacidosis, an initial intravenous injection of 20 units to 50 units of regular insulin is indicated. This can be followed by continuous intravenous infusion of insulin. Since insulin receptors become fully saturated at moderate levels of circulating insulin, small amounts of intravenous insulin given continuously are effective. Indeed, continuous infusion of 1 U·hr^{-1} to 10 U·hr^{-1} of regular insulin have been reported to be effective in the management of ketoacidosis.[12] With a maximum insulin effect, blood glucose concentrations will decrease 100 mg·dl^{-1}·hr^{-1} to 200 mg·dl^{-1}·hr^{-1}. This decrease, however can be even larger and more rapid, secondary to rehydration in the presence of low intravascular fluid volume. Isotonic saline and, in severe cases, plasma or albumin are necessary to reestablish extracellular fluid volume. Sodium bicarbonate is indicated when the arterial pH falls below 7.1, the plasma bicarbonate concentration is less than 10 mEq·L^{-1} or the patient is too weak to hyperventilate sufficiently to reduce the arterial carbon dioxide partial pressure to below 20 mmHg. As ketoacidosis resolves and the plasma glucose concentrations decline, potassium reenters intracellular fluid spaces and hypokalemia can develop. Therefore, plasma potassium concentrations should be monitored and supplemental intravenous potassium (40 mEq·hr^{-1}) administered when plasma concentrations fall below 3.0 mEq·L^{-1}.

NEUROPATHIES

Most diabetics have demonstrable neuropathic changes after several years of the disease. Segmental demyelination leads to the development of neuropathy. The exact pathogenesis of this demyelination is unclear. Excesses of sorbitol or glucose, or inadequate amounts of inositol, in cell membranes of the nerves may be responsible. Microangiopathy of the vasa nervorum has also been implicated as a cause of demyelination.

Autonomic Nervous System Dysfunction. Autonomic nervous system dysfunction (neuropathy) reflects neurologic changes associated with diabetes.[13–15] Cardiovascular manifestations of autonomic nervous system dysfunction include orthostatic hypotension, resting tachycardia, and reduction or absence of beat-to-beat variation of the heart rate during voluntary deep breathing. The basic defect in orthostatic hypotension associated with diabetes is lack of vasoconstriction due to sympathetic nerve dysfunction. Plasma concentrations of norepinephrine increase less when diabetics with symptoms of orthostatic hypotension assume the standing position. Cardiac parasympathetic dysfunction appears to be more prevalent than sympathetic dysfunction as evidenced by loss of beat-to-beat variability of heart rate. Indeed, compared with nondiabetic patients, diabetics with evidence of autonomic nervous system neuropathy manifest small heart rate responses after the administration of atropine and propranolol.[15] Bradycardia that does not respond to atropine has been observed after reversal of nondepolarizing muscle relaxants or in the presence of renal failure, suggesting co-existing damage to the cardiac vagal nerve.[16,17] Autonomic nervous system dysfunction may also interfere with control of ventilation, making patients with diabetes more susceptible to respiratory depressant effects of drugs. Delayed gastric emptying (gastroparesis) is another manifestation of autonomic nervous system dysfunction. Bowel dysfunction, characterized as intermittent diarrhea, and bladder dysfunction may be elicited from the medical history. Finally, painless myocardial infarction and unexplained cardiorespiratory arrest (some occurring intraoperatively and in the recovery room) have been reported in diabetic patients with autonomic nervous system dysfunction.[18] Indeed, unexplained hypotension may reflect silent myocardial infarction in these patients. It seems the prevalence of cardiac autonomic nervous system dysfunction in unselected diabetic patients is greater than appreciated (20 percent to 40 percent depending on the sensitivity of tests employed). Once this form of dysfunction develops, the prognosis is poor, with mortality exceeding 50 percent over a 5 year period.[19]

Peripheral Somatic Nervous System Dysfunction. Peripheral somatic nervous system dysfunction (neuropathy) may be manifest as nocturnal sensory discomfort of the lower extremities. There is a high incidence of carpal tunnel syndrome among diabetics. Local trauma and toxins such as alcohol can enhance the neuropathies in these patients. Autonomic nervous system dysfunction and somatic nervous system dysfunction may develop in parallel in diabetic patients.

ATHEROSCLEROSIS

Atherosclerosis can appear at an early age in association with diabetes. Indeed, accelerated coronary artery disease accounts for much of the morbidity and mortality associated with diabetes. Cerebral vascular accidents, myocardial infarctions, and peripheral vascular disease are twice as common in patients with diabetes. Cardiomyopathy is not an uncommon event in diabetics.

MICROANGIOPATHY

Microangiopathy is characterized by a thickened and leaky capillary wall. These changes are present in all organs of the body. The most common manifestations of this pathologic change are in the eyes and kidneys. For example, diabetic patients are prone to blindness from a proliferating retinopathy. Cataracts and glaucoma are frequent. Hyperglycemia can also produce visual impairment due to osmotic changes in the lens. Changes in the glomerulus, afferent and efferent arterioles, and interlobular arteries of the kidneys are characterized by a thickened basement membrane. There may be associated proteinuria and increasing plasma creatinine concentrations.

INFECTION

Leukocyte function is not optimal in diabetic patients. Indeed, diabetics are prone to infection. Furthermore, infection is often the cause of sudden increases in insulin requirements.

Management of Anesthesia

There are two goals in the management of anesthesia for patients with diabetes. First, hypoglycemia is prevented by insuring an adequate supply of exogenous glucose. Second, ketoacidosis, with associated hyperglycemia, dehydration, and electrolyte abnormalities, is prevented by the administration of exogenous insulin.

PREOPERATIVE EVALUATION

Preoperative evaluation of diabetic patients is influenced by whether patients are insulin-dependent and likely to develop ketoacidosis or whether the diabetes is the maturity-onset type, with little likelihood of ketoacidosis. Preoperative evaluation should include the adequacy of blood glucose control. Good control of blood glucose concentrations reduces the need for gluconeogenesis and provides a favorable setting for protein synthesis and wound healing. Absence of ketoacidosis must be confirmed before undertaking any elective operative procedure. Indeed, elective surgery should never be undertaken in known diabetics who show evidence of ketoacidosis in the preoperative period. Manifestations of coronary artery disease, cerebral vascular disease, hypertension, or renal dysfunction should also be sought. Signs of peripheral neuropathies and autonomic nervous system dysfunction should be noted. Juvenile-onset diabetes occasionally is associated with nonfamilial short stature and joint contractures that may make direct laryngoscopy difficult. Likewise, obesity is frequent in adult onset diabetics and may introduce similar concerns for the technical ease of intubation of the trachea. Finally, operations are ideally scheduled for early in the morning.

It should be remembered that ketoacidosis can mimic an acute abdomen such as appendicitis. However, in contrast to an intra-abdominal surgical emergency, ketoacidosis is associated with nausea and vomiting, which precedes the onset of abdominal pain. Nevertheless, emergency surgery in insulin-dependent diabetics may require active treatment of ketoacidosis and decreased intravascular fluid volume with regular insulin and intravenous infusion of balanced salt solutions during the operative procedure. Supplemental potassium may be necessary to treat hypokalemia, which occurs when insulin-stimulated glucose entry into cells also carries potassium into cells.

MANAGEMENT OF DAILY INSULIN DOSE

No available data confirm that close control of blood glucose concentrations in the relatively brief intraoperative period benefits diabetic patients. Nevertheless, understanding metabolic responses to surgery and how those responses are altered by insulin provides approaches to minimize derangements in blood glucose concentrations in the perioperative period. A frequent approach is to administer one-fourth to one-half of the usual daily intermediate-acting dose of insulin. If regular insulin is part of the morning schedule, the intermediate-acting insulin dose should be increased 0.5 units for each unit of regular insulin; remember that the stress of anesthesia and surgery increases the need for insulin. If oral hypoglycemic drugs are being used, they can be continued until the evening before surgery. It must be remembered, however, that these drugs may produce hypoglycemia as long as 24 hours to 36 hours after their administration.

Administration of a partial dose of long-acting insulin on the morning of surgery has been questioned.[20] Indeed, compared with patients receiving a partial dose of insulin before the induction of anesthesia, the intraoperative control of plasma glucose concentrations was better in patients not given preoperative insulin but receiving regular insulin or glucose on the basis of blood glucose determinations (Fig. 24-1).[20] Therefore, an acceptable alternative to routine administration of preoperative insulin is to withhold insulin and measure blood glucose concentrations frequently during the intraoperative period. Based on these measurements, blood glucose concentrations can be maintained between 100 mg·dl^{-1} to 250 mg·dl^{-1} during the intraoperative period by intravenous infusion of additional glucose or regular insulin (Table 24-7).[20]

Another alternative to the preoperative administration of a portion of the normal daily dose of insulin is the continuous intravenous infusion of low doses of regular insulin during the operation. For example, 1 unit of regular

TABLE 24-7. Recommendations for Perioperative Management of Diabetes Mellitus

1. Do not use arbitrary insulin regimens in the preoperative period.
2. Begin intravenous infusion of glucose (5–7 g·hr^{-1}) in the preoperative period.
3. Measure blood glucose concentrations before induction of anesthesia and every 1–2 hours during surgery and the immediate postoperative period.
4. Administer 5–10 units of regular insulin intravenously if blood glucose concentrations are above 250 mg·dl^{-1}.
5. Increase rate of glucose infusion if blood glucose concentrations are below 100 mg·dl^{-1}.

(Data from Walts LF, Miller J, Davidson MB, Brown J. Perioperative management of diabetes mellitus. Anesthesiology 1981;55:104–9)

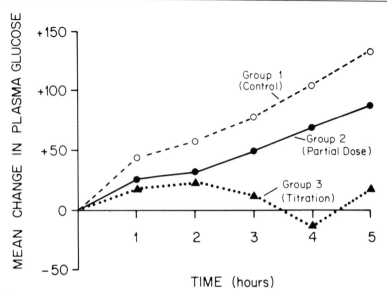

FIG. 24-1. Changes in plasma glucose concentrations were determined during the intraoperative period in insulin-dependent adult diabetic patients. Group 1 patients received no preoperative insulin or glucose. Group 2 patients received one-fourth to one-half of their usual dose of insulin at 7 A.M. on the morning of surgery. In addition, intravenous infusions of glucose-containing solutions were started at the same time the insulin was administered. The rate of intravenous infusions were adjusted to deliver about 6.25 g·hr^{-1} of glucose. Group 3 patients received no insulin or glucose preoperatively but were treated with intravenous regular insulin if blood glucose concentrations measured at the induction of anesthesia or intraoperatively exceeded 200 mg·dl^{-1}. (Walts LF, Miller J, Davidson MB, Brown J. Perioperative management of diabetes mellitus. Anesthesiology 1981;55:104–9)

insulin administered intravenously, followed by continuous intravenous infusion of 1 U·hr^{-1} of regular insulin, results in blood glucose concentrations during the operative period similar to blood glucose levels measured in patients receiving two-thirds of their normal daily dose of insulin subcutaneously as part of the preoperative medication.[21]

PREPARATION IN THE OPERATING ROOM

Upon arrival in the operating room, an intravenous infusion of glucose is started. A logical selection is an intravenous solution containing 5 percent glucose and electrolytes. Since lactate is converted to glucose by gluconeogenesis, it is reasonable to consider lactated Ringer's solution as a glucose infusion with electrolytes. Determination of blood glu-

cose concentrations before the induction of anesthesia is recommended (Table 24-7).[20] Comparison of the glucose concentration in this blood sample, as reported from the laboratory, with that glucose value estimated by using a Dextrostix confirms the accuracy of this latter approach. Estimation of blood glucose concentrations using a Dextrostix can then be repeated with confidence as to their accuracy during the operative procedure. Simultaneous estimates of blood glucose concentrations and the presence or absence of ketone bodies in the blood can be determined using a Keto-Diastix.

Measurement of urine glucose concentrations and the use of a sliding scale for management of insulin requirements in the perioperative period are not optimal. For example, a urinary catheter would be necessary to obtain a urine specimen from a sedated or anesthetized patient. In view of the potential for infection, a urinary catheter should probably not be placed only to monitor glycosuria in diabetics. Furthermore, a high renal threshold for glucose, as often present in maturity-onset diabetics, can result in undertreatment of hyperglycemia. Conversely, a low renal threshold for glucose, as often present in juvenile-onset diabetics, can result in overtreatment and potential hypoglycemia. Therefore, measurement of glucose concentrations in blood is the best indicator of the need for additional insulin in diabetic patients.

INDUCTION AND MAINTENANCE

Choice of drugs for induction and maintenance of general anesthesia is less important than monitoring and treating potential physiologic derangements associated with diabetes. Indeed, effects of anesthetic drugs on blood glucose concentrations and insulin release are varied and probably clinically insignificant with respect to the total management of anesthesia in diabetic patients. Intubation of the trachea with a cuffed tube seems prudent in view of the prolonged gastric emptying associated with autonomic nervous system dysfunction. Hypoglycemia must be considered whenever delayed awakening occurs in the postoperative period.

Epidural anesthesia has been advocated on the basis of preservation of glucose tolerance and insulin release during surgery, but this remains an unconfirmed benefit in diabetics.[22] The high incidence of peripheral neuropathy must be considered in choosing regional anesthetic techniques in patients with diabetes. Conversely, there is an increased risk of nerve injury in diabetic patients who are rendered unconscious, emphasizing the importance of proper positioning while these patients are still awake. Local anesthetic dose requirements may be decreased if arteriosclerosis accompanies diabetes.[23]

TREATMENT OF INTRAOPERATIVE HYPERGLYCEMIA

Additional regular insulin is indicated during the intraoperative period whenever blood glucose concentrations exceed 250 mg·

dl^{-1} or ketones are detected in the blood. The route of administration for this additional regular insulin is controversial. Subcutaneous injection may not give the rapid absorption and onset of effect desired when blood glucose concentrations are above 250 mg·dl^{-1}. Conversely, adding regular insulin to intravenous solutions is complicated by absorption of unknown amounts of insulin onto the glass or plastic used to package and deliver the intravenous fluid.[24] Addition of 1 ml human albumin to each liter of fluid will greatly reduce this absorption. Another criticism of adding insulin to intravenous solutions is that variations in the rate of intravenous infusion will alter the speed of insulin delivery to patients. Considering all these factors, an alternative may be to inject 5 units to 10 units of regular insulin at the hub of a catheter placed in a peripheral vein. Blood glucose concentrations should be redetermined 30 minutes to 45 minutes after administration. The same dose of insulin can be repeated if these determinations reveal blood glucose concentrations are still above 250 mg·dl^{-1}. Indeed, more important than knowing how much insulin is administered or remains attached to the delivery system is the presence of rapid and accurate methods to measure blood glucose concentrations.

NONKETOTIC HYPEROSMOLAR HYPERGLYCEMIC COMA

Nonketotic hyperosmolar hyperglycemic coma has been observed as a complication of many primary illnesses in both diabetic and nondiabetic patients.[25,26] In fact, two-thirds of patients have no history of diabetes mellitus and do not require insulin after recovery from this syndrome. A precipitating event, such as infection or dehydration, is present in about 50 percent of patients. Elderly patients or otherwise incapacitated patients whose thirst mechanisms are ineffective are vulnerable to the development of this type of coma.

TABLE 24-8.   Nonketotic Hyperosmolar Hyperglycemic Coma

Hyperglycemia (above 600 mg·dl^{-1})
Osmotic diuresis
Electrolyte deficiency and decreased intravascular fluid volume
Absence of ketosis
Plasma osmolarity (above 330 mOsm·L^{-1})
Central nervous system dysfunction

Symptoms

Typical findings in patients with nonketotic hyperosmolar coma are listed in Table 24-8. Blood glucose concentrations usually exceed 600 mg·dl^{-1}. This hyperglycemia results in a marked osmotic diuresis, which leads to loss of sodium, potassium, and intravascular fluid. Reductions in intravascular fluid volume are associated with hypotension, metabolic acidosis, hemoconcentration, and increases in blood urea nitrogen concentrations. Absence of ketoacidosis may reflect the antiketogenic effects of severe hyperglycemia or effects of insulin on fat and carbohydrate metabolism. Plasma osmolarity is usually greater than 330 mOsm·L^{-1}. This extreme hyperosmolality leads to decreases in intracellular brain water, with subsequent central nervous system dysfunction. Indeed, the first manifestation of this syndrome can be altered mentation, culminating in seizures and coma.

Treatment

Treatment of nonketotic hyperosmolar hyperglycemic coma is directed at correction of hypovolemia and hyperosmolality. Intravenous fluids such as lactated Ringer's solution or 0.45 percent saline should be given until the blood pressure and urine output are stabilized. Potassium supplementation may be required to replace that lost due to osmotic diuresis. Hyperglycemia responds initially to small doses of intravenous regular insulin (10 U·hr^{-1} to 20 U·hr^{-1}). The average patient requires 300 units to 400 units of insulin during the first 24 hours.

Insulin therapy is necessary until blood glucose concentrations decreases to about 300 mg·dl^{-1}. It must be appreciated that these patients can be very sensitive to the effects of insulin. Indeed, rapid lowering of blood glucose concentrations can lead to cerebral edema.

HYPOGLYCEMIA

The actual level below which blood glucose concentrations are insufficient to meet energy requirements is not precisely defined. Indeed, symptoms of hypoglycemia appear at widely differing blood glucose levels and vary from patient to patient. For example, patients with a long-standing insulin secreting tumors may remain asymptomatic despite blood glucose levels of 30 mg·dl^{-1} to 40 mg·dl^{-1}. Conversely, rapid lowering of blood glucose concentrations from 300 mg·dl^{-1} to 100 mg·dl^{-1} with the administration of insulin may precipitate hypoglycemic reactions in diabetic patients. Nevertheless, in normal patients, signs of hypoglycemia begin to appear when blood glucose levels decrease to about 50 mg·dl^{-1}.

There are a number of compensatory mechanisms to offset hypoglycemia. For example, liver glycogen is the source of glucose during the first 12 hours of fasting. Subsequently, gluconeogenesis in the liver produces glucose from amino acids derived from skeletal muscles. Severe liver disease interferes with these compensatory responses and makes patients with cirrhosis of the liver vulnerable to hypoglycemia. An important hormonal response to hypoglycemia is release of glucagon from alpha cells of the pancreas. Glucagon subsequently stimulates liver glycogenolysis, so as to maintain blood glucose concentrations. Finally, release of epinephrine in response to hypoglycemia stimulates breakdown of glycogen in the liver. Hypoglycemia can be classified as fasting and postprandial.

Fasting Hypoglycemia

The most important cause of fasting hypoglycemia is an insulinoma (insulin-secreting tumor) of pancreatic beta cells. Fasting hypoglycemia can also be produced by liver failure, congestive heart failure, or diffuse carcinomatosis. In elderly patients, fasting hypoglycemia can result from large, usually mesodermally derived, tumors such as fibrosarcomas and mesotheliomas. The mechanism is not known.

INSULINOMA

Failure of plasma insulin concentrations to decrease as blood glucose concentrations fall is suggestive of the presence of an insulinoma. Angiography, computed tomography, and selective venous catheterization, with simultaneous measurements of plasma concentrations of insulin, can be used to confirm the diagnosis and to localize the tumor. About 10 percent of these tumors are malignant. Therefore, a preoperative liver scan is indicated to exclude the presence of hepatic metastases.

The major challenge during anesthesia for surgical excision of an insulinoma is the maintenance of normal blood glucose concentrations.[27] For example, profound hypoglycemia can occur, particularly during manipulation of the tumor. Since signs of hypoglycemia (hypertension, tachycardia, diaphoresis) may be masked during anesthesia, it is probably wise to include glucose in the intravenous fluids administered intraoperatively. Conversely, marked hyperglycemia can follow successful surgical removal of the tumor. The ability to estimate rapidly blood glucose concentrations with a Dextrostix is important. An artificial pancreas (Biostater), which continuously analyzes blood glucose concentrations and automatically infuses insulin or glucose, has been used for the intraoperative management of these patients.[28] Nevertheless, intermittent sampling of blood glucose concentrations every 15 minutes has been proposed as an acceptable alternative to the artificial pancreas

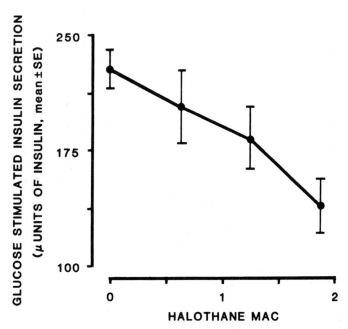

FIG. 24-2. In vitro secretion of insulin from isolated pieces of rat pancreas is inhibited by halothane in a dose-dependent manner. Halothane concentrations equivalent to 0.63 MAC, 1.25 MAC, and 1.88 MAC produce 8 percent, 19 percent, and 37 percent reductions in the secretion of insulin respectively. (Data adapted from Gingerick R, Wright PH, Paradise RR. Inhibition by halothane of glucose-stimulated insulin secretion in isolated pieces of rat pancreas. Anesthesiology 1974;40:449–52)

in these patients assuming glucose levels are maintained above 60 mg·dl^{-1}.[29]

Effects of anesthetic drugs on insulin dynamics are not well-defined. In vitro studies with halothane (Fig. 24-2)[30] and enflurane [31] have shown a concentration-dependent suppression of glucose-stimulated insulin release. Indeed, administration of glucose loads to patients anesthetized with halothane results in the release of less insulin into the circulation than that which occurs when the same glucose loads are administered to awake patients (Fig. 24-3).[32] Nevertheless, it is likely that blood glucose concentrations will increase during surgery, regardless of the drugs used to produce anesthesia. This increase presumably reflects intraoperative increases in sympathetic nervous system activity and release of epinephrine, glucagon, and cortisol. Finally, there is a suggestion that general anesthetics can induce a state of relative glucose intolerance, which is most likely due to inhibitory effects of anesthetics on glucose transport across cell membranes.

Monitoring blood glucose concentrations has been advocated as a method to confirm complete removal of the insulinoma.[29] For example, blood glucose concentrations should increase at least 40 mg·dl^{-1} (hyperglycemic re-bound) in the first 30 minutes after complete removal of the tumor. Failure of blood glucose concentrations to increase promptly may imply that surgical resection of hyperfunctioning islet tissues is not complete. Nevertheless, hyperglycemic responses are variable and unpredictable, making them an unreliable clinical indicator of the completeness of surgical removal of the insulinoma.[29,33]

Postprandial Hypoglycemia

After glucose loads (meals), there is a brisk release of insulin, which may cause blood glucose levels to fall below 40 mg·dl^{-1}. This overload occurs frequently in patients who have undergone gastric surgery and in whom gastric emptying is rapid. When symptoms of hypoglycemia occur in the absence of prior gastric surgery, the diagnosis of reactive hypoglycemia is a consideration. Despite the frequent claim that emotional disorders are related to low blood glucose concentrations, the true incidence of reactive hypoglycemia is rare.

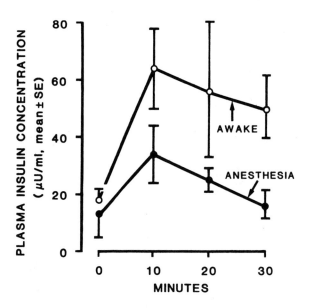

FIG. 24-3. Increases in plasma concentrations of insulin after the intravenous administration of glucose (25 g) are less during halothane-nitrous oxide anesthesia than during the awake state. Data during anesthesia were obtained before surgical stimulation. (Data adapted from Merin RG, Samuelson PN, Schalch DS. Major inhalation anesthetics and carbohydrate metabolism. Anesth Analg 1971;50:625–31 Reprinted with permission from IARS.)

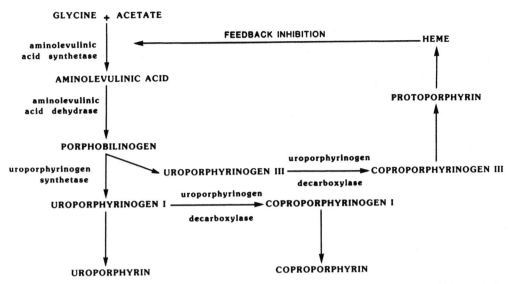

FIG. 24-4. The first step in the synthesis of heme is the formation of aminolevulinic acid from glycine and acetate. The first step is catalyzed by aminolevulinic acid synthetase and inhibited by heme. The formation of porphobilinogen is catalyzed by aminolevulinic acid dehydrase. Excess amounts of both aminolevulinic acid and porphobilinogen, as seen in acute intermittent porphyria, occur as a result of stimulation of aminolevulinic acid synthetase activity, and decreased uroporphyrinogen synthetase activity. Decreased activity of uroporphyrinogen decarboxylase can lead to an accumulation of uroporphyrin, which is believed to cause porphyria cutanea tarda.

PORPHYRIA

Porphyria refers to a group of specific disease entities that result from an abnormality of porphyrin metabolism. The production of porphyrins from glycine and acetate ultimately leads to formation of heme (Fig. 24-4). Abnormalities of enzyme activity along this pathway are responsible for the adverse manifestations that characterize the porphyrias. Porphyrias are categorized as hepatic or erythropoietic (Table 24-9). Regardless of the classification or manifestations, all forms of porphyria are characterized by excessive excretion of porphyrin pigments in the urine.

Acute Intermittent Porphyria

Acute intermittent porphyria is the most serious form of the hepatic porphyrias. This disease is an inborn error of porphyrin metab-

olism, affecting both central and peripheral nervous systems. Transmission is as a nonsex-linked autosomal dominant gene. The metabolic defect is most likely due to an increase in the activity of the aminolevulinic acid synthetase enzyme and a decrease in uroporphyrinogen synthetase activity (Fig. 24-4). As a result of these changes in enzyme activity, there is an accumulation of excessive amounts of porphobilinogen.

Diagnosis of acute intermittent porphyria is suggested by the demonstration of increased urinary excretion of aminolevulinic acid and

TABLE 24-9. Classification of Porphyria

Hepatic Porphyrias
    Acute intermittent porphyria
    Porphyria cutanea tarda
    Variegate porphyria
    Hereditary coproporphyria

Erythropoietic Porphyrias
    Erythropoietic uroporphyria
    Erythropoietic protoporphyria

porphobilinogen during an acute attack. It must be appreciated that urinary excretion of these substances may not be elevated between attacks. Definitive biochemical diagnosis is made by demonstrating reduced levels of uroporphyrinogen synthetase in erythrocytes. Clinically, it may be observed that the urine turns black on standing, reflecting the increased urinary excretion of porphobilinogen.

MANIFESTATIONS

Classic manifestations of acute intermittent porphyria are severe abdominal pain plus variable neurologic deficits occurring in young to middle-aged females.[34] Abdominal pain associated with attacks of acute intermittent porphyria is commonly mistaken for acute cholecystitis, acute pancreatitis, appendicitis, or renal colic. Indeed, these patients often have a history of previous negative surgical explorations of the abdomen.

The principal neurologic lesion produced is demyelination, leading to motor weakness, diminished peripheral reflex responses, and dysfunction of the autonomic nervous system and cranial nerves. Dysfunction of the autonomic nervous system manifests as labile hypertension, orthostatic hypotension, diaphoresis, and arterial vasospasm. Bulbar paralysis and cerebellar dysfunction have been observed. Death can occur from paralysis of the muscles of respiration. Emotional disturbances or psychoses may persist between attacks.

PROPHYLAXIS

It is important for these patients to avoid events and medications capable of provoking an attack of acute intermittent porphyria. For example, starvation, dehydration, and sepsis may trigger an acute attack. A role for female hormones is suggested by the greater severity and frequency of this disease in females, its almost total absence before puberty, and its frequent exacerbation during pregnancy. Classically, barbiturates have been associated with provoking an attack. It is speculated that these drugs increase activity of aminolevulinic acid synthetase enzyme, leading to stimulation of

TABLE 24-10. Drugs Alleged Capable of Precipitating Acute Intermittent Porphyria in Susceptible Individuals

Barbiturates	Pentazocine
Benzodiazepines	Etomidate
Ethyl alcohol	Meprobamate
Phenytoin	Glutethimide
Ketamine	Corticosteroids

porphyrin synthesis in susceptible individuals. A number of drugs in addition to the barbiturates have also been alleged to act as precipitating agents for attacks (Table 24-10).

TREATMENT

Treatment of acute intermittent porphyria involves hydration, infusion of hematin, infusion of glucose, and administration of drugs to reduce pain. Hematin (3 mg·kg^{-1}·day^{-1} to 4 mg·kg^{-1}·day^{-1}) is specific therapy, as it provides substrate for cytochrome production and, at the same time, suppresses activity of aminolevulinic acid synthetase.[35] Glucose is thought to be beneficial by virtue of suppressing activity of enzymes involved in the production of aminolevulinic acid and porphobilinogen. Abdominal pain is often well controlled with oral phenothiazines, such as chlorpromazine. Opioids may be necessary for management of severe pain, but these drugs must be used sparingly, as there is an increased risk that these patients will develop drug dependence with repeated attacks.

MANAGEMENT OF ANESTHESIA

Management of anesthesia in patients with the diagnosis of acute intermittent porphyria is designed not to provoke an attack with drugs used in the perioperative period. Barbiturates are most often incriminated, but even the safety of benzodiazepines[36] and ketamine[37] has been questioned. Nevertheless, ketamine has been used safely in these patients.[38] Furthermore, it is equally well documented that attacks do not always follow administration of barbiturates to patients who are subsequently diagnosed as having acute intermittent por-

TABLE 24-11. Drugs Alleged Safe for Use in Patients with Acute Intermittent Porphyria

Chlorpromazine	Opioids
Promethazine	Droperidol
Anticholinergics	Nitrous oxide
Anticholinesterases	Volatile anesthetics
Depolarizing and nondepolarizing muscle relaxants	

phyria.[36,39,40] Drugs considered safe for use in these patients include opioids, with the possible exception of pentazocine, inhaled anesthetics, and muscle relaxants (Table 24-11). It would seem prudent to provide anesthesia with these "safe" drugs, even though barbiturates do not always evoke attacks. Likewise, the use of regional anesthesia is questionable, since neurologic deficits produced by porphyria might be incorrectly attributed to the anesthetic technique. Perioperative monitoring of these patients should consider the frequent presence of autonomic nervous system dysfunction and the possibility of labile blood pressure. Frequent neurologic evaluation will aid in the ventilatory management of patients with bulbar involvement.

Porphyria Cutanea Tarda

Porphyria cutanea tarda is the only form of hepatic porphyria not associated with neurologic involvement. Transmission of the enzymatic defect responsible is as an autosomal dominant trait. Increased urinary excretion of uroporphyrin may reflect decreased hepatic activity of the uroporphyrinogen decarboxylase enzyme (Fig. 24-4). Symptoms manifest most often in men, after 35 years of age. Alcohol abuse is frequently present in these patients. Indeed, abstinence from alcohol can produce dramatic remissions in symptomatic patients. Photosensitivity is prominent, and the skin is very friable. Porphyrin accumulation in the liver is associated with hepatocellular necrosis.

Anesthesia is not a hazard in these patients, assuming protection from ultraviolet light is provided and excessive pressure on the skin from face masks and tape is avoided. Choice of drugs for anesthesia should take into consideration the likely presence of co-existing liver disease.

Variegate Porphyria

Variegate porphyria affects both sexes, with an onset between the ages of 10 years and 30 years. Transmission occurs as an autosomal dominant trait. Photosensitivity and neurologic sequelae are characteristic. The skin is fragile, and bullae frequently develop. As with acute intermittent porphyria, barbiturates should be avoided. Glucose infusion is effective in treating acute attacks.

Hereditary Coproporphyria

Hereditary coproporphyria, like variegate porphyria, is associated with neurologic deficits. Inheritance is as an autosomal dominant trait. Increased fecal excretion of coproporphyrinogen III is characteristic. Treatment and implications for management of anesthesia are similar to those detailed for acute intermittent porphyria.

Erythropoietic Uroporphyria

Erythropoietic uroporphyria is a rare form of erythropoietic porphyria, transmitted as an autosomal recessive trait. Hemolytic anemia, bone marrow hyperplasia, and splenomegaly are often present. Repeated infections are common, and photosensitivity is severe. The urine of these patients turns red when exposed to light. There are no neurologic or abdominal symptoms, and barbiturates do not influence the course of the disease. Death usually occurs early in childhood.

Erythropoietic Protoporphyria

Erythropoietic protoporphyria is a more common but less debilitating form of erythropoietic porphyria. Manifestations include photosensitivity, vesicular eruptions, urticaria, and edema. Some individuals develop cholelithiasis secondary to increased protoporphyrin excretion. Barbiturates do not produce adverse effects, and survival to adulthood is common.

GOUT

Gout is a disorder of purine metabolism, which may be classified as primary or secondary. Normally, purines are converted to uric acid by the action of the enzyme xanthine oxidase. Uric acid is subsequently filtered at the glomerulus, some is reabsorbed at proximal convoluted renal tubules, and additional uric acid is secreted by distal renal tubules.

Primary Gout

Primary gout is due to an inherited metabolic defect of purine metabolism, leading to an overproduction of uric acid. Renal excretion of uric acid can also be defective, contributing to hyperuricemia.

Secondary Gout

Secondary gout is due to identifiable causes of excess uric acid production. For example, cancer chemotherapeutic drugs, as used in the treatment of leukemia, can produce such rapid lysis of purine-containing tissues that acute hyperuricemia results. Excess purine production leading to hyperuricemia and gout

can also occur in the presence of polycythemia. Thiazide diuretics, aspirin, and alcohol can increase plasma uric acid concentrations by interfering with the renal excretion of uric acid. Finally, carbohydrate deprivation and ketosis in normal individuals can lead to hyperuricemia.

Manifestations

Gout is characterized by plasma uric acid concentrations above 7.5 mg·dl^{-1}, in association with recurrent episodes of acute arthritis due to deposition of urate crystals in joints. Fever, leukocytosis, and an elevated sedimentation rate are often present during the acute attack. Deposition of urate crystals typically initiates inflammatory responses that cause pain and limitation of motion of the joint. At least one-half of the initial attacks of gout are confined to the first metatarsophalangeal joint. In addition, the ankle and knee are commonly involved. Destruction of bone and cartilage may be seen as radiolucent areas on radiographs of the joint. Overall, gouty arthritis accounts for about 5 percent of all cases of arthritis.

Persistent hyperuricemia is also associated with deposits of urate crystals in extraarticular locations. For example, nephrolithiasis due to urate crystal deposition in renal tubules occurs in 10 percent to 15 percent of patients with primary gout and 35 percent to 40 percent of those with secondary gout. Uric acid stones can cause chronic obstructive renal disease, with hydronephrosis and pyelonephritis. Renal parenchymal damage is due to deposition of urate crystals in the interstitium of the kidneys, with development of chronic inflammation. Urate crystal deposition can also occur in the myocardium, aortic valve, and extradural spinal regions.

A number of diseases are associated with gout. Hypertension is frequently present in these patients. Indeed, chronic hypertension may contribute to the high incidence of renal disease in patients with gout. There is an increased incidence of coronary artery disease.

Diabetes mellitus may be present in as many as 80 percent of patients with gout.

Treatment

Treatment of gout is designed to maintain plasma uric acid concentrations below 6 mg·dl^{-1}.[41] This goal is often accomplished by using uricosuric drugs, such as probenecid, to decrease renal tubular reabsorption of uric acid and thus facilitate renal excretion, leading to reductions in plasma uric acid concentrations. It should be appreciated that aspirin antagonizes uricosuric effects of probenecid.

Reduction in plasma concentrations of uric acid can also be accomplished by inhibiting activity of xanthine oxidase, which is the enzyme necessary for conversion of purines to uric acid. Allopurinol, one drug that inhibits this enzyme, is useful for treatment of patients with uric acid stones. It is also indicated for patients with leukemia who have an increased production of uric acid due to breakdown of cells secondary to the effects of cancer chemotherapeutic drugs.

Colchicine is the drug of choice for treatment of acute gouty arthritis. Colchicine has no specific effect on purine metabolism but is effective in relieving pain of gouty arthritis by modifying leukocyte migration and phagocytosis. This drug can be given orally or intravenously. Side effects of colchicine include vomiting and diarrhea. Large doses of colchicine can produce hepatorenal dysfunction and agranulocytosis. Other drugs used in management of acute gouty arthritis include indomethacin, phenylbutazone, and corticosteroids.

Management of Anesthesia

Management of anesthesia in the presence of gout is designed to facilitate continued renal elimination of uric acid. Therefore, adequate hydration, beginning several hours before operative procedures, is important. Sodium bicarbonate to alkalinize the urine also facilitates excretion of uric acid. As lactate can decrease the renal tubular secretion of uric acid, the use of lactated Ringer's solution may not be wise, although this is unproven. Despite these precautions and for reasons that are not clear, acute attacks of gout often follow surgical procedures in afflicted patients.

Extra-articular manifestations of gout, as well as side effects of drugs used to control this disease, should be considered when formulating plans for management of anesthesia. Renal function should be carefully evaluated. Indeed, clinical manifestations of gout usually increase as renal function deteriorates. Abnormalities detected on the electrocardiogram might reflect urate deposits in the myocardium. The high incidence of hypertension, coronary artery disease, and diabetes mellitus should be remembered. Although rare, adverse renal and hepatic effects can be associated with both probenicid and colchicine. Finally, limited temporomandibular joint motion from gouty arthritis can make direct laryngoscopy for intubation of the trachea a difficult procedure.

PSEUDOGOUT

Pseudogout is the acute onset of arthritis, typically in the knee, associated with the presence of synovial fluid crystals that are not urate. Mild fever and leukocytosis can occur. Attacks seem to be precipitated in some patients by surgical procedures, including parathyroidectomy. The mechanism of this acute synovitis syndrome is not known, and colchicine does not produce dramatic relief. Salicylates, indomethacin, and corticosteroids are occasionally effective in relieving symptoms.

LESCH-NYHAN SYNDROME

Lesch-Nyhan syndrome is a genetically determined disorder of purine metabolism, which occurs exclusively in males. Biochemically, the defect is reduced or absent activity of hypoxanthine-guanine phosphoribosyl transferase, which leads to excess purine production and elevation of uric acid concentrations throughout the body. Clinically, patients are often mentally retarded and exhibit a characteristic spasticity and self-mutilation pattern. Self-mutilation usually involves trauma to perioral tissues and subsequent scarification may present difficulties with direct laryngoscopy for endotracheal intubation. Seizure disorders are associated with this syndrome. Drug therapy often includes benzodiazepines. Athetoid dysphagia may increase the likelihood of aspiration should vomiting occur. Malnutrition is often present. Hyperuricemia is associated with nephropathy, urinary tract calculi, and arthritis. Death is often due to renal failure.

Management of anesthesia is influenced by co-existing renal dysfunction and possible impaired metabolism of drugs administered during anesthesia.[42] The presence of a spastic skeletal muscle disorder suggests caution in the use of succinylcholine. The sympathetic nervous system response to stress is enhanced, suggesting caution in the administration of exogenous catecholamines to these patients.

HYPERLIPIDEMIA

Hyperlipidemia can be due to increases in plasma concentrations of cholesterol or triglycerides. The electrophoretic pattern produced by lipoproteins in the plasma is used to classify hyperlipidemia into six categories (Table 24-12).[43,44] The four classes of lipoproteins present in plasma are chylomicrons, very low density lipoproteins, low density lipoproteins, and high density lipoproteins. It should be remembered that lipid blood levels show a normal age-related increase, which is greater for cholesterol than for triglycerides (Tables 24-13).

Genetic factors that determine the presence of low density lipoprotein receptors can influence plasma concentrations of cholesterol that may be further influenced by dietary intake (see Chapter 1).[44] Secondary causes of hyperlipidemia include untreated diabetes mel-

litus, hypothyroidism, excessive ingestion of alcohol, and corticosteroid therapy. Regardless of the cause, hyperlipidemia is often associated with cardiovascular disease, particularly coronary artery atherosclerosis (Table 24-12) (see Chapter 1).[43,44]

Characteristics of the Lipoprotein Fractions

The very low density lipoprotein fraction carries a high risk for atherosclerosis. Diabetes mellitus, obesity, hypertension, and hyperuricemia all have in common predictable increases in plasma fractions of the very low density lipoproteins. Low density lipoprotein fractions are also considered to be atherogenic.

High density lipoprotein fractions appear to protect against atherosclerosis. This observation is consistent with the probable transporting of cholesterol from peripheral tissues to the liver, for eventual elimination as bile acids. Plasma fractions of high density lipoproteins are reduced in patients with diabetes mellitus or premature atherosclerosis. Cigarette smoking and obesity are also associated with reduced fractions of high density lipoproteins in the plasma. In contrast, moderate consumption of alcohol (one drink daily) and/or physical exercise are associated with an increased plasma fraction of high density lipoprotein.[45]

Treatment

Treatment for all the hyperlipidemias is initially diet control plus weight reduction. Patients with hypercholesterolemia should substitute polyunsaturated for saturated fats. When plasma cholesterol levels remain elevated despite diet and weight reduction, institution of therapy with cholestyramine may be indicated. Cholestyramine sequesters and binds bile salts, leading to the gastrointestinal excretion of cholesterol. Adverse responses to

TABLE 24-12. Characteristics of Hyperlipidemias

	Cholesterol	Triglyceride	Xanthomas	Risk of Coronary Artery Disease
Familial lipoprotein lipase deficiency (Hyperchylomicronemia)	Normal	Increased	Eruptive	Very low
Familial dysbetalipoproteinemia	Increased	Increased	Palmar Planar Tendon	Very High
Familial hypercholesterolemia	Increased	Normal to increased	Tendon	Very high
Familial hypertriglyceridemia	Normal	Increased	Eruptive	Low
Familial combined hyperlipidemia	Markedly increased	Markedly increased	Palmar Planar Tendon	High
Polygenic hypercholesterolemia	Increased	Normal	Tendon	Moderate

cholestyramine include hyperchloremic acidosis and loss of fat soluble vitamins, with resultant reductions in the circulating levels of prothrombin. In addition to binding cholesterol, this drug also combines with other fat soluble drugs, including barbiturates, anticoagulants, and certain antibiotics.

Clofibrate is effective in lowering plasma triglyceride concentrations, presumably reflecting the ability of this drug to decrease synthesis of very low density lipoproteins. Despite plasma triglyceride reductions, a prolongation of survival has not been confirmed when therapy with this drug is initiated after a myocardial infarction occurs. Side effects of clofibrate include vomiting, diarrhea, alopecia, and skin rash. Occasionally, skeletal muscle weakness and cramping occur in association with increased plasma creatine kinase concentrations. Finally, therapy with this drug has been shown to increase the incidence of biliary tract disease.

TABLE 24-13. Normal Plasma Concentrations of Cholesterol and Triglyceride

Population	Cholesterol (mg·dl^{-1})	Triglyceride (mg·dl^{-1})
Newborn	100	100
Children	215–265	120–170
Adult males	270	160
Adult females	240	140

Management of Anesthesia

Management of anesthesia is influenced by the possibility that patients with hyperlipidemia have coronary artery disease (Table 24-12).[43,44] Familial lipoprotein lipase deficiency is not associated with an increased risk of coronary artery disease, but these patients develop hepatosplenomegaly. The likelihood of adverse events or drug interactions in the perioperative period can be minimized by reviewing the pharmacology of the drugs used to treat hyperlipidemia (see the section Treatment of Hyperlipidemia). Finally, the risk of thrombosis and tissue necrosis in association with an indwelling arterial catheter may be increased in these patients.[46]

DISORDERS OF CARBOHYDRATE METABOLISM

Disorders of carbohydrate metabolism usually reflect a genetically-determined enzymatic defect. The defect can result in deficiencies or excesses of precursors or end-products of metabolism, which are normally involved in the formation of glycogen from glucose. In some instances, an alternate metabolic pathway is used. Ultimately, clinical manifestations of specific disorders of carbohydrate metabolism reflect the effects produced by alterations in the amounts of precursors or end-products of metabolism, which occur as a result of the enzymatic defects.

von Gierke's Disease

von Gierke's disease is due to the enzymatic lack of glucose-6-phosphatase. As a result of this defect, the liver cannot convert glycogen to glucose, and hypoglycemia occurs. Oral feedings are required every 2 hours to 3 hours to prevent hypoglycemia and associated seizures. Other clinical manifestations include hyperuricemia, mental retardation, and growth retardation. Hepatomegaly is due to the accumulation of glycogen in the liver. A hemorrhagic diathesis can be due to platelet dysfunction. Survival beyond 2 years of age is unusual, although the surgical creation of a portocaval shunt may be of benefit in some patients.

Management of anesthesia includes monitoring the arterial pH and provision of exogenous glucose to prevent unrecognized intraoperative hypoglycemia.[47] Acidosis is commonly present, presumably reflecting the inability of these patients to convert lactic acid to glycogen. For this reason, it is wise not to use intravenous solutions that contain lactate. Indeed, metabolic acidosis can occur from lactate administration during the perioperative period.[48]

Pompe's Disease

Pompe's disease is due to a specific glucosidase enzyme deficiency that results in glycogen deposits in smooth, striated, and cardiac muscle. Myocardial involvement is the most prominent feature, often manifesting clinically as congestive heart failure. Echocardiography may reveal cardiac hypertrophy and outflow tract obstruction (i.e., subaortic stenosis) due to interventricular septal enlargement. A large,

protuding, glycogen-infiltrated tongue and poor skeletal muscle tone predisposes these patients to upper airway obstruction. Impaired neurologic function manifests as decreased cough and gag reflexes and incoordination of swallowing. Aspiration and atelectasis are common.

Management of anesthesia must consider potential airway obstruction when these patients are rendered unconscious.[49] Volatile anesthetics may produce excess cardiac depression, especially if congestive heart failure co-exists. Decreases in either preload or afterload and/or increases in heart rate and myocardial contractility may precipitate subaortic stenosis. In view of skeletal muscle involvement, it may be wise to avoid administration of succinylcholine to these patients. Diagnostic skeletal muscle biopsies in the lower extremities have been performed using regional anesthesia.[49]

Forbes' Disease

Forbes' disease results from the absence of a debranching glucosidase enzyme. Hypoglycemia is the primary concern during anesthesia. In addition, the possibility of decreased cardiac function due to glycogen deposition in the heart should be considered.

Andersen's Disease

Andersen's disease is due to the absence of an enzyme that results in deposition of abnormal glycogen in various tissues. There is progressive cirrhosis of the liver, leading to hepatic failure. Death usually occurs by 3 years of age.

McArdle's Disease

McArdle's disease is caused by a selective deficiency of phosphorylase enzyme in skeletal muscle. Myoglobinuria leading to renal failure can occur. In view of this potential, it is prudent to monitor urine output and maintain good hydration during the perioperative period. Mannitol may be indicated if urine output is reduced despite adequate volume replacement. The propensity for developing myoglobinuria also raises a question regarding the use of succinylcholine, though problems have not been substantiated by clinical experience. Since repeated episodes of skeletal muscle ischemia can lead to muscle atrophy, the use of an intraoperative tourniquet on an extremity is not recommended. Finally, infusion of glucose-containing solutions is indicated to prevent adverse effects from unrecognized intraoperative hypoglycemia.

Galactosemia

Galactosemia is due to a deficiency of galactokinase and an inability to convert galactose to glucose. As a result, galactose accumulates in various tissues, as manifested by the development of cataracts, cirrhosis of the liver, and mental retardation. Furthermore, elevated plasma galactose levels can suppress release of glucose from the liver, leading to hypoglycemia.

Galactosemia can be mild, with no symptoms until childhood, or can result in hepatic failure and death in infancy. Treatment consists of avoiding foods, such as milk, which are high in lactose content. In the absence of hypoglycemia or hepatic dysfunction, there are no specific considerations for the management of anesthesia.

Fructose-1, 6-Diphosphatase Deficiency

Deficiency of fructose-1, 6-diphosphatase enzyme means that the liver is unable to convert efficiently fructose, lactate, glycerol, and amino acids to glucose. When liver glycogen stores are depleted by starvation, the occurrence of hypoglycemia and metabolic acidosis is likely. Hepatomegaly, fatty liver infiltration, and skeletal muscle hypotonia are common.

Administration of sufficient glucose during the perioperative period is essential.[50] The use of intravenous solutions containing lactate is questionable, since these patients cannot convert lactate to glucose. As a result, metabolic acidosis could be produced by infusion of lactated Ringer's solution.

Pyruvate Dehydrogenase Deficiency

Pyruvate dehydrogenase deficiency results in the inability to convert pyruvate to acetyl coenzyme A with the subsequent development of chronic metabolic (lactic) acidosis due to accumulation of pyruvate and lactate (Fig. 24-5).[51] Management of anesthesia includes avoidance of events that could contribute to lactic acidosis such as hyperventilation of the lungs, reductions in cardiac output, or hypothermia. Lactate containing intravenous solutions are questionable, as their adminis-

FIG. 24-5. Enzymatic reactions involving pyruvate, lactate, pyruvate dehydrogenase (PDH), and pyruvate carboxylase (PC). (Dierdorf SF, McNiece WL. Anaesthesia and pyruvate dehydrogenase deficiency. Can Anaesth Soc J 1983;30: 413–6)

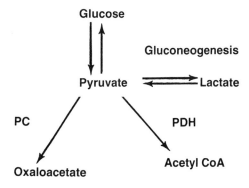

tration would increase lactate concentrations. Lactic acidosis may be accentuated by carbohydrate loads as delivered by glucose-containing solutions. Selection of drugs for induction and maintenance of anesthesia is influenced by possible drug-induced inhibitory effects on gluconeogenesis, which could enhance co-existing metabolic acidosis. In this regard, thiopental and halothane may inhibit gluconeogenesis. Opioids have been recommended for these patients, but excessive depression of ventilation persisting into the postoperative period is possible. Overall, experience is too limited to justify recommendations as to optimal selection of drugs for anesthesia.

DISORDERS OF AMINO ACID METABOLISM

Although there are more than 70 known disorders of amino acid metabolism, the majority are rare. Classic manifestations include mental retardation, seizures, and amino aciduria (Table 24-14). Metabolic acidosis, hyperammonemia, hepatic failure, and thromboembolism can also occur. Management of anesthesia in patients with these types of disorders is directed toward maintenance of intravascular fluid volume and acid-base homeostasis. Use of anesthetics, such as

enflurane and ketamine, has been questioned, in view of the likely presence of seizure disorders in these patients.

Phenylketonuria

Phenylketonuria is the prototype of disorders due to abnormal amino acid metabolism. Phenylalanine accumulates due to an enzymatic deficiency of phenylalanine hydroxylase. Clinical features include mental retardation and seizures. The skin may be friable and vulnerable to damage from pressure or friction created by adhesive materials.

Homocystinuria

Homocystinuria is due to failure of transsulfuration of precursors of cysteine, an important constituent of cross-linkages in collagen. Manifestations of the disease reflect weakened collagen and include dislocation of the lens, osteoporosis, kyphoscoliosis, brittle light-colored hair, and malar flush.[52] Mental retardation may be prominent. Diagnosis is confirmed by demonstration of homocystine in the urine as evidenced by development of a characteristic magenta color when nitroprus-

TABLE 24-14.   Disorders of Amino Acid Metabolism

	Retardation	Seizures	Metabolic Acidosis	Hyperammonemia	Hepatic Failure	Thromboembolism	Other
Phenylketonuria	Yes	Yes	No	No	No	No	
Homocystinuria	Yes/No	Yes	No	No	No	Yes	
Hypervalinemia	Yes	Yes	Yes	No	No	No	Hypoglycemia
Homocystinuria	Yes/No	Yes	No	No	No	Yes	
Citrullinemia	Yes	Yes	No	Yes	Yes	No	
Branched chain ketoaciduria	Yes	Yes	Yes	No	Yes	Yes	
Isoleucinemia	Yes	Yes	Yes	Yes	Yes	No	
Methioninemia	Yes	No	No	No	No	No	Thermal instability
Histidinuria	Yes	Yes/No	No	No	No	No	Erythrocyte fragility
Neutral aminoaciduria (Hartnup disease)	Yes/No		Yes	No	No	No	Dermatitis
Arginemia	Yes		No	Yes	Yes	No	

side is added. Thromboembolism can be life-threatening and is presumed to reflect activation of Hageman factor by homocystine, resulting in increased platelet adhesiveness. Attempts to minimize the likelihood of thromboembolism in the perioperative period include administration of pyridoxine, which reduces platelet adhesiveness, preoperative hydration, infusion of dextran, and early ambulation.[52]

Hypervalinemia (Maple Syrup Urine Disease)

Hypervalinemia results from defects in oxidative decarboxylation of metabolites of branched chain amino acids, which include valine, leucine and isoleucine. This defective decarboxylation leads to accumulation of ketoacids and amino acids in the blood and urine. These materials give the urine the odor of maple syrup. Elevated blood levels of ketoacids contribute to the production of metabolic acidosis. Another significant hazard is the development of hypoglycemia, probably as a reflection of the ability of excessive blood levels of leucine to stimulate the release of insulin. Mental retardation occurs if the disease is not recognized promptly in infants who initially appear normal.

Surgery and anesthesia introduce a number of hazards in patients with this metabolic defect.[53] For example, catabolism of body proteins produced by surgery or infection results in elevated blood concentrations of branched chain amino acids. Even blood in the gastrointestinal tract, as can occur after a tonsillectomy, produces an added metabolic load in these patients. Accumulation of branched chain amino acids in the circulation can produce neurologic deterioration in the perioperative period. The danger of hypoglycemia in these patients is further enhanced by the period of starvation, which precedes elective operations. Therefore, it is important to begin intravenous infusions of glucose preoperatively and to measure blood glucose concentrations intraoperatively. Finally, measurement of ar-

terial pH is necessary to detect metabolic acidosis due to the accumulation of ketoacids. Significant metabolic acidosis in the perioperative period should be treated with sodium bicarbonate.

MUCOPOLYSACCHARIDOSES

Mucopolysaccharidoses are inherited disorders due to deficiencies of enzymes that influence their metabolism (Table 24-15). Clinical manifestations reflect organ dysfunction, which results from accumulation of abnormal mucopolysaccharide materials in cells of practically every organ in the body. The brain, heart, liver, and spleen are most severely affected. Since deposition of mucopolysaccharides is a function of time, the magnitude of organ involvement increases with age.

Preoperative evaluation of patients with these diseases involves assessment of pulmonary, cardiac, and hepatic function. Pulmonary infections are common and should be vigorously treated before elective surgery. Airway obstruction due to accumulation of mucopolysaccharides in the tongue is a common problem. Intubation of the trachea can be technically difficult for this reason. Digitalis and diuretics are indicated if cardiac dysfunction is marked.

General anesthesia is preferred over regional anesthetic techniques, considering the likely presence of mental retardation and the usual young age of these patients. Experience is too limited to recommend a specific drug or drug combination for maintenance of anesthesia. Avoidance of large doses of opioids, however, would seem wise in view of the high

---

TABLE 24-15. Mucopolysaccharidoses

Hurler's syndrome (Mucopolysaccharidosis I)
Hunter's syndrome (Mucopolysaccharidosis II)
Sanfilippo's syndrome (Mucopolysaccharidosis III)
Morquio's syndrome (Mucopolysaccharidosis IV)
Scheie's syndrome (Mucopolysaccharidosis V)
Maroteaux-Lamy syndrome
        (Mucopolysaccharidosis VI)
I cell disease (Mucopolysaccharidosis VII)

incidence of respiratory disease in these patients.

Hurler's Syndrome (Gargoylism)

Clinical manifestations of Hurler's syndrome include dwarfism, severe mental retardation, hepatosplenomegaly, cardiac valvular abnormalities (mitral valve most often involved), and coronary artery disease. These patients are prone to respiratory tract infections. Inguinal hernia, diastasis recti, and umbilical hernia are frequent. Intubation of the trachea may be difficult due to the large tongue and short neck. Abnormalities of tracheal cartilages and cervical vertebrae must be kept in mind when performing direct laryngoscopy and intubation of the trachea. Most patients die before 10 years of age from pulmonary infections or congestive heart failure.

Hunter's Syndrome

Hunter's syndrome is similar to Hurler's syndrome but is clinically less severe. Patients often survive to the fourth decade.

Sanfilippo's Syndrome

Sanfilippo's syndrome is characterized by progressive mental retardation. Cardiac abnormalities have not been described. Patients often survive to the fifth decade.

Morquio's Syndrome

The basic defect in Morquio's syndrome is an abnormality of mucopolysaccharide metabolism most apparent in cartilage and bone. Re-

sulting skeletal deformities include shortening of the trunk and limbs, curvature of the spine, and pectus carinatum (pigeon breast). There is a high incidence of instability of the cervical spine and hypoplasia of the odontoid. Indeed, atlantoaxial subluxation, leading to spinal cord compression and paralysis, is a potential complication of this syndrome.[54,55] Inguinal hernia is common in these patients. Likewise, aortic regurgitation is frequently present. Widely spaced teeth with defective enamel, prominent maxilla, and short nose result in a characteristic facial appearance. Most of these patients die before 30 years of age, usually from chronic pulmonary infections.

Management of anesthesia must consider the possible instability of the cervical spine. Excessive extension of the head and neck during direct laryngoscopy should be avoided.[55] Heavy sedation is not recommended, in view of the high incidence of chronic lung disease due to severe chest deformity. The impact of co-existing aortic regurgitation on the conduct of anesthesia and choice of drugs must be remembered (see Chapter 2).

Scheie's Syndrome

Patients with Scheie's syndrome present with nearly normal intelligence. Aortic regurgitation and carpal tunnel syndrome are frequently associated with this disorder. Skeletal abnormalities are not severe.

Maroteaux-Lamy Syndrome

This syndrome is characterized by normal intelligence and severe skeletal abnormalities.

I Cell Disease

I cell disease is characterized by increases in intracellular lipid content, which exceeds the accumulation of mucopolysaccharides.

TABLE 24-16. Gangliosidoses

Tay-Sachs disease
Niemann-Pick disease
Gaucher's disease

Management of anesthesia is complicated by thick secretions and airway obstruction. Indications for surgery are usually for the repair of inguinal or umbilical hernias.

GANGLIOSIDOSES

Gangliosidoses are diseases characterized by an abnormality in sphingolecithin metabolism, which results in damage to nerve membranes (Table 24-16). Dementia, seizures, and cerebellar and pyramidal tract signs reflect neurodegeneration. The course is that of progressive deterioration with no known treatment. There are no unique anesthetic considerations in these patients.

MORBID OBESITY

Obesity is the most common nutritional disorder in the United States. A body weight 20 percent above ideal weight is defined as obesity. Morbid obesity is present when body weight is twice the ideal weight. Another definition of obesity employs the calculation of body mass index (Table 24-17). A body mass index greater than 30 indicates significant obesity.

Although long sought, metabolic defects

TABLE 24-17. Calculation of Body Mass Index

$$\text{Body Mass Index (BMI)} = \frac{\text{Weight (kg)}}{\text{Height}^2 \text{ (m)}}$$

Example: A 150 kg, 1.8 m tall patient has a BMI of 47. A similar patient but weighing 80 kg has a BMI equal to 25.

to explain obesity have not been found. A genetic influence is suggested by studies in adopted individuals demonstrating a correlation of body weight with biologic but not adoptive parents.[56] In adults, the final common pathway leading to obesity is a positive caloric intake, with subsequent increases in the size of adipose cells to accommodate the excess of triglycerides. Obesity occurring in early childhood is due to increases in the number of adipose cells. In addition to a positive caloric intake, hormonal abnormalities, such as hypothyroidism or an excess of cortisol, can lead to obesity. Finally, psychological disturbances are often associated with obesity.

Obesity increases the risk for developing medical and surgical disease. Manifestations of these changes are metabolic, respiratory, cardiovascular, and hepatic. Management of anesthesia is influenced by these obesity-induced alterations in physiologic function.

Metabolic

Obese individuals are resistant to effects of insulin.[4] Glucose tolerance curves are frequently abnormal, and the incidence of maturity-onset diabetes mellitus is increased severalfold in obese patients. Oxygen consumption and carbon dioxide production are increased. This increased metabolic demand places a significant stress on cardiopulmonary reserves. Other metabolic consequences of obesity include hypercholesterolemia and hypertriglyceridemia.

Respiratory

The respiratory system undergoes considerable change in obese patients. For example, the enlarged abdomen produces thoracic kyphosis and lumbar lordosis, which limits rib movement and produces a relative fixation of the thorax. The diaphragm is elevated and its excursion is markedly limited due to the weight of the abdominal wall. Chest wall compliance is decreased secondary to the massive quantities of fat. Furthermore, chest wall muscles are unable to participate fully in chest wall excursion. As a result, work of breathing is increased, and ventilation becomes diaphragmatic and position-dependent.

Pulmonary function studies suggest a restrictive pattern of lung disease. The most consistent changes are reductions in the expiratory reserve volume, inspiratory capacity, vital capacity, and functional residual capacity. These alterations are accentuated by the supine position. Obese patients typically breathe rapidly and shallowly. This breathing pattern is useful at rest because the oxygen cost of breathing is lower than it would be with other combinations of volume and rate.

Arterial oxygen partial pressure is predictably decreased by obesity. The presumed mechanism for decreased arterial oxygenation is overperfusion of underventilated areas of the lung. Closing volume is increased in obese patients, and increased closing volumes combined with decreased expiratory reserve volumes result in underventilation of dependent lung regions.[57] These changes are reversible with weight loss. For example, obese patients who lose weight sufficient to decrease body mass index by at least 20 percent manifest increased expiratory reserve volumes and improved arterial oxygenation.[58]

In contrast to decreases in arterial oxygenation, the arterial carbon dioxide partial pressure, as well as ventilatory responses to carbon dioxide, remain in normal ranges in obese individuals, reflecting the high diffusing capacity and favorable characteristics of the dissociation curve for carbon dioxide. The margin of reserve, however, is small. Administration of ventilatory depressant drugs or the assumption of the head-down position can lead to accumulation of carbon dioxide in obese patients.

Cardiovascular

The increased oxygen demand of obese individuals results in increased work loads on the heart. For example, cardiac output and blood volume are increased. This is not surprising, as each kilogram of fat contains nearly 3,000 meters of blood vessels.[59] It is estimated that cardiac output increases about 0.1 $L \cdot min^{-1}$ for every kilogram of weight gain related to adipose tissue. This elevated output is due to an increased stroke volume, as resting heart rates in obese individuals remain normal or even low. Indeed, cardiomegaly due to left ventricular hypertrophy is common in obese patients and most likely reflects chronic increases in stroke volume. Increases in cardiac output with exercise are normal, but pulmonary artery pressure often increases above normal with exercise in obese patients.

There is a positive correlation between increases in blood pressure and weight gain. The cause of elevated blood pressure is presumably the increased cardiac output. Therefore, normotension in obese patients implies that systemic vascular resistance is decreased. Pulmonary hypertension is common and most likely reflects the effects of chronic arterial hypoxemia and/or increased pulmonary blood volume. The risk of coronary artery disease is doubled in obese patients. Finally, the increased demands placed on the cardiovascular system by obesity reduce the reserve of the cardiovascular system and limit exercise tolerance.

Hepatic

Abnormal liver function tests and fatty infiltration of the liver occur frequently in obese patients. There is evidence that fluorinated volatile anesthetics are metabolized to a greater extent in obese individuals. For example, plasma concentrations of fluoride increase more after administration of halothane or enflurane to obese individuals than after administration of these drugs to nonobese individuals (Figs. 24-6 and 24-7).[60-63] Reductive metabolism of halothane must occur for fluoride to appear as a metabolite. This introduces the concern that fatty liver infiltration, which occurs in the presence of morbid obesity, can result in hepatocyte hypoxia and favor reductive pathways for halothane metabolism, lead-

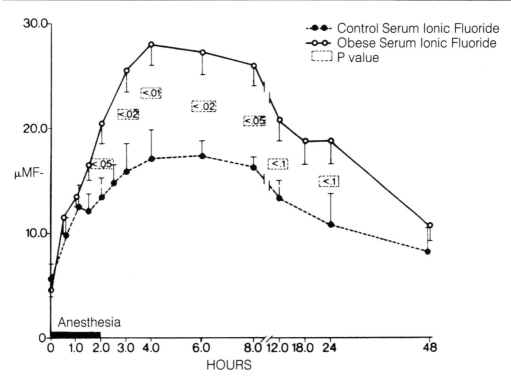

FIG. 24-6. Plasma ionic fluoride (F^-) concentrations ($\mu M \cdot L^{-1}$, Mean ± SE) in obese (128 ± 6 kg) and nonobese adults (67 ± 1 kg) were measured during and after anesthesia with enflurane plus 50 percent nitrous oxide. All patients were undergoing elective abdominal surgery. F^- levels were significantly higher during and after anesthesia in obese patients. (Bentley JB, Vaughn RW, Miller MS, et al. F^- levels in obese patients during and after enflurane anesthesia. Anesth Analg 1979;58:409–12 Reprinted with permission from IARS.)

ing to the production of hepatotoxic reactive intermediary metabolites. Nevertheless, there is no evidence of increased hepatocellular damage in obese patients receiving halothane based on measurement of plasma concentrations of transaminase enzymes.[63]

Hepatic dysfunction is particularly likely to occur after jejunoileal small bowel bypass operations for the treatment of morbid obesity. Indeed, liver biopsies obtained several months after this operation often show fatty infiltration and fibrosis.[64] Other complications associated with this operation include diarrhea and electrolyte disturbances, decreased plasma concentration of folate and/or vitamin B_{12}, nephrolithiasis and cholelithiasis. In contrast, gastric bypass is associated with fewer complications.

The risk for developing gallbladder and biliary tract disease is increased threefold in obese patients. Abnormal cholesterol metabolism in obese patients may be responsible for an increased incidence of gallstones.

Management of Anesthesia

Obese patients pose a number of problems in the perioperative period. Possible interactions of medications used to treat obesity with drugs used during anesthesia must be considered. For example, amphetamines are commonly used as appetite suppressants. Volume of distribution of drugs may be altered since fat contains less water than other tissues, leading to decreases in total body water content in obese patients.

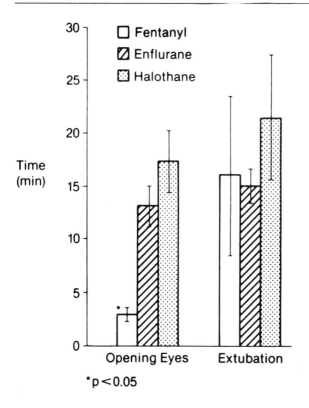

FIG. 24-7. Awakening time (Mean ± SE), as defined by the time from the last skin stitch until opening the eyes on command, and by the time from the last skin stitch until extubation of the trachea, was measured in obese patients anesthetized with nitrous oxide plus fentanyl, enflurane, or halothane for gastric stapling operations. Criteria for extubation of the trachea included sustained responses to tetanus for 5 seconds and the ability to maintain head lift for 5 seconds. The time to opening eyes on command was shortest in patients anesthetized with nitrous oxide-fentanyl. Nevertheless, time to extubation of the trachea was similar in all three anesthesia study groups. (Cork RC, Vaughn RW, Bentley JB. General anesthesia for morbidly obese patients—an examination of postoperative outcomes. Anesthesiology 1981;54:310–3)

PULMONARY ASPIRATION

Obese patients should be considered at increased risk for inhalation of gastric contents. For example, obese patients have an increased incidence of gastroesophageal reflux and hiatal hernia. Furthermore, gastric acidity, gastric fluid volume, and intragastric pressure are increased.[65] Preoperative administration of an H-2 receptor antagonist and metoclopramide can be used to increase gastric fluid pH and decrease gastric fluid volume in obese patients.[66] Other maneuvers, including rapid induction of anesthesia during cricoid pressure and intubation of the trachea with a cuffed tube, are indicated to minimize the risk of pulmonary aspiration.

INDUCTION

It must be remembered that mandibular and cervical mobility can be decreased in obese patients because of the massive amount of soft tissue. This limitation of motion can make airway maintenance and intubation of the trachea difficult. After induction of anesthesia, the low functional residual capacity reduces mixing time for inhaled drugs in the lungs. As a result, the rate of increase in the alveolar concentration of an inhaled drug may be accelerated. Furthermore, low functional residual capacity predisposes obese patients to rapid reductions in arterial oxygen partial pressures during any period of apnea, such as may accompany direct laryngoscopy for intubation of the trachea.

MAINTENANCE

The best choice of drugs or techniques for maintenance of anesthesia in obese patients has not been defined. The high incidence of fatty liver infiltration and co-existing liver disease must be appreciated when selecting volatile anesthetics. Although volatile drugs have not been shown to cause liver or renal damage in obese patients, it has been demonstrated that defluorination of methoxyflurane, halothane, and enflurane are greater in obese as compared with nonobese patients (Figs. 24-6 and 24-7).[60-63] The possibility of prolonged responses to drugs stored in fat, including volatile anesthetics, opioids, and barbiturates, should be considered in obese patients. Nevertheless, there is no evidence that the high lipid solubility of volatile anesthetics results in delayed postanesthesia awakening or prolonged recovery time in morbidly obese subjects (Fig. 24-7).[61] In view of present evidence, it is not possible to recommend a specific drug or drug combination for maintenance of anesthesia in obese patients.

Spinal and epidural anesthesia may be technically difficult in obese patients, as bony landmarks are obscured. Increased epidural pressure secondary to engorged epidural veins makes predictability of anesthetic level difficult. It would seem prudent to reduce initial doses of local anesthetics used for regional anesthesia when body weight is greatly increased due to excess adipose tissue.

MANAGEMENT OF VENTILATION

Known pulmonary abnormalities associated with obesity can be accentuated by anesthesia. After induction of anesthesia, further decreases in functional residual capacity often occur, with airway closure and increased perfusion of unventilated alveoli. Therefore, controlled ventilation of the lungs using large tidal volumes is recommended during the intraoperative period. Responses of obese patients to positive end-expiratory pressure is unpredictable. In one report, addition of positive end-expiratory pressure to a ventilation pattern using large tidal volumes did not improve arterial oxygenation during the intraoperative period.[67] Conceivably, positive end-expiratory pressure could so reduce cardiac output that the benefits of improved matching of ventilation to perfusion are offset. The prone and head-down positions can further decrease chest wall compliance and arterial oxygenation in obese patients. Assumption of the supine position in obese patients breathing spontaneously can seriously impair arterial

oxygenation and result in cardiac and ventilatory arrest.[67] Finally, monitoring of arterial blood gases and pH is helpful in evaluating the adequacy of oxygenation and ventilation in the perioperative period.

POSTOPERATIVE COMPLICATIONS

Postoperative morbidity and mortality in obese patients are increased compared to nonobese patients. Wound infection is twice as common. The likelihood of deep vein thrombosis and the risk of pulmonary embolism are increased, emphasizing the importance of early postoperative ambulation. Pulmonary complications are frequent, particularly after abdominal surgery. The semisitting position should be employed in the postoperative period, so as to minimize the development of arterial hypoxemia. Arterial oxygenation should be closely monitored and supplemental oxygen provided as indicated by the arterial oxygen partial pressure. The maximum reduction in arterial oxygenation typically occurs 2 days to 3 days postoperatively.[68]

OBESITY-HYPOVENTILATION SYNDROME

Obesity-hypoventilation or Pickwickian syndrome occurs in about 8 percent of obese patients.[69] These patients exhibit massive obesity, episodic daytime somnolence, and hypoventilation. Documentation of increased arterial carbon dioxide partial pressures in obese patients should suggest either the presence of this syndrome or severe underlying lung disease. Ultimately, hypoventilation leads to respiratory acidosis, arterial hypoxemia, polycythemia, pulmonary hypertension, and right ventricular failure. Weight loss is associated with decreases in arterial carbon dioxide partial pressures. The etiology of the obesity-hypoventilation syndrome is not clear but may represent a disorder of the central nervous system regulation of ventilation and/or inability of muscles of respiration to respond to neural impulses. Obstructive sleep apnea associated with this syndrome has been effectively treated by continuous positive airway pressure applied via a nasal airway.[70]

MALNUTRITION

Malnutrition is a medically definable syndrome, which is responsive to therapy.[71,72] Critically ill patients are often undergoing progressive starvation (that is, negative caloric intake), complicated by hypermetabolic states due to increased caloric needs produced by trauma, fever, sepsis, and wound healing. It is estimated that 1,500 calories·day^{-1} to 2,000 calories·day^{-1} are necessary for maintenance of basic energy requirements. An elevation of body temperature by 1 degree Celsius will increase daily energy requirements by about 15 percent. For example, patients who are expending 2,000 calories·day^{-1} in the hospital while afebrile, will consume about 3,000 calories·day$^-$ in the presence of elevations in body temperature to 40.5 degrees Celsius. Multiple fractures increase energy needs about 25 percent and major burns 100 percent. Finally, it should be appreciated that a large tumor, by virtue of its growth and metabolism, requires fuels that can exceed by 100 percent basal energy requirements of the host.

Carbohydrate is the major fuel source for energy needs. Carbohydrate stores, however, in the form of circulating glucose and glycogen in the liver and skeletal muscle are limited. For example, only about 80 calories are available from circulating glucose, 250 calories to 300 calories stored as liver glycogen, and up to 600 calories stored as glycogen in skeletal muscles. Carbohydrate energy stores of skeletal muscles, however, are not generally available because skeletal muscles do not contain glucose-6-phosphatase. This enzyme is necessary for the release of glucose from skeletal muscles into the circulation. Therefore, glucose stores are rapidly depleted in the presence of decreased or absent caloric intake.

Proteins can serve as alternative sources of energy when glucose supplies are depleted. For example, cells have the ability to produce glucose from amino acids by gluconeogenesis. It must be appreciated, however, that proteins are not stored for use as a source of energy. Indeed, conversion of proteins to glucose inevitably leads to deterioration of organ function. For example, skeletal muscle mass decreases as amino acids are mobilized for conversion to glucose. This decrease in skeletal muscle mass may involve muscles of respiration, leading to a reduced ventilatory reserve. The amount of cardiac muscle may also decrease when proteins are mobilized for energy requirements. Furthermore, immunocompetence is impaired when patients become protein malnourished. Protein malnutrition is significant when plasma albumin concentrations are below 3 g·dl^{-1}.

Fat, like proteins, can serve as an alternative to glucose for energy supplies. For example, fat, in the form of triglycerides, is broken down in the liver to glycerol and free fatty acids. Glycerol is converted to glucose. Free fatty acids are partially oxidized to produce ketones, which can be used for energy by the brain and peripheral tissues. Unlike amino acids, free fatty acids cannot be converted to glucose.

ANOREXIA NERVOSA

Anorexia nervosa is a psychiatric disease characterized by striking increases in physical activity and marked diminution of food intake in the obsessive pursuit of thinness. Females in adolescence or early adulthood are most often affected and weight loss is equal to or greater than 25 percent of normal body weight. In some patients, hypothalamic-pituitary dysfunction is suggested by amenorrhea, hypothermia, and impaired ability to concentrate urine.[73] Orthostatic hypotension and bradycardia may reflect alterations in autonomic nervous system activity. Occasional patients manifest hepatic dysfunction related to fatty liver infiltration. Leukopenia occurs in nearly one-half the patients, but infection is uncommon. The hemoglobin level is usually normal. Dehydration and electrolyte abnormalities are the result of malnutrition. Gastric hydrogen ion secretion is reduced. Treatment consists of psychotherapy. Drug therapy with amitriptyline or chlorpromazine has been of variable success. When starvation is severe, it is mandatory to institute enteral nutrition. Mortality is 7 percent to 10 percent and is usually the result of starvation.

The presence of electrolyte disturbances, bradycardia, and hypothermia should be remembered when considering management of anesthesia. Starvation could decrease lung elasticity, which would manifest as decreased pulmonary compliance during the intraoperative period. Furthermore, spontaneous pneumomediastinum has been observed in patients with anorexia nervosa.[74] Finally, it has been observed that prolonged fasting in animals is associated with decreased cardiac dysrhythmic thresholds for epinephrine during halothane anesthesia.[75] This observation suggests that administration of halothane to patients with anorexia nervosa could be associated with an increased incidence of ventricular dysrhythmias.

DISORDERS RELATED TO VITAMIN IMBALANCE

Vitamin deficiencies are largely of historic interest. Nevertheless, it is conceivable that administration of anesthesia for surgery will be required in patients with co-existing nutritional deficiencies of one or more of the essential vitamins. This is most likely to occur in chronic alcoholic patients. Although no specific anesthetic drug or techniques can be recommended, it is important to appreciate the changes related to vitamin deficiencies to insure proper medical judgments in the perioperative period.

Thiamine (Vitamin B₁)

Classic symptoms due to thiamine deficiency are known as beriberi. Beriberi is most frequently seen in chronic alcoholic patients who have a reduced dietary intake of thiamine. In addition, carbohydrate metabolism, and thus the need for thiamine, is increased in alcoholic patients. Signs and symptoms of thiamine deficiency are manifest on the cardiovascular system, central nervous system, peripheral nervous system, and gastrointestinal tract.

CARDIOVASCULAR SYSTEM

The principal cardiovascular effects of thiamine deficiency are decreased systemic vascular resistance and increased cardiac output. The resulting increased workload imposed on the heart may be so great that high output cardiac failure occurs. This form of cardiac failure is similar to the hyperdynamic heart failure that occurs in patients with large arterial-to-venous shunts. It may be difficult to differentiate heart failure due to thiamine deficiency from the cardiomyopathy that results from chronic alcoholism.

CENTRAL NERVOUS SYSTEM

Central nervous system changes due to thiamine deficiency can intially manifest as loss of recent memory and emotional changes. Korsakoff's psychosis is characterized by antegrade amnesia and confabulation. Loss of deep tendon reflexes, skeletal muscle weakness, and cranial nerve impairment, particularly of the 6th cranial nerve (nystagmus), herald the onset of Wernicke's encephalopathy.

PERIPHERAL NERVOUS SYSTEM

Polyneuropathy, with wasting of skeletal muscles and impairment of sensory modalities, is common in patients with thiamine deficiency. Peripheral nerves show evidence of demyelination. Foot drop, paraesthesias, and sensory deficits (glove and stocking distribution) are characteristic. There may be destruction of peripheral sympathetic nervous system fibers, which could impair compensatory vasomotor responses during anesthesia. This impaired ability might manifest as exaggerated reductions in blood pressure in response to hemorrhage, positive pressure ventilation of the lungs, or sudden changes in body position.

GASTROINTESTINAL TRACT

Decreased bowel motility, nausea, and vomiting are signs of gastrointestinal tract dysfunction due to thiamine deficiency.

TREATMENT

Treatment of thiamine deficiency is with intravenous preparations of this vitamin. This rapidly corrects decreased peripheral vascular tone, but sudden increases in systemic vascular resistance can also increase the magnitude of cardiac failure. Digitalis, which is not usually helpful in the treatment of high output cardiac failure, may be of value in maintaining myocardial contractility when systemic vascular resistance is abruptly restored to normal.

Ascorbic Acid (Vitamin C)

Deficiency of ascorbic acid produces a clinical picture known as scurvy. Ascorbic acid is required for the conversion of proline to hydroxyproline in the production of normal collagen. When ascorbic acid is deficient, manifestations of abnormal ground substance are seen in all tissues. Indeed, capillary fragility, as manifested by petechial hemorrhages, is prominent in patients with ascorbic acid deficiency. There can be hemorrhage into joints and skeletal muscles. Failure of odontoblastic activity results in loosened teeth and gangrenous alveolar margins. Fibroblast activity is deficient, resulting in poor wound healing and decreased strength of new surgical wounds. A catabolic state associated with a negative nitrogen balance and potassium deficiency is also characteristic. Iron deficiency anemia is frequent, but the presence of macrocytic anemia suggests a concomitant folic acid deficiency. There are no special considerations for the management of anesthesia.

Nicotinic Acid (Niacin)

A deficiency of nicotinic acid produces pellagra (black tongue). Nicotinic acid is part of nicotinamide adenine dinucleotide phosphate, which is an important component of cellular oxidation-reduction reactions. The body does not depend on exogenous nicotinic acid, as this vitamin can be manufactured from tryptophan. Patients with a carcinoid tumor can develop pellagra, since available tryptophan is diverted to formation of serotonin rather than nicotinic acid. A diet with high contents of maize can lead to a nicotinic acid deficiency, as corn contains large amounts of leucine, which interferes with metabolism of tryptophan. Other causes of pellagra include malabsorption syndromes and chronic alcoholism.

Mental confusion, irritability, and peripheral neuropathy are characteristic of nicotinic acid deficiency. Administration of nicotinic acid usually reverses central nervous system dysfunction in less than 24 hours. Gastrointestinal symptoms include achlorhydria and severe diarrhea, which can lead to hypovolemia and loss of electrolytes. Vesicular dermatitis that involves the mucous membranes is also characteristic. Manifestations of dermatitis include stomatitis, glossitis, excessive salivation, and urethritis. There are no specific recommendations regarding the management of anesthesia.

Vitamin A

A deficiency of vitamin A can result from dietary lack of foodstuffs that contain this vitamin (leafy vegetables, animal liver), or from malabsorption syndromes. Clinical manifestations of vitamin A deficiency include loss of night vision, conjunctival drying, and corneal destruction. Anemia from depressed hemoglobin synthesis is frequent. Management of anesthesia requires frequent application of artificial tears and keeping the eyes closed during the intraoperative period.

An excess of vitamin A can produce irritability, hydrocephalus, hepatosplenomegaly, and anemia. Cranial symptoms can be caused by intracranial hypertension secondary to cerebral sinus obstruction.

Vitamin D

Nutritional rickets is due to decreased availability of the active from of vitamin D. Gastrointestinal absorption of calcium is impaired when vitamin D is absent, and there is a tendency to develop hypocalcemia. This tendency is balanced by parathyroid hormone activity, which increases in response to low plasma calcium concentrations. The osteolytic activity of parathyroid hormone restores plasma calcium concentrations to near normal levels at the expense of older bone, which becomes demineralized. New bone formation, which is dependent on plasma calcium concentrations, takes place in a normal manner. Therefore, changes in the skeleton characteristic of rickets reflect unimpaired formation of new bone and the breakdown of old bone. Thoracic kyphosis from this mechanism may be so severe as to produce respiratory embarrassment. Laboratory studies in the presence of vitamin D deficiency show normal or low plasma calcium concentrations, low plasma phosphate levels, increased plasma alkaline phosphatase concentrations, and low urinary excretion of calcium.

Vitamin K

Vitamin K is synthesized by bacteria, which reside in the gastrointestinal tract. Prolonged antibiotic therapy can eliminate these bacteria, leading to prolonged prothrombin times. Since vitamin K is fat soluble, a deficiency of this substance is likely whenever there is failure of fat absorption from the gastrointestinal tract. Decreased absorption of vitamin K from the gastrointestinal tract is most likely to occur when bile salts are excluded from the intestine.

ENTERAL AND PARENTERAL NUTRITION

Caloric support in the presence of increased energy requirements is best provided by enteral or total parenteral nutrition (hyperalimentation).[76,77] It is recommended that patients who have lost more than 20 percent of their body weight be treated nutritionally before operation.[77] Patients who are still unable to eat or absorb food 1 week postoperatively require parenteral nutrition. More than 90 percent of malnourished patients are identified by plasma albumin concentrations below 3 g·dl^{-1} and transferrin levels below 200 mg·dl^{-1}. Skin test anergy (i.e., immunosuppression) also accompanies malnutrition. Other indications for supplemental caloric support may include severe trauma, burns, sepsis, carcinoma, renal, and hepatic failure.

Enteral Nutrition

The gastrointestinal tract should be the site used for nutritional supplementation whenever possible. When the gastrointestinal tract is functioning, enteral nutrition can be provided by means of nasogastric or gastrostomy tube feedings. Continuous-drip infusion techniques are the simplest and safest way to administer enteral feedings. The rate of infusion is usually 100 ml·hr^{-1} to 120 ml·hr^{-1}.

Several liquid diets are available for enteral nutrition. Meal replacement formulas are used in patients who have almost normal proteolytic and lipolytic activity in their gastrointestinal tract. Elemental diets are helpful in patients who have an abnormal gastrointestinal tract (inflammatory bowel disease, enterocutaneous fistula, pancreatic insufficiency) because the proteolytic and lipolytic capacity is not required for absorption. Furthermore, elemental diets have low viscosity, which allows their infusion through needle-catheter jejunostomy tubes. Feeding modules are concentrated sources of one nutrient that can be added to a formula diet to increase specific components that are deficient, or to yield a small-volume, high-caloric mixture for patients in whom fluids should be restricted.

Complications of enteral feedings are infrequent but can include hyperglycemia, leading to osmotic diuresis and hypovolemia. Therefore, blood glucose concentrations should be monitored and exogenous insulin administered when levels exceed 250 mg·dl^{-1}. High osmolarity (550 mOsm·L^{-1} to 850 mOsm·L^{-1}) of elemental diets is often a cause of diarrhea. The reasons for occasional elevations of the plasma bilirubin, transaminase, or alkaline phosphatase concentrations in patients receiving enteral feedings are not known. Critically ill patients, however, often manifest hepatic dysfunction unrelated to nutrition. Furthermore, fatty liver infiltration is commonly associated with malnutrition.

Total Parenteral Nutrition (Hyperalimentation)

Total parenteral nutrition is indicated when the gastrointestinal tract is not functioning. Total parenteral nutrition using isotonic solutions delivered through peripheral veins is acceptable when patients require less than 2,000 calories·day^{-1} and the anticipated need for nutritional support is less than 2 weeks. When caloric requirements exceed 2,000 calories·day^{-1} or prolonged nutritional support is required, a venous catheter is placed in the subclavian vein, so as to permit infusion of a hypertonic parenteral nutrition solution (1,900 mOsm·L^{-1}). The daily volume of infusion is about 40 ml·kg^{-1}. Solutions infused through these cannulae can support growth of bacteria and fungi, and infection at infusion sites is a serious hazard. In view of the hazards of contamination, use of central venous hyperalimentation catheters for administration of medications, as during the perioperative period, or for sampling of blood is not recommended.

Essential fatty acid requirements can be provided by isotonic preparations administered through peripheral veins. Furthermore,

TABLE 24-18. Complications Associated with Total Parenteral Nutrition

Hyperglycemia
Nonketotic hyperosmolar hyperglycemic coma
Hypoglycemia
Hyperchloremic metabolic acidosis
Fluid overload
Increased production of carbon dioxide
Catheter-related sepsis
Electrolyte abnormalities
Renal dysfunction
Hepatic dysfunction
Thrombosis of central veins

fat emulsions can provide up to 2,000 calories·day^{-1}, which can be used to supplement nutritional contributions of hyperalimentation in patients with dramatically increased energy requirements.

Potential complications of total parenteral nutrition are numerous (Table 24-18). Hyperglycemia can lead to osmotic diuresis and hypovolemia. Therefore, blood glucose concentrations should be carefully monitored during the perioperative period. Exogenous insulin should be provided when blood glucose concentrations exceed 250 mg·dl^{-1}. Nonketotic hyperosmolar hyperglycemic coma is a potential complication of this form of nutrition. Coma due to this mechanism is usually precipitated by latent or undiagnosed diabetes mellitus, pancreatitis, sepsis, or concomitant use of phenytoin.[77] Persistence of increased circulating levels of endogenous insulin can contribute to hypoglycemia if total parenteral nutrition is abruptly discontinued. Indeed, episodes of hypoglycemia are often related to sudden decreases in the rate of infusion, due to mechanical obstruction or kinking of venous delivery tubes. Hyperchloremic metabolic acidosis may occur because of the liberation of hydrochloric acid during the metabolism of amino acids present in most parenteral nutrition solutions. This complication can be prevented by the routine addition of 15 mEq to 30 mEq of acetate to each liter of solution. Parenteral feeding of patients with compromised cardiac function is associated with the risk of congestive heart failure due to fluid overload. Increased production of carbon dioxide resulting from the metabolism of large quantities of glucose may result in the need to initiate mechanical ventilation of the lungs or in failure to wean patients from long-term ventilation support.[78] Catheter-related sepsis is a constant threat. Other adverse effects include hypokalemia, hypomagnesemia, hypocalcemia, hypophosphatemia, renal dysfunction, hepatic dysfunction, and thrombosis of central veins. If intravenous hyperalimentation is present during surgery, there should be appropriate reductions in the infusion rates of other intravenous fluids.

ENDOCRINE AND METABOLIC CHANGES IN THE PERIOPERATIVE PERIOD

Surgical stimulation produces profound endocrine and metabolic responses, which parallel the magnitude of operative trauma.[79] Inhaled or injected drugs used to produce anesthesia result in minimal effects on hormone secretion in the absence of surgical stimulation.

Endocrine Responses

Initial endocrine response is characterized by an increase in circulating concentrations of catabolic hormones, including catecholamines, glucagon, and cortisol. At the same time, there are decreases in plasma concentrations of the anabolic hormones, insulin, and testosterone. For example, circulating insulin concentrations are decreased despite co-existing hyperglycemia. This emphasizes that normal hormonal regulation of the blood glucose concentrations is suppressed in response to surgical stimulation. Indeed, increased blood glucose levels during anesthesia and surgery are predictable. As a result, excessive amounts of glucose delivered in the intravenous maintenance fluids can result in intraoperative hyperglycemia. The most likely mechanism for decreased insulin release and associated increases in the blood glucose concentrations

during general anesthesia is a nonspecific response to stress, mediated by increased sympathetic nervous system activity and epinephrine secretion. Epinephrine produces hyperglycemia by stimulation of glycogenolysis and gluconeogenesis, as well as by directly inhibiting release of insulin from the pancreas.

Metabolic Responses

Increases in protein degradation are a major response of the body to surgical trauma. Urinary secretion of nitrogen is increased for 4 days to 6 days after abdominal surgery. A male with an average body build can lose 0.5 kg of lean tissue each day after a major abdominal operation. The main effect of protein degradation is release of amino acids, particularly alanine. Alanine is transported to the liver for conversion to glucose by gluconeogenesis. In addition, surgical stimulation often activates the renin-angiotensin-aldosterone system and results in release of antidiuretic hormone, as evidenced by sodium and water retention and urinary excretion of potassium. Inappropriate secretion of antidiuretic hormone in the postoperative period combined with intravenous infusion of sodium deficient solutions may result in life-threatening hyponatremia.[80]

Mechanisms for Endocrine and Metabolic Responses

Afferent nerve impulses from the operative area are the most likely explanation for endocrine and metabolic changes, which occur in response to surgical stimulation. A variety of other disturbances, including the effect of hemorrhage, fasting, dehydration, and apprehension, can contribute to the overall hormonal responses. In the postoperative period, infection, prolonged best rest, arterial hypoxemia, and even alterations in the usual day-night physiologic cycles can contribute to changes in endocrine function.

Modification of Endocrine and Metabolic Responses

Modification of endocrine responses to surgery can be produced by afferent neuronal blockade, as with regional anesthesia, or by inhibition of hypothalamic function with large doses of opioids. For example, epidural analgesia (T4 sensory level) reduces or abolishes the usual increases in blood glucose, cortisol, and catecholamine concentrations produced by lower abdominal surgery.[81] It is likely that extradural analgesia merely postpones hyperglycemia and adrenocorticol responses until the postoperative period. Large doses of morphine (4 mg·kg^{-1}), fentanyl (75 μg·kg^{-1}) and sufentanil (20 μg·kg^{-1}) have also been shown to inhibit endocrine and metabolic responses to surgery.[82] These doses of opioids, however, are not sufficient to prevent the endocrine response evoked by institution of cardiopulmonary bypass. Increases in plasma norepinephrine concentrations and stimulation of the cardiovascular system associated with surgical skin incision are prevented in 50 percent of adult patients by the administration of 60 percent nitrous oxide and a volatile anesthetic (1.45 MAC halothane, 1.60 MAC enflurane) or morphine (1.13 mg·kg^{-1}).[83] Furthermore, a subarachnoid block sufficient to prevent the pain of skin incision eliminates both adrenergic and cardiovascular responses to surgical stimulation in all patients.[84]

Although it is difficult to quantitate total adverse effects produced by endocrine and metabolic responses to surgical stimulation, it would seem prudent to minimize the magnitude and duration of these changes whenever possible. This is ideally achieved by rapid correction of adverse physiologic disturbances, provision of necessary metabolic substrates, and assurance of adequate depths of anesthesia relative to the magnitude of surgical stimulation. Indeed, the concept that administration of the lowest possible amount of anesthetic is best may not be valid during periods of acute surgical stimulation.[83]

It should be appreciated that exogenous glucose administered to critically ill patients undergoing major surgery makes little or no difference in the magnitude of protein catabolism. Indeed, there is no basis for the recommendation that administration of 100 g·day^{-1} of exogenous glucose will provide optimal sparing of body proteins.[71]

REFERENCES

1. Cahill GF, McDevitt HO. Insulin-dependent diabetes mellitus: The initial lesion. N Engl J Med 1981;304:1454–65
2. Eisenbarth GS. Type I diabetes mellitus. A chronic autoimmune disease. N Engl J Med 1986;314:1360–8
3. Stiller CR, Dupre J, Gent M, et al. Effects of cyclosporine immunosuppression in insulin-dependent diabetes mellitus of recent onset. Science 1984;223:1362–7
4. Archer JA, Garden P, Roth J. Defect in insulin binding to receptors in obese man: Amelioration with caloric restriction. J Clin Invest 1975;55:166–74
5. Elliott MJ, Gill GV, Home PD, et al. A comparison of two regimens for the management of diabetes during open-heart surgery. Anesthesiology 1984;60:364–8
6. Shen S-W, Bressler R. Clinical pharmacology of oral antidiabetic agents. N Engl J Med 1977;296:493–7
7. UGDP hypoglycemic agents. Diabetes 1970; 19:747–88
8. Stewart WJ, McSweeney SM, Kellett MA, et al. Increased risk of severe protamine reactions in NPH insulin-dependent diabetics undergoing cardiac catheterization. Circulation 1984; 70:788–92
9. Moorthy SS, Pond W, Rowland RG. Severe circulatory shock following protamine (an anaphylactic reaction). Anesth Analg 1980;59:77–8
10. Borland LM, Cook DR. Anesthesia for organ transplantation. In: Stoelting RK, Barash PG, Gallagher TJ, eds. Advances in Anesthesia. Chicago. Year Book Medical Publishers 1986:1–6
11. Mordes D, Kreutner K, Metzger W, Colwell JA. Dangers of intravenous ritodrine in diabetic patients. JAMA 1982;248:973–5
12. Page MM, Alberti KGMM, Greenwood R, et al.

Treatment of diabetic coma with continuous low dose infusion of insulin. Br Med J 1974;2:687–90

13. Ewing DJ. Cardiovascular reflexes and autonomic neuropathy. Clin Sci Mol Med 1978;55:321–7

14. Ewing DJ, Campbell IW, Clarke BF. Assessment of cardiovascular effects in diabetic autonomic neuropathy and prognostic implications. Ann Intern Med 1980;92:308–11

15. Lloyd-Mostyn RH, Watkins PJ. Defective innervation of heart in diabetic autonomic neuropathy. Br Med J 1975;3:15–7

16. Triantafillou AN, Tsueda K, Berg J, Wieman TJ. Refractory bradycardia after reversal of muscle relaxant in a diabetic with vagal neuropathy. Anesth Analg 1986;65:1237–41

17. Ciccarelli LL, Ford CM, Tsueda K. Autonomic neuropathy in a diabetic patient with renal failure. Anesthesiology 1986;64:283–7

18. Page MM, Watkins PJ. Cardiorespiratory arrest and diabetic autonomic neuropathy. Lancet 1978;1:14–6

19. Ewing DJ, Campbell IW, Clarke BF. The natural history of diabetic autonomic neuropathy. Q J Med 1980;49:95–108

20. Walts LF, Miller J, Davidson MB, Brown J. Perioperative management of diabetes mellitus. Anesthesiology 1981;55:104–9

21. Taitelman U, Reece EA, Bessman AN. Insulin in the management of the diabetic surgical patient. Continuous intravenous infusion vs. subcutaneous administration. JAMA 1977;237:658–60

22. Houghton A, Hickey JB, Ross SA, Dupre J. Glucose tolerance during anaesthesia and surgery: Comparison of general and extradural anesthesia. Br J Anaesth 1978;50:494–9

23. Bromage PR. Exaggerated spread of epidural analgesia in arterisclerotic patients. Dosage in relation to biological and chronological aging. Br Med J 1962;1:1634–8

24. Petty C, Cunningham NL. Insulin absorption by glass infusion bottles, polyvinylchloride infusion containers, and intravenous tubing. Anesthesiology 1974;40:400–4

25. Wulfson HD, Dalton B. Hyperosmolar hyperglycemic nonketotic coma in a patient undergoing emergency cholecystectomy. Anesthesiology 1974;41:286–90

26. Podolsky S. Hyperosmolar nonketotic coma in the elderly diabetic. Med Clin North Am 1978;62:815–28

27. VanHeerden JA, Edis AJ, Service FJ. The surgical aspects of insulinomas. Ann Surg 1979;189:677–82

28. Pulver JJ, Cullen BF, Miller DR, Valenta LJ. Use of the artificial beta cell during anesthesia for surgical removal of an insulinoma. Anesth Analg 1980;59:950–2

29. Muier JJ, Endres SM, Offord K, et al. Glucose management in patients undergoing operation for insulinoma removal. Anesthesiology 1983;59:371–5

30. Gingerich R, Wright PH, Paradise PR. Inhibition by halothane of glucose-stimulated insulin secretion in isolated pieces of rat pancreas. Anesthesiology 1974;40:449–52

31. Ewart RBL, Rusy BF, Bradford MW. Effects of enflurane on release of insulin by pancreatic islets in vitro. Anesth Analg 1981;60:878–84

32. Merin RG, Samuelson PN, Schalch DS. Major inhalation anesthetics and carbohydrate metabolism. Anesth Analg 1971;50:625–31

33. Tutt GO, Edis AJ, Service FJ, VanHeerden JA. Plasma glucose monitoring during operation for insulinoma: A critical reappraisal. Surgery 1980;88:351–6

34. Sergay SM. Management of neurologic exacerbations of hepatic porphyria. Med Clin North Am 1979;63:453–63

35. Watson CJ, Pierach CA, Bossenmaier I, Cardinal R. Use of hematin in acute attack of the inducible hepatic porphyrias. Adv Intern Med 1978;23:265–86

36. Allen SC, Rees GAD. A previous history of acute intermittent porphyria as a complication of obstetric anesthesia. Br J Anaesth 1980;52:835–8

37. Kostrzewska E, Gregor A. Ketamine in acute intermittent porphyria-dangerous or safe? (letter). Anesthesiology 1978;49:376–7

38. Bancroft GH, Lauria JI. Ketamine induction for cesarean section in a patient with acute intermittent porphyria and achondroplastic dwarfism. Anesthesiology 1983;59:143–4

39. Mustajoki P, Heinonen J. General anesthesia in "inducible" porphyrias. Anesthesiology 1980;53:15–20

40. Salvin SA, Christoforides C. Thiopental administration in acute intermittent porphyria without adverse effect. Anesthesiology 1976;44:77–9

41. Simkin PA. Management of gout. Ann Intern Med 1979;90:812–6

42. Larson LO, Wilkins RG. Anesthesia and the Lesch-Nyhan syndrome. Anesthesiology 1985;63:197–9

43. Motulsky AG. The genetic hyperlipidemias. N Engl J Med 1976;294:823–7

44. Grundy SM. Cholesterol and coronary heart disease. A new era. JAMA 1986;256:2849–58

45. Willett W, Hennekens CH, Siegel AJ, et al. Alcohol consumption and high-density lipoprotein cholesterol in marathon runners. N Engl J Med 1980;303:1159–61

46. Cannon BW, Meshier WT. Extremity amputation

following radial artery cannulation in a patient with hyperlipoproteinemia Type V. Anesthesiology 1982;56:222–3

47. Edelstein G, Hirshman CA. Hyperthermia and ketoacidosis during anesthesia in a child with glycogen-storage disease. Anesthesiology 1980;52:90–2

48. Casson H. Anaesthesia for portocaval bypass in patients with metabolic diseases. Br J Anaesth 1975;47:969–75

49. Rosen KR, Broadman LM. Anaesthesia for diagnostic muscle biopsy in an infant with Pompe's disease. Can Anaesth Soc J 1986;33:790–4

50. Hashimoto Y, Watanabe H, Satou M. Anaesthetic management of a patient with hereditary fructose-1, 6-diphosphate deficiency. Anesth Analg 1978;57:503–6

51. Dierdorf SF, McNiece WL. Anaesthesia and pyruvate dehydrogenase deficiency. Can Anaesth Soc J 1983;30:413–6

52. Parris WCV, Quimby CW. Anesthetic considerations for the patient with homocystinuria. Anesth Analg 1982;61:70–1

53. Delaney A, Gal TJ. Hazards of anesthesia and operation in maple-syrup-urine disease. Anesthesiology 1976;44:83–6

54. Birkinshaw KJ. Anaesthesia in a patient with an unstable neck: Morquio syndrome. Anaesthesia 1975;30:46–9

55. Jones AEP Croley TF. Morquio syndrome and anesthesia. Anesthesiology 1979;51:261–2

56. Stunkard AJ, Sorensen TIA, Hanis C, et al. An adoption study of human obesity. N Engl J Med 1986;314:193–8

57. Hedenstierns G, Santesson J, Norlander O. Airway closure and distribution of inspired gas in the extremely obese breathing spontaneously and during anaesthesia with intermittent positive pressure ventilation. Acta Anaesthesiol Scand 1976;20:334–42

58. Vaughn RW, Cork RC, Hollander D. The effect of massive weight loss on arterial oxygenation and pulmonary function tests. Anesthesiology 1981;54:325–8

59. Fisher A, Waterhouse TD, Adams AP. Obesity: Its relation to anaesthesia. Anaesthesia 1975;30:633–47

60. Bentley, JB, Vaughan RW, Miller MS, et al. Serum inorganic fluoride levels in obese patients during and after enflurane anesthesia. Anesth Analg 1979;58:409–12

61. Cork RC, Vaughan RW, Bentley JB. General anesthesia for morbidly obese patients—an examination of postoperative outcomes. Anesthesiology 1981;54:310–3

62. Bentley JB, Vaughan RW, Gandolfi AJ, Cork RC.

Halothane biotransformation in obese and nonobese patients. Anesthesiology 1982;57:94–7

63. Nawaf K, Stoelting RK. SGOT values following evidence of reductive biotransformation of halothane in man. Anesthesiology 1979;51:185–6

64. Hocking MP, Duerson MC, O'Leary JP, Woodward ER. Jejunoileal bypass for morbid obesity. Late follow-up in 100 cases. N Engl J Med 1983;308:995–9

65. Vaughan RW, Baker S, Wise L. Volume and pH of gastric juice in obese patients. Anesthesiology 1975;43:686–9

66. Wilson SL, Mantena NR, Salverson JD. Effects of atropine, glycopyrrolate, and cimetidine on gastric secretions in morbidly obese patients. Anesth Analg 1981;60:37–40

67. Salem MR, Dald FY, Zygmunt MP, et al. Does PEEP improve intraoperative arterial oxygenation in grossly obese patients? Anesthesiology 1978;48:280–1

68. Vaughan RW, Wise, L. Postoperative arterial blood gas measurements in obese patients: Effect of position on gas exchange. Ann Surg 1975;182:705–9

69. Rochester DF, Enson V. Current concepts in the pathogenesis of the obesity-hypoventilation syndrome. Am J Med 1974;57:402–20

70. Rapoport DM, Sorkin B, Garay SM, Goldring RM. Reversal of the "Pickwickian syndrome" by longterm use of nocturnal nasal-airway pressure. N Engl J Med 1982;307:931–3

71. Steffee WP. Malnutrition in hospitalized patients. JAMA 1980;244:2640–5

72. Bassili HR, Deitel M. Nutritional support in longterm intensive care with special reference to ventilator patients: A review. Can Anaesth Soc J 1981;28:17–20

73. Gold PW, Kaye W, Robertson GL, Ebert M. Abnormalities in plasma and cerebrospinal-fluid arginine vasopressin in patients with anorexia nervosa. N Engl J Med 1983;308:1117–23

74. Donley AJ, Kemple TJ. Spontaneous pneumomediastinum complicating anorexia nervosa. Br Med J 1978;2:1604–5

75. Miletich DJ, Albrecht RF, Seals C. Responses to fasting and lipid infusion of epinephrine-induced dysrhythmias during halothane anesthesia. Anesthesiology 1978;48:245–9

76. Powell-Tuck J, Goode AW. Principles of enteral and parenteral nutrition. Br J Anaesth 1981;53:169–80

77. Michel L, Serrano A, Malt RA. Nutritional support of hospitalized patients. N Engl J Med 1981;304:1147–52

78. Askanazi J, Nordenstrom J, Rosenbaum SH, et al. Nutrition for the patient with respiratory failure: Glucose vs. fat. Anesthesiology 1981;54:373–7

79. Traymor C, Hall GM. Endocrine and metabolic changes during surgery: Anaesthetic implications. Br J Anaesth 1981;53:153–60

80. Arieff AI. Hyponatremia, convulsions, respiratory arrest, and permanent brain damage after elective surgery in healthy women. N Engl J Med 1986;314:1529–35

81. Engquist A, Brandt MR, Fernandes A, Kehlet H. The blocking effect of epidural analgesia on the adrenocortical and hyperglycaemic responses to surgery. Acta Anaesthesiol Scand 1977;21:330–5

82. Bovill JG, Sebel PS, Fiolet JWT, et al. The influence of sufentanil on endocrine and metabolic responses to cardiac surgery. Anesth Analg 1983;62:391–7

83. Roizen MF, Horrigan RW, Frazer BM. Anesthetic doses blocking adrenergic (stress) and cardiovascular responses to incision-MAC BAR. Anesthesiology 1981;54:390–8

84. Pflug AE, Halter JB. Effect of spinal anesthesia on adrenergic tone and the neuroendocrine responses to surgical stress in humans. Anesthesiology 1981;55:120–6

25

Anemia

Anemia is a numerical deficiency of erythrocytes caused by either too rapid loss or too slow production of the cells. As a result, numerical concentrations of hemoglobin are reduced and the oxygen carrying capacity of blood is decreased. Indeed, the most important adverse effect of anemia is reduced oxygen delivery to peripheral tissues. A history of decreased exercise tolerance, often characterized as exertional dyspnea, is a frequent clinical sign of chronic anemia. A functional heart murmur and evidence of cardiomegaly may be detected during performance of the physical examination.

Assessment of erythrocyte production can be made from the reticulocyte count in peripheral blood. For example, low reticulocyte count in the presence of a low hematocrit suggests an erythrocyte production defect, rather than blood loss or hemolysis, as a cause of anemia. Bone marrow examination may be indicated if an erythrocyte production defect is suspected. Decreases in hematocrit that exceed 1 percent·day^{-1} can be explained only by acute blood loss or intravascular hemolysis. In chronic blood loss, patients often cannot absorb sufficient iron from the gastrointestinal tract to form hemoglobin as rapidly as erythrocytes are lost. As a result, erythrocytes are produced with too little hemoglobin, giving rise to microcytic hypochromic anemia.

ARTERIAL OXYGEN CONTENT

Calculation of arterial oxygen content is important for appreciating the impact of re-ductions in hemoglobin concentrations on tissue oxygen availability (Table 25-1). For example, in the presence of normal concentrations of hemoglobin and arterial oxygen partial pressures, the oxygen content of arterial blood is about 20 ml·dl^{-1}. Reductions in the concentration of hemoglobin from 15 g·dl^{-1} to 10 g·dl^{-1} results in a 33 percent decrease in the arterial content of oxygen. Conversely, increasing the arterial partial pressure of oxygen above 100 mmHg has a minor impact on increasing the arterial content of oxygen.

Normal arterial-to-venous content differences for oxygen in blood are 5 ml·dl^{-1}, reflecting the basal oxygen use of peripheral tissues. When tissue oxygen consumption remains unchanged, arterial-to-venous differences for oxygen vary directly with cardiac output. For example, reductions in cardiac output result in increased arterial-to-venous differences for oxygen, reflecting the need for peripheral tissues to extract the same amount of oxygen from a decreased total blood flow.

COMPENSATION FOR CHRONIC ANEMIA

Compensation for the decreased oxygen carrying capacity of arterial blood that occurs in the presence of chronic anemia is accomplished by a shift to the right of the oxyhemoglobin dissociation curve (Fig. 25-1) and an increase in the cardiac output. This shift of the

557

TABLE 25-1. Calculation of Arterial
Content of Oxygen

CaO_2	= $(Hb \times 1.39)Sat + PaO_2(0.003)$
CaO_2	= arterial content of oxygen, $ml \cdot dl^{-1}$
Hb	= hemoglobin, $g \cdot dl^{-1}$
1.39	= oxygen bound to hemoglobin, $ml \cdot g^{-1}$
Sat	= saturation of hemoglobin with oxygen, %
PaO_2	= arterial partial pressure of oxygen, mmHg
0.003	= dissolved oxygen, $ml \cdot mmHg^{-1} \cdot dl^{-1}$
Example	Hb = 15 $g \cdot dl^{-1}$, Sat 100%, PaO_2 100 mmHg
	CaO_2 = $(15 \times 1.39)100 + 100(0.003)$
	CaO_2 = 20.85 + 0.3
	CaO_2 = 21.15 $ml \cdot dl^{-1}$
Example	Hb = 10 $g \cdot dl^{-1}$, Sat 100%, PaO_2 100 mmHg
	CaO_2 = $(10 \times 1.39)100 + 100(0.003)$
	CaO_2 = 13.9 + 0.3
	CaO_2 = 14.2 $ml \cdot dl^{-1}$
Example	Hb = 10 $g \cdot dl^{-1}$, Sat 100%, PaO_2 100 mmHg
	CaO_2 = $(10 \times 1.39)100 + 100(0.003)$
	CaO_2 = 13.9 + 0.3
	CaO_2 = 14.2 $ml \cdot dl^{-1}$
Example	Hb = 10 $g \cdot dl^{-1}$, Sat 100%, PaO_2 500 mmHg
	CaO_2 = $(10 \times 1.39)100 + 500(0.003)$
	CaO_2 = 13.9 + 1.5
	CaO_2 = 15.4 $ml \cdot dl^{-1}$

curve is due in part to increased concentrations of 2,3-diphosphoglycerate in erythrocytes. A shift to the right of the oxyhemoglobin dissociation curve facilitates release of oxygen from hemoglobin to tissues at higher arterial oxygen partial pressures and reduces the need for increases in cardiac output (Fig. 25-1). An increased P_{50} value from a normal of about 26 mmHg confirms a rightward shift of the oxyhemoglobin dissociation curve. Increases in cardiac output as a compensatory mechanism to maintain tissue oxygen delivery becomes increasingly important when hemoglobin concentrations are less than 9 $g \cdot dl^{-1}$. In addition, decreases in viscosity of blood, due to decreased concentrations of erythrocytes, contribute to increases in tissue blood flow. Furthermore, when oxygen delivery to peripheral tissues is inadequate, the kidneys release erythropoietin, which subsequently stimulates erythroid precursors in the bone marrow to produce additional erythrocytes. Fatigue and decreased exercise tolerance reflect the inability of cardiac output to increase further and maintain tissue oxygenation when anemic patients become physically active.

CHRONIC ANEMIA AND THE MANAGEMENT OF ANESTHESIA

Minimum acceptable hemoglobin concentrations that should be present before proceeding with elective surgery cannot be stated. Although concentrations of 10 $g \cdot dl^{-1}$ are frequently used as a guideline, there is no evidence that significant hazards are introduced when surgery is performed in the presence of hemoglobin values below this level.[1,2] The decision to proceed with surgery in the presence of low hemoglobin concentrations must be individualized, taking into consideration the urgency of the surgery, etiology of the anemia, and ability of the cardiovascular system to compensate for the decreased arterial oxygen content. Preoperative transfusion of erythrocytes (i.e., packed erythrocytes) can be used to increase hemoglobin concentrations, but it should be remembered that about 24 hours are necessary to restore intravascular fluid volume and blood viscosity. Compared with a similar volume of whole blood, erythrocytes produce about twice the increase in hemoglobin concentration.

If elective surgery is performed in the presence of chronic anemia, it would seem prudent to minimize the likelihood of changes that could interfere with tissue oxygen delivery. For example, decreases in myocardial contractility as produced by volatile drugs may reduce cardiac output and thus impair an important compensatory mechanism. Likewise, shifts to the left of the oxyhemoglobin dissociation curve, as produced by hyperventilation of the lungs and resulting respiratory alkalosis, can impair release of oxygen from hemoglobin to the tissues (Fig. 25-1). Maintenance of body temperature in the perioperative period is important, since hypothermia also shifts the ox-

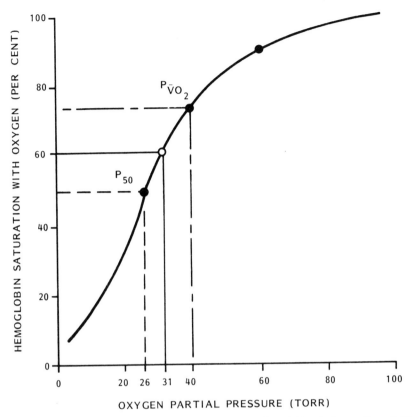

FIG. 25-1. The oxyhemoglobin dissociation curve describes the relation between the saturation of hemoglobin with oxygen and the partial pressures of oxygen. The arterial partial pressures of oxygen at which hemoglobin saturation with oxygen is 50 percent is designated the P_{50}. In the presence of a normal pH (7.4) and body temperature (37 degrees Celsius), the P_{50} is about 26 mmHg. An increase to 31 mmHg reflects a shift to the right of the curve and decreased affinity of hemoglobin for oxygen. This means that oxygen can be released from hemoglobin to peripheral tissues at higher arterial oxygen partial pressures. Events that shift the curve to the right and thus facilitate availability of oxygen to peripheral tissues include increased levels of 2,3-diphosphoglycerate in erythrocytes, acidosis, and elevations of body temperature. Opposite changes move the curve to the left, reflecting increased affinity of hemoglobin for oxygen. This increased affinity will impair release of oxygen from hemoglobin to peripheral tissues. Normal venous blood has oxygen partial pressures (PvO_2) near 40 mmHg and associated saturation of hemoglobin of about 75 percent. Saturation of hemoglobin with oxygen is about 90 percent when the arterial partial pressures of oxygen are 60 mmHg. Oxygen saturation of hemoglobin can be considered to be 100 percent when the arterial partial pressures of oxygen are 100 mmHg or greater.

yhemoglobin dissociation curve to the left. It should be appreciated that inhaled anesthetics may be less soluble in blood deficient in lipid rich erythrocytes.[3,4] As a result, establishment of arterial partial pressures of these drugs in anemic patients might be accelerated. Nevertheless, the effect of decreased solubility of inhaled anesthetic drugs in blood due to anemia is probably offset by the impact of increased

cardiac output. Therefore, it seems unlikely that clinically detectable differences in the rate of induction of anesthesia or vulnerability to overdoses of inhaled anesthetics would occur in anemic patients, as compared with patients having normal hemoglobin concentrations. Hemodynamic responses to volatile anesthetics, as reflected by measurements in chronically anemic animals, are characterized by a higher

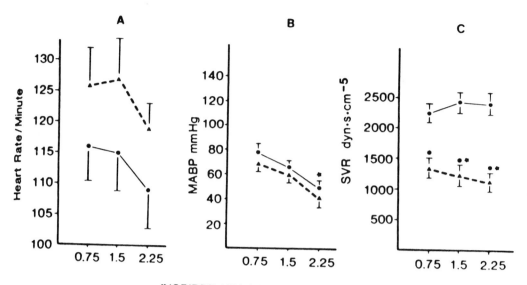

FIG. 25-2. Hemodynamic effects of increasing doses of halothane were determined in chronically anemic (hemoglobin 3.4 g·dl⁻¹, broken lines) and normal (hemoglobin 13.7 g·dl⁻¹, solid lines) dogs. Heart rate and mean arterial blood pressure (MABP) were not significantly different between anemic and control animals. Anemic dogs showed a significantly lower systemic vascular resistance (SVR) at each dose of halothane when compared with controls. (Barrera M, Miletich DJ, Albrecht RF, Hoffman WE. Hemodynamic consequences of halothane anesthesia during chronic anemia. Anesthesiology 1984;61:36–42)

heart rate, lower systemic vascular resistance, and unchanged mean arterial pressure when compared with normal animals (Fig. 25-2).[5] Intraoperative blood loss should be promptly replaced with whole blood or erythrocytes when there is co-existing anemia. Finally, in the postoperative period, it is important to minimize the occurrence of shivering or increases in body temperature, since these changes can greatly increase total body oxygen requirements.

ACUTE BLOOD LOSS

Sites of acute blood loss leading to anemia are usually obvious. On occasion, however, the site may not be apparent, as in the presence of an ectopic pregnancy, fracture of the femur, or bleeding from an abdominal aortic aneurysm.

TABLE 25-2. Clinical Signs Associated with Acute Blood Loss

Percent of Blood Volume Lost	Clinical Signs
10	None
20–30	Orthostatic hypotension
	Tachycardia
40	Tachycardia
	Hypotension
	Tachypnea
	Diaphoresis

Signs and Symptoms

Signs and symptoms of anemia due to acute blood loss depend on the percent of the total blood volume that is lost (Table 25-2).[1] Typically, when 20 percent or more of the blood volume is lost, clinical signs include orthostatic hypotension, tachycardia and low central venous pressure. Hematocrit may not reflect anemia due to acute blood loss, since mechanisms for restoring plasma volume operate slowly. For example, after acute hemorrhage, the body replaces plasma in 1 day to 3 days, whereas production of erythrocytes to restore hemoglobin concentrations to normal may require 3 weeks to 4 weeks. A peripheral blood smear is of no value in the diagnosis. The obvious treatment of anemia due to acute blood loss is correction of the cause leading to hemorrhage and prompt restoration of intravascular fluid volume with erythrocytes plus colloid and·or crystalloid solutions.

Shock

Hemorrhagic shock is a potential complication of acute blood loss. The fundamental defect in hemorrhagic shock is decreased intravascular fluid volume, leading to decreased cardiac output and inadequate tissue perfusion. Although myocardial contractility ultimately decreases, it does not appear that cardiac failure is prominent even in early hemorrhagic shock. During hemorrhage, there are increases in sympathetic nervous system activity, which are beneficial in redirecting blood flow to the brain and heart. Prolonged increases in sympathetic nervous system activity, however, with associated arteriolar vasoconstriction, result in detrimental reductions in renal and splanchnic blood flow, as reflected by reductions in urine output. Furthermore, there is an increase in anaerobic metabolism in tissues, which manifests as metabolic (lactic) acidosis.

Treatment of hemorrhagic shock is with infusion of whole blood. Crystalloid solutions are also indicated, since interstitial fluid shifts accompany acute hemorrhage. Vasopressors should be used sparingly in the treatment of hemorrhagic shock; however, it may be necessary to support cerebral and cardiac perfusion pressures with vasopressors until intravascular fluid volume can be replaced. Dopamine in low doses (usually less than 5 $\mu g \cdot kg^{-1} \cdot min^{-1}$) is a useful drug when goals of therapy include a mild inotropic effect plus increased renal blood flow. Persistent metabolic acidosis is almost always an indication of inadequate intravascular fluid volume replacement.

Induction and maintenance of anesthesia in the presence of hemorrhagic shock often includes administration of ketamine. Use of ketamine is supported by the known ability of this drug to stimulate the sympathetic nervous system and a study in which evidence of tissue ischemia was less and survival was greater in acutely hemorrhaged rats anesthetized with ketamine as compared with volatile anesthetics.[6] Nevertheless, other animal evidence suggests that ketamine, in contrast to volatile anesthetics, is associated with inadequate tissue perfusion, as reflected by the development of metabolic acidosis.[7] Clinically, adverse metabolic effects of ketamine may be offset by the benefit of maintaining perfusion pressure to vital organs until intravascular fluid volume can be restored.

CHRONIC BLOOD LOSS

Iron deficiency anemia due to persistent blood loss is the most frequent form of chronic anemia. Hemoglobin synthesis is impaired when iron deficiency is severe. Resulting iron deficiency anemia is usually mild, with hemoglobin values ranging from 9 $g \cdot dl^{-1}$ to 10 $g \cdot dl^{-1}$. Iron therapy should increase hemoglobin concentrations 2 $g \cdot dl^{-1}$ in 3 weeks or restore hemoglobin concentration to normal in 6 weeks. Clinical symptoms of a chronic anemia depend on the hemoglobin concentration (Table 25-3).[1]

In adults, iron deficiency anemia typically reflects depletion of body iron stores due to chronic blood loss, either from the gastroin-

TABLE 25-3. Clinical Symptoms of Chronic Anemia

Hemoglobin Concentration ($g \cdot dl^{-1}$)	Clinical Symptoms
9–10	Tachycardia
	Pallor
7–8	Dyspnea or exertion
5–6	Weakness
Less than 5	Dyspnea at rest
	Congestive heart failure

testinal tract or from the female genital tract during menstruation. Pregnant women are prone to development of iron deficiency anemia because of the increased erythrocyte mass present during gestation plus needs of the fetus for iron. Young children have increased demands for erythrocyte production during periods of rapid growth, when dietary deficiencies of iron introduces the likelihood of iron deficiency anemia. In contrast, dietary deficiencies of iron may contribute to iron deficiency anemia in adults but are rarely the primary cause.

CHRONIC DISEASES AND IRON DEFICIENCY

Persistent infections, neoplastic processes, connective tissue disorders, and renal and hepatic disease are examples of disease states often associated with chronic anemia. Anemia is typically due to a lack of sufficient iron for new erythropoiesis. Management of anemia due to chronic diseases requires treatment of the underlying disorders.

Renal Disease

Chronic renal disease results in a severe form of anemia. Hemoglobin concentrations are often in the range of 5 $g \cdot dl^{-1}$ to 8 $g \cdot dl^{-1}$. Deficiency of erythropoietin production is the primary problem. This decreased production may be due to reduced renal mass or to an inability of diseased kidneys to produce adequate amounts of erythropoietin in response to increased demand. Inhibitors of erythropoiesis present in plasma and urine of uremic patients may also contribute to anemia. Finally, uremic toxins result in decreased erythrocyte life spans. Anemia of chronic renal failure improves with dietary supplementation and hemodialysis.

Liver Disease

Anemia in the presence of liver disease can reflect alcohol-induced inhibition of erythrocyte production, dietary deficiency of folic acid, or chronic blood loss due to gastritis. In addition, congestive splenomegaly associated with chronic cirrhosis of the liver is associated with hemolysis of erythrocytes. Zieve's syndrome is acute hemolysis, jaundice, and hyperlipidemia in the presence of fatty infiltration of the liver due to alcohol abuse.

APLASTIC ANEMIA

Aplastic anemia refers to bone marrow failure characterized by destruction of rapidly growing cells normally present in the marrow. Pancytopenia is the most frequent presentation. The most common etiology is destruction of bone marrow stem cells by cancer chemotherapeutic drugs. This form of bone marrow depression usually responds to removal of the offending drug and supportive treatment with transfusions of erythrocytes until surviving stem cells can repopulate the bone marrow. Other causes of aplastic anemia, which are less responsive to this treatment, include solvents, radiation, viral infections, and immunologic disorders. Chloramphenicol causes aplastic anemia in approximately 1 of every 10,000 to 20,000 treated patients, possibly reflecting a unique genetic susceptibility. Bone marrow transplantation as treatment of aplastic anemia may be considered in selected patients (see Chapter 30).

Variations

Variations of aplastic anemia occur in pediatric patients. For example, Fanconi's syndrome is congenital aplastic anemia plus numerous associated anomalies, including patchy hyperpigmentation, microcephaly, exaggerated tendon reflexes, strabismus, and short stature. Defects of the bones of the radial sides of the forearm and hand are frequent. Cleft palate may be present. Cardiac defects and abnormalities of the genitourinary tract have been observed. There is an increased incidence of malignancy in these patients. Treatment of Fanconi's syndrome is with erythrocytes, corticosteroids, and androgens.

Diamond-Blackfan syndrome is a form of pure erythrocyte aplasia, which presents as severe anemia in the first few months of life. Leukocyte and platelet production is normal. Anomalies associated with this syndrome include neck webbing and abnormalities of the first digit of the hand. These infants are treated with erythrocytes and corticosteroids. Splenectomy may be required for patients resistant to corticosteroids. An infant form of erythrocyte aplasia is associated with thymomas and myasthenia gravis.[8] This association may reflect an immunologic mechanism or the presence of erythropoietic inhibitory factors. Thymectomy will cure about 30 percent of patients with this form of anemia.

Management of Anesthesia

Management of anesthesia for patients with aplastic anemia requires an understanding of the disease process and the drugs being used in its treatment.[9] For example, supplementation with corticosteroids may be necessary in the perioperative period. Anemia may be profound, requiring transfusions of erythrocytes before the induction of anesthesia. Vulnerability of these patients to infections in the presence of pancytopenia must be appreciated, and care must be taken to avoid iatrogenic infections from equipment used during the perioperative period. Thrombocytopenia introduces the risk of hemorrhage with even minor trauma. Intubation of the trachea should be performed when indicated, but it must be appreciated that excessive trauma associated with this procedure could produce hemorrhage in the airway. Choice of drugs used to produce anesthesia is not influenced by the presence of aplastic anemia, although the possible depres-

sant effects of nitrous oxide on bone marrow are a consideration. Maintenance of arterial oxygen partial pressures near 100 mmHg and avoidance of anesthetic-induced reductions in cardiac output are important goals during anesthesia to assure optimal tissue oxygenation.

MEGALOBLASTIC ANEMIA

Megaloblastic anemias are most often due to deficiencies of vitamin B_{12} or folic acid. Both of these vitamins must be supplied by the diet, as neither is produced in adequate amounts by intrinsic synthesis. These vitamin deficiencies are reflected in peripheral blood smears as macrocytic anemia with hypersegmented polymorphonuclear leukocytes and large platelets.

Vitamin B_{12} Deficiency

Vitamin B_{12} is released from ingested proteins in the stomach by enzymatic proteolysis. Absorption of released B_{12} is dependent on a glycoprotein produced by the gastric parietal cells. This glycoprotein is known as intrinsic factor. Malabsorption of B_{12} from the small intestine, due to disease or surgical resection, is the usual cause of vitamin B_{12} deficiency. In addition, atrophy of the gastric mucosa, presumably due to an autoimmune response, results in the absence of intrinsic factor and subsequent inability to absorb vitamin B_{12}. Pernicious anemia refers to megaloblastic anemia that reflects B_{12} deficiency due to atrophy of the gastric mucosa and subsequent lack of intrinsic factor. Demonstration of decreased plasma B_{12} concentrations confirms the diagnosis of pernicious anemia.

PERIPHERAL NEUROPATHY

In addition to megaloblastic anemia, deficiency of vitamin B_{12} is associated with a bilateral peripheral neuropathy due to degeneration of the lateral and posterior columns of the spinal cord. There are symmetrical paresthesias with loss of proprioceptive and vibratory sensations, especially in the lower extremities. Gait is unsteady and deep tendon reflexes are diminished. These neurologic deficits are progressive unless parenteral vitamin B_{12} is provided.

MANAGEMENT OF ANESTHESIA

Management of anesthesia in patients with megaloblastic anemia due to vitamin B_{12} deficiency must consider the need to maintain delivery of oxygenated arterial blood to peripheral tissues. Presence of neurologic changes may detract from selection of regional anesthetic techniques or use of peripheral nerve blocks. Use of nitrous oxide is questionable, since this drug has been shown to inhibit activity of methionine synthetase by oxidizing the cobalt atom of vitamin B_{12} from an active to inactive state.[10] Indeed, prolonged inhalation of nitrous oxide results in megaloblastic anemia and neurologic changes indistinguishable from pernicious anemia[11-13] (see Chapter 31).

Folic Acid Deficiency

Folic acid deficiency is the most common of the vitamin deficiencies. Since folic acid is essential for maturation of erythrocytes, it is not surprising that megaloblastic anemia develops when there is dietary deficiency of this vitamin. Manifestations of folic acid deficiency include a smooth tongue, hyperpigmentation, and peripheral edema. Peripheral neuropathy may or may not accompany these changes. Liver dysfunction frequently occurs. Severely ill patients, alcoholics, and pregnant women are most likely to develop megaloblastic anemia due to deficiencies of folic acid in the diet. Phenytoin and other anticonvulsant drugs, including barbiturates, are on rare occasions associated with megaloblastic anemia, presumably reflecting impaired gastrointestinal absorption of folate. Oral folic acid is effective

in reversing megaloblastic anemia due to deficiencies of this substance.

ANEMIA DUE TO HEMOLYSIS

Anemia due to intravascular hemolysis of erythrocytes is characterized by rapid reductions in the hematocrit and elevated plasma concentrations of bilirubin. Normal erythrocyte survival time of 90 days to 120 days is greatly shortened in patients with hemolytic anemia. Peripheral blood smears reveal increased numbers of reticulocytes. Causes of hemolysis include abnormalities of erythrocyte membranes, enzyme defects, and alterations in the normal structure of hemoglobin. These changes make erythrocytes fragile so that they rupture easily as they pass through capillaries, especially in the spleen. Therefore, even though the number of erythrocytes formed is normal, the life span is so shortened by intravascular hemolysis that anemia results.

Hereditary Spherocytosis

Hereditary spherocytosis is characterized by abnormalities of erythrocyte membranes that allows sodium to enter erythrocytes at enhanced rates.[13] Water also enters erythrocytes, resulting in swollen or spherocytic cells. These spherical cells, in contrast to normal biconcave erythrocytes, cannot be compressed and are vulnerable to rupture (hemolysis) with even slight compression as they pass through the spleen. Anemia, reticulocytosis, and mild jaundice are characteristic expressions of hereditary spherocytosis. Anemia and hyperbilirubinemia may be manifestations of this disease in neonates. Children with this defect may present with chronic mild anemia plus episodic falls in hematocrit, particularly during bacterial infections. Elderly patients who have previously been able to compensate may develop anemia as the ability to produce erythrocytes declines with age. Cholelithiasis secondary to chronic hemolysis and elevation of plasma bilirubin concentrations is frequent in patients with hereditary spherocytosis.

Treatment of patients with hereditary spherocytosis includes splenectomy if anemia is severe. Splenectomy greatly reduces hemolysis, returning erythrocyte survival to 80 percent of normal. Splenectomy, however, may be followed by an increased incidence of bacterial infections (especially pneumococcal) in these patients. Prophylactic pneumococcal vaccine may be indicated for these patients.

Paroxysmal Nocturnal Hemoglobinuria

Paroxysmal nocturnal hemoglobinuria is characterized by acute episodes of hemolysis superimposed on a background of chronic hemolysis. The defect is an abnormal sensitivity of erythrocyte membranes to destruction by complement proteins. The peak incidence of this disease is in young adults. Clinical manifestations are variable and consist primarily of anemia, neutropenia, and jaundice. Classically, patients note hemoglobinuria on first voiding after awakening. Anemia is frequently so severe that patients need transfusions of erythrocytes. There is an increased risk of thrombosis involving the hepatic, splenic, portal, and cerebral veins. Surgery with associated stasis and trauma may accentuate hemolysis and thrombosis. Prophylactic anticoagulation should be considered in the postoperative period.

Glucose-6-Phosphate Dehydrogenase Deficiency

Glucose-6-phosphate dehydrogenase deficiency is the most common of the inherited erythrocyte enzyme disorders.[14] Indeed, this deficiency affects about 8 percent of black male adults in the United States. Patients with this deficiency have chronic hemolytic anemia of varying severity. Drugs that form peroxides by

TABLE 25-4. Drugs Which May Induce Hemolysis in Patients with Glucose-6-Phosphate Dehydrogenase Deficiency

Nonopioid Analgesics or Antipyretics
  Phenacetin
  Acetaminophen

Antibiotics
  Nitrofurans
  Penicillin
  Streptomycin
  Chloramphenicol
  Isoniazid

Sulfonamides

Antimalarials

Miscellaneous
  Probenecid
  Quinidine
  Vitamin K analogs
  Methylene blue
  Nitroprusside (?)

interaction with oxyhemoglobin can trigger hemolysis in these patients (Table 25-4). Normally, these peroxides are inactivated by nicotinamide-adenine dinucleotide phosphate and glutathione, which are ordinarily produced via metabolic processes dependent on glucose-6-phosphate dehydrogenase enzyme activity. Although drugs used during anesthesia have not been incriminated as triggering agents, the onset of hemolysis and jaundice in the early postoperative period, particularly in black men, should suggest this diagnosis.[15]

Pyruvate Kinase Deficiency

Pyruvate kinase deficiency is the most common of the enzyme defects in the anaerobic glycolytic pathway of erythrocytes. The result of this enzyme deficiency is erythrocyte membranes that are highly permeable to potassium and susceptible to rupture, as evidenced by hemolytic anemia. There is accumulation of 2,3-diphosphoglycerate in these erythrocytes, causing a shift of the oxyhemoglobin dissociation curve to the right and facilitation of oxygen release from hemoglobin to peripheral tissues. Splenectomy does not prevent hemolysis but does serve to reduce greatly the rate of erythrocyte destruction. Despite increased permeability of erythrocyte membranes to potassium, the administration of succinylcholine has not been associated with hyperkalemia.

Immune Hemolytic Anemias

Immune hemolytic anemias are characterized by immunologic alterations of erythrocyte membranes. An important aspect of the evaluation of patients with suspected immune hemolytic anemias is performance of the Coombs' test. Coombs' antiserum is an antibody to human immunoglobulin G. The direct Coombs' test is the addition of antiserum to a sample of blood from the patient. The indirect Coombs' test is the addition of antiserum to a sample of plasma from the patient, to which has been added a sample of erythrocytes of known antigenicity. Clumping of erythrocytes in response to addition of antiserum indicates the presence of antibodies to erythrocytes and is designated as a positive direct or indirect Coombs' test. Immune hemolytic anemia may be due to drugs, diseases, or sensitization of erythrocytes.

DRUG-INDUCED HEMOLYSIS

Alpha-methyldopa causes a time- and dose-dependent production of immunoglobulin G antibodies, which are directed against Rh antigens on the surfaces of erythrocytes. Indeed, a positive direct Coombs' test is often present in patients being treated with alpha-methyldopa, but hemolysis occurs in less than 1 percent of patients receiving this drug. The mechanism for drug-induced stimulation of antibody production by alpha-methyldopa is unknown. Treatment is withdrawal of the drug, which results in rapid increases in hemoglobin concentrations, although the direct Coombs' test may remain positive for as long as 2 years.

High-dose penicillin therapy can also lead to hemolysis, by attaching to erythrocytes to form haptens that lead to production of anti-

bodies. Levodopa is another drug that occasionally produces an autoimmune hemolytic anemia. Finally, some drugs can cause hemolysis by stimulating production of antibodies that activate the complement system.

DISEASE-INDUCED HEMOLYSIS

Hypersplenism is an example of a disease process that can be associated with hemolysis, anemia, leukopenia, and thrombocytopenia. It is thought that an enlarged spleen has an increased blood flow and vascular surface area, which exposes an unusually large proportion of erythrocytes and platelets to attack by phagocytes. For unknown reasons, hypersplenism produces marked increases in plasma volume, which result in dilutional anemia in addition to hemolytic anemia. Splenectomy may be necessary when anemia due to hemolysis is severe. If thrombocytopenia is present, it may be desirable to infuse platelets intraoperatively, after the splenic pedicle has been surgically clamped.

SENSITIZATION OF ERYTHROCYTES

Sensitization of erythrocytes most often manifests as hemolytic disease of the newborn (erythroblastosis fetalis). Hemolysis of fetal erythrocytes occurs when maternal antibodies against fetal erythrocytes are produced and cross the placenta. Differences in the maternal and fetal ABO blood groups can cause this form of hemolysis. Severe anemia, however, does not usually occur because ABO antibodies are of the immunoglobin M class, and as such do not readily cross the placenta. More often, maternal development of antibodies to Rh antigens occurs after delivery of an Rh-positive infant. During subsequent pregnancies, erythrocytes of an Rh-positive fetus may undergo significant hemolysis from maternal antibodies directed against Rh antigens. The incidence of the development of maternal anti-Rh antibodies has decreased to less than 1 percent since the introduction of Rh-immune globulin (RhoGAM). This substance, when given to the mother within 72 hours of delivery, destroys fetal erythrocytes in the maternal circulation and thus prevents subsequent development of sensitization.

Clinical features of hemolytic disease of the newborn are related to anemia and hyperbilirubinemia. The fetus can be examined indirectly during gestation by periodic measurement of bilirubin levels in amniotic fluid samples. A fetus determined to be experiencing severe hemolysis may require intrauterine transfusion or induced delivery. Hemolysis may continue after delivery, requiring transfusion of the infant with erythrocytes. In addition, exchange transfusions of blood may be necessary to reduce plasma levels of bilirubin in the newborn. Eventually, maternal immunoglobulins against Rh antigens are excreted by the newborn, and hemolysis of the erythrocytes ceases.

Sickle Cell Disease

Sickle cell disease represents an inherited group of disorders, ranging in severity from the usually benign sickle cell trait to the debilitating and often fatal sickle cell anemia.[16] All the variants of sickle cell disease share in the possession of various quantities of hemoglobin S. Hemoglobin S differs from normal adult hemoglobin A by the substitution of valine for glutamic acid at the sixth position on the beta chain of hemoglobin molecules. Confirmation of the presence of hemoglobin S is dependent on electrophoretic studies.

SICKLE CELL TRAIT

Sickle cell trait is the heterozygote manifestation of sickle cell disease containing the hemoglobin genotype AS. Erythrocytes of patients with the sickle cell trait contain 20 percent to 40 percent hemoglobin S, with the remainder being hemoglobin A. The incidence among the black population of the United States is about 10 percent. Affected individuals are usually asymptomatic.

SICKLE CELL ANEMIA

Sickle cell anemia is present when patients are homozygous for hemoglobin S. Approximately 0.3 percent to 1.0 percent of the black population in the United States are homozygous for hemoglobin S. In the homozygous state, 70 percent to 98 percent of hemoglobin is the S type, resulting in severe hemolytic anemia.

PATHOPHYSIOLOGY

Deoxygenated forms of hemoglobin S result in deformation of erythrocytes into sickle shapes. Molecularly, the substitution of valine for glutamic acid provides two reactive sites when hemoglobin S releases oxygen. As a result, hemoglobin S molecules tend to bond with each other at these reactive sites, forming long aggregates or tactoids. Tactoids of sickle cells increase the viscosity of blood, leading to stasis of blood flow. An infarctive crisis occurs when localized or generalized vascular occlusion occurs due to formation of sickle cells. In addition, low oxygen concentrations cause hemoglobin S to precipitate into long crystals inside erythrocytes, causing cells to assume a sickle rather than biconcave shape. This precipitated hemoglobin damages erythrocyte membranes, leading to their rupture and chronic hemolytic anemia.

Formation of sickle cells is exaggerated by low oxygen partial pressures. Arterial oxygen partial pressures below 40 mmHg are likely to result in formation of sickle cells in patients who are homozygous for hemoglobin S. Sickling of erythrocytes in patients with sickle cell trait probably does not occur until arterial oxygen partial pressures decrease to about 20 mmHg. Formation of sickle cells tends to be greater in veins than in arteries, emphasizing the importance of pH. Indeed, the presence of acidosis favors the formation of sickle cells, regardless of prevailing oxygen partial pressures. Reduction in body temperature also promotes formation of sickle cells by virtue of vasoconstriction, which leads to stasis of blood flow and deoxygenation of hemoglobin S. Likewise, dehydration and resulting stasis of blood flow favor formation of sickle cells.

Sickle cells may undergo retransformation to biconcave forms upon oxygenation if cellular metabolic processes controlling membrane rigidity have not been irreversibly altered. Nevertheless, variable numbers of erythrocytes in the circulation of patients with sickle cell anemia remain irreversibly in the sickle state.

CLINICAL MANIFESTATIONS

Clinical manifestations of sickle cell anemia are those of infarctive events due to occlusion of blood vessels with sickle cells and anemia due to hemolysis. These chronic events are periodically interrupted by acute exacerbations of the disease. In the steady state, hemoglobin concentrations are 5 $g \cdot dl^{-1}$ to 10 $g \cdot dl^{-1}$. Cardiac output is generally increased, in compensation for the prevailing chronic anemia. Furthermore, the oxyhemoglobin dissociation curve for hemoglobin S is shifted to the right (P_{50} about 31 mmHg), reflecting increased erythrocyte concentrations of 2,3-diphosphyglycerate. This shift facilitates unloading of oxygen from hemoglobin S but also places hemoglobin S-containing erythrocytes in greater jeopardy of undergoing sickle cell formation, since the critical degree of deoxygenation is reached at higher arterial oxygen partial pressures.

Infarctive events are responsible for widespread organ damage. For example, cardiomegaly most likely reflects cor pulmonale due to repeated pulmonary emboli. Increased alveolar-to-arterial differences for oxygen are often present, presumably reflecting previous pulmonary infarctive events produced by sickle cells. Total lung capacity and vital capacity are frequently decreased. The renal medulla, because of its low oxygen partial pressures, is a frequent site of vascular occlusion with sickle cells. Infarctive events in the renal medulla lead to papillary necrosis with hematuria, impaired ability to concentrate urine, and ultimately renal failure. The liver is mildly enlarged, and has varying amounts of focal necrosis and fibrosis due to previous vascular occlusions. Chronic hemolysis of erythrocytes is reflected by elevated plasma concentrations of bilirubin. Increased bilirubin loads are associated with a high incidence of cholelithiasis. The need for periodic transfusion with erythrocytes increases the risk of viral hepatitis. In severe cases requiring frequent transfusions of erythrocytes, the resulting increased load of iron may be deposited in the liver as hemosiderin leading to cirrhosis. Left ventricular dysfunction may reflect deposition of excess iron in the heart. Splenomegaly is often present in infants with sickle cell anemia. A gradual reduction in the size of the spleen, however, occurs secondary to repeated thrombosis and infarction. Indeed, by 6 years of age most patients with sickle cell anemia are, for all practical purposes, asplenic. The absence of splenic function is associated with decreased production of antibodies and an increased risk for developing bacterial infections. Neurologic dysfunction is likely in patients with sickle cell anemia, manifesting most often as cerebral infarction in children and as intracranial hemorrhage in adults. Multiple organ dysfunction produced by infarctive events in patients with sickle cell anemia is the major reason that survival beyond 30 years of age is unlikely in these patients.

An infarctive crisis may be triggered by trauma or infection, with associated elevations in body temperature. The acute onset of pain, often abdominal in location, may signal the beginning of an infarctive crisis. Episodes of abdominal pain associated with fever and vomiting can mimic surgical disease. Treatment of a painful infarctive crisis is with hydration and mild alkalinization of the blood. Partial exchange transfusions with erythrocytes containing hemoglobin A will reduce concentrations of hemoglobin S and thus decrease the likelihood of further infarctive damage.[17] The goal of exchange transfusions is to increase hemoglobin A concentrations to at least 40 percent. Patients with sickle cell anemia are at risk for bacterial infection. Streptococcal bacteremia predominates in children less than 6 years of age.[17] In older children with sickle cell anemia, *Escherichia coli* urinary tract infections and *Salmonella* osteomyelitis often develop.

In addition to acute and chronic problems caused by infarctive events and hemolysis, patients with sickle cell anemia are susceptible to the development of aplastic and sequestration crises. Aplastic crises are characterized by bone marrow depression and are most often associated with viral infections. Sequestration crises are due to depletion of circulating erythrocytes, by virtue of pooling of these cells in the liver and spleen. Patients experiencing sequestration crises may become acutely hypovolemic and die.

MANAGEMENT OF ANESTHESIA

The possible presence of sickle cell disease must be considered in the preoperative evaluation of every black patient. Patients with sickle cell trait probably are not at increased risk during the perioperative period. Conversely, patients with sickle cell anemia must be given special consideration in the management of anesthesia.

Orthopedic conditions requiring surgical correction are frequent in patients with sickle cell anemia. For example, necrosis of the head of the femur is common. The incidence of *Salmonella* osteomyelitis is increased. Leg ulcers are often present, requiring skin grafting. Presence of gallstones is reflected by the frequent need for cholecystectomy in these patients. Priapism is a common occurrence in patients with sickle cell anemia. Cardiopulmonary bypass, with its attendant low peripheral blood flow plus hypothermia and acidosis, poses a special peril to patients with sickle cell anemia.[18]

Preoperative preparation should include correction of co-existing infections and achievement of adequate states of hydration and stable hematologic states. The need for preoperative transfusion of erythrocytes is determined by the severity of co-existing anemia and the magnitude of the planned surgery. The goal of preoperative infusion of erythrocytes is to increase the concentration of hemoglobin A to at least 40 percent. Hazards of preoperative transfusions include depression of hyperactive bone marrow and increased blood viscosity.

Goals in management of anesthesia include avoidance of acidosis due to hypoventilation of the lungs, maintenance of optimal oxygenation, prevention of circulatory stasis due to improper body positioning or use of tourniquets, and maintenance of normal body temperature. Preoperative medication must not produce excessive depression of ventilation. Concentrations of inspired oxygen should be increased to insure maintenance of normal to increased arterial oxygen partial pressures. Monitoring of mixed venous oxygen partial pressures may be helpful in recognizing patients vulnerable to developing sickle cells and in whom therapeutic measures to increase oxygenation are indicated. Administration of supplemental oxygen may be prudent if regional anesthetic techniques are selected. Prevention of circulatory stasis requires (1) maintenance of cardiovascular stability by the appropriate adjustment of the depth of anesthesia, (2) anticipation and rapid correction of hypotension, and (3) maintenance of intravascular fluid volume by intravenous infusion of crystalloid solutions. An orthopedic tourniquet is indicated only when optimal surgical results depend on its use.[19] Hazards introduced by the use of tourniquets include stasis of blood flow, acidosis, and hypoxemia, with subsequent formation of sickle cells. Overzealous transfusion of erythrocytes can lead to undesirable increases in viscosity of the blood and predispose to stasis of blood flow. Maintenance of normal body temperature is important to prevent vasoconstriction and stasis of blood flow.

There is no evidence that one anesthetic drug or combination of drugs is superior for administration to patients with sickle cell anemia. Indeed, there may be a decrease in the number of circulating sickle cells during and immediately after general anesthesia, regardless of the drugs employed.[20] Use of succinylcholine is modified by occasional occurrences of decreased plasma cholinesterase activity in these patients.[21] Regional anesthetic techniques have been advocated in preference to general anesthesia, but the same precautions regarding ventilation, oxygenation, hypotension, and stasis of blood flow must be appreciated. Regional blocks, including axillary, epidural, or subarachnoid, produce compensatory vasoconstriction and decreased arterial oxygen partial pressures in the nonblocked areas, making these areas possible sites for infarction.[22]

The postoperative period is a crucial time for patients with sickle cell anemia. Incisional pain, use of analgesics, a high incidence of pulmonary infections, and expected reductions in arterial oxygen partial pressures will all predispose to the formation of sickle cells. Depending on the operative site, arterial oxygen partial pressures may not return to preoperative levels for several days. Supplemental oxygen and maintenance of intravascular fluid volume and body temperature are important considerations.

Thalassemia

Thalassemia is a collective term used to designate a number of inherited disorders characterized by reduced rates of synthesis or failure of synthesis of structurally normal hemoglobin.[23]

BETA-THALASSEMIA

Beta-thalassemia is due to relative or absolute lack of formation of beta globulin chains of hemoglobin. As a result, normal adult hemoglobin A is not formed. Newborn infants with thalassemia, however, are initially normal, because fetal hemoglobin is composed of two alpha and two gamma chains. Thalassemia manifests as the child grows and is unable to produce hemoglobin A.

Beta-thalassemia is categorized as minor, intermedia, and major (Cooley's anemia). Patients with thalassemia minor develop a mild hypochromic and microcytic anemia but are otherwise asymptomatic. Thalassemia intermedia is associated with increased levels of hemoglobin F and decreased erythrocyte levels of 2,3-diphosphoglycerate, resulting in an anemia functionally more severe than is apparent from absolute levels of hemoglobin.

Thalassemia major is a severe form of anemia, which appears in infancy and is associated with multiple organ system changes and dysfunction. For example, increased production of erythrocytes results in characteristic skeletal changes, including cephalofacial deformities and thinning of cortical bone. Overgrowth of the maxillae can make visualization of the glottis difficult during direct laryngos-

copy. The liver is enlarged from extramedullary hematopoiesis. Deficiencies of hepatic production of procoagulants may reflect liver damage. Spinal cord compression secondary to massive extramedullary hematopoiesis and destruction of vertebral bodies can occur.[24] Splenomegaly is predictably present. Cardiac abnormalities in these patients include supraventricular cardiac dysrhythmias and pericarditis. Congestive heart failure is a frequent complication.[25] In this regard, it must be appreciated that these patients are unusually sensitive to the effects of digitalis.

Treatment of thalassemia major is with transfusion of erythrocytes to maintain hemoglobin concentrations above 9 g·dl^{-1}. The rationale for this approach is to reduce endogenous hematopoiesis and to prevent problems associated with excessive activity of the bone marrow. Chronic transfusion of erythrocytes, however, can lead to hemosiderosis, requiring concomitant treatment with drugs to chelate excess iron. Manifestations of hemosiderosis can include left ventricular dysfunction. In some patients, splenectomy may be necessary to control hemolysis and thrombocytopenia.

ALPHA-THALASSEMIA

Alpha-thalassemia is due to lack of production of alpha chains of normal adult hemoglobin. Patients who are heterozygous for alpha-thalassemia (thalassemia trait) characteristically develop mild hypochromic and microcytic anemia. On occasion, transfusion of erythrocytes or splenectomy may be necessary to control hemolysis. A homozygous genotype for alpha-thalassemia is incompatible with life, resulting in intrauterine demise or early neonatal death.

Methemoglobinemia

Methemoglobin is hemoglobin A in which iron exists in the ferric rather than normal ferrous state. The ferric form of iron is not able to bind oxygen; as a result, oxygen carrying capacity of arterial blood is greatly reduced. In addition to an inability to combine reversibly with oxygen, methemoglobin shifts the oxyhemoglobin dissociation curve to the left, making it more difficult for hemoglobin to release oxygen to tissues. Normally, some iron in hemoglobin exists in the ferric state, but methemoglobin concentrations do not become excessive because of the presence of methemoglobin reductase enzyme. Congenital absence of this enzyme may predispose to the development of methemoglobinemia in patients being treated with nitrate-containing compounds such as nitroglycerin.[26-28]

Methemoglobinemia is suggested by cyanosis in the presence of adequate arterial oxygen partial pressures and low measured saturations of hemoglobin with oxygen. It must be appreciated that calculation of arterial oxygen saturations of hemoglobin using a nomogram and measurement of arterial oxygen partial pressures will not detect the discrepancy between these two values. Indeed, when cyanosis due to methemoglobinemia is suspected, it is important to measure directly both the arterial oxygen partial pressure and the saturation of hemoglobin with oxygen. Cyanosis is usually present when plasma concentrations of methemoglobin exceed 1.5 $g \cdot dl^{-1}$, whereas 5 $g \cdot dl^{-1}$ of deoxygenated hemoglobin are necessary to produce cyanosis. Treatment of cyanosis due to methemoglobinemia is with intravenous infusion of 1 $mg \cdot kg^{-1}$ to 2 $mg \cdot kg^{-1}$ of methylene blue over 5 minutes. This dose may be repeated every 60 minutes if cyanosis persists, but it must be appreciated that doses in excess of about 7 $mg \cdot kg^{-1}$ may oxidize hemoglobin to methemoglobin.

Sulfhemoglobinemia

Sulfhemoglobinemia resembles methemoglobinemia in that neither form of hemoglobin can carry oxygen, and both conditions are associated with cyanosis, despite the presence of adequate arterial oxygen partial pressures.[29] Drugs that stimulate formation of methemoglobin are also capable of leading to the production of sulfhemoglobin. Indeed, the most common cause of sulfhemoglobinemia is

oxidation of iron in hemoglobin by drugs.[27,28] The reason some patients develop sulfhemoglobinemia and others methemoglobinemia is not known. In contrast to methemoglobin, sulfhemoglobin cannot be reconverted to hemoglobin by methylene blue. The only means for removing sulfhemoglobin is via eventual destruction of the erythrocyte.

Miscellaneous Hemoglobinopathies

Heinz body anemias are a group of hemoglobinopathies characterized by accelerated rates of hemolysis. Hemoglobin Koln is the most common form of abnormal hemoglobin associated with this type of anemia. This form of hemoglobin has an increased affinity for oxygen, resulting in reduced P_{50} values. Hemoglobin Yakima is also characterized by increased affinity for oxygen, having P_{50} values of about 12 mmHg. These patients compensate by increasing production of erythrocytes, resulting in increased concentrations of hemoglobin. Examples of abnormal hemoglobins with decreased affinity for oxygen include hemoglobin Kansas (P_{50} 70 mmHg) and hemoglobin Seattle (P_{50} = 41 mmHg).

LEUKOCYTES

Leukocytes are categorized as neutrophils (polymorphonuclear leukocytes), lymphocytes, eosinophils, basophils, and monocytes (Table 25-3). Total leukocyte concentrations in blood are 4,500 mm^3 to 10,000 mm^3, with a predominance of neutrophils (Table 25-5).

Neutrophils

Neutrophils are the first line of defense against bacterial infections. Production of humoral chemotactic factors by the host is re-

TABLE 25-5. Classification of Leukocytes

	Total mm³ (Range)	% of Total Differential Count (Range)
Neutrophils	3,000–6,000	55–65
Lymphocytes	1,500–3,500	25–35
Eosinophils	0–300	1–3
Basophils	0–100	0–1
Monocytes	300–500	3–6

sponsible for attracting neutrophils to infected sites. The rate at which neutrophils move toward a chemotactic stimulus is reduced by drugs used during anesthesia, including halothane, enflurane, and morphine. Reduced motility of neutrophils toward a chemotactic stimulus could increase the risk of bacterial infections. Nevertheless, there is no evidence that general anesthesia increases the risk of postoperative infections (see Chapter 29). Neutrophil motility is also inhibited by catecholamines. In addition, patients with diabetes mellitus and rheumatoid arthritis manifest reduced neutrophil motility. After neutrophils reach sites of infection, they release lysosomal enzymes and perform phagocytosis. As with neutrophil motility, general anesthesia depresses phagocytosis, but there is no evidence that this contributes to bacterial infections.

NEUTROPHILIA

Neutrophilia is most frequently a reflection of bacterial infections. Drug-induced increases in the peripheral neutrophil count can also be due to lithium and corticosteroids. Corticosteroids increase the number of circulating neutrophils by prolonging the survival of these cells in blood. Occasionally, myeloproliferative disorders stimulate production of neutrophils.

NEUTROPENIA

Neutropenia is present when circulating neutrophil counts are less than 1,800 mm³. Neutrophil counts less than 1,000 mm³ are likely to be associated with bacterial infections. Neutropenia may occur in patients with anemia or thrombocytopenia. Likewise, as many as 30 percent of patients with infectious mononucleosis develop neutropenia.

Lymphocytes

Lymphocytes are important in the production of immunoglobulins and the recognition of foreign antigens. Lymphocytosis is typically associated with viral infections.

Eosinophils and Basophils

The role of eosinophils is not well defined. Increased circulating levels of eosinophils are associated with allergic reactions, fungal infections, and diseases such as polyarteritis nodosa and sarcoidosis. Loeffler's syndrome is eosinophilia plus pulmonary infiltrates, cough, dyspnea, and elevations in body temperature. Treatment of this syndrome is with corticosteroids. Conversely, reductions in circulating eosinophil counts are not a common sign of underlying disease.

Basophils contain granules that release histamine in response to stimulation, as produced by antigen-antibody reactions. In addition, degranulation of basophils results in release of platelet activating factors.

REFERENCES

1. Kowalyshyn TJ, Prager D, Young J. A review of the present status of preoperative hemoglobin requirements. Anesth Analg 1972;51:75–9
2. Szer LSC, Shoemaker WC. Optimal hematocrit value in critically ill postoperative patients. Surg Gynecol Obstet 1978;147:363–8
3. Ellis DE, Stoelting RK. Individual variations in fluroxene, halothane, and methoxyflurane

blood-gas partition coefficients, and the effect of anemia. Anesthesiology 1975;42:748–50

4. Lerman J, Gregory GA, Eger EI. Hematocrit and the solubility of volatile anesthetics in blood. Anesth Analg 1984;63:911–4

5. Barrera M, Miletich DJ, Albrecht RF, Hoffman WE. Hemodynamic consequences of halothane anesthesia during chronic anemia. Anesthesiology 1984;61:36–42

6. Longnecker DE, Sturgill BC. Influence of anesthetic agent on survival following hemorrhage. Anesthesiology 1976;45:516–21

7. Weiskopf RB, Townsley MI, Riordan KK, et al. Comparison of cardiopulmonary responses to graded hemorrhage during enflurane, halothane, isoflurane, and ketamine anesthesia. Anesth Analg 1981;160:481–91

8. Houghton JB, Toghill PJ. Myasthenia gravis and red cell aplasia. Br Med J (Clin Res) 1978;2:1402–3

9. Bruce DL, Koepke JA. Anesthetic management of patients with bone-marrow failure. Anesth Analg 1972;51:597–606

10. Koblin DD, Watson JE, Deady JE, et al. Inactivation of methionine synthetase by nitrous oxide in mice. Anesthesiology 1981;54:318–24

11. Kripke BJ, Talarico L, Shah NK, Kelman AD. Hematologic reaction to prolonged exposure to nitrous oxide. Anesthesiology 1977;47:342–8

12. Layzer RB. Myeloneuropathy after prolonged exposure to nitrous oxide. Lancet 1978;2:1227–30

13. Spence AA. Environmental pollution by inhalation anaesthetics. Br J Anaesth 1987;59:96–109

14. Burka ER, Weaver Z, Marks PA. Clinical spectrum of hemolytic anemia associated with glucose-6-phosphate dehydrogenase deficiency. Ann Intern Med 1966;64:817–25

15. Shapley JM, Wilson JR. Post-anesthetic jaundice due to glucose-6-phosphate dehydrogenase deficiency. Can Anaesth Soc J 1973;20:390–2

16. Lessin LS, Jensen WN. Sickle cell anemia 1910–1973. An overview. Arch Intern Med 1974;133:529–43

17. Zarkowsky HS, Gallagher D, Gill FM, et al. Bacteremia in sickle hemoglobinopathies. J Pediatr 1986;109:579–85

18. Heiner M, Teasdale SJ, David T, et al. Aorto-coronary bypass in a patient with sickle cell trait. Can Anaesth Soc J 1979;26:428–34

19. Stein RE, Urbaniak J. Use of the tourniquet during surgery in patients with sickle cell hemoglobinopathies. Clin Orthop 1980;151:231–3

20. Maduska AL, Guinee WS, Heaton JA, et al. Sickling dynamics of red blood cells and other physiologic studies during anesthesia. Anesth Analg 1975;54:361–5

21. Hilkovitz G, Jacobson A. Hepatic dysfunction and abnormalities of the serum proteins and serum enzymes in sickle-cell anemia. J Lab Clin Med 1961;57:856–67

22. Bridenbaugh PO, Moore DC, Bridenbaugh LD. Alterations in capillary and venous blood gases after regional-block anesthesia. Anesth Analg 1972;51:280–6

23. Niehius AW. Thalassemia major: Molecular and clinical aspects. Ann Intern Med 1979;91:883–97

24. Cross JN, Morgan OS, Gibbs WN, Cheruvanky I. Spinal cord compression in thalassemia. J Neurol Neurosurg Psychiatry 1977;40:1120–2

25. Leon MB, Borer JJ, Bacharach SL, et al. Detection of early cardiac dysfunction in patients with severe beta-thalassemia and chronic iron overload. N Engl J Med 1979;301:1143–8

26. Gabel RA, Bunn HF. Hereditary methemoglobinemia as a cause of cyanosis during anesthesia. Anesthesiology 1974;40:516–8

27. Fibuch EE, Cecil WT, Reed WA. Methemoglobinemia associated with organic nitrate therapy. Anesth Analg 1979;58:521–3

28. Zurick AM, Wagner RH, Starr NJ, et al. Intravenous nitroglycerin, methemoglobinemia, and respiratory distress in a postoperative cardiac surgical patient. Anesthesiology 1984;61:464–6

29. Schmitter CR. Sulfhemoglobinemia and methemoglobinemia—uncommon causes of cyanosis. Anesthesiology 1975;43:586–7

26

Disorders of Coagulation

An understanding of the coagulation system is necessary for recognizing and evaluating defects in hemostasis that occur during the perioperative period. Likewise, an appreciation of normal clotting mechanisms facilitates management of anesthesia in patients with known co-existing defects of coagulation.

PHYSIOLOGY OF COAGULATION

Physiology of coagulation may be considered to consist of vascular, platelet, and procoagulant phases. When the integrity of a blood vessel is broken, the proper function and interaction of each phase is necessary to assure effective hemostasis. Many of the events of coagulation take place on the surface of platelets and injured walls of blood vessels, so as to assure that the hemostatic process is precisely localized to the damaged area.

Vascular Phase

The vascular phase of coagulation is characterized by vasoconstriction in the area of the break in the blood vessel, which is due to contraction of vascular wall smooth muscle, and represents the initial phase of coagulation. With breaks in small blood vessels or injury due to puncture wounds, this phase can be sufficient to provide hemostasis.

Vasoconstriction is most intense in traumatized or crushed blood vessels. Conversely, sharply transected blood vessels, as occur during surgery, undergo less vasospasm and blood loss is greater.

Platelet Phase

The platelet phase of coagulation is initiated by exposure of platelets to subendothelial substances on walls of injured blood vessels.[1] The ability of platelets to adhere to vascular collagen is the crucial first step leading to the primary aggregation of platelets and the subsequent release of vasoactive substances from storage granules in platelets. Release of vasoactive substances, such as serotonin, contributes to localized vasoconstriction of the vascular phase. In addition, platelets release adenosine diphosphate and thromboxane A_2 in response to exposure to collagen. This release serves as an additional potent stimulus for attracting more platelets to the site of vascular injury (secondary aggregation) and for the subsequent releasing of their granular contents.

Aggregation of platelets at the site of vascular injury forms a hemostatic plug and also serves as the activating surface for a number of circulating procoagulants. The platelet plug mechanism is crucial for closing minute breaks in small blood vessels that occur daily. When the number of platelets is reduced, small hemorrhagic areas appear under the skin and internally. Typically, platelet plugs do not occlude lumens of blood vessels.

Platelets are derived from megakaryocytes in bone marrow. After entering the circulation, platelets survive about 10 days. Nearly one-third of the platelets are found in the spleen, as a pool that can freely exchange with the circulation. Under circumstances of platelet need, production of these cells can increase as much as eightfold.

Procoagulant Phase

The procoagulant phase of coagulation leading to formation of fibrin consists of the extrinsic coagulation pathway, the intrinsic coagulation pathway, and the common pathway of coagulation (Fig. 26-1). Procoagulants are designated as a factor plus a Roman numeral, or by a synonym (Table 26-1). Procoagulants are numbered in the order of discovery and not in order of activation.

Thromboplastin release by tissue trauma activates the extrinsic pathway; diverse events, including collagen on damaged vascular walls and antigen-antibody complexes, are responsible for initiating activity of the intrinsic pathway. These pathways converge at the step where active factor X is formed. Factor X initiates events via the common pathway of coagulation, culminating in formation of fibrin. Fibrin is the fundamental structural constituent of blood clots. Continued clot formation occurs only where blood is not flowing. Otherwise, blood flow dilutes procoagulants released during the clotting process, thus preventing their concentrations from rising high enough to sustain continued formation of clot. Clot retraction, which acts to pull walls of the blood vessels together, begins soon after clot is formed and requires platelets. In addition, the procoagulant system contains natural inhibitors of clot formation and a fibrinolytic system that is mediated by plasmin. Plasmin causes breakdown of fibrin into small segments known as fibrin degradation (split) products, which are normally removed by the reticuloendothelial system. High plasma concentrations of fibrin degradation products inhibit cross-linking of fibrin monomers and produce platelet dysfunction.

All circulating procoagulants are synthe-

TABLE 26-1.   Plasma Procoagulants

Factor Synonyms	Plasma Concentration ($\mu g \cdot ml^{-1}$)	Half-Time (Hours)	Minimal Level for Surgical Hemostasis (% of normal)	Stability on Storage in Whole Blood (4 degrees Celsius, 21 days)
I Fibrinogen	2000–4000	95–150	50–100	No change
II Prothrombin	150	65–90	20–40	No change
III Thromboplastin				
IV Calcium				
V Proaccelerin	10	15–24	5–20	Half-time 7 days
VII Proconvertin	0.5	4–6	10–20	No change
VIII Antihemophilic factor	15	10–12	30	Half-time 7 days
IX Christmas factor	3	18–30	20–25	No change
X Stuart-Prower factor	15	40–60	10–20	No change
XI Plasma thromboplastin antecedent	<5	45–60	20–30	Half-time 7 days
XII Hageman factor	<5	50–70	0	No change
XIII Fibrin-stabilizing factor	20	72–120	1–3	No change

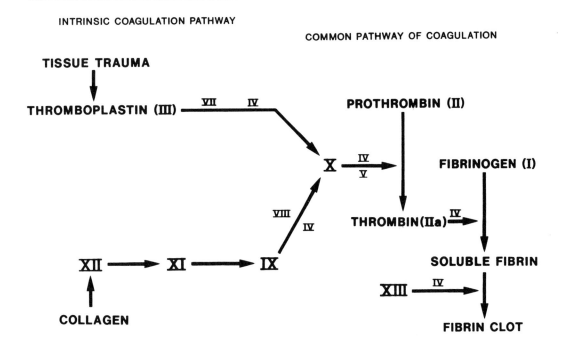

INTRINSIC COAGULATION PATHWAY

COMMON PATHWAY OF COAGULATION

EXTRINSIC COAGULATION PATHWAY

FIG. 26-1. Schematic diagram of the procoagulant phase of coagulation, depicting the cascade sequence in three steps designated as the extrinsic coagulation pathway, intrinsic coagulation pathway, and common pathway of coagulation. Tissue trauma activates the extrinsic pathway; the intrinsic pathway is stimulated by the presence of collagen on walls of damaged vessels. The extrinsic and intrinsic pathways converge at the formation of activated factor X. This formation initiates a series of cascade steps in the common pathway, culminating in the formation of a fibrin clot.

sized in the liver, with the exception of factor VIII, which is produced in the reticuloendothelial system. Procoagulants dependent on the presence of vitamin K for their normal synthesis in the liver include factors II, VII, IX, and X.

LABORATORY TESTS OF COAGULATION

Laboratory tests of coagulation must evaluate platelet and procoagulant phases. A knowledge of those tests useful for evaluation of the adequacy of coagulation is crucial for

confirming the status of coagulation preoperatively and for facilitating the differential diagnosis of inadequate hemostasis in the perioperative (Table 26-2). Tests of the platelet phase include the bleeding time and platelet count. Evaluation of platelet aggregation in response to adenosine diphosphate, epinephrine, or collagen may be useful for defining an abnormality in platelet function in the presence of normal platelet counts but prolonged bleeding times. Tests of the procoagulant phase include measurement of the prothrombin time, partial thromboplastin time, thrombin time, plasma fibrinogen concentration, and level of circulating fibrin degradation products. Measurement of prothrombin time and partial thromboplastin time provides an assessment of activity of all procoagulants.

TABLE 26-2. Tests of Coagulation

	Normal Value	Measures
Bleeding time (Ivy)	3–10 minutes	Platelet function, Vascular integrity
Platelet count	150,000–400,000 mm^3	
Prothrombin time	12–14 seconds	Factors I, II, V, VII, X
Partial thromboplastin time	25–35 seconds	Factors I, II, V, VIII, IX, X, XI, XII
Thrombin time	12–20 seconds	Factors I, II
Fibrinogen	200–400 mg·dl^{-1}	
Fibrin degradation products	4 μg·ml^{-1}	
Thrombelastography		Procoagulants and platelets

Bleeding Time

Bleeding time is the best measure of platelet function. The hallmark of a defect in platelet function is a prolonged bleeding time (greater than 10 minutes) despite platelet counts above 100,000 mm^3. Performance of bleeding time in the intraoperative period may be helpful when excessive bleeding develops. A blood pressure cuff placed on the arm to be tested is inflated to a pressure of 40 mmHg, and an incision 9 mm long and 1 mm deep is made with a special scalpel on the volar surface of the midforearm. The incision is made with a special scalpel to insure reproducible results. The incision is touched at 30 second intervals with an absorbant paper. Bleeding time is the interval between the incision and when blood no longer moistens the paper. A normal bleeding time is less than 5 minutes.

Platelet Count

Platelet count estimates only the number and not the function of these cells. On a normal stained peripheral blood smear, 8 to 12 platelets will be visible in each magnification (1,000 ×) field. This corresponds to a normal platelet count of 150,000 mm^3 to 450,000 mm^3. Platelet counts below 100,000 mm^3 are associated with prolonged bleeding times. A minimum platelet count of 50,000 mm^3 to 100,000 mm^3 is suggested before undertaking elective surgical procedures.[1] The risk of spontaneous hemorrhage is increased with platelet counts below 30,000 mm^3. The risk of spontaneous intracranial hemorrhage occurs with platelet counts below 10,000 mm^3.

Prothrombin Time

Prothrombin time is a reflection of events occurring in the extrinsic coagulation pathway. A normal prothrombin time is 12 seconds to 14 seconds. Curves based on commercial standards can be used to express this result in terms of a percentage of a normal response.

Reductions in the activities of factors II (prothrombin), V, VII, and X are reflected by prolongation of the prothrombin time. Prothrombin time does not reflect the presence or absence of factor VIII activity. Small doses of heparin (5,000 units administered to an adult) are unlikely to alter prothrombin time (Table 26-3). Likewise, prothrombin time is not influenced by plasma concentrations of factor I (fibrinogen), until the level of this procoagulant in the circulation decreases to less than 100 mg·dl^{-1}. Large doses of heparin or small doses of a coumarin anticoagulant inhibit activity of factor VII and prolong the prothrombin time (Table 26-3).

Partial Thromboplastin Time

Partial thromboplastin time is a reflection of events occurring in the intrinsic and common coagulation pathway.[2] A normal partial thromboplastin time is 25 seconds to 35 sec-

TABLE 26-3. Impact of Anticoagulants on Tests of Coagulation

	Factors Inhibited	Prothrombin Time	Partial Thromboplastin Time
Heparin (low dose)	IX	Normal	Prolonged
Heparin (high dose)	II, IX, X	Prolonged	Prolonged
Coumarin (low dose)	VII	Prolonged	Normal
Coumarin (high dose)	II, VII, IX, X	Prolonged	Prolonged

onds. Prolongation occurs in the presence of a plasma deficiency of all the procoagulants, with the exception of factors VII and XIII. For example, small doses of a coumarin anticoagulant inhibit factor VII, and partial thromboplastin time is not prolonged (Table 26-3). Conversely, small doses of heparin inhibit activity of factor IX, and partial thromboplastin time is prolonged (Table 26-3). Ideally, therapeutic doses of heparin are adjusted to maintain the partial thromboplastin time at about double the pretreatment value.

Thrombin Time

Thrombin time measures the rate of conversion of fibrinogen to fibrin. A normal thrombin time is 12 seconds to 20 seconds. Thrombin time is prolonged in the presence of decreased plasma activity of factors I and II. Prolongation of the thrombin time also occurs in the presence of heparin and increased plasma concentrations of fibrin degradation products.

Fibrinogen

Fibrinogen is present in chemically measurable amounts in the circulation. Normal concentrations are 200 mg·dl^{-1} to 400 mg·dl^{-1}. Low plasma levels of fibrinogen may reflect consumption of this procoagulant by diffuse and excessive clotting.

Fibrin Degradation Products

Fibrin degradation products are a result of the breakdown of fibrinogen and fibrin by plasmin. Normal plasma concentrations of fibrin degradation products are less than 4 µg·ml^{-1}. Elevated circulating levels are evidence of increased fibrinolysis. Primary fibrinolysis is an uncommon disorder but has been observed in association with cardiopulmonary bypass, cirrhosis of the liver, and carcinoma of the prostate. More common is secondary fibrinolysis, typically due to disseminated intravascular coagulation.

Specific Procoagulant Assays

In special circumstances, it is appropriate to measure plasma concentrations or activity of specific procoagulants. These tests usually involve addition of the patient's blood to test plasma known to be deficient for a specific procoagulant. The deficiency or absence of this procoagulant in the patient's blood is confirmed by the demonstration of prolonged times to clot formation, or by its absence.

Thrombelastography

Thrombelastography is a test that evaluates overall clot formation, allowing diagnosis of procoagulant deficiency, platelet abnormalities, disseminated intravascular coagulation, and fibrinolysis within 30 minutes of obtaining a blood sample. Using this technique, it has been demonstrated that progressive blood loss during surgery is associated with a trend toward increased coagulability.[3] It is likely that surgical stress, tissue trauma with release of tissue thromboplastin, and elevations in plasma concentrations of catecholamines offset any hypocoagulable tendency resulting from hemodilution and loss of procoagulants during progressive blood loss. A decrease in coagulation activity after induction of general anesthesia but before surgical stimulation may reflect decreased levels of stress and lower plasma concentrations of catecholamines compared to the awake state.[3] Clearly, there is no justification for empiric use of fresh frozen plasma or platelets during moderate to massive blood loss without first documentation of defects in coagulation as can be provided by laboratory tests.

PREOPERATIVE EVALUATION OF A PATIENT FOR ABNORMAL COAGULATION

Preoperative evaluation of patients for the presence of abnormal coagulation includes the history, physical examination, and performance of appropriate laboratory tests. Careful exclusion of defects of coagulation before induction of anesthesia facilitates the differential diagnosis of intraoperative bleeding.

History

A properly taken history is vital for detecting coagulation disorders in the preoperative period. One of the most important questions deals with hemostatic responses to prior surgery. Challenges to the coagulation system during infancy include umbilical cord separation and circumcision. Two common surgical procedures that test the coagulation system

during childhood are tonsillectomy and dental extractions. Bleeding problems that manifest in infancy or childhood suggest a congenital deficiency of an essential procoagulant. The response of the coagulation system to episodes of nonsurgical trauma should also be elicited. Questions as to relatives with bleeding disorders should be pursued. A detailed record of drug ingestion, as well as questions regarding occupation and possible exposure to toxic substances, should be included.

Physical Examination

Physical examination may reveal petechiae, which are suggestive of abnormalities of platelet function, decreased numbers of platelets, or defects in the integrity of vascular walls. In contrast, subcutaneous bleeding that occurs in the presence of deficiencies of procoagulants typically manifests as ecchymoses. Likewise, hemarthrosis or deep bleeding into skeletal muscles is more likely to reflect procoagulant deficiencies than defects of platelet function or a reduced number of platelets.

Laboratory Tests

Preoperative laboratory tests that constitute a screening coagulation profile are useful whenever the history or physical examination suggests the presence of a coagulation abnormality. Examples of patients who may benefit from preoperative coagulation evaluation include those with liver disease, malabsorption, malnutrition, and those undergoing procedures that may interfere with normal coagulation. Baseline coagulation studies are useful in patients being treated with anticoagulants. Laboratory tests should evaluate all phases of coagulation. A coagulation profile that will detect most abnormalities includes measurements of bleeding time, platelet count, prothrombin time, partial thromboplastin time, and plasma fibrinogen concentrations (Table 26-2).

CONGENITAL DISORDERS OF COAGULATION

Congenital disorders of coagulation are usually due to the absence or decreased presence of a single procoagulant.[4] The three most common congenital disorders of coagulation are hemophilia A (factor VIII deficiency, classic hemophilia), hemophilia B (factor IX deficiency, Christmas disease), and von Willebrand's disease. Knowledge of the missing factor, the elimination half-time of this factor after exogenous administration, and products available for treatment of the coagulation disorder are important in the preoperative preparation of these patients (Table 26-1).

Hemophilia A

Hemophilia A is due to the absence of adequate activity of factor VIII. It is estimated that hemophilia A is present in about 12,000 patients in the United States.[5] The gene for factor VIII activity is carried on X chromosomes, explaining the manifestation of this disease in males, while females usually remain asymptomatic carriers.

DIAGNOSIS

Diagnosis of hemophilia A is made by family history and by measurement of plasma concentrations of factor VIII. There is a direct relationship between plasma concentrations of factor VIII and the severity of bleeding (Table 26-4). For example, spontaneous hemorrhage is likely when factor VIII concentrations are less than 3 percent of the normal value.

A useful screening test for hemophilia A is the partial thromboplastin time. This test will be prolonged in all but those with very

TABLE 26-4. Factor VIII Concentrations Necessary for Hemostasis

Hemostasis	Factor VIII Concentration (% of normal)
Spontaneous hemorrhage	1–3
Moderate trauma	4–8
Hemarthrosis and deep skeletal muscle hemorrhage	10–15
Major surgery	>30

mild disease; it is, for example, likely to be prolonged when plasma concentrations of factor VIII are less than 50 percent of normal. Prothrombin time is normal in patients with hemophilia A, as this test does not measure factor VIII activity.

CLINICAL MANIFESTATIONS

Deep tissue bleeding, hemarthrosis, and hematuria are common forms of clinical bleeding associated with hemophilia A. Central nervous system bleeding is the major cause of death in patients with hemophilia A. Femoral neuropathy can occur secondary to hemorrhage into surrounding skeletal muscles.

PREOPERATIVE PREPARATION

The goal of preoperative preparation of patients with hemophilia A is to establish plasma concentrations of factor VIII that will assure hemostasis in the perioperative period (Table 26-4). Calculations of factor VIII replacement therapy are based on the convention that 100 percent of a procoagulant means there is 1 unit of procoagulant ml^{-1} plasma and that the plasma volume is 40 $ml \cdot kg^{-1}$. Therefore, a 50 kg patient with less than 1 percent of procoagulant activity would require 2,000 units of factor VIII to raise the concentration of this procoagulant to 100 percent of normal (40 $ml \cdot kg^{-1} \times$ 50 kg $\times$ 1 unit of factor VIII·ml^{-1}). This dose will need to be repeated twice daily, as the elimination half-time of factor VIII is 10 hours to 12 hours. Ideally, levels of factor VIII should be raised to nearly 100 percent before elective surgery to assure that activity does not decrease below 30 percent of normal during surgery.[4] Plasma factor VIII concentrations greater than 30 percent of normal are considered to be adequate for hemostasis after major surgery. Despite achievement of optimal plasma concentrations of factor VIII, postoperative hemorrhage often occurs, suggesting that other factors may be important.[6] For example, the high incidence of postoperative hemorrhage after knee surgery may reflect the presence of a large surface area of inflamed synovium. Approximately 5 percent to 15 percent of patients with hemophilia A develop antibodies to factor VIII, resulting in rapid inactivation of infused material.[7] As a result, there may be difficulty in achieving normal plasma levels of factor VIII. Replacement of factor VIII can be with cryoprecipitate or specific concentrates of factor VIII. Fresh frozen plasma is no longer considered a therapy of choice for patients with hemophilia A.[8] Cryoprecipitate contains 5 units to 10 units of factor VIII·ml^{-1}, but its use is associated with an increased risk for the transmission of viral diseases. Factor VIII concentrates contain up to 40 units·ml^{-1}, providing a significant advantage in terms of infusion volume. However, the risk of transmission of viral hepatitis and acquired immune deficiency syndrome is substantial (see Chapter 29). An alternative to blood products may be administration of the synthetic androgen, danazol, which has been shown to increase factor VIII activity and decrease the incidence of hemorrhage in some but not all patients with hemophilia A.[9] Finally, drugs that interfere with normal platelet function, such as aspirin, must be avoided in patients with hemophilia A.

MANAGEMENT OF ANESTHESIA

Preoperative medication of patients with hemophilia A is ideally achieved with drugs administered orally. Although intramuscular injection of drugs is alleged to be safe when factor VIII levels are at least 35 percent of normal, it would seem prudent to avoid this route whenever possible.[10] An anticholinergic drug can be administered intravenously before the induction of anesthesia, if it is deemed a necessary part of the anesthetic. Maintenance of anesthesia is most often with general anesthesia, as the risk of uncontrolled bleeding detracts from selection of regional anesthetic techniques. Nevertheless, the uncomplicated use of an axillary block in two patients with hemophilia A has been described.[10] Selection of anesthetic drugs should consider the likely presence of co-existing liver disease due to hepatitis from prior blood or factor VIII transfusions. Likewise, the virus responsible for transmission of acquired immune deficiency syndrome may be present (see Chapter 29). Intubation of the trachea need not be avoided, but care must be taken to minimize trauma during direct laryngoscopy. Superficial hemorrhage can be controlled by the application of external pressure until treatment with solutions containing factor VIII can be initiated.

Hemophilia B

Hemophilia B is due to absent or decreased activity of factor IX. The inheritance pattern and clinical features are indistinguishable from those of hemophilia A. Diagnosis of hemophilia B depends on the demonstration of a low or absent plasma factor IX concentration in the presence of normal factor VIII activity. Partial thromboplastin time will be prolonged in patients with hemophilia B.

Treatment of hemophilia B is with specific procoagulant concentrates to raise plasma concentrations of factor IX. Fresh frozen plasma is no longer considered a therapy of choice for patients with hemophilia B.[8] The therapeutic goal before elective surgery is to raise plasma concentrations of factor IX to levels that will assure maintenance of levels of at least 30 percent of normal during the perioperative period. Dosing intervals of solutions used to increase plasma concentrations of factor IX are based on an elimination half-time of about 24 hours. Preoperative preparation and management of anesthesia are as described for hemophilia A.

von Willebrand's Disease

The coagulation defect known as von Willebrand's disease is transmitted as an autosomal dominant characteristic affecting both sexes. The specific defect has not been identified, but it is most likely due to the deficiency of a protein (von Willebrand's factor) important for adequate activity of factor VIII and optimal function of platelets. The classic expression of this disease is a prolonged bleeding time, impaired aggregation of platelets, and decreased plasma concentrations of factor VIII. Epistaxis, bleeding from mucosal surfaces, and superficial bruising are common. Hemarthrosis and bleeding into skeletal muscles are uncommon. Trauma or surgical procedures performed in previously undiagnosed patients can result in excessive bleeding, which is localized to the site of injury. Pregnancy produces an increase in factor VIII and von Willebrand's factor in parturients with mild to moderate forms of this coagulation disorder. Consequently, vaginal delivery can usually be performed without the need for transfusions. Treatment before surgery is with cryoprecipitate (40 U·kg^{-1}), which provides von Willebrand's factor, as well as factor VIII. Alternatively, the synthetic analog of antidiuretic hormone, desmopressin, is effective in inducing the release of von Willebrand's factor in these patients. Surprisingly, factor VIII concentrates alone are not effective.[11] As with hemophilia A and B, these patients should be warned to avoid drugs that interfere with the optimal aggregation of platelets.

Afibrinogenemia

Congenital absence of fibrinogen activity may first present as continued bleeding from the stump of the umbilical cord. Minor trauma can precipitate severe hemorrhage, but hemarthroses do not occur. Bleeding time, prothrombin time, partial thromboplastin time, and thrombin time are usually prolonged. Quantitative determination of plasma fibrinogen concentrations reveals only trace amounts or total absence of this procoagulant. Treatment is with fibrinogen or cryoprecipitate to increase plasma concentrations of fibrinogen to at least 50 mg·dl^{-1}

Hypoprothrombinemia

Congenital absence or deficiency of prothrombin activity is characterized by prolonged bleeding times and prolonged prothrombin times. Treatment is with fresh frozen plasma or specific prothrombin concentrates.

Factor V Deficiency

Factor V deficiency is inherited as an autosomal recessive characteristic and can affect both sexes. Bleeding time, prothrombin time, and partial thromboplastin time are prolonged. Bleeding is most often from mucous membranes. Severe menorrhagia may be a manifestation of this coagulation disorder. Hemorrhage from accidental trauma or surgery can be extreme. Treatment is with fresh frozen plasma to maintain plasma concentrations of factor V in the range of 5 percent to 20 percent of normal.[8]

Factor XIII Deficiency

Deficiency of factor XIII results in an inability to form insoluble fibrin, which can manifest at birth as persistent bleeding from the stump of the umbilical cord. In later life, this factor deficiency can result in delayed hemorrhage after accidental trauma or surgery.[12] Central nervous system hemorrhage is common. The position of factor XIII in the coagulation pathway results in normal values of all the routine tests for coagulation (Fig. 26-1). The urea clot lysis time is specific for deficiencies of factor XIII. Treatment is with fresh frozen plasma or cryoprecipitate.[8]

Protein C Deficiency

Protein C is a vitamin K-dependent anticoagulant synthesized in the liver, which inhibits activated clotting factors V and VIII and stimulates fibrinolysis. A deficiency of this protein may be inherited or acquired (liver disease, disseminated intravascular coagulation, postoperative adult respiratory distress syndrome). Congenital protein C deficiency manifests in infancy as life-threatening venous thrombosis and cutaneous necrosis. Mild protein C deficiency, either acquired or inherited as a heterozygous trait, usually presents in adults. Such deficiencies are often associated with a tendency for thromophlebitis, which may include pulmonary embolism. In addition, thrombi may result in cerebral, myocardial, or renal infarction. Thrombosis may be initiated by events that accompany the perioperative period, including endothelial damage, immobility, and stasis of blood flow.

Management of anesthesia introduces the concern that pressure from the tracheal tube could compromise tracheal blood flow. In this regard, use of a tube with an audible air leak has been recommended for management of neonates.[13] Preoperative replacement of protein C is accomplished by transfusion of fresh frozen plasma. Regional anesthetic techniques may be useful alternatives to general anesthesia in these patients.

ACQUIRED DISORDERS OF COAGULATION

Acquired disorders of coagulation, in contrast to congenital disorders, are usually due to multiple abnormalities in the coagulation process. Causes of acquired deficiencies include (1) major organ system disease, (2) vitamin K deficiency, (3) ingestion of anticoagulant drugs, (4) massive blood transfusions, (5) disseminated intravascular coagulation, and (6) drug-induced platelet dysfunction. In addition, pure thrombocytopenia can be disease-induced, drug-induced, idiopathic, or due to the presence of thrombogenic catheters in the vascular system.

Major Organ System Disease

Vitamin K is necessary in the liver to facilitate production of gamma-carboxylglutamic acid, required for the biologic function of factors II, VII, IX, and X. Specifically, coumarin anticoagulants prevent carboxylation of vitamin K from its inactive oxidized form. Bile salts are necessary for absorption of vitamin K from the gastrointestinal tract. Therefore, obstructive jaundice is likely to be associated with acquired defects of coagulation due to deficiencies of vitamin K. Other causes of vitamin K deficiencies include malnutrition, intestinal malabsorption, and antibiotic-induced elimination of intestinal flora necessary for the synthesis of vitamin K. Neonates lack stores of vitamin K and can develop deficiencies of this vitamin in the absence of supplemental therapy.

Vitamin K deficiencies are reflected by prolonged prothrombin times in the presence of normal partial thromboplastin times. Treatment of coagulation disorders due to vitamin K deficiencies depends on the urgency of the situation. For example, parenteral vitamin K requires 3 hours to 6 hours to exert beneficial effects. If active hemorrhage is present, the infusion of fresh frozen plasma is rapidly effective.[8]

Ingestion of Anticoagulant Drugs

Heparin acts indirectly as an anticoagulant by acceleration of the formation of antithrombin III, which is an alpha-2 globulin normally present in the plasma. Antithrombin III forms complexes with activated thrombin, resulting in neutralization of thrombin activity and prevention of the conversion of fibrinogen to fibrin (Fig. 26-1). Antithrombin III also neutralizes activated factor X, thus preventing conversion of prothrombin to thrombin (Fig. 26-1). An overdose of heparin manifests as subcutaneous hemorrhages and deep tissue hematomas. Prothrombin and partial thromboplastin time is prolonged; bleeding time is normal. Heparin is inactivated in the liver and excreted by the kidneys, explaining prolonged anticoagulant effects in patients with hepatorenal disease. Reductions in body temperature are also associated with prolonged anticoagulant effects of heparin. Antagonism of heparin effect is with intravenous administration of protamine.

Coumarin anticoagulants interfere with hepatic synthesis of vitamin K dependent procoagulants, which include factors II, VII, IX, and X. Ecchymosis formation, mucosal hemorrhage, and subserosal bleeding into the wall of the gastrointestinal tract are manifestations of hemorrhage due to overdoses of coumarin anticoagulants. Large doses result in prolongation of the prothrombin time and partial thromboplastin time. Rapid reversal of anticoagulant effects produced by these drugs is achieved by the intravenous infusion of fresh frozen plasma.[8] Parenteral vitamin K will not produce effective antagonism for at least 3 hours to 6 hours.

Massive Blood Transfusion

Massive transfusion of stored whole blood (10 units or more) can lead to acquired disorders of coagulation. The mechanism for this coagulation disorder is dilutional thrombocytopenia and/or dilution of plasma concentrations of factors V and VIII.

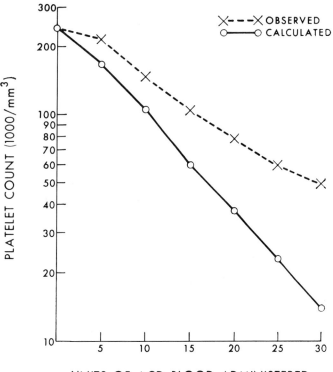

FIG. 26-2. Platelet counts observed in patients receiving whole blood stored for longer than 24 hours are compared with predicted platelet counts if platelet-free solutions had been administered. The approximation of the curves suggests that the observed thrombocytopenia is dilutional, resulting from the infusion of whole blood that is essentially platelet-free. (Miller RD, Robbins TO, Tong MJ. Coagulation defects associated with massive blood transfusions. Ann Surg 1971;174:794–801)

DILUTIONAL THROMBOCYTOPENIA

Dilutional thrombocytopenia occurs in many patients who receive more than 10 units of whole blood. This reflects the virtual absence of viable platelets in whole blood, which has been stored at 4 degrees Celsius for more than 24 hours. For example, it is likely that platelet counts will fall below 100,000 mm^3 in most adult patients receiving 10 units to 15 units of whole blood (Fig. 26-2).[14] Bleeding has been shown to occur frequently at platelet levels below 100,000 mm^3. In addition to dilution, consumption of platelets often occurs in patients receiving massive blood transfusions. Treatment of dilutional thrombocytopenia is with infusion of platelet concentrates. In a 70 kg patient, each unit of platelet concentrate infused can be expected to increase platelet counts by 5,000 mm^3 to 10,000 mm^3. Each unit of platelets contains 50 ml to 70 ml of plasma, emphasizing the likely simultaneous delivery of procoagulants with this therapy.

DILUTION OF PROCOAGULANTS

Levels of factors V and VIII in whole blood decrease to 20 percent to 50 percent of normal after 21 days of storage (Table 26-1). Nevertheless, infusion of large amounts of stored whole blood rarely dilutes plasma concentrations of these factors below 50 percent of normal. Only 5 percent to 20 percent of the normal amount of factor V and 30 percent of factor VIII are necessary for hemostasis in patients undergoing surgery. As a result, it is unlikely that a hemorrhagic diathesis due to dilution of these factors would occur during massive transfusion of stored whole blood. Abnormalities of coagulation due to dilution of circulating levels of factors V and VIII are more likely to occur with infusion of erythrocytes that include minimal plasma volume. Fresh frozen plasma is the indicated treatment when objective measurements confirm inadequate hemostasis due to reduced plasma concentrations of these factors.[8] Dilution of plasma procoagulants other than factors V and VIII does not occur during massive transfusions of whole blood, since all the other factors are stable in stored blood (Table 26-1).

Disseminated Intravascular Coagulation

Disseminated intravascular coagulation is characterized by uncontrolled activation of the coagulation system, with consumption of platelets and procoagulants.[15] Thrombi develop in the microcirculation and bleeding results due to loss of coagulation factors into these thrombi. This disorder is highly variable in its presentation and may accompany many abnormalities, including (1) low cardiac output with hemorrhagic shock, sepsis, or burns; (2) retained placenta after delivery; (3) trauma to the central nervous system; and (4) prolonged extracorporeal circulation.

PATHOPHYSIOLOGY

Under normal conditions, deleterious effects of uncontrolled intravascular coagulation are modulated by (1) dilutional effects of blood flow (2) circulating antithrombins, and (3) breakdown of activated clotting factors in the liver. These carefully controlled mechanisms can be overwhelmed when extensive tissue damage delivers large amounts of thromboplastic material into the circulation, with subsequent activation of the extrinsic coagulation pathway (Fig. 26-1). Consumption of platelets and procoagulants, including factors I, II, V, VIII, and XIII, reflects generalized activation of the entire coagulation system (Fig. 26-1). In addition, shock, with reduced blood flow, reduces beneficial dilutional effects on concentrations of procoagulants. Furthermore, impaired perfusion of the liver interferes with optimal hepatic extraction of activated clotting factors.

DIAGNOSIS

Diagnosis of disseminated intravascular coagulation is based on the clinical picture and on tests of coagulation. The clinical picture is characterized by hemorrhage from wound sites and around sites of placement of intravascular catheters. Platelet counts are often reduced to below 150,000 mm³ due to consumption of platelets. Prothrombin time and partial thromboplastin time are prolonged, reflecting consumption of procoagulants by uncontrolled continuation of intravascular clotting. Decreased plasma concentrations of fibrinogen (less than 150 mg·dl⁻¹) reflect consumption of this procoagulant. Elevated levels of fibrin degradation products in the circulation are characteristic.

TABLE 26-5. Drugs Associated with Platelet Dysfunction

Nonsteroidal Anti-Inflammatory Drugs
Aspirin
Phenylbutazone
Indomethacin
Antihistamines
Tricyclic Antidepressants
Local Anesthetics
Licocaine
Cocaine
Alpha-Adrenergic Antagonists

TREATMENT

The goal in treatment of disseminated intravascular coagulation is correction of the underlying disorder responsible for initiating the widespread clotting process. For example, improvement of cardiac output, restoration of intravascular fluid volume, or treatment of sepsis may be sufficient therapy. Improvement is indicated by stabilization of platelet counts and plasma concentrations of fibrinogen, plus decreases in circulating concentrations of fibrin degradation products. Platelet concentrates and fresh frozen plasma are administered, as indicated by measurement of platelet counts and determination of the prothrombin time and partial thromboplastin time. Heparin has been recommended as therapy, but its use in this situation is controversial and ill-defined. Aminocaproic acid or fibrinogen should not be given in the presence of continuing intravascular coagulation. Aminocaproic acid would inhibit secondary fibrinolysis, which is an intrinsic protective mechanism in patients with persistent disseminated intravascular coagulation.

Drug-Induced Platelet Dysfunction

Drugs associated with inhibition of platelet function include nonsteroidal anti-inflammatory agents such as aspirin (Table 26-5). In contrast to aspirin, acetaminophen or sodium salicylate have minimal effects on platelet function. Aspirin irreversibly acetylates platelet cyclo-oxygenase, the enzyme responsible for conversion of arachidonic acid to prostaglandin endoperoxidases and thromboxane A2. As a result, platelet release reactions normally evoked by collagen or adenosine diphosphate do not occur, platelet aggregation is absent and bleeding times become prolonged. Indeed, prolongation of bleeding times is detectable within 2 hours after the ingestion of 300 mg of aspirin.[16] Platelet dysfunction induced by aspirin persists for the life of the cells. Therefore, management of aspirin-induced hemorrhage involves transfusion of platelets, which can release adenosine diphosphate. In response to such release, platelets, which have been inhibited by aspirin, can aggregate.

A logical recommendation would be to defer elective operations that can be associated with significant blood loss until effects of aspirin on platelet function have waned. Nevertheless, perioperative blood loss is not increased in patients receiving 1.2 g·day⁻¹ to 3.6 g·day⁻¹ of aspirin and undergoing total hip replacement.[16] The effect of aspirin on platelet function should be appreciated when considering the selection of regional anesthetic techniques. Certainly, measurement of bleeding times would seem prudent before performing epidural blocks in patients being treated with aspirin. Nevertheless, there is no evidence that regional anesthesia should be avoided in patients who manifest prolonged bleeding times due to aspirin.

Volatile anesthetics and nitrous oxide studied using in vitro models produce dose-related decreases in adenosine diphosphate-induced platelet aggregation.[17] It is thought that anesthetics may change the surface characteristics of platelet cell membranes and thus interfere with their cohesion. The clinical importance of this effect on platelet aggregation, if any, is not known.

ANTICOAGULATION AND PERFORMANCE OF SPINAL OR EPIDURAL BLOCK

A controversial question deals with performance of spinal or epidural blocks in patients who will subsequently receive heparin. The obvious concern is delayed hemorrhage from blood vessels damaged during performance of the block leading to formation of a subarachnoid or epidural hematoma. Nevertheless, symptomatic hematomas did not occur in any of 847 patients receiving spinal or epidural blocks followed 1 hour later by sufficient heparin to maintain activated clotting times at approximately twice baseline.[18] Likewise, subarachnoid morphine administered 50 minutes before heparinization for cardiopulmonary bypass was not followed by subarachnoid hematoma.[19] Despite these reports involving large numbers of patients, caution seems indicated in performing regional anesthesia in patients who will subsequently receive heparin. Indeed, spontaneous subarachnoid or epidural hematomas may occur in such patients.[20] Certainly, it would seem prudent to delay surgery for 24 hours should a traumatic needle insertion result in aspiration of blood at the time of performance of the block.

Even more controversial is performance of spinal or epidural blocks in patients who are already anticoagulated. Many are reluctant to perform regional blocks on these patients, although one large series describes 1,000 uneventful epidural anesthetics administered to 950 patients receiving oral anticoagulants preoperatively followed by intraoperative administration of heparin.[21] In another report, caudal epidural blocks administered to anticoagulated

patients (prothrombin time or partial thromboplastin time 1.5 or more times above control levels) or in the presence of thrombocytopenia (platelet counts less than 50,000 mm^3 due to radiation and/or chemotherapy) were not followed by complications due to excessive bleeding.[22] Likewise, neurologic complications have not been reported after administration of spinal or epidural anesthetics to patients being treated with low-dose heparin preoperatively. Nevertheless, many feel it is prudent to avoid spinal or epidural anesthesia in the presence of anticoagulant therapy unless these techniques offer clear advantages over general anesthesia.

Drug- or Disease-Induced Thrombocytopenia

Drugs that have been associated with thrombocytopenia include heparin, quinine, quinidine, thiazide diuretics, and medications derived from sulfa. The mechanism for accelerated platelet destruction leading to thrombocytopenia is presumed to be immunologic, due to platelet absorption of drug-antibody complexes. Drugs responsible should be discontinued as soon as thrombocytopenia is recognized. Infusion of platelet concentrates will not result in the anticipated increase in platelet counts, because of increased rates of destruction of these cells.

Autoimmune diseases are associated with an increased incidence of thrombocytopenia. For example, about 10 percent of patients with systemic lupus erythematosus manifest decreased platelet counts. Thrombocytopenia has also been observed in patients with Raynaud's phenomenon, rheumatoid arthritis, and hyperthyroidism. Finally, thrombocytopenia has been associated with a wide variety of bacterial and viral infections.

Extracorporeal Circulation

Patients who undergo heart surgery requiring extracorporeal circulation (cardiopulmonary bypass) are at risk for excessive bleeding due to surgical damage to blood vessels and acute defects in hemostasis. Studies of patients following cessation of extracorporeal circulation demonstrate decreased plasma concentrations of procoagulants (especially factor V) compared with preoperative values, but the magnitude of these decreases is usually not sufficient to cause bleeding.[23] Furthermore, fibrinogen dysfunction or activation of the fibrinolytic system with appearance of fibrin degradation products in the plasma do not seem to contribute to bleeding in these patients. Improved protocols for administration of protamine assure neutralization of heparin activity without heparin rebound and without protamine-related coagulopathy. Excessive doses of protamine may impair platelet aggregation.

In contrast to the apparent minor importance of the above mechanisms in causing bleeding, there is persuasive evidence that hemorrhage, which occurs after cessation of extracorporeal circulation, is most often due to acute acquired defects in formation of platelet plugs.[24] Transient impairment of platelet function is mediated by platelet activation during passage through the oxygenator of the cardiopulmonary bypass machine. The degree of impairment of platelet function is directly proportional to the duration of extracorporeal circulation and is also probably related to the level of hypothermia and to the prophylactic use of semisynthetic penicillins and possibly other drugs. In most patients, this platelet dysfunction is rapidly reversible within 1 hour, but if bleeding persists, the treatment is infusion of platelet concentrates. Alternatives to platelet transfusions and their associated risks are drugs such as prostacyclin and desmopressin. Prostacyclin is not likely to be useful, however, because of associated hypotensive effects. Desmopressin is a synthetic analog of antidiuretic hormone, which lacks vasoconstrictive activity but evokes release of von Willebrand's factor necessary for adequate activity of factor VIII and optimal function of platelets. Indeed, intraoperative administration of desmopressin reduces blood loss after extracorporeal circulation without associated adverse effects.[25] Whether desmopressin increases the possibility of occlusion of vein grafts is not known. Previous suggestions that positive end-expiratory pressure reduce mediastinal bleeding were not confirmed by a controlled study.[26] Likewise, prophylactic administration of platelets is of no proven value (see Chapter 27).

Idiopathic Thrombocytopenic Purpura

Idiopathic thrombocytopenic purpura is a syndrome characterized by persistent thrombocytopenia caused by circulating antiplatelet factors, which result in platelet destruction by the reticuloendothelial system.[27] Antiplatelet factors are most likely immunoglobulin G antibodies directed toward platelet-associated antigens.

CLINICAL MANIFESTATIONS

Clinical manifestations of idiopathic thrombocytopenic purpura can closely mimic drug-induced thrombocytopenic purpura. Idiopathic thrombocytopenic purpura typically manifests in young females, in the absence of a history of drug ingestion. The hallmark of thrombocytopenia is the presence of petechiae. With severe thrombocytopenia, there may be purpura, epistaxis, vaginal bleeding in females, and hemorrhage from the mucosa, especially that in the upper respiratory tract. Intracranial hemorrhage is the principal hazard of idiopathic thrombocytopenic purpura, whereas adenopathy and splenomegaly are unusual findings.

Transplacental transfer of maternal antibodies to platelets frequently causes neonatal thrombocytopenia. This predisposes infants to spontaneous bleeding, including intracranial hemorrhage. Therefore, cesarean section may be recommended to avoid risks of cerebral trauma to infants and hemorrhage in parturients during vaginal delivery.

TREATMENT

Treatment of idiopathic thrombocytopenic purpura associated with bleeding is with corticosteroids such as prednisone. Presumably, corticosteroids are effective by interfering with the macrophagic attack on immunoglobulin G-coated platelets. In addition, these drugs are likely to slow endogenous production of autoantibodies. Other immunosuppressant drugs that have been used in the treatment of these patients include cyclophosphamide, vincristine, and azathioprine (see Chapter 30).

Transfusion of platelet concentrates should be given as often as necessary to control hemorrhage. It should be appreciated, however, that survival of platelets is shortened in patients with idiopathic thrombocytopenic purpura. Indeed, infused platelets may be destroyed so rapidly that detectable increases in platelet counts do not occur.

Splenectomy is indicated when high doses of corticosteroids are required or when relapse occurs when the dose of these drugs is tapered. Splenectomy is rarely performed in children, but if this method of treatment is selected, it is ideally deferred until after the age of 6 years because of the increased risk of bacterial infections after removal of the spleen. Ideally, surgery for splenectomy is not performed until corticosteroid therapy has induced an increase in platelet counts. When surgery must be performed in the presence of active hemorrhage and platelet counts below 50,000 mm³, it is helpful to administer platelet concentrates at the time of induction of anesthesia and after ligation of the splenic pedicle. Management of anesthesia in these patients must include minimization of trauma to the upper airway, as during direct laryngoscopy for intubation of the trachea. Regional anesthesia is rarely selected because of the potential for spontaneous hemorrhage. Corticosteroids should be continued in the postoperative period. Beneficial effects of splenectomy are reflected by increases in platelet counts in the postoperative period.

Thrombotic Thrombocytopenic Purpura

Thrombotic thrombocytopenic purpura is characterized by disseminated intravascular aggregation of platelets.[28] This response is presumed to be due to the presence of an abnormal platelet aggregating factors. Clinical manifestations include fever, altered states of consciousness, severe anemia (hemoglobin concentrations often less than 6 g·dl⁻¹), and thrombocytopenia. The most common hemorrhagic manifestations are retinal, genitourinary, and gastrointestinal. Renal manifestations include proteinuria, hematuria, and azotemia. Hepatosplenomegaly is often present, and increased unconjugated fractions of bilirubin in plasma may lead to jaundice.

Treatment of thrombotic thrombocytopenic purpura is with antiplatelet drugs, such as aspirin, plus exchange plasmapheresis. High doses of corticosteroids are commonly used, in combination with antiplatelet drug therapy. Splenectomy is often performed, but the reasons for its beneficial effects are not known. Mortality from thrombotic thrombocytopenic purpura can exceed 80 percent.

Thrombogenesis and Thrombocytopenia Due to Intravascular Catheters

Thrombus formation on catheters placed in the systemic or pulmonary circulations is a predictable event.[29] Catheter thrombogenicity is presumed to reflect an interaction of blood with physicochemical and textural properties of the catheters. Catheters fabricated from polyvinylchloride are particularly thrombogenic. For example, it has been demonstrated that pulmonary artery catheters induce thrombus formation within 1 hour to 2 hours after placement, despite use of continuous infusions of heparinized saline through the catheter. In contrast, use of pulmonary artery catheters with heparin incorporated into the plastic material does not induce thrombus formation.[29] Although symptomatic pulmonary embolism is not a predictable event associated with use of thrombogenic pulmonary artery catheters, it would seem prudent to minimize the likelihood of thrombus formation if possible. Therefore, use of heparin-bonded pulmonary artery catheters may be a useful consideration.

Pulmonary artery catheters have been associated with thrombocytopenia.[30] Conceivably, increased platelet consumption due to thrombus formation on pulmonary artery catheters is responsible for decreases in platelet counts. Therefore, when thrombogenic catheters are present in patients who develop thrombocytopenia, it would seem prudent to consider sequestration of platelets on the catheter as a possible explanation.

REFERENCES

1. Barrer MJ, Ellison N. Platelet function. Anesthesiology 1977;46:202–11
2. Suchman AL, Mushlin AI. How well does the activated partial thromboplastin time predict postoperative hemorrhage. JAMA 1986;256:750–3
3. Tuman KJ, Spiess BD, McCarthy RJ, Ivankovich AD. Effects of progressive blood loss on coagulation as measured by thrombelastography. Anesth Analg 1987;66:856–63
4. Ellison N. Diagnosis and management of bleeding disorders. Anesthesiology 1977;47:171–80
5. Roberts HR. Hemophiliacs with inhibitors: Therapeutic options. N Engl J Med 1981;305:757–8
6. Kasper CK, Boylen AL, Ewing NP, et al. Hematologic management of hemophilia A for surgery. JAMA 1985;253:1279–83
7. Syamsoedin LJM, Heijnen L, Mauser-Bunschoten EP, et al. The effect of activated prothrombin-complex concentrate (FEIBA) on joint and muscle bleeding in patients with hemophilia A and antibodies to factor VIII. N Engl J Med 1981;305:717–21
8. Fresh frozen plasma. Indications and risks. JAMA 1985;253:551–3
9. Gralnick HR, Maisonneuve P, Sultan Y, Rick ME. Benefits of danazol treatment in patients with hemophilia A (classic hemophilia). JAMA 1985;253:1151–3
10. Sampson JF, Hamstra R, Aldrete JA. Management of hemophiliac patients undergoing surgical procedures. Anesth Analg 1979;58:133–5
11. Nilsson IM, Bergentz SE, Larsson SA. Surgery in von Willebrand's disease. Ann Surg 1970;190:746–52
12. Kitchens CS, Newcomb TF. Factor XIII. Medicine 1979:58:413–29
13. Wetzel RC, Marsh BR, Yaster M, Casella JF. Anesthetic implications of protein C deficiency. Anesth Analg 1986;65:982–4
14. Miller RD, Robbins TO, Tong MJ. Coagulation defects associated with massive blood transfusions. Ann Surg 1971;174:794–801
15. Mant MJ, Kind EG. Severe, acute disseminated intravascular coagulation. Am J Med 1979;67:557–63
16. Amrein PC, Ellman L, Harris WH. Aspirin-induced prolongation of bleeding time and perioperative blood loss. JAMA 1981;245:1825–8
17. Fauss BG, Meadows JC, Bruni CY, Qureshi GD. The in vitro and in vivo effects of isoflurane and nitrous oxide in platelet aggregation. Anesth Analg 1986;65:1170–4
18. Rao TLK, El-Etr AA. Anticoagulation following placement of epidural and subarachnoid catheters. Anesthesiology 1981;55:618–20
19. Matthews ET, Abrams LD. Intrathecal morphine in open heart surgery. Lancet 1980;2:543
20. Owens EL, Kasten GW, Hessel EA. Spinal subarachnoid hematoma after lumbar puncture and heparinization. A case report, review of the literature, and discussion of anesthetic implications. Anesth Analg 1986;65:1201–7
21. Odoom JA, Sih IL. Epidural analgesia and anticoagulant therapy. Experience with one thousand cases of continuous epidurals. Anaesthesia 1983;38:254–9
22. Waldman SD, Feldstein GS, Waldman HJ, et al. Caudal administration of morphine sulphate in anticoagulated and thrombocytopenic patients. Anesth Analg 1987;66:267–8
23. Harker LA. Bleeding after cardiopulmonary bypass. N Engl J Med 1986;314:1446–8
24. Harker LA, Malpass TW, Branson HE, et al. Mechanism of abnormal bleeding in patients undergoing cardiopulmonary bypass: Acquired transient platelet dysfunction associated with selective alpha-granule release. Blood 1980;56:824–34
25. Salzman EW, Weinstein MJ, Weintraub RM, et al. Treatment with desmopressin acetate to reduce blood loss after cardiac surgery. A double-blind randomized trial. N Engl J Med 1986;314:1402–6
26. Murphy DA, Finlayson DC, Craver JM, et al. Effect of positive end-expiratory pressure on excessive mediastinal bleeding after cardiac operations. A controlled study. J Thorac Cardiovasc Surg 1983;85:864–9
27. McMillan R. Chronic idiopathic thrombocytopenic purpura. N Engl J Med 1981;304:1135–7
28. Crain SM, Choudhury AM. Thrombotic thrombocytopenia. A reappraisal. JAMA 1981;246:1243–6
29. Hoar PF, Wilson RM, Mangano DT, et al. Heparin bonding reduces thrombogenicity of pulmonary-artery catheters. N Engl J Med 1981;305:993–5
30. Richman KA, Kim YL, Marshall BE. Thrombocytopenia and altered platelet kinetics associated with prolonged pulmonary-artery catheterization in the dog. Anesthesiology 1980;53:101–5

27

Transfusion Therapy

Most bleeding disorders encountered in the perioperative period are due to surgical transection of blood vessels. Replacement of blood loss due to this mechanism is with stored whole blood or erythrocytes (i.e., packed erythrocytes). Use of blood components is usually reserved for treatment of specific defects of coagulation.[1] The importance of recognizing adverse reactions associated with transfusion therapy is emphasized by the estimate that over one-half of all transfusions of blood products are given during anesthesia.[1,2]

PRETRANSFUSION TESTING

Pretransfusion testing for compatibility between donor and recipient blood assures the safety of administering stored blood to patients. Complete pretransfusion testing includes determination of the blood type (group) of the donor and recipient and the cross match between donor and recipient blood.

Blood Type

Determination of the blood type of the recipient and donor is the first step in selecting blood for transfusion therapy. Routine typing of blood is done to identify the category of antigens present on the membranes of erythrocytes. Categorization of blood as group A, B, AB, or O is based on the antigen makeup of erythrocyte membranes (Table 27-1). Naturally occurring antibodies (anti-B, anti-A) are formed whenever erythrocyte membranes lack A and/or B antigens (Table 27-1). These antibodies are capable of causing rapid intravascular destruction of erythrocytes that contain the corresponding antigens. Erythrocyte membranes are typed for the presence of the Rh antigen, also referred to as the D antigen (Table 27-1). Eighty-five percent of patients have erythrocytes that contain Rh antigens. These patients are classified as Rh-positive. In contrast to the naturally occurring antibodies to the A and B antigens, a patient who is Rh-negative will lack naturally occurring anti-Rh antibodies in the plasma. Nevertheless, recipients can develop anti-Rh antibodies in the plasma when given a transfusion with Rh-positive blood. Another frequent stimulus for the production of anti-Rh antibodies is the transfer of Rh-positive erythrocytes from the fetus into the circulation of a Rh-negative mother. Antibodies to A and B antigens do not cross the placenta, explaining the absence of hemolysis in the fetus when maternal and fetal blood types differ.

TABLE 27-1.   Major Blood Groups and Associated Antibodies

Blood Group	Antigen on Erythrocyte	Plasma Antibodies (Naturally Occurring)	Approximate Incidence in United States (%)			
			Whites	Blacks	American Indians	Orientals
A	A	Anti-B	40	27	16	28
B	B	Anti-A	11	20	4	27
AB	AB	None	4	4	1	5
O	None	Anti-A Anti-B	45	49	79	40
Rh	Rh(D)	None	42	17	44	70

Cross Match

Cross match for compatibility of recipient and donor erythrocytes and plasma is performed after determination of the blood type. This test is an in vitro simulation of what will happen on transfusing donor erythrocytes into a recipient. A complete cross match can be completed in 45 minutes to 60 minutes.

The major cross match is when the donor's erythrocytes are incubated with the plasma of the recipient. Agglutination confirms that the plasma of the recipient contains antibodies to antigens on cell membranes of donor erythrocytes. Incubation of the plasma of the donor with the erythrocytes of the recipient is a minor cross match. Agglutination results if the plasma of the donor contains antibodies to antigens on cell membranes of erythrocytes of the recipient.

The third phase of the cross match involves addition of antihuman globulin or Coombs' serum to donor erythrocytes or the plasma of the recipient. This phase of the cross match detects immunoglobulin G antibodies, including those directed against the Kell, Kidd, and Duffy blood group systems (Table 27-2).

TABLE 27-2.   Blood Groups Detected by Antihuman Globulin (Coombs') Serum

Blood Group	Approximate Incidence in United States (%)	
	Whites	Blacks
Kell	9	3.5
Kidd	73	>90
Duffy	65	

Inheritance of these factors is independent of the other blood group systems. Among these factors, Kell antigens are the most antigenic; the Kidd and Duffy antigens are less likely to elicit antibody responses.

Type and Screen

Type and screen denotes blood that has been typed for A, B, and Rh antigens and screened for antibodies.[3] This screening procedure is similar to a major cross match and requires the same amount of time (45 minutes to 60 minutes). This approach is used when the scheduled surgical procedure is unlikely to require transfusion of blood but is one for which blood should be available. Examples of such operations are cholecystectomy and hysterectomy.[4] When an emergency transfusion is needed, a partial cross match (recipient plasma plus donor erythrocytes) can be completed in 5 minutes to 10 minutes. Providing blood in this manner (type specific, antibody screen, and partial cross match) is 99 percent effective in preventing incompatible transfusions.[4] Type and screen without a complete cross match does not protect against transfusion reactions due to antibodies against antigens of low incidence, not represented in screening cell samples but present on cell membranes of donor erythrocytes.

Use of a type and screen permits more efficient use of stored blood and is cost-effective. For example, a type and cross match, in contrast to a type and screen, makes that blood unavailable to other patients, resulting in the possible loss of storage time if the blood is not used. Furthermore, use of a complete cross match makes it necessary to have more blood available than is actually transfused. This results in an increase in the amount of blood that becomes outdated before use. Therefore, use of type and screen for operative procedures that routinely necessitate transfusions of less than 0.5 units of blood seems acceptable.[3]

Predeposited Autologous Blood

Patients scheduled for elective surgery that may require transfusion of blood may elect to donate blood preoperatively (i.e., predeposit) for possible retransfusion in the perioperative period.[5] In contrast to homologous blood, autologous blood does not transmit disease or cause sensitization reactions and thus represents the safest source for blood transfusion. Donations may be made approximately every 3 days to 7 days, with the last unit collected 72 hours or more before surgery to permit restoration of plasma volume. Ferrous sulfate is often administered to these patients between blood donations. Most patients are able to easily donate 3 units of blood assuming the preoperative hematocrit is greater than 30 percent. Autologous blood transfusions can also be accomplished through intraoperative salvage serving as an alternative to transfusion of homologous blood.

Designated Donors

Designated donors are typically friends or relatives who donate blood to be saved for a specific patient. There is no evidence that such blood is safer and the logistics of collecting and distributing blood from designated donors are complex. Most important, donors so coerced to donate may withhold social or medical information that would otherwise preclude their donation, thereby placing the recipient at potential risk for transfusion-transmitted diseases.[1]

EMERGENCY BLOOD TRANSFUSION

The urgent need to replace intravascular fluid volume may require use of blood that has not undergone a type and cross match. Alternatively, crystalloid or colloid solutions (i.e., asanguinous fluids) can be administered to maintain intravascular fluid volume. Indeed, healthy patients can sustain acute blood losses equivalent to 30 percent of their blood volume and require replacement with only asanguinous fluids. Nevertheless, when the hemotocrit is acutely reduced to below 25 percent, it may become necessary to transfuse blood before completion of all the compatibility tests. In this situation, available approaches in order of preference are the administration of (1) type-specific, partially cross matched blood; (2) type-specific, uncrossmatched blood; and (3) O-Rh-negative, uncrossmatched blood.

Type-Specific, Partially Cross Matched Blood

A partial cross match is performed by adding the plasma of the recipient to the erythrocytes of the donor and observing the specimen for agglutination after centrifugation. This procedure takes only 5 minutes to 10 minutes and will eliminate hemolytic transfusion reactions due to ABO incompatibility. Antibodies directed against Rh and Kell antigens are not detected.

Type-Specific Uncrossmatched Blood

Use of type-specific but uncrossmatched blood is safe in the majority of patients who have not been pregnant or previously exposed to foreign erythrocytes. The relative risk of experiencing a hemolytic transfusion reaction increases from 1:1000 in unsensitized patients to about 1:100 in potentially sensitized patients receiving type-specific blood without an antibody screen.[1]

O-Rh-Negative Uncrossmatched Blood

Type O erythrocytes lack A and B antigens. Therefore, these erythrocytes are not hemolyzed by anti-A and anti-B antibodies that may be present in the plasma of the recipient. As such, type O blood has been designated as a "universal donor," and recommended for use when time is not available for performance of a type and complete cross match. Plasma of type O blood, however, does contain antibodies capable of destroying type A or B erythrocytes. Therefore, uncrossmatched O-Rh-negative erythrocytes should be used in preference to O-Rh-negative whole blood since infusion of erythrocytes introduces only a small volume of plasma that could contain dangerous antibodies. The administration of O-Rh-positive blood to Rh-negative patients is acceptable in an emergency but should be avoided if possible in women of childbearing age.

After emergency transfusion of more than 2 units of type O-Rh-negative or Rh-positive uncrossmatched blood, the patient should not be given blood of the correct blood type. This precaution is necessary to avoid hemolysis of erythrocytes with A or B antigens by anti-A or anti-B antibodies introduced with the transfusion of type O blood. Type specific A, B, or AB blood can be safely administered only when it can be documented that transfused plasma levels of anti-A or anti-B antibodies have decreased to levels that will permit such infusion. Continued administration of O-Rh-negative blood results in only minor hemolysis of recipient erythrocytes, with associated hyperbilirubinemia as the major complication.

COMPONENT THERAPY

Advantages of component therapy include (1) the ability to achieve a selective therapeutic effect by replacement of only the deficient procoagulant; (2) storage of specific procoagulants under optimal conditions to allow use at a later date; (3) minimization of the chance of circulatory overload; and (4) avoidance of the transfusion of unnecessary donor plasma, which may contain undesirable antigens or antibodies.[1,6] A unit of whole blood (500 ml) can be subdivided into a number of fractions (Table 27-3).

Erythrocytes (Packed Erythrocytes)

Erythrocytes (volume 250 ml to 300 ml, hematocrit 70 percent to 80 percent) are used for treatment of anemia that is not associated with acute reductions in intravascular fluid volume. The goal is to increase the oxygen-carrying capacity of blood. One unit of infused erythrocytes will increase the average adult hemoglobin concentration about 1 $g\cdot dl^{-1}$. Mixing of erythrocytes with 50 ml to 100 ml of saline

TABLE 27-3. Components Derived from Whole Blood

Erythrocytes (previously termed packed erythrocytes)
Leukocyte poor blood
Leukocyte concentrates
Platelet concentrates
Heat treated plasma (derived from outdated whole blood)
    Albumin—5 percent and 25 percent (Albumisol)
    Plasma protein fraction (Plasmanate)
Fresh plasma (derived from fresh whole blood)
    Fresh frozen plasma
    Cryoprecipitate
    Factor VIII
    Fibrinogen
    Other specific procoagulant concentrates—factors II, VII, IX, X (Proplex, Konyne)
    Antibody concentrates

decreases the viscosity of this blood component and allows more rapid infusion. Glucose solutions may cause hemolysis and calcium, as in lactated Ringer's solution, may cause clotting if mixed with erythrocytes. The principal disadvantage of using erythrocytes to replace acute blood loss is the difficulty associated with rapid infusion of these highly viscous solutions. Nevertheless, a common recommendation is that erythrocytes should be used to replace blood loss in adults that is less than 1500 ml.[7]

Preparation of erythrocytes from whole blood just before transfusion results in the infusion of less sodium, potassium, ammonia, citrate, and lactic acid. As a result, erythrocytes so prepared are useful for patients with renal or hepatic dysfunction. Most erythrocytes, however, are prepared on the day the blood is collected from the donor and therefore, are subject to the same storage lesions as whole blood. Still, regardless of when erythrocytes are prepared, the amount of plasma infused is less than when whole blood is transfused. As a result, less anti-A and anti-B antibodies are transferred, permitting safer transfusion in emergency situations of type O cells to patients with type A or B blood. Because less plasma-containing proteins are transfused, there is also a decreased incidence of allergic transfusion reactions associated with the use of erythrocytes, as compared with whole blood. No data document a reduced risk of post-transfusion hepatitis when erythrocytes are used instead of whole blood.

Frozen Erythrocytes

Long-term preservation of erythrocytes is accomplished by the addition of glycerol, which permits storage at −85 degrees Celsius without damage to cells. The major advantage of frozen erythrocytes is long-term storage, with almost normal function and viability upon thawing. This normal function reflects maintenance of concentrations of 2,3-diphosphoglycerate and adenosine triphosphate in erythrocytes at levels near those present at the time the cells were frozen; therefore, erythrocytes frozen soon after collection will maintain nearly normal concentrations of 2,3-diphosphoglycerate. Additional advantages include a decreased incidence of nonhemolytic transfusion reactions, since these cell preparations are almost entirely free of both leukocytes and plasma proteins. Frozen erythrocytes have been alleged to be less likely to be associated with post-transfusion hepatitis. Nevertheless, transmission of viral hepatitis still can occur after administration of frozen erythrocytes.

Disadvantages of frozen erythrocytes include cost, the 45 minutes required for thawing, and the need to remove the glycerol before infusion of these cells. Furthermore, the possibility of bacterial contamination during processing required for thawing necessitates that a unit of thawed erythrocytes be used within 24 hours. Indeed, advantages of prolonged storage of frozen erythrocytes may become less important as improvements in anticoagulant preservative solutions (citrate-phosphate-dextrose plus adenine) prolong the viability of erythrocytes maintained at 4 degrees Celsius. At present, the major indication for frozen erythrocytes is a source of rare blood types.

Leukocyte-Poor Blood

Leukocyte-poor blood is indicated for patients in whom severe febrile transfusion reactions are known to have occurred during a previous administration of blood. Leukocyte antibodies responsible for febrile transfusion reactions are common in patients who have received multiple transfusions of whole blood, multiparous women, and patients who have received a kidney transplant. Leukocyte-poor blood is prepared by removing the buffy coat from fresh whole blood after its centrifugation. Micropore filters remove 40 percent to 85 percent of leukocytes and when combined with centrifugation before administration up to 90 percent of these cells are removed.[1] Frozen erythrocytes are also a source of leukocyte-poor blood.

Platelet Concentrates

Patients with thrombocytopenia or abnormal platelet function may benefit from administration of platelets if the platelet disorder is likely to be causing or contributing to bleeding. For nonsurgical patients, platelet counts less than 10,000 mm^3 to 30,000 mm^3 are associated with spontaneous hemorrhage. Therefore, counts in this range are indications for the transfusion of platelets. Prophylactic therapy is probably not indicated for patients with platelet counts between 30,000 mm^3 and 100,000 mm^3, except when major surgical procedures are planned, when it is desirable to increase platelet counts to between 50,000 mm^3 and 100,000 mm^3. Platelet-function-related prolongation of the bleeding time to at least twice normal is usually an indication for transfusion of platelets. The majority of patients who receive rapid replacement of one to two blood volumes do not develop microvascular bleeding as a result of thrombocytopenia.[8] Therefore, platelets should not be administered in the absence of documented thrombocytopenia and evidence of abnormal bleeding. Controlled studies have demonstrated no correlation between platelet counts and bleeding after cardiopulmonary bypass and no detectable benefit from the prophylactic administration of platelets to such patients.[8]

Platelet concentrates are preferred over such other sources of platelets as fresh, whole blood and platelet-rich plasma because the same therapeutic effect can be achieved more rapidly, with administration of less volume. One unit of platelet concentrate will increase the platelet count 5,000 mm^3 to 10,000 mm^3 as documented by platelet counts obtained 1 hour after infusion. A standard 170 micron filter is recommended for administration of platelets.[8]

Platelets that have been stored at 20 degrees Celsius to 24 degrees Celsius and infused within 24 hours of being drawn are viable for as long as 8 days.[9] This compares with a normal platelet life span of 9 days to 11 days. For unknown reasons, however, storage of platelets at 22 degrees Celsius results in a storage lesion that prevents effective hemostatic function for the first 8 hours to 24 hours after administration of these cells.[9] In contrast, platelets that have been stored at 4 degrees Celsius are viable for only 2 days to 3 days, but platelet function is better preserved than in those cells stored at 20 degrees Celsius to 24 degrees Celsius.

The major risks associated with administration of platelet concentrates are sensitization reactions and transmission of disease, especially if pooled donor products are administered. Platelets possess HLA antigens on their cell membranes. Patients who are sensitized to these antigens will destroy infused platelets, which manifests as the absence of a therapeutic response. Sensitization to platelet antigens is common in patients who have received multiple prior platelet transfusions. Fever and respiratory distress may accompany sensitization reactions and reflect the release of serotonin and other vasoactive substances during the immune destruction of platelets. In these sensitized patients, administration of type-specific HLA platelets is the only acceptable approach. Sensitization reactions observed in donors undergoing automated plateletpheresis have been attributed to ethylene oxide gas used to sterilize plastic components in disposable apheresis kits.[10]

Viruses transmitted by platelet transfusions are similar to those transmitted by other blood components and include hepatitis virus, cytomegalovirus, Epstein-Barr virus, and human immunodeficiency virus. These are of special concern because platelet concentrates are often prepared by pooling from multiple donors and frequently administered to immunodepressed patients. An unusual, but sometimes life-threatening complication of platelet transfusions is sepsis from infusion of bacteria that have proliferated during storage at 20 degrees Celsius to 24 degrees Celsius.[8]

Albumin

Albumin is available as 5 percent and 25 percent solutions. The risk of transmission of viral hepatitis by albumin is eliminated by heating these solutions to 60 degrees Celsius for 10 hours. The 5 percent solution is isotonic with pooled plasma and is most often used when rapid expansion of intravascular fluid volume is indicated.

The 25 percent solution of albumin is osmotically equivalent to about five times its volume. Furthermore, this concentration contains only about one-seventh the amount of sodium present in the same volume of plasma. Hypoalbuminemia is the most frequent indication for the administration of 25 percent albumin. Its administration will draw 3 ml to 4 ml of fluid from the interstitial space into the intravascular fluid space for every 1 ml administered. This increase in intravascular fluid volume is the reason 25 percent albumin is not recommended for patients with anemia or congestive heart failure. Simultaneous infusion of crystalloid solutions is necessary to prevent dehydration due to administration of 25 percent albumin.

It should be appreciated that albumin does not provide coagulation factors. In fact, albumin-induced increases in intravascular fluid volume may dilute plasma concentrations of procoagulants.

Plasma Protein Fractions

Plasma protein fractions are a 5 percent solution of plasma proteins in saline solutions, which are osmotically equivalent to an equal volume of plasma. These proteins are obtained by fractionating a large pool of human plasma. Like albumin, this blood component is heat-treated to eliminate the risk of transmission of viral hepatitis. Plasma protein fractions contain at least 83 percent albumin and no more than 17 percent globulins of which 1 percent or less are gamma globulins. Sodium concentrations are 130 mEq·L^{-1} to 160 mEq·L^{-1}, whereas potassium concentration is no more than 2 mEq·L^{-1}. In addition, plasma protein fraction may contain a prekallikrein activator that stimulates the kallikrein system, resulting in peripheral vasodilation and hypotension during rapid infusion of these solutions.[11] The most frequent use of this blood component is to increase acutely the intravascular fluid volume. No cross matching is necessary and the absence of cellular elements removes the risk of sensitization with repeated infusions. It must be appreciated that plasma protein fractions do not contain coagulation factors and are thus of no value for treating bleeding disorders.

Fresh Frozen Plasma

Fresh frozen plasma is the fluid portion obtained from a single unit of whole blood that is centrifuged, separated and frozen within 6 hours of collection. Risks of administration of fresh frozen plasma include transmission of disease (viral hepatitis, acquired immunodeficiency syndrome), allergic reactions and fluid overload. Fresh frozen plasma contains all procoagulants except platelets and has been extensively used to treat specific, as well as multiple procoagulant deficiencies. Despite the presence of procoagulants, fresh frozen plasma is not considered to be superior to other blood components (cryoprecipitate, factor VIII concentrates, factor IX concentrates, immune globulin) that provide greater efficacy and safety.[12,13] There is no documentation that fresh frozen plasma has beneficial effects when used as part of the management of massively hemorrhaging patients in the absence of a documented procoagulant defect.[12] Immediate reversal of warfarin anticoagulation in patients who require emergency surgery can be achieved with administration of fresh frozen plasma. Nevertheless, vitamin K is the preferred therapy for reversal of warfarin in patients who do not require immediate surgery. All factors considered, there is little scientific evidence to support the increasing use of fresh frozen plasma in clinical medicine.[12] As a volume expander fresh frozen plasma is less effective than albumin solutions.

Cryoprecipitate

Cryoprecipitate is that fraction of plasma that precipitates when fresh frozen plasma is thawed. This fraction can then be frozen and stored for future use. Cryoprecipitate is useful for treating hemophilia A, since it contains high concentrations of factor VIII in a small plasma volume. For example, each unit of cryoprecipitate contains about 80 units to 120 units of factor VIII activity in a volume of only about 10 ml. Hemolytic anemia may occur if type specific (A, B, AB, or O) cryoprecipitate is not administered. This component should be infused through a 170 micron filter. About 15 percent of patients with hemophilia develop an inhibitor that inactivates factor VIII. The presence of this inhibitor should be determined before treatment of patients with hemophilia, especially before surgery. Cryoprecipitate is also useful for treatment of von Willebrand's disease. Cryoprecipitate contains nearly 25 percent of the fibrinogen normally present in a unit of blood and can be administered to patients with hypofibrinogenemia. Multiple transfusions of cryoprecipitate in the absence of low fibrinogen concentrations may result in hyperfibrinogenemia. The presence of fibrinogen introduces the risk of transmission of viral diseases.

Immune Globulin

Immune globulin is a concentrated solution of globulins prepared from pooled human plasma. This preparation protects against clinical manifestations of hepatitis A and is useful as replacement therapy for patients with hypogammaglobulinemia. Hepatitis B immune globulin is a specific preparation with a high antibody titer against hepatitis B.

Factor VIII Concentrates

Factor VIII concentrates are useful for treatment of hemophilia A. In contrast to cryoprecipitate, this blood component is more expensive and carries a greater risk of transmission of viral diseases due to its preparation from pooled plasma.

Factor IX Concentrates

Factor IX concentrates are prepared from pooled plasma. This blood component is useful for the treatment of hemophilia B but carries the risk of transmission of viral diseases. There is a high risk of thrombotic complications associated with infusion of factor IX concentrates, presumably reflecting the high concentrations of prothrombin and factor X that result from this factor.[14]

Specific Procoagulant Concentrates

Concentrates of vitamin-K-dependent procoagulants (the prothrombin complex) are available for the treatment of bleeding due to deficiencies of factors II, VII, IX, and X. Because of their pooled sources, these preparations introduce the risk for transmission of viral diseases.

DEXTRANS

Dextrans are branched polysaccharides, which can be used for acute expansion of the intravascular fluid volume. Advantages of dextrans include absence of the ability to transmit viral diseases and ready availability. The molecular weight of dextran solutions ranges from 40,000 (Rheomacrodex) to 70,000 (Macrodex). Low molecular weight dextran is acceptable for expansion of the intravascular fluid volume, but the effect is transient, as this substance leaks out of the vascular bed in 2 hours to 4 hours. This form of dextran is used most often to prevent thromboembolism by reducing blood viscosity and preventing platelet aggregation. Indeed, dextran in initial doses of 10 $ml \cdot kg^{-1}$ appears to be equally effective to low-dose heparin for prevention of pulmonary embolism (see Chapter 13). Dextran with an average molecular weight of 70,000 is capable of expanding the intravascular fluid volume for a prolonged time. This form of dextran, however, has minimal beneficial effect on the microcirculation. This form of dextran may also be used in hysteroscopy to help distend and irrigate the uterine cavity and to prevent tubal adhesions after reconstructive tubal surgery for infertility. Disadvantages of dextrans include coagulation defects due to platelet dysfunction when the amount of infused dextran exceeds 1500 ml. Dextrans can also cause erythrocytes to agglutinate, resulting in difficulty in performing a cross match of blood. Allergic reactions may occur in association with administration of dextrans. Elimination of dextrans is primarily by the kidneys.

STROMA-FREE HEMOGLOBIN SOLUTIONS

Stroma-free hemoglobin solutions may be useful as plasma volume expanders, with the potential capacity to transport oxygen to and carry carbon dioxide from tissues.[15] The value of stroma-free solutions for expanding the intravascular fluid volume is related to the high molecular weight (68,000) of hemoglobin. The ability of hemoglobin in solution to transport oxygen and maintain tissue oxygenation, however, has been questioned, since free hemoglobin has an increased affinity for oxygen, as reflected by a decreased P_{50} value. Nevertheless, stroma-free solutions administered to animal models have been shown to deliver oxygen adequately to the peripheral tissues.[16,17] Other advantages of stroma-free solutions, as compared with blood products, include the lack of need for performing a type and cross match and longer storability. Renal dysfunction during infusion of hemoglobin does not occur when stromal contents of the erythrocytes and lipids are removed from the hemoglobin solution.[15] This observation suggests that renal dysfunction associated with intravascular hemolysis, as occurs during transfusion reactions, is due to the deposition of stromal contents of erythrocytes in renal tubules, rather than the precipitation of free he-

moglobin at these sites. It is possible that stroma-free solutions will emerge in the future as alternatives to blood or blood components for the treatment of acute reductions in intravascular fluid volume that occur during the perioperative period.

FLUOSOL

Fluosol is an emulsion of perfluorochemicals with oxygen-carrying capability. Intravenous administration of this emulsion may be followed by improvement in arterial oxygenation and cardiac output due to improved venous return. Fluosol, therefore, has the potential to serve both as a volume expander and a method to improve arterial oxygenation, especially in patients with life-threatening anemia who refuse treatment with blood products. Adverse effects of fluosol infusion may include complement activation with resultant hypotension and pulmonary infiltrates.[18,19]

HETASTARCH

Hetastarch (hydroxyethyl starch) is a synthetic colloid solution, which is as effective as 5 percent albumin as an intravascular fluid volume expander. In this regard, hetastarch solutions (20 ml·kg^{-1}) are used to expand intravascular fluid volume in the management of acute hypovolemia.[20] Excessive doses of hetastarch decrease the hematocrit and dilute plasma concentrations of platelets and procoagulants. Hetastarch solutions have about the same risk as dextrans for producing allergic reactions. Unlike dextrans, hetastarch solutions do not interfere with crossmatching of blood. Hypervolemia is a potential adverse effect, particularly in patients with impaired renal function, since hetastarch is excreted primarily by the kidneys.

COMPLICATIONS OF BLOOD TRANSFUSION

Complications that can accompany administration of blood or blood components include transfusion reactions, metabolic abnormalities, transmission of viral diseases, and infusion of microaggregates, which accumulate during the storage of blood. Accidental infusion of outdated blood may produce increases in pulmonary vascular resistance and renal damage due to hemolysis.[21]

Transfusion Reactions

Transfusion reactions are categorized as allergic, febrile, hemolytic, and delayed hemolytic.[1,22]

ALLERGIC REACTIONS

Allergic reactions initiated by transfusion of correctly typed and crossmatched blood occur in about 3 percent of patients. Incompatible plasma proteins are the presumed mechanism. Manifestations include pruritus, erythema, and urticaria, often accompanied by increases of body temperature and eosinophilia. Occasionally, laryngospasm and bronchospasm are also present. During anesthesia the first manifestation of an allergic reaction due to blood administration may be the appearance of erythema along the pathway of the vein receiving the blood plus urticaria, particularly on the chest, neck, and face. Changes in blood pressure or heart rate rarely occur. Severe allergic reactions are most likely to occur in patients who lack immunoglobulin A in the plasma. Indeed, infusion of as little as 10 ml of blood into immunoglobulin A deficient patients can result in life-threatening anaphylaxis. Immunoglobulin A deficiency occurs in 1 in every 700 patients and these individuals should receive transfusions obtained only from immunoglobulin A deficient donors (see Chapter 31).

Treatment of mild allergic reactions, manifested only by erythema, urticaria, and minimal elevations of body temperature, is with the intravenous administration of 0.5 mg·kg^{-1} to 1.0 mg·kg^{-1} of diphenhydramine. More severe reactions mandate discontinuation of the transfusion, as well as the administration of diphenhydramine. Subsequent transfusions should be with washed erythrocytes or platelets to assure removal of plasma proteins. Patients with a previous history of allergic reactions to blood or with known allergies seem to be more susceptible to this type of adverse blood reaction. In these at-risk patients, prophylactic administration of histamine receptor antagonists, such as diphenhydramine, may be helpful in reducing the incidence of this complication.

A rare manifestation of allergic reactions to blood is the development of an acute pulmonary hypersensitivity response, characterized by the abrupt onset of fever, dry nonproductive cough, and pulmonary edema, in the absence of any evidence of intravascular fluid overload or congestive heart failure.[1,23] Radiographs of the chest reveal congestion of the pulmonary vasculature. There may be associated urticaria and eosinophilia. Hypotension and arterial hypoxemia have been observed on rare occasions. The mechanism has not been confirmed, but it is thought that leukocyte antibodies in the plasma of the donor react with leukocytes of the recipient producing cellular aggregation, microvascular occlusion, and pulmonary capillary leakage.[23] Serologic studies performed after the reaction may confirm the presence of HLA-specific leukocyte antibodies in the plasma of the donor or recipient, suggesting that pulmonary edema was caused by a leukoagglutination reaction. Treatment is symptomatic and includes discontinuation of the transfusion and administration of diphenhydramine.

FEBRILE REACTIONS

Febrile reactions are the most common adverse nonhemolytic response to the transfusion of blood accompanying 0.5 percent to 1 percent of transfusions.[1] Body temperature usually begins to increase within 4 hours after starting the transfusion but rarely increases above 38 degrees Celsius. Since temperature elevation may also be an early sign of hemolytic transfusion reactions, the diagnosis of nonhemolytic febrile transfusion reactions is based on the absence of signs of hemolysis. The most likely explanation for febrile reactions is an interaction between recipient antibodies and antigens present on the leukocytes and/or platelets of the donor. Incriminated antibodies are presumed to have been formed as a result of previous blood transfusions or pregnancy. Fever is thought to result from release of pyrogenic substances from injured cells. Headache, nausea, vomiting, and chest or back pain may accompany the elevation of body temperature. On rare occasions, development of bilateral perihilar infiltrates can be seen on the radiograph of the chest.

Treatment of mild febrile reactions is by slowing the rate of infusion of blood and by administering aspirin or acetaminophen. Meperidine, 25 mg administered intravenously to adults, is useful for treatment of shivering, which may accompany these reactions. Severe febrile reactions may require discontinuation of the blood infusion. Diphenhydramine and corticosteroids are of doubtful value in treatment of febrile reactions. Patients who experience two or more febrile reactions are candidates for receipt of leukocyte-poor erythrocytes, frozen erythrocytes, or type-specific platelets administered through micropore filters. Since only one of eight patients who experience a febrile reaction will have a similar reaction to subsequent transfusions, it is not appropriate to request leukocyte-poor erythrocytes unless more than one prior febrile reaction has occurred.[1] Bacterial contamination is a rare cause of fever during transfusion of blood.

HEMOLYTIC REACTIONS

Hemolytic reactions occur when specific antibodies in the plasma of the recipient interact with antigens on cell membranes of donor erythrocytes (i.e., incompatible blood). The common factor in the production of intravascular hemolysis and development of spontaneous hemorrhage is activation of the complement system, which also causes release of histamine and enhances capillary permeability.

In awake patients, immediate manifestations of acute hemolytic reactions include lumbar and substernal pain, fever with or without shivering, restlessness, nausea, dyspnea, skin flushing, and hypotension. It should be remembered that erythema and urticaria are manifestations of allergic and not hemolytic reactions. With the exception of hypotension, the immediate signs of hemolytic reactions are masked in an anesthetized patient.

Immediate manifestations of hemolytic reactions are followed by hemoglobinuria, oliguria, anuria, intractable hemorrhage, anemia, and jaundice. Acute renal failure is presumed to reflect precipitation of stromal and lipid contents of erythrocytes in distal renal tubules. It should be appreciated that free hemoglobin in plasma is unlikely to be responsible for the renal dysfunction that accompanies intravascular hemolysis[15] (see the section Stroma-Free Hemoglobin Solutions). Decreased renal cortical blood flow, due to histamine-induced vasomotor changes, and deposition of fibrin in the microcirculation may also contribute to renal dysfunction. Disseminated intravascular coagulation is initiated by material released from hemolyzed erythrocytes, leading to thrombocytopenia and increased circulating concentrations of fibrin degradation products. Elevations of unconjugated fractions of bilirubin in the plasma are maximal 3 hours to 6 hours after the onset of hemolytic reactions.

Treatment of acute hemolytic reactions begins with the immediate discontinuation of the infusion of blood. Indeed, severity of hemolytic reactions are directly proportional to the amount of incompatible blood infused. The donor blood and a blood sample from the patient should be sent to the laboratory for a repeat type and cross match. It is imperative to maintain renal function, as the magnitude of deposition of erythrocyte stroma and lipids in renal tubules is inversely related to urinary output. Urine output is maintained by liberal intravenous infusion of crystalloid solutions and administration of mannitol or furosemide. Intravenous administration of sodium bicarbonate to alkalinize the urine has been recommended to prevent deposition of foreign material in distal renal tubules by improving the solubility of hemoglobin degradation products resulting from hemolysis. Nevertheless, the value of alkalinization of the urine has not been confirmed. Finally, the value of corticosteroids in the management of hemolytic reactions is unproven.

DELAYED HEMOLYTIC REACTIONS

Delayed hemolytic reactions occur when the amount of antibody in plasma of the recipient is insufficient to cause immediate hemolysis of the correctly typed and cross matched donor erythrocytes. Since antibodies are below detectable levels, these reactions are not preventable. Clinically, jaundice becomes manifest up to 14 days after administration of the blood, and the hematocrit may decrease. A positive indirect Coombs' test indicates that plasma of the recipient contains antibodies against antigens present on transfused but not on autologous cells. Treatment is supportive.

Metabolic Abnormalities

Metabolic abnormalities produced by administration of blood are related to changes that occur during storage (Table 27-4). For example, hydrogen ions, carbon dioxide, and potassium increase; erythrocyte concentrations of 2,3-diphosphoglycerate decrease during storage of whole blood at 4 degrees Celsius. Furthermore, the presence of citrate anticoagulant

in stored blood has important potential implications when transfused into recipients. A unit of whole blood contains about 450 ml of blood and 65 ml of citrate-containing preservative. The maximum allowable storage time is determined by the type of preservative. Blood collected in citrate-phosphate-dextrose (CPD) may be stored for 21 days, whereas that collected in citrate-phosphate-dextrose adenine (CPDA-1) has a shelf life of 35 days. Storage time is defined by the requirement for 70 percent viability of transfused erythrocytes 24 hours after transfusion.

HYDROGEN IONS

Hydrogen ion content of stored blood is initially increased by the addition of acid-citrate-dextrose (pH 5.0) or citrate-phosphate-dextrose (pH 5.6). Continued metabolic function of erythrocytes results in additional production of hydrogen ions, such that pH of stored blood is usually less than 7 after 14 days to 21 days. Furthermore, arterial carbon dioxide partial pressures increase to between 150 mmHg and 200 mmHg since this gas cannot diffuse through glass or plastic materials used as blood containers. Despite these changes, metabolic acidosis is not a consistent occurrence, even with the rapid infusion of large volumes of stored blood. Therefore, intravenous administration of sodium bicarbonate to patients receiving transfusions of whole blood should be determined by measurement of arterial pH and not based on arbitrary regimens.

Metabolic alkalosis, rather than metabolic acidosis, is a frequent accompaniment of massive blood transfusions.[24] This alkalosis is presumed to be partly due to metabolism of infused citrate to bicarbonate, which could be

TABLE 27-4. Changes that Occur During Storage of Whole Blood in Citrate-Phosphate-Dextrose

	Days of Storage at 4 Degrees Celsius				
	0	7	14	21	28
Viable cells 24 hours after transfusion (%)	100	98	85	80	75
Plasma pH at 37 degrees Celsius	7.20	7.00	6.90	6.84	6.78
2,3-diphosphoglycerate ($\mu M \cdot ml^{-1}$)	4.8	1.2	1	1	1
P_{50} (mmHg)	24	23	20	17	17
Plasma potassium ($mEq \cdot L^{-1}$)	4	12	17	21	23

further exaggerated by administration of lactated Ringer's solution. Obviously, routine administration of sodium bicarbonate to treat a presumed metabolic acidosis could accentuate a co-existing and unrecognized alkalosis. Post-transfusion metabolic alkalosis is most likely to occur in patients who have diminished renal function, since the kidneys are responsible for elimination of bicarbonate.

POTASSIUM

Potassium content of acid-citrate-dextrose blood reaches about 14 mEq·L^{-1} by 7 days of storage and increases further to 21 mEq·L^{-1} to 24 mEq·L^{-1} after 21 days. Potassium levels of blood stored in citrate-phosphate-dextrose are about 20 percent lower. Nevertheless, massive transfusions of stored blood rarely increase plasma concentrations of potassium. For example, after massive transfusions, 78 percent of patients remain normokalemic, 12 percent become hypokalemic, and 10 percent become hyperkalemic.[25] Transfusion of frozen erythrocytes is often associated with hypokalemia. Failure of plasma concentrations of potassium to predictably increase most likely reflects the small amount of potassium actually present in a unit of stored whole blood. For example, since a unit of whole blood contains only 300 ml of plasma, a measured plasma potassium concentration of 21 mEq·L^{-1} would represent less than 7 mEq of potassium. Transfusion of 10 units of stored whole blood would result in the addition of only about 70 mEq of potassium, an amount unlikely to elevate plasma concentrations. In addition, it must be appreciated that production of metabolic alkalosis by massive transfusions of whole blood will favor transfer of potassium from extracellular fluid into intracellular spaces, further offsetting any tendency toward hyperkalemia. Nevertheless, it must be appreciated that potassium present in stored blood could produce hyperkalemia in patients with impaired or absent renal function.

The major value of warming stored blood to near 37 degrees Celsius before infusion is to minimize reductions in body temperature that can accompany the administration of blood. As a guideline, blood warmers should be used in adults receiving two or more units of rapidly infused blood.[1] Previous suggestions that warming of stored blood before infusion was important for restoring integrity of erythrocyte cell membranes and favoring entry of potassium back into cells have not been confirmed. Indeed, there is evidence that warming stored blood does not change concentrations of potassium in plasma that accompanies this blood (Fig. 27-1).[26]

DECREASED 2,3-DIPHOSPHOGLYCERATE

Storage of blood is associated with progressive reductions in concentrations of 2,3-diphosphoglycerate in erythrocytes, resulting in increased affinity of hemoglobin for oxygen. The resulting shift in the oxyhemoglobin dissociation curve of recipients to the left, after massive blood transfusions, is manifested by decreased P$_{50}$ values. Conceivably, this change could jeopardize tissue oxygen delivery, particularly in the presence of anemia. Nevertheless, the clinical significance of decreased 2,3-diphosphoglycerate concentrations in erythrocytes has not been confirmed. Furthermore, the higher pH of citrate-phosphate-dextrose anticoagulant, as compared with acid-citrate dextrose anticoagulant, prevents rapid depletion of 2,3-diphosphoglycerate concentrations in erythrocytes. Indeed, the P$_{50}$ of citrate-phosphate-dextrose preserved blood is maintained at near normal levels for the first 2 weeks of storage, and the P$_{50}$ of acid-citrate-dextrose preserved blood decreases below normal during the first week of storage.

CITRATE ANTICOAGULANT

Citrate metabolism to bicarbonate may contribute to metabolic alkalosis, whereas binding of calcium by citrate could result in hypocalcemia. Although of questionable clinical importance, citrate-phosphate-dextrose contains 15 percent to 20 percent less citrate than does acid-citrate-dextrose.

Manifestations of hypocalcemia due to citrate intoxication include hypotension and prolonged Q-T intervals on the electrocardi-

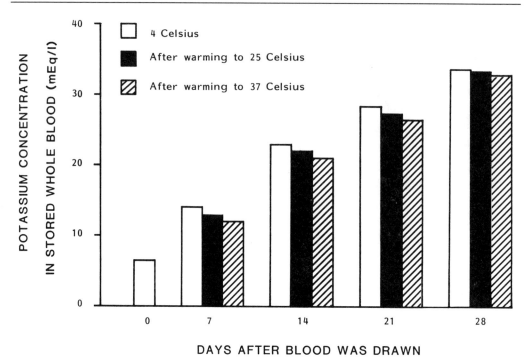

DAYS AFTER BLOOD WAS DRAWN

FIG. 27-1. Plasma potassium concentrations were measured in whole blood (acid-citrate-dextrose) at three different temperatures over a 28-day period. Warming whole blood from 4 degrees Celsius to 25 degrees Celsius or 37 degrees Celsius did not alter potassium concentrations in plasma. Each bar represents the mean concentration of potassium, as determined from 10 units of stored blood. (Data adapted from Eurenius S, Smith RM. The effect of warming on the serum potassium content of stored blood. Anesthesiology 1973;38:482–4)

ogram. Nevertheless, hypocalcemia due to citrate binding of calcium is rare, reflecting mobilization of calcium stores in bone, and the ability of the liver to metabolize rapidly citrate to bicarbonate. Indeed, the rate of whole blood transfusion to adults had to exceed 50 ml·min^{-1} before reductions in plasma ionized calcium concentrations could be documented (Fig. 27-2).[27] Therefore, arbitrary administration of calcium, in the absence of objective indications of hypocalcemia, such as changes in the electrocardiogram or measurement of plasma ionized calcium concentrations, is not indicated. Reversal of hypotension when calcium is administered does not confirm the existence of citrate intoxication, since dose-related positive inotropic effects of calcium can be expected to improve left ventricular stroke volume and blood pressure.

Although hypocalcemia due to citrate binding of calcium is unlikely in adults the same is probably not true in neonates receiving transfusions of blood. In neonates, supplemental calcium administration may be necessary. Likewise, in the presence of hypothermia or marked liver dysfunction, the ability to metabolize citrate to bicarbonate may be reduced. When selecting a calcium preparation for intravenous administration, it must be recognized that calcium chloride contains about four times more available ion than calcium gluconate. The usual dose of calcium chloride is 3 mg·kg^{-1} to 6 mg·kg^{-1}, administered over 5 minutes to 15 minutes during continuous monitoring of the electrocardiogram. For infusion through peripheral veins, however, calcium gluconate may be preferred because it is less likely to produce venous irritation. Further-

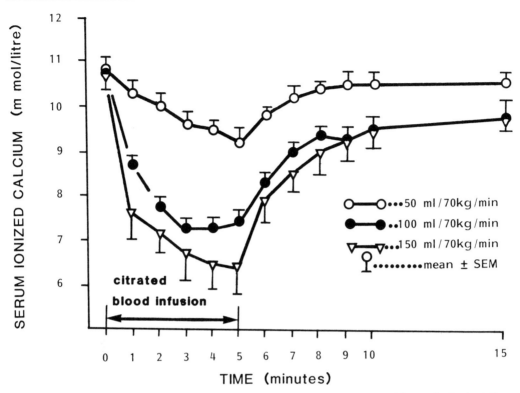

FIG. 27-2. Plasma (serum) ionized calcium concentrations were measured in 30 anesthetized adult patients receiving citrated whole blood at three different rates of infusion over a 5 minute period. Measured reductions in calcium concentrations were dependent on the total dose of citrate administered and the rate of infusion. Maximum reductions, as compared with control, were measured at the completion of the 5 minute infusion of blood and represented 14 percent, 31 percent, and 41 percent decreases, at infusion rates of 50 ml, 100 ml, and 150 ml·70 kg^{-1}·min^{-1} respectively. All these changes were statistically significant ($P < 0.01$), but significant cardiovascular changes did not occur. The transient nature of the citrate-induced hypocalcemia is emphasized by the rapid return to normal of plasma calcium concentrations after completion of blood transfusions. (Denlinger JK, Nahrwold ML, Gibbs PS, Lecky JH. Hypocalcemia during rapid blood transfusion in anaesthetized man. Br J Anaesth 1976;48:995–1000)

more, tissue irritation is more likely to accompany accidental extravasation of calcium chloride than calcium gluconate.

Viral Diseases

Transmission of viral hepatitis by the administration of blood or blood components is a major hazard of transfusion therapy. Mandatory screening of donors since 1972 for the presence of the hepatitis B antigen is helpful but will not eliminate the hazard of hepatitis due to transfusion on non-A, non-B hepatitis virus. Indeed, non-A, non-B hepatitis accounts for 85 percent to 90 percent of transfusion-related hepatitis and occurs in 5 percent to 10 percent of patients receiving multiple blood transfusions.[28] Other viruses that can be transmitted by transfusion of whole blood or blood products include cytomegalovirus, Epstein-Barr virus, and human immunodeficiency virus (see Chapter 29). Criteria for the diagnosis of non-A, non-B hepatitis include at least two plasma alanine aminotransaminase determinations equal to or more than twice the normal level, occurring 2 weeks to 26 weeks after transfusion.[29] Approximately 75 percent of cases are anicteric and symptoms are usually minor (anorexia, fatigue), emphasizing that the majority of cases occurring in transfused patients go unrecognized.[1] Cytomegalovirus has also been implicated as a cause of post-transfusion hepatitis.

Microaggregate Infusion

Microaggregates consisting of platelets and leukocytes form during storage of whole blood. Accumulation of these microaggregates becomes significant after 3 days to 5 days (Fig. 27-3).[30] For example, whole blood that has been stored for 21 days may contain 50 million to 100 million microaggregates, with diameters between 10 microns and 170 microns. Approximately 90 percent have diameters in the 10 micron to 40 micron range.

Infusion of whole blood containing microaggregates has been implicated as a cause of post-transfusion pulmonary dysfunction. As a result, micropore filters have been developed to remove particles with diameters in the 10 micron to 40 micron range. Advocates for routine use of micropore filters believe that infusion of microaggregates causes pulmonary vascular obstruction, with subsequent release

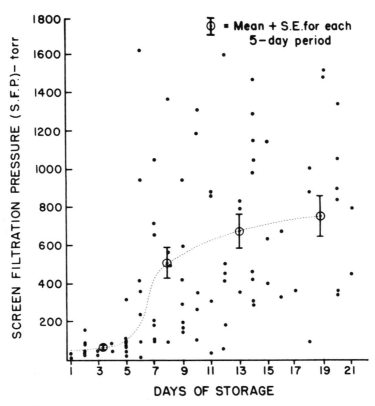

FIG. 27-3. Screen filtration pressures, as a reflection of the presence of microaggregates, were measured in whole blood that had been stored for 1 day to 21 days in acid-citrate-dextrose solutions under standard blood bank conditions. Values for screen filtration pressures remained low during the first 5 days, suggesting the absence of significant amounts of microaggregates. During the second 5 days, screen filtration pressures increased greatly, presumably reflecting time-dependent accumulation of microaggregates. (Harp JR, Wyche MQ, Marshall BE, Wurzel HA. Some factors determining rate of microaggregate formation in stored blood. Anesthesiology 1974;40:398–400)

of vasoactive substances. It is presumed that these substances damage capillary and alveolar membranes, with subsequent transudation of fluid into the alveoli. Nevertheless, use of micropore filters has not been conclusively documented to alter the incidence of pulmonary dysfunction after multiple blood transfusions, emphasizing that factors other than microaggregates may be important.[31]

Centrifuged erythrocytes administered through micropore filters may be recommended for patients with histories of repeated febrile transfusion reactions.[1] Micropore filters placed on the arterial side of the cardiopulmonary bypass machine may be useful for preventing microaggregate emboli in patients undergoing cardiac surgery. An extension of this logic would be the use of micropore filters in patients with right-to-left intracardiac shunts in whom blood not passing through the lungs could be the vehicle for transmission of microaggregate emboli to the arterial circulation. Micropore filters are not necessary for whole blood less than 3 days old and perhaps not even when large volumes of blood are administered regardless of age (Fig. 27-3).[1,31] Resistance to flow is increased and hemolysis can occur when blood more than 14 days old is forced through micropore filters.[32] It must be appreciated, however, that whole blood or erythrocytes should always be administered through 170 micron filters.

REFERENCES

1. Stehling LC. Recent advances in transfusion therapy. In: Stoelting RK, Barash PG, Gallagher TJ, eds. Advances in Anesthesia. Chicago. Year Book Medical Publishers 1987;4:213–52
2. Hilgard P. Immunological reactions to blood and blood products. Br J Anaesth 1979;51:45-9
3. Kelton JG, Perrault RA, Blajchman MA. Substitution of the "group-and-screen" for the full crossmatch in elective operations. Can Anaesth Soc J 1983;30:641–5
4. Reisner LS. Type and screen for cesarean section: A prudent alternative. Anesthesiology 1983;58:476–8
5. Pearl TCY, Strauss RG, Stehling LC, et al. Predeposited autologous blood for elective surgery.
6. A national multicenter study. N Engl J Med 1987;316:517–20
6. Blajchman MA, Herst R, Perrault RA. Blood component therapy in anaesthetic practice. Can Anaesth Soc J 1983;30:382-9.
7. Grindon AJ, Tomasulo PS, Bergin JJ, et al. The Hospital Transfusion Committee, guidelines for improving practice. JAMA 1985;253:540–3
8. Consensus Conference. Platelet transfusion therapy. JAMA 1987;257:1777–80
9. Barrer MJ, Ellison N. Platelet function. Anesthesiology 1977;46:202–11
10. Leitman SF, Boltansky H, Alter HJ, et al. Allergic reactions in healthy plateletpheresis donors caused by sensitization to ethylene oxide. N Engl J Med 1986;315:1192–6
11. Isbister JP, Fisher M McD. Adverse effects of plasma volume expanders. Anaesth Intensive Care 1980;8:145–51
12. Consensus Conference. Fresh frozen plasma. Indications and risks. JAMA 1985;253:551–3
13. Bove JR. Fresh frozen plasma: Too few indications—too much use. Anesth Analg 1985;64:849–50
14. Fuerth JH, Mahrer P. Myocardial infarction after factor IX therapy. JAMA 1981;245:1455–6
15. Rabiner SF, Helbert JR, Lopas H, Friedman LH. Evaluation of a stroma-free hemoglobin solution for use as a plasma expander. J Exp Med 1967;126:1127–41
16. Bonhard K. Acute oxygen supply by infusion of hemoglobin solutions. Fed Proc 1975;34:1466–7
17. Moss GS, DeWiskin R, Rosen AL, et al. Transport of oxygen and carbon dioxide by hemoglobin-saline solution in the red cell-free primate. Surg Gynecol Obstet 1976;142:357–62
18. Tremper KK, Vercellotti GM, Hammerschmidt DE. Hemodynamic profile of adverse clinical reactions to fluosol-DA 20%. Crit Care Med 1984;123:428–31
19. Police AM, Waxman K, Tominaga G. Pulmonary complications after fluosol administration to patients with life-threatening blood loss. Crit Care Med 1985;13:96–8
20. Puri VK, Howard M, Paidipaty BB, Singh S. Resuscitation in hypovolemia and shock: A prospective study of hydroxyethyl starch and albumin. Crit Care Med 1983;11:518–23
21. Gossinger H, Laggner A, Druml W, et al. Hemodynamic, pulmonary and renal reactions to inadvertent transfusion of outdated blood. Crit Care Med 1986;14:70–1
22. Rush B, Lee NLY. Clinical presentation of non-haemolytic transfusion reactions. Anaesth Intensive Care 1980;8:125–31
23. De Wolf AM, Van Den Berg BW, Hoffman HJ, Van Zundert AA. Pulmonary dysfunction during

one-lung ventilation caused by HLA-specific antibodies against leukocytes. Anesth Analg 1987;66:463–7

24. Miller RD, Tong MJ, Robbins TO. Effects of massive transfusion of blood on acid-base balance. JAMA 1971;216:1762–5

25. Wilson RF, Mannen E, Walt AJ. Eight years experience with massive blood transfusions. J Trauma 1971;11:275–85

26. Eurenius S, Smith RM. The effect of warming on the serum potassium content of stored blood. Anesthesiology 1973;38:482–4

27. Denlinger JK, Nahrwold ML, Gibbs PS, Lecky JH. Hypocalcemia during rapid blood transfusion in anaesthetized man. Br J Anaesth 1976;48:995–1000

28. Wick MR, Moore S, Taswell HR. Non-A, non-B hepatitis associated with blood transfusion. Transfusion 1985;25:93–101

29. Aach RD, Kahn RA. Post-transfusion hepatitis: Comment and perspectives. Ann Intern Med 1980;92:539–42

30. Harp JR, Wyche MQ, Marshall BE, Wurzel HA. Some factors determining rate of microaggregate formation in stored blood. Anesthesiology 1974;40:398–400

31. Snyder EL, Hazzey A, Barash PG, Palermo G. Microaggregate blood filtration in patients with compromised pulmonary function. Transfusion 1982;22:21–5

32. Schmidt WF III, Kim HC, Tomassini N, Schwartz E. RBC destruction caused by a micropore blood filter. JAMA 1982;248:1629–32

28

Skin and Musculoskeletal Diseases

EPIDERMOLYSIS BULLOSA (ACANTHOLYSIS BULLOSA)

Epidermolysis bullosa is a rare hereditary disorder of the skin. In addition, mucous membranes, particularly of the oropharynx and esophagus, can be involved. The disease is characterized by bullae formation (blistering) due to separation within the epidermis, followed by fluid accumulation. The basic defect is thought to be the loss of intercellular bridges, resulting in separation of epidermal cells with even minor trauma. Bullae formation is typically initiated when lateral shearing forces are applied to the skin. Pressure applied perpendicular to the skin is not as great a hazard. Bullae formation may also occur spontaneously.

Classification

Epidermolysis bullosa is classified as epidermolysis bullosa simplex, epidermolysis bullosa dystrophica (hyperdysplastic and polydysplastic), and junctional epidermolysis bullosa. The simplex form is characterized by a benign course and normal development. In contrast, patients with the junctional form rarely survive beyond early childhood, usually dying from sepsis. Other features that distinguish junctional epidermolysis bullosa from other forms are generalized blistering beginning at birth, absence of scar formation, and generalized mucosal involvement (skin, gastrointestinal, genitourinary, and respiratory). The dystrophic variety has an incidence of about 1 in every 300,000 births. In contrast to the junctional form, manifestations of epidermolysis bullosa dystrophica include severe scarring with fusion of the digits (pseudosyndactyly), constriction of the oral aperature (microstomia) and esophageal strictures. Teeth are often dysplastic. Malnutrition, anemia, electrolyte derangements and hypoalbuminemia are common, most likely reflecting chronic infection and debilitation. Survival beyond the second decade is unusual. Diseases associated with epidermolysis bullosa include porphyria, amyloidosis, multiple myeloma, diabetes mellitus, and hypercoagulable states.

Treatment

Treatment of epidermolysis bullosa is symptomatic. Many of these patients will be receiving corticosteroids. Phenytoin has been reported to reduce the frequency and magnitude of bullae formation in some patients.[1] Infection of bullae with *Staphylococcus aureus* or beta-hemolytic streptococci is common.

611

Management of Anesthesia

Management of anesthesia in patients with epidermolysis bullosa must consider the drugs being used to treat the disease. For example, supplemental corticosteroids may be indicated during the perioperative period, if patients have been chronically treated with these drugs. Avoidance of trauma to the skin and mucous membranes is important. Trauma from tape; blood pressure cuffs; tourniquets; adhesive electrodes, as used to monitor the electrocardiogram or activity at the neuromuscular junction; and rubbing with alcohol wipes may cause bullae formation. A blood pressure cuff, if used, should be padded with a loose cotton dressing. Intravenous and intra-arterial catheters should be sutured, or held in place with a gauze wrap rather than taped in place. Pulse oximetry using a nonadhesive sensor is indicated.

Trauma from an anesthetic face mask must be minimized by gentle application against the skin. Lubrication of the patient's face and mask with cortisol ointment can be helpful. Upper airway instrumentation should be minimized, as the squamous epithelium that lines the oropharynx and esophagus is more susceptible to trauma than is the columnar epithelium of the trachea. Frictional trauma to the oropharynx, as produced by an oral airway, may result in large intraoral bullae formation and extensive hemorrhage from denuded mucosa. A nasal airway is equally hazardous. Esophageal stethoscopes should be avoided as they may lead to formation of intraoral or esophageal bullae. Hemorrhage from ruptured oral bullae has been treated successfully by epinephrine-soaked gauze applied to the bullae.

Intubation of the trachea, despite theoretical hazards, has not been associated with laryngeal or tracheal complications in patients with epidermolysis bullosa dystrophica and its more routine use in these patients has been recommended.[2] Indeed, laryngeal involvement with this form of the disease is rare and tracheal bullae have not been reported. This is consistent with the greater resistance of the columnar epithelium that lines the trachea to disruption compared with the fragile squamous epithelium in the oral cavity. Generous lubrication of the laryngoscope blade and an undersized endotracheal tube is recommended. Chronic scarring of the oral cavity can result in a narrow oral aperature and immobility of the tongue, while esophageal bullae may lead to strictures. Safety of tracheal intubation in patients with junctional epidermolysis bullosa that involves all mucosa including the respiratory epithelium is unproven.[3]

Selection of drugs for anesthesia must consider the increased incidence of porphyria in patients with epidermolysis bullosa.[4] For this reason, use of barbiturates has been questioned. Even ketamine has been alleged to be capable of triggering an attack of porphyria, but this remains controversial. Indeed, ketamine is a useful drug for operative procedures that permit spontaneous ventilation by not requiring skeletal muscle relaxation or intra-abdominal manipulation. There are no known contraindications to the use of inhaled anesthetic drugs in these patients.

PEMPHIGUS

Pemphigus is a vesiculobullous disease, which may involve extensive areas of the skin and mucous membranes. Buccal pemphigus closely resembles the oral manifestations of epidermolysis bullosa dystrophica. Involvement of the oropharynx is present in about 50 percent of patients with pemphigus. Extensive oropharyngeal involvement makes eating painful, and patients may reduce oral intake to the point that severe malnutrition develops. Skin denudation and bullae formation can result in significant fluid and protein loss. The risk of secondary infection is great.

Etiology

Pemphigus is most likely an autoimmune disorder in which circulating antibodies attack antigenic sites on the epidermal cell surface, resulting in destruction of the cell. As with epidermolysis bullosa, there may be an absence of intercellular bridges that normally prevent the separation of epidermal cells. Therefore, frictional trauma may result in bullae formation. Occasionally, infection or drug sensitivity appear to be the inciting event for bullae formation.

Treatment

Treatment with corticosteroids has reduced mortality from this disease to less than 40 percent. Drugs, such as azathioprine and methotrexate, have also been successfully used in early treatment of pemphigus.

Management of Anesthesia

Preoperative drug therapy and fragility of the mucous membranes must be considered in the management of anesthesia. Supplementation of the usual corticosteroid dose may be necessary. Methotrexate produces immunosuppression, hepatorenal dysfunction, and depression of bone marrow activity but is unlikely to alter activity of plasma cholinesterase enzyme. Azathioprine has been reported to antagonize nondepolarizing neuromuscular blockade, presumably reflecting inhibition of phosphodiesterase enzyme by this drug.[5] Such inhibition would result in the accumulation of cyclic adenosine monophosphate and presumably result in more available acetylcholine for release in response to nerve action potentials. Management of the upper airway and intubation of the trachea is as described for patients with epidermolysis bullosa. Ketamine has been successfully used in these patients.[6]

PSORIASIS

Psoriasis is a common dermatologic disorder characterized by accelerated epidermal growth, resulting in a typical erythematous papule covered with loosely adherent scales. Synthesis of deoxyribonucleic acid in the epidermis of these patients is four times that present in normal epidermis. The skin lesions are symmetrically distributed, and typically involve the elbows, knees, hairlines, and presacral regions. An inflammatory asymmetric arthropathy occurs in about 20 percent of patients with psoriasis. Uveitis and sacroilitis associated with ascending vertebral body disease are common. High cardiac output congestive heart failure has also been observed. Generalized pustular psoriasis is a rare form of the disease, which may be complicated by decreased plasma concentrations of albumin and renal failure.

Treatment

Treatment of psoriasis is directed at slowing the rapid proliferation of epidermal cells. Crude coal tar is effective because of its antimitotic action and ability to inhibit enzymes. Topical corticosteroids are also effective, but the disease promptly recurs when treatment is discontinued. Application of corticosteroids under occlusive dressings can result in significant systemic absorption, with associated suppression of endogenous adrenal cortex activity. Methotrexate has been used for the treatment of psoriasis when topical therapy has not been effective.

Management of Anesthesia

Management of anesthesia must consider the drugs being used for the treatment of psoriasis. Skin trauma such as venipuncture and surgical incision may accentuate psoriasis in some individuals. Patients with psoriasis can have a marked increase in skin blood flow, which could contribute to altered thermoregulation.

MASTOCYTOSIS

Mastocytosis is characterized by an abnormal proliferation of mast cells, which contain histamine and heparin.[7] When the increase of mast cells occurs in the skin as small red-brown maculae on the trunk and upper extremities, the condition is known as urticaria pigmentosa, usually a benign and asymptomatic form of the disease that accounts for about 90 percent of the patients with mastocytosis. Children are most often afflicted, and in nearly half of patients the lesions disappear by adulthood. Systemic mastocytosis is present when sites other than skin, most commonly the skeleton, liver, spleen, and lymph nodes, are invaded by mast cells. These abnormal aggregations of cells are primarily secretory and can abruptly release vasoactive substances.

Signs and Symptoms

Degranulation of mast cells, with release of histamine and heparin into the systemic circulation, can be initiated by trauma, changes in body temperature, or exposure to drugs that stimulate the release of histamine. Often the precipitating event is unknown. The classic symptoms of mastocytosis are felt to be anaphylactoid in origin, with manifestations of mast cell degranulation being pruritus, urticaria, and cutaneous flushing. These changes are frequently accompanied by hypotension and tachycardia. Hypotension may be so severe as to be life-threatening.

Symptoms of mastocytosis have traditionally been attributed to the release of histamine from mast cells. Nevertheless, there is a low incidence of respiratory distress seen in patients with this syndrome. Furthermore, H-1 and H-2 histamine receptor antagonists may not be protective, suggesting that vasoactive substances in addition to histamine may be involved. For example, there is evidence in some patients that symptoms may be due to overproduction of prostaglandin D_2.[8] Finally, a

bleeding tendency in these patients is unusual, despite the fact that mast cells contain heparin.

Management of Anesthesia

There is insufficient information available to permit recommendations for specific anesthetic regimens or techniques for patients with mastocytosis. Although the intraoperative period is usually benign, there are reports of life-threatening anaphylactoid reactions occurring with even minor surgical procedures, emphasizing the need to have resuscitation drugs such as epinephrine immediately available when anesthetizing these patients.[9,10] Preoperative administration of both H-1 and H-2 antagonists would block receptor uptake of histamine. Nevertheless, these drugs would not influence histamine release from the mast cells. If prostaglandins are thought to be playing a role in a specific patient, it might be helpful to add a prostaglandin inhibitor such as aspirin to the preoperative preparation.[8] Conversely, aspirin is considered to be contraindicated by some on the basis of an alleged ability of this drug to initiate mast cell degranulation. An obvious goal during the perioperative period is to avoid administering drugs known to be potent stimuli for the release of histamine. Nevertheless, both meperidine and succinylcholine have been administered without adverse effects.[9] Inhaled anesthetic drugs are considered to be acceptable for administration to patients with mastocytosis.

ATOPIC DERMATITIS

Atopic dermatitis is the cutaneous manifestation of the atopic state. It is characterized by dry, scaly, eczematous, pruritic patches on the face, neck, and flexor surfaces of the arms or legs. Pruritus is the primary symptom. Systemic antihistamines may be effective in reducing pruritus. Corticosteroids may be indicated for short-term treatment of severe cases.

URTICARIA

Urticaria (hives) is characterized by circumscribed wheals and localized areas of edema produced by extravasation of fluid through the walls of blood vessels. Angioedema describes urticaria involving the mucous membranes, particularly those of the mouth, pharynx, and larynx. Mast cells and basophils regulate the urticarial reaction. When stimulated by certain immunologic (drugs, inhaled allergens) or nonimmunologic events, storage granules in these cells release histamine and other vasoactive substances such as bradykinins. These substances result in the localized vasodilation and transudation of fluid that is characteristic of urticarial lesions.

Antihistamine drugs are the mainstay of treatment of mild cases of urticaria. Severe urticarial attacks, especially if accompanied by angioedema, may require aggressive treatment with intravenous epinephrine and diphenhydramine.

COLD URTICARIA

Cold urticaria is a rare disease characterized by relatively innocuous cutaneous lesions, which develop on exposure to cold. The pathophysiology appears to be the result of the release of histamine. Symptoms are usually limited to local erythematous and pruritic urticarial lesions. Highly sensitive individuals, however, on exposure to severe cold, may develop laryngeal edema, bronchospasm, and hypotension.[11]

Management of anesthesia should include avoidance of drugs that are likely to cause the release of histamine. Drugs that have been safely administered to these patients include volatile anesthetics, nitrous oxide, and fentanyl.[11] Preoperative intravenous administration of diphenhydramine (1 mg·kg^{-1} to 1.5 mg·kg^{-1}) and cimetidine (4 mg·kg^{-1} to 5 mg·kg^{-1}) has been recommended when an intraoperative reduction in body temperature is unavoidable, as in patients undergoing cardiac surgery requiring cardiopulmonary bypass.[11] This drug combination will block H-1 and H-2 receptors and thus minimize circulatory effects of cold-induced histamine release. Finally, the administration of unwarmed intravenous solutions and the use of any sort of external cooling equipment, such as a surface blanket, would seem unwise.

ERYTHEMA MULTIFORME

Erythema multiforme is an acute and recurrent disorder of the skin and mucous membranes characterized by lesions ranging from edematous macules and papules to vesicular or bullous lesions, which may ulcerate. Attacks are associated with viral diseases (especially herpes simplex), hemolytic streptococcal infections, neoplastic processes, collagen vascular diseases, and drug-induced hypersensitivity.

Stevens-Johnson Syndrome

Stevens-Johnson syndrome is a severe manifestation of erythema multiforme associated with multisystem involvement. High fever, tachycardia, and tachypnea may occur. Corticosteroids are effective in the management of severe cases.

Hazards of administering anesthesia to patients with Stevens-Johnson syndrome are similar to those encountered in patients with epidermolysis bullosa.[12] For example, involvement of the respiratory tract can make management of the upper airway and intubation of the trachea difficult. The presence of pulmonary blebs can make these patients vulnerable to pneumothorax, particularly with positive intrathoracic pressure. In addition, the presence of pulmonary blebs might detract from the use of nitrous oxide. Ketamine has been used successfully for anesthesia in these patients.

SCLERODERMA

Scleroderma or progressive systemic sclerosis is characterized by inflammation, vascular sclerosis and fibrosis of the skin and viscera.[13] In some patients, the disease may evolve into the CREST syndrome (calcinoses, Raynaud's phenomenon, esophageal hypomotility, sclerodactyly and telangiectasias). Prognosis is poor and related to the extent of visceral rather than cutaneous involvement. There is no known effective treatment for this disease. Corticosteroids should not be administered to patients with scleroderma.

The etiology of scleroderma is unknown, but the disease process has characteristics of both a collagen disease and an autoimmune process. The typical time of onset is between 20 years and 40 years of age, and women are most often afflicted. Significant manifestations of scleroderma occur in the skin and musculoskeletal system, peripheral nervous system, heart, lungs, kidneys, and gastrointestinal tract. Pregnancy accelerates progression of scleroderma in about half of patients. The incidence of spontaneous abortion, premature labor, and perinatal mortality is high.

Skin and Musculoskeletal System

The skin exhibits a mild thickening and a diffuse nonpitting edema. As scleroderma progresses, the skin becomes taut, leading to limited mobility and flexion contractures, especially of the fingers.

Skeletal muscles may exhibit a myopathy, which manifests as weakness of the proximal muscle groups. Plasma creatinine kinase levels are typically elevated. Mild inflammatory arthritis may occur, but most of the joint movement limitation is due to the thickened and taut overlying skin. Avascular necrosis of the femoral head may be present.

Nervous System

Peripheral or cranial nerve neuropathy in the presence of scleroderma has been ascribed to nerve compression by thickened connective tissue that surrounds nerve sheaths. Facial pain of trigeminal neuralgia may also occur as a result of this thickening. Keratoconjunctivitis sicca exists in some patients and may predispose to corneal abrasions.

Cardiovascular System

Changes in the myocardium associated with scleroderma reflect sclerosis of smaller coronary arteries and the conduction system, replacement of cardiac muscle with fibrous tissue, and the indirect effects of systemic and pulmonary hypertension. These changes result in cardiac dysrhythmias, cardiac conduction abnormalities, and congestive heart failure.[14] Intimal fibrosis of the pulmonary artery walls is associated with a high incidence of pulmonary hypertension, which may progress to cor pulmonale. Pulmonary hypertension is often present even in asymptomatic patients.[15] Pericarditis and pericardial effusion, with or without cardiac tamponade, are not an infrequent occurrence. Changes in the peripheral vascular system are common and characterized by intermittent vasospasm in the small arteries to the digits (see Chapter 12). Oral or nasal telangiectasias may be present.

Lungs

Effects of scleroderma on the lungs are of major significance. Diffuse interstitial pulmonary fibrosis may occur independently of the vascular changes that lead to pulmonary hypertension. Pulmonary fibrosis causes decreased inspiratory capacity and increased residual volume. Although dermal sclerosis does not decrease chest wall compliance, pulmonary compliance is diminished by fibrosis and increased airway pressures may be required for adequate ventilation. Arterial hypoxemia resulting from decreased diffusion capacity is not unusual in these patients even at rest.

Kidneys

Renal artery obstruction as a result of arteriolar intimal proliferation leads to reductions in renal blood flow and hypertension. Indeed, sudden development of accelerated hypertension and irreversible renal failure is the most common cause of death in patients with scleroderma. Captopril may improve impaired renal function that accompanies hypertension seen in these patients.

Gastrointestinal Tract

Involvement of the gastrointestinal tract by scleroderma may manifest as dryness of the oral mucosa (xerostomia). Progressive fibrosis of the gastrointestinal tract causes hypomotility of the lower esophagus and small intestine. Dysphagia is a common complaint, due to hypomotility of the esophagus. Lower esophageal sphincter tone is reduced, with subsequent reflux of acidic gastric fluid into the esophagus. Symptoms from the resulting esophagitis can be treated with antacids. Bacterial overgrowth due to intestinal hypomotility can produce a malabsorption syndrome. Indeed, a coagulation disorder may reflect malabsorption of vitamin K from the gastrointestinal tract. Broad-spectrum antibiotics are effective in the treatment of this type of malabsorption syndrome.

Management of Anesthesia

Preoperative evaluation of patients with scleroderma should focus attention on the multiple organ systems likely to be involved by the progressive changes associated with this disease.[16,17] Decreased mandibular motion and narrowing of the oral aperature due to taut skin must be appreciated before the induction of anesthesia. Use of a fiberoptic layrngoscope may facilitate endotracheal intubation through a small oral opening. Oral or nasal telangiectasias may bleed profusely if traumatized during placement of a tube in the trachea. Intravenous access may be impeded by dermal thickening. Vasoconstriction may interfere with blood pressure monitoring by auscultation necessitating the use of an ultrasonic blood pressure device. Catheterization of a peripheral artery introduces the same concerns as present in patients with Raynaud's phenomenon. Cardiac evaluation, including auscultation of the chest and review of the electrocardiogram, may provide evidence of pulmonary hypertension. Because of chronic systemic hypertension and vasomotor instability, patients with scleroderma can have a contracted intravascular fluid volume, which manifests as hypotension, with vasodilation induced by drugs used for anesthesia. Relaxation of the lower esophageal sphincter makes these patients vulnerable to regurgitation and subsequent pulmonary aspiration, should protective laryngeal reflexes be depressed. For this reason, efforts to increase gastric fluid pH with antacids or histamine receptor antagonists before the induction of anesthesia would seem logical.

Intraoperatively, decreased pulmonary compliance may necessitate increased positive airway pressures to assure adequate ventilation of the lungs. Supplemental oxygen is indicated in view of impaired diffusion capacity and vulnerability to develop arterial hypoxemia. Indeed, events known to increase pulmonary vascular resistance, such as respiratory acidosis and arterial hypoxemia, must be prevented. An acute increase in central venous pressure during administration of nitrous oxide could reflect pulmonary artery vasoconstriction due to effects of this drug. The eyes should remain protected at all times in view of the possibility of co-existing keratoconjunctivitis. The role of renal function should be considered in the selection of drugs dependent on this route for clearance from the plasma. Prolonged responses to local anesthetics have been reported, but the explanation or significance of this observation is unclear. Furthermore, regional anesthesia may be technically difficult because of skin and joint changes that accompany scleroderma. Attractive features of regional anesthesia include postoperative analgesia and peripheral vasodilation that improve perfusion to the lower extremities. Other measures to minimize peripheral vasoconstriction include maintenance of operating room temperature above 21 degrees Celsius and administration of warm intravenous fluids. Finally, these patients may be sensitive to the ventilatory depressant effects of opioids and postoperative support of ventilation may be required, especially if severe co-existing pulmonary disease is present.

PSEUDOXANTHOMA ELASTICUM

Pseudoxanthoma elasticum is a rare hereditary disorder of elastic tissue.[18] Elastic fibers degenerate and calcify with time. The most striking feature of this condition, and often the basis for the diagnosis, is the appearance of angioid streaks in the retina. Substantial loss of visual acuity may result from these changes. Additional impairment of vision may occur when vascular changes predispose to vitreous hemorrhage. Skin changes, consisting of yellowish, rectangular, elevated xanthoma-like lesions, occurring primarily in the neck, axilla, and inguinal regions, are often the earliest recognized clinical features. It is surprising that those tissues most rich in elastic fibers, such as the lungs, aorta, palms, and soles, are not affected by the disease process.

Gastrointestinal hemorrhage is a frequent occurrence in these patients. It is thought that degenerative changes in the walls of arteries supplying the gastrointestinal tract prevent constriction of these vessels in response to even minimal mucosal damage. The incidence of hypertension and coronary artery disease is increased in these patients. Endocardial calcification may involve the conduction system

of the heart, predisposing these patients to cardiac dysrhythmias and sudden death. Involvement of cardiac valves with this disease process is frequent. Calcification of peripheral vessels, particularly of the radial or ulnar arteries, is common. Finally, pyschiatric disturbances often accompany this disease.

Management of Anesthesia

Management of anesthesia in the presence of pseduoxanthoma elasticum is based on an appreciation of the abnormalities associated with this disease.[18] Cardiovascular derangements that may occur in these patients are probably the most important considerations. The high incidence of coronary artery disease should be remembered when establishing limits for acceptable changes in blood pressure and heart rate. Monitoring of the electrocardiogram is particularly important, in view of the potential for the development of cardiac dysrhythmias. Use of an ultrasonic sensor to monitor blood pressure is an acceptable alternative to placement of an intra-arterial catheter. Trauma to the mucosa of the upper gastrointestinal tract, as may be produced by instrumentation with a gastric tube or esophageal stethoscope, should be minimized. There are no specific recommendations regarding the choice of anesthetic drugs or techniques.

EHLERS-DANLOS SYNDROME

Ehlers-Danlos syndrome is an inherited connective tissue disorder characterized by hypermobility of the joints and increased extensibility of the skin.[19] These patients tend to manifest extensive ecchymosis, with even minimal trauma. Nevertheless, a specific coagulation defect has not been identified. Dilation of all parts of the gastrointestinal and respiratory tract, including the esophagus and trachea, is often present. The incidence of pneumothorax is increased in these patients. Mitral regurgitation and cardiac conduction abnormalities are frequent. Premature labor and excessive bleeding with delivery are common obstetrical problems.

Management of Anesthesia

Management of anesthesia in patients with Ehlers-Danlos syndrome must consider the cardiorespiratory manifestations of this disease and the propensity for these patients to bleed excessively with interruption of vascular integrity. Prophylactic antibiotics to protect against infective endocarditis may be indicated, if a cardiac murmur suggestive of mitral regurgitation is present. Avoidance of intramuscular injections or instrumentation of the nose or esophagus is important in view of the bleeding tendency. Trauma during direct laryngoscopy for intubation of the trachea must be minimized. Likewise, placement of arterial or central venous catheters must be tempered with the realization that hematoma formation may be extensive. Extravasation of intravenous fluids due to a displaced venous cannula may go unnoticed because of the extreme distensibility of the skin. Maintenance of low airway pressures during assisted or controlled ventilation of the lungs would seem prudent in view of the increased incidence of pneumothorax in these patients. There are no specific recommendations for drug choices to provide anesthesia. Regional anesthesia, however, is not recommended, because of the tendency of these patients to bleed and form extensive hematomas. Surgical complications include uncontrollable hemorrhage and postoperative wound dehiscence.

POLYMYOSITIS (DERMATOMYOSITIS)

Polymyositis is a multisystem disease of unknown etiology, which manifests as nonsuppurative inflammation of skeletal muscle. Cutaneous changes include discoloration of the upper eyelids, periorbital edema, a scaly erythematous malar rash, and symmetric erythematous atrophic changes over the extensor surfaces of joints. This characteristic rash has led to the alternate designation of this disease as dermatomyositis. It is speculated that an abnormality of the immune response may be responsible for slowly progressive skeletal muscle damage.

Skeletal Muscles

Weakness of skeletal muscles typically involves proximal muscle groups, including the flexors of the neck, shoulders, and hips. Patients may have difficulty climbing stairs. Dysphagia, pulmonary aspiration, and pneumonia may result from paresis of pharyngeal and respiratory muscles. Weakness of the intercostal muscles and diaphragm can contribute to ventilatory insufficiency. Necrosis of skeletal muscles result in elevations of plasma creatine kinase levels, which parallels the extent and rapidity of muscle destruction. Electromyography may reveal a triad consisting of spontaneous fibrillation potentials, reduced amplitude of voluntary contraction potentials, and repetitive potentials on needle insertion. Skeletal muscle biopsy adds support to the clinical diagnosis.

Systemic Manifestations

Heart block, left ventricular dysfunction, and myocarditis can occur. Polymyositis, developing after the age of 40 years, is associated with an occult neoplasm in nearly 10 percent of patients. Carcinoma of the breast, lung, gastrointestinal tract, and uterus are the most frequently associated tumors. Polymyositis can also be associated with systemic lupus erythematosus, scleroderma, and rhematoid arthritis. A widespread necrotizing vasculitis may be present in the childhood form of this disease.

Diagnosis and Treatment

The diagnosis of polymyositis is confirmed by proximal skeletal muscle weakness, elevated plasma creatine kinase concentrations and the presence of the characteristic skin rash. Muscular dystrophy or myasthenia gravis can mimic polymyositis. Corticosteroids are considered the treatment of choice, although their efficacy has not been proven in carefully controlled trials. Methotrexate may be effective when the response to corticosteroids is inadequate.

Management of Anesthesia

Management of anesthesia must consider the vulnerability of patients with polymyositis to pulmonary aspiration.[20] In view of co-existing skeletal muscle weakness, it is not surprising that these patients may manifest prolonged responses to nondepolarizing muscle relaxants.[21] The response to succinylcholine may resemble that observed in patients with myotonic dystrophy. The possibility of postoperative skeletal muscle weakness, which can lead to ventilatory insufficiency, must be appreciated.

SYSTEMIC LUPUS ERYTHEMATOSUS

Systemic lupus erythematosus is a chronic disease of unknown etiology, which involves many organ systems. One hypothesis for its pathogenesis is a genetically determined lack of suppression of B-lymphocyte function by T-lymphocytes, such that antibodies are produced against host antigens. Stresses such as infection, pregnancy, or surgery may exacerbate the disease.

The onset of systemic lupus erythematosus may also be drug-induced. Drugs most frequently associated with this syndrome are hydralazine, procainamide, isoniazid, D-penicillamine, and occasionally nonbarbiturate anticonvulsants. Susceptibility to the development of systemic lupus erythematosus, as induced by hydralazine or procainamide, is related to the acetylator phenotype of the patient. Patients who metabolize these drugs slowly (slow acetylators) are more likely to develop the disease.

Clinical manifestations of systemic lupus erythematosus are articular and systemic. The clinical picture of the drug-induced syndrome is similar to the spontaneous form of the disease, but progression of the disease is usually much slower and symptoms are milder.

Articular Manifestations

Symmetric arthritis involving the hands, wrists, elbows, knees, and ankles is the most common manifestation of systemic lupus erythematosus, occurring in 90 percent of patients. Another form of skeletal involvement is avascular necrosis, which most often involves the femoral head or condyle.

Systemic Manifestations

Systemic manifestations affect the heart, lungs, kidneys, liver, neuromuscular system, and skin.

HEART

Pericarditis resulting in chest pain and a friction rub is the most common cardiac manifestation of systemic lupus erythematosus. Myocarditis may result in abnormalities of cardiac conduction. Persistent tachycardia and congestive heart failure can develop with extensive cardiac involvement. Left ventricular dysfunction has been demonstrated in young patients. A noninfectious endocarditis (Libman-Sacks endocarditis) may involve the aortic and mitral valves.

LUNGS

Pulmonary involvement of systemic lupus erythematosus may manifest as lupus pneumonia, characterized by diffuse pulmonary infiltrates, pleural effusion, dry cough, dyspnea, and arterial hypoxemia. Pulmonary function studies in these patients commonly show a restrictive type of pulmonary disease.

RENAL

The most common renal abnormality is glomerulonephritis with proteinuria, resulting in hypoalbuminemia. Hematuria is a frequent finding. Severe reductions in glomerular filtration rate can terminate in oliguric renal failure.

LIVER

Abnormalities of liver function tests may be present in a large number of patients with systemic lupus erythematosus. Some patients develop lupoid hepatitis, which is characterized by recurrent jaundice, hepatomegaly, abnormal liver function tests, and hyperglobulinemia. This form of hepatitis may be fatal. In addition, patients may develop signs of an acute abdomen secondary to intestinal ischemia.

NEUROMUSCULAR

Psychologic changes ranging from mood disturbances suggestive of schizophrenia to signs of organic psychosis with deterioration of intellectual capacity occur in nearly half the patients with systemic lupus erythematosus. Myopathy, with weakness of proximal skeletal muscle groups and elevated plasma creatine kinase concentrations, is often present.

SKIN

The typical skin lesion associated with systemic lupus erythematosus is an erythematous rash, which develops over the nasal malar area (butterfly rash). This rash is usually transient and often accompanies exacerbations of the disease. Alopecia is another frequent manifestation of an exacerbation of the disease.

Laboratory Findings

In addition to the predictable laboratory findings associated with liver and renal dysfunction, patients with systemic lupus erythematosus manifest unexpected laboratory alterations. For example, over 90 percent of patients with this disease have a positive antinuclear antibody test. Circulating anticoagulants can be reflected by a prolonged prothrombin time and activated partial thromboplastin time. Patients with circulating anticoagulants often manifest a biologic false-positive test for syphilis. Anemia, thrombocytopenia, and leukopenia are common.

Treatment

Anti-inflammatory therapy with aspirin is the usual initial treatment of systemic lupus erythematosus. After initiation of this therapy, some patients develop elevated plasma transaminase concentrations, presumably reflecting aspirin-induced hepatitis. Corticosteroids are effective for suppressing glomerulonephritis and adverse changes in the cardiovascular system. Immunosuppressive drugs are often used when patients do not respond to corticosteroids. Antimalarial drugs, in small doses, may be effective in treating arthritis and the skin rash.

Management of Anesthesia

Management of anesthesia is influenced by drugs used in the treatment of systemic lupus erythematosus and by the magnitude of dysfunction of those organs damaged by the disease.

MUSCULAR DYSTROPHY

Muscular dystrophy is a hereditary disease characterized by painless degeneration and atrophy of skeletal muscles.[22,23] There is progressive skeletal muscle weakness but no evidence of muscle denervation. Mental retardation is often present. There is increased permeability of skeletal muscle membranes, which precedes clinical evidence of the disease. Muscular dystrophy can be categorized as pseudohypertrophic, facioscapulohumeral, limb-girdle and nemaline rod myopathy.

Pseudohypertrophic Dystrophy (Duchenne Muscular Dystrophy)

Pseudohypertrophic dystrophy is the most common (3 per 10,000 births) and severe form of childhood progressive muscular dystrophy.[23] The disease is caused by an X-linked recessive gene becoming apparent in boys between 2 years and 6 years of age. Initial symptoms (waddling gait, frequent falling, difficulty climbing stairs) reflect involvement of the proximal muscle groups of the pelvis. Affected skeletal muscles may become large as a result of fatty infiltration, accounting for designation of this disorder as pseudohypertrophic. There is steady deterioration in skeletal muscle strength, resulting in confinement to a wheelchair by 8 years to 11 years of age. Kyphoscoliosis may develop reflecting unopposed action of antagonists of the dystrophic muscles. Skeletal muscle atrophy can predispose to long bone fractures. Plasma creatine kinase concentrations are 30 times to 300 times normal even early in the disease, reflecting skeletal muscle necrosis and increased permeability of skeletal muscle membranes. Approximately 70 percent of female carriers for this disease also manifest elevated plasma creatine kinase concentrations. Skeletal muscle biopsies early in the course of the disease reveal necrosis and phagocytosis of muscle fibers. Death usually occurs between 15 years and 25 years of age due to congestive heart failure and/or pneumonia.

CARDIOPULMONARY DYSFUNCTION

Degeneration of cardiac muscle invariably accompanies muscular dystrophy. Characteristic changes on the electrocardiogram include tall R waves in V_1, deep Q waves in limb leads, short P-R intervals, and sinus tachycardia. Mitral regurgitation may be due to papillary muscle dysfunction and decreased myocardial contractility.

Chronic weakness of inspiratory respiratory muscles and decreased ability to cough can result in loss of pulmonary reserve and accumulation of secretions that predisposes to recurrent pneumonia. Respiratory insufficiency often remains covert because impaired skeletal muscle function prevents patients from exceeding their limited breathing capacity. As the disease progresses, kyphoscoliosis can contribute further to a restrictive pattern of lung disease. Sleep hypoxemia is possible and may contribute to development of pulmonary hypertension. Seventy percent of deaths among patients with this form of muscular dystrophy is due to respiratory causes.[22]

MANAGEMENT OF ANESTHESIA

Preparations for anesthesia in patients afflicted with pseudohypertrophic dystrophy must take into consideration the implications of increased permeability of skeletal muscle membranes and decreased cardiopulmonary reserve. Succinylcholine may be associated with exaggerated potassium release leading to life-threatening cardiac dysrhythmias. Indeed, ventricular fibrillation occurring during induction of anesthesia that included succinylcholine has been observed in patients later discovered to have pseudohypertrophic dystrophy.[24] Rhabdomyolysis manifesting as myoglobinemia can occur. Nondepolarizing muscle relaxants can result in prolonged responses when co-existing skeletal muscle weakness is prominent. Dantrolene should be immediately available as there is an increased incidence of malignant hyperthermia in these patients.[25-27] Malignant hyperthermia has been observed after only a brief period of administration of halothane alone, although most cases have been triggered by succinylcholine or with prolonged inhalation of halothane.[28] Hypomotility of the gastrointestinal tract may delay gastric emptying, which in the presence of weak laryngeal reflexes will increase the risk of pulmonary aspiration. Depressant effects of volatile anesthetics on myocardial contractility can be exaggerated in these patients.[27] Monitoring should be directed at early detection of malignant hyperthermia and cardiac depression. Postoperative pulmonary dysfunction must be anticipated and attempts made to facilitate clearance of secretions. Delayed pulmonary insufficiency may occur 5 hours to 36 hours postoperatively despite apparent recovery to the preoperative level of skeletal muscle strength. Regional anesthesia avoids many of the unique risks of general anesthesia in these patients and in the postoperative period provides analgesia, which may facilitate chest physiotherapy.[29]

Facioscapulohumeral Dystrophy

Facioscapulohumeral dystrophy is characterized by slowly progressive wasting of facial, pectoral, and shoulder-girdle muscles that begins in adolescence. Eventually, the lower limbs are involved. Early symptoms include difficulty in raising the arms above the head and smiling. The heart is not involved, and plasma creatine kinase concentrations are seldom elevated. The course is slow, and longevity is likely.

Limb-Girdle Dystrophy

Limb-girdle dystrophy is a slowly progressive and relatively benign disease. The age of onset varies from the second to fifth decades. The shoulder girdle or hip girdle may be the only skeletal muscle group involved.

Nemaline Rod Myopathy

Nemaline rod myopathy is an autosomal dominant disease characterized by nonprogressive symmetrical skeletal muscle weakness affecting principally proximal skeletal muscles. Diagnosis is confirmed by histologic examination of skeletal muscle demonstrating the presence of rods between normal myofibrils. Affected infants may present with hypotonia, dysphagia, respiratory distress, and cyanosis. Micrognathia and dental malocclusion are common. Other skeletal deformities include kyphoscoliosis and pectus excavatum. Restrictive lung disease may result from myopathy and scoliosis. Cardiac failure has been described.

Intubation of the trachea may be difficult due to associated anatomic abnormalities.[30] Respiratory depressant effects of drugs may be exaggerated in these patients. Bulbar palsy may further complicate anesthetic management due to regurgitation and pulmonary aspiration. Resistance to the effects of succinylcholine has been described in a patient who responded normally to pancuronium.[31] There has been no reported association of nemaline rod myopathy with malignant hyperthermia.

MYOTONIC DYSTROPHY

Myotonic dystrophy designates a group of hereditary degenerative diseases of skeletal muscles characterized by persistent contracture of skeletal muscles after their stimulation. Inability of skeletal muscles to relax after stimulation is diagnostic and results from abnormal calcium metabolism as the cellular–adenosine triphosphatase system fails to return calcium to the sarcoplasmic reticulum. Unsequestered calcium then remains available to produce sustained skeletal muscle contraction. This is the reason contraction of skeletal muscles is not prevented or relieved by general anesthesia, regional anesthesia, or muscle relaxants. Infiltration of contracted skeletal muscles with local anesthetics may induce relaxation. Quinine, 300 mg to 600 mg administered intravenously, has been reported to be effective in some cases.[32] Warming the ambient air temperature in the operating room reduces the severity of myotonia, as well as the incidence of postoperative shivering, which may precipitate contraction of skeletal muscles. The three important syndromes of myotonic dystrophy are myotonia dystrophica, myotonia congenita, and paramyotonia.

Myotonia Dystrophica (Myotonia Atrophica, Steinert's Disease)

Myotonia dystrophica is the most common (2.4 to 5.5 per 100,000 of the population) and serious form of myotonic dystrophy that afflicts adults.[32–35] This disease is inherited as an autosomal dominant trait, with the onset of symptoms occurring in the second to third decades of life. Treatment is symptomatic, and may include phenytoin, quinine, or procainamide. Death from pneumonia and/or cardiac failure usually occurs by the sixth decade. There is progressive involvement of skeletal, cardiac, and smooth muscles.

SIGNS AND SYMPTOMS

Myotonia dystrophica is a multiple system disease, although skeletal muscles are principally afflicted. Typically, patients manifest early facial weakness (expressionless facies), wasting and weakness of sternocleidomastoid muscles, ptosis, dysarthria, and inability to relax the grip (myotonia). A triad of characteristic features is mental retardation, frontal baldness, and cataract formation. Involvement of endocrine glands is manifested as gonadal atrophy, diabetes mellitus, decreased thyroid function, and adrenal insufficiency. Occurrence of central sleep apnea in patients with

myotonic dystrophy is well known and probably accounts for their hypersomnolence.[22] There is an increased incidence of cholelithiasis especially in males. Exacerbation of symptoms during pregnancy is common, and it is not unusual for uterine atony and retained placenta to accompany vaginal delivery.[36]

Cardiac dysrhythmias and conduction abnormalities presumably reflect myocardial involvement by the myotonic process.[37] First degree atrioventricular heart block is a common finding on the electrocardiogram before the clinical onset of the disease. Up to 20 percent of these patients have evidence of mitral valve prolapse on echocardiography. Reports of sudden death may reflect third-degree atrioventricular heart block. Weakness of thoracic, pharyngeal, and thoracic muscles renders these patients vulnerable to pulmonary aspiration of acidic gastric fluid.

MANAGEMENT OF ANESTHESIA

Management of anesthesia in these patients must consider the likely presence of cardiomyopathy, respiratory muscle weakness, and abnormal responses to drugs used during anesthesia. It should be assumed that even asymptomatic patients have some degree of cardiomyopathy. Therefore, myocardial depression from volatile anesthetic drugs may be exaggerated.[38,39] The need to control cardiac dysrhythmias must be anticipated. Anesthesia and surgery could theoretically aggravate co-existing cardiac conduction blockade by increasing vagal tone or causing transient hypoxia of the conduction system.

The most important potential adverse reaction in these patients is prolonged skeletal muscle contraction after the injection of succinylcholine (Fig. 28-1).[33] Contraction of skeletal muscles can last 2 minutes to 3 minutes and can be so severe as to make adequate ventilation of the lungs difficult. Conversely, responses to nondepolarizing muscle relaxants are normal. Theoretically, reversal of neuromuscular blockade could precipitate skeletal muscle contraction, by facilitating depolarization of the neuromuscular junction. Nevertheless, adverse responses do not occur when

Succinylcholine (mg/kg)

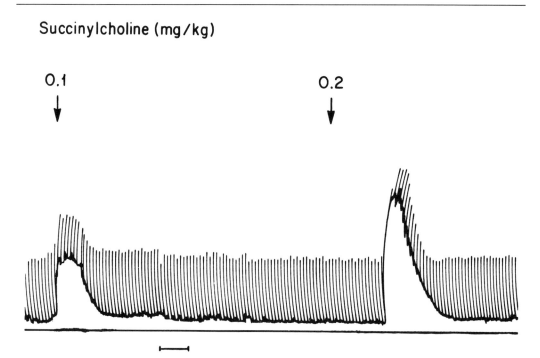

FIG. 28-1. Administration of succinylcholine to patients with myotonia dystrophica results in contraction of skeletal muscles. Contraction is evidenced by the dose-related upward shift of the baseline produced by even small doses of succinylcholine. (Mitchell MM, Ali HH, Savarese JJ. Myotonia and neuromuscular blocking agents. Anesthesiology 1978;49:44–8)

neostigmine is used to reverse neuromuscular blockade in patients with myotonic dystrophy.[38] Careful titration of neuromuscular blockade and administration of intermediate-acting muscle relaxants, such as atracurium or vecuronium, may obviate the need for pharmacologic reversal in selected patients.[40]

These patients are very sensitive to the respiratory depressant effects of barbiturates, opioids, and diazepam.[34] This most likely reflects central nervous system depression of ventilation by the drug, superimposed on an already weak and atrophic peripheral respiratory musculature. Furthermore, the co-existing hypersomnolence and vulnerability to central sleep apnea may contribute to increased sensitivity to depressant drugs. Although there is an association between this syndrome and malignant hyperthermia, there are no data to confirm a definite relationship.[34] Postoperatively, local or regional anesthesia is useful for pain relief and careful nursing surveillance is indicated for several hours.

Myotonia Congenita (Thomsen's Disease)

Myotonia congenita is transmitted as a Mendelian dominant characteristic and manifests at birth or early in childhood. Skeletal muscle involvement is widespread, but there is usually no involvement of other organ systems. The disease does not progress or result in a decreased life expectancy. Patients with myotonia congenita respond to quinidine therapy.

Paramyotonia

Paramyotonia is the rarest of the myotonic syndromes. Signs and symptoms are identical to those of myotonia congenita, except that paramyotonia develops only on exposure to cold. Treatment of skeletal muscle contracture is removal to a warm environment and administration of quinidine if symptoms persist. The possibility of initiating skeletal muscle contraction by exposure to a decreased ambient temperature in the operating rooms is undocumented. Nevertheless, logic would suggest that reduced ambient temperatures should be avoided when patients with this diagnosis require operation.

HYPEREKPLEXIA

Hyperekplexia (stiff-baby syndrome) is a rare genetic syndrome characterized by intense skeletal muscle rigidity manifesting immediately after birth. Similarities between this syndrome and hyperexplexia (exaggerated startle response to sudden noises or movement) are remarkable and they may be the same disease. Electromyography in individuals with hyperexplexia demonstrates continuous skeletal muscle activity, with only rare periods of quiescence. Choking, vomiting, and difficulty with swallowing are common; motor development is delayed but intelligence is normal. Skeletal muscle stiffness or hyperekplexia disappears gradually during the first years of life.

Experience with this syndrome is too limited to make recommendations regarding anesthesia. In a single affected infant, resistance to succinylcholine was observed, whereas responses to pancuronium and neostigmine were considered normal.[41] In this same patient, a substantial increase in the resting tension of skeletal muscles was observed during the onset of action of succinylcholine. Release of potassium was not enhanced after administration of succinylcholine. Responses to volatile anesthetics and nitrous oxide seem to be predictable in these patients.

TRACHEOMEGALY

Tracheomegaly is characterized by marked dilation of the trachea and bronchi, which is due to a congenital defect of elastic and smooth muscle fibers of the tracheobronchial tree or their destruction after radiotherapy, especially to the head and neck.[42] Diagnosis is confirmed by a tracheal diameter greater than 30 mm on a radiograph of the chest. Symptoms include chronic productive cough and frequent pulmonary infections, most likely reflecting chronic aspiration. Tracheal and bronchial walls are abnormally flaccid and may collapse, especially during vigorous coughing. Aspiration is a possibility during general anesthesia, especially if maximal inflation of the tracheal tube cuff fails to provide an airtight seal. Careful use of the laryngoscope, tracheal tubes, and suction catheters is necessary.

MYASTHENIA GRAVIS

Myasthenia gravis is a chronic autoimmune disease involving the neuromuscular junction. The hallmark of the disease is weakness and rapid fatigability of voluntary skeletal muscles with repetitive use, followed by partial recovery with rest.[43] The incidence is about 1 in every 20,000 adults. Women between 20 years and 30 years of age are most often affected.

Pathophysiology

The basic defect resulting in skeletal muscle weakness and easy fatigability is a decrease in the number of available receptors for acetylcholine at the postsynaptic neuromuscular junction (Fig. 28-2).[44] This decrease is due to their inactivation or destruction by circulating antibodies. Attachment of these antibodies to receptors for acetylcholine either blocks access of neurotransmitter to receptors or accelerates degradation of receptors. It is estimated that 70 percent to 80 percent of functional acetylcholine receptors are lost.[44] This explains the easy fatigability of patients with myasthenia gravis and their marked sensitivity to nondepolarizing muscle relaxants.

Receptor binding antibodies are present in the plasma of more than 80 percent of patients

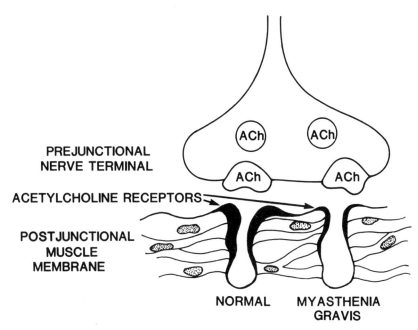

PREJUNCTIONAL
NERVE TERMINAL

ACETYLCHOLINE RECEPTORS

POSTJUNCTIONAL
MUSCLE
MEMBRANE

NORMAL   MYASTHENIA
GRAVIS

FIG. 28-2. Schematic diagram of the neuromuscular junction, depicting the density of acetylcholine (ACh) receptors on the folds of postjunctional muscle membranes. Compared with normal folds, the density of ACh receptors is greatly reduced in the presence of myasthenia gravis. (Adapted from Drachman DB. Myasthenia gravis. N Engl J Med 1978;298:136–42)

with myasthenia gravis. Indeed, identification of circulating antibodies is a reliable diagnostic test for myasthenia gravis. The origin of this autoimmune type of response is not known, but a role for the thymus gland is suggested by the association of myasthenia gravis with thymus gland abnormalities. For example, hyperplasia of the thymus gland is present in over 70 percent of patients with myasthenia gravis, and 10 percent to 15 percent of these patients have thymomas. Indeed, about 75 percent of patients undergo a remission of their myasthenia gravis after thymectomy.

Clinical Manifestations

The clinical course of myasthenia gravis is marked by periods of exacerbations and remissions. Ptosis and diplopia from extraocular muscle weakness are the most common initial complaints. Weakness of pharyngeal and laryngeal muscles (bulbar muscles) results in dysphagia, dysarthria, and difficulty in eliminating oral secretions. Skeletal muscle strength may be normal in well-rested patients, but weakness occurs promptly with exercise. Arm, leg, or trunkal weakness can occur in any combination and is usually asymetrical in distribution. Skeletal muscle atrophy is unlikely. Patients with myasthenia gravis are at high risk for pulmonary aspiration of gastric contents. Myasthenia gravis may be associated with cardiomyopathy. Other diseases often considered autoimmune in origin can occur in association with myasthenia gravis. For example, decreased thyroid function is present in about 10 percent of patients with myasthenia gravis and rheumatoid arthritis, systemic lupus erythematosus, and pernicious anemia occur more commonly than in patients without myasthenia gravis. About 15 percent of infants born to mothers with myasthenia gravis demonstrate transient skeletal muscle weakness. Infection, electrolyte abnormalities, pregnancy, emotional stress, and surgery may precipitate skeletal muscle weakness or exacerbate co-existing weakness. Antibiotics, particularly the aminoglycosides, can aggravate skeletal muscle weakness associated with myasthenia gravis.

Classification

Myasthenia gravis may be classified on the basis of the skeletal muscles involved and the severity of the symptoms. Type I is limited to involvement of the extraocular muscles. About 20 percent of patients show signs and symptoms confined to the extraocular muscles and are considered to have ocular myasthenia gravis. Any extension beyond the ocular muscles is likely to involve bulbar muscles. Patients in whom the disease has been confined to ocular muscles for greater than 3 years are unlikely to experience any progression in their disease.[43] Type IIA is a slowly progressive and mild form of skeletal muscle weakness, which spares the muscles of respiration. The response to anticholinesterase drugs and occasionally corticosteroids is good in these patients. Type IIB is a more severe and rapidly progressive form of skeletal muscle weakness than that which occurs with type IIA. Response to drug therapy is not as good, and muscles of respiration may be involved. Type III is characterized by an acute onset and rapid deterioration of skeletal muscle strength (within 6 months) that is associated with a high mortality. Type IV is a severe form of skeletal muscle weakness that results from progression of type I or II.

Treatment

Modalities of therapy for myasthenia gravis include anticholinesterase drugs, corticosteroids, immunosuppressants other than corticosteroids, thymectomy, and plasmapheresis. These therapies may be employed singly or in combination. Cyclosporine may be an effective therapy in some patients with myasthenia gravis.

ANTICHOLINESTERASE DRUGS

Neostigmine or pyridostigmine are the anticholinesterase drugs most often selected to treat myasthenia gravis. Presumably, these drugs are effective because they inhibit the enzyme responsible for the hydrolysis of acetylcholine, which serves to increase the amount of neurotransmitter available at the neuromuscular junction. Neostigmine, 15 mg orally, is equivalent to an intramuscular dose of 1.5 mg, and an intravenous dose of 0.5 mg. Oral pyridostigmine lasts longer (3 hours to 6 hours) and produces fewer muscarinic side effects than neostigmine. An oral dose of pyridostigmine, 60 mg, is equivalent to an intramuscular or intravenous dose of 2 mg. Phospholine iodide is an extremely potent anticholinesterase drug reserved for patients with severe myasthenia gravis.

Excessive anticholinesterase drug effect may result in skeletal muscle weakness known as a cholinergic crisis. The presence of muscarinic side effects (salivation, miosis, bradycardia) plus accentuated skeletal muscle weakness after intravenous administration 1 mg to 2 mg of endrophonium confirms the diagnosis.

CORTICOSTEROIDS

Various corticosteroids have been used to treat myasthenia gravis, but the best success has been attained with prednisone. The usual daily dose is 50 mg to 100 mg. Presumably, corticosteroids interfere with production of antibodies, which are responsible for degradation of cholinergic receptors. Corticosteroids may also facilitate neuromuscular transmission. Azothioprine, cyclophosphamide, or plasmapheresis may also be effective by virtue of their ability to prevent the production or reduce the circulating concentrations of antibodies to the neuromuscular junction. Assessment of the efficacy of drug therapy is difficult because of the natural variability of the disease.

THYMECTOMY

Thymectomy is recommended for patients with drug-resistant myasthenia gravis. About 75 percent of these patients demonstrate a marked improvement in skeletal muscle strength after thymectomy, and drug therapy is no longer required.[44] Those patients who fail to show substantial improvement in skeletal muscle strength after thymectomy can often be managed with reduced doses of anticholinesterase drugs, compared with preoperative requirements.

Management of Anesthesia

Management of anesthesia for patients with myasthenia gravis must take into account preoperative drug therapy and the potential impact of this drug therapy on responses to muscle relaxants. In addition, it is likely that these patients will require ventilatory support in the postoperative period.

PREOPERATIVE PREPARATION

Depressant drugs should be used with caution if at all in the preoperative medication. The interaction between anticholinesterase drugs administered to treat myasthenia gravis and muscle relaxants must be considered before the administration of either succinylcholine or nondepolarizing muscle relaxants. For example, anticholinesterase drugs not only inhibit true cholinesterase but also impair activity of plasma cholinesterase. Therefore, the dose of succinylcholine administered to these patients should be reduced to avoid a potentially prolonged response due to slowed hydrolysis of the drug. This recommendation is particularly appropriate if anticholinesterase drug therapy is with phospholine iodide. For example, 0.05 mg·kg^{-1} to 0.1 mg·kg^{-1} of succinylcholine may produce profound paralysis in patients who have been receiving phospholine iodide to treat myasthenia gravis. Anticholinesterase drugs would theoretically antagonize the effects of nondepolarizing muscle relaxants. Nevertheless, this response does not seem to occur clinically.

Corticosteroid therapy probably does not alter dose requirements for succinylcholine, but it has been reported that these drugs can reduce the dose requirements for nondepolarizing muscle relaxants.[45] This potentiation, however, if it does occur, seems to be of minor significance.

It must be remembered that patients with undiagnosed myasthenia gravis will be exquisitely sensitive to the effects of nondepolarizing muscle relaxants. In this situation, a defasciculating dose of d-tubocurarine (30 µg·kg^{-1} to 50 µg·kg^{-1}) could result in respiratory muscle paralysis. Conversely, it has been suggested that undiagnosed patients will be resistant to the effects of succinylcholine. The mechanism for this resistance, and its clinical significance, are unclear.

It is likely that patients with myasthenia gravis will require ventilatory support after surgery. Preoperatively, criteria that correlate with the likely need for controlled ventilation of the lungs in the postoperative period after transsternal thymectomy include (1) duration of the disease greater than 6 years, (2) presence of chronic obstructive airways disease unrelated to myasthenia gravis, (3) dose of pyridostigmine greater than 750 mg daily in the 48 hours preceding surgery, and (4) preoperative vital capacity less than 2.9 L.[46,47] These criteria are less predictive of the need for postoperative ventilatory support after transcervical thymectomy, suggesting this less invasive surgical approach has a respiratory sparing effect. It is wise to advise these patients during the preoperative interview that they will most likely have an endotracheal tube in place when they awaken.

INDUCTION OF ANESTHESIA

There are no contraindications to the use of barbiturates or benzodiazepines for the induction of anesthesia in patients with myasthenia gravis. Logic would suggest, however, that respiratory depressant effects of these drugs could be accentuated. Intubation of the trachea can be accomplished without muscle relaxants in many patients by taking advantage of co-existing skeletal muscle weakness and the relaxing effect of volatile anesthetics on skeletal muscle. Succinylcholine or intermediate-acting nondepolarizing muscle relaxants can be used to facilitate intubation of the trachea, keeping in mind the need to decrease the initial dose until the response at the neuromuscular junction can be documented with a peripheral nerve stimulator.

MAINTENANCE OF ANESTHESIA

Maintenance of anesthesia is ideally provided with nitrous oxide plus a volatile anesthetic. Use of volatile anesthetics may decrease the necessary dose of muscle relaxants or even eliminate the need for their intraoperative administration. Should administration of nondepolarizing muscle relaxants be necessary, the initial dose should be reduced at least one-half to two-thirds, and the response observed, using a peripheral nerve stimulator. The inherent short duration of action of atracurium or vecuronium are desirable characteristics when muscle relaxants are administered to these patients either to facilitate intubation of the trachea or to provide maintenance skeletal muscle relaxation.[48] The ability to dissipate the effects of inhaled drugs at the conclusion of anesthesia is important for evaluation of skeletal muscle strength in the early postoperative period. Prolonged effects of opioids, especially on ventilation, detracts from the use of these drugs for the maintenance of anesthesia. At the conclusion of surgery, it is wise to leave the tracheal tube in place until patients demonstrate an ability to maintain an adequate level of ventilation. Skeletal muscle strength often seems adequate in the early stages after anesthesia and surgery only to deteriorate a few hours later. The need to support ventilation of the lungs in the postoperative period should be anticipated for those patients who demonstrate findings in the preoperative evaluation known to correlate with inadequate ventilation after surgery (see the section Preoperative Preparation).

MYASTHENIC SYNDROME (EATON-LAMBERT SYNDROME)

The myasthenic syndrome is a rare disorder of neuromuscular transmission most often associated with carcinoma of the lung.[49]

Complaints of weakness of the limb-girdle muscles may be erroneously confused with myasthenia gravis. In contrast to myasthenia gravis, this skeletal muscle weakness is not reliably reversed with anticholinesterase drugs or corticosteroids. Furthermore, exercise improves, rather than reduces, muscle strength.

These patients are sensitive to the effects of both depolarizing and nondepolarizing muscle relaxants. The mechanism for this sensitivity is not known but is most likely due to a defect in the prejunctional release of acetylcholine. Indeed, 4-aminopyridine, which has a presynaptic site of action, attenuates skeletal muscle weakness seen in patients with this syndrome.[50]

The potential presence of myasthenic syndrome and the need to reduce the dose of muscle relaxants should be considered in patients with known carcinoma. Furthermore, this syndrome should be considered in those patients undergoing diagnostic procedures such as bronchoscopy, mediastinoscopy, or exploratory thoracotomy for the suspected diagnosis of carcinoma of the lung.

FAMILIAL PERIODIC PARALYSIS

Familial periodic paralysis is characterized by intermittent but acute attacks of skeletal muscle weakness or paralysis, which usually spares only the muscles of respiration (that is, bulbar musculature). Attacks may last hours or days. Familial periodic paralysis is characterized as hypokalemic, normokalemic, or hyperkalemic (Table 28-1). The hypokalemic form is transmitted as an autosomal dominant trait.

The fundamental defect in patients with familial periodic paralysis is unknown. Each form of this disease, however, is associated with abnormal flux of potassium between plasma and skeletal muscle cells, plus alterations in skeletal muscle membrane potentials, which tend to render muscles inexcitable during acute attacks. For example, a sudden shift of potassium into cells results in hyperpolar-

TABLE 28-1. Clinical Features of Familial Periodic Paralysis

Type	Plasma Potassium Concentrations During Symptoms	Precipitating Factors	Other Features
Hypokalemic	3 mEq·L^{-1}	Large glucose meals Strenuous exercise Glucose-insulin infusions	Cardiac dysrhythmias Electrocardiogram signs of hypokalemia Sensitive to nondepolarizing muscle relaxants
Normokalemic	3–5.5 mEq·L^{-1}	Alcohol Exercise Emotional stress	Skeletal muscle weakness persists up to 14 days
Hyperkalemic	5.5 mEq·L^{-1}	Exercise Potassium infusions Exposure to cold	Skeletal muscle weakness often localized to tongue and eyelids Sensitive to succinylcholine

ization of cell membranes leading to resistance to the effects of acetylcholine at the neuromuscular junction. Potassium is not lost in the urine or feces. Cardiac dysrhythmias are frequent. In this situation, there is increased sensitivity (similar to myasthenia gravis) to the effects of nondepolarizing muscle relaxants, and presumably resistance to the effects of succinylcholine. Conversely, acute increases in plasma potassium concentrations result in hypopolarized membranes and produce a depolarizing type of neuromuscular blockade. Theoretically, these patients would be sensitive to succinylcholine and resistant to the effects of nondepolarizing muscle relaxants.

Management of Anesthesia

The principal emphasis for management of anesthesia in patients with familial periodic paralysis is avoidance of events that will precipitate skeletal muscle weakness.[51,52] Large carbohydrate meals should be avoided the day before surgery since glucose that enters cells may also facilitate intracellular migration of potassium. Indeed, a reliable method for inducing skeletal muscle weakness for diagnostic purposes in suspected patients is administration of glucose and insulin. For this reason glucose-containing intravenous fluid solutions should be avoided in the perioperative period. Exposure to a cold environment or trauma associated with the operative procedure can also produce skeletal muscle weakness. Increasing the ambient temperature of the operating room and warming inhaled gases and intravenous fluids will minimize reductions in body temperature, which could accentuate hypokalemia. Regardless of the predicted response of these patients to muscle relaxants, the prudent approach may be to avoid administering these drugs during anesthesia.[51] When muscle relaxants are necessary, it would seem logical to reduce greatly the initial dose and to monitor the response produced at the neuromuscular junction with a peripheral nerve stimulator. Prolonged postoperative monitoring of these patients is indicated, even in the presence of an uneventful intraoperative course.

Treatment of all three types of familial periodic paralysis is with acetazolamide. This drug is thought to produce acidosis, which protects against hypokalemic paralysis and is thought to promote renal excretion of potassium in hyperkalemic paralysis.

PSEUDOHYPERKALEMIA

Pseudohyperkalemia is characterized by elevated serum concentrations of potassium (as high as 7 mEq·L^{-1}) due to release of this ion from platelets, leukocytes, or erythrocytes during the clotting or separation process.[53] This abnormal in vitro leakage of potassium may reflect an inherited trait. Clinically, pseudohyperkalemia is distinguished from hyperkalemia by measuring both plasma and serum levels of potassium. In pseudohyperkalemia, only the serum levels of potassium are elevated, while plasma levels remain normal. These patients are asymptomatic and lack detectable adrenal or renal abnormalities. Failure to recognize this syndrome may result in hyperkalemia if aggressive pharmacologic attempts to lower plasma potassium concentrations are instituted. Confirmation of the presence of this syndrome preoperatively removes concerns typically expressed for management of anesthesia in the presence of hyperkalemia.

ALCOHOLIC MYOPATHY

Acute and chronic forms of proximal skeletal muscle weakness occur frequently in alcoholics. Distinction of alcoholic myopathy from alcoholic neuropathy is based on proximal rather than distal skeletal muscle involvement, elevation of plasma creatine kinase concentrations, myoglobinuria in acute cases, and rapid recovery after cessation of alcohol consumption.

FREEMAN-SHELDON SYNDROME

Freeman-Sheldon syndrome is a generalized myopathy transmitted as an autosomal dominant trait.[54] Increased tone and fibrosis of facial muscles results in microstomia, which may be accompanied by micrognathia. Skeletal muscle contractures lead to a short neck and cephalad positioning of the larynx, restrictive lung disease, and kyphoscoliosis. Chronic upper airway obstruction reflects involvement of oral and nasal pharyngeal muscles. Difficulty with swallowing may lead to malnourishment.

Anesthetic considerations include potential difficulty in exposing the glottic opening for intubation of the trachea.[54] Muscle relaxants may not improve intubating conditions if microstomia is due to hypoplasia of facial muscles. Thickening of subcutaneous tissues may interfere with achievement of intravenous access.

PRADER-WILLI SYNDROME

The Prader-Willi syndrome manifests at birth as muscular hypotonia, which may be associated with weak swallowing and cough reflexes and upper airway obstruction. Nasogastric feeding may be necessary in infancy. The syndrome progresses during childhood and is characterized by hyperphagia leading to obesity, plus endocrine abnormalities including hypogonadism and diabetes mellitus. The Pickwickian syndrome develops in some patients. There is little growth in height and patients remain of short stature. Mental retardation is often severe. There is a high frequency of chromosome 15 deficiency in patients with this syndrome, and an autosomal-recessive mode of inheritance has been proposed. It has been suggested that the incidence of the Prader-Willi syndrome is not greatly different from the occurrence of the trisomy 21 defect.

Management of Anesthesia

The principal concerns relevant to management of anesthesia for these patients are skeletal muscle hypotonia and altered metabolism of carbohydrates and fat.[55] Weak skeletal musculature is associated with an ineffective cough and an increased incidence of pneumonia. Intraoperative monitoring of blood glucose concentrations and provision of exogenous glucose are necessary, as these patients continue to use circulating glucose to manufacture fat rather than to meet basal energy needs. Calculation of doses of drugs should consider decreased skeletal muscle mass and increased fat content of these patients. Although not substantiated, it is predictable that muscle relaxant requirements could be reduced in the presence of skeletal muscle hypotonia. Succinylcholine has been administered without incident to these patients.[55]

Micrognathia, high arched palate, strabismus, a straight ulnar border, and congenital dislocation of the hip may be present. Dental caries associated with enamel defects are common. Disturbances in thermoregulation, often characterized as intraoperative rises in body temperature and metabolic acidosis, have been observed, although a relation to malignant hyperthermia has not been established.[55] Seizures are associated with this syndrome, suggesting caution in the use of drugs known to stimulate the central nervous system. Cardiac dysfunction does not seem to accompany this syndrome. Halothane has been used for anesthesia, although isoflurane or enflurane would also seem to be acceptable selections.

PRUNE-BELLY SYNDROME

Prune-belly syndrome is characterized by congenital agenesis of the lower central abdominal musculature and the presence of urinary tract anomalies.[56] Recurrent respiratory infections reflect the impaired ability of these patients to cough effectively. It is unlikely that muscle relaxants will be necessary during management of anesthesia.

RHEUMATOID ARTHRITIS

Rheumatoid arthritis is a chronic inflammatory disease of unknown etiology, characterized by symmetric polyathropathy and significant systemic involvement (Table 28-2). Terminal interphalangeal joints are spared, which helps distinguish this disease from osteoarthritis. Rheumatoid arthritis predominates in females, and the onset is typically between the ages of 30 years to 50 years. Its course is often that of exacerbations and remissions. Rheumatoid nodules are typically present at pressure points, particularly below the elbow. Rheumatoid factor is an immunoglobulin present in nearly 80 percent of patients with classic rheumatoid arthritis. The etiology of rheumatoid arthritis is unknown, but an immunologic mechanism is suggested by the presence of rheumatoid factor.

Joint Manifestations

Multiple joints, particularly the hands, wrists, and knees, are afflicted at the same time in a symmetric distribution. Fusiform swelling is typical of the involvement of the proximal interphalangeal joints. Characteristically, these joints are painful, swollen, and warm on arising and remain stiff for up to 3 hours after the start of daily activity. Histologically, the synovium of the involved joint exhibits an increased number of lining cells, which may progress into a proliferative and infiltrative phase, forming a pannus. Joints of the thoracic, lumbar, and sacral spine are rarely involved, but involvement of the cervical spine is common and may result in neurologic complications. For example, atlantoaxial subluxation and consequent separation of the atlanto-odontoid articulation may result in protrusion of the odontoid process into the foramen magnum. This protrusion can exert pressure on the spinal cord or impair blood flow through the vertebral arteries. Synovitis of the temporomandibular joint may lead to marked limitation of mandibular motion. Cricoarytenoid arthritis is common and is manifested by hoarseness, painful speech, dysphagia, and stridor.

Systemic Manifestations

Many of the systemic manifestations of rheumatoid arthritis are most likely a consequence of vasculitis due to deposition of immune complexes in the walls of small vessels, with a subsequent inflammtory reaction. Sys-

TABLE 28-2. Comparison of Rheumatoid Arthritis and Ankylosing Spondylitis

	Rheumatoid Arthritis	Ankylosing Spondylitis
Positive family history	Rare	Frequent
Onset	Female (30–50 years old)	Male (20–30 years old)
Joint involvement	Symmetric polyarthropathy	Asymmetric oligoarthropathy
Sacroiliac involvement	No	Yes
Vertebral involvement	Cervical	Total (ascending)
Cardiac changes	Pericardial effusion	Cardiomegaly
	Arteritis of coronary arteries	Cardiac conduction
	Cardiac valve fibrosis	abnormalities
	Cardiac conduction abnormalities	Aortic regurgitation
	Aortic regurgitation	
Pulmonary changes	Pleural effusion	Pulmonary fibrosis (upper lobe)
	Pulmonary fibrosis	
Eyes	Keratoconjunctivitis sicca	Conjunctivitis
		Uveitis
Rheumatoid factor	Positive	Negative
HLA-B27	Negative	Positive

temic involvement is most obvious in patients with severe articular disease.

HEART

Pericardial thickening or effusion is present in about one-third of patients with rheumatoid arthritis. Pericardectomy may be necessary to relieve cardiac tamponade. Cardiac involvement may also manifest as pericarditis, myocarditis, arteritis involving the coronary arteries, cardiac valve fibrosis, and formation of rheumatoid nodules in the cardiac conduction system. Aortitis with dilation of the aortic root may result in aortic regurgitation.

LUNGS

The most common pulmonary manifestation of rheumatoid arthritis is a pleural effusion. Rheumatoid nodules occur in the pulmonary parenchyma and on pleural surfaces. These nodules may mimic tuberculosis or neoplasia. Progressive pulmonary fibrosis, associated with cough, dyspnea, and diffuse changes on the chest radiograph, is a rare manifestation.

Costochondral involvement may cause restrictive pulmonary changes, with decreased lung volumes and vital capacity. These changes may be accentuated by pulmonary fibrosis. The resulting mismatch of ventilation to perfusion leads to decreased arterial oxygenation.

NEUROMUSCULAR

Neurologic complications are common and include peripheral nerve compression (carpal tunnel syndrome) and cervical nerve root compression. Mononeuritis multiplex occurs with severe disease and is presumed to be caused by deposition of immune complexes in the walls of blood vessels supplying the nerve. Weakness of skeletal muscles adjacent to the diseased joint is common.

BLOOD

Mild anemia is almost always present and is most likely due to hemodilution or chronic blood loss related to aspirin therapy. Felty's syndrome is rheumatoid arthritis with leukopenia (less than 2,000 mm^3) and hepatosplenomegaly.

EYE

Keratoconjunctivitis sicca (Sjögren's syndrome) occurs in about 10 percent of patients with rheumatoid arthritis. The cause is lack of tear formation due to impairment of lacrimal gland function. The same process may involve the salivary glands, resulting in dryness of the mouth.

Treatment

Drugs effective in treatment of rheumatoid arthritis produce analgesic, anti-inflammatory, and immunosuppressive effects. Aspirin is the most important drug for initial treatment. Optimum therapeutic blood levels of 12 mg·dl^{-1} to 25 mg·dl^{-1} can be achieved with a daily dose of 3 g to 5 g. Limiting factors in the use of aspirin are gastrointestinal bleeding and interference with platelet function. Aspirin may also cause hepatic dysfunction.[57]

Corticosteroids are used extensively for the management of rheumatoid arthritis and are presumably effective in providing symptomatic relief because of their potent anti-inflammatory effects. Nevertheless, these drugs probably do not alter the course of rheumatoid arthritis or change the ultimate degree of damage to the joints. Significant side effects of corticosteroid therapy include suppression of endogenous cortisol release, poor wound healing, increased susceptibility to infection, osteoporosis, gastrointestinal bleeding, and myopathy. Useful nonsteroidal but anti-inflammatory drugs include indomethacin, phenylbutazone, ibuprofen, fenoprofen, naproxen, tolmetin, and culindac. Complications due to phenylbutazone therapy include gastrointestinal bleeding and bone marrow depression.

Gold salts or D-penicillamine may be efficacious in patients with severe rheumatoid arthritis. Gold salts decrease phagocytic activity at inflammatory sites, but a detectable symptomatic improvement may require several months. D-pencillamine, an amino acid constituting part of the penicillin molecule, presumably acts by its ability to dissociate macroglobulins, although confirmatory evidence is not available. Side effects due to both drugs include anemia, leukopenia, and thrombocytopenia. Azathioprine may be effective when other forms of drug therapy do not produce a satisfactory response.

Surgical treatment of rheumatoid arthritis, such as synovectomy or total replacement of severely diseased joints, may relieve pain and restore function. Release of carpal tunnel compression usually produces relief of symptoms related to median nerve compression.

Management of Anesthesia

Multiple organ involvement and side effects of drugs used in the treatment of rheumatoid arthritis must be appreciated in planning management of anesthesia. Preoperatively, patients should be evaluated for airway problems due to the disease process. Compromise of the airway may occur at the cervical spine, temporomandibular joints, and cricoarytenoid joints. For example, flexion deformity of the cervical spine may make it impossible to straighten the neck, and upper airway obstruction is likely when these patients are rendered unconscious. Atlantoaxial subluxation may be present, particularly in those with severe hand deformities and subcutaneous nodules. Radiologic demonstration that the distance from the anterior arch of the atlas to the odontoid process exceeds 3 mm confirms the presence of atlantoaxial subluxation. The importance of atlantoaxial subluxation lies in the fact that the displaced odontoid process can compress the cervical spinal cord or medulla, in addition to occluding the vertebral arteries. In its presence even minimal trauma, as may be associated with movement of the neck during intubation of the trachea, may cause further displacement of the odontoid process and damage to the underlying spinal cord. Certainly, patients should be evaluated before the induction of anesthesia to determine if there is interference with vertebral artery blood flow during flexion, extension, or rotation of the head. Limitation of movement at the temporomandibular joints must be appreciated before the induction of anesthesia. The combination of limited mobility of these joints and of the cervical spine may make visualization of the glottis by direct laryngoscopy difficult or impossible. Intubation of the trachea before induction of anesthesia, using a fiberoptic laryngoscope, may be indicated when preoperative evaluation suggests that direct visualization of the glottis will be difficult. Finally, involvement of the cricoarytenoid joints by arthritic changes is suggested by the presence of hoarseness or stridor preoperatively and the observation of erythema and edema of the vocal cords during direct laryngoscopy. There may be diminished or even absent movement of these joints, which results in narrowing of the glottic opening.

Preoperative pulmonary function studies plus arterial blood gases and pH may be indicated if severe lung disease is suspected. The effect of aspirin on clotting should be evaluated. The need for exogenous corticosteroid supplementation must be considered when these drugs are being used for chronic therapy. The presence and implications of anemia should be appreciated. The need for postoperative ventilatory support should be anticipated if there is severe restrictive lung disease present preoperatively. Postextubation laryngeal obstruction may occur in patients with cricoarytenoid arthritis.

SPONDYLARTHROPATHIES

Spondylarthropathies are a group of non-rheumatic arthropathies, which include ankylosing spondylitis (Marie-Strümpell disease), Reiter's syndrome, juvenile chronic polyarthropathy, and enteropathic arthropathies. These diseases are characterized by involvement of the sacroiliac joints, peripheral inflammatory arthropathy, and the absence of rheumatoid nodules or rheumatic factor (e.g., seronegative). Causes of these seronegative spondylarthropathies are not known, but there is often an association with the human leukocyte antigen (HLA) designated as B27.

Ankylosing Spondylitis

A patient with back pain characterized by morning stiffness that improves with exercise, plus radiographic evidence of sacroilitis, has ankylosing spondylitis (Table 28-2). This disease occurs predominately in men between 20 years and 30 years of age. The strong familial incidence is supported by the finding that 90 percent of patients with this diagnosis are HLA-B27 positive, compared with an incidence of 6 percent in the normal population. The disease is often erroneously diagnosed as back pain due to lumbar disc degeneration. Examination of the spine may reveal skeletal muscle spasm, loss of lordosis, and decreased mobility involving the entire vertebral column.

SYSTEMIC MANIFESTATIONS

Systemic involvement is manifested as weight loss, fatigue, and low grade fever. Conjunctivitis and uveitis occur in about 25 percent of patients. Pulmonary fibrosis is particularly common in the upper lobes, where it mimics tuberculosis. Aortic regurgitation due to thickening and shortening of the valve cusps and dilation of the valve annulus, cardiomegaly, and cardiac conduction abnormalities may be present in about 10 percent of patients.

TREATMENT

Treatment of this disease is with exercises designed to maintain joint mobility, plus anti-inflammatory drugs. Indomethacin or phenylbutazone are commonly used. Bone marrow depression is a potential adverse effect of these drugs. Prognosis is good with early detection and treatment.

Management of Anesthesia. Management of anesthesia in the presence of ankylosing spondylitis is related to the (1) magnitude of upper airway involvement, (2) presence of a restrictive pattern of lung function due to costochondral rigidity and flexion deformity of the thoracic spine, and (3) degree of cardiac involvement. Awake intubation of the trachea, either blindly or with the aid of a fiberoptic laryngoscope, may be necessary if spinal column deformity is extensive.[58] Excessive manipulation of the cervical spine could injure the spinal cord. Intraoperatively, ventilation of the lungs should be supported, since the chest wall is stiff and breathing is diaphragmatic. Regional anesthesia is acceptable for peripheral or lower abdominal operative procedures but may be technically difficult due to limited joint mobility and closed interspinous spaces. Sudden or excessive reductions in systemic vascular resistance are poorly tolerated when aortic regurgitation is present.

Reiter's Disease

Reiter's disease occurs in young males and consists of nonspecific urethritis, uveitis, and arthritis. Predisposing factors are a unique genetic makeup (HLA-B27 positive) plus a bacterial infection with *Shigella* or *Chlamydia* organisms. Most of the signs of this disease persist for only a few days, but arthritis progresses to sacroilitis and spondylitis in about 20 percent of patients. Cricoarytenoid arthritis can also occur. Hyperkeratotic skin lesions cannot be distinguished from psoriasis, and the two diseases frequently appear to overlap. There is no cure for Reiter's disease. Symptomatic management is with indomethacin or phenylbutazone.

Juvenile Chronic Polyarthropathy

Pathology of chronic juvenile polyarthropathy is similar to adult rheumatoid arthritis. Growth abnormalities may occur if the arthritis appears before puberty. Hepatic dysfunction may be present, but cardiac involvement is unusual. An acute form of polyarthritis, which presents as fever, rash, lymphadenopathy, and splenomegaly in young children who are negative for rheumatoid factor and HLA-B27, is designated Still's disease.

Aspirin is the treatment of choice. Corticosteroids are also effective, but these drugs can produce growth retardation when administered to young patients.

Enteropathic Arthropathies

Approximately 20 percent of patients with granulomatous ileocolitis or ulcerative colitis develop an acute migratory inflammatory polyarthritis, most often involving the large joints of the lower extremities. Remissions occur spontaneously, although subsequent recurrence may parallel exacerbation of the underlying disease. Treatment is directed at control of the underlying gastrointestinal disorder.

Inflammatory bowel disease may also be associated with sacroilitis and occasionally severe ankylosing spondylitis. There is no correlation between the severity of the bowel disorder and spondylitis. Treatment is as described for ankylosing spondylitis.

A postintestinal bypass syndrome consisting of arthropathy and dermatitis is well documented. The cause is unknown, although immune mechanisms have been implicated.

OSTEOARTHRITIS

Osteoarthritis is a degenerative process affecting articular cartilage. This process differs from rheumatoid arthritis in that there is minimal inflammatory reaction. The pathogenesis is unclear but may be related to joint trauma. Advancing age and a genetic predisposition are important associated factors. Pain is usually present on motion and relieved by rest. Stiffness tends to disappear rapidly with joint motion, in contrast to the morning stiffness associated with rheumatoid arthritis, which may last several hours.

Characteristically, one joint to several joints are affected by osteoarthritis. The knees and hips are common sites of involvement. Bony enlargements referred to as Heberden's nodes are seen at the distal interphalangeal joints. There may be degenerative disease of the vertebral bodies and intervertebral discs, which may be complicated by protrusion of the nucleus pulposus and compression of nerve roots. Degenerative changes are most significant in the middle to lower cervical spine and in the lower lumbar area. Spinal fusion is unusual, in contrast to its common occurrence in ankylosing spondylitis. Radiographic findings may reveal narrowing of the intervertebral disc spaces and osteophyte formation.

Treatment of osteoarthritis is symptomatic and includes application of heat and administration of drugs (aspirin, indomethacin) known for their analgesic and anti-inflammatory effects. Symptomatic improvement with application of heat may be due to an increased pain threshold in warm compared with cold tissues. Corticosteroids are not recommended, as they may contribute to degenerative joint changes. Reconstructive joint surgery (total hip or knee replacement) may be recommended when pain is persistent and disabling.

OSTEOPOROSIS

Osteoporosis is a generalized decrease in bone mass, which results from a rate of bone resorption that exceeds the rate of bone formation. Radiographs reveal a decline in density of bone. The most common association of osteoporosis is with advancing age, and women are afflicted more often than men. Other causes of osteoporosis include endocrine abnormalities (thyrotoxicosis, hyperadrenocorticism), intestinal malabsorption, immobilization, and drugs, especially corticosteroids.

Clinical problems introduced by osteoporosis are pathologic fractures, pain, and skeletal deformity. Fractures are most common in the lower thoracic and lumbar vertebral bodies. With each fracture, there is sudden severe pain; anterior compression of the vertebral body results in loss of height and the development of a kyphotic deformity, typically in the region of the thoracic spine. Shortening of the vertebral column leads to relaxed anterior abdominal musculature and protuberant abdomen. There are no characteristic laboratory abnormalities. Plasma calcium, phosphate, and alkaline phosphatase concentrations are normal.

Treatment of osteoporosis is designed to produce a positive calcium balance. Estrogens decrease bone resorption and may be effective in the treatment of women with osteoporosis.

Use of estrogens, however, may increase the risk of endometrial carcinoma. Alternatives to estrogens are supplements of calcium and vitamin D. Calcium supplements have not been documented to prevent postmenopausal bone loss.[59]

OSTEOMALACIA

Osteomalacia is a term applied to diseases in which there is a failure to mineralize adequately newly formed bone. Rickets is the analogous disease in children. Elderly patients whose diet is deficient in dairy products and who are not exposed to enough sunlight to synthesize their own vitamin D may have an element of osteomalacia superimposed on osteoporosis. Chronic use of anticonvulsant drugs, including barbiturates and phenytoin, has been associated with altered vitamin D metabolism and osteomalacia. Osteomalacia and osteoporosis may be indistinguishable by history and radiographic findings, but hypophosphatemia suggests osteomalacia.

PAGET'S DISEASE

Paget's disease is characterized by excessive osteoblastic and osteoclastic activity, resulting in abnormally thickened but weak bone. The cause is unknown but may reflect an excess of parathyroid hormone or a deficiency of calcitonin. Radiographic findings include lytic and sclerotic changes, which may involve the skull. There is cortical thickening of long bones. A familial tendency is present, with white men over the age of 40 years being most frequently affected. Increased bone formation and resorption are associated with elevated plasma alkaline phosphatase levels. In addition to pain and deformity, complications include pathologic fractures, nerve compression, renal calculi, high output cardiac failure, and hypercalcemia.

Calcitonin, which appears to act as a primary inhibitor of bone resorption, is an effective therapeutic agent. Sodium etiodronate, which suppresses osteoblastic and osteoclastic activity, is effective in decreasing pain and the rate of bone turnover. When Paget's disease involves the hip, a replacement arthroplasty may be considered.

OSTEOGENESIS IMPERFECTA

Osteogenesis imperfecta is a rare, autosomal dominant, inherited disease of connective tissue in which bones are extremely brittle because of defective collagen production. The incidence is higher in females. Clinically, the disease manifests as one of two forms designated osteogenesis imperfecta congenita and osteogenesis imperfecta tarda. In the congenita form, fractures occur in utero, and death usually occurs in the perinatal period. The tarda form typically manifests in childhood or early adolescence with the presence of blue sclera (due to defective collagen production), fractures with trivial trauma, kyphoscoliosis as a reflection of collapse of vertebral bodies, bowing of the femur and tibia, and the gradual onset of otosclerosis and deafness. Impaired platelet function in these patients may manifest as a mild bleeding tendency. Increased body temperature with hyperhydrosis may occur in patients with osteogenesis imperfecta.

Management of Anesthesia

Management of anesthesia is influenced by co-existing orthopedic deformities and vulnerability to additional fractures during the perioperative period.[60] Intubation of the trachea must be accomplished with minimal manipulation and trauma, as cervical and mandibular fractures may occur. Dentition is defective and may be vulnerable to easy damage, as during direct laryngoscopy. Awake intubation of the trachea with use of a fiberoptic laryngoscope may be prudent if co-existing orthopedic deformities could make visualization of the glottic opening difficult by direct lar-

yngoscopy. Associated kyphoscoliosis and pectus excavatum may reduce vital capacity, decrease chest wall compliance, and result in arterial hypoxemia due to maldistribution of ventilation relative to perfusion. Regional anesthesia may be acceptable in selected patients but technically difficult because of kyphoscoliosis. Coagulation status should be evaluated, especially before selecting regional anesthetic techniques. In view of the potential for increases in body temperature, it is important to monitor temperature continuously.

MC CUNE-ALBRIGHT SYNDROME

McCune-Albright syndrome consists of a triad of physical signs characterized as osseous lesions termed polyostotic fibrous dysplasia, melanotic cutaneous macules called café au lait spots, and sexual precocity. Conductive and neural deafness occurs when osseous lesions involve the temporal bone with resultant ossicular or cochlear impingement. Osseous fractures are likely in childhood. In addition to the classic triad some patients manifest endocrine dysfunction, especially hyperthyroidism, hypercortisolism, growth hormone excess, and hypophosphatemia.[61]

MYOSITIS OSSIFICANS

Myositis ossificans is a rare inherited autosomal dominant disease, which usually manifests before 6 years of age and is characterized clinically by interstitial myositis and proliferation of connective tissue. Connective tissue undergoes cartilaginous and osteoid transformation, eventually leading to displacement of skeletal muscle mass by ectopic bone formation. Ectopic bone formation typically affects skeletal muscles of the elbow, hip, and knee leading to serious limitation of joint movement. Temporomandibular joint involvement with obvious implications for intubation of the trachea may occur.[62] Skeletal muscles of the face, larynx, eye, anterior abdominal wall, diaphragm, and heart usually escape involvement.

In early stages of the disease, fever may occur at the same time localized lumps appear in affected skeletal muscles. Alkaline phosphatase activity is increased during active phases of the disease. A restrictive pattern of breathing reflects limitation of rib movement. Progression to respiratory failure is rare, although pneumonia is a common complication. Abnormalities on the electrocardiogram may include ST-segment changes and right bundle branch block. Deafness may occur but mental retardation is unlikely.

MARFAN'S SYNDROME

Marfan's syndrome is a disorder of connective tissue, inherited as an autosomal dominant trait.[63] The incidence is 4 to 6 per 100,000 births, and the mean age of survival is 32 years. The biochemical defect responsible is unknown. Manifestations are primarily on the skeletal system, but important changes may also take place in the cardiovascular system, lungs, and eyes.

Skeletal System

Characteristically, these patients have long tubular bones, giving them a tall stature and an "Abe Lincoln" appearance. Additional skeletal abnormalities include a high arched palate, pectus excavatum, kyphoscoliosis, and hyperextensibility of the joints.

Cardiovascular System

There is progressive cystic medial necrosis in the wall of the aorta, leading to an increased incidence of aneurysms of the aorta, usually involving the ascending thoracic aorta. Dissec-

tion of an aneurysm of the aorta may cause acute aortic regurgitation. Extension of this dissection through the sinus of Valsalva into the pericardium can lead to sudden cardiac tamponade (see Chapter 11).

Mitral valve prolapse is present in the majority of patients with Marfan's syndrome (see Chapter 4). The risk of bacterial endocarditis is increased in the presence of valvular heart disease. Cardiac conduction abnormalities, especially bundle branch block, are common.

Lungs

Patients with Marfan's syndrome are prone to the early development of pulmonary emphysema. This change will accentuate the impact of restrictive lung disease that may be present, due to the development of kyphoscoliosis. There is a high incidence of spontaneous pneumothorax in these patients.

Eyes

Ocular changes characterized by lens dislocation, myopia, and detachment of the retina occur at some time in more than one-half of patients with Marfan's syndrome.

Management of Anesthesia

Preoperative evaluation of patients with Marfan's syndrome should concentrate on cardiopulmonary abnormalities. Prophylactic antibiotics are appropriate if valvular heart disease is present. In most patients, skeletal abnormalities have little impact on the upper airway. Care should be exercised, however, to avoid extreme movements of the mandible, as these patients are prone to temporomandibular joint dislocation. In view of the possibility of a weakened wall of the thoracic aorta, it is prudent to avoid excessive elevations of blood pressure, as can occur during laryngoscopy for intubation of the trachea or in response to painful surgical stimulation. A high index of suspicion must be maintained for the development of pneumothorax.

SCOLIOSIS

Scoliosis is a disease manifested as a lateral curve of the spine and an accompanying rotation of the vertebrae, resulting in distortion of the rib cage. Scoliosis may be idiopathic, or due to neuromuscular disease (meningomyelocele, poliomyelitis, cerebral palsy, muscular dystrophy). Alternatively, scoliosis could reflect inability of the central nervous system to sense and control spinal alignment at a subconscious level. Idiopathic scoliosis has an incidence of about 4 per 1,000 population. There seems to be a familial predisposition, with the disease onset occurring most often in females during the rapid growth phase of adolescence. The curve is usually right-sided and involves seven to ten vertebral bodies. A curve greater than 40 degrees is considered to be severe and most likely to be associated with physiologic derangements in cardiac and pulmonary function.

Physiologic Derangement

Restrictive lung disease and pulmonary hypertension progressing to cor pulmonale are the major causes of mortality in patients with scoliosis. Lung volumes and pulmonary compliance are reduced, and the alveolar-to-arterial difference for oxygen is increased. Arterial carbon dioxide partial pressure is usually normal. Pulmonary hypertension reflects increased pulmonary vascular resistance due to compression of lung vasculature by the curve in the spine and to the pulmonary vascular response to arterial hypoxemia.

Management of Anesthesia

Preoperatively, it is important to assess the severity of the physiologic derangement produced by the skeletal deformity. Pulmonary function tests, with special attention to the vital capacity and forced exhaled volume in 1 second, will reflect the magnitude of restrictive lung disease. Arterial blood gases and pH are helpful for detecting unrecognized hypoxemia or acidosis that could be contributing to pulmonary hypertension. Patients with scoliosis due to neuromuscular disease may enter the preoperative period with pneumonia due to chronic aspiration of acidic gastric fluid. Certainly, any reversible component of pulmonary dysfunction, such as bacterial infection or bronchospasm, should be corrected before elective operations. Preoperative medication with depressant drugs must be done with caution, if at all, in view of the narrow margin of ventilatory reserve in these patients, plus adverse effects on the pulmonary vascular resistance that would occur with respiratory acidosis from hypoventilation.

Intraoperatively, ventilation of the lungs should be controlled to facilitate adequate arterial oxygenation and elimination of carbon dioxide. Adequacy of oxygenation should be confirmed by measurements of the arterial oxygen partial pressure. Although no specific drug or drug combination can be recommended as superior, it should be remembered that nitrous oxide may increase pulmonary vascular resistance, presumably by direct vasoconstrictive effects on the pulmonary vasculature. Monitoring of central venous pressure may provide an early warning of increased pulmonary vascular resistance produced by nitrous oxide. Signs of malignant hyperthermia (tachycardia, hypercapnia, acidosis, and increased body temperature) must be appreciated, as it has been suggested that there is an increased incidence of this syndrome in patients with scoliosis.[64]

If the surgical procedure is for correction of the spinal curvature, special consideration must be given to intraoperative blood loss and recognition of spinal cord injury. Controlled hypotension, with a combination of a volatile anesthetic and a peripheral vasodilator such as nitroprusside, is effective in reducing blood loss. As the spinal curve is straightened, excess traction on the spinal cord may manifest as paralysis in the postoperative period. An intraoperative maneuver to detect spinal cord injury is to reverse neuromuscular blockade and discontinue the inhaled anesthetics until the patient is sufficiently awake to move both legs on request and thus confirm that the spinal cord is intact (i.e., wake up test).[65] Inhalation anesthesia is then reestablished and the operation completed. Somatosensory cortical-evoked potential monitoring is also useful to confirm an intact spinal cord. The advantage of evoked potentials is that patients need not be awakened intraoperatively. If this approach is used, it must be appreciated that many drugs, including volatile anesthetics, interfere with interpretation of evoked potentials. Therefore, a nitrous oxide-opioid technique is often recommended. In this regard, continuous infusion of the opioid maintains any drug-induced change on evoked potentials at a constant level, making it easier to interpret changes due to spinal cord damage.[66] Furthermore, dose requirements for opioids are less during continuous infusion compared with intermittent injections. Even wake up tests may be achieved without use of opioid antagonists after discontinuation of continuous infusion of opioids.

Postoperatively, the major concern is restoration of adequate ventilation. It is likely that slow weaning from the ventilator will be necessary in most patients with severe scoliosis, regardless of the operative procedure.

ACHONDROPLASIA

Achondroplasia is the most common cause of dwarfism, occurring most often in females, with an incidence of 1 in every 26,000 births. Transmission is by an autosomal dominant gene, although an estimated 80 percent of cases represent spontaneous mutation. Indeed, fertility among achondroplastic dwarfs is low. The basic defect is thought to be a decrease in the rate of endochondral ossification, which, coupled with normal periosteal bone formation, leads to short tubular bones. The pre-

dicted height for achondroplastic males is 132 cm and for females 122 cm. Kyphoscoliosis and genu varum are common. Premature fusion of the bones at the base of the skull occurs in achondroplasia, resulting in a shortened skull base and small stenotic foramen magnum. This change may result in infantile hydrocephalus or damage to the cervical cord. For example, achondroplastic dwarfs who experience sleep apnea may be manifesting brain stem compression from foramen magnum stenosis. Mental and skeletal muscle development is normal, as is life expectancy for those who survive the first year of life.

Management of Anesthesia

Achondroplastic dwarfs characteristically require a number of specific procedures, including suboccipital craniectomy for foramen magnum stenosis, laminectomy for spinal column stenosis, or nerve root compression and ventricular peritoneal shunts. Abnormal bone growth is responsible for several potential anesthetic problems[67,68] Facial features characterized by a large protruding forehead, short maxilla, large mandible, flat nose, and large tongue suggest difficulty in attaining a suitable fit with the anesthetic face mask and maintenance of a patent upper airway. Despite these characteristics, clinical experience has not confirmed difficulty in maintaining the upper airway or intubation of the trachea.[67] Certainly, hyperextension of the neck during direct laryngoscopy for intubation of the trachea should be avoided, considering the likely presence of foramen magnum stenosis. Weight rather than age is the best guide for predicting the proper size endotracheal tube for these patients.[67] Excess skin and subcutaneous tissue may make establishment of peripheral intravenous lines more difficult. Achondroplastic dwarfs undergoing suboccipital craniectomy, especially in the sitting position, are at high risk for venous air embolism, emphasizing the potential value of a right atrial catheter.[69] Placement of a right atrial catheter, however, is technically difficult because of the short neck and difficulty identifying landmarks that may be obscured by excess soft tissues. Monitoring of somatosensory evoked potentials is useful during operations that may be associated with brain stem or spinal cord injury. Achondroplastic dwarfs seem to respond normally to drugs used for anesthesia and skeletal muscle relaxation. An anesthetic technique that permits rapid awakening may be desirable for prompt evaluation of neurologic function.

Regional anesthesia in achondroplastic dwarfs may be considered for cesarean section, which is mandated by the small and contracted pelvis in these patients combined with near normal infant birth weights.[70] Technical difficulties may occur because of kyphoscoliosis and a narrow epidural space and spinal canal. Indeed, the small space present may make it difficult to introduce a catheter or obtain a free flow of cerebrospinal fluid. Neurologic changes may occur in later life because of compression of the spinal cord by osteophytes, prolapsed intervertebral discs, or deformed vertebral bodies. There are no data confirming the appropriate dose of local anesthetic for epidural or spinal anesthesia in these patients. For this reason, epidural anesthesia may be preferable to spinal anesthesia, as it permits titration of the local anesthetic dose to achieve a desired sensory level of blockade.

HALLERMANN-STREIFF SYNDROME

Hallermann-Streiff syndrome is characterized by oculomandibulodyscephaly and dwarfism. The nose and mandible are hypoplastic, the teeth brittle, and the temporomandibular joints weak and easily dislocated. These airway abnormalities make direct laryngoscopy for intubation of the trachea both hazardous and difficult. Awake nasotracheal intubation can be difficult if the nares are hypoplastic.[71]

DUTCH-KENTUCKY SYNDROME

Dutch-Kentucky syndrome is a rare inherited disorder characterized by decreased ability to open the mouth due to trismus plus flex-

ion deformity of the fingers, which occurs with wrist extension (pseudocampodactyly). Enlarged coronoid processes may be the cause of trismus. Foot deformities and shorter than normal stature are frequently present. When these patients require surgery, management of the airway may be facilitated by fiberoptic laryngoscopy.[72]

WILLIAMS-BEUREN SYNDROME

Williams-Beuren syndrome is a rare entity characterized by mental retardation, hypercalcemia with associated kidney dysfunction and corneal opacities, kyphoscoliosis, and skeletal muscle hypotonia. Characteristic facies include broad forehead, pointed chin, flattened nasal bridge, large upper lip, and prognathism. Aortic regurgitation is present in over one half of these patients. Presence of stenosis of the left subclavian artery can result in unequal blood pressure measurements in the upper extremities.

KLIPPEL-FEIL SYNDROME

Klippel-Feil syndrome is characterized by shortness of the neck, resulting from reduction in the number of cervical vertebrae or fusion of several vertebrae into an osseous mass. Movement of the neck is limited and associated skeletal abnormalities include spinal canal stenosis or scoliosis. Mandibular malformations and micrognathia may be present. There is an increased incidence of cardiac and genitourinary anomalies in these patients. Management of anesthesia must consider the risk of neurologic damage during direct laryngoscopy in the presence of cervical spine instability.[73] Preoperative lateral neck radiographs will help evaluate stability of the cervical spine.

REFERENCES

1. Bauer EA, Cooper TW, Tucker DR, Esterly NB. Phenytoin therapy of recessive dystrophic epidermolysis bullosa. Clinical trial and proposed mechanism of action on collagenase. N Engl J Med 1980;303:776–81

2. James I, Wark H. Airway management during anesthesia in patients with epidermolysis bullosa dystrophica. Anesthesiology 1982;56:323–6

3. Holzman RS, Worthen HM, Johnson K. Anaesthesia for children with junctional epidermolysis bulloas (letalis). Can J Anaesth 1987;34:395–9

4. Broster T, Placek R, Eggers GWN. Epidermolysis bullosa: Anesthetic management for cesarean section. Anesth Analg 1987;66:341–3

5. Dretchen KL, Morgenroth VH, Standaert FG, Walts LF. Azathioprine: Effects on neuromuscular transmission. Anesthesiology 1976;45:604–9

6. Jeyaram C, Torda TA. Anesthetic management of cholecystectomy in a patient with buccal pemphigus. Anesthesiology 1974;40:600–1

7. Kovenblat PE, Wedner HJ, Whyte MP, et al. Systemic mastocytosis. Arch Intern Med 1984;144:2249–59

8. Roberts LJ, Sweetman BJ, Lewis RA, et al. Increased production of prostaglandin D_2 in patients with systemic mastocytosis. N Engl J Med 1980;303:1400–4

9. Coleman MA, Liberthson RR, Crone RK, Levine FH. General anesthesia in a child with urticaria pigmentosa. Anesth Analg 1980;59:704–6

10. Hosking MP, Warner MA. Sudden intraoperative hypotension in a patient with asymptomatic urticaria pigmentosa. Anesth Analg 1987;66:344–6

11. Johnston WE, Moss J, Philbin DM, et al. Management of cold urticaria during hypothermic cardiopulmonary bypass. N Engl J Med 1982;306:219–21

12. Cucchira RF, Dawson B. Anesthesia in Stevens-Johnson syndrome: Report of a case. Anesthesiology 1971;35:537–9

13. Siegel RC. Scleroderma. Med Clin North Am 1977;61:283–97

14. Bulkey BH, Ridolfi RL, Salyar WR, Hutchins GM. Myocardial lesions of progressive systemic sclerosis: A cause of cardiac dysfunction. Circulation 1976;53:483–90

15. Young RH, Mark GJ. Pulmonary vascular changes in scleroderma. Am J Med 1978;64:998–1000

16. Younker D, Harrison B. Scleroderma and pregnancy: Anaesthetic considerations. Br J Anaesth 1985;57:1136–9

17. Thompson J, Conklin KA. Anesthetic management of a pregnant patient with scleroderma. Anesthesiology 1983;59:69–71

18. Krechel SLW, Ramirez-Inawant RC, Fabian LW. Anesthetic considerations in pseudoxanthoma elasticum. Anesth Analg 1981;60:344–7

19. Dolan P, Sisko F, Riley E. Anesthetic considerations for Ehlers-Danlos syndrome. Anesthesiology 1980;52:266–9

20. Johns RA, Finhold DA, Stirt JA. Anaesthetic management of a child with dermatomyositis. Can Anaesth Soc J 1986;33:71–4

21. Flusche G, Unger-Sargon J, Lambert DH. Prolonged neuromuscular paralysis with vecuronium in a patient with polymyositis. Anesth Analg 1987;66:188–90

22. Smith PEM, Calverley PMA, Edwards RHT, et al. Practical problems in the respiratory care of patients with muscular dystrophy. N Engl J Med 1987;316:1197–1204

23. Smith CL, Bush GH. Anaesthesia and progressive muscular dystrophy. Br J Anaesth 1985;57:1113–8

24. Seay AR, Ziter FA, Thompson JA. Cardiac arrest during induction of anesthesia in Duchenne's muscular dystrophy. J Pediatr 1978;93:88–90

25. Rosenberg H, Heiman-Patterson T. Duchenne's muscular dystrophy and malignant hyperthermia: Another warning. Anesthesiology 1983;59:362

26. Brownell AKW, Paasuke RT, Elash A, et al. Malignant hyperthermia in Duchenne's muscular dystrophy. Anesthesiology 1983;58:180–2

27. Wang JM, Stanley TH. Duchenne muscular dystrophy and malignant hyperthermia-two case reports. Can Anaesth Soc J 1986;33:492–7

28. Sethna NF, Rockoff MA. Cardiac arrest following inhalation induction of anaesthesia in a child with Duchenne's muscular dystrophy. Can Anaesth Soc J 1986;799–802

29. Murat I, Esteve C, Montay G, et al. Pharmacokinetics and cardiovascular effects of bupivacaine during epidural anesthesia in children with Duchenne muscular dystrophy. Anesthesiology 1987;67:249–52

30. Cunliffe M, Burrows FA. Anaesthetic implications of nemaline rod myopathy. Can Anaesth Soc J 1985;32:543–7

31. Heard SO, Kaplan RF. Neuromuscular blockade in a patient with nemaline myopathy. Anesthesiology 1983;59:588-90

32. Hook R, Anderson EF, Noto P. Anesthetic management of a parturient with myotonia atrophica. Anesthesiology 1975;43:689–92

33. Mitchell MM, Ali HH, Savarese JJ. Myotonia and neuromuscular blocking agents. Anesthesiology 1978;49:44–8

34. Mudge BJ, Taylor PB, Vanderspek AFL. Periop-

erative hazards in myotonic dystrophy. Anaesthesia 1980;35:492–5

35. Aldridge LM. Anaesthetic problems in myotonic dystrophy. A case report and review of the Aberdeen experience comprising 48 general anaesthetics in a further 16 patients. Br J Anaesth 1985;57:1119–30

36. Cope DK, Miller JN. Local and spinal anesthesia for cesarean section in a patient with myotonic dystrophy. Anesth Analg 1986;65:687–90

37. Heymsfield SB, McNish T, Perkins JV, Felner JM. Sequence of cardiac changes in Duchenne's muscular dystrophy. Am Heart J 1978;95:283–94

38. Ravin M, Newmark Z, Saviello G. Myotonia dystrophica-an anesthetic hazard: Two case reports. Anesth Analg 1975;54:216–8

39. Meyers MB, Barash PG. Cardiac decompensation during enflurane anesthesia in a patient with myotonia atrophica. Anesth Analg 1976;55:433–6

40. Nightingale P, Healy TEJ, McGuinness K. Dystrophia myotonica and atracurium. Br J Anaesth 1985;57:1131–5

41. Cook WP, Kaplan RF. Neuromuscular blockade in a patient with stiff-baby syndrome. Anesthesiology 1986;65:525–8

42. Parris WCV, Johnson AC. Tracheomegaly. Anesthesiology 1982;56:141–3

43. Seybold ME. Myasthenia gravis. A clinical and basic science review. JAMA 1983;250:2516–21

44. Drachman DB. Myasthenia gravis. N Engl J Med 1978;298:136–42

45. Lake CL. Curare sensitivity in steroid-treated myasthenia gravis: A case report. Anesth Analg 1978;57:132–4

46. Leventhal SR, Orkin FK, Hirsh RA. Prediction of the need for postoperative mechanical ventilation in myasthenia gravis. Anesthesiology 1980;53:26–30

47. Eisenkraft JB, Papatestas AE, Kahn CH, et al. Predicting the need for postoperative mechanical ventilation and myasthenia gravis. Anesthesiology 1986;65:79–82

48. Baraka A, Dajani A. Atracurium in myasthenics undergoing thymectomy. Anesth Analg 1984;63:1127–30

49. Wise RP. A myasthenia syndrome complicating bronchial carcinoma. Anaesthesia 1962;17:488–90

50. Agoston S, vanWeerden T, Westra P, Broekert A. Effects of 4-aminopyridine in Eaton-Lambert syndrome. Br J Anaesth 1978;50:383–5

51. Melnick B, Chang J-L, Larson CE, Bedger RC. Hypokalemic familial periodic paralysis. Anesthesiology 1983;58:263–5

52. Rollman JE, Dickson CM. Anesthetic management of a patient with hypokalemic familial periodic paralysis for coronary artery bypass surgery. Anesthesiology 1985;63:526–7

53. Naidu R, Steg NL, MacEwen GD. Hyperkalemia: Benign, hereditary, autosomal dominant. Anesthesiology 1982;56:226–8

54. Laishley RS, Roy WL. Freeman-Sheldon syndrome: Report of three cases and the anaesthetic implications. Can Anaesth Soc J 1986;33:388–93

55. Yamashita M, Koishi K, Yamaya R, et al. Anaesthetic considerations in the Prader-Willi syndrome: Report of four cases. Can Anaesth Soc J 1983;30:179–84

56. Hannington-Kiff JG. Prune-belly syndrome and general anesthesia: Case report. Br J Anaesth 1970;42:649–52

57. Seaman WE, Plotz PH. Effects of aspirin on liver tests in patients with RA or SLE and in normal volunteers. Arthritis Rheum 1976;19:155–60

58. Munson ES, Cullen SC. Endotracheal intubation in a patient with ankylosing spondylitis of the cervical spine. Anesthesiology 1965;26:365

59. Riis B, Thomsen K, Christiansen C. Does calcium supplementation prevent postmenopausal bone loss? A double-blind, controlled clinical study. N Engl J Med 1987;316:173–7

60. Cunningham AJ, Donnelly M, Comerford J. Osteogenesis imperfecta: Anesthetic management of a patient for cesarean section: A case report. Anesthesiology 1984;61:91–3

61. Lee PA, VanDop C, Migeon CJ. McCune-Albright syndrome. Long-term follow-up. JAMA 1986;256:2980–4

62. Shipton EA, Retief LW, Theron HDUT, DeBruin FA. Anaesthesia in myositis ossificans progressiva. SAMJ 1985;67:26–8

63. Pyeritz RE, McKusick VA. The Marfan syndrome. Diagnosis and management. N Engl J Med 1979;300:772–7

64. Kafer ER. Respiratory and cardiovascular functions in scoliosis and the principles of anesthetic management. Anesthesiology 1980;52:339–51

65. Waldman J, Kaufer H, Hensinger RV, et al. Wake-up technique to avoid neurological sequelae during Harrington rod procedure. A case report. Anesth Analg 1977;56:733–5

66. Pathak KS, Brown RH, Nash CL, Cascorbi HF. Continuous opioid infusion for scoliosis fusion surgery. Anesth Analg 1983;62:841–5

67. Mayhew JF, Katz J, Miner M, et al. Anaesthesia for the achondroplastic dwarf. Can Anaesth Soc J 1986;33:216–21

68. Kalla GN, Fening E, Obiaya MD. Anaesthetic management of achondroplasia. Br J Anaesth 1986;58:117–9

69. Katz J, Mayhew JF. Air embolism in the achondroplastic dwarf. Anesthesiology 1985;63:205–7

70. Cohen SE. Anesthesia for cesarean section in

achondroplastic dwarfs. Anesthesiology 1980;52:264–6

71. Ravindran R, Stoops CM. Anesthetic management of a patient with Hallermann-Streiff syndrome. Anesth Analg 1979;58:254–5

72. Browder FH, Lew D, Shahbazian TS. Anesthetic management of a patient with Dutch-Kentucky syndrome. Anesthesiology 1986;65:218–9

73. Naguib M, Farag H, Ibrahim AEW. Anaesthetic considerations in Klippel-Feil syndrome. Can Anaesth Soc J 1986;33:66–70

29

Infectious Diseases

An understanding of diseases caused by infectious organisms and of the appropriate treatment of these diseases is important for optimal patient care during surgery and anesthesia. Although infectious diseases are rarely the primary indications for surgery, not infrequently a co-existing infection influences management of patients during the perioperative period. Certainly, postoperative infections are significant causes of morbidity in hospitalized patients.

INFECTIONS DUE TO GRAM-POSITIVE BACTERIA

Organisms categorized as gram-positive bacteria include pneumococci, streptococci, and staphylococci. These organisms are frequently implicated as causes of infections that may contribute to significant morbidity in hospitalized patients.

Pneumococci

There are more than 80 distinct serotypes of the pneumococcus genus (*Streptococcus pneumoniae*).[1] These serotypes differ from each other by virtue of the polysaccharide polymers forming their outer capsules. These capsules are crucial to the virulence of pneumococci, since they allow these bacteria to resist phagocytosis. Capsular polysaccharides from the 14 most prevalent serotypes of pneumococci have been incorporated into a pneumococcal vaccine. Pneumococci remain the most important cause of bacterial pneumonia, accounting for about 60 percent of these infections. Acute otitis media, due to spread of pneumococci from the nasopharynx is one of the most frequent bacterial infections in children. Indeed, the nasopharynx is the natural habitat of pneumococci. In rare instances, meningitis may reflect spread of pneumococcal organisms from the middle ear or nasal sinuses. An uncommon pneumococcal syndrome is overwhelming infection after surgical splenectomy.

Penicillin or another antibiotic with a similar spectrum of activity remains the drug of choice for treatment of infections due to pneumococci. Pneumococcal vaccine is indicated in patients at risk for developing infections, including those with chronic cardiopulmonary disease, cirrhosis of the liver, nephrosis, and sickle cell anemia. The vaccine may also be useful in the management of patients with Hodgkin's disease, who are at risk for developing pneumococcal sepsis after staging laparotomy and splenectomy. It should be appreciated that responses to this vaccine are poor after chemotherapy and radiotherapy.

Streptococci

Streptococci are a diverse group of gram positive bacteria that reside in humans as part of the normal flora. Based on the composition of their carbohydrate cell walls, streptococci are divided into 18 groups designated as A through H and K through T.

GROUP A STREPTOCOCCI

Group A streptococci (*Streptococcus pyogens*) are important human pathogens, responsible for several common bacterial infections (Table 29-1). The most important mode of spread is by droplets, originating either from asymptomatic nasopharyngeal carriers, or from patients with pharyngitis. Group A streptococci elaborate enzymes that account for the ability of these organisms to produce inflammation and to spread rapidly to adjacent tissues. Among these enzymes are streptolysin O and streptolysin S, which are responsible for hemolysis (i.e., beta-hemolytic streptococci) and inactivation of leukocytes. A streptokinase enzyme elaborated by certain streptococci is responsible for promoting fibrinolysis. Elaboration of hyaluronidase enzyme by streptococci facilitates spread of infection into adjacent tissues, due to the ability of this substance to digest hyaluronic acid present in connective tissues.

Group A streptococci are the most common causes of bacterial pharyngitis and tonsillitis. Elaboration of an exotoxin known as erythrogenic toxin is responsible for scarlet fever. Acute rheumatic fever occurs only after pharyngitis caused by group A streptococci. Patients in the 5- to 15-year-old age group are most likely to develop rheumatic fever. Typi-

TABLE 29-1. Infections Due to Group A Streptococci

Pharyngitis and tonsillitis
Scarlet fever
Rheumatic fever
Superficial skin infections (impetigo)
Deep skin infections (cellulitis, erysipelas)
Bacteremia (endocarditis, meningitis, osteomyelitis)

cally, symptoms of acute rheumatic fever manifest 1 week to 3 weeks after streptococcal infection. Antibodies formed against streptococcal antigens are the most likely mechanism by which prior infection with group A streptococci produces delayed tissue damage. This damage may manifest as pericarditis, myocarditis, or endocarditis. The mitral and aortic valves are often involved in this disease process. An acute migratory arthritis occurs in over one-half the patients who develop rheumatic fever. Early treatment of pharyngitis due to infection with group A streptococci will prevent subsequent attacks of acute rheumatic fever.[1] Aspirin is effective in controlling the febrile and articular manifestations associated with acute rheumatic fever.

Superficial infections of the epidermis due to group A streptococci are known as impetigo. Impetigo is highly contagious and predisposes to the poststreptococcal infection syndrome known as glomerulonephritis. Surgical wound infections due to streptococci often manifest as acute elevations of body temperature despite a relatively benign appearing incision site.

Deep skin infections due to group A streptococci are known as erysipelas and cellulitis. Osteomyelitis, meningitis, and endocarditis are potential complications of group A streptococcal bacteremia. Group A streptococci are the classic cause of postpartum infection.

Penicillin is the drug of choice for treatment of infections due to group A streptococci. Alternative drugs to penicillin include erythromycin and clindamycin. Tetracyclines should not be relied upon, since many strains of group A streptococci are resistant to this antibiotic.

GROUP B STREPTOCOCCI

Group B streptococci are the most common cause of bacterial sepsis in neonates. Infections due to this organism are most often associated with prematurity and prolonged rupture of the membranes. Pneumonia or meningitis are present in about one-half of the neonates who develop infection with this organism. Mortality ranges from 20 percent to 75 percent, despite aggressive treatment with antibiotics. Neurologic sequelae are often present in those neonates who survive. Despite the demonstration of a decreased incidence of necrotizing enterocolitis in high-risk infants treated with prophylactic antibiotics, the routine use of this approach is not popular because of the rapid emergence of resistant organisms.

GROUP D STREPTOCOCCI

Group D streptococci reside in the gastrointestinal and genitourinary tract. These enterococci are relatively common causes of superficial wound infections, urinary tract infections, peritonitis, endocarditis, and bacteremia. Infections with group D streptococci are most likely in patients with co-existing disease of the genitourinary or gastrointestinal tract. Treatment of infections due to group D streptococci is difficult, since these organisms are unique among the streptococci in being resistant to penicillin.

Staphylococci

The two important species of staphylococci are *Staphylococcus aureus* and *Staphylococcus epidermidis* (formerly albus). Unlike pneumococci and streptococci, there is not a satisfactory serologic classification of staphylococci.

S. AUREUS

S. aureus are widely distributed organisms, with asymptomatic carriers or individuals with staphylococcal lesions acting as reservoirs of infection. The incidence of nasal carriage is 15 percent to 50 percent in hospital populations. The incidence is even greater in drug addicts and patients with insulin-dependent diabetes mellitus. Contamination of the hands with nasal secretions is the primary mode of transmission.

The most frequent manifestations of *S. aureus* are superficial (conjunctivitis, furuncle, paronychia) and soft tissue (cellulitis, mastitis, surgical incision) infections. These organisms are among the principal causes of septic arthritis and osteomyelitis. Staphylococcal bacteremia may result in endocarditis and meningitis. Staphylococci do not cause pharyngitis and are responsible for less than 10 percent of all bacterial pneumonias.

Staphylococcal invasion of the gastrointestinal tract may take two forms. In one form, ingestion of staphylococcal enterotoxin results in vomiting and diarrhea within 3 hours to 6 hours after consumption of food contaminated with *S. aureus*. Characteristically, these symptoms are not accompanied by an increase in body temperature. In the second form, staphylococcal enterocolitis is caused by the intestinal overgrowth of *S. aureus* in patients receiving broad-spectrum oral antibiotics.

S. aureus is usually resistant to penicillin. Effective antibiotics include aminoglycoside and cephalosporin antibiotics, oxacillin, and nafcillin. In addition to therapy with antibiotics, other measures, including removal of such portals of entry as indwelling venous catheters and surgical drainage, may be necessary.

Toxic Shock Syndrome.   Toxic shock syndrome is a potentially fatal multisystem illness due to *S. aureus* infection and production of toxins. This syndrome is associated with tampon use during menstruation and with use of vaginal contraceptive sponges. Toxic shock syndrome may be a complication of staphylococcal pneumonia that follows an influenza-like illness (i.e., postinfluenza toxic shock syndrome).[2] Other nonmenstrual cases of toxic shock syndrome have been related to nasal packing, childbirth and abortion, surgical wound infections, and vaginal infections.

Criteria for diagnosis of toxic shock syndrome include fever, diffuse macular erythroderma, and hypotension. Desquamation is a characteristic feature of this syndrome but is not an early finding. Evidence of multisystem involvement may include diarrhea, skeletal muscle myalgia (elevated plasma concentrations of creatine kinase), renal dysfunction (elevated plasma creatinine concentrations), hepatic dysfunction (elevated plasma concentrations of transaminase enzymes and bilirubin), disseminated intravascular coagulation and thrombocytopenia. Isolation of toxin producing *S. aureus* from secretions of affected patients further supports the diagnosis of toxic shock syndrome.

S. EPIDERMIDIS

S. epidermidis are organisms of low pathogenic potential, universally present as part of the normal flora of the skin. Because of their ubiquity, *S. epidermidis* are frequently isolated from clinical specimens, including blood cultures. Nevertheless, these organisms are most often skin contaminants rather than true pathogens, producing infections only in patients with severe underlying medical problems.

A frequent manifestation of infection with *S. epidermidis* is bacteremia resulting from infection of intravenous catheters. Many of these patients have associated persistent low-grade fevers, with periodic marked elevations in body temperature. Signs of thrombophlebitis may or may not be present. Removing the contaminated intravenous catheters is the most important aspect of therapy.

The most difficult therapeutic problems caused by *S. epidermidis* are infections of prosthetic heart valves. This infection typically has a subacute course, but eradication of organisms is difficult, due to their resistance to many of the available antibiotics.

INFECTIONS DUE TO GRAM-NEGATIVE BACTERIA

Clinically important diseases caused by infections with gram-negative bacteria include salmonellosis, shigellosis, *Escherichia coli*-induced diarrhea, and cholera. Manifestations of these diseases are predominantly on the gastrointestinal tract.

Salmonellosis

Gastroenteritis accounts for about two-thirds of all infections with salmonella. Ingestion of these organisms is followed in 8 hours to 48 hours by abdominal cramps, vomiting, and diarrhea. Abdominal pain is typically periumbilical, or localized to the right lower quadrant. As such, this pain can mimic acute appendicitis, cholecystitis, or a ruptured viscus. Antibiotics are not effective.

Enteric fever (typhoid fever) is characterized by sustained gram-negative bacteremia and persistent elevations of body temperature. There may be associated dysfunction of multiple organ systems. Chloramphenicol is the treatment of choice.

Shigellosis

Shigellosis is an acute inflammatory disease of the gastrointestinal tract that ranges in severity from mild nonspecific diarrhea to classic dysentery. Initial manifestations of infection with these gram-negative organisms include fever, abdominal cramps, and watery diarrhea. Treatment is with antibiotics from the tetracycline class.

Cholera

Cholera is an acute diarrheal disease produced by enterotoxin secreted by *Vibrio cholerae* organisms. Humans are the only known hosts, so transmission can occur only via infected human excreta. These organisms are exquisitely sensitive to gastric acid; thus, individuals who are achlorhydric or taking antacids are most susceptible to cholera.

Diarrhea is massive and watery. Fluid loss may be equivalent to 1 L·hr^{-1} of isotonic fluid at the peak of the disease. Hypotension and metabolic acidosis reflect the large fluid and electrolyte losses. Fever is characteristically absent. Treatment is with fluid and electrolyte replacement and eradication of gram-negative organisms with a tetracycline antibiotic.

E.coli-induced Diarrhea

E. coli are important constituents of normal flora of the gastrointestinal tract. Some strains of *E. coli*, however, are not part of the normal flora and produce diarrhea (traveler's disease) when introduced into the gastrointestinal tract via contaminated food or water. Clinical manifestations include abrupt onset of abdominal cramps and watery diarrhea. Absence of a temperature elevation is in keeping with failure of these organisms to invade other tissues or to produce inflammation. This form of diarrhea cannot be distinguished clinically from shigellosis. The most important aspect of treatment is fluid and electrolyte replacement. A single daily dose of the tetracycline antibiotic doxycycline may be effective in preventing this disease.[3]

INFECTIONS DUE TO SPORE-FORMING ANAEROBES

Spore-forming gram-positive anaerobes that cause invasive infections are normally found in the lower gastrointestinal tracts of humans and animals and in soil contaminated with their excrement. These organisms are strict anaerobes and are protected from lethal effects of oxygen by formation of spores. Introduction of spores into wounds (puncture wounds, burns, uterine instrumentation, subcutaneous infections in drug addicts) sets the stage for the conversion of spores to exotoxin-producing vegetative forms. The species most often responsible for disease in humans are *Clostridium perfringens*, *C. tetani*, and *C. botulinum*. Exotoxins elaborated by vegetative forms of these organisms are the causes of clostridial myonecrosis, tetanus, and botulism, respectively.

Clostridial Myonecrosis

Clostridial myonecrosis (gas gangrene) is due to infection with *C. perfringens*. The incubation period after inoculation with clostridial spores is 8 hours to 72 hours, after which there is a sudden onset of localized skeletal muscle pain and swelling. Necrosis of skeletal muscles and alterations in integrity of the capillary membranes are caused by elaboration of an exotoxin (lecithinase) by these organisms. A brownish discharge with a foul odor is characteristic. In addition to the exotoxin, these organisms liberate hydrogen and carbon dioxide, which is responsible for crepitus over involved skeletal muscles, while associated swelling can cause compression of surrounding blood vessels.

SYSTEMIC EFFECTS

Systemic effects of infections with *C. perfringens* are prominent. Tachycardia and fever are followed by hypotension and oliguria. Presumably, these responses reflect reductions in intravascular fluid volume due to massive tissue edema. Anemia, jaundice, and hemoglobinuria are due to intravascular hemolysis in association with clostridial bacteremia. Renal failure may be a consequence of hemoglobinuria.

TREATMENT

Treatment of clostridial myonecrosis is immediate surgical debridement of infected tissues. Penicillin or an equivalent antibiotic is administered to eradicate organisms not removed by debridement, and to control bacteremia.

MANAGEMENT OF ANESTHESIA

Management of anesthesia for surgical debridement must take into account the multiple physiologic derangements produced by infections with this organism.[4] Preoperatively, important considerations include status of the intravascular fluid volume, oxygen-carrying capacity of the blood, and renal function. Ketamine is a useful drug for induction and maintenance of anesthesia. A theoretical hazard to the use of nitrous oxide would be expansion of gas pockets produced by clostridial infection. This seems unlikely, however, since these gas pockets are relatively avascular. Likewise, the release of potassium from necrotic skeletal muscles after administration of succinylcholine seems unlikely, since involved skeletal muscles are avascular and thus effectively isolated from the circulation. In vitro oxygen exposures to less than 2.5 atmospheres pressure do not inhibit release of the clostridial exotoxin. Therefore, delivery of oxygen concentrations during surgery, which are greater than those needed to maintain adequate arterial oxygenation, is of no advantage. Renal function needs to be considered if long-acting nondepolarizing muscle relaxants are administered during surgical debridement. Use of electrocautery must be questioned, in view of the production of hydrogen gas by clostridial organisms. Regional anesthesia is not recommended because clostridial organisms may be introduced into other sites by the needle used to perform the block. Furthermore, blockade of the peripheral sympathetic nervous system would be undesirable in the presence of an unstable cardiovascular system.

Postoperatively, these patients are not likely to be sources of cross-infection to other patients, since *C. perfringens* organisms are neutralized when exposed to air. Therefore, strict isolation of these patients is not mandatory.

Tetanus

Tetanus is caused by the gram-positive anaerobic bacillus *C. tetani*. Elaboration of the neurotoxin tetanospasmin by vegetative forms of these organisms is responsible for clinical manifestations of tetanus. With the exception of botulinum toxin, tetanospasmin is the most powerful poison to humans.

Tetanospasmin, when elaborated into wounds, spreads centrally along motor nerves to the spinal cord or enters the systemic circulation to reach the central nervous system. This toxin affects the nervous system in several areas. At the neuromuscular junction, there is inhibition of the release of acetylcholine. In the spinal cord, toxin suppresses inhibitory internuncial neurons. As a result, generalized

spasm of skeletal muscles occurs. In the brain, there is fixation of toxin by gangliosides. The fourth cerebral ventricle is believed to have a selective permeability for tetanospasmin, resulting in early manifestations of trismus and neck rigidity.[5] Sympathetic nervous system hyperactivity may manifest as the disease progresses.[6]

SIGNS AND SYMPTOMS

Trismus is the presenting symptom of tetanus in 75 percent of patients. The greater strength of the masseter muscles, compared with the opposing digastric and mylohyoid muscles, results in "lockjaw." Indeed, these patients are often first seen by a dentist. Rigidity of facial muscles results in the characteristic appearance described as the sardonic smile (risus sardonicus). Spasm of laryngeal muscles can occur at any time. Dysphagia may be due to spasm of the pharyngeal muscles. Spasm of intercostal muscles and the diaphragm interferes with adequate ventilation. Rigidity of abdominal and lumbar muscles accounts for the opisthotonic posture. Skeletal muscle spasms are tonic and clonic in nature, and are excruciatingly painful. Furthermore, the increased skeletal muscle work is associated with dramatic increases in oxygen consumption, and peripheral vasoconstriction can contribute to elevations in body temperature. External stimulation, including sudden exposures to bright light, unexpected sounds, or tracheal suction, can precipitate generalized skeletal muscle spasm, which leads to ineffective ventilation and death. Hypotension has been attributed to myocarditis. Isolated and unexplained tachycardia may be an early manifestation of hyperactivity of the sympathetic nervous system. More often, this hyperactivity is manifest as a transient hypertension. Sympathetic nervous system responses to external stimuli are exaggerated, as demonstrated by cardiac tachydysrhythmias and labile blood pressure changes. In addition, excessive sympathetic nervous system activity is associated with intense peripheral vasoconstriction, diaphoresis, and increased urinary excretion of catecholamines. Inappropriate secretion of antidiuretic hormone manifesting as hyponatremia and decreases in plasma osmolarity may occur.[7]

TREATMENT

Treatment of patients with tetanus is directed at (1) control of skeletal muscle spasms, (2) prevention of sympathetic nervous system hyperactivity, (3) support of ventilation of the lungs, (4) neutralization of circulating exotoxin, and (5) surgical debridement to eliminate the source of exotoxin. Intravenous administration of diazepam (40 mg·day^{-1} to 200 mg·day^{-1}) is useful to control skeletal muscle spasms. If spasms are not controlled by diazepam, administration of nondepolarizing muscle relaxants and control of ventilation of the lungs via a tube placed in the trachea is necessary. Indeed, early and aggressive protection of the airway is mandatory, as laryngospasm may accompany generalized skeletal muscle spasm. Overactivity of the sympathetic nervous system is best managed with intravenous administration of beta-adrenergic antagonists such as propranolol. Continuous epidural block has also been used to control tetanus-induced sympathetic nervous system activity.[8] Neutralization of circulating exotoxin is provided with use of intramuscular human hyperimmune globulin. This neutralization does not alter the already present symptoms but does prevent additional exotoxin from reaching the central nervous system. Penicillin is effective in destroying exotoxin-producing vegetative forms of *C. tetani*. Surgical debridement should be delayed until several hours after patients receive antitoxin because free tetanospasmin is mobilized into the circulation during surgical manipulation. General anesthesia with intubation of the trachea is a useful approach for surgical debridement. Monitoring should include continuous recording of arterial blood pressure from a catheter in a peripheral artery, and measurement of central venous and/or pulmonary artery occlusion pressures. Volatile anesthetics are useful for the maintenance of anesthesia if excessive sympathetic nervous system activity is present. In view of potential cardiac irritability, it might be prudent to select enflurane or isoflurane rather than halothane. Drugs such as lidocaine, propranolol, and nitroprusside should be readily available for treatment of excess sympathetic nervous system activity in the perioperative period.

Botulism

Botulism is due to effects of a neurotoxin elaborated by *C. botulinum*. This neurotoxin interferes with presynaptic release of acetylcholine from preganglionic nerve endings and at the neuromuscular junction. Diagnosis of botulism must be considered in patients who present with acute and symmetrical skeletal muscle weakness or paralysis leading to ventilatory failure. The incubation period is 18 hours to 36 hours after oral ingestion of food contaminated with these organisms.

INFECTIONS DUE TO TREPONEMA PALLIDUM

Syphilis is a sexually transmitted infection caused by *Treponema pallidum*. Humans are the only known hosts. Disease of more than 4 years duration is rarely transmissible. An untreated pregnant woman, however, can pass syphilis to her fetus regardless of the stage of her disease.

Signs and Symptoms

Clinical manifestations of syphilis depend on the chronologic stage of the disease. The first clinical sign is the chancre, which develops at the inoculation site after 3 weeks to 4 weeks of incubation. Secondary syphilis, characterized by widespread mucocutaneous lesions, lymphadenopathy, and splenomegaly, develops about 6 weeks after the chancre has healed. During the latent stage, there are no clinical or cerebrospinal fluid abnormalities, but serologic tests are positive. The tertiary stage of syphilis is characterized by destructive lesions in the central nervous system, peripheral nervous system, and cardiovascular system.

NERVOUS SYSTEM

Tables dorsalis (locomotor ataxia) develops 15 years to 20 years after the initial infection with syphilis. Posterior root dysfunction and posterior column degeneration result in ataxia with a broad-based gait, hypotonic bladder, and jabbing pains that typically occur in the legs. Sudden attacks of abdominal pain may mimic a surgical abdomen.

CARDIOVASCULAR SYSTEM

Cardiovascular syphilis is most often manifested as aortitis, with dilation of the aortic ring and subsequent aortic regurgitation. Aneurysms due to syphilis almost always involve the ascending thoracic aorta, and only rarely the abdominal aorta. Diagnosis of aortitis due to syphilis should be considered in adults with isolated aortic regurgitation and positive serologic tests. Linear calcification in the wall of the ascending aorta that is visible on chest radiographs plus positive serologic tests suggest an aneurysm due to syphilis.

LYME DISEASE

Lyme disease is an immune-mediated multisystem disorder caused by spirochetes, which are transmitted primarily by tick bites.[9] Like other spirochetal infections, Lyme disease usually occurs in clinically distinct stages with manifestations that undergo remissions and exacerbations. Erythema chronicum migrans is the initial unique clinical marker for Lyme disease. This classic cutaneous manifestation begins as an area of redness, which expands to a diameter ranging from 3 cm to 68 cm. Malaise and fatigue, headache, fever, and chills often accompany skin involvement. Some patients

have evidence of meningeal irritation, encephalopathy, lymphadenopathy, and hepatitis. Cranial neuritis including bilateral facial palsy may occur. Neurologic abnormalities typically last for months but usually resolve completely. Within several weeks after the onset of illness, about 8 percent of patients develop cardiac involvement, most often manifesting as fluctuating degrees of atrioventricular heart block lasting 7 days to 10 days. Rarely, mild left ventricular dysfunction may manifest. Duration of cardiac involvement is usually brief (3 days to 6 weeks), but it may recur. From a few weeks to as long as 2 years after the onset of illness, about 60 percent of patients develop arthritis. Typically this arthritis consists of migratory musculoskeletal pain, which may recur for years. In about 10 percent of patients with arthritis, involvement of large joints becomes chronic with erosion of cartilage and bone.

Laboratory abnormalities early in the course of Lyme disease include a high erythrocyte sedimentation rate, elevated plasma concentrations of liver transaminase enzymes, and immunoglobulin M proteins. These levels generally return to normal within several weeks. Mild anemia may be present. Renal function tests are not altered. Treatment is initially with tetracyclines followed by penicillin and erythromycin. Despite antibiotic therapy nearly one-half of patients continue to experience minor complications such as headache, fatigue, or musculoskeletal pain.

INFECTIONS DUE TO MYCOBACTERIA

Mycobacterium tuberculosis is an obligate aerobe responsible for tuberculosis. These organisms grow most successfully in tissues with high oxygen concentrations, explaining the increased incidence of tuberculosis in the apices of the lungs. Although clinical tuberculosis is uncommon, an estimated 7 percent of the population has a positive tuberculin skin test, indicating previous infections. These individuals harbor viable tubercle bacilli unless they have received antituberculous chemotherapy.

Transmission

Almost all cases of tuberculosis are acquired via aerosol transmission. Since most infectious patients discharge few organisms, there is a low risk of infection in casual contacts. Infectivity is greatest from patients who have pulmonary cavitary disease or tuberculosis of the larynx. After infected particles have settled on surfaces exposed to ambient conditions, they become essentially noninfectious.

More than 90 percent of patients remain asymptomatic during the initial infection and can be identified only by conversion of the tuberculin skin test. Among symptomatic patients, the most frequent manifestations are fever and nonproductive cough. These symptoms resemble pneumonia caused by infection with *Mycoplasma pneumoniae* (see the section Infections Due to Mycoplasma).

Treatment

Patients who manifest positive skin tests should receive antituberculous chemotherapy with isoniazid. The major toxicities of isoniazid are on the peripheral nervous system, liver, and possibly the kidneys. Neurotoxicity can be prevented by daily administration of pyridoxine. Hepatotoxicity is most likely to be related to metabolism of isoniazid by hepatic acetylation. Depending on a genetically determined trait, patients may be characterized as slow or rapid acetylators. Hepatitis seems more common in rapid acetylators, which is consistent with greater production of hydrazine, a potentially hepatotoxic metabolite of isoniazid. Persistent elevations of plasma transaminase concentrations mandate that isoniazid be discontinued; mild and transient elevations do not require discontinuation. In addition to toxic effects on the liver, metabolites of isoniazid, which contain a hydrazine moiety, may also increase defluorination of volatile anesthetics. Indeed, elevated plasma fluoride levels have been observed after enflurane anesthesia

administered to patients who were also being treated with isoniazid.[10]

Other drugs used in the treatment of tuberculosis include streptomycin and rifampin. Adverse effects of rifampin include thrombocytopenia, leukopenia, hemolytic anemia, and renal failure. Hepatitis associated with elevation of plasma transaminase concentrations occurs in about 10 percent of patients receiving rifampin.

SYSTEMIC MYCOTIC INFECTIONS

The three most common systemic mycotic infections are blastomycosis, coccidioidomycosis, and histoplasmosis. All three diseases are caused by a specific fungus, which gains entry into the host via inhalation into the lungs. Clinical manifestations resemble tuberculosis and include pulmonary cavitary lesions. Intravenous amphotericin B is the drug of choice for eradication of invading organisms that cause these three fungal diseases. Amphotericin B can produce adverse renal and hematologic reactions. For example, decreases in glomerular filtration rate are unavoidable during therapy with this drug. It may be necessary to discontinue amphotericin temporarily so as to maintain plasma creatinine concentrations below 3 mg·dl^{-1}. Renal tubular acidosis, hypokalemia, and hypomagnesemia occur frequently, and exogenous electrolyte replacement is usually necessary. Ventricular fibrillation and asystole after infusion of amphotericin have been observed.[11] Adverse hematologic effects are typically manifested as anemia. Fever, chills, and hypotension frequently occur in the first few hours after intravenous administration of amphotericin B. Hepatotoxicity is not produced by this drug.

Sporotrichosis differs from other systemic fungal infections because of its wide geographic distribution. Furthermore, the portal of entry and major site of infection is the skin. Pulmonary cavitary disease is rarely present. Treatment is with oral iodides.

Blastomycosis

Blastomycosis is caused by the fungus *Blastomyces dermatitidis*, which is endemic in the southeastern and south central portions of the United States. Pulmonary involvement manifests as cavitary disease of the upper lobes. Fever, productive cough, hemoptysis, and simultaneous involvement of other organ systems, particularly the skin and skeleton, are present in many patients. Surgery may be necessary for treatment of persistent pulmonary cavities or to correct deforming orthopedic lesions.

Coccidioidomycosis

Coccidioidomycosis is caused by the fungus *Coccidioides immitis*, which is endemic in the southwestern United States. Positive skin tests may be the only evidence of systemic infection with this fungus. Pulmonary cavitary disease is often discovered on routine chest radiographs. The most serious extrapulmonary manifestation of coccidioidomycosis is meningitis. Meningitis due to this organism is an indication for intrathecal administration of amphotericin B. Surgical intervention may be necessary to treat hydrocephalus that has occurred as a result of meningitis. Finally, arthralgia develops in 10 percent to 20 percent of patients with coccidioidomycosis.

Histoplasmosis

Histoplasmosis is infection of phagocytic cells of the reticuloendothelial system, caused by the fungus *Histoplasma capsulatum*. This fungus is endemic in the eastern and central portions of the United States and grows particularly well in soil contaminated with fecal material from birds. The majority of individuals infected with this fungus are asymptomatic or develop symptoms indistinguishable from the common cold. Presence of positive skin tests confirms infection with these organisms.

Chronic cavitary histoplasmosis is predominantly a disease of middle-aged and elderly men who also have chronic obstructive airways disease. Surgical ablation of the pulmonary cavity, combined with intravenous administration of amphotericin B, may be necessary in the presence of cavitary lung disease. Disseminated histoplasmosis is most likely to occur in elderly or immunosuppressed patients.

INFECTIONS DUE TO MYCOPLASMA

Mycoplasma pneumoniae, formerly designated pleuropneumonia-like organisms, are the smallest known living organisms. Infection with these organisms produces *Mycoplasma pneumoniae* pneumonia, also known as primary atypical pneumonia. In urban populations, about 20 percent of all pneumonias are due to these organisms.[12]

Mycoplasma pneumoniae pneumonia is characterized by subacute onset of a nonproductive cough and pharyngitis. Headache, chills, and fever up to 40 degrees Celsius are present in the majority of patients. Congested tympanic membranes are present in 10 percent to 20 percent of patients. The peripheral leukocyte count is normal in most patients, and helps rule out pneumonia due to bacteria. About 50 percent of patients show a fourfold or greater increase in the cold agglutinin titer (1:128 or higher). In contrast, low titers (less than 1:32) may occur with infectious mononucleosis, and with pneumonias caused by adenovirus or influenza viruses. Infection characteristically spreads slowly throughout a family. Erythromycin or tetracyclines are the antibiotics of choice for eradication of these organisms.

INFECTIONS DUE TO RICKETTSIAL ORGANISMS

Rocky mountain spotted fever and Q fever are diseases caused by rickettsial organisms.

Antibiotics of choice for eradication of these organisms are chloramphenicol or tetracyclines.

Rocky Mountain Spotted Fever

Rocky mountain spotted fever is an acute tick-borne illness caused by *Rickettsia rickettsii*. The disease is characterized by the sudden onset of fever, headache, and a rash that begins on the extremities and spreads to the trunk. Rash is the most valuable diagnostic sign. Abdominal pain may be prominent, suggesting the need for surgical exploration. Thrombocytopenia occurs in nearly one-half of patients with this infection. Involvement of the myocardium by rickettsial organisms can be manifested on the electrocardiogram as nonspecific ST segment and T-wave changes.

Q Fever

Q fever is an acute systemic infection caused by rickettsial organisms known as *Coxiella burnetii*. Infection with these organisms produces a clinical picture similar to *mycoplasma pneumoniae* pneumonia. Q fever differs from other diseases caused by rickettsial organisms in that a rash is absent. Furthermore, infection is airborne from infected feces and not via injection from tick bites. Hepatosplenomegaly, jaundice, abnormal liver function tests, and endocarditis may occur.

INFECTIONS DUE TO ADULT RESPIRATORY VIRUSES

Influenza viruses, rhinoviruses, corona viruses, and adenoviruses are responsible for infections of the respiratory tract. These infections can occur in all age groups but are most frequent in adult populations. Transmission of viruses is a common event in hospitals.[13]

Influenza Virus

Infection with influenza virus produces an acute febrile illness associated with myalgia, malaise, and headache. This syndrome is commonly referred to as influenza. The most important reservoir of viral particles are nasopharyngeal secretions of infected persons. Thus, anesthesia personnel can have frequent contact and contribute to spread of influenza among the surgical population. Influenza is usually self-limited, unless it is complicated by bacterial infections or the presence of coexisting chronic pulmonary disease. Indeed, pneumonia from secondary bacterial infections is the most common complication occurring after influenza. In this regard, it seems likely that influenza causes damage to mucosal surfaces of the tracheobronchial tree, which, together with impaired mucociliary transport, promotes colonization with bacteria such as *Pseudomonas aeruginosa*.[14] Severe myositis can be associated with myocarditis. Rarely, Guillain-Barré syndrome can follow infections with influenza A.

Risk of transmission of influenza to patients is reduced by vaccination of staff as reflected by less virus being shed in nasal secretions of vaccinated personnel.[15] Another form of protection is prophylactic use of amantadine, which results in an 80 percent reduction in the incidence of influenza A.[16] Amantadine is not effective against influenza B. This drug may accumulate when renal function is impaired.

Administration of general anesthesia to patients with respiratory tract infections is traditionally avoided. Nevertheless, experimental justification for this practice is not supported by animal data describing effects of anesthetics on viral pathogenesis. For example, mortality was reduced in animals inoculated with influenza virus during anesthesia with halothane or enflurane, perhaps reflecting anesthetic-induced inhibition of viral replication.[13]

Rhinovirus

Rhinovirus is responsible for one-third or more of adult common colds. Transmission is most likely by inoculation from contaminated environmental surfaces or from skin of infected individuals. Airborne transmission via cough or sneeze is unlikely. The classic syndrome includes acute coryza, slight fever, and malaise. Infection occurs most often in the winter, but the reason for this seasonal incidence is not known. Postexposure prophylaxis with intranasal interferon may prevent respiratory symptoms in those exposed to infected individuals.[17]

Avoidance of general anesthesia because of the presence of mild upper respiratory tract infections is a common practice. The conservative approach is to postpone operations until the illness and its symptoms have resolved. Conversely, there is no evidence that postoperative complications are increased in children with upper respiratory viral infections undergoing myringotomy and tympanoplasty with halothane anesthesia delivered by mask.[18] In this regard, it would seem that general anesthesia for minor operations need not be postponed if patients have an uncomplicated upper respiratory infection and if intubation of the trachea is not planned.[13] Exceptions might be patients requiring abdominal or hernia procedures who might jeopardize the postoperative integrity of the surgical incision should coughing become excessive.

Adenovirus

Adenovirus produces an acute febrile disease associated with pharyngitis and cough, which most commonly affects children or semiclosed populations, such as military recruits. Another illness caused by adenovirus is highly contagious pharyngoconjunctival fever characterized by pharyngitis, conjunctivitis, and fever, which usually affects children and young adults. Epidemic keratoconjunctivitis is easily transmitted by contaminated fingers.

When caring for patients known to have adenoviral disease, handwashing and use of gloves should reduce the risk of iatrogenic spread of these organisms.

Respiratory Syncytial Virus

Respiratory syncytial virus is the most frequent cause for infant pneumonia and bronchiolitis. Hospital personnel act as transmitters of infection to children by carrying contaminated secretions on their hands and clothes.

Parainfluenza Virus

Parainfluenza virus is the principal cause of laryngotracheobronchitis in children. Transmission occurs by person-to-person contact or large droplet spread.

Herpes Simplex Virus

Herpes simplex virus is a common infection with breaks in the oral mucosa (fever blister) mucous membranes or skin serving as the portal of entry. The virus remains in the individual throughout life in a dormant form residing in sensory ganglia that innervate the site of primary infection. Various stimuli will reactivate the virus, which will appear near the site of original infection or track along nerves to more distant sites.

The most common and significant infection caused by herpes simplex virus is keratitis, which may lead to destruction of the cornea. Herpetic infection of the digits (whitlow) is possible in personnel who experience sustained direct contact with oral, pharyngeal, or tracheal secretions of infected individuals. Despite pain that occurs with paronychial involvement, it is stressed that treatment should not include surgical drainage, as this may cause entrance of the virus into the deep pulp space and secondary bacterial infections. Infected personnel should refrain from dealing with chronically ill, debilitated, or immunosuppressed patients until the lesions resolve. Vidarabine and acyclovir are antiviral drugs effective in the treatment of infections due to herpes simplex virus. Oral acyclovir also shortens the duration of lesions in patients with genital herpes.[19]

Varicella-Zoster Virus

Varicella-zoster virus is highly contagious and causes varicella (chickenpox) and zoster (shingles). Herpes zoster follows endogenous reactivation of the virus, particularly in immunosuppressed patients. It is assumed that spinal sensory ganglia become infected during varicella or zoster and that herpes zoster represents a recurrence of infection within these ganglia during periods of low host resistance. Varicella in one patient does not lead to zoster in another, but the reverse may occur.

Cytomegalovirus

Infection with cytomegalovirus is usually asymptomatic, except in immunosuppressed patients and infants. For example, this virus may cause destruction of the immature central nervous system during the neonatal period. The most frequent manifestation of infection is a heterophil-negative mononucleosis syndrome, characterized by fever, adenopathy, splenomegaly, hepatitis, and atypical lymphocytes in the blood. Hepatitis is mild and only rarely progresses to chronic liver disease. Blood should be tested for antibodies to this virus before administration to seronegative infants or kidney transplant recipients. Posttransfusion mononucleosis due to cytomegalovirus is a complication of surgery requiring cardiopulmonary bypass.[20] There is no evidence of a risk of transmission of cytomegalovirus from infected patients to hospital personnel.[21]

Epstein-Barr Virus

Epstein-Barr virus infects most humans and about one-third develop heterophil-positive infectious mononucleosis. The most common symptoms are fever, pharyngitis, lymphadenopathy, and hepatosplenomegaly. Hyperplasia of tonsils and adenoids, or edema of the uvula or epiglottis, can compromise the patency of the upper airway.[22] Mild hepatitis can occur as evidenced by moderate elevations in plasma concentrations of transaminase enzymes and jaundice develops in 10 percent to 20 percent of patients. A relationship between chronic fatigue syndromes and infections with this virus has been considered but not documented. Transmission is via oral-to-oral contact and the incubation period is about 28 days. Fewer than 1 percent of patients with infectious mononucleosis develop encephalitis, meningitis, or Gullain-Barré syndrome. This virus persists for life in salivary glands and B lymphocytes and in the presence of deficient immunocompetence may present as life threatening B-cell proliferative disorders.

RUBELLA

Rubella is highly contagious being spread by airborne transmission. The teratogenic potential of rubella emphasizes the importance for susceptible hospital personnel to become vaccinated.

CREUTZFELDT-JAKOB DISEASE

Creutzfeldt-Jakob disease is a subacute degenerative disease of the central nervous system caused by a transmissible virus. The virus is resistant to physical and chemical inactivation and fails to produce any detectable immune reaction.[13] Inactivation of the virus is reliably achieved by steam and ethylene oxide sterilization as well as sodium hypochlorite (bleach).

Patients with this disease manifest progressive presenile dementia, with death almost always occurring within 6 months of onset. It would seem prudent to avoid contact with body fluids and clearly label specimens of patients undergoing brain biopsies for diagnosis of unknown central nervous system diseases. Instruments used for surgery in these patients should be carefully sterilized to avoid transmission of the virus with subsequent use. Despite these concerns, the disease is only remotely contagious and there seems no justification for hospital personnel to avoid participation in the care of these patients, including the administration of anesthesia.[13]

VIRAL HEPATITIS
(see Chapter 19)

VIRAL ENTERIC INFECTIONS

Viral enteric infections are probably second only to the common cold as causes of human illness. Viruses responsible for most symptomatic enteric diseases include rotaviruses, Norwalk agent, and hepatitis A and B viruses. Rotavirus is an important cause of diarrhea in infants. Norwalk virus typically produces vomiting and diarrhea in children and adults, particularly during the winter months.

Additional enteroviruses include echoviruses and coxsackieviruses. Spread of these viruses is primarily by the fecal-oral route, and only rarely by the airborne route. Serious disease is rare, but on occasion these viruses can cause aseptic meningitis, pneumonia, pericarditis, and myocarditis. Coxsackieviruses have been associated epidemiologically with diabetes mellitus.

ACQUIRED IMMUNODEFICIENCY SYNDROME

Acquired immunodeficiency syndrome (AIDS) is not a single disease but rather the appearance of various opportunistic infections and malignancies due to generalized depression of the immune system, as well as subacute encephalitis.[23] Immunodeficiency is caused by infection of helper T-lymphocytes with a retrovirus known as human immunodeficiency virus (HIV) (also known as human T-cell lymphotropic virus type III and the lymphadenopathy virus).[24] This virus selectively replicates in and destroys T-lymphocytes, leaving the host unable to cope with a variety of infections and neoplastic diseases. In addition to those with AIDS, there are estimated to be hundreds of thousands of asymptomatic carriers of HIV who may constitute an unrecognized threat of infection to others.

Transmission

Since HIV preferentially infects lymphocytes, concentrations of the virus are probably highest in secretions containing lymphocytes such as semen, vaginal secretions, and blood. Indeed, transmission of HIV is by sexual contact, especially between homosexuals, inoculation by other body secretions, and transfusion of blood or blood products, especially factor VIII concentrates.[24,25] As a result of these modes of transmission, those individuals most likely to contract AIDS are homosexuals with multiple partners, drug addicts who share needles, and hemophiliacs, especially those treated with factor VIII concentrates. Among adult patients with AIDS over 90 percent are men, and 70 percent of these individuals are homosexual or bisexual males.[26] Heterosexual intravenous drug users comprise 15 percent of males with AIDS and 51 percent of affected females. Persons with hemophilia/coagulation disorders represent 1 percent of all cases of AIDS, and recipients of transfused blood account for 2 percent of all cases. Disruption of mucous membranes very likely facilitates systemic entry of HIV as emphasized by the fragility of the columnar epithelium lining the rectum and the association of AIDS with rectal intercourse. AIDS may also be transmitted by heterosexual contact and passed from mother to fetus. Nevertheless, HIV seems less likely to be transmitted during a single heterosexual contact than other sexually transmitted diseases such as gonorrhea and syphilis. Furthermore, hepatitis B virus is much more infectious than is HIV. There is no evidence of airborne transmission of AIDS and spread to health care workers even after accidental exposure to infected blood is highly unlikely.[27] Many body fluids including saliva, tears, urine, and cerebrospinal fluid contain lymphocytes; but transmission by these routes has not been documented.

The only certain barrier to further spread of AIDS is development of a vaccine.[23] Because many strains of HIV may exist, a vaccine must be developed that has an antigen common to all strains. Risk of transmission by transfusion of blood is reduced by voluntary deferral of those in high risk groups from donating blood. More important, since March 1985, all blood and blood products have undergone serologic testing for antibodies to HIV.[28] The enzyme immunoassay for antibodies to HIV is highly specific and has virtually eliminated the use of blood or blood products from infected donors.[29] Nevertheless, there may be a period of low sensitivity with the enzyme assay during seroconversion.[30] Heat treatment of factor VIII concentrates will reduce transmission of HIV by this route. Modification of sexual practices and avoidance of nonmedical use of injected drugs have obvious implications in control of the spread of AIDS. Use of condoms may provide protection against sexual transmission of HIV.[24]

HIV may survive for prolonged periods outside the host. Nevertheless, HIV is quite sensitive to mycobactericidal disinfectants or sodium hypochlorite, as well as low levels of heat (10 minutes at 56 degrees Celsius). Common hospital sterilization techniques using ethylene oxide, steam, and boiling water kill HIV.

Manifestations

The immune system becomes devastated after selective infection of T-lymphocytes, resulting in opportunistic infections due to protozal, helminthic, fungal, bacterial, and viral organisms. Pneumonia due to the parasite *Pneumocystis carinii* is the most frequently encountered opportunistic life-threatening infection. The most common malignant condition encountered in patients with AIDS is Kaposi's sarcoma. Other opportunistic infections include candida esophagitis, cytomegalovirus infections, cryptococcosis, and chronic herpes simplex. There is lymphopenia and reduction in the ratio of helper T-lymphocytes to suppressor T-lymphocytes. A reduction in antibody response to polysaccharide and protein antigens indicates these patients have an acquired B-lymphocyte, as well as T-lymphocyte immunodeficiency. Central nervous system dysfunction ranging from apathy and psychomotor retardation to full-blown subacute encephalitis and dementia occurs in over 50 percent of patients.[23] Weight loss, chronic diarrhea, fatigue, idiopathic thrombocytopenia, and anemia are nonspecific findings. In addition to development of overt AIDS, there is a wide range of milder manifestations including a (1) transient mononucleosis-like syndromes with fever, fatigue, and weight loss; and (2) persistent generalized lymphadenopathy. There is no precise estimate as to what percentage of patients with mild manifestations of AIDS will progress to the overt disease.

Detection of antibodies to HIV using an enzyme-linked immunoassay (EIA) indicates the patient has been infected with the virus and may still harbor the virus. To increase reliability, a positive EIA test is confirmed by a Western blot test. Sensitivity of these tests exceeds 99 percent. Persons infected with HIV usually develop antibody (seroconvert) against the virus within 6 weeks to 12 weeks after infection. A positive antibody test does not mean the individual has AIDS or will develop the syndrome. It is estimated that less than 20 percent of individuals infected with the virus will develop overt AIDS. The primary purpose of the antibody test is to screen blood and plasma that are donated for transfusion or production of blood products.

The incubation period for AIDS may be 7 years or longer.[28] Transfusion-transmitted AIDS has an average incubation period of 27 months.[31] Mortality approaches 70 percent within 2 years after diagnosis. Death is a result of overwhelming sepsis or uncontrolled tumor growth with wasting debility.

Drug Treatment

Oral administration of zidovudine (azidothymidine, AZT) inhibits replication of some retroviruses, including HIV, and therefore may be useful in reducing the risk of developing opportunistic infections associated with AIDS. This drug is primarily eliminated by renal excretion following glucuronidation in the liver. Drugs such as probenecid, acetaminophen, aspirin, and indomethacin may competitively inhibit glucuronidation of zidovudine. Anemia and granulocytopenia may accompany treatment with zidovudine, especially if therapy is prolonged or if predrug levels of erythrocytes and leukocytes were reduced. Blood cell counts are recommended at biweekly intervals in patients being treated with zidovudine. Concomitant administration of drugs which are nephrotoxic or that interfere with erythrocyte or leukocyte production may increase the risk of zidovudine-induced toxicity.

Management of Anesthesia

Management of anesthesia must assume that all patients are potentially infected with HIV or other blood born pathogens.[27,32] In this regard, appropriate barrier precautions should include gloves, masks, and protective eyewear to prevent contact with blood and body fluids during invasive procedures, including placement of intravascular catheters and intubation of the trachea. Barrier precautions are particularly important in emergency care settings in which the risk of blood exposure is increased and the infection status of the patient is unknown. Although saliva has not been implicated in HIV transmission it is appropriate to minimize the need for emergency mouth-to-mouth resuscitation by providing equipment (mouthpieces, resuscitation bags) in areas

where the need for resuscitation is predictable. Attempts to cap needles after use are not recommended as accidental needle sticks are a potential risk of this procedure. Health care workers with breaks in normal skin integrity (cuts, dermatitis, acne) should be particularly careful to cover these sites when dealing with AIDS patients. Hands and other contaminated surfaces should be immediately washed if accidental contamination with blood or secretions from these patients occurs. There is no evidence that gowns, hoods, or strict patient isolation are of value; and patients with AIDS may be transported to the operating rooms by the usual routes and personnel. Patients wear masks only if it is felt transmission of opportunistic infections will be reduced by this approach.

Lack of evidence for spread of HIV by the respiratory tract does not eliminate concern regarding anesthesia equipment since airway secretions can be mixed with blood, which is a medium for transmission. Disposable anesthetic circuits, soda lime canisters, and ventilator bellows seem prudent although routine sterilization should kill HIV. Laryngoscopes and other nondisposable items that have touched mucosal membranes or contacted blood or secretions from infected patients should remain separated from clean equipment, be thoroughly washed with a detergent and water, and either gas or steam sterilized or subjected to appropriate disinfection.[32] Surgeons use disposable drapes and gowns that are discarded in the usual manner for contaminated material. Surgical specimens are labeled to indicate the patient has AIDS. Instruments are sterilized in the usual manner and the room is cleaned with a dilute (1:10) solution of sodium hypochlorite, which destroys HIV. Care should be taken to avoid spillage of undiluted sodium hypochlorite, which generates fumes when it contacts proteins as present in dried blood.

Choice of anesthetic drugs, techniques, and monitors is influenced by accompanying systemic manifestations of AIDS and associated opportunistic infections. For example, oxygenation may be impaired by pneumonia due to *Pneumocystis carinii*. Nutrition may be inadequate and blood volume deficient. Anemia from chronic infection is predictable. Care should be taken in placing vascular catheters and tracheal tubes so as to avoid introduction of bacteria. Postoperatively, these patients are managed in the recovery room using criteria reserved for management of patients with communicable diseases. Nurses assigned to care of patients with AIDS should not take care of other patients at the same time.

Cardiopulmonary resuscitation raises obvious concerns that can best be circumvented by avoidance of mouth-to-mouth ventilation. Early use of protective airway devices and intubation of the trachea is indicated. As in the operating room and recovery room masks, gloves, and glasses are recommended for health care workers.

Should a health care worker experience a needle stick from a patient with AIDS it is recommended that serologic testing be conducted.[32] If the worker is initially seronegative, tests should be repeated every 6 weeks to determine if transmission has occurred. Most infected persons will seroconvert in 6 weeks to 12 weeks. At the same time as serologic testing, counseling about the risk of infection and prevention of transmission of HIV to others is undertaken. In addition, the health care worker should be reassured that transmission by a single needle stick is unlikely.[27]

NOSOCOMIAL INFECTION

Nosocomial infections are those that occur in the course of a hospital stay. Common sites and causes include the urinary tract (*E. coli*), respiratory tract (*Klebsiella pneumoniae, Pseudomonas aeruginosa*), and surgical incision sites. Nosocomial pneumonias are an important cause of morbidity and mortality in hospitalized patients, accounting for about 15 percent of all hospital-acquired infections. Nosocomial infections are often resistant to treatment with antibiotics. Transmission of viruses is a common event in hospitals and most of these infections involve the respiratory tract. Thorough handwashing between patients is an effective way to reduce the role of hospital personnel in transmitting bacterial and viral infections. Use of gloves, likewise, protects both patients and hospital personnel.

Anesthesia Equipment

The role of bacterial contamination of anesthesia machines and equipment, and subsequent development of pulmonary infections and of cross-infection between patients, is controversial.[33] It is assumed that equipment used to deliver anesthesia is a potential source of bacterial contamination to patients. Based on this assumption, use of disposable anesthetic delivery circuits containing built-in bacterial filters has been advocated. Nevertheless, their routine use has not been shown to alter the incidence of postoperative pneumonia or other types of infections, as compared to similar surgical patients receiving anesthesia via circuits without bacterial filters. Furthermore, anesthesia administered to patients with known colonization of gram-negative bacteria does not result in contamination of the anesthesia machine with significant levels of bacteria.[34] These observations suggest that basic hygienic management of equipment used to deliver anesthetic gases will provide safety from the standpoint of cross-infections between patients, and prevent development of nosocomial infections from this source. Finally, it has been shown that bacteria placed in vaporizers containing volatile anesthetics do not survive.[35] The role of anesthesia equipment in transmitting viral illness has not been determined, but airborne transmission of intracellular viruses seems less likely than extracellular bacteria.[13] High humidity in the anesthesia circuit will speed inactivation of viruses. Furthermore, anesthetic concentrations of halogenated volatile anesthetics may inhibit viral replication.[36]

Gram-Negative Bacteremia

About one-half of all primary nosocomial bacteremias are associated with gram-negative bacteria. The most frequent presentation of gram-negative bacteremia is fever, chills, and leukocytosis, without hypotension. Chills and fever may not be significant in elderly, debilitated, or immunosuppressed patients.

SEPTIC SHOCK

Septic shock occurs most commonly after trauma or operative procedures on the genitourinary tract. Aggressive oncologic chemotherapy, immunosuppressive therapy for organ transplantation, and use of surgical prostheses have contributed to an increase in the incidence of blood stream invasion by bacteria. About 70 percent of cases are due to gram-negative bacteremia. Septic shock can be divided into early (hyperdynamic) and late (hypovolemic) phases (Fig. 29-1).[37,38]

Early Phase

The early phase of septic shock is characterized by hypotension associated with reductions in systemic vascular resistance and an increased cardiac output. Fever and hyperventilation are frequently present. Vasodilation is presumed to be due to an endotoxin derived from cell walls of bacteria. This endotoxin acts as an antigenic stimulus, causing release of such vasoactive substances as histamine and bradykinin. This phase can last up to 24 hours.

Late Phase

In the late phase of septic shock, cardiac output is reduced. Lactic acidosis develops, reflecting impaired tissue oxygenation, presumably due to decreased cardiac output as well as dilation of peripheral vessels that permits shunting of blood across tissues. There may be damage to vascular smooth muscle, causing substantial loss of intravascular fluid volume. Oliguria is characteristically present. Hematologic abnormalities invariably accompany severe septic shock. For example, there is typically a reduction in the platelet count and prolongation of prothrombin time and partial thromboplastin time. Elevations in the concentrations of fibrin degradation products mirror the presence of disseminated intravascular coagulation.

Diagnosis

Diagnosis of septic shock is suggested by development of hypotension in the presence of peripheral vasodilation. This diagnosis should be particularly suspected if these symptoms occur following operations or instrumentation of the genitourinary tract. Changes in the state of consciousness, including confusion and disorientation, can occur as manifestations of gram-negative bacteremia. Measurements of cardiac output and calculation of systemic vascular resistance are helpful in confirming the diagnosis in the early phase. Positive blood cultures are diagnostic but are not always present.

Treatment

Treatment of septic shock is with intravenous administration of antibiotics and repletion of intravascular fluid volume. Antibiotics should be started immediately after blood is drawn for culture and sensitivity. Most often two antibiotics are selected, with one effective against gram-positive and another against gram-negative bacteria. Clindamycin (25 mg·kg^{-1}) is often chosen for protection against gram-positive organisms, and gentamicin (5 mg·kg^{-1}) is a frequent choice for eradication of gram-negative bacteria. Antibiotics can be changed if necessary after the results of the blood culture are known. Aggressive intravenous fluid replacement is necessary to restore intravascular fluid volume. Fluid replacement is ideally guided by measurement of right or left heart filling pressures and urine output. Dopamine is an effective inotropic drug when pharmacologic support of both blood pressure and renal function is necessary.

A role for endorphins in the manifestations of septic shock is suggested by reversal

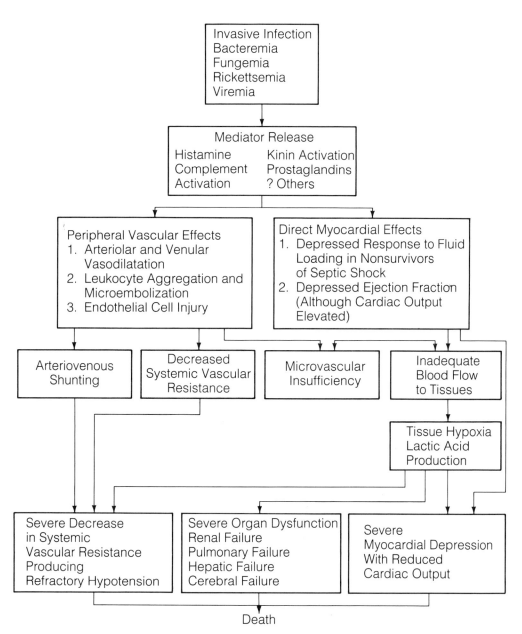

FIG. 29-1. Flow diagram of pathogenesis of septic shock in humans. (Parker MM, Parrillo JE. Septic shock. Hemodynamics and pathogenesis. JAMA 1983;250:3324–7. Copyright 1983, American Medical Association)

of endotoxin-induced hypotension and decreased mortality in animals treated with naloxone. Likewise, intravenous administration of naloxone, 0.4 mg to 1.2 mg, to patients with sepsis often resulted in elevations of blood pressure, which were accompanied by improved mentation, increased cardiac output, and decreased systemic vascular resistance.[39] The mechanism may be related to simultaneous release of adrenocorticotrophic hormone and beta-endorphins from a common molecule (beta-lipotropin) present in the pituitary gland. It is thought that beta-endorphins are producing vasodilation and that this response is antagonized by naloxone. Presumably, large doses of corticosteroids would inhibit the release of beta-endorphins as well as adrenocorticotrophic hormone. If this is correct, it is likely that large doses of corticosteroids would be helpful if adverse circulatory changes during septic shock were due to the release of endorphins. Nevertheless, administration of high doses of methylprednisolone or other corticosteroids for treatment of septic shock have not been shown to be beneficial and thus cannot be recommended as adjunctive therapy.[40]

Surgical intervention may be necessary to treat the source of bacteremia. No specific anesthetic drug has been shown to be ideal in the presence of septic shock. However, administration of ketamine to animals with hemorrhagic shock was associated with less damage to splanchnic organs and increased survival as compared with animals anesthetized with volatile anesthetics.[41] Conversely, another animal study implies that ketamine-induced peripheral vasoconstriction jeopardizes tissue blood flow as reflected by the development of metabolic acidosis.[42] Despite these conflicting studies, clinical experience suggests that ketamine is an acceptable drug for induction of anesthesia in patients requiring emergency operative procedures in the presence of hypovolemia due to bacteremia.

INFECTIVE ENDOCARDITIS

Infective endocarditis is a microbial infection that implants on a heart valve or on the wall of the endocardium. Streptococcal organisms account for nearly one-half the cases. Gram-negative bacteria and fungi are rare causes. Morbidity and mortality remain significant despite improvements in antibiotic therapy.

Predisposing Factors

Infective endocarditis cannot occur without preceding bacteremia. Operative procedures predictably associated with transient bacteremia include dental treatments resulting in bleeding of the gingiva and surgical procedures or instrumentation of the upper airway, gallbladder, lower gastrointestinal tract, and genitourinary tract. Parenteral injection of drugs, as in the drug addict, or prolonged placement of indwelling venous catheters, as used for hyperalimentation, can also lead to bacteremia. Patients with prosthetic heart valves are at the greatest risk for developing infective endocarditis when transient bacteremia occurs. The incidence of infective endocarditis is also increased in patients with acquired or congenital heart defects that produce turbulent blood flow. For example, mitral regurgitation, aortic regurgitation, bicuspid aortic valves, and ventricular septal defects as present with tetralogy of Fallot, produce turbulent blood flow, and are associated with an increased incidence of infective endocarditis. Patients with aortic or pulmonary stenosis have a lower probability of infection; patients with mitral stenosis or atrial septal defects rarely develop infective endocarditis.

Antibiotic Prophylaxis

Prophylactic use of antibiotics is recommended in susceptible patients when surgical procedures associated with bacteremia are planned (Table 29-2). Even in the absence of known heart disease, presence of diastolic heart murmurs must be assumed to represent organic heart disease requiring prophylactic antibiotic therapy in the perioperative period.

TABLE 29-2. Procedures in Susceptible Patients for Which Antibiotic Prophylaxis Is Recommended

Dental operations associated with gingival bleeding

Operations or procedures performed on the respiratory tract associated with disruption of the respiratory mucosa
Tonsillectomy and adenoidectomy
Nasotracheal intubation
Bronchoscopy

Instrumentation of the gastrointestinal tract or genitourinary tract

Cardiac surgery

Noncardiac surgery in patients with prosthetic vascular grafts or heart valves

Operations on infected tissues

Patients who are receiving chronic antibiotic therapy because of prior rheumatic fever should also receive additional antibiotics, since doses of antibiotics used for rheumatic fever prophylaxis are probably not adequate to protect against development of infective endocarditis.

Bacteriocidal antibiotics are typically chosen to provide prophylaxis against infective endocarditis. Prophylactic antibiotic therapy must be initiated before surgery, as the drug needs to be present in tissues, as well as blood, to provide protection. Furthermore, antibiotic therapy must be continued for 48 hours to 72 hours after surgery. Specific antibiotic regimens selected should consider the type of bacteria likely to enter the systemic circulation during the operative procedure (Table 29-3).

ALPHA-HEMOLYTIC STREPTOCOCCI

Alpha-hemolytic streptococci are most likely to enter the circulation during dental procedures or surgical manipulations of the upper respiratory tract. Penicillin is highly effective against these organisms (Table 29-3). Vancomycin or erythromycin is selected for patients with histories of allergy to penicillin. Combined use of penicillin and streptomycin

is recommended for patients with prosthetic heart valves, as these individuals are at greatest risk.

ENTEROCOCCI

Bacteremia due to enterococci is most likely to follow instrumentation or surgery on the gallbladder, lower gastrointestinal tract, or genitourinary tract. Gram-negative bacteremia may also enter the circulation after procedures are performed in these areas, but such organisms rarely produce infective endocarditis. Therefore, prophylaxis is with antibiotics effective against enterococci (Table 29-3).

STAPHYLOCOCCI

Staphylococci are the organisms most likely to invade the circulation during surgery requiring cardiopulmonary bypass. Antibiotics effective against staphylococci include penicillinase resistant penicillins and cephalosporins (Table 29-3).

Clinical Manifestations

Diagnosis of infective endocarditis must be considered in patients with heart murmurs, anemia, and fever, particularly if there is a history of co-existing cardiac disease and/or recent surgical procedures. Evidence of systemic embolization, including cerebral vascular occlusion and hematuria, may reflect dissemination of emboli from vegetations present on cardiac valves. Congestive heart failure is the most frequent cardiac complication. Acute aortic or mitral regurgitation can reflect destruction or perforation of cardiac valve leaflets. Mitral regurgitation can also be due to rupture of chordae tendineae. Cardiac conduction abnormalities may indicate extension of valvular infection into the ventricular septum. Cardiac rhythm disturbances, such as premature ventricular beats, may reflect myocarditis.

Operative intervention for valve replacement must be performed when patients de-

TABLE 29-3. Infective Endocarditis Prophylaxis

Procedure	Organism	Routine	Antibiotics* Allergic to Penicillin	Prosthetic Heart Valve
Dental treatment Tonsillectomy Adenoidectomy Nasotracheal intubation Bronchoscopy	Alpha-hemolytic streptococci	Penicillin	Vancomycin or erythromycin	Penicillin plus streptomycin
Gallbladder	Enterococci (*Streptococcus fecalis*)	Penicillin or ampicillin plus gentamicin or streptomycin	Vancomycin	As for Routine
Cardiac surgery	Staphylococci	Penicillinase resistant penicillins or cephalosporins	As for Routine	As for Routine

* Administered intravenously or intramuscularly 30–60 minutes before start of operation.

velop intractable congestive heart failure. Ideally surgery is delayed until high doses of appropriate antibiotics can be administered, so as to reduce the likelihood of infection of the new valve.

INFECTIONS OF THE UPPER RESPIRATORY TRACT

Bacterial infections of the upper respiratory tract frequently follow processes that impair normal host defense mechanisms. For example, clearance of pulmonary secretions can be impaired due to reduced activity of cilia or decreased cough reflexes. Viral respiratory tract infections are often the cause of impaired respiratory defense mechanisms.

Sinusitis

Acute sinusitis is characterized by nasal discharge, fever, leukocytosis, and facial pain, which typically increases when patients lean forward. Nasopharyngeal instrumentation (nasotracheal tubes, nasogastric tubes, nasal packing) in traumatized patients may predispose to sinusitis.[43] Nasal polyps or deviation of the nasal septum may also predispose to sinusitis by obstructing sinus drainage. Maxillary and frontal sinusitis are more frequent in adults, whereas infection of the ethmoid sinus predominates in children. Maxillary sinusitis is characterized by pain and tenderness over the cheeks. This pain is often referred to the teeth. Frontal sinusitis produces pain and tenderness over the forehead. Patients with ethmoid sinusitis typically complain of pain behind the orbit.

Acute sinusitis responds well to decongestants and analgesics. Most patients do not need antibiotics. Sinusitis that leads to intracranial infection, either by bony spread or via venous channels, requires treatment with high doses of antibiotics and surgical drainage.

Otitis Media

Otitis media results when bacteria spread from the nasopharynx to the normally sterile middle ear. The most frequent cause of purulent otitis media are pneumococci, followed by *Hemophilus influenzae*. Diagnosis is suggested by bulging tympanic membranes and obscured bony landmarks. Treatment is with analgesics, decongestants, and antibiotics. Myringotomy does not hasten recovery but is indicated for patients with progressive deafness or poor responses to medical therapy. Acute mastoiditis was once a frequent sequelae but is now, with the routine use of antibiotics, an unusual complication.

Serous otitis media differs from the purulent form in that fever and pain are absent. In contrast to purulent otitis media, tympanic membranes are retracted and bony landmarks are preserved.

Chronic otitis media is characterized by hearing loss and perforation of the tympanic membrane. Marginal or peripheral perforations may be associated with invasive cholesteatomas.

Pharyngitis

Viruses are the most frequent cause of pharyngitis. Among bacterial causes, group A streptococci account for 20 percent to 30 percent of all cases. A throat culture is necessary to distinguish viral from streptococcal pharyngitis. Pneumococci and staphylococci do not cause pharyngitis.

Peritonsillar Abscess

Peritonsillar abscess (quinsy) is a complication of streptococcal tonsillitis. Dysphagia results in drooling, and edema produces a characteristic muffled voice. The soft palate is edematous and trismus may be present. Treatment is with antibiotics and surgical drainage.

Retropharyngeal Infections

Retropharyngeal infections occur almost exclusively in childhood, as lymph nodes in this region atrophy during adulthood. Penicillin is the antibiotic of choice. Surgical drainage is necessary to prevent airway obstruction or extension of the infection to the mediastinum.

Ludwig's Angina

Ludwig's angina is cellulitis of the submandibular, sublingual, and submental regions. It is most frequently caused by streptococci and is characterized by fever and a rapidly progressive edema of the anterior neck and floor of the mouth. Elevation of the tongue impedes swallowing, and upper airway obstruction is a potentially fatal complication. Intubation of the trachea may not be possible, necessitating tracheostomy to preserve the airway.

Epiglottitis

Epiglottitis (supraglottitis) is a rapidly progressive and potentially lethal infection of the upper airway, most frequently caused by *Hemophilus influenzae*, type B. This infection is most common in boys between 2 years and 6 years of age (see Chapter 35).

PULMONARY PARENCHYMAL INFECTIONS

Pulmonary parenchymal infections typically develop after an event that impairs normal host defense mechanisms, such as viral infections that alter the physical and chemical characteristics of the normally protective mucous secretions in the airway. Indeed, the seasonal increase in viral infections during winter months is typically associated with an increased incidence of bacterial pneumonia. Patients with chronic obstructive pulmonary disease are vulnerable to bacterial infection in the lungs because of impaired mucociliary transport and inefficient cough mechanisms. Cigarette smoke may contribute to an increased incidence of pulmonary infection, by virtue of inhibition of ciliary activity by smoke.

Bacterial Pneumonia

Pneumococci remain the most frequent cause of bacterial pneumonia in adults. Streptococci are also a common cause of bacterial pneumonia. Inhalation of oropharyngeal secretions containing these bacteria, rather than droplet spread from person to person, is responsible for most pneumococcal pneumonias. Inhalation of oropharyngeal secretions often occurs during normal sleep. Nevertheless, bacterial pneumonia is uncommon in healthy patients because of efficient host defense mechanisms. In contrast, alcoholism, drug abuse, and neurologic disorders are examples of conditions that can impair consciousness and predispose to inhalation of bacteria-containing secretions and pneumonia. Bacterial pneumonia due to gram-negative organisms occurs most often in chronically ill and debilitated patients who are confined to bed.

DIAGNOSIS AND TREATMENT

Bacterial pneumonia is characterized by an initial chill, followed by an abrupt elevation of body temperature and copious sputum production. Segmental distribution of the infective process results in bronchopneumonia. Lobar pneumonia is present when infection includes more than one segment of a pulmonary lobe, or when multiple lobes are involved. Nevertheless, classic physical and radiographic findings of lobar consolidation may be absent. Indeed, dehydration can minimize abnormalities seen on the radiograph of the chest in the presence of bacterial pneumonia. Polymorphonuclear leukocytosis is typical, and arterial hypoxemia may occur in severe cases of bacterial pneumonia. Arterial hypoxemia reflects shunting due to perfusion of alveoli filled with inflammatory exudate. Microscopic examination of sputum, plus a culture and sensitivity, is necessary for the etiologic diagnosis of pneumonia and the selection of appropriate antibiotic treatment. In addition to antibiotic therapy, adequate hydration via systemic administration of fluids or local humi-dification of the airways is important for optimizing clearance of secretions.

BACTERIAL VERSUS VIRAL ETIOLOGY

It is important to distinguish between bacterial and nonbacterial pneumonia. Nonbacterial pneumonia, such as *Mycoplasma pneumoniae* pneumonia, occurs most frequently in previously healthy and young patients. In contrast to bacterial pneumonia, the presence of a nonbacterial pulmonary infections are suggested by nonproductive cough and the absence of leukocytosis. An interstitial infiltrate on the radiograph of the chest also suggests a nonbacterial etiology.

ACUTE BRONCHITIS VERSUS PNEUMONIA

The distinction between acute bronchitis and bacterial pneumonia is anatomic rather than etiologic, since the same organisms may cause both diseases. Patients with bacterial pneumonia are more likely to develop high temperatures, bacteremia, and arterial hypoxemia. Radiographs of the chest typically show infiltrates in patients with pneumonia. Changes associated with chronic lung disease and bronchitis, however, can mimic pulmonary infiltrations.

Legionnaires' Disease

Legionnaires' disease is a form of pneumonia caused by a filamentous gram-negative bacillus designated *Legionella pneumophilia*. The disease caused by this organism is characterized by a prodromal myalgia, malaise, and headache, followed within 24 hours by an acute elevation of body temperature, tachypnea, nonproductive cough, oliguria, and often obtundation. Clinical and radiographic features are not specific. Mild cases of this disease resemble *Mycoplasma pneumoniae* pneumonia. Erythromycin is the antibiotic of choice for treatment of this disease.

Bronchiectasis

Bronchiectasis is characterized by dilation of bronchi and destruction of bronchial walls. In severe cases, cor pulmonale and respiratory failure may occur. Treatment of bronchiectasis is with pulmonary physiotherapy and intermittent antibiotics, as required by recurrence of pulmonary infections.

Lung Abscess

Lung abscesses typically develop after bacterial pneumonia. Alcoholism and poor dental hygiene are frequently present in patients who develop lung abscesses. Septic pulmonary embolization, which is most common in drug addicts, may also result in formation of lung abscesses.

A radiograph of the chest is required to establish the presence of a lung abscess. The finding of an air-fluid level signifies rupture of the abscess into the bronchial tree. Foul smelling sputum is also characteristic when the lung abscess drains into the bronchial tree.

Antibiotics are the mainstay of treatment of lung abscesses. Surgery is indicated only when such complications as an empyema occur. Thoracentesis is necessary to establish the diagnosis of empyema, and treatment requires chest tube drainage and antibiotics. Surgical drainage is necessary for treatment of chronic empyema.

INTRA-ABDOMINAL INFECTIONS

Peritonitis and subphrenic abscess are examples of intra-abdominal infections that can present in the perioperative period. Both these processes can be confused with pulmonary infections.

Peritonitis

Peritonitis is a localized to diffuse inflammatory process involving the peritoneum. Diffuse inflammation of the peritoneum typically follows a breakdown in the integrity of the gastrointestinal tract, as can occur with appendicitis or diverticulitis, or following trauma. Multiple organisms are likely contributing to the disease process when peritonitis is due to these events. Acute pancreatitis can also mimic bacterial peritonitis. Likewise, abdominal pain associated with an acute peptic ulcer, cholecystitis, mesenteric artery occlusion, acute porphyria, and diabetic acidosis may suggest peritonitis. Occasionally, patients with systemic lupus erythematosus develop bacterial peritonitis.

Peritonitis has also been observed in patients with alcoholic cirrhosis of the liver. The most common causative organism in these patients is *E. coli*. For this reason, examination of ascitic fluid is indicated in any patient with cirrhosis who develops abdominal pain or unexplained fever. Gentamicin is the drug of choice when *E. coli* is the cause of peritonitis.

Subphrenic Abscess

Subphrenic abscess should be suspected in patients who have undergone abdominal surgery and subsequently develop unexplained fever. The frequent presence of pleural effusion in association with a subphrenic abscess can be attributed incorrectly to bacterial pneumonia. A wide separation between the upper margin of the gastric air bubble and diaphragm, as demonstrated on the radiograph of the chest, suggests a subphrenic abscess. Leukocytosis is almost always present. Treatment of a subphrenic abscess is with surgical drainage plus antibiotics. The antibiotic can be changed if indicated when results of the culture of the abscess fluid are available.

INFECTIONS OF THE URINARY TRACT

Urinary tract infections are the most common of all bacterial infections affecting humans. During the first 50 years of life, this is a disease that predominates in females. Symptoms range from asymptomatic bacteriuria to acute pyelonephritis. Most patients complain of dysuria and frequency. Urinalysis reveals hematuria and the presence of protein. The most frequent etiologic organisms are gram-negative bacteria such as *E. coli.*

Acute bacterial prostatitis is a febrile illness associated with fever, chills, pelvic pain, dysuria, and urinary frequency. The most common causative organism is *E. coli.* Chronic bacterial prostatitis may require surgical removal of the gland.

FEVER OF UNDETERMINED ORIGIN

Fever of undetermined origin is characterized by temperature elevations exceeding 38 degrees Celsius on several occasions during at least a 3 week period. The majority of patients manifesting fever of undetermined origin are subsequently shown to have infections, neoplasms, or connective tissue disorders. The two major systemic infections to consider are tuberculosis and infective endocarditis. Localized infections to consider include hepatic abscess, subphrenic abscess, and urinary tract infection. Viral infections usually do not produce fevers lasting 3 weeks or longer, the one important exception being infection due to cytomegalovirus.

MUCOCUTANEOUS LYMPH NODE SYNDROME

Mucocutaneous lymph node syndrome (Kawasaki syndrome) is an acute febrile illness of unknown origin recognized predominately

in children under 9 years of age.[44] The incidence of this disease is increased in Asian-American children and affects boys more than girls (approximately 1.5:1). Fever lasting 5 days or longer is associated with conjunctivitis, pharyngitis, erythematous tongue, truncal rash, and cervical lymphadenopathy. The most serious complications of this syndrome are cardiovascular. Coronary artery aneurysms develop in 15 percent to 25 percent of children with this disease and may lead to sudden death from cardiac dysrhythmias or myocardial infarction. High dose intravenous gamma globulin is effective in reducing the incidence of coronary artery abnormalities when administered early in the course of the disease.[45] Management of anesthesia in these children should consider the possibility of intraoperative myocardial ischemia.[46]

INFECTION IN THE IMMUNOSUPPRESSED HOST

Therapeutic programs that can have effects on the ability of patients to withstand infections include antibiotics, radiation therapy, corticosteroids, and cancer chemotherapeutic drugs. The major adverse effects of antibiotics are to create a selection process for colonization with organisms resistant to antibiotics. Radiation therapy and treatment with corticosteroids or cancer chemotherapeutic drugs adversely affect host immune mechanisms by impairing the function of neutrophils. For example, decreases in neutrophil counts to less than 1,000 mm³ are the most important factor predisposing to bacterial infections after organ transplantation or in the presence of cancer.

Bacterial Infections

Pneumococcal pneumonia is the most common cause of bacterial infections and death in patients who are immunosuppressed. Gram-negative organisms are also a frequent cause of pneumonia in these patients. Fever without localizing signs is a common manifestation of bacterial infections in the immunosuppressed host. In these same patients, potentially fatal bacteremia may be associated with a trivial appearing pulmonary infiltrate on the radiograph of the chest.

Fungal Infections

Immunosuppressed patients are prone to invasion by a variety of fungal organisms.

CANDIDA ALBICANS

Candida albicans is the fungus responsible for the disease known as candidiasis (moniliasis). The most common opportunity for infection with this fungus is via intravenous fluid therapy, as during total parenteral nutrition. Prolonged urethral catheterization can also be a portal of entry for *Candida albicans*. Treatment consists of removing the offending catheter, plus administration of specific antifungal drugs such as amphotericin B or miconazole.

ASPERGILLUS

Necrotizing bronchopneumonia may reflect invasion of the compromised host by the fungus known as *Aspergillus*. The treatment of choice is amphotericin B.

CRYPTOCOCCOSIS

Cryptococcosis is a systemic fungal infection, which can cause meningitis in the immunosuppressed host. Treatment is with amphotericin B.

PNEUMOCYSTIS CARINII

Pneumocystis carinii is a part of the normal respiratory flora. Pneumonia due to this organism is a major hazard for immunosup-

pressed patients, particularly in those individuals with leukemia or AIDS (see the section Acquired Immunodeficiency Syndrome). Rapid onset of nonproductive cough, dyspnea, and tachypnea, accompanied by diffuse bilateral perihilar infiltrates visible on the radiograph of the chest, is typical of pneumonia due to these organisms. A thoracotomy to obtain a lung biopsy is usually necessary to establish the diagnosis. During anesthesia, these patients require controlled ventilation of the lungs with high inspired concentrations of oxygen. In addition, use of positive end-expiratory pressure may be necessary to insure optimal arterial oxygenation. Treatment of pneumocystis pneumonia is with the fixed drug combination of trimethoprim and sulfamethoxazole.[47]

Pittsburgh pneumonia agent has also been identified as a cause of pneumonia in immunosuppressed patients.[48] Pleural involvement is prominent, with scanty sputum production. Consolidation is visible on the radiograph of the chest. Antibiotics effective in treatment of this infection include erythromycin, rifampin, trimethoprim, and sulfamethoxazole.

ADVERSE REACTIONS TO ANTIBIOTICS

Adverse reactions to antibiotics include microbial superinfections (see the section Infection in the Immunosuppressed Host), allergic reactions, altered neuromuscular conduction, and direct organ toxicity.

Allergic Reactions

It is mandatory that a history of drug allergy be sought in every patient before initiating treatment with antibiotics. Severe allergic reactions are more likely to follow parenteral rather than oral administration of antibiotics. Penicillin is the antibiotic most often associated with immune-mediated hypersensitivity reactions. Indeed, allergic reactions to penicillin develop in up to 10 percent of patients receiving this drug. Furthermore, penicillins and cephalosporins may share major antigenic determinants.

Altered Neuromuscular Conduction

Antibiotics act at multiple sites to interfere with neuromuscular conduction (Fig. 29-2).[49] For example, antibiotics classified as aminoglycosides interfere with neuromuscular conduction by inhibiting the presynaptic release of acetylcholine, as well as by decreasing sensitivity of postjunctional membranes to the neurotransmitter. Other antibiotics may produce local anesthetic effects on postjunctional membranes or direct relaxant effects on skel-

etal muscles. Skeletal muscle weakness due to effects of antibiotics on the neuromuscular junction is possible but not often seen in otherwise healthy patients. Patients with co-existing disease at the neuromuscular junction (myasthenia gravis), however, may be susceptible to antibiotic-induced neuromuscular blockade.

The important effect of antibiotic-induced changes in neuromuscular conduction is the potentiation of skeletal muscle paralysis produced by depolarizing and nondepolarizing muscle relaxants. Indeed, the only antibiotics not associated with this potentiation are the penicillins, cephalosporins, and erythromycin.[49] Oral neomycin, as used to sterilize the gastrointestinal tract before abdominal surgery, is unlikely to potentiate neuromuscular blockade, since this antibiotic is not absorbed into the systemic circulation. Nevertheless, prolonged oral administration of neomycin has been associated with antibiotic-induced neuromuscular blockade.[50]

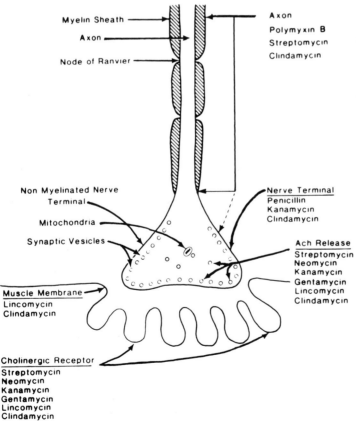

FIG. 29-2. Schematic diagram of possible sites of action of antibiotics on neuromuscular conduction. (Sokoll MD, Gergis SD. Antibiotics and neuromuscular function. Anesthesiology 1981;55:148–159)

Potentiation of neuromuscular blockade is most likely to occur when high blood levels of an antibiotic are present. Therefore, intravenous administration of antibiotics is most likely to produce potentiation. The likelihood for developing prolonged neuromuscular blockade after irrigation of operative sites with antibiotic-containing solutions depends on the total dose of antibiotic retained within the body. Thus, irrigation of an extremity incision would be expected to have little effect, since only small amounts of drug would be retained. Conversely, irrigation of the peritoneal or pleural cavities with large volumes of antibiotic-containing solutions may have significant effects.

It is important to appreciate that neostigmine- or calcium-produced antagonism of antibiotic-potentiated neuromuscular blockade may be incomplete. Therefore, it is essential to confirm the adequacy of recovery from neuromuscular blockade when the possibility of antibiotic-induced potentiation exists. This goal is best achieved by observing the responses elicited by a peripheral nerve stimulator, as well as by evaluating skeletal muscle strength as reflected by hand grip and head lift. Indeed, neuromuscular blockade in the presence of streptomycin or neomycin can be characterized by sustained responses to continuous electrical stimulation delivered by a peripheral nerve stimulator, and a train-of-four ratio near 1.0, despite a markedly decreased twitch response.[51] This emphasizes the necessity for clinical evaluation of neuromuscular blockade, as well as for the use of electrophysiologic criteria. In addition, a high index of suspicion for the possibility of recurarization must be maintained when administering antibiotics in the postoperative period to patients who have previously received muscle relaxants. In view of the unreliable reversal of neuromuscular blockade produced by combination of muscle relaxants and antibiotics, it may be best to mechanically support ventilation of the lungs via a tube in the trachea until clearance of the muscle relaxant from the body has occurred.

Antibiotic-potentiated neuromuscular blockade has been successfully reversed by 4-aminopyridine. Usefulness of this approach is questionable, however, as this drug is not available for clinical administration. There is no evidence that reversal of antibiotic-potentiated neuromuscular blockade with calcium or 4-aminopyridine alters the antimicrobial effect of the antibiotic.[52]

Direct Organ Toxicity

Antibiotics that are potentially nephrotoxic include the aminoglycosides, vancomycin, polymyxins, and amphotericin B. Azotemia due to co-existing renal disease can be accentuated by tetracyclines, since these drugs contribute to the breakdown of protein. Finally, penicillins, cephalosporins, aminoglycosides, and tetracyclines are excreted to a large extent unchanged by the kidneys. This dependence on renal excretion must be remembered when determining doses of antibiotics to be administered to patients with renal insufficiency.

Occurrence of hypotension during intravenous administration of vancomycin may reflect drug-induced histamine release or a direct myocardial depressant effect of this antibiotic.[53,54] Conceivably, deep anesthesia with volatile anesthetics could potentiate these adverse effects of vancomycin. Ototoxicity is an adverse effect of all aminoglycoside antibiotics, and vancomycin especially, in elderly patients who have age-related reductions in the glomerular filtration rate. Hepatotoxicity is most likely to occur with antibiotics used to treat tuberculosis. Pseudomembranous colitis is a potential complication of therapy with clindamycin. Chloramphenicol can produce bone marrow suppression, and in occasional patients aplastic anemia develops.

REFERENCES

1. Mufson MA. Pneumococcal infections. JAMA 1981;246:1942–8
2. MacDonald KL, Osterholm MT, Hedberg CW, et al. Toxic shock syndrome. A newly recognized complication of influenza and influenzalike illness. JAMA 1987;157:1053–8
3. Merson MH, Morris GK, Sack DA, et al. Traveler's diarrhea in Mexico: A prospective study of phy-

sicians and family members attending a Congress. N Engl J Med 1976;294:1299–1305

4. Laflin MJ, Tobey RE, Reves JG. Anesthetic considerations in patients with gas gangrene. Anesth Analg 1976;55:247–51

5. Alfrey DD, Rauscher LA. Tetanus: A review. Crit Care Med 1979;7:176–81

6. Tsueda K, Oliver OB, Richter RW. Cardiovascular manifestations of tetanus. Anesthesiology 1974;40:588–92

7. Potgieter PD. Inappropriate ADH secretion in tetanus. Crit Care Med 1983;11:417–8

8. Southorn PA, Blaise GA. Treatment of tetanus-induced autonomic nervous system dysfunction with continuous epidural blockade. Crit Care Med 1986;14:251–2

9. Malawista SE, Steere AC. Lyme disease: Infectious in origin, rheumatic in expression. In: Stollerman GH, Harrington WJ, LaMont JT, et al. eds. Advances in Internal Medicine. Chicago. Year Book Medical Publishers 1986;147–66

10. Rich SA, Sbordone L, Mazze RI. Metabolism by rat hepatic microsomes of fluorinated ether anesthetics following isoniazid administration. Anesthesiology 1980;53:489–93

11. Craven PC, Gremillion DH. Risk factors of ventricular fibrillation during rapid amphotericin B infusion. Antimicrob Agents Chemother 1985;27:868–71

12. Foy HM, Kenny GE, McMahan R, et al. Mycoplasma pneumoniae pneumonia in an urban area: Five years of surveillance. JAMA 1970;214:1666–72

13. duMoulin GC, Hedley-Whyte J. Hospital-associated viral infection and the anesthesiologist. Anesthesiology 1983;59:51–65

14. Nugent KN, Pesanti E. Tracheobronchial colonization with bacteria during influenza. Am Rev Respir Dis 1982;125:173–85

15. Hoffman DC, Dixon RE. Control of influenza in the hospital. Ann Intern Med 1977;87:725–8

16. Hirsch MS, Swartz MN. Antiviral agents. N Engl J Med 1980;302:949–53

17. Hayden FG, Albrecht JK, Kaiser DL, Givaltney JM. Prevention of natural colds by contact prophylaxis with intranasal alpha$_2$-interferon. N Engl J Med 1986;71–5

18. Tait AR, Narhwold ML, LaBond VA, Knight PR. Anesthesia and upper respiratory viral infections. Anesthesiology 1982;57:A450

19. Reichman RC, Badger GJ, Mertz GJ, et al. Treatment of recurrent genital herpes simplex infections with oral acyclovir. JAMA 1984;251:2103–7

20. Drew WL, Miner RC. Transfusion-related cytomegalovirus infection following noncardiac surgery. JAMA 1982;247:2389–91

21. Balfour CL, Balfour HH. Cytomegalovirus is not an occupational risk for nurses in renal transplant and neonatal units. Results of a prospective surveillance study. JAMA 1986;256:1909–14

22. Meyers EF, Krupin B. Anesthetic management of emergency tonsillectomy and adenoidectomy in infectious mononucleosis. Anesthesiology 1975;42:490–1

23. Ho DD, Pomerantz RJ, Kaplan JC. Pathogenesis of infection with human immunodeficiency virus. N Engl J Med 1987;317:278–86

24. Peterman TA, Curran JW. Sexual transmission of human immunodeficiency virus. JAMA 1986;256:2222–5

25. Curran JW, Lawrence DN, Jaffe H, et al. Acquired immunodeficiency syndrome (AIDS) associated with transfusions. N Engl J Med 1984;310:69–75

26. Update: Acquired immunodeficiency syndrome-United States. JAMA 1986;257:433–7

27. Recommendations for prevention of HIV transmission in health-care settings. JAMA 1987;258:1293–1305

28. Peterman TA, Jaffe HW, Feorino PM, et al. Transfusion-associated acquired immunodeficiency syndrome in the United States. JAMA 1985;254:2913–7

29. Ward JW, Grindon AJ, Feorino PM, et al. Laboratory and epidemiologic evaluation of an enzyme immunoassay for antibodies to HTLV-III. JAMA 1986;256:357–61

30. Marlink RG, Allan JS, McLane MF, et al. Low sensitivity of ELISA testing in early HIV infection. N Engl J Med 1986;315:1549

31. Feorino PM. Transfusion-associated AIDS. Evidence for persistent infection in blood donors. N Engl J Med 1985;312–27

32. Kunkel SE, Warner MA. Human T-cell lymphotropic virus type III (HTLV-III) infection: How it can affect you, your patients, and your anesthetic practice. Anesthesiology 1987;66:195–207

33. Feeley TW, Hamilton WK, Xavier B, et al. Sterile anesthetic breathing circuits do not prevent postoperative pulmonary infection. Anesthesiology 1981;54:369–72

34. DuMoulin GC, Saubermann AJ. The anesthesia machine and circle system are not likely to be sources of bacterial contamination. Anesthesiology 1977;47:353–8

35. Johnson BH, Eger EI. Bactericidal effects of anesthetics. Anesth Analg 1979;58:136–8

36. Knight PR, Bedows E, Nahrwold ML, et al. Alterations in influenza virus pulmonary pathology induced by diethy ether, halothane, enflurane, and pentobarbital anesthesia in mice. Anesthesiology 1983;58:209–15

37. Sheagren JN. Septic shock and corticosteroids. N Engl J Med 1981;305:456–8

38. Parker MM, Parrillo JE. Septic shock. Hemody-

namics and pathogenesis. JAMA 1983;250:3324–7

39. Peters WP, Johnson MW, Friedman PA, Mitch WE. Pressor effects of naloxone in septic shock. Lancet 1981;529–32

40. Bone RC, Fisher CJ, Clemmer TP, Slotman GJ, Metz CA, Balk RA et al. A controlled clinical trial of high-dose methylprednisolone in the treatment of severe sepsis and septic shock. N Engl J Med 1987;317:653–8

41. Longnecker DE, Ross DC. Influence of anesthetic on microvascular responses to hemorrhage. Anesthesiology 1979;51:S142

42. Weiskopf RB, Townsley MI, Riordan KK, et al. Comparison of cardiopulmonary responses to graded hemorrhage during enflurane, halothane, isoflurane, and ketamine anesthesia. Anesth Analg 1981;60:481–91

43. Caplan ES, Hoyt NJ. Nosocomial sinusitis. JAMA 1982;247:639–42

44. Feigin RD, Barron KS. Treatment of Kawasaki syndrome. N Engl J Med 1986;315:388–90

45. Newburger JW, Takahashi M, Burns JC, et al. The treatment of Kawasaki syndrome with intravenous gamma globulin. N Engl J Med 1986;315:341–7

46. McNiece WL, Krishna G. Kawasaki disease—a disease with anesthetic implications. Anesthesiology 1983;58:269–71

47. Hughes WT, Feldman S, Chaudhary SC, et al. Comparison of pentamidine isethionate and trimethorprim-sulfamethoxazole in the treatment of Pneumocystis carinii pneumonia. J Pediatr 1978;92:285–91

48. Myerowitz RL, Pasculle AW, Dowling JN, et al. Opportunistic lung infection due to Pittsburgh pneumonia agent. N Engl J Med 1979;301:954–8

49. Sokoll MD, Gergis SD. Antibiotics and neuromuscular function. Anesthesiology 1981;55:148–59

50. Pittinger CP, Eryasa T, Adamson R. Antibiotic-induced paralysis. Anesth Analg 1970;49:487–501

51. Lee C, Chen D, Barnes A, Katz RL. Neuromuscular block by neomycin in the cat. Can Anaesth Soc J 1976;23:527–33

52. Booij LHDJ, vanderPloeg GCJ, Crul JF, Muytjens HL. Do neostigmine and 4-aminopyridine inhibit the antibacterial activity of antibiotics? Br J Anaesth 1980;52:1097–9

53. Mayhew JF, Deutsch S. Cardiac arrest following administration of vancomycin. Can Anaesth Soc J 1985;32:65–6

54. Symons NLP, Hobbes AFT, Leaver HK. Anaphylactoid reactions to vancomycin during anaesthesia: Two clinical reports. Can Anaesth Soc J 1985;32:178–81

30

Cancer

Cancer is the second most frequent cause of mortality in the United States, accounting for about 400,000 deaths annually.[1] An estimated 5 million Americans currently are afflicted with cancer and by the year 2,000 this number will likely increase to 6.2 million reflecting the anticipated aging of the population. The economic cost of cancer in the United States was estimated to be about 51 billion dollars in 1980, about 11 percent of the total cost of illness of all types.[2]

Cancer reflects the uncontrolled growth and spread of cells due to mutations in their genetic complement (genome). The probability of such mutations is increased by ionizing radiation; chemical substances (carcinogens as may be present in tobacco smoke); physical irritants, such as continued abrasion of the gastrointestinal mucosa by certain types of food; and viruses. Diet may be responsible for many forms of cancer. In this regard there is an association between low plasma concentrations of vitamin E and the risk of any type of lung cancer and between low levels of plasma beta-carotene and the risk of squamous cell carcinoma of the lung.[3] In some families, there is a hereditary tendency to develop cancer.

Most mutant cells form abnormal proteins because of their altered genes. These abnormal proteins cause the immune system to form antibodies that destroy cancer cells. In support of a protective role of the immune system is an increased incidence of cancer in immunosuppressed patients, such as those undergoing organ transplantation. Cancer cells compete with normal tissues for nutrients and may eventually cause nutritive death of slowly proliferating or nonproliferating noncancerous cells.

Water suppressed proton nuclear magnetic resonance spectroscopy of plasma may be useful in detection of cancer and the monitoring of chemotherapy. For example, compared with normal patients, those with cancer manifest a narrowing of plasma lipoprotein-lipid proton line widths (Fig. 30-1).[4] This narrowing of lipoprotein-lipid resonances in patients with cancer is consistent with metabolic responses of hosts to tumor growth.

Management of anesthesia for patients with cancer requires an appreciation of pathophysiologic disturbances, which frequently accompany malignant diseases. Furthermore, it is important to be aware of potential adverse effects produced by cancer chemotherapeutic drugs. For example, drug-induced toxicity may influence management of anesthesia, as well as the patient's physiologic response to the stress of the operative period.

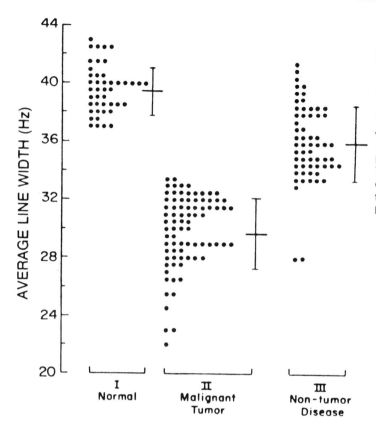

FIG. 30-1. Patients with cancer manifest a narrowing of plasma lipoprotein-lipid proton line widths compared with normal individuals and those with nontumor disease. Each symbol represents an individual patient. Mean ± SD. (Fossel ET, Carr JM, McDonagh J. Detection of malignant tumors. Water-suppressed proton nuclear tumors. Water-suppressed proton nuclear magnetic resonance spectroscopy of plasma. N Engl J Med 1986;315:1369–76)

PATHOPHYSIOLOGIC DISTURBANCES ASSOCIATED WITH CANCER

Many pathophysiologic disturbances accompany cancer (Table 30-1). These manifestations are referred to as paraneoplastic syndromes.

Fever

Fever may accompany any type of cancer but is particularly likely when metastases to the liver have occurred. Elevations of body temperature are also common with lymphomas, particularly Hodgkin's disease. Proposed mechanisms include tumor necrosis, inflammation, the release of toxic products by the tumor cells, and the production of endogenous pyrogens.[5]

Anorexia and Weight Loss

Anorexia and weight loss are frequent occurrences in patients with cancer. These disturbances may be a direct consequence of tumors or result from the psychological impact of the malignancy.

Lactic Acidosis

Severe lactic acidosis may occur with diseases that involve rapidly proliferating tumors, such as the acute leukemias and lymphomas.

TABLE 30-1. Pathophysiologic Manifestations of Cancer

Fever
Anorexia and weight loss
Lactic acidosis
Anemia or polycythemia
Thrombocytopenia
Coagulopathies
Neuromuscular abnormalities
Ectopic hormone production
Hypercalcemia
Hyperuricemia
Adrenal insufficiency
Nephrotic syndrome
Ureteral obstruction
Pulmonary osteoarthropathy
Obstruction of superior vena cava
Pericardial effusion and tamponade
Spinal cord compression
Brain metastases

Acidosis results from increased anaerobic glycolysis of the hypoxic proliferating tumor cells, especially when hepatic function is concomitantly impaired. Tumors that cause lactic acidosis are often responsive to chemotherapy, if the life-threatening acidosis is first corrected with appropriate fluids and electrolytes.

Anemia or Polycythemia

The most likely causes of anemia are direct effects of the cancer, such as gastrointestinal ulceration with bleeding, or tumor replacement of bone marrow. Cancer chemotherapeutic drugs that depress activity of bone marrow are another frequent cause. Other causes include shortened erythrocyte survival time, hypersplenism, autoimmune hemolysis, and nutrient deficiencies. In contrast to anemia, increased amounts of erythropoietin produced by hypernephromas or hepatomas can increase red cell mass.

Thrombocytopenia

Thrombocytopenia can be due to unrecognized cancers. Indeed, unexplained thrombocytopenia is an indication to search for occult neoplasms. Thrombocytopenia that cannot be attributed to therapy with chemotherapeutic drugs may reflect hypersplenism or disseminated intravascular coagulation.

Coagulopathies

Disseminated intravascular coagulation may occur in patients with advanced cancer, especially in the presence of hepatic metastases. Recurrent venous thrombosis due to unknown mechanisms is associated with pancreatic neoplasms.

Neuromuscular Abnormalities

Neuromuscular abnormalities occur in 5 percent to 10 percent of patients with cancer. The most common manifestations are skeletal muscle weakness (myasthenic syndrome) associated with carcinoma of the lung (see Chapter 28).[6] Prolonged responses to depolarizing and nondepolarizing muscle relaxants have been observed in patients with co-existing skeletal muscle weakness, particularly when weakness is associated with undifferentiated small cell carcinomas of the lung.

Ectopic Hormone Production

Physiologically active hormones are produced by a number of cancers. These hormones produce predictable physiologic effects (Table 30-2).

Hypercalcemia

Hypercalcemia is most likely to occur as a result of metastases to bone, with subsequent release of calcium. Bone metastases with as-

TABLE 30-2. Ectopic Hormone Production

Hormone	Associated Cancer	Manifestation
Adrenocorticotrophic hormone	Lung (small cell)	Cushing's syndrome
	Thyroid (medullary)	
	Thymoma	
	Carcinoid	
	Non-beta islet cell of pancreas	
Antidiuretic hormone	Lung (small cell)	Water intoxication
	Pancreas	
	Lymphomas	
Gonadotropin	Lung (large cell)	Gynecomastia
	Ovary	Precocious puberty
	Adrenal	
Melanocyte stimulating hormone	Lung (small cell)	Hyperpigmentation
Parathormone	Renal	Hyperparathyroidism
	Lung (squamous)	
	Pancreas	
	Ovary	
Thyroid stimulating hormone	Choriocarcinoma	Hyperthyroidism
	Testicular (embryonal)	
Thyrocalcitonin	Thyroid (medullary)	Hypocalcemia
Insulin	Retroperitoneal tumors	Hypoglycemia

sociated hypercalcemia are often from carcinoma of the breast. Occasionally, hypercalcemia is the result of ectopic parathormone production, most often associated with tumors that arise from the kidneys, lung, pancreas, or ovaries. Hypercalcemia may be precipitated or aggravated when painful bone lesions lead to decreased patient mobility. Hypercalcemia may be further accentuated if opioids taken for relief of pain result in further immobility, vomiting, or dehydration.

Hyperuricemia

Hyperuricemia is characteristically associated with leukemia in which there is a large tumor and cancer chemotherapeutic drugs have produced destruction of malignant cells. Acute renal failure can accompany hyperuricemia, particularly if plasma uric acid concentrations exceed 15 mg·dl^{-1}. Allopurinol, systemic hydration, and alkalinization of the urine are important aspects of prevention and treatment of hyperuricemia.

Adrenal Insufficiency

Adrenal insufficiency caused by complete replacement of the adrenal glands by metastatic tumor are rare. More often there is a relative adrenal insufficiency, due to partial replacement of the adrenal cortex by tumor, or suppression of adrenal cortex function by prolonged treatment with corticosteroids. Adrenal insufficiency is most often seen in patients with metastatic disease due to melanoma, retroperitoneal tumors, carcinoma of the lung, and carcinoma of the breast.

The stress of the perioperative period may unmask adrenal insufficiency. Clinical manifestations include fatigue, dehydration, oliguria, and cardiovascular collapse. Treatment of acute adrenal insufficiency is with the rapid intravenous administration of cortisol, followed by a continuous infusion of cortisol until oral replacement can be initiated.

Nephrotic Syndrome

It is thought that tumor antigen-antibody complexes are deposited on the glomerular capillary membrane, resulting in findings typical of the nephrotic syndrome.[7]

Ureteral Obstruction

Unilateral obstruction of the ureter is most likely to occur as a consequence of retroperitoneal tumors, including lymphomas and testicular cancers. Bilateral ureteral obstruction is rare and usually accompanies known pelvic neoplasms, such as carcinoma of the ovaries, bladder, or prostate. Ureteral obstruction by neoplasms is often asymptomatic until renal failure begins. Percutaneous nephrostomy is indicated if a ureter is totally obstructed.

Pulmonary Osteoarthropathy

Pulmonary osteoarthropathy, in its more limited manifestations, such as clubbing of the fingers, is often associated with neoplasms arising from the lung.

Obstruction of the Superior Vena Cava

The first evidence of the spread of cancer into the mediastinum may be obstruction of the superior vena cava. The principal manifestation is engorgement of veins above the waist, particularly jugular veins and those veins in the upper extremities. Airway obstruction may accompany invasion of the mediastinum with tumor. Treatment is immediate radiation of the mediastinal mass to reduce the size of the tumor and thus relieve venous and airway obstruction.

Pericardial Effusion and Tamponade

Metastatic cardiac involvement occurs most often in patients with leukemia, melanoma, carcinoma of the breast, and carcinoma of the lung. Clinical manifestations are related to pericardial metastases, which produce pericardial effusions. Malignant pericardial effusions are the most common cause of electrical alternans on the electrocardiogram. Paroxysmal atrial fibrillation or flutter is an early manifestation of malignant involvement of the pericardium or myocardium. Cardiac tamponade may result if accumulation of effusion fluid is rapid or the volume large. Thoracotomy and removal of part of the pericardium may be necessary to relieve cardiac tamponade (see Chapter 10).

Spinal Cord Compression

Spinal cord compression results from tumor infiltration of the epidural space. Lymphomas, multiple myeloma, carcinoma of the breast, and carcinoma of the lung are the tumors most likely to invade this space. A myelogram is essential when spinal cord compression is suggested by motor weakness or sensory deficits. Radiation therapy is the treatment of choice when neurologic deficits are partial. Corticosteroids are also administered to minimize inflammatory reactions and edema, which can result from radiation directed to tumors in the epidural space. Once total paralysis has developed, results of a surgical laminectomy to decompress the spinal cord or of radiation to the epidural space are equally poor.[8]

Brain Metastases

It is common for cancer cells to spread from primary sites to the brain. The incidence of brain metastases is between 25 percent and

50 percent for malignancies originating in the breast, kidneys, and thyroid gland. Whole brain radiation and administration of dexmethasone to relieve cerebral edema may be effective in reducing the size and subsequent neurologic effects produced by brain metastases. Surgical excision of an isolated metastasis is indicated when the brain scan shows no other lesions.

COMMON CANCERS ENCOUNTERED IN CLINICAL PRACTICE

The most frequently encountered cancers in adults are carcinoma of the breast, lung, gastrointestinal tract, prostate, and testicle. Lymphomas and leukemias represent neoplastic disease, which can afflict children as well as adults.

Carcinoma of the Breast

Carcinoma of the breast is the most common form of malignancy in women in the United States. It is estimated that about 5 percent of women in the United States will develop this form of cancer. Indeed, carcinoma of the breast is the most frequent medically related cause of death in women between the ages of 40 and 45 years.

Initial treatment includes surgery and administration of cancer chemotherapeutic drugs. Chemotherapy repeated every 4 weeks to 6 weeks for 1 year to 2 years after mastectomy is beneficial in premenopausal women with positive axillary lymph nodes at the time of surgery.[9] Drugs employed include melphalan or combination therapy with cyclophosphamide, methotrexate, and 5-fluorouracil.

An important concept in the management of patients with metastases from carcinoma of the breast relates to the discovery that cancer cells may contain significant amounts of estrogen-binding receptor protein.[10] Most patients with estrogen-binding receptor protein respond to endocrine ablative procedures or exogenously administered antiestrogen drugs. Surgical adrenalectomy or hypophysectomy are equally effective palliative procedures for patients with tumors that are estrogen-binding receptor protein-positive.

Carcinoma of the Lung

Primary cancers of the lung are bronchogenic carcinoma, bronchiolar or alveolar cell carcinoma, and pleural mesothelioma. Bronchogenic carcinomas account for about 90 percent of these cancers. The four histologic categories of bronchogenic carcinomas are squamous or epidermoid, undifferentiated small cell or oat cell, adenocarcinoma, and undifferentiated large cell. Squamous cell tumors account for about 50 percent of bronchogenic carcinomas. Undifferentiated small cell tumors are present in about 20 percent of patients with carcinoma of the lung. The remaining cell types are nearly evenly distributed between adenocarcinoma and undifferentiated large cell tumors.

Patients with chronic obstructive airways disease have a fourfold higher risk of lung cancer as compared with smokers without airway obstruction.[11,12] This suggests the possibility of a genetic susceptibility (an inherited recessive mutation similar to those described for retinoblastoma and Wilms' tumor) for the development of chronic obstructive airways disease and lung cancer. Identification of the responsible gene or genes could be used to counsel persons at risk against unnecessary exposure to known or suspected carcinogens.

Surgical excision and radiation of the tumor are the principal treatment modalities. There is no evidence that preoperative or postoperative radiation to the tumor site improves the surgical cure rate. Only about 5 percent of patients with carcinoma of the lung are cured by these treatments. Virtually none of the patients with undifferentiated small cell carcinoma are curable with surgery, although an occasional patient may benefit from surgery plus chemotherapy.[13] Combination chemotherapy may be of some benefit, particularly in patients with undifferentiated small cell tumors. Furthermore, median survival in patients with undifferentiated small cell carcinomas was increased from 24 weeks to 50 weeks when warfarin was added to combination chemotherapy plus radiation therapy.[14] These data support the hypothesis that the blood coagulation mechanism may be involved in the growth and spread of cancers in humans. Patients with cured lung cancer have an increased propensity toward the development of a second cancer.

Carcinoma of the Colon and Rectum

Carcinomas of the colon and rectum represent the most common malignancies afflicting both men and women. This type of cancer usually spreads initially to regional lymph nodes and then to the lungs and liver. Evaluation of the liver should include isotope scans and determination of plasma concentrations of alkaline phosphatase. Surgery is the primary curative modality for patients with lower gastrointestinal tract cancers. Chemotherapy has only limited value.

There is evidence that the transfusion of blood during surgical resection for colorectal cancer results in decreased survival times.[15] If true, this could reflect immunosuppression produced by blood that allows previously controlled cancer cells to more rapidly proliferate. Use of plasma volume expanders, rather than blood and reliance on anesthetic techniques that lower blood pressure and thus intraoperative blood loss, have been proposed in these patients.[16]

Carcinoma of the Prostate

Carcinoma of the prostate is the second most frequent cause of cancer-related death in men. Elevation of plasma acid phosphatase concentrations are indicative of spread of the tumor beyond the confines of the capsule of the prostate gland, usually indicating metastases of the tumor to bone. Osteoblastic lesions may be visible on radiographs of the skeleton.

Surgery is the principal curative treatment, while radiation is most useful for palliation. The most effective treatment for metastatic lesions originating from carcinoma of the prostate is hormonal manipulation via surgical orchiectomy, or estrogen treatment using diethylstilbestrol. Cancer chemotherapeutic drugs have not been widely used.

Testicular Cancer

Testicular carcinoma is one of the few epithelial tumors controllable with cancer chemotherapeutic drugs, as well as by surgery and radiation. These tumors are categorized as embryonal cell carcinoma, teratocarcinoma, choriocarcinoma, and teratoma. Tumors of the testes usually spread first to the retroperitoneal lymph nodes via the lymphatics.

Hodgkin's Disease

There is highly suggestive evidence that Hodgkin's disease and some other lymphomas have an infectious, possibly viral, origin. A typical onset of Hodgkin's disease is a painless enlarging mass that classically appears in the neck. Pruritus can be generalized and severe. Cyclic elevations of body temperature and unexplained weight loss may occur. Superior vena cava obstruction reflects invasion of the mediastinum by tumor. Moderately severe anemia is often present. Radiographs of the chest reflect frequent involvement of the lungs in Hodgkin's disease. Hodgkin's disease can also invade the liver and spleen. Peripheral neuropathies and spinal cord compression may occur as a direct result of tumor growth.

Exploratory laparotomy and splenectomy are performed as the initial treatment. Exploration of the abdomen allows evaluation of the spread of the disease and is the basis for classifying it in preparation for selection of the appropriate treatment. Combination chemotherapy has been used to achieve prolonged disease-free intervals. Frequently used drugs are nitrogen mustard, vincristine, procarbazine, and prednisone.

Leukemias and Myeloproliferative Disorders

Leukemia is uncontrolled production of leukocytes due to cancerous mutation of lymphogenous cells or myelogenous cells. As such, leukemias are commonly divided into lymphocytic leukemias and myeloid leukemias. Lymphocytic leukemias begin in lymph nodes or other lymphogenous tissues and then spread to other areas of the body. Myeloid leukemias begin as cancerous production of myelogenous cells in bone marrow, with spread to extramedullary organs. Occasionally, cancerous cells are well differentiated but more often are undifferentiated, not resembling other leukocytes and lacking the usual functional characteristics of white cells.

Pathophysiology of leukemias and myeloproliferative disorders relates to the impact of the expanding white blood cell line, which infiltrates bone marrow, rendering patients functionally aplastic. Anemia may be profound. Eventually, bone marrow failure is the cause of fatal infection or hemorrhage due to thrombocytopenia. In addition to bone marrow, leukemic cells may infiltrate the liver, spleen, lymph nodes, and meninges, to produce signs of dysfunction at these sites. Extensive use of nutrients by rapidly proliferating cancerous cells depletes amino acids and vitamins, leading to extreme patient fatigue and metabolic starvation of normal tissues.

A kilogram of leukemic cells (about 10^{12} cells) appears to be a lethal mass. However, symptoms leading to the diagnosis of leukemia are unlikely until the tumor load is about 10^{9} cells. Cancer chemotherapeutic drugs are given to reduce the number of tumor cells so that organomegaly will regress and function of bone marrow will improve. Drugs used for chemotherapy are predominantly those that depress activity of bone marrow, such that hemorrhage and infection become the determinants of maximum acceptable doses. Destruction of leukemic cells by cancer chemotherapeutic drugs produces a uric acid load, which may result in urate nephropathy and gouty arthritis.

ACUTE LYMPHOBLASTIC LEUKEMIA

Acute lymphoblastic leukemia accounts for about 15 percent of all leukemia in adults. Central nervous system dysfunction is common. These patients are highly susceptible to life-threatening infections, including those produced by *Pneumocystitis carinii* and cytomegalovirus.

CHRONIC LYMPHOCYTIC LEUKEMIA

Chronic lymphocytic leukemia comprises about 25 percent of all leukemias and is seen most often in elderly males. Diagnosis is confirmed by the presence of lymphocytosis (greater than 15,000 mm^3) and lymphocytic infiltrates in bone marrow. There may be neutropenia, with an associated increased susceptibility to bacterial infections. Treatment is with cancer chemotherapeutic drugs classified as alkylating agents.

ACUTE MYELOID LEUKEMIA

This form of leukemia is among the most aggressive malignant disease known to humans, resulting in death in about 3 months if untreated. Fever, weakness, bleeding, and hepatosplenomegaly are characteristic. Chemotherapy produces a temporary remission in about one-half the patients.

CHRONIC MYELOID LEUKEMIA

Massive hepatosplenomegaly and white blood cell counts greater than 50,000 mm^3 are characteristic of chronic myeloid leukemia.

Fever and weight loss reflect the presence of hypermetabolism. Anemia may be severe. Splenectomy is routinely performed in these patients.

POLYCYTHEMIA VERA

Polycythemia vera is a myeloproliferative disease, which classically occurs in patients between 60 years and 70 years of age. Hyperactivity of myeloid progenitor cells results in increased production of erythrocytes, leukocytes, and platelets. Hemoglobin concentrations typically exceed 18 g·dl^{-1}, and platelet counts can be greater than 400,000 mm^3. Clinical symptoms are due to hyperviscosity of the blood, which leads to stasis of blood flow and an increased incidence of vascular thrombosis, particularly in the cardiovascular and central nervous systems. Defective platelet function is the most likely mechanism for spontaneous hemorrhage occasionally observed in these patients. Treatment of this disease is by repeated phlebotomy to reduce the viscosity of the blood.

Hemoglobin concentrations should be reduced to near normal levels by phlebotomy before elective surgery. Surgery in the presence of uncontrolled polycythemia vera is associated with a high incidence of perioperative hemorrhage and postoperative venous thromboses. In emergency situations, viscosity of the blood can be reduced by intravenous infusions of crystalloid solutions or low molecular weight dextrans.

CANCER CHEMOTHERAPY

Cancer chemotherapy is the best available therapy for eradication of cancerous cells, which can occur anywhere in the body. Effectiveness of cancer chemotherapy requires that there be complete destruction of all cancer cells, since a single surviving clonogenic cell can give rise to sufficient progeny to ultimately kill the host. Recognition for the need of total destruction of cancerous cells has led to the frequent use of combinations of cancer chemotherapeutic drugs or their administration in planned sequences over short periods. This approach is based on the empiric observation that normal cells usually recover from pulses of maximal chemotherapy more rapidly than do tumor cells. Furthermore, immunosuppression is less with intermittent chemotherapy.

An important principle of combination chemotherapy is the administration of the largest possible doses of drugs as each works by different mechanisms and does not share similar toxic effects. Using combinations of drugs with different mechanisms of action also reduces chances that drug-resistant tumor cell populations will emerge. Bone marrow transplant is also becoming an increasingly successful therapy for leukemia.

Patients receiving drugs for treatment of cancer are frequently subjected to elective and emergency surgery. Rational management of anesthesia for these patients requires a clear understanding of the mechanisms of action, potential interactions, and likely toxicities associated with the use of cancer chemotherapeutic drugs.[17-19]

Most cancer chemotherapeutic drugs act by interfering with the action of enzymes, which are important in the synthesis or function of deoxyribonucleic acid (DNA). Consequently, these drugs exert their therapeutic and toxic effects by inhibiting cells undergoing synthesis of DNA. Vulnerability of normal cells to such chemotherapeutic drugs is expected, as many normal tissues (bone marrow, gastrointestinal mucosa, hair follicle cells) have turnover rates, which exceed proliferative rates of malignant cells. With this in mind, it is predictable that adverse clinical effects of cancer chemotherapeutic drugs can include bone marrow suppression (susceptibility to infection, thrombocytopenia, leukopenia, and anemia), nausea, vomiting, diarrhea, ulceration of gastrointestinal mucosa, and alopecia. Suppression of bone marrow function is the most frequent dose-limiting factor for cancer chemotherapeutic drugs. Slow-growing cancerous cells with slow rates of division, such as carcinoma of the lung and colon, are often unresponsive to cancer chemotherapeutic drugs.

Cancer chemotherapeutic drugs can be

TABLE 30-3.   Adverse Side Effects Produced by Cancer + Chemotherapeutic Drugs.
(Table continues.)

	Immuno-suppression	Thrombo-cytopenia	Leuko-penia	Anemia	Cardiac Toxicity	Pulmo-nary Toxicity	Renal Toxicity
Alkylating agents							
Busulfan (Myleran)	+	+++	+++	+++		++	++
Chlorambucil (Leukeran)	+	++	++	++		+	
Cyclophosphamide (Cytoxan)	++++	+	++	+		+	+
Melphalan (Alkeran)	+	++	++	++		+	
Thiotepa (Thiotepa)	+	+++	+++	+++		+	
Antimetabolites							
Methotrexate (Methotrexate)	+++	+++	+++	+++		+	++
6-Mercapt-opurine (Purinethol)	+++	++	++	++			++
Thioguanine (Thioguanine)	+++	+	++	++			
5-Fluorouracil (Fluorouracil)	++++	+++	+++	+++			
Plant alkaloids							
Vinblastine (Velban)	++	+	+++	+			
Vincristine (Oncovin)	++	+	++	+			+
Antibiotics							
Doxorubicin (Adriamycin)		+	+++	++	+++		
Daunorubicin (Daunomycin)	+	++	+++	++	+++		
Bleomycin (Blenoxane)		+	+	+		+++	
Mithramycin (Mithracin)	+	++++	++++	+++			++
Nitrosoureas							
Carmustine (BiCNU)		++	++ / +++	++		+	+
Lomustine (CeeNU)		+++		++			
Enzymes							
L-asparaginase (Elspar)	++	+	+	+			+

+ = minimal; ++ = mild; +++ = moderate; ++++ = marked.
(Adapted from Selvin BL. Cancer chemotherapy: Implications for the anesthesiologist. Anesth Analg 1981;60:425–34. Reprinted with permission from IARS.)

TABLE 30-3 (Continued).

Hepatic Toxicity	CNS Toxicity	Peripheral Nervous System Toxicity	Autonomic Nervous System Toxicity	Stomatitis	Plasma Cholin-esterase Inhibition	Other
				+	+	Adrenocortical-like effect (+) Hemolytic anemia (+ +)
+	+				+	Hemolytic anemia (+ +)
+				+	+ +	Hemolytic anemia (+ +)
					+	Hemorrhagic cystitis (+ + +) Inappropriate ADH secretion (+)
					+ +	Hemolytic anemia (+ +)
						Hemolytic anemia (+ +)
+				+ + +		
+ + +				+		
+ + +				+		
		+		+ + +		
		+	+	+		Inappropriate ADH secretion (+)
	+	+ +	+ +			
+				+ +		Red urine (+)
				+ +		Red urine (+)
				+ + +		
+ +	+			+ + +		Coagulation defects (+ + +) Hypocalcemia (+) Hypokalemia (+)
				+		
+				+		
+ + +	+			+		Hemorrhagic pancreatitis (+) Coagulation defects (+)

classified as alkylating agents, antimetabolites, plant alkaloids, antibiotics, nitrosoureas, enzymes, and random synthetics.[17] Adverse side effects produced by these drugs may be common to all chemotherapeutic drugs or unique to specific classes of drugs (Table 30-3).[17]

Alkylating Agents

Alkylating agents most likely act by alkylation of nucleic acids. Suppression of bone marrow activity is the most important dose-limiting factor for these drugs. Hemolytic anemia and increased skin pigmentation are common. Mucosal ulceration of the gastrointestinal tract is less common than with other classes of cancer chemotherapeutic drugs. Inhibition of plasma cholinesterase by alkylating agents could result in prolonged responses to succinylcholine. Nevertheless, succinylcholine has been administered to these patients without unusually prolonged effects.[18] Alkylating agents also introduce the potential for pneumonitis and pulmonary fibrosis. Damage to hair follicles leading to alopecia is common. Increased skin pigmentation is likely to occur, as is nausea and vomiting. Skeletal muscle weakness and seizures may be present.

Rapid destruction of tumor cells secondary to chemotherapy with these drugs can result in accelerated breakdown of purine and lead to development of uric acid nephropathy. Adequate fluid intake, alkalinization of the urine, and concomitant administration of allopurinol reduces the likelihood of renal dysfunction.

Antimetabolites

Antimetabolite drugs are structural analogs of normal endogenous metabolites essential for cell function and reproduction. Antimetabolites interact with specific enzymes, resulting in production of metabolites that cannot be used by cells. Rapidly proliferating bone marrow cells and cells of the gastrointestinal tract are most susceptible to antimetabolite drugs. Immunosuppression often accompanies therapy with antimetabolites. Diarrhea, hemorrhagic enteritis, and perforation of the intestine may occur. The possibility of liver and/or renal dysfunction should be determined preoperatively. Ulceration of the buccal mucosa and stomatitis are potential side effects of these drugs.

Plant Alkaloids

Plant alkaloids exert therapeutic and toxic effects by binding with microtubular proteins within cells, leading to arrest of cellular mitosis. These drugs also interact with nucleic acids. Bone marrow suppression, characterized by leukopenia, is a prominent side effect. Neurologic toxicity is evidenced by encephalopathies and peripheral neuropathies. Dysfunction of the autonomic nervous system most often manifests as abdominal pain and decreased gastrointestinal tract activity, leading to constipation and occasionally perforation of the colon. Neurotoxicity may be associated with inappropriate secretion of antidiuretic hormone.

Antibiotics

Antibiotics effective in treatment of cancer act by forming stable complexes with DNA. These drugs have a major role in the effective treatment of acute leukemia. Hodgkin's disease, carcinoma of the breast, carcinoma of the lung, and soft-tissue sarcomas. Successful use of these drugs has been hampered by conventional (bone marrow depression) and unique (cardiac) toxicities. Cardiac toxicity manifests as cardiomyopathy or as nonspecific changes on the electrocardiogram. Pulmonary toxicity is another side effect observed in patients treated with bleomycin.[19] Mithramycin is a highly toxic drug, producing coagulation defects and hepatorenal dysfunction.

CARDIOMYOPATHY

Severe cardiomyopathy leading to congestive heart failure occurs in nearly 2 percent of patients treated with doxorubicin or daunorubicin. The initial appearance of symptoms suggestive of an upper respiratory tract infection (nonproductive cough) is followed by rapidly progressive congestive heart failure, often refractory to cardiac inotropic drugs or mechanical cardiac assistance. Death occurs in about 60 percent of patients. Cardiomegaly and/or pleural effusions may be apparent on radiographs of the chest. Voltage of QRS complexes on the electrocardiogram may be decreased. Patients who have received high doses of radiation therapy, particularly to the mediastinum, and those who are on concurrent cyclophosphamide therapy, are particularly susceptible to developing cardiomyopathy.[18] Marked impairment of left ventricular function for as long as 3 years after discontinuation of doxorubicin has been observed.[20]

Electrocardiogram Changes. Nonspecific and usually benign changes on the electrocardiogram have been observed in about 10 percent of patients. Frequently, observed changes are supraventricular tachydysrhythmias, premature atrial beats, premature ventricular beats, abnormalities of conduction of the cardiac impulse, left axis deviation, decreased QRS voltage, and a variety of nonspecific ST segment and T-wave abnormalities. These changes do not seem to be dose related, nor do they necessarily reflect underlying cardiomyopathy.

PULMONARY TOXICITY

Bleomycin is an antibiotic particularly useful in the treatment of metastatic testicular carcinomas. Pulmonary toxicity, however, occurs in 10 percent to 25 percent of patients.[21] This toxicity ranges from decreased pulmonary function to severe pulmonary fibrosis. Approximately 1 percent to 2 percent of patients treated with this drug have died from pulmonary toxicity. Geriatric patients, those receiving more than 200 U to 400 U of drug, and those with co-existing lung disease are at an increased risk. Prior radiotherapy also predisposes patients to pulmonary toxicity.[19]

The gradual and often insidious appearance of dyspnea and nonproductive cough are typical initial manifestations. Pulmonary function testing typically demonstrates changes characteristic of restrictive pulmonary disease. Alveolar-to-arterial differences for oxygen are often increased, and pulmonary diffusing capacity may be reduced. Appearance of radiographic changes (bilateral diffuse interstitial infiltrates) often means irreversible pulmonary fibrosis has occurred.[19]

The possibility that bleomycin treatment could render patients more susceptible to toxic pulmonary effects of oxygen has been suggested by an apparent increased incidence of postoperative acute respiratory failure in those receiving enriched inhaled concentrations of oxygen (average 39 percent) during surgery.[22] One speculation is that increased inhaled concentrations of oxygen facilitate production of superoxide and other free radicals in the presence of bleomycin. For this reason, it has been recommended that inhaled concentrations of oxygen during surgery be maintained below 30 percent.[19,22] Nevertheless, data from animals and patients do not demonstrate increased pulmonary toxicity in the presence of bleomycin therapy and high concentrations of oxygen.[23-25] The prudent approach would seem to be administration of sufficient inhaled concentrations of oxygen to assure adequate arterial oxygenation. Accumulation of interstitial pulmonary fluid in bleomycin-treated patients receiving crystalloids, rather than colloids, during surgery may reflect impaired lymphatic drainage due to drug-induced pulmonary fibrosis.[22]

Nitrosoureas

Nitrosoureas appear to act by alkylation of nucleic acids. Pulmonary toxicity, manifesting as fibrosis, may be related to this alkylation. Hepatotoxicity and renal tubular damage are possible but rare complications. Streptozocin may cause hypoinsulinism due to its selective destruction of pancreatic beta cells.

Enzymes

The enzyme L-asparaginase is thought to act by destroying extracellular supplies of asparagine, leading to the death of cancer cells lacking enzymatic ability to make this amino acid. Hepatotoxicity is a major side effect of this drug, with about 50 percent of treated patients demonstrating evidence of liver dysfunction. Hemorrhagic pancreatitis occurs in about 5 percent of patients. Patients treated with L-asparaginase may exhibit lethargy and somnolence. Bone marrow suppression is usually mild, but clotting abnormalities may be present.

Random Synthetics

CISPLATIN

Suppression of bone marrow function and renal toxicity are the dose-limiting factors for this drug. Neurotoxicity may manifest as seizures and peripheral neuropathies. Cardiotoxicity is a rare adverse effect. Hypercalcemia has been observed as a side effect of this drug.

PROCARBAZINE

Suppression of bone marrow activity is the most important side effect of this drug. Procarbazine is also a weak monoamine oxidase inhibitor, with implications for the use of sympathomimetics, opioids, and barbiturates in the perioperative period (see Chapter 23). Hypersensitivity reactions characterized by pleural-pulmonary changes can occur.

Management of Anesthesia

Management of anesthesia for patients taking cancer chemotherapeutic drugs requires an awareness of the potential adverse side effects produced by these drugs. Routine clinical tests to detect dysfunction related to treatment with these drugs should include hematocrit, platelet count, white blood cell count, plasma electrolytes, blood glucose concentration, renal and liver function tests, plasma amylase concentration, coagulation profile, radiograph of the chest, and electrocardiogram. Transfusion of erythrocytes to correct anemia may be necessary before surgery. Blood components may be necessary to prevent perioperative coagulopathy. Correction of electrolyte and fluid balance and nutrient deficiencies may be required preoperatively.

Attention to aseptic technique is important, since immunosuppression occurs with most cancer chemotherapeutic agents. A history of dyspnea, nonproductive cough, and fever may reflect pulmonary fibrosis from these drugs. Signs of central nervous system depression, autonomic nervous system dysfunction, and peripheral neuropathies should be sought in the preoperative evaluation.

Selection of drugs for use during the intraoperative period may be influenced by adverse effects related to cancer chemotherapeutic drugs. For example, volatile anesthetics may be associated with exaggerated reductions in myocardial contractility in patients with cardiotoxicity due to cancer chemotherapeutic drugs. The presence of renal or hepatic dysfunction may influence the choice of anesthetic drugs and muscle relaxants. Although not a consistent observation, the possibility of prolonged responses to succinylcholine must be considered in patients taking alkylating agents.[18] Operative and postoperative monitoring of central venous pressure and urinary output is important.

It is particularly important to monitor arterial oxygen partial pressures in patients with co-existing pulmonary fibrosis. Intraoperative fluid replacement must be guided carefully in these patients and consideration given to administering colloid rather than crystalloid solutions. Support of ventilation of the lungs in the postoperative period is likely to be required in many of these patients, particularly after invasive and/or prolonged operations. A preoperative history of congestive heart failure due to cancer chemotherapeutic drugs increases the likelihood of postoperative cardiovascular complications.[20]

BONE MARROW TRANSPLANTATION

Bone marrow transplantation may be indicated in the treatment of leukemia or aplastic anemia. Patients with diseases that may be successfully treated by irradiation or immunosuppression that would destroy the bone marrow may undergo removal of their bone marrow before treatment for reinfusion post-therapy (e.g., autologous marrow rescue). Long-term survival after bone marrow transplantation is often greater than 50 percent in patients with acute lymphoblastic or myeloblastic leukemia and may exceed 70 percent in patients with aplastic anemia.

Donor bone marrow (300 ml to 1,000 ml) is obtained from multiple punctures of the anterior and posterior iliac crests and sternum during general anesthesia.[26] Usually the donor is related to the recipient and has matched HLA antigens. Nitrous oxide is often avoided in these patients because of potential drug-induced adverse effects on bone marrow. Brief heparinization before removal of bone marrow may influence use of spinal or epidural anesthesia for this procedure. One to 2 weeks before bone marrow removal, the donor may undergo venesection as autotransfusion of blood is often necessary. Postoperative complications are rare, although discomfort at puncture sites is predictable. Bone marrow regeneration occurs in a few weeks.

The bone marrow of the recipient is destroyed by drugs (cyclophosphamide) or irradiation before transplantation. These patients experience nausea and are susceptible to sepsis during this time. During bone marrow transplantation fat embolism may occur, although the incidence of this complication is rare. After the transplant infusion patients are maintained on immunosuppressant drug therapy and nursed in environments designed to minimize sources of infection.

REFERENCES

1. Silverberg E, Lubera J. Cancer statistics. CA 1986;36:9–25
2. Rice DP, Hodgson TA, Kopstein AN. The economic cost of illness: A replication and update. Health Care Finance Review 1985;7:61–80
3. Menkes MS, Comstock GW, Vuilleumier JP, et al. Serum beta-carotene, vitamins A and E, selenium, and the risk of lung cancer. N Engl J Med 1986;315:1250–4
4. Fossel ET, Carr JM, McDonagh J. Detection of malignant tumors. Water suppressed proton nuclear magnetic resonance spectroscopy of plasma. N Engl J Med 1986;315:1369–76
5. Bodel P. Tumors and fever. Ann N Y Acad Sci 1974;230:6–13
6. Wise RP. A myasthenic syndrome complicating bronchial carcinoma. Anaesthesia 1962;17:488–90
7. Kaplan BS, Klassen J, Gault MH. Glomerular injury in patients with neoplasia. Annu Rev Med 1976;27:117–25
8. Gilbert RW, Kim J-H, Posner JB. Epidural spinal cord compression from metastatic tumor: Diagnosis and treatment. Ann Neurol 1978;3:40–51
9. Bonadonna G, Valagussa P, Rossi A, et al. Are surgical adjuvant trials altering the course of breast cancer? Semin Oncol 1978;5:450–64
10. McGuire WL, Horwitz KB, Pearson OH, et al. Current status of estrogen and progesterone receptors in breast cancer. Cancer 1977;39:2934–47
11. Skillrud DM, Offord KP, Miller RD. Higher risk of lung cancer in chronic obstructive pulmonary disease: A prospective, matched, controlled study. Ann Intern Med 1986;105:503–7
12. Harris CC. Tobacco smoke and lung disease: Who is susceptible? Ann Intern Med 1986;105:607–9
13. Minna JD, Ihde DC, Glatstein EJ. Lung cancer: Scalpels, beams, drugs and probes. N Engl J Med 1986;315:1411–4
14. Azcharski LR, Henderson WG, Rickles FR, et al. Effect of warfarin on survival in small cell carcinoma of the lung. Veterans Administration Study No. 75. JAMA 1981;245:831–5
15. Fielding LP. Red for danger: Blood transfusion and colorectal cancer. Br Med J 1985;291:841–3
16. Hunter AR. Colorectal surgery for cancer: The anaesthetist's contribution. Br J Anaesth 1986;58:825–6
17. Selvin BL. Cancer chemotherapy: Implications for the anesthesiologist. Anesth Analg 1981;60:425–34
18. Dillman JB. Safe use of succinylcholine during

repeated anesthetics in a patient treated with cyclophosphamide. Anesth Analg 1987;66:351–3

19. Klein DS, Wilds PR. Pulmonary toxicity of antineoplastic agents: Anaesthetic and postoperative implications. Can Anaesth Soc J 1983;30:399–405

20. Burrows FA, Hickey PR, Colan S. Perioperative complications in patients with anthracycline chemotherapeutic agents. Can Anaesth Soc J 1985;32:149–57

21. Batist G, Andrews JL. Pulmonary toxicity of antineoplastic drugs. JAMA 1981;246:1449–53

22. Goldiner PL, Schweizer O. The hazards of anesthesia and surgery in bleomycin-treated patients. Semin Oncol 1979;6:121–4

23. Douglas MJ, Coppin CML. Bleomycin and subsequent anaesthesia: A retrospective study at Vancouver General Hospital. Can Anaesth Soc J 1980;27:449–52

24. La Mantia KR, Glick JH, Marshall BE. Supplemental oxygen does not cause respiratory failure in bleomycin-treated surgical patients. Anesthesiology 1984;60:65–7

25. Matalon S, Harper WV, Nickerson PA, Olszowka J. Intravenous bleomycin does not alter the toxic effects of hyperoxia in rabbits. Anesthesiology 1986;64:614–9

26. Borland LM, Cook DR. Anesthesia for organ transplantation. In: Stoelting RK, Barash PG, Gallagher TJ, eds. Advances in Anesthesia. Chicago. Year Book Medical Publishers 1986:1–36

31

The Immune System

Functions of the immune system have important implications for the administration of anesthesia.[1] For example, patients may experience allergic reactions to drugs administered during anesthesia. Anesthetic drugs may alter resistance to infection or malignancy. Chronic exposure to trace concentrations of anesthetic gases may have important effects on functions of the immune system. Finally, incidental diseases involving immunoglobulins may be present in patients requiring surgery.

BASIC CONCEPTS

The primary function of the immune system is to recognize the presence of foreign substances (antigens), which might be harmful to the host. Such recognition sets into motion a series of steps designed ultimately to destroy the antigens. Traditionally, function of the immune system is divided into nonspecific and specific immune mechanisms.

Nonspecific Immune Mechanisms

Nonspecific immune mechanisms include (1) the ciliary action of respiratory epithelium,

(2) the antibacterial action of mucus secreted by cells, and (3) the acute local inflammatory response that increases capillary permeability and facilitates transfer of cells necessary for phagocytosis into the inflamed area. Events in the perioperative period may alter the effectiveness of these responses. For example, mucociliary flow in the trachea can be decreased by reductions in body temperature or fluid deprivation. Halothane and perhaps other anesthetic drugs produce dose-dependent decreases in mucociliary flow (Fig. 31-1).[2] Decreased clearance of mucus due to reductions in mucociliary flow could predispose to atelectasis and pneumonia, especially in patients with chronic bronchitis, who already have excessive secretions that often contain infective organisms.

Specific Immune Mechanisms

Specific immune mechanisms are superimposed on nonspecific immune responses. The most important cells involved are lymphocytes. Lymphocytes derived from a common bone marrow stem cell are designated as B-lymphocytes (bursa dependent) or T-lymphocytes (thymus dependent). B-lymphocytes,

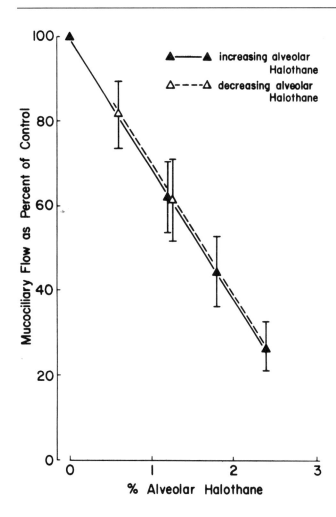

FIG. 31-1. Halothane produces dose-dependent decreases in mucociliary flow. Each value is the Mean ± SE for six dogs expressed as a percent of control. Control values were obtained during anesthesia produced with thiopental. (Forbes AR. Halothane depresses mucociliary flow in the trachea. Anesthesiology 1976;45:59–63)

on contact with specific antigens, become plasma cells and produce antibodies. Antibodies are a heterogenous group of plasma proteins with structural specificity for the stimulating antigen. Examples of antibody-mediated immunity include allergic reactions (anaphylaxis), elimination of bacteria, neutralization of toxins, and prevention of viral reinfection (vaccination).

T-lymphocytes, also known as helper T-lymphocytes, do not produce antibodies but instead regulate antibody production by B-lymphocytes (see Chapter 29). T-lymphocytes are also genetically programmed to distinguish "self" from "non-self," and are thus responsible for cell-mediated immunity, which can lead to rejection of transplanted foreign tissues. Activity of helper T-lymphocytes is counter-balanced by suppressor T-lymphocytes; which in turn dampen immune responses.

ANTIGENS

Antigens are any substance capable of interacting with lymphocytes to stimulate formation of antibodies. Proteins are almost always antigenic. For example, the protein composition of cell membranes determines histocompatibility antigens, which serve to differentiate host cells from foreign tissues. Haptens are small molecules, such as drugs (penicillin) that combine with a protein to induce antibody formation. Indeed, many drug reactions are caused by binding to a self-protein. Polysaccharides, when coupled to proteins, can also stimulate antibody formation, as demonstrated by the successful development of a pneumococcal vaccine. Characteristic of specific immune responses is the accelerated production of antibody-producing lymphocytes, following antigenic stimulus.

ANTIBODIES

Antibodies produced by the B-lymphocytes are referred to as immunoglobulins (Ig). Immunoglobulins are classified as IgG, IgA, IgM, IgD, and IgE, depending on their structure and function (Table 31-1). Ordinarily, specific B-lymphocytes produce only one class of immunoglobulin.

The most prevalent immunoglobulin in the plasma is IgG, the major antibody produced to provide defense against infection. The fetus does not produce IgG, but maternal antibody readily crosses the placenta to provide neonatal immunity. IgG is also referred to as gamma globulin, or complement-fixing gamma globulin. IgA is the predominant antibody in secretions (tears and mucus), serving as a topical defense mechanism. The primary function of IgM is bacterial cell wall lysis, which is facilitated by activation of complement. The function of IgD is not known. IgE (previously referred to as reagin) is present in only trace amounts in plasma. Nevertheless, this is the antibody responsible for immune-mediated hypersensitivity reactions, which are a reflection of antigen interaction with IgE. Levels of IgE are often elevated in individuals who manifest allergic phenomena such as asthma.[1]

COMPLEMENT

The complement system consists of more than 20 individual plasma proteins, which interact in a highly specific manner to generate elements of the inflammatory response.[3] Patients deficient in various complement proteins manifest an increased susceptibility to infection. The majority of complement proteins are synthesized in the liver.

Stimulation of the complement system classically requires an antigen-antibody interaction, which initiates a sequential cascading process by activating the normally inactive C_1 complement protein present in plasma (Fig. 31-2). Complement proteins, designated as C_1 through C_9, are typically described in the cascade process. An enzyme in the serum known as C_1 inhibitor protein regulates the progression of the complement cascade. A deficiency of this protein leads to uncontrolled accumulation of the components of the complement system (see the section Hereditary Angioedema). The complement system can also be activated by an alternate pathway that involves bacterial polysaccharides. The products of complement activation are responsible for a number of events, including release of vasoactive substances from mast cells, that leads to increased capillary permeability. This increased permeability permits more antibody to gain access to the site of inflammation. In addition, active components of the complement system attract polymorphonuclear leukocytes to the inflamed area, facilitating phagocytosis and lysis of bacterial cell walls.

TABLE 31-1. Properties of Human Immunoglobulins

	IgG	IgA	IgM	IgD	IgE
Location	Plasma Amniotic fluid	Plasma Saliva Tears	Plasma	Plasma	Plasma
Plasma concentration (mg·dl^{-1})	550–1900	60–333	45–145	0.3–30	Trace
Half-time (days)	23	6	5	3	2.5
Function	Immunity and defense against systemic infection	Topical defense against infection	Lysis of bacterial cell walls	Not known	Immune-mediated hypersensitivity (anaphylaxis)

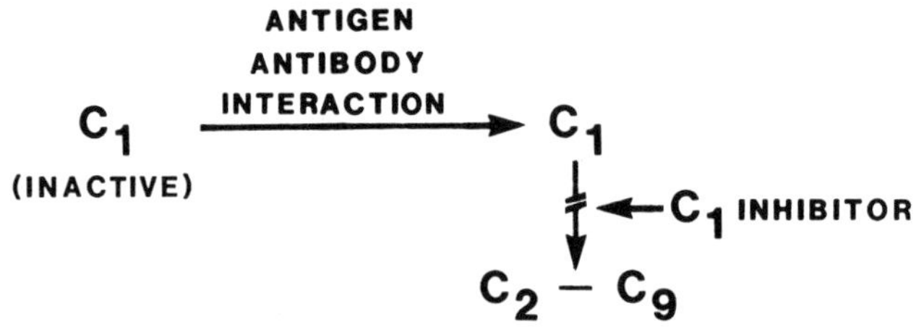

FIG. 31-2. The first component (C_1) of the complement cascade is a protein normally present in the plasma in an inactive form. Inactive C_1 protein is converted to active C_1 by an antigen-antibody interaction. Active C_1 is subsequently responsible for initiating the complement cascade, leading to the production of complement proteins designated as C_2 through C_9. Another enzyme in the plasma (C_1 inhibitor protein) closely regulates the first step in the progression of the complement cascade.

ALLERGIC REACTIONS TO DRUGS

Allergic reactions to drugs may reflect antigen-antibody interactions (anaphylaxis, immune-mediated), direct release of histamine (anaphylactoid), or activation of the complement system.[4–6] In the same patient, more than one mechanism may be involved in production of an allergic reaction. It has been estimated that one of every six patients requiring medical treatment has suffered a true or suspected allergic reaction to a drug at one time.[7] Furthermore, the incidence of allergic reactions to drugs administered during the perioperative period seems to be increasing, presumably reflecting the frequent administration of several drugs to the same patient and cross-sensitivity between drugs. Regardless of the mechanism responsible for allergic reactions, the manifestations and immediate treatment are identical.

Anaphylaxis

Anaphylaxis (immune-mediated hypersensitivity, type 1 hypersensitivity) is possible when prior exposure to an antigen (drug) has evoked the production of antigen-specific IgE antibodies and has thus sensitized the host.

Most of the IgE antibodies attach to receptor sites on cell membranes of mast cells in tissues and basophils in plasma. It is estimated each cell membrane contains 40,000 to 100,000 receptor sites potentially available to interact with IgE antibodies.[6] Subsequent exposure of the sensitized host to the same or chemically similar antigens (drugs) results in antigen-antibody interactions that initiate degranulation of mast cells and basophils. Degranulation releases vasoactive substances responsible for signs and symptoms of anaphylaxis (Table 31-2). Histamine is often considered the most important cause of manifestations of allergic reactions, although the role of leukotrienes may also be important. Indeed, leukotrienes may be 3,000- to 10,000-fold more potent in producing bronchoconstriction than histamine.[6]

PREDICTION OF ANAPHYLAXIS

It is not possible to predict reliably which patient is likely to experience anaphylaxis after administration of drugs, which are usually innocuous. Nevertheless, the likelihood of an allergic reaction to a drug increases with the number of exposures to the drug and duration between exposures. A period of about 14 days between repeat exposures is associated with the greatest potential for anaphylaxis. Patients with a history of allergy (asthma, foods, drugs, family history) have an increased incidence of anaphylaxis, primarily as a reflection of a ge-

TABLE 31-2. Vasoactive Substances Released During Antigen-Antibody
Induced Degranulation

Vasoactive Substance	Physiologic Effect
Histamine	Increased capillary permeability
	Peripheral vasodilation
	Bronchoconstriction
Leukotrienes (slow-reacting substance of anaphylaxis)	Increased capillary permeability
	Intense bronchoconstriction
	Negative inotropic effects
	Coronary vasoconstriction
Prostaglandins	Bronchoconstriction
Eosinophil chemotatic factor of anaphylaxis	Attraction of eosinophils
Neutrophil chemotatic factor	Attraction of neutrophils
Platelet activating factor	Platelet aggregation and release of vasoactive amines

netic predisposition to form increased amounts of IgE antibodies.[1] A history of allergy to specific drugs is obviously helpful, but it must be appreciated that prior uneventful exposure to those drugs does not eliminate the possibility of anaphylaxis after a subsequent exposure. Initial injection of a small test dose of drug is more likely to unmask an idiosyncratic response than to prevent anaphylaxis. For example, 5 mg of protamine is equivalent to 60×10^{15} molecules. Although the severity of anaphylaxis is likely to be related to the total dose of antigen injected, the rarity of allergic reactions does not support the routine use of test doses of drugs.

A positive intradermal test (wheal and flare greater than 4 mm in diameter) confirms the presence of specific IgE antibodies to the injected antigen.[8] This test, however, has an inherent risk, emphasizing the need to start with injection of dilute preservative-free solutions of the suspected antigen (10 μl to 20 μl of a solution containing 5 μg·ml^{-1} of the drug).[8] A false-positive intradermal test may occur if drugs capable of causing local release of histamine (morphine, meperidine, d-tubocurarine) are tested. The radioallergosorbent test (RAST) and enzyme-linked immunoadsorbent assay (ELISA) are commercially available antigen preparations, which detect specific IgE antibodies in plasma of sensitized patients. The limiting factor in the use of these tests is the availability of preparations of antigens to the suspected drug. It has been suggested, however, that these more sophisticated tests add little information to that gained from intra-

dermal testing when dealing with drugs that do not release histamine.[9]

MANIFESTATIONS OF ANAPHYLAXIS

In sensitized individuals, symptoms of anaphylaxis usually develop within 5 minutes of injection of the offending drug, although delayed reactions occasionally occur.[8] Hypotension and tachycardia are invariable accompaniments of anaphylaxis. Bronchospasm, laryngeal edema, periorbital edema, arterial hypoxemia, and cardiac dysrhythmias may occur. Extravasation of fluid into the extracellular fluid space reflects marked increases in capillary permeability. Indeed, hypovolemia is a principal cause of hypotension in these patients, although negative inotropic actions of leukotrienes could also play a role. Cutaneous flushing with or without urticaria are common. Coagulation defects and leukopenia occur in some patients. General or regional anesthesia do not protect against the occurrence of anaphylaxis. It is conceivable, however, that blockade of the innervation of the adrenal glands by regional anesthetics could accentuate symptoms of anaphylaxis by preventing the endogenous release of catecholamines, especially epinephrine (as explained in the next section).[10]

The initial in vivo response of plasma IgE concentrations during anaphylaxis is a sharp reduction (Fig. 31-3).[11] This reduction reflects the complexing of IgE antibody with newly in-

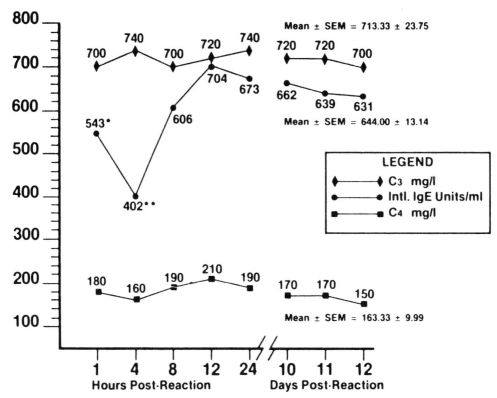

FIG. 31-3. A patient experiencing an anaphylactic reaction to thiopental manifested a decline followed by an overshoot in the plasma concentration of immunoglobulin E (IgE). Concentrations of complement proteins C_3 and C_4 were unchanged. (Lilly JK, Hoy RH. Thiopental anaphylaxis and reagin involvement. Anesthesiology 1980;53:335–7)

jected antigens. After this initial decrease, there is often an overshoot of the plasma concentration of antibodies. Absence of changes in plasma concentrations of complement proteins further supports an allergic reaction due to an anaphylaxis mechanism.

TREATMENT

The three immediate goals in treatment of anaphylaxis are reversal of arterial hypoxemia, replacement of intravascular fluid, and inhibition of further degranulation with release of vasoactive substances (Table 31-3). Often, 1 L to 4 L of balanced salt solutions and/or colloid solutions must be infused rapidly to restore intravascular fluid volume and blood pressure. Drug-induced beta-adrenergic effects increase intracellular concentrations of cyclic adeno-

sine monophosphate (cAMP) and thus decrease degranulation, explaining the rapid and often life-saving effect of epinephrine (Fig. 31-4). Beta-adrenergic effects of epinephrine also serve to relax bronchial smooth muscle, whereas drug-induced hyperglycemia attenuates the release of histamine from mast cells.[5] When anaphylaxis is life-threatening in an adult, epinephrine should be injected intravenously in initial doses of 10 μg to 100 μg.[12]

TABLE 31-3. Treatment of Allergic Reactions

Supplemental oxygen
Balanced salt solutions or colloid
Epinephrine
Diphenhydramine
Aminophylline
Corticosteroids

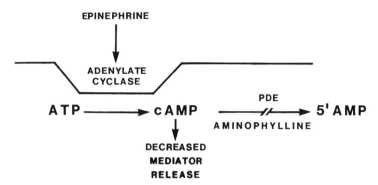

FIG. 31-4. Epinephrine attaches to receptors that face the external surface of cell membranes and act as recognition sites for ligands. Adenylate cyclase is an enzyme facing the interior of the cell and functions as an effector to catalyze the conversion of adenosine triphosphate (ATP) to cyclic adenosine monophosphate (cAMP). Interposed between the receptors and effector are guanine nucleotide regulatory proteins (G proteins) that are necessary for receptor-mediated effects on effector enzymes. Phosphodiesterase (PDE) is the enzyme responsible for converting cAMP to an inactive form (5′ AMP). Intracellular accumulation of cAMP is responsible for initiating events that decrease the release of vasoactive substances (mediators) from mast cells and basophils. (Koblin DD, Watson JE, Deady JE, et al. Inactivation of methionine synthetase by nitrous oxide in mice. Anesthesiology 1981;54:318–24)

The dose of epinephrine should be doubled and repeated every 1 minute to 3 minutes until a satisfactory blood pressure response is obtained. This titration approach with epinephrine reduces the likelihood of undesirable overshoots in blood pressure produced by alpha-adrenergic effects of the drug. When anaphylaxis is not life-threatening, subcutaneous epinephrine 0.3 mg to 0.5 mg of a 1:1000 dilution is the standard adult dose.

An antihistamine, such as diphenhydramine 50 mg to 100 mg administered intravenously to an adult, will compete for membrane receptor sites normally occupied by histamine and perhaps reduce manifestations of anaphylaxis such as hypotension, edema, pruritus, and bronchospasm. In contrast, bronchospasm or negative inotropic effects due to leukotrienes will not be influenced by antihistamines. Sympathomimetic drugs with alpha-adrenergic effects may be necessary to maintain perfusion pressure during the acute phase of anaphylaxis.

Aminophylline 3 mg·kg^{-1} to 5 mg·kg^{-1} administered intravenously is often effective in treating bronchospasm in these patients, presumably because of its ability to inhibit receptors normally responsible to adenosine. Corticosteroids (cortisol or methylprednisolone 10 mg·kg^{-1} to 15 mg·kg^{-1}) are often ad-

ministered intravenously to patients experiencing allergic reactions, although these drugs have no known action on degranulation or antigen-antibody interaction. Favorable effects of corticosteroids may reflect an enhancement of beta effects of other drugs and inhibition of pathways responsible for production of leukotrienes and prostaglandins. Corticosteroids may be uniquely beneficial in patients experiencing allergic reactions due to activation of the complement system.

Anaphylactoid Reactions

Anaphylactoid reactions reflect massive release of histamine from mast cells and basophils in response to administration of drugs.[5,6] This histamine release is independent of antigen-antibody interactions, but its manifestations are indistinguishable from those that accompany anaphylaxis. Anaphylactoid reactions may occur with the first exposure to a drug in contrast to anaphylaxis, which requires previous sensitization. The magnitude of histamine release produced on reexposure to a drug that previously resulted in an anaphylactoid reaction can be reduced by decreasing the dose of drug and slowing the rate of its intravenous infusion.

Treatment of anaphylactoid reactions is identical to that described for anaphylaxis (Table 31-3). Since histamine is the principal cause of anaphylactoid reactions, it would seem logical to provide prophylaxis in the preoperative period to patients, who, on the basis of history, are deemed likely to develop this reaction. Prophylaxis should include pretreatment with both H-1 and H-2 receptor antagonists.[5,6] Cromolyn is also effective in preventing release of histamine from cells and the subsequent development of bronchospasm. This drug, however, is of no value after an anaphylactoid reaction is established.

INHERENT DRUG-INDUCED HISTAMINE RELEASE

Primarily, basic drugs, including opioids and long-acting muscle relaxants, have an inherent ability to displace directly another basic molecule such as histamine from cells. Manifestations of drug-induced histamine release include erythema along the vein into which the drug is injected, cutaneous flushing, and reductions in blood pressure. It is estimated that plasma histamine concentrations must double before blood pressure reductions occur. This degree of drug-induced histamine release is insufficient, however, to be considered an anaphylactoid reaction; and the patient should not be considered to be allergic to the drug. Pretreatment with histamine receptor antagonists is more effective in controlling symptoms associated with drug-induced histamine release than those accompanying anaphylactoid reactions. Presumably, fewer vasoactive substances are involved in drug-induced responses and histamine is relatively more important.

DRUGS ASSOCIATED WITH ALLERGIC REACTIONS

Allergic reactions have been reported to virtually all drugs that may be injected during the administration of anesthesia.[5,6,13] These include muscle relaxants, drugs used for induction of anesthesia, local anesthetics, opioids, chymopapain, antibiotics, protamine, intravascular contrast media, blood, and plasma volume expanders. Although clinical manifestations of allergic reactions may be modified by the effects of anesthetics, there is no evidence that anesthetics alter the incidence of anaphylaxis.[1,10]

Muscle Relaxants

Anaphylactic and anaphylactoid reactions have been most frequently reported after the administration of muscle relaxants.[13–16] Furthermore, there may be cross-sensitivity between muscle relaxants. It is estimated that 50 percent of patients who experience an allergic reaction to a muscle relaxant will also be allergic to one or more of the other muscle relaxants.[17] Cross-sensitivity between muscle relaxants emphasizes structural similarities of these drugs, especially the presence of one or more antigenic quaternary ammonium groups. Indeed, IgE antibodies to choline have been detected in patients who have experienced allergic reactions to succinylcholine and other muscle relaxants.[18] Drug-induced histamine release from mast cells and basophils is also a possibility with all muscle relaxants, although this effect is least likely after administration of vecuronium (see the section Inherent Drug-Induced Histamine Release).

Anaphylaxis that occurs after the first exposure to a muscle relaxant may reflect sensitization that occurs from prior contact with cosmetics and soaps, which also contain quaternary ammonium groups. In this regard, the majority of reported allergic reactions to muscle relaxants have been in females. The liquid, but not powder, form of succinylcholine contains methylparaben, introducing the possibility that the preservative could be responsible for stimulating antibody production (see the section Local Anesthetics). Although structural similarities are not present, many patients who experience allergic reactions to succinylcholine are also allergic to penicillin.[15]

Drugs Used for Induction of Anesthesia

Allergic reactions after administration of barbiturates for the induction of anesthesia are rare (1 in 30,000 administrations) but often life-threatening.[5,6] The majority of reported cases are in patients with a history of allergy and previous uneventful anesthetics that included barbiturates.[11,19,20] In one report, an allergic reaction occurred after induction of anesthesia with thiamylal, despite the chronic uneventful use of oral barbiturates.[21] Anaphylaxis is the most frequent mechanism for allergic reactions evoked by barbiturates. Indeed, reduction of IgE levels was demonstrable within 40 minutes after the intravenous administration of 10 µg of thiopental to a patient with suspected hypersensitivity to this drug.[19] Allergic reactions may occur after administration of both thiobarbiturates or oxybarbiturates, although in vitro data suggest methohexital is least likely to evoke the release of histamine (Fig. 31-5).[22]

Allergic reactions to etomidate differ from those of other drugs used for the induction of

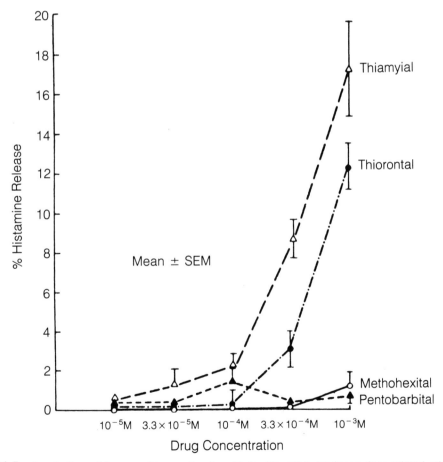

FIG. 31-5. Incubation of human skin mast cells with barbiturates produces dose-related release of histamine in the presence of thiamylal and thiopental. Histamine release did not occur at any concentration of methohexital or pentobarbital. (Hirshman CA, Edelstein RA, Ebertz JM, Hanifin JM. Thiobarbiturate-induced histamine release in human skin mast cells. Anesthesiology 1985;63:353–6)

anesthesia in that symptoms are predominantly cutaneous or gastrointestinal in the absence of cardiopulmonary manifestations.[6] Likewise, life-threatening allergic reactions after administration of ketamine are unlikely, although cutaneous rashes have been reported.[23]

Local Anesthetics

Allergic reactions to local anesthetics are rare, despite the frequent use of these drugs. Furthermore, adverse responses due to excessive plasma concentrations of local anesthetic (systemic toxicity) are often incorrectly labeled allergic reactions. Indeed, it is estimated that only about 1 percent of all reactions to local anesthetics have an allergic mechanism.[24]

DIFFERENTIAL DIAGNOSIS

The mechanism for adverse responses to local anesthetics can often be determined by careful questioning of the patient and review of past medical records describing the event. For example, the occurrence of hypotension and seizures is characteristic of a systemic reaction due to excessive blood levels of local anesthetics. Conversely, patients who manifest urticaria, conjunctivitis, and bronchospasm are most likely having an allergic reaction. These initial allergic phenomena may be followed later by laryngeal edema. A vagal response to injection of local anesthetics is suggested by the presence of a slow heart rate and syncope. Finally, tachycardia and hypertension associated with injection of local anesthetics most likely reflect systemic absorption of epinephrine that was combined with the anesthetics.

ALLERGIC POTENTIAL

Ester local anesthetics that produce metabolites related to the highly antigenic compound para-aminobenzoic acid are more likely than amide local anesthetics to produce allergic reactions. Indeed, reports of amide-induced allergic reactions are rare.[25] Local anesthetic solutions may also contain methylparaben or propylparaben as preservatives with bacteriostatic and fungistatic properties. The structural similarity of these preservatives to para-aminobenzoic acid renders them antigenic. As a result, anaphylaxis may be due to prior stimulation of antibody production by the preservative and not local anesthetics.

A common clinical problem deals with the safety of administering local anesthetics to patients with a history of allergy to these types of drugs. It is generally agreed that cross-sensitivity does not exist between ester and amide local anesthetics. Therefore, it should be acceptable to administer amide local anesthetics to patients with an allergic history for ester local anesthetics. The reverse of this recommendation would also be true. It must be remembered, however, that use of preservative-free local anesthetics is important, since these compounds may have been the etiology of allergic reactions incorrectly attributed to local anesthetics.

DOCUMENTATION OF ALLERGY

Documentation of allergy to local anesthetics is difficult. Intradermal testing may give false-positive results due to needle trauma or from local histamine release after skin puncture. Furthermore, protein in the skin may not be the protein with which local anesthetics have complexed to initiate the formation of antibodies. Metabolites of local anesthetics could also be the offending stimulus, in which case skin tests would not be reliable indicators of the true allergic potential of local anesthetics. Despite these disadvantages, others believe that safe local anesthetics can be identified in patients with an allergic history, using intradermal testing as part of a progressive challenge protocol.[24] All factors considered, it would seem reasonable to recommend intradermal testing with preservative-free alternative local anesthetics in occasional patients who describe a convincing allergic history and in whom failure to document a safe drug would prevent use of local anesthesia.

Opioids

Anaphylaxis occurring after administration of opioids is rare but possible.[26] Delayed manifestations of anaphylaxis have been observed after administration of fentanyl.[8] In this report, a second injection of fentanyl, administered about 2 hours after the first, failed to evoke symptoms of an allergic reaction, suggesting the initial challenge had produced nearly complete degranulation such that immediate rechallenge failed to produce any significant additional release of vasoactive substances. Opioids, especially morphine, may directly evoke release of histamine from mast cells and basophils to produce anaphylactoid reactions in susceptible patients.

Chymopapain

Allergic reactions that may be life-threatening occur in about 0.82 percent of patients undergoing chemonucleolysis with chymopapain. These allergic reactions appear to be more common in females, patients with multiple allergies, and individuals with known allergies to papaya. The principal manifestation of an allergic reaction is hypotension; only about one-fourth of patients develop bronchospasm. Manifestations of allergic reactions may be immediate or delayed up to 2 hours after injection of chymopapain. Pretreatment with H-1 and H-2 receptor antagonists, as well as corticosteroids, has been recommended; but allergic reactions may still occur.[27]

Antibiotics

Anaphylaxis and anaphylactoid reactions may occur after intravenous administration of antibiotics, especially penicillins, in the perioperative period. The most common manifestations of allergy to penicillins are maculopapular rashes and urticaria. In occasional patients, life-threatening bronchospasm and angioedema manifesting as marked swelling of the face, lips, and tongue, with or without laryngeal edema, occurs. In addition to the well-recognized potential for penicillin to evoke allergic reactions, the aminoglycoside derivative, vancomycin has been associated with a high incidence of allergic reactions.[28] Slow administration of vancomycin may reduce the magnitude of drug-induced histamine release in susceptible patients, although anaphylaxis has also been observed. Cross-sensitivity between penicillins and cephalosporins, as well as between aminoglycosides and other para-aminobenzoic acid derivatives (ester local anesthetics), should be considered.

Protamine

Anaphylactic reactions to protamine may occur in patients allergic to seafood, emphasizing the derivation of this drug from salmon sperm.[29] Another group at increased risk for anaphylaxis after administration of protamine in large doses to neutralize heparin are patients treated with protamine-containing insulin preparations.[30,31] Presumably, small amounts of protamine in insulin preparations (0.7 mg of protamine in 25 units of protamine zinc insulin) stimulate production of antibodies such that anaphylaxis occurs when large doses of protamine are administered to neutralize the effects of heparin. Vasectomized or infertile males may have circulating antibodies to spermatozoa, but an increased risk for allergic reactions to protamine is undocumented and seems unlikely since the antibody levels are very low. Protamine is also capable of directly evoking the release of histamine from cells and in susceptible patients producing an anaphylactoid reaction (see the section Drug-Induced Histamine Release). Patients known to be allergic to protamine present a therapeutic dilemma when neutralization of heparin is required since hexadimethrine, the alternative drug to protamine, is not commercially available. Spontaneous dissipation of the anticoagulant effects of heparin is prolonged and may be associated with large amounts of blood loss, especially after successful weaning from cardiopulmonary bypass.[32] In patients considered to be at increased risk for protamine allergy, it is prudent to begin with a small intravenous test dose (1 mg to 10 mg) of the drug. Bronchoconstriction and pulmonary hypertension, which occasionally accompanies protamine neutralization of heparin, may reflect complement activation and release of thromboxane.[33]

Intravascular Contrast Media

Iodine in intravascular contrast media, as injected intravenously for radiologic studies, evokes systemic reactions in about 5 percent of patients. Patients at greatest risk are those with co-existing allergies to other drugs or foods. Many reactions appear to be anaphylactoid and can be modified with pretreatment including H-1 and H-2 receptor antagonists and corticosteroids and limitation of the dose of iodine.

Blood and Plasma Volume Expanders

Allergic reactions to properly cross matched blood occur in about 3 percent of patients with manifestations ranging from pruritus, urticaria, and raised body temperature to noncardiogenic pulmonary edema. Incompatible plasma proteins may initiate the release of histamine from mast cells and basophils. Synthetic plasma protein solutions (dextran, gelatin, hydroxyethyl starch solutions) have been implicated in anaphylaxis and anaphylactoid reactions, with manifestations ranging from only a cutaneous rash and modest hypotension to shock and bronchospasm. Low molecular weight dextrans cannot induce formation of antibodies but may react with preformed antidextran IgG or IgM antibodies produced in response to prior exposure to polysaccharides of viral or bacterial origin. Dextran may also activate the complement system to produce signs of an allergic reaction. Although the incidence of allergic reactions is very rare plasma substitutes should be administered with caution to patients with allergic histories.

RESISTANCE TO INFECTION AND CANCER

There is abundant evidence that exposure to anesthesia and surgery alters many facets of immunocompetence.[1] Conceivably, depression of the immune system by anesthesia could increase the likelihood that patients would develop postoperative infections or that co-existing infections might be augmented. Also, anesthetic-induced depression of the immune system could interfere with the normal protective role of this system in the suppression of malignant cell proliferation.

Resistance to Infection

Inflammatory responses to infection require production and mobilization of polymorphonuclear leukocytes, and subsequent migration of these cells, for phagocytosis. Evidence suggests that local and general anesthetics (especially nitrous oxide) produce dose-dependent depression of all these functions.[1,34] Nevertheless, effects produced by these drugs are probably clinically insignificant, considering the usual duration of anesthesia and the dose used. Indeed, the incidence of postoperative infections seems more likely to be related to surgical trauma and associated release of cortisol and catecholamines that are known to inhibit phagocytosis.[1] Anesthetic drugs, in the absence of surgical stimulation, are not predictably associated with increased circulating levels of cortisol or catecholamines. The consensus, based on available information, is that effects of anesthetics on resistance to infection are transient, reversible, and of minor importance, when compared with the prolonged immunosuppressive effects of cortisol and catecholamines released as part of the hormonal response to surgery.[1]

If the hormonal response to surgical stimulation is undesirable with respect to vulnerability to infection, it could be reasoned that light anesthesia, which does not reliably attenuate activity of the sympathetic nervous system, is less desirable than a deeper level of anesthesia. Evidence suggests that about 1.5 MAC halothane or enflurane, or greater than 1 mg·kg^{-1} of morphine, is necessary to prevent the sympathetic nervous system response to surgical skin incision in 50 percent of patients.[35] Sternal incisions requiring cutting of bone seem to need even more anesthesia to block sympathetic nervous system responses. Regional anesthesia may also reduce hormonal responses to surgical stimulation.[34] Despite these observations, there is no evidence that the incidence of postoperative infections can be altered by the depth of anesthesia or by the techniques selected to produce anesthesia.

Possible bacteriostatic effects of anesthetic drugs must also be considered. Local anesthetics have been shown to have such effects on a wide variety of organisms at concentrations achievable with topical application.[34] Clinical implications of this observation are that topical anesthesia, as used for bronchoscopy, could reduce the incidence of positive cultures. Conversely, concentrations of local anesthetics in the circulation, in association with regional anesthesia or after intravenous administration, do not alter bacterial growth. Likewise, volatile anesthetics do not have bacteriostatic effects.[34] Liquid volatile anesthetics, however, may be bactericidal. Volatile anesthetics in doses as low as 0.2 MAC produce dose-dependent inhibition of measles virus replication and reduce mortality in mice receiving intranasal influenza virus.[36]

Resistance to Cancer

Immune competence is essential for host resistance to cancer. It is a clinical impression that some patients with the preoperative di-agnosis of cancer experience a rapid growth of the tumor after anesthesia and surgery. Conceivably, drugs administered to produce anesthesia could enhance tumor initiation or spread, by depressing host resistance. Despite this concern, there is no evidence that short-term effects of anesthetic drugs are of any significance in the resistance of the host to cancer.[37] As with infections, the more important concern is immunosuppression produced by hormonal responses to surgical stimulation. If hormonal responses are indeed undesirable from the aspect of host resistance to cancer, it would seem logical to suppress these responses with either regional or deep general anesthesia. It should be emphasized, however, that there is no evidence to support the validity of this speculation.

In contrast to the concern in patients with cancer, immunosuppression secondary to hormonal responses produced by surgical stimulation could be beneficial for patients undergoing organ transplants. Nevertheless, if such benefit does occur, it is probably too small or transient to be of any significance in the early period after administration of anesthesia and surgery.

TOXIC EFFECTS OF ANESTHETICS IN THE NONPATIENT POPULATION

Health hazards documented to occur with employment in the operating room include an increased rate of spontaneous abortion and birth defects in the offspring of women either working in the operating room or married to men who work in this environment.[38-40] The most invoked explanation is chronic exposure to trace concentrations of waste anesthetic gases, particularly nitrous oxide. Efficient scavenging systems can remove over 90 percent of waste anesthetic gases. In view of the strong suggestion that these gases may be responsible for health hazards, it would seem prudent to recommend scavenging in all areas in which the administration of anesthesia is undertaken. Nevertheless, data to support beneficial effects of scavenging are not available. Indeed, animal studies employing intermittent exposure to trace concentrations of nitrous oxide, halothane, enflurane, and isoflurane have not revealed harmful reproductive effects.[41] Conversely, exposure of pregnant rats to 75 percent nitrous oxide for 6 hours daily on three consecutive days is associated with increased fetal resorptions (abortions).[42] In view of these data, the advisability of not working in the operating room if a woman is contemplating pregnancy is an unsettled question.

Exposure of animals to nitrous oxide has also been shown to produce reversible dose-dependent inhibition of the activity of the vitamin B_{12} containing enzyme, methionine synthetase (Fig. 31-6).[40,43] For example, nitrous oxide (0.8 atm) administered for 30 minutes can decrease enzyme activity by more than 50 percent. Conversely, low concentrations of nitrous oxide (0.5 atm) or volatile anesthetics (1 MAC) do not alter activity of methionine syn-

thetase. Nitrous oxide inhibits methionine synthetase activity by oxidizing the cobalt atom in vitamin B_{12} from an active to an inactive state. Inhibition of enzyme activity results in decreased availability of tetrahydrofolate, which is necessary for the synthesis of deoxyribonucleic acid. Interference with synthesis of deoxyribonucleic acid is consistent with the development of anemia and leukopenia in patients with tetanus who were treated with nitrous oxide [44] and may play a role in the polyneuropathy observed in dentists who administer nitrous oxide to patients for dental analgesia, [45] or in individuals who periodically inhale high concentrations of nitrous oxide for nonmedical purposes.[46,47] Nevertheless, onset of nitrous oxide-induced inhibition of methionine synthetase activity seems to be much slower in humans than in animals. For example, administration of 60 percent to 70 percent nitrous oxide to patients for 25 minutes to 217 minutes (average 88 minutes) produces no de-

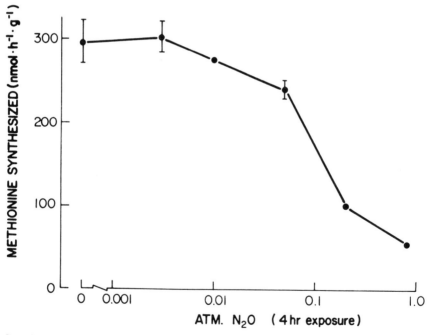

FIG. 31-6. Nitrous oxide produces dose-dependent inhibition of methionine synthetase activity in liver preparations taken from mice. All exposures lasted 4 hours. Each point represents the Mean ± SE for eight mice. For the points for which the error bars are not exhibited, the errors are within the size of the symbols. (Koblin DD, Watson JE, Deady JE, et al. Inactivation of methionine synthetase by nitrous oxide in mice. Anesthesiology 1981;54:318–24)

tectable effects on methionine synthetase activity.[40,48] Furthermore, absence of changes in activity of this enzyme during chronic exposure to trace concentrations of nitrous oxide does not support a role for this mechanism in the production of spontaneous abortion or birth defects.[43]

DISORDERS OF THE IMMUNOGLOBULINS

X-Linked Agammaglobulinemia

X-linked agammaglobulinemia (congenital agammaglobulinemia, panhypoglobulinemia) is a genetically transmitted disease characterized by recurrent bacterial infections starting in infancy or early childhood, decreased plasma concentrations, or absence of all classes of immunoglobulins (plasma IgG concentrations less than 100 mg·dl^{-1}) and inability to produce antibodies, even in response to intense antigenic stimulation.[49] As the name implies, only males are affected, although rare cases with similar clinical features have been described in females. The defect in these patients appears to be failure of B-lymphocyte maturation such that antibodies cannot be produced. In contrast, T-lymphocytes are normal and cell-mediated immunity is intact.

In addition to recurrent bacterial infections, patients with X-linked agammaglobulinemia often have persistent viral or parasitic infections. They are at risk for development of vaccine-associated poliomyelitis and an unusual form of enterovirus encephalitis. *Pneumocystis carinii* pneumonia may be the presenting manifestation of this disease. Recurrent infections may lead to chronic sinusitis and bronchiectasis.

Treatment of X-linked agammaglobulinemia is with intramuscular injections of gamma globulin or infusions of plasma. The limiting factor for use of gamma globulin is the large volume required for intramuscular injection; hepatitis is a risk of plasma administration. Immunoglobulin preparations appropriate for intravenous use will provide a needed alternative. The usual monthly intramuscular dose of gamma globulin is 100 mg·kg^{-1}, which provides an increase of about 200 mg·dl^{-1} in plasma concentrations of IgE. Antibiotics are indicated when bacterial infection occurs.

Acquired Hypoimmunoglobulinemia

Acquired hypoimmunoglobulinemia does not appear to be genetically determined and is usually not manifested until after puberty. Symptoms and treatment are the same as for X-linked agammaglobulinemia. This syndrome is associated with autoimmune diseases and malabsorption syndromes.

Selective Immunoglobulin A Deficiency

An absence or marked reduction in plasma concentrations of IgA (below 5 mg·dl^{-1}) is not uncommon being present in as many as 1 of 700 people in the general population.[49] The majority of such persons are asymptomatic and remain undetected until they are screened as potential blood donors.[50] Although this defect may be without adverse effects, there may be an increased incidence of sinus and pulmonary infections, autoimmune disorders, allergy, and malabsorption syndromes. Drugs such as phenytoin may result in induction of suppressor T-lymphocytes, which interferes with maturation of B-lymphocytes and production of antibodies including IgA.[51] Some of these patients produce anti-IgA antibodies and will develop anaphylactic reactions when given solutions containing IgA. Therefore, these patients should receive blood or blood components only from IgA-deficient donors.

Wiskott-Aldrich Syndrome

Wiskott-Aldrich syndrome is inherited on an X-linked recessive basis, thus affecting only males. The syndrome is characterized by thrombocytopenia, eczema, and increased susceptibility to infections. Thrombocytopenia is the result of rapid platelet destruction caused by an intrinsic defect in platelets. Presenting features are usually related to thrombocytopenia and associated hemorrhage. Therapy is with platelet transfusions as thrombocytopenia is resistant to corticosteroids and is not improved by splenectomy. Plasma concentrations of IgM are often reduced.

Ataxia Telangiectasia

Ataxia telangiectasia is characterized by progressive cerebellar ataxia beginning in childhood, recurrent sinus and pulmonary infections, and subsequent development of telangiectasia of the bulbar conjunctivae. A familial incidence suggests this disease is inherited in an autosomal recessive manner. Skin manifestations may include café au lait spots and sclerodermoid changes. Disorders of glucose metabolism may be present. Most patients manifest absent or reduced plasma concentrations of IgA and IgE. Function of T-lymphocytes may also be impaired in these patients. There is a high incidence of terminal lymphoma.

Chronic Mucocutaneous Candidiasis

Chronic mucocutaneous candidiasis is an infection with *Candida albicans* involving skin, nails, scalp, buccal, and vaginal membranes. Endocrinopathies, including hypoparathyroidism and hypoadrenocorticism, are commonly associated with this infection. Defects in cell-mediated immunity are likely.

Conversely, humoral immunity appears intact as evidenced by increased plasma concentrations of antibodies for *Candida albicans*.

Cryoglobulinemia

Cryoglobulinemia is a disorder in which circulating abnormal immunoglobulins (cold agglutinins) cause agglutination of erythrocytes in the presence of decreased body temperatures.[52] Normally, symptoms occur only at temperatures below 32 degrees Celsius. On rare occasions, however, abnormal immunoglobulins can cause agglutination in areas such as the renal vasculature, despite a nearly normal body temperature. Acute renal failure may accompany this microvascular thrombosis.[52] Indeed, renal dysfunction eventually occurs in more than 20 percent of patients. Acrocyanosis, Raynaud's phenomenon, and gangrene may also occur.

Management of anesthesia in patients with cryoglobulinemia should include maintenance of body temperature above 35 degrees Celsius during the perioperative period. This goal is best achieved by an increased ambient temperature of the operating room, use of a warming blanket, and ventilation of the lungs with warmed and humidified gases. Passing intravenous fluids through blood warmers before delivery to patients should also reduce the loss of body heat during anesthesia.

Patients scheduled for operations requiring cardiopulmonary bypass with hypothermia present special problems.[53] Preoperative screening for cold agglutinins will identify susceptible patients. In these patients, preoperative plasmapheresis may be used to reduce circulating levels of cold agglutinins. Maintenance of blood temperature above the critical temperature determined for agglutination to occur is indicated.

Plasma Cell Myeloma

Immunoglobulins are secreted by plasma cells, with each individual cell producing a single type of protein. Plasma cell myeloma is present when there is poorly controlled growth of a single line of plasma cells.

Multiple Myeloma

Multiple myeloma is characterized by a neoplastic proliferation of plasma cells. These cells invade bone marrow, resulting in thrombocytopenia, neutropenia, anemia, and increased susceptibility to infections. Malignant plasma cells can also infiltrate the liver, spleen, and lymph nodes. These cells have a special predilection for the nasopharynx and paranasal sinuses. Plasma cell tumors may invade the epidural space and produce symptoms of spinal cord compression, requiring emergency laminectomy.

Plasmacytomas are plasma cell tumors in bone that result in painful fractures, particularly of the vertebrae. Hypercalcemia from destruction of bone by plasma cells can lead to central nervous system depression and renal dysfunction.

Immunoglobulins associated with multiple myeloma can inactivate circulating procoagulants, including factors I, II, and XI. In addition, abnormal immunoglobulins can interfere with platelet function. Deposition of Bence Jones proteins in renal tubules may result in renal dysfunction. Approximately 70 percent of patients with myelomatous proteinuria manifest renal disease, characterized by casts in the renal tubules.

DIAGNOSIS

Diagnosis of multiple myeloma is suggested by increased circulating levels of immunoglobulins, especially IgG or IgA. Conversely, plasma albumin concentrations are often reduced in these patients.

TREATMENT

Treatment of multiple myeloma is with chemotherapeutic drugs and corticosteroids, in an effort to reduce proliferation of plasma cells. Prevention of dehydration is important if plasma calcium levels are elevated. Bed rest must be avoided, as inactivity leads to increased mobilization of calcium and predisposes to urinary tract infections and formation of venous thrombi due to venous stasis. Localized radiotherapy is beneficial for treatment of isolated bone lesions due to plasma cell invasion. Plasmapheresis before transfusion of blood is indicated if there is co-existing hyperviscosity of the plasma.

The presence of compression fractures emphasizes the need for caution in positioning these patients during anesthesia and surgery. Postoperatively, pathologic fractures of the ribs may impair ventilation and predispose to the development of pneumonia. Finally, it is an undocumented speculation that the presence of abnormal circulating immunoglobulins, plus decreased plasma albumin concentrations, could result in altered responses to drugs normally bound to protein.

Waldenström's Macroglobulinemia

Waldenström's macroglobulinemia is due to neoplastic proliferation of cells, which produce abnormal immunoglobulins related to the IgM class. Plasma viscosity is increased by increased circulating levels of immunoglobulins. Lymphadenopathy and hepatosplenomegaly reflect infiltration of these tissues by abnormal proteins. Anemia and an increased incidence of spontaneous hemorrhage are frequent findings in these patients. In contrast to multiple myeloma, Waldenström's macroglobulinemia rarely involves the skeletal system. As a result, renal dysfunction due to hypercalcemia is unlikely to occur.

Treatment of Waldenström's macroglobulinemia is with plasmapheresis to diminish the viscosity of the plasma, particularly if transfusion of blood is planned. Cancer chemotherapeutic drugs are administered to reduce the proliferation of the cells responsible for production of abnormal immunoglobulins.

Amyloidosis

Amyloidosis is characterized by deposition of glycoproteins in various tissues, including the heart, vascular smooth muscle, kidneys, spleen, adrenal glands, small intestine, peripheral nerves, and skin. The frequent finding of these abnormal proteins in the wall of the rectum makes rectal biopsy an important diagnostic test.

Symptoms associated with amyloidosis reflect invasion of tissues by glycoproteins. For example, renal failure, carpal tunnel syndrome, and macroglossia are manifestations. Development of amyloidosis is frequently associated with multiple myeloma, rheumatoid arthritis, and prolonged antigenic challenges, as produced by chronic infections.

DISORDERS OF THE COMPLEMENT SYSTEM

Hereditary Angioedema

Hereditary angioedema is a rare autosomal dominant disorder, which is associated with abnormally low plasma concentrations of C_1 esterase inhibitor or by the presence of functionless C_1 esterase inhibitor.[3] This inhibitor protein is necessary for regulation of the complement cascade system (Fig. 31-2). In the absence of C_1 esterase inhibitor, initial activation of C_1 is followed by uncontrolled and excessive activation of the complement cascade with depletion of C_2 and C_4 and ultimate release of vasoactive substances that increase vascular permeability and lead to edema formation. The disease often presents at puberty in an accelerated state.

MANIFESTATIONS

Hereditary angioedema is characterized by episodic and painless edema of the skin (face and limbs) and mucous membranes of the respiratory and gastrointestinal tracts. Attacks typically last 48 hours to 72 hours. Edema involving the larynx is the most serious manifestation of this syndrome. Abdominal cramps may reflect edema of the small intestine and, on occasion, falsely suggest the need for an exploratory laparotomy. An attack may occur spontaneously but is more often initiated by trauma, particularly dental procedures. Diagnosis of hereditary angioedema is on the basis of family history, clinical picture, and documentation of low or absent plasma levels of C_1 inhibitor protein. About 15 percent of patients with this disease have normal levels of C_1 inhibitor protein, but the activity of this protein is zero.

PROPHYLAXIS BEFORE SURGERY

The most effective long-term control of this disease is with the androgen derivative danazol. This drug induces a threefold to fivefold increase in plasma C_1 inhibitor protein levels, presumably by stimulating synthesis of this enzyme in the liver. Prophylaxis initiated with danazol at least 10 days before a surgical procedure is of vital importance, especially if trauma to the airway is likely as during intubation of the trachea.[54] A useful alternative to this approach is the administration of 2 units to 4 units of fresh frozen plasma within 24 hours preoperatively.[55] Fresh frozen plasma is a natural source of C_1 inhibitor protein producing sustained increases (1.25 $mg \cdot dl^{-1}$ for each unit infused) in plasma concentrations that last 1 day to 4 days. Viral hepatitis is a hazard of treatment with fresh frozen plasma.

TREATMENT OF ACUTE ATTACK

Treatment of an acute attack of hereditary angioedema is with fresh frozen plasma, which produces evidence of clinical improvement within 40 minutes. It is theoretically possible that fresh frozen plasma in addition to providing C_1 inhibitor protein would also provide substrates such as C_2 and C_4, thus enhancing the acute attack. In practice this does not seem to occur.[56] Alternatively, a purified preparation of C_1 inhibitor protein has been reported to be effective in abating symptoms when administered intravenously during an acute attack.[57] This preparation is also effective as prophylaxis and does not introduce the risk of viral hepatitis. Should airway obstruction develop during an acute attack of hereditary angioedema, a tube should be placed in the trachea until the edema involving the airway subsides. Antihistamines, corticosteroids, or epinephrine are not effective in therapy.

MANAGEMENT OF ANESTHESIA

Management of anesthesia for patients with hereditary angioedema is based on proper prophylaxis in the preoperative period (danazol for 10 days to 14 days plus fresh frozen plasma the evening before surgery) and availability of appropriate drugs and equipment to treat an acute attack, should edema develop intraoperatively.[56] Intramuscular injections do not seem to cause any unique problems in these patients. Trauma to the upper airway, as with placement of an oropharyngeal airway or during direct laryngoscopy for intubation of the trachea, must be minimized. Indeed, regional anesthetic techniques are reasonable considerations, if their selection will eliminate the need for intubation of the trachea. Nevertheless, intubation of the trachea with a cuffed tube should not be avoided in these patients, if its placement will contribute to the safe conduct of the anesthetic. Choice of drugs to provide general or regional anesthesia is not influenced by the presence of hereditary angioedema.

Deficiency of C_2 Complement Protein

Deficiency of C_2 complement protein occurs in approximately 1 in every 10,000 individuals.[3] About one-half of the C_2 deficient patients described have had systemic lupus erythematosus or a related disorder such as Henoch-Schönlein purpura. This association

may reflect a viral origin for these diseases and complement participation in viral neutralization.

Deficiency of C_3 Complement Protein

Deficiency of C_3 complement protein is associated with increased susceptibility to life-threatening bacterial infections. Complement-mediated functions such as bactericidal activity, chemotaxis, and opsonization are absent in C_3-deficient plasma. Patients who are homozygous for a deficiency in C_5, C_6, C_7, or C_8 complement proteins also manifest increased susceptibility to infections; in contrast to patients with a deficiency in C_3, they are also subject to disseminated gonococcal disease.[3]

AUTOIMMUNE DISEASE

Autoimmune disease implies antigen-antibody responses in which host tissues act as antigens and binding with antibodies is deleterious. Resulting tissue injury may be due to release of destructive enzymes or may reflect antigen-antibody interactions in vascular smooth muscles, producing vasculitis. Vasculitis may be limited to specific organs (often the kidneys) or may be generalized, involving diverse areas of the vascular system.

In healthy patients, T-lymphocytes are probably responsible for blocking antibody production to host antigen. Failure of suppressor T-lymphocytes to prevent such antibody production results in autoimmune diseases. The mechanism for initiating an autoimmune process is not known but may be genetically determined. For example, infection with beta-hemolytic streptococci may be the triggering event in genetically susceptible hosts.

REFERENCES

1. Walton B. Effects of anesthesia and surgery on immune status. Br J Anaesth 1979;51:37–43
2. Forbes AR. Halothane depresses mucociliary flow in the trachea. Anesthesiology 1976;45:59–63
3. Colten HR, Alper CA, Rosen FS. Genetics and biosynthesis of complement proteins. N Engl J Med 1981;304:653–6
4. Beamish D, Brown DT. Adverse responses to IV anaesthetics. Br J Anaesth 1981;53:55–7
5. Beaven MA. Anaphylactoid reactions to anesthetic drugs (Editorial). Anesthesiology 1981;55:3–5
6. Moudgil GC. Anaesthesia and allergic drug reactions. Can Anaesth Soc J 1986;33:400–14
7. Van Arsdel PP. Diagnosing drug allergy. JAMA 1982;247:2576–81
8. Bennett MJ, Anderson LK, McMillan JC, et al. Anaphylactic reaction during anaesthesia associated with positive intradermal skin test to fentanyl. Can Anaesth Soc J 1986;33:75–8
9. Fisher M. Intradermal testing after anaphylactoid reaction to anaesthetic drugs: Practical aspects of performance and interpretation. Anaesth Intensive Care 1984;12:115–20
10. Hirshman CA, Peters J, Cartwright-Lee I. Leukocyte histamine release to thiopental. Anesthesiology 1982;56:64–7
11. Lilly JK, Hoy RH. Thiopental anaphylaxis and reagin involvement. Anesthesiology 1980;53:335–7
12. Barach EM, Nowak RM, Lee TG, Tomlanovich MC. Epinephrine for treatment of anaphylactic shock. JAMA 1984;251:2118–22
13. Fisher M McD, Munro I. Life-threatening anaphylactoid reactions to muscle relaxants. Anesth Analg 1983;62:559–64
14. Farmer BC, Sivarajan M. An anaphylactoid response to a small dose of d-tubocurarine. Anesthesiology 1979;51:358–9
15. Ravindran RS, Klemm JE. Anaphylaxis to succinylcholine in a patient allergic to penicillin. Anesth Analg 1980;59:944–5
16. Mishima S, Yamamura T. Anaphylactoid reaction to pancuronium. Anesth Analg 1984;63:865–6
17. Harle DG, Baldo BA, Fisher MM. Cross-reactivity of metocurine, atracurium, vecuronium and fazadinium with IgE antibodies from patients unexposed to these drugs but allergic to other myoneural blocking drugs. Br J Anaesth 1985;57:1073–6
18. Harle DG, Baldo BA, Fisher MM. Detection of IgE antibodies to suxamethonium after anaphylactoid reactions during anaesthesia. Lancet 1984;1:930
19. Etter MS. Helrich M. Mackenzie CF. Immunoglobulin E fluctuation in thiopental anaphylaxis. Anesthesiology 1980;52:181–3
20. Wyatt R, Watkins J. Reaction to methohexitone. Br J Anaesth 1975;47:119–20
21. Thompson DS, Eason CN, Flacke JW. Thiamylal anaphylaxis. Anesthesiology 1973;39:556–8
22. Hirshman CA, Edelstein RA, Ebertz JM, Hanifin JM. Thiobarbiturate-induced histamine release in human skin mast cells. Anesthesiology 1985;63:353–6
23. Mathieu A, Goudsouzian N, Snider MT. Reaction to ketamine: Anaphylactoid or anaphylactic? Br J Anaesth 1975;47:624–7
24. DeShazo RD, Nelson HS. An approach to the patient with a history of local anesthetic hypersensitivity: Experience with 90 patients. J Allergy Clin Immunol 1979;63:387–94
25. Brown DT, Beamish D, Wiedsmith JAW. Allergic reaction to an amide local anaesthetic. Br J Anaesth 1981;53:435–7
26. Levy JH, Rockoff MA. Anaphylaxis to meperidine. Anesth Analg 1982;61:301–3
27. Bruno LA, Smith DS, Bloom MJ, et al. Sudden hypotension with a test dose of chymopapain. Anesth Analg 1984;63:533–5
28. Symons NLP, Hobbes AFT, Leaver HK. Anaphylactoid reactions to vancomycin during anaesthesia: Two clinical reports. Can Anaesth Soc J 1985;32:178–81
29. Knape JTA, Schuller JL, deHaan P, et al. An anaphylactic reaction to protamine in a patient allergic to fish. Anesthesiology 1981;55:324–5
30. Moorthy SS, Pond W, Rowland RG. Severe circulatory shock following protamine (an anaphylactic reaction). Anesth Analg 1980;59:77–8
31. Stewart WJ, McSweeney SM, Kellett MA, et al. Increased risk of severe protamine reactions in NPH insulin-dependent diabetics undergoing cardiac catheterization. Circulation 1984;70:788–92
32. Campbell FW, Goldstein MF, Akins PC. Management of the patient with protamine hypersensitivity for cardiac surgery. Anesthesiology 1984;61:761–4
33. Morel DR, Zapol WM, Thomas ST, et al. C5a and thromboxane generation associated with pulmonary vaso- and broncho-constriction during protamine reversal of heparin. Anesthesiology 1987;66:597–604
34. Duncan PG, Cullen BF. Anesthesia and immunology. Anesthesiology 1976;45:522–38
35. Roizen MF, Horrigan RW, Frazer BM. Anesthetic doses blocking adrenergic (stress) and cardio-

vascular responses to incision—MAC BAR. Anesthesiology 1981;54:390–8

36. Knight PR, Bedows E, Nahrwold ML, et al. Alterations in influenza virus pulmonary pathology induced by diethyl ether, halothane, enflurane, and pentobarbital anesthesia in mice. Anesthesiology 1983;58:209–15

37. Lewis RE, Cruse JM, Hazelwood J. Halothane-induced suppression of cell-mediated immunity in normal and tumor-bearing C3H$_f$/He mice. Anesth Analg 1980;59:666–71

38. Spence AA, Cohen EN, Brown BW. Occupational hazards for operating room-based physicians. JAMA 1977;238:955–9

39. Cohen EN, Brown BW, Wu ML, et al. Occupational disease in dentistry and chronic exposure to trace anesthetic gases. J Am Dent Assoc 1980;101:21–31

40. Spence AA. Environmental pollution by inhalation anaesthetics. Br J Anaesth 1987;59:96–109

41. Mazze RI. Fertility, reproduction, and postnatal survival in mice chronically exposed to isoflurane. Anesthesiology 1985;63:663–7

42. Mazze RI, Fujinaga M, Rice SA, et al. Reproductive and teratogenic effects of nitrous oxide, halothane, isoflurane, and enfurane in Sprague-Dawley rats. Anesthesiology 1986;64:339–44

43. Koblin DD, Watson JE, Deady JE, et al. Inactivation of methionine synthetase by nitrous oxide in mice. Anesthesiology 1981;54:318–24

44. Lassen HCA, Henrickson E, Neukirch F, Fristensen HS. Treatment of tetanus. Severe bone-marrow depression after prolonged nitrous oxide anaesthesia. Lancet 1956;1:527–30

45. Brodsky JB, Cohen EN, Brown BW, et al. Exposure to nitrous oxide and neurologic disease among dental professionals. Anesth Analg 1981;60:297–301

46. Layzer RB, Fishman RA, Schafer JA. Neuropathy following abuse of nitrous oxide. Neurology 1978;28:504–6

47. Layzer RB. Myeloneuropathy after prolonged exposure to nitrous oxide. Lancet 1978;2:1227–30

48. Nunn JF, Sharer NM, Bottiglieri T, Rossiter J. Effect of short-term administration of nitrous oxide on plasma concentrations of methionine, tryptophan, phenylalanine and s-adenosyl methionine in man. Br J Anaesth 1986;58:1–10

49. Rosen FS, Cooper MD, Wedgwood RJP. The primary immunodeficiencies. N Engl J Med 1984;311:235–42

50. Ropars C, Muller A, Paint N, et al. Large scale detection of IgA deficient blood donors. J Immunol Methods 1982;54:183–9

51. Dosch H-M, Jason J, Gelfand EW. Transient antibody deficiency and abnormal T suppressor cells induced by phenytoin. N Engl J Med 1982;306:406–9

52. Carloss HW, Tavassoli M. Acute renal failure from precipitation of cryoglobulins in a cold operating room. JAMA 1980;244:1472–3

53. Diaz JH, Cooper ES, Ochsner JL. Cardiac surgery in patients with cold autoimmune diseases. Anesth Analg 1984;63:349–52

54. Pitts JS, Donaldson VH, Forristal J, Waytt RJ. Remission induced in hereditary angioneurotic edema with an attenuated androgen (danazol): Correlation between concentrations of C_1-inhibitor and the fourth and second components of complement. J Lab Clin Med 1978;92:501–7

55. Jaffe CJ, Atkinson JP, Gelfand JA, Frank MM. Hereditary angioedema: The use of fresh frozen plasma for prophylaxis in patients undergoing oral surgery. J Allergy Clin Immunol 1975;55:386–93

56. Poppers PJ. Anaesthetic implications of hereditary angioneurotic oedema. Can J Anaesth 1987;34:76–8

57. Gadek JE, Hosea SW, Gelfand JA, et al. Replacement therapy in hereditary angioedema. Successful treatment of acute episodes of angioedema with partly purified C_1 inhibitor. N Engl J Med 1980;302:542–6

32

Psychiatric Illness

MENTAL DEPRESSION

Mental depression sufficient to warrant medical attention affects 2 percent to 4 percent of the general population.[1] Functional deficiency of two central nervous system neurotransmitters, norepinephrine and serotonin (5-hydroxytryptamine), is presumed to be responsible for many of the clinical manifestations of mental depression. Drugs effective in treating mental depression most likely act by increasing the amounts of neurotransmitters available in the central nervous system. Drugs most often used include tricyclic and tetracyclic antidepressants and monoamine oxidase inhibitors. Electroconvulsive therapy may be useful initial treatment in certain patients.

Tricyclic Antidepressants

Tricyclic antidepressants are often administered as initial treatment of mental depression. These drugs potentiate the action of norepinephrine in the central nervous system by prevention of uptake (reuptake) back into postganglionic sympathetic nerve endings. The role of this effect in reversing mental depression remains unsubstantiated despite its frequent proposal as a mechanism. Prevention of uptake of serotonin may also contribute to the efficacy of these drugs.

ADVERSE EFFECTS

Adverse effects of tricyclic antidepressants are numerous and include sedation, anticholinergic effects (tachycardia, dry mouth, blurred vision, urinary retention, prolonged gastric emptying time), and cardiovascular changes (Table 32-1). With the exception of doxepin, tricyclic antidepressants slow conduction of cardiac impulses through the atria and ventricles manifesting on the electrocardiogram as prolongation of the P-R intervals, widening of QRS complexes, and flattening or inversion of T-waves. Nevertheless, these electrocardiographic changes in the absence of excessive plasma concentrations of drug are probably benign and may gradually disappear with continued therapy.[2] Previous suggestions that tricyclic antidepressants increase the risk of cardiac dysrhythmias and sudden death have not been substantiated in the absence of drug overdose. Furthermore, even in the presence of co-existing cardiac dysfunction tricyclic antidepressants lack adverse effects on left ventricular function and may even possess cardiac antidysrhythmic properties.[3,4] Orthostatic hypotension, however, is more common in patients treated with imipramine than with nortriptyline.[4]

TABLE 32-1. Characteristics of Tricyclic Antidepressant Drugs

Generic Drug (Trade Name)	Dose Range (mg·day^{-1})	Sedative Potency	Affected Neurotransmitter	Anticholinergic Potency
Amitriptyline (Elavil)	75–300	High	Serotonin	High
Nortriptyline (Aventyl)	40–150	Moderate	Norepinephrine Serotonin	Moderate
Imipramine (Tofranil)	75–300	Low	Norepinephrine Serotonin	Moderate
Desipramine (Norpramin)	75–300	Low	Norepinephrine	Low
Doxepin (Sinequan)	75–300	High	Unknown	Moderate

DRUG CHOICE

The choice of specific tricyclic antidepressants is designed to match side effects of these drugs with the clinical symptoms of patients (Table 32-1). For example, drugs with sedative properties (amitriptyline, doxepin) are ideal for agitated patients. When tachycardia would be undesirable, the drug of choice is desipramine because it has the least anticholinergic properties. Prolongation of cardiac conduction is produced by amitriptyline, nortriptyline, and imipramine, but not by doxepin. Therefore, doxepin is the logical drug choice for administration to patients with evidence of cardiac conduction defects on the electrocardiogram.

MANAGEMENT OF ANESTHESIA

Treatment with tricyclic antidepressants need not be discontinued before administration of anesthesia for elective operations. Alterations in responses to drugs administered during the perioperative period, however, should be anticipated in these patients. For example, increased availability of neurotransmitters in the central nervous system can lead to increased anesthetic requirements.[5] Likewise, increased availability of norepinephrine at postsynaptic receptors in the peripheral sympathetic nervous system can be responsible for exaggerated blood pressure responses after administration of indirect-acting vasopressors such as ephedrine. If vasopressors are required during the perioperative period, a direct-acting drug such as methoxamine or phenylephrine would seem useful. Should hypertension require treatment, alpha-adrenergic blockers, such as phentolamine, would be specific pharmacologic antagonists. Potent peripheral vasodilators, such as nitroprusside, would also be effective.

Continuous monitoring of the electrocardiogram is important in the perioperative period, in view of the potential for tricyclic antidepressant drugs to produce cardiac conduction abnormalities. Atropine would be appropriate for management of atrioventricular heart block.

Chronic therapy with tricyclic antidepressants may alter responses to pancuronium. For example, tachydysrhythmias have been observed after administration of pancuronium to patients anesthetized with halothane who were also receiving imipramine.[6] In dogs chronically treated with imipramine, administration of pancuronium resulted in tachycardia and ventricular dysrhythmias (Fig. 32-1).[6] Similar cardiac dysrhythmias in dogs did not occur when anesthesia was maintained with enflurane. The dose of exogenous epinephrine necessary to produce ventricular dysrhythmias during anesthesia with volatile drugs may be reduced by prior acute treatment with imipramine.[7] Therefore, it is conceivable that treatment with tricyclic antidepressants could also accentuate the arrhythmogenic potential of absorbed epinephrine, as used with local anesthetics in the performance of peripheral nerve blocks. Conversely chronic imipramine ther-

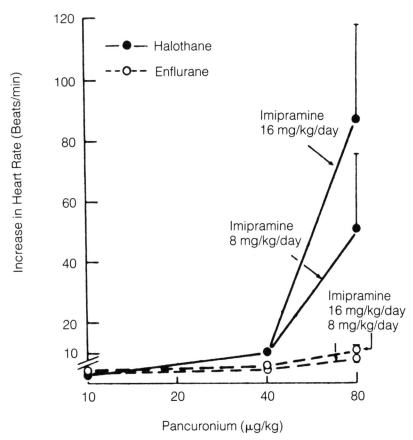

FIG. 32-1. Chronic administration of imipramine is associated with dose-related increases in heart rate after administration of pancuronium to dogs anesthetized with halothane but not enflurane. (Edwards RP, Miller RD, Roizen MF, et al. Cardiac responses to imipramine and pancuronium during anesthesia with halothane or enflurane. Anesthesiology 1979;50:421–5)

apy does not alter cardiac dysrhythmia potential, presumably because of compensatory mechanisms occurring at the sympathetic nerve endings.[8] In addition, it should be remembered that catecholamine stores in the heart can be decreased by chronic treatment with tricyclic antidepressants. Therefore, cardiac depressant effects of drugs used to produce anesthesia could be exaggerated; however, this remains an unconfirmed speculation.

Maintenance of anesthesia with enflurane in patients taking tricyclic antidepressants is questionable since both drugs produce electroencephalographic evidence of seizure activity. Indeed, clonic movements during administration of low inspired concentrations of enflurane have been observed in patients receiving amitriptyline.[9] It was speculated that enflurane-induced seizure activity in these patients was enhanced by the presence of amitriptyline. In animals, tricyclic antidepressants augment analgesic and ventilatory depressant effects of opioids, as well as sedative effects of barbiturates. If these responses also occur in patients, it is predictable that doses of these drugs should be reduced so as to avoid exaggerated and/or prolonged effects.[10] Postoperatively, the likelihood of delerium and confusion might be increased by the additive anticholinergic effects of tricyclic antidepressants and centrally active anticholinergic drugs used for preoperative medication.

Monoamine Oxidase Inhibitors

Monoamine oxidase inhibitors comprise a heterogenous group of drugs that have in common the ability to prevent oxidative deamination of exogenous and endogenous monoamines. As a result, these drugs lead to increased intraneuronal concentrations of amine neurotransmitters including dopamine, norepinephrine, epinephrine, and serotonin (5-hydroxytryptamine). It is this intraneuronal accumulation of neurotransmitters in the central nervous system that is presumed to produce antidepressant effects. Indeed, these drugs may be used to treat mental depression in patients who do not show therapeutic responses to tricyclic antidepressants. Clinically used monoamine oxidase inhibitors are classified as hydrazine or nonhydrazine derivatives with a further subdivision based on the presence or absence of selectivity for the A or B form of the enzyme (Fig. 32-2) (Table 32-2).[11] Theoretically, use of selective monoamine oxidase-A inhibitors could reduce the incidence of adverse effects of nonselective monoamine

oxidase inhibitors. Indeed, adverse effects greatly limit the clinical use of monoamine oxidase inhibitors. In contrast to tricyclic antidepressants, monoamine oxidase inhibitors have negligible anticholinergic effects and do not produce sedation or sensitize the heart to arrhythmogenic effects of epinephrine.[7]

ADVERSE EFFECTS

Adverse effects produced by monoamine oxidase inhibitors include hepatotoxicity and undesirable responses that reflect the impact of these drugs on peripheral sympathetic nervous system activity. For example, inhibition of the activity of the monoamine oxidase enzyme present in the cytoplasm of all peripheral sympathetic nerve endings results in increased availability of norepinephrine to postsynaptic receptor sites. Therefore, sympathomimetic drugs, such as ephedrine, that act by stimulating the release of norepinephrine can precipitate severe hypertension. Likewise, foods containing tyramine (cheeses, wines) have been associated with hypertensive crises in patients receiving monoamine oxidase inhibitors. This

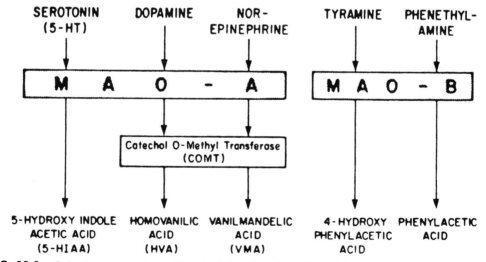

FIG. 32-2. Selective monoamine oxidase inhibitors interfere with activity of either the monoamine oxidase A (MAO-A) or B forms (MAO-B) of the enzyme. Nonselective monoamine oxidase inhibitors interfere with both forms of the enzyme. (Michaels I, Serrins N, Shier NW, Barash PG. Anesthesia for cardiac surgery in patients receiving monoamine oxidase inhibitors. Anesth Analg 1984;63:1041–4. Reprinted with permission from IARS)

TABLE 32-2. Classification of Monoamine Oxidase Inhibitors

	MAO-A	MAO-B
Hydrazine Compounds		
Phenelzine	+	+
Isocarboxazid	+	+
Iproniazid	+	+
Nonhydrazine Compounds		
Tranylcypromine	+	+
Pargyline	?	+
Clorgyline	+	0
Deprenyl	?	+

occurs because tyramine is normally inactivated by monoamine oxidase. However, tyramine becomes a potent stimulus for the release of norepinephrine from postganglionic sympathetic nerve endings when activity of the monoamine oxidase enzyme is inhibited.

Orthostatic hypotension has been observed in patients receiving monoamine oxidase inhibitors. The mechanism for this hypotension is not known but may reflect accumulation of false neurotransmitters such as octopamine. Octopamine is a less active neurotransmitter than norepinephrine at postsynaptic receptor sites. As a result, evidence of decreased sympathetic nervous system activity occurs. This mechanism may also explain antihypertensive effects observed with chronic use of monoamine oxidase inhibitors.

Although uncommon, adverse interactions between monoamine oxidase inhibitors and opioids must be appreciated.[12] Specifically, hypertension, hypotension, tachycardia, diaphoresis, respiratory depression, hyperthermia, seizures, and coma have been observed after administration of opioids to patients being treated with monoamine oxidase inhibitors. Meperidine has been the most often incriminated drug, but the same syndrome can occur with other opioids. Explanations for these adverse responses include reduced metabolism of opioids, mass sympathetic nervous system discharge caused by opioids, and formation of toxic metabolites. A speculated mechanism for the elevation in body temperature after administration of opioids to these patients is increased central nervous system concentrations of serotonin. Indeed, the effects

of serotonin are potentiated by meperidine, which inhibits the neuronal uptake of this neurotransmitter.

MANAGEMENT OF ANESTHESIA

Since enzyme inhibition of monoamine oxidase is often irreversible, it is frequently recommended that monoamine oxidase inhibitors be discontinued at least 14 days to 21 days before elective surgery to permit synthesis of new enzyme. Regeneration of new enzyme, however, may be more rapid after discontinuation of tranylcypromine or pargyline, as these drugs do not bind irreversibly to monoamine oxidase. Even patients receiving irreversible enzyme inhibitors may be safely anesthetized (e.g., electroconvulsive therapy) without waiting 14 days to 21 days for regeneration of new enzyme to occur.[11,13]

Measurement of liver function tests would seem prudent before induction of anesthesia. Indeed, prolonged apnea after administration of succinylcholine has been attributed to decreased plasma cholinesterase activity, presumably reflecting reduced production of this enzyme due to drug-induced hepatic dysfunction.[14]

When anesthesia and operation cannot be delayed, it is important to adjust the choice and doses of drugs used during anesthesia. Opioids should be avoided in the preoperative and intraoperative period. Induction of anesthesia with intravenous barbiturates or benzodiazepines is acceptable, but central nervous system and respiratory depression are likely to be accentuated. Succinylcholine should be used with caution, in view of the possibility of decreased plasma cholinesterase activity. Nitrous oxide combined with volatile anesthetics is acceptable for maintenance of anesthesia. Selection of specific volatile anesthetics, however, should consider the possibility of co-existing drug-induced liver disease. It is possible that anesthetic requirements would be elevated due to increased concentrations of norepinephrine present in the central nervous system, although this theory is unsubstantiated.

During anesthesia and operation, avoidance of stimulation of the sympathetic nervous system, as produced by arterial hypoxemia, hypercarbia, hypotension, or indirect-acting vasopressors, is essential to reduce the incidence of hypertension and/or cardiac dysrhythmias. Should vasopressors be required, direct-acting drugs such as methoxamine or phenylephrine are recommended. Even with these drugs, the doses should be reduced to minimize the likelihood of exaggerated hypertensive responses.

Morphine is the preferred drug for postoperative analgesia, but the dose should be the least amount necessary to produce pain relief. Furthermore, a high index of suspicion for adverse effects produced by the opioid should be maintained. An alternative to opioids is provision of postoperative analgesia with regional block procedures, intraspinal opioids, or transcutaneous electrical nerve stimulation.

Neuroleptic Malignant Syndrome

Neuroleptic malignant syndrome occurs in 0.5 percent to 1 percent of all patients treated with antipsychotic drugs.[15] The syndrome typically develops over 24 hours to 72 hours and is characterized by hyperthermia, hypertonicity of skeletal muscles, autonomic nervous system instability with alterations in blood pressure, and heart rate plus cardiac dysrhythmias and fluctuating levels of consciousness.[15] Skeletal muscle spasm may so reduce chest wall compliance that mechanical support of ventilation becomes necessary. Creatine kinase is often elevated and liver transaminase enzymes are increased. The cause of neuroleptic malignant syndrome is not known and, as a result, treatment is symptomatic. Skeletal muscle rigidity is treated with dantrolene, nondepolarizing muscle relaxants and dopamine agonists. Mortality may approach 30 percent with common causes of death including cardiac failure and/or dysrhythmias, ventilatory failure, renal failure, and thromboembolism. In vitro skeletal muscle contracture testing reveals responses similar to those present in malignant hyperthermia susceptible patients.[16]

Electroconvulsive Therapy

Electroconvulsive therapy is typically reserved for treatment of severe mental depression in patients who have not responded to drugs, those jeopardized by drug side effects, and acutely suicidal patients.[17–19] It is estimated that 4 percent of psychiatric admissions are given electroconvulsive therapy and that 75 percent to 85 percent of these patients respond favorably. Although the mechanism of action of electroconvulsive therapy is unknown, it is generally agreed that grand mal seizures lasting 25 seconds to 60 seconds, rather than the electricity, produce the therapeutic benefits. The electrical stimulus produces a grand mal seizure consisting of a tonic phase lasting 10 seconds to 12 seconds and a 30 second to 50 second clonic phase. The electroencephalogram shows changes similar to those present during spontaneous grand mal seizures.

PHYSIOLOGIC SIDE EFFECTS OF ELECTROCONVULSIVE THERAPY

Physiologic side effects of electroconvulsive therapy manifest principally on the cardiovascular and central nervous systems (Table 32-3).[19] For example, an initial central vagal discharge may lead to bradycardia with a fall in blood pressure lasting about 60 seconds followed by sympathetic nervous system activation and an increase in heart rate and blood pressure. Ventricular premature beats presumably reflect excess sympathetic nervous system activity. Venous return to the heart is reduced by raised intrathoracic pressure accompanying the seizure and/or positive pressure ventilation of the lungs. Cardiovascular changes produced by electroconvulsive therapy detract from the use of this therapy in patients with coronary artery disease. Cerebral blood flow increases up to sevenfold, reflecting increases in cerebral oxygen consumption that accompany the seizures. This increased cerebral blood flow gives rise to dramatic but transient increases in intracranial pressure. For this reason electroconvulsive therapy is not

TABLE 32-3. Physiologic Effects of Electroconvulsive Therapy

Parasympathetic nervous system stimulation
  Bradycardia
  Hypotension

Sympathetic nervous system stimulation
  Tachycardia
  Hypertension
  Cardiac dysrhythmias

Increased cerebral blood flow

Increased intracranial pressure

Decreased alveolar ventilation

Increased intraocular pressure

Increased intragastric pressure

Memory impairment

considered in patients with known co-existing increases in intracranial pressure. Elevations in intraocular pressure are inevitable side effects of electrically-induced seizures and may detract from the use of this therapy in patients with glaucoma. Likewise, increased intragastric pressure occurs during seizure activity. Transient apnea plus postictal confusion may follow seizures. The most frequent reported long-term effects of electroconvulsive therapy are memory disturbances. Memory impairment may be less with unilateral electrode placement on the nondominant hemisphere.

MANAGEMENT OF ANESTHESIA

Anesthesia is usually administered to ensure patient comfort and safety during the electrically induced seizure.[17] Patients should be in fasted states before this treatment. Preanesthetic medication is not recommended, as drug-produced sedation could prolong the period of recovery after electroconvulsive therapy. Intravenous administration of anticholinergic drugs (atropine or glycopyrrolate) may be included 1 minute to 2 minutes before the induction of anesthesia and delivery of the electrical current to decrease the likelihood of bradycardia, which can be associated with electrically-induced seizures. Intravenous ad-

ministration of anticholinergic drugs is more effective than subcutaneous injection for the prevention of bradycardia and spares patients from the discomfort of dry mouths. Centrally acting anticholinergic drugs may have additive effects with central and peripheral anticholinergic actions produced by tricyclic antidepressants manifesting as delirium and confusion in the postanesthetic period.[19] For this reason, glycopyrrolate may be preferred to atropine when electroconvulsive therapy is administered to patients being treated with tricyclic antidepressants. Nevertheless, many patients have safely undergone electroconvulsive therapy without prior administration of anticholinergic drugs.[19] Nitroglycerin ointment applied 45 minutes before electroconvulsive therapy minimizes the magnitude of treatment-induced hypertension and thus may be useful in patients at risk for developing myocardial ischemia.[20] Certainly, monitoring of the electrocardiogram is indicated, in view of the occasional occurrence of cardiac dysrhythmias in association with electroconvulsive therapy.

Anesthesia is most often provided with an intravenous barbiturate plus succinylcholine. It is important to keep doses of barbiturates to a minimum, since these drugs can increase central nervous system seizure thresholds, as well as decrease the duration of electrically induced seizures. This effect is undesirable, as it is thought that the efficacy of electroconvulsive therapy is at least partially determined by the duration of the grand mal seizure (ideally 25 seconds to 60 seconds). Intravenous administration of methohexital, 0.5 mg·kg^{-1} to 1.0 mg·kg^{-1}, is a frequent choice to produce unconsciousness before electroconvulsive therapy. Thiopental has no advantage over methohexital and might be associated with a longer recovery time. It is also important to recognize that prior treatment of patients with tricyclic antidepressants or monoamine oxidase inhibitors may augment the depressant effects of barbiturates. Intravenous injection of succinylcholine immediately following the induction of anesthesia is designed to attenuate the potentially dangerous skeletal muscle contractions and subsequent fractures, which could be associated with the seizures. Although the amount of succinylcholine administered varies, a dose of 0.3 mg·kg^{-1} to 0.5 mg·kg^{-1} is usually sufficient to attenuate adequately contractions of skeletal muscles and still permit visual confirmation that seizures are occurring. Pretreatment with nondepolarizing muscle relaxants before administration of succinylcholine has not been evaluated in these patients. Support of ventilation of the lungs with increased inspired concentrations of oxygen is necessary, both before the production of seizures and until the effects of succinylcholine have dissipated. Denitrogenation of the lungs with oxygen before production of seizures minimizes the likelihood for the development of arterial hypoxemia, should it become difficult to support ventilation of the lungs during the period of seizure activity. Furthermore, it should be appreciated that apnea (usually lasting about 2 minutes) can occur after electroconvulsive therapy, in the absence of succinylcholine. Use of a peripheral nerve stimulator will confirm the degree of neuromuscular blockade produced by succinylcholine and will also identify patients with previously unrecognized atypical cholinesterase enzyme. Since repeated anesthetics will be necessary, it is possible to establish a dose of methohexital and succinylcholine that produces the most predictable and desirable effects in each patient. Myalgia is remarkably uncommon (about 2 percent) after administration of succinylcholine to these patients.[19]

Muscle relaxants may obscure evidence that grand mal seizures have occurred. In this regard, the surest way to document electrically induced seizures is to record the electroencephalogram. An alternative method is to observe movement in an arm isolated from the circulation with a tourniquet before administration of succinylcholine. Arm movements persisting for at least 25 seconds are regarded as evidence that a seizure has occurred.

Occasionally, electroconvulsive therapy will be necessary in patients with permanently implanted artificial cardiac pacemakers. Fortunately, most artificial pacemakers do not seem to be adversely influenced by the electrical current used to produce seizures. Nevertheless, it would seem prudent to have an appropriate external magnet available to ensure the capability for converting the pacemaker to an asynchronous mode should malfunction

occur. In addition, continuous monitoring of the electrocardiogram, use of a Doppler sensor, and palpation of a peripheral arterial pulse document the uninterrupted function of the artificial pacemaker.

MANIA

Clinical manifestations of mania most likely reflect functional excesses of neurotransmitters in the central nervous system. Lithium is the drug of choice for the treatment of mania, as well as for prophylaxis against its recurrence.[21]

Lithium

The reason for the calming effects of lithium during manic phases of manic-depressive illness is not known. Conceivably, lithium acts by decreasing the excitability of cells. Indeed, lithium mimics sodium by entering cells during depolarization. Subsequent extrusion of lithium from cells is slow, which is consistent with decreased cell activity. In addition, lithium appears to interfere with the ability of several different hormones to stimulate adenylate cyclase. Reduced activity of adenylate cyclase would be associated with decreased responses of postsynaptic receptor sites to norepinephrine.

Lithium is efficiently absorbed following oral administration. Therapeutic plasma levels of lithium are 0.5 mEq·L^{-1} to 1.5 mEq·L^{-1}. These concentrations produce no significant effects on ventilation or the cardiovascular system. However, leukocytosis in the range of 10,000 mm^3 to 14,000 mm^3 may occur. Lithium inhibits release of thyroid hormones and may lead to hypothyroidism in a small number of patients. Long-term administration of lithium occasionally results in a vasopressin-resistant diabetes insipidus-like syndrome, which resolves when the drug is discontinued. Prolonged use of lithium causes benign and reversible depression of T-waves on the electrocardiogram.

RENAL EXCRETION

Lithium is almost exclusively eliminated via the kidneys with a half-time of 24 hours. Reabsorption of lithium occurs at proximal convoluted tubules and is inversely related to the concentrations of sodium in the glomerular filtrate. For this reason, the administration of diuretics, which lead to increased renal excretion of sodium, will facilitate reabsorption of lithium, with corresponding elevations in its blood level. Conversely, administration of sodium or osmotic diuretics will favor the renal excretion of lithium.

TOXICITY

The therapeutic range for lithium is narrow, with plasma concentrations below 0.8 mEq·L^{-1} often being ineffective and levels above 1.5 mEq·L^{-1} producing toxicity. Early and mild signs of lithium toxicity include sedation, skeletal muscle weakness, and changes on the electrocardiogram characterized by widening of the QRS complexes. Atrioventricular heart block, hypotension, and seizures may occur when plasma lithium concentrations exceed 2 mEq·L^{-1}. Treatment of lithium toxicity is with the intravenous administration of sodium-containing solutions and osmotic diuretics in efforts to speed renal excretion of the drug.

MANAGEMENT OF ANESTHESIA

Treatment with lithium need not be discontinued before elective surgery. It is helpful, however, to understand the interactions between sodium and lithium, and the potential elevations in plasma lithium concentrations that can be produced by the administration of diuretics that stimulate the loss of sodium. Therefore, it is important to include sodium in the intravenous fluids administered during the perioperative period. In addition, caution must be used in stimulating urine output with loop diuretics such as furosemide, as this treatment could increase plasma lithium concentrations. The association of sedation with lithium therapy suggests that anesthetic requirements for

injected and inhaled drugs may be reduced. Indeed, sedative effects of lithium, plus the absence of cardiopulmonary depression, is the rationale for considering the use of this drug for preoperative medication.[22] Responses to muscle relaxants must be monitored, as the duration of action of succinylcholine and pancuronium, but not d-tubocurarine, may be prolonged in the presence of lithium.[23]

SCHIZOPHRENIA

Schizophrenia accounts for about 20 percent of all persons treated for mental illness.[1] The hallmark of schizophrenia is psychosis characterized by delusions or hallucinations. Treatment of schizophrenia is with antipsychotic drugs (Table 32-4). These drugs are not addicting, tolerance does not occur, and safety is emphasized by the wide margin between therapeutic and lethal doses. The mechanism of action of antipsychotic drugs is not well established, but is most likely due to inhibition of the action of neurotransmitters such as dopamine at postsynaptic receptor sites. Indeed, prolactin secretion is stimulated by phenothiazines, presumably reflecting inhibition of the actions of dopamine at the hypothalamus and pituitary.

Sedation and extrapyramidal symptoms are potential responses that can accompany treatment with antipsychotic drugs. Acute dystonia (contraction of the muscles of the neck, mouth, and tongue; rigidity; tremor) responds to the intravenous administration of 25 mg to 50 mg of diphenhydramine. The most serious side effect of therapy with antipsychotic drugs is tardive dyskinesia, which is characterized by involuntary choreoathetoid movements. Tardive dyskinesia usually develops after several months of treatment with antipsychotic drugs and may be irreversible. Geriatric patients are most susceptible to developing this complication.

Cardiovascular effects of antipsychotic drugs are minimal, but high doses may produce alpha-adrenergic blockade, with subsequent decreases in systemic vascular resistance and reductions in blood pressure. This effect on the

TABLE 32-4. Drugs Used in Treatment of Schizophrenia

Classification	Generic Name	TradeName	Dose (mg·day^{-1})
Phenothiazines	Chlorpromazine	Thorazine	100
	Triflupromazine	Vesprin	30
	Mesoridazine	Serentil	50
	Thioridazine	Mellaril	95
	Fluphenazine	Prolixin	2
	Perphenazine	Trilafon	10
	Trifluoperazine	Stelazine	5
Thioxanthenes	Chlorprothixene	Taractan	65
	Thiothixene	Navane	5
Butyrophenones	Haloperidol	Haldol	2
Indolones	Molindone	Moban	10

sympathetic nervous system may be an important consideration when planning management of anesthesia. For example, intraoperative reductions in blood pressure, especially with blood loss or positive pressure ventilation of the lungs, may be exaggerated, since compensatory sympathetic nervous system-mediated vasoconstriction is attenuated by the alpha-adrenergic blockade. The presence of sedation preoperatively may parallel reduced anesthetic requirements. Cholestasis was observed early in the clinical use of chlorpromazine but rarely seems to occur with current use of this drug. Nevertheless, preoperative evaluation of liver function would exclude even rare patients manifesting adverse hepatic effects from antipsychotic drugs.

ALCOHOLISM

Disulfiram may be administered as an adjunctive drug along with psychiatric counseling to decrease consumption of alcohol.[24] The unpleasantness of symptoms (flushing, vertigo, diaphoresis, nausea, vomiting, tachycardia) that accompanies ingestion of alcohol in the presence of disulfiram is the basis for use of this drug. These symptoms reflect the accumulation of acetaldehyde from oxidation of alcohol, which cannot be further oxidized because of disulfiram-induced inhibition of acetaldehyde dehydrogenase activity. Compliance with long-term oral disulfiram therapy is often poor.

Management of anesthesia in patients being treated with disulfiram should consider the potential presence of disulfiram-induced sedation and hepatotoxicity. Decreased drug requirements could reflect additive effects with co-existing sedation or the ability of disulfiram to inhibit metabolism of drugs other than alcohol. For example, disulfiram may result in potentiation of the effects of benzodiazepines. Acute and unexplained hypotension during general anesthesia could reflect inadequate stores of norepinephrine due to disulfiram-induced inhibition of dopamine beta-hydroxylase.[24] This hypotension may respond to ephedrine, but direct-acting sympathomimetics, such as phenylephrine, would seem more logical for treatment of hypotension due to depletion of norepinephrine. Use of regional anesthesia may be influenced by occasional patients treated with disulfiram who develop polyneuropathy. Alcohol-containing solutions, as used for skin cleansing, should be avoided in these patients.

AUTISM

Autism is a developmental disorder characterized by disturbances in the rate of development before 30 months of age of physical, social, and language skills, although specific cognitive capacities may be present. Abnormal responses to sensory inputs manifest with hyper-reactivity that alternates with hyporeactivity. The prevalence of this syndrome is estimated as 4.7 per 10,000 live births, and males are affected five times as often as females. Enlarged cerebral ventricles may be present and seizures frequently begin during late childhood. The cause of this syndrome is not known but proposed etiologic factors include viral encephalitis and metabolic disorders. Congenital or familial factors are suggested by the occurrence of autism in twins or siblings. No treatment alters the natural history of the disease and life expectancy is normal. Long-range prognosis is poor and many patients are classified as mentally retarded. Drug therapy is symptomatic and works best when aimed at controlling specific behaviors.

REFERENCES

1. Cassem NH. Psychiatry. In: Federman E, Rubenstein DD, eds. Scientific American Medicine. New York. Scientific American 1981:1–18
2. Thompson TL, Moran MG, Nies AS. Psychotropic drug use in the elderly. N Engl J Med 1983;308:194–8
3. Veith RC, Raskind MA, Caldwell JH, et al. Cardiovascular effects of tricyclic antidepressants in depressed patients with chronic heart disease. N Engl J Med 1982;306:954–9
4. Roose SP, Glassman AH, Giardina E-GV, et al. Nortriptyline in depressed patients with left ventricular impairment. JAMA 1986;256:521–6
5. Miller RD, Way WL, Eger EI. The effects of alphamethyldopa, reserpine, guanethidine and iproniazid on minimum alveolar anesthetic requirement (MAC). Anesthesiology 1968;29:1153–8
6. Edwards RP, Miller RD, Roizen MF, et al. Cardiac responses to imipramine and pancuronium during anesthesia with halothane or enflurane. Anesthesiology 1979;50:421–5
7. Wong KC, Puerto AX, Puerto BA, Blatnick RA. Influence of imipramine and pargyline on the arrhythmogenicity of epinephrine during halothane, enflurane or methoxyflurane anesthesia in dogs. Anesthesiology 1980;53:S25
8. Spiss CK, Smith CM, Maze M. Halothane-epinephrine arrhythmias and adrenergic respon-

siveness after chronic imipramine administration in dogs. Anesth Analg 1984;63:825–8
9. Sprague DH, Wolf S. Enflurane seizures in patients taking amitriptyline. Anesth Analg 1982;61:67–8
10. Frommer DA, Kulig KW, Marx JA, Rumack B. Tricyclic antidepressant overdose. A review. JAMA 1987;257:521–6
11. Michaels I, Serrins M, Shier NQ, Barash PG. Anesthesia for cardiac surgery in patients receiving monoamine oxidase inhibitors. Anesth Analg 1984;63:1014–4
12. Brown TCK, Cass NM. Beware—the use of MAO inhibitors is increasing again. Anaesth Intensive Care 1979;7:65–8
13. El-Ganzouri AR, Ivankovich AD, Braverman B, McCarthy R. Monoamine oxidase inhibitors: Should they be discontinued preoperatively? Anesth Analg 1985;64:592–6
14. Wong KC. Preoperative discontinuation of monoamine oxidase inhibitor therapy: An old wives' tale. Seminars in Anesthesiology 1986;5:145–8
15. Guze BH, Baxter LR. Neuroleptic malignant syndrome. N Engl J Med 1985;313:163–6
16. Caroff SN, Rosenberg H, Fletcher JE, et al. Malignant hyperthermia susceptibility in neuroleptic malignant syndrome. Anesthesiology 1987;67:20–5
17. Marks PJ. Electroconvulsive therapy: physiological and anesthetic considerations. Can Anaesth Soc J 1984;31:541–8
18. Selvin BL. Electroconvulsive therapy—1987. Anesthesiology 1987;67:367–85
19. Gaines GY, Rees EI. Electroconvulsive therapy and anesthetic considerations. Anesth Analg 1986;65:1345–56
20. Lee JT, Erbguth PH, Stevens WC, Sack RL. Modification of electroconvulsive therapy induced hypertension with nitroglycerin ointment. Anesthesiology 1985;62:793–6
21. Havdala HS, Borison RL, Diamond BI. Potential hazards and applications of lithium in anesthesiology. Anesthesiology 1979;50:534–7
22. Diamond BI, Havdala HS, Borison RL. Potential of lithium as an anesthetic premedicant. Lancet 1977;2:1229–30
23. Hill GE, Wong KC, Hodges MR. Lithium carbonate and neuromuscular blocking agents. Anesthesiology 1977;46:122–6
24. Diaz JH, Hill GE. Hypotension with anesthesia in disulfiram-treated patients. Anesthesiology 1979;51:366–8

33

Substance Abuse and Drug Overdose

Substance abuse and drug overdose represent potential complicating aspects of management of anesthesia.[1-3] Patients who present with substance abuse histories may be chronically dependent on drugs or some type of substitution (clonidine, methadone) or antagonist (disulfiram, naltrexone) therapy or presently drug-free (i.e., rehabilitated). Similarly, anesthesiologists may be asked to participate in resuscitation of, or to anesthetize, traumatized, acutely drug-intoxicated patients.

SUBSTANCE ABUSE

Substance abuse may be defined as self-administration of drugs that deviates from accepted medical or social use which if sustained can lead to tolerance, physical dependence, and in some instances life-threatening withdrawal symptoms when the substance is not continuously available.[1] Addiction to drugs represents combinations of tolerance, psychologic dependence, and physical dependence.

Tolerance is a state in which tissues become accustomed to the presence of a drug such that increased quantities of that drug become necessary to produce effects observed with original doses. Acquired tolerance often occurs with chronic substance abuse second-ary to increased rates of metabolism of the drug due to stimulation of microsomal enzymes in the liver by the drug itself (i.e., enzyme induction or pharmacokinetic changes). This accelerated rate of breakdown means that less pharmacologically active drug is available to act at receptors. Likewise, receptors, may become less responsive (i.e., adapt) to the effects of given blood levels of an abused drug (i.e., pharmacodynamic changes). Additionally, substance abuse patients can manifest clinically significant cross-tolerance to drugs. As a result, it is difficult to predict analgesic or anesthetic requirements. Most often, chronic substance abuse results in greater than normal analgesic and anesthetic requirements. In contrast, additive or even synergistic depressant drug interactions among drugs of the same class should be anticipated in the presence of acute substance abuse. It must also be appreciated that levels of tolerance are dynamic phenomena. In the case of certain classes of drugs (barbiturates, opioids) relatively normal responses may occur to usual doses soon after completion of the withdrawal syndrome from that particular drug. Failure to appreciate this phenomenon can lead to relative overdoses with dramatic adverse consequences.

Physical dependence has developed when presence of the drug in the body is necessary for normal physiologic function. In the case of a number of substances (barbiturates, opioids) an altered physiologic state develops in which continued administration of drug is necessary to prevent appearance of withdrawal symptoms characteristic for that particular drug. In general, the withdrawal syndrome consists of a rebound in the physiologic systems modified by the drug itself. Knowing the physiologic impact of abused substances on specific organ systems allows prediction of the manifestations of withdrawal symptoms from a given drug. Failure to recognize withdrawal symptoms not only can confuse the diagnosis of perioperative events but also may be life-threatening.

Timing and severity of withdrawal is dependent on the specific drug abused and the amount, duration, and continuity of abuse, as well as the health and personality of the patient. In general, abrupt discontinuation of drugs with short elimination half-times, which are metabolized to inactive compounds, results in brief, intense withdrawal syndromes. Conversely, drugs with longer elimination half-times and active metabolites are associated with more prolonged, milder withdrawal syndromes. It is important to recognize signs of drug withdrawal in the perioperative period. Certainly, acute drug withdrawal should not be attempted at this time.

CHRONIC SUBSTANCE ABUSE

Opioids

Opioids are well absorbed from the gastrointestinal tract, as well as subcutaneous and intramuscular injection sites. First pass hepatic extraction and metabolism primarily account for the less intense effects of oral doses of opioids, such as morphine, as compared with their parenteral administration. Opioids are abused orally, subcutaneously (i.e., skin popping), or intravenously for either their euphoric or analgesic effects. Numerous medical problems can be encountered in opioid addicts, particularly intravenous abusers. These problems include cellulitis, superficial skin abscesses and septic thrombophlebitis; tetanus

(additives such as quinine used to adulterate heroin lower the redox potential of tissues and promote growth of anaerobes); bacterial or fungal endocarditis, which may be associated with both right and left sided valvular heart lesions and pulmonary emboli (may result in pulmonary hypertension); systemic septic emboli and infarctions; chronic atelectasis and aspiration pneumonitis; hepatitis; acquired immunodeficiency syndrome; suppression of adrenal cortical function; varying states of malnutrition; a high incidence of both positive and false-positive serologies; pancytopenia; and rarely, transverse myelitis. Evidence for these medical problems should be sought in opioid addicts entering the perioperative period.

Tolerance may develop to some of the effects of opioids (analgesic, sedative, emetic, euphoric, and respiratory depression) but not to others (miotic, constipating). Fortunately, as tolerance increases, lethal doses of opioids also increase. In general, there is a high degree of cross-tolerance between drugs with morphine-like actions: however, tolerance can wane rapidly when addicts are withdrawn from opioids.

Physical dependence also occurs with chronic opioid abuse, making it important to recognize symptoms and signs of opioid withdrawal in the perioperative period. Failure to provide opioid addicts with their usual daily doses of opioids can result in development of abrupt withdrawal symptoms. Times of onset, peak intensity, and duration of withdrawal after abrupt discontinuation of commonly abused opioids are important considerations in the perioperative period (Table 33-1).[4] Opioid withdrawal symptoms develop within seconds after intravenous administration of opioid antagonists.

Opioid withdrawal symptoms often include manifestations of excess activity of the sympathetic nervous system (diaphoresis, mydriasis, hypertension, tachycardia). Craving for the drug and anxiety are followed by yawning, lacrimation, and rhinnorhea. As these symptoms worsen, piloerection (origin of the term "cold turkey"), tremors, hot and cold flashes, skeletal muscle and bone discomfort, and anorexia ensue. Insominia, hyperthermia, abdominal cramps, and diarrhea may manifest. Skeletal muscle spasms and jerking of the legs

TABLE 33-1. Time Course of Opioid Withdrawal Syndrome

Drug	Onset	Peak Intensity	Duration
Meperidine Dihydromorphine	2–6 hours	8–12 hours	4–5 days
Codeine Morphine Heroin	6–18 hours	36–72 hours	7–10 days
Methadone	24–48 hours	3–21 days	6–7 weeks

(origin of the term "kicking the habit") follow and cardiovascular collapse is possible. Seizures are rare and their occurrence should introduce the consideration of other etiologies. Metabolic alterations that may occur during opioid withdrawal include dehydration and metabolic acidosis.

Although withdrawal from opioids is rarely life-threatening, it is unpleasant and confuses the diagnosis of perioperative events. It is usually possible, however, to abort withdrawal syndromes by reinstituting administration of the abused opioid or by substituting methadone (2.5 mg equivalent to about 10 mg of morphine). Indeed, administration of methadone orally or intramuscularly every 2 hours to 6 hours as needed to control and reverse withdrawal symptoms is recommended.[4] Usually 20 mg to 40 mg of methadone are required in the first 24 hours.

Clonidine has also proven to serve a beneficial role in opioid withdrawal syndromes.[5] It is thought that clonidine acts by replacing opioid-mediated inhibition (absent during withdrawal syndromes) with alpha-2 agonist-mediated inhibition of the sympathetic nervous system in the brain. This has led to self-administered withdrawal trials by addicts, which may result in patients who present manifesting significant side effects of clonidine (bradycardia, cardiac dysrhythmias, hypotension, congestive heart failure, and sedation) (see Chapter 6).

Patients addicted to opioids or receiving methadone or clonidine should have their drug maintained during the perioperative period. These patients should receive generous preoperative medication that includes their usual opioid or equivalent doses of methadone.[6]

There is no advantage in trying to maintain anesthesia with opioids in opioid addicts, as doses of opioids greatly in excess of normal are likely to be required to suppress sympathetic nervous system responses to noxious stimulation. Volatile anesthetics would seem better choices, remembering, however, that these patients are likely to have underlying liver disease. Similarly, mixed agonist-antagonist opioids and opioid antagonists should be avoided in these patients, as their administration may precipitate acute withdrawal syndromes.[7]

As many as 20 percent of these patients may exhibit symptoms of opioid withdrawal in the perioperative period.[6] There is a tendency for perioperative hypotension to occur, which might reflect (1) inadequate intravascular fluid volume secondary to chronic infections and fever or malnutrition, (2) adrenocortical insufficiency, and (3) inadequate levels of opioids in the central nervous system.[8] Although acute administration of opioids reduces anesthetic requirements, chronic opioid usage leads to cross-tolerance to other central nervous system depressants. For example, rats made tolerant to morphine exhibit decreased analgesic responses to nitrous oxide (Fig. 33-1).[9] Reports that opioid addicts need higher doses of anesthetic drugs than nonaddicted adults lends support to these animal findings.[8]

Management of anesthesia for rehabilitated opioid addicts, as well as patients on antagonist therapy such as naltrexone, is best achieved with volatile anesthetics. Regional anesthesia may have a role in some patients, but it is important to remember (1) the tendency for hypotension to occur, (2) the in-

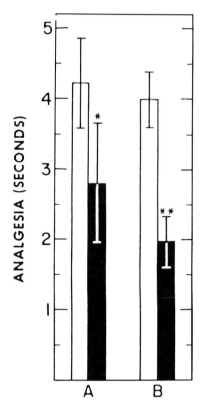

FIG. 33-1. Rats tolerant to morphine (darkened bars) are cross tolerant to 80 percent nitrous oxide as reflected by analgesia determined by tail flick latency. Clear bars represent control (nontolerant) rats untreated with morphine. A are Long-Evans rats and B are Sprague-Dawley rats. Mean ± SE. *P < 0.05 compared with nontolerant rats. **P < 0.005 compared with nontolerant rats. (Berkowitz BA, Finck AD, Hynes MD, Ngai SH. Tolerance to N_2O anesthesia in rats and mice. Anesthesiology 1979;51:309–14)

creased incidence of positive serology, (3) the occasional presence of peripheral neuritis and phlebitis, and (4) the rare occurrence of transverse myelitis.

These patients seem to have exaggerated degrees of postoperative pain. For reasons that are not clear, satisfactory postoperative analgesia is often achieved when average doses of meperidine are administered in addition to usual daily doses of methadone or other opioids.[10] Serious consideration should be given to the use of transcutaneous electrical nerve stimulation or continuous regional an-

esthetic techniques to provide postoperative pain relief. Conceivably, epidural or subarachnoid opioids should be tried in lieu of parenterally administered opioids.

Barbiturates

Barbiturates, as well as nonbarbiturate sedative-hypnotics (meprobamate, glutethimide, methaqualone), differ primarily in their lipid solubilities and elimination half-times. These central nervous system depressant drugs produce similar effects on mood and consciousness, presumably via either direct gamma-aminobutyric acid-like actions or by enhancing effects of this inhibitory neurotransmitter in the central nervous system.[3] These drugs are most commonly abused orally for their euphoric effects, for production of sleep, or to counteract central nervous system stimulatory effects of other drugs. Tolerance occurs to most of the actions of these drugs, as well as cross-tolerance to other central nervous system depressants. Although doses of barbiturates required to produce sedative or euphoric effects increase rapidly, lethal doses do not increase at the same rate or magnitude.[3] Thus, a barbiturate abuser's margin of error decreases as they increase their dose to produce desired effects.

Physical dependence occurs with barbiturates, as well as most other nonbarbiturate sedative-hypnotic drugs. In contrast to opioids, withdrawal symptoms from barbiturates are potentially life-threatening.[11] Times of onset, peak intensity, and duration of withdrawal symptoms for barbiturates are delayed compared with opioids (Table 33-2). Barbiturate withdrawal symptoms manifest as anxiety, restlessness, tremors, weakness, hyperreflexia, insomnia, nausea and vomiting, tachycardia, diaphoresis, and orthostatic hypotension. The most serious problem associated with barbiturate withdrawal is the occurrence of grand mal seizures. Toxic delerium (disorientation, hallucinations) often develops if barbiturate withdrawal is inadequately treated. Hyperthermia and cardiovascular collapse have been observed. Many of the manifestations of bar-

TABLE 33-2. Time Course of Barbiturate Withdrawal Syndrome

Drug	Onset	Peak Intensity	Duration
Pentobarbital Secobarbital	12–24 hours	2–3 days	7–10 days
Phenobarbital	2–3 days	6–10 days	10 days to weeks

biturate withdrawal, and in particular seizures, are difficult to abort once they develop, which contrasts with opioid withdrawal syndromes.

Maintenance of barbiturate requirements is the mainstay of treatment in the perioperative period.[10,11] If withdrawal symptoms develop, replacement therapy with barbiturates such as pentobarbital in initial oral doses of 200 mg to 400 mg with subsequent doses titrated to effect (sedation, slurred speech, ataxia) are recommended. These doses should be titrated carefully as tolerance has been reported to disappear very rapidly in these patients.[3] Phenobarbital and diazepam may also be useful in suppressing barbiturate withdrawal syndromes.

Chronic barbiturate abuse is not associated with major pathophysiologic changes in most organ systems. Exceptions include an increased incidence of emotional problems and respiratory disorders that may co-exist in these patients. In addition to the many problems that accompany intravenous abuse of any drug, intravenous barbiturate abuse also results in significant sclerosis of the venous system, secondary to the high alkalinity of these compounds.

Although little data exist concerning management of anesthesia in chronic barbiturate abusers, it is predictable that cross-tolerance to sedative effects of anesthetic drugs will occur. Mice tolerant to thiopental awaken at higher tissue levels of barbiturates than control animals.[12] Similarly, anecdotal reports describe needs for increased doses of barbiturates for induction of anesthesia and shorter duration of sleep in chronic barbiturate abusers.[13] Although acute administration of barbiturates has been shown to decrease anesthetic requirements, there are no reports of increased MAC requirements in chronic barbiturate abusers.[3] Another concern is that chronic barbiturate abuse leads to significant induction of hepatic microsomal enzymes, introducing the potential for drug interactions with concomitantly administered medications (warfarin, digitalis, phenytoin, volatile anesthetics).

Benzodiazepines

As with barbiturates, tolerance and physical dependence occur with chronic benzodiazepine abuse. Symptoms of withdrawal syndromes generally occur later than with barbiturates and are less severe due to prolonged elimination half-times of most benzodiazepines, as well as the fact that many of these drugs are metabolized to pharmacologically active metabolites that also have prolonged elimination half-times. Benzodiazepines do not significantly induce microsomal enzymes. Anesthetic considerations in chronic benzodiazepine abusers are similar to those described for chronic barbiturate abusers.

Amphetamines

Amphetamines exert pharmacologic effects by stimulating release of catecholamines from nerve terminals in the central nervous system and from peripheral sympathetic nerve endings.[3,14] As such, acute administration of amphetamines increases cortical alertness and electrical activity throughout the brain. Such alerting effects on the central nervous system result in decreased needs for sleep and appetite suppression—two of the primary reasons for abuse of these drugs. Similarly, amphetamines can produce feelings of increased ability and well-being. Amphetamines are most commonly abused orally or, in the case of methamphetamine, intravenously. Amphetamines are usually slowly metabolized by hepatic enzymes.

Chronic amphetamine abuse is associated with tolerance (particularly as regards appetite suppression, euphoric and sympathomimetic effects) and psychologic dependence.[3] Although physical dependence probably does not occur, abrupt discontinuation of administration after chronic use of amphetamines results in mental depression, prolonged sleep, fatigue, suicidal ideations, and hyperphagia. Neither fatalities nor seizures, however, occur as the result of abrupt amphetamine withdrawal.[3] Chronic abuse of amphetamines results in depletion of body stores of catecholamines. Such depletion may manifest in the form of somnolence or other abnormal sleeping disorders and anxiety or psychotic-like states. Other physiologic abnormalities reported with long-term amphetamine abuse include hypertension, cardiac dysrhythmias, and malnutrition. A rare medical problem associated with amphetamine abuse is that of necrotizing angiitis with microvascular damage to several organ systems.[15] Intravenous amphetamine abuse may be associated with the same problems common to intravenous opioid or barbiturate abuse.

Intraoperatively, patients who are acutely intoxicated from ingestion of amphetamines may manifest hypertension, tachycardia, increased body temperature, and elevated requirements for volatile anesthetics. Indeed, in animals, acute intravenous administration of dextroamphetamine produces dose-related increases in body temperature and anesthetic requirements for halothane.[16] Based on these observations, it would seem prudent to monitor body temperature during the perioperative period. Furthermore, direct-acting vasopressors and drugs that sensitize the heart to catecholamines must be used with caution in these patients.

Chronic use of amphetamines depletes body stores of catecholamines. This depletion may attenuate responses to indirect-acting vasopressors and be responsible for somnolence characteristic of chronic abuse. Indeed, anes-

thetic requirements for halothane are decreased in animals that have been chronically treated with dextroamphetamine.[16]

Cocaine

Cocaine use for nonmedical purposes has evolved from a relatively minor problem into a major public health threat with important economic and social consequences.[17,18] It is estimated that 30 million Americans have used cocaine and that 5 million use it regularly. Myths associated with cocaine abuse are that its use is sexually stimulating, nonaddicting, and physiologically benign. Deaths have occurred after administration of cocaine by all routes (intranasal, orally, intravenous, and inhalation by smoking). Smoking delivers large quantities of cocaine to the circulation, producing effects comparable to intravenous injection. Acute myocardial infarction, cardiac dysrhythmias, cerebrovascular accidents, hyperthermia, seizures, and gastrointestinal ischemia represent life-threatening side effects of cocaine, presumably reflecting the ability of this drug to enhance sympathetic nervous system activity principally due to inhibition of norepinephrine uptake into postganglionic nerve endings and/or direct actions on dopamine receptors.[17,18] Cocaine abuse among parturients is associated with spontaneous abortion, abruptio placenta, and congenital malformations. Lung damage and pulmonary edema have been observed in individuals who smoke cocaine. Most cocaine is metabolized in the liver within 2 hours to its principal metabolite, which is promptly excreted in the urine. Persons with decreased plasma cholinesterase enzyme activity (geriatric patients, parturients, severe liver disease) are at risk for sudden death when using cocaine because this enzyme is also essential for metabolizing the drug. Deaths from cocaine are usually due to seizures, respiratory paralysis, or cardiac dysrhythmias.[19] Diazepam may be effective in terminating cocaine-induced seizures. Ventricular cardiac dysrhythmias have been successfully managed with propranolol. Increased body temperature is thought to result from generalized vasoconstriction, increased skeletal muscle activity, and possibly central effects on temperature regulation.

Tolerance can develop to the euphoric effects of cocaine, although this is an inconsistent observation. Psychologic dependence develops with chronic use but physical dependence does not occur. Symptoms associated with withdrawal from cocaine include prolonged sleep, fatigue, increased hunger, and mental depression.

Medical problems associated with chronic cocaine abuse include nasal septal atrophy, nervousness, agitated behavior, paranoid thinking, heightened reflexes, and resting tachycardia. In the absence of acute intoxication, chronic abuse of cocaine has not been shown to be associated with adverse anesthetic interactions. This likely reflects rapid metabolism of cocaine so that acutely intoxicated patients rarely present in the operating room. It would seem prudent, however, to avoid administration of sympathomimetic drugs to these patients. Similarly, arrhythmogenic doses of epinephrine are significantly reduced in dogs receiving intravenous injections of cocaine, 2 mg·kg^{-1}, during halothane-nitrous oxide anesthesia.[20] Altered anesthetic requirements may be present in acutely intoxicated patients. Indeed, halothane MAC is increased in animals after intravenous administration of cocaine, presumably reflecting elevated levels of catecholamines in the central nervous system (Fig. 33-2).[21] Cocaine 1.5 mg·kg^{-1} administered topically before initiating nasotracheal intubation and followed by nitrous oxide-halothane anesthesia was not associated with detectable cardiovascular effects.[22]

Lysergic Acid Diethylamide

Lysergic acid diethylamide (LSD) and similar drugs (mescaline, diethyltryptamine) produce signs of sympathetic nervous system stimulation including hallucinations, mydriasis, hypertension, and tachycardia. These changes may reflect multiple sites of action in the central nervous system, although stimulation of the hypothalamus by LSD seems likely. Ability of the brain to suppress relatively unimportant stimuli is impaired by LSD.

Onset of sympathomimetic effects occur about 20 minutes to 40 minutes after oral ingestion of LSD and last about 6 hours. Psychic effects become evident 1 hour to 2 hours after ingestion and may last up to 8 hours to 12 hours.[23] LSD has a relatively short elimination half-time (3 hours) and is almost totally inactivated in the liver.

Tolerance to behavioral effects of LSD occurs rapidly, whereas tolerance to cardiovas-

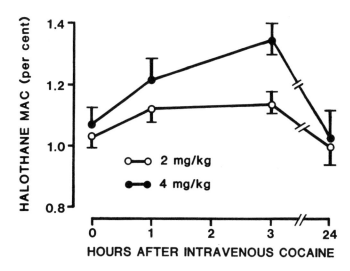

FIG. 33-2. Intravenous injection of cocaine (2 mg·kg^{-1} and 4 mg·kg^{-1}) produces dose-related increases in dog halothane MAC as measured 1 hour and 3 hours later. Anesthetic requirements were not different from control measurements 24 hours after administration of cocaine. (Data adapted from Stoelting RK, Creasser CW, Martz RC. Effect of cocaine administration on halothane MAC in dogs. Anesth Analg 1975;54:422–4 Reprinted with permission from IARS)

cular effects are less pronounced. Although there is a high degree of psychological dependence, there is no evidence of physical dependence or withdrawal symptoms when LSD is acutely discontinued.

No major physiologic derangements associated with chronic LSD abuse have been described. An exception is the immune system, where chronic LSD abuse may inhibit or disrupt antibody formation. It has also been recognized that LSD has anticholinesterase effects.[24] It has thus been suggested that succinylcholine and ester local anesthetics should be used with caution in such patients, although data to support this notion are scant.[10] Exaggerated responses to sympathomimetic drugs would seem likely. Analgesic and presumably ventilatory effects of opioids are prolonged by LSD. Flashbacks are known to occur in about 1 percent to 2 percent of LSD users. Anesthesia and surgery have been reported to precipitate such responses, the mechanism of which is unclear.[3] In the event flashback or panic reactions occur, diazepam is likely to be efficacious.

Marijuana

Marijuana is a generic term indicating any part of the hemp plant with psychoactive compounds. Hashish more specifically refers to the resin extracted from the tops of hemp plants, which contain a higher percentage of active constituents. Tetrahydrocannabinol (THC) is the primary psychoactive constituent of marijuana. Marijuana is metabolized in the liver and eliminated in the feces.

Marijuana is usually abused by smoking the plant, although it may be taken orally and retain its effects. Smoking increases bioavailability five times to ten times over that of ingestion. Pharmacologic effects occur within minutes after smoking of marijuana begins and plasma concentrations of THC peak within 20 minutes to 30 minutes. Effects rarely persist more than 2 hours to 3 hours. Oral ingestion of marijuana delays onset of effects for 30 min-

utes to 60 minutes, but the duration of effects is prolonged to 3 hours to 5 hours. Inhalation of marijuana smoke produces euphoria and signs of increased sympathetic nervous system activity and inhibition of the parasympathetic nervous system. The most consistent cardiovascular change is an increased resting heart rate. Orthostatic hypotension may occur. THC potentiates depression of ventilation produced by opioids (Fig. 33-3).[25] Barbiturate and ketamine sleeping times are prolonged in THC-treated animals.[26,27] There is dilation of the efferent blood vessels in the iris, which may reduce intraocular pressure. Theoretically, this response should be beneficial in patients with glaucoma. Conjunctival reddening is evidence of dilation of blood vessels in the iris. Drowsiness is a frequent side effect, and animal studies have documented decreases in anesthetic requirements after intravenous injection of THC.[28,29] An accepted medical use of THC is the oral administration of this drug to provide antiemetic activity in patients receiving cancer chemotherapy.[30] Side effects of oral THC are similar to those observed after inhalation of smoke containing marijuana.

Chronic marijuana abuse leads to increased tar deposits in the lung, impaired pulmonary defense mechanisms, and decreased pulmonary function. As such, an increased incidence of sinusitis and bronchitis is likely. Additionally, chronic marijuana abuse may provoke seizures in predisposed individuals.

Tolerance to most of the psychoactive effects of THC has been observed. Although physical dependence is not believed to occur, abrupt cessation after chronic use is characterized by mild symptomatology including irritability, restlessness, anorexia, insomnia, diaphoresis, nausea, vomiting, and diarrhea.

Cyclohexylamines

Cyclohexylamines (phencyclidine, ketamine) are abused because of their euphoric and mood-altering effects. These compounds are easily manufactured in clandestine laboratories and are available in forms usually taken

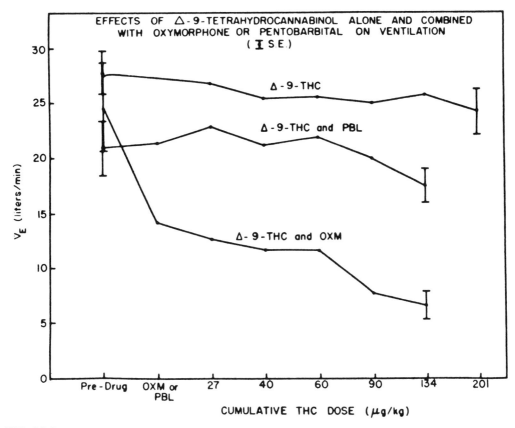

FIG. 33-3. Effects of tetrahydrocannabinol (THC) on minute ventilation (V_E) in awake volunteers when administered alone or preceded by oxymorphone (OXM) or pentobarbital (PBL). (Johnstone RC, Lief PL, Kulp RA, Smith TC. Combination of delta-9-tetrahydrocannabinol with oxymorphone or pentobarbital. Anesthesiology 1974;42:674–9)

orally, smoked, or injected intravenously. Mechanisms of action are unknown, although it is believed they interact with several neurotransmitters. Cyclohexylamines are metabolized by the liver and excreted in the urine. Likewise, these compounds can undergo significant enterohepatic circulation.

Tolerance to cyclohexylamines does occur with chronic abuse. Physical dependence does not seem to occur. Chronic abuse has not been reported to result in organ system dysfunction. Decreased anesthetic requirements and enhanced responses to sympathomimetics are predictable. Likewise, patients acutely intoxicated with cyclohexylamines may be difficult to manage during regional anesthetic techniques.

Alcoholism (see Chapter 32)

DRUG OVERDOSE

Drug overdose is the leading cause of unconsciousness observed in patients brought to emergency rooms.[31] Unconsciousness due to drug overdose lacks localizing signs. Conditions other than drug overdose may result in unconsciousness, emphasizing the importance of laboratory testing (electrolytes, blood glucose concentrations, arterial blood gases, renal, and liver function tests) in these patients.

Depth of central nervous system depression can be estimated on the basis of the (1) response to painful stimulation, (2) activity of the gag reflex, (3) presence or absence of hypotension, (4) breathing rate, and (5) size and responsiveness of the pupils.[31,32]

Clinical manifestations and principles of management of drug overdoses are similar, regardless of the drug or drugs ingested. Clinical assessment and treatment should proceed simultaneously. The first step is securement of the airway and support of ventilation and circulation. Absence of a gag reflex is confirmatory evidence that protective laryngeal reflexes are dangerously depressed. In this situation, a cuffed tube should be placed in the trachea to protect the lungs from aspiration. The presence of hypotension may reflect direct cardiac depression from ingested drugs, venous pooling, or decreased intravascular fluid volume due to increased capillary permeability. Treatment of hypotension due to drug overdose is determined by the suspected cause for the decreased blood pressure; it may include administration of positive inotropic drugs, sympathomimetic drugs, or fluids. Body temperature should be monitored, as hypothermia frequently accompanies unconsciousness due to drug overdose. In contrast, life-threatening hyperthermia may accompany overdoses of central nervous system stimulants.

Decisions to attempt removal of the ingested substance or to facilitate its renal excretion depends on the drug ingested, the time since ingestion, and the degree of central nervous system depression.[31,32] Analeptics have no place in the treatment of drug overdose. Gastric lavage may be beneficial if less than 4 hours have elapsed since drug ingestion. Tricyclic antidepressant drugs prolong gastric emptying time because of their anticholinergic effects. Therefore, recovery of tricyclic antidepressant drugs with gastric lavage may occur for as long as 12 hours after ingestion. Stimulation of vomiting with syrup of ipecac or apomorphine may also be effective in eliminating contents from the upper gastrointestinal tract. It must be emphasized, however, that gastric lavage or pharmacologic stimulation of vomiting is contraindicated when ingested substances are hydrocarbon materials or corrosive substances, or when protective laryngeal reflexes are not intact. After emesis or gastric lavage activated charcoal can be administered to absorb drug remaining in the gastrointestinal tract. Charcoal binds organic compounds and creates stable complexes that do not dissociate. These characteristics may be particularly useful in treating drug overdose that slows gastrointestinal motility.

Forced diuresis produced by intravenous administration of fluids and diuretics has limited application, since few drugs are significantly excreted by the kidneys in the unchanged form. Renal excretion of certain drugs, however, may be enhanced by appropriate manipulation of urine pH to increase ionized fractions of drugs in the urine. For example, salicyclic acid excretion can be increased by alkalinization of the urine. Conversely, acidification of the urine would theoretically facilitate renal excretion of amphetamines and LSD. Forced diuresis introduces the risk of fluid overload and electrolyte abnormalities, especially hypokalemia.

Hemodialysis may be considered when a potentially fatal dose of drug has been ingested, when there is progressive deterioration of cardiovascular function, or when normal routes of metabolism and renal excretion are impaired. Hemodialysis is of little value in treating patients who have ingested drugs that are highly bound to protein or avidly stored in tissues. For example, hemodialysis is not effective in lowering total body concentrations of tricyclic antidepressant drugs since only small proportions of these highly lipid soluble drugs will be present in the plasma.

Opioid Overdose

Manifestations of opioid overdose most often occur in the central nervous system and cardiovascular system.[3,33] Central nervous system manifestations range from dysphoria to unconsciousness. Seizures are rare but can occur, especially after overdoses of meperidine or pentazocine. The most obvious manifestations of opioid overdose (usually heroin) are slow breathing rates, with normal to increased tidal volumes. The pupils are usually miotic, although mydriasis may occur if apnea results in severe arterial hypoxemia.

The principal cardiovascular manifestations of opioid overdose are orthostatic hypotension and syncope due to opioid-induced bradycardia and peripheral vasodilation of capacitance vessels. Additionally, in heroin abusers, significant myocardial depression may result from the commonly used adulterant, quinine. Pulmonary edema occurs in a high proportion of patients who take overdoses of opioids, especially heroin. The etiology is poorly understood, but arterial hypoxemia, hypotension, neurogenic mechanisms, and drug-related pulmonary endothelial damage are considerations. Gastric atony is a predictable accompaniment of acute opioid overdose. Fatal opioid overdoses are most frequently accidental outcomes of fluctuations in the purity of street products or to the combination of opioids with other central nervous system depressants.

Naloxone is a specific opioid antagonist that should be administered intravenously (0.2 mg to 0.4 mg every 2 minutes to 5 minutes; 0.01 mg·kg^{-1} in infants) up to three doses or until breathing rates increase to at least 12 breaths·min^{-1}.[33] When naloxone is given, however, it must be titrated to effect to avoid over-reversal and subsequent sympathetic nervous system hyperactivity. Likewise, it must be remembered that elimination half-times of naloxone (1 hour to 2 hours) are shorter than that of most opioids, such that repeated administrations or continuous infusions of naloxone may be necessary.

Barbiturate Overdose

Central nervous system depression is the primary pharmacologic effect of barbiturate overdose.[1] Barbiturate blood levels correlate with the degree of central nervous system depression. Such depression may manifest as somnolence, slurred speech, ataxia, and disinhibition (lability of mood, irritability, and combativeness). High blood levels result in loss of pharyngeal and deep tendon reflexes and coma. No specific pharmacologic antagonist exists to reverse this central nervous system depression and use of nonspecific stimulants is discouraged. Barbiturates also cause significant depression of ventilation, particularly if taken in large doses or by patients with co-existing lung disease. As with opioid overdoses, control of the airway and support of ventilation of the lungs are essential.

Acute overdoses of barbiturates may also be associated with cardiovascular depression due to central vasomotor depression, direct myocardial depression and increases in venous capacitance. Barbiturate-induced hypotension usually responds to correction of co-existing arterial hypoxemia or hypercarbia, to head-down positioning and infusion of fluids. Occasionally, administration of vasopressors or positive inotropic drugs may be required. Hypothermia is a frequent occurrence and may necessitate aggressive attempts to restore normothermia. Acute renal failure due to hypotension and rhabdomyolysis may also occur.

Forced diuresis and alkalinization of the urine promote elimination of phenobarbital but are of lesser value with many of the other barbiturates. Induced emesis or gastric lavage is indicated if less than 6 hours have elapsed since the time of barbiturate ingestion. This should be followed by the administration of activated charcoal and cathartics.

Benzodiazepine Overdose

Acute benzodiazepine overdose is much less likely to produce depression of ventilation as compared with barbiturate overdose. It should be recognized, however, that combinations of benzodiazepines and other central nervous system depressants, such as alcohol, have proven to be potentially lethal. Supportive measures suffice as adequate treatment for most benzodiazepine overdoses. Physostigmine has proven at times to be efficacious in reversing disorientation or hallucinations resulting from benzodiazepine overdose.

Specific benzodiazepine antagonists, as currently available for opioids, provide an obvious method of treatment of benzodiazepine overdose.

Amphetamine Overdose

Amphetamine overdose causes anxiety, psychotic states, and progressive central nervous system irritability manifesting as hyperactivity, hyperreflexia, and occasionally seizures.[1] Other physiologic effects include increases in blood pressure and heart rate, cardiac dysrhythmias, decreases in gastrointestinal motility, mydriasis, diaphoresis, and hyperthermia. Metabolic imbalances such as dehydration, lactic acidosis, and ketosis may occur.

Treatment of oral amphetamine overdose is with induced emesis or gastric lavage followed by administration of activated charcoal and cathartics. Phenothiazines may antagonize many of the acute central nervous system effects of amphetamines. Similarly, diazepam may be useful to control amphetamine-induced seizures. Acidification of the urine will promote elimination of amphetamines.

Cocaine Overdose

Many of the manifestations arising from acute cocaine overdose are similar to acute amphetamine overdose.[34] Marked hyperthermia can follow cocaine overdose and results from generalized vasoconstriction, increased skeletal muscle activity, and possibly central effects on temperature regulation. Benzodiazepines should be effective against cocaine-induced seizures. Acute cocaine administration can result in decreases in coronary artery blood flow.[19] Presumably, cocaine-induced coronary artery vasospasm is responsible for angina pectoris and acute myocardial infarctions that may occur in patients experiencing cocaine overdoses.

Lysergic Acid Diethylamine (LSD) Overdose

LSD, in addition to its euphoric and hallucinogenic properties, causes stimulatory effects on the sympathetic nervous system (via stimulation of the hypothalamus) including mydriasis; piloerection; tremor; hyperreflexia; and increases in body temperature, heart rate, and blood pressure. On rare occasions, LSD produces seizures and apnea. LSD can likewise produce acute panic reactions characterized by hyperactivity, extreme lability of mood, and illogical reasoning patterns. This syndrome typically lasts 24 hours to 48 hours. Overt psychosis can also occur where patients lose touch with reality.

LSD overdose has not been associated with mortality, although patients often suffer traumatic injuries which may go undetected due to intrinsic analgesic activity of LSD. Benzodiazepines may be useful to control patients' anxiety. Blood pressure, heart rate, cardiac rhythm, and body temperature should be monitored; and abnormalities may need to be aggressively treated.

Cyclohexylamine Overdose

Cyclohexylamine (phencyclidine, ketamine) overdose produces dose-related effects, often manifesting as agitation and combativeness. Speech is often slowed and slurred. The patients' eyes are open and have a "blank stare." Nystagmus and ataxia are common. Skeletal muscle tone is increased and rigidity can occur. Other features include flushing, hypersalivation, and facial grimacing. Signs of increased sympathetic nervous system activity predominate including tachycardia, hypertension, diaphoresis, and hyperthermia. More severe overdoses can result in profound central nervous system and ventilatory depression and unconsciousness. Seizures may occur. Rhabdomyolysis may result from skeletal muscle spasm and hyperthermia.

Patients should be placed in calm and

quiet environments with minimal external stimuli. No specific antidote exists. Benzodiazepines may be used to control agitation. Supportive care in the form of airway management, support of ventilation, treatment of seizures, and control of manifestations of sympathetic nervous system hyperactivity when appropriate is warranted. Forced diuresis and acidification of the urine promote elimination of phencyclidine.

Salicylic Acid Overdose

Symptoms of salicylic acid overdose may occur from doses greater than 100 mg·kg^{-1} to 150 mg·kg^{-1}.[31] Salicylic acid overdose results in (1) uncoupling of oxidative phosphorylation, (2) impairment of carbohydrate metabolism, (3) direct stimulation of the central nervous system, and (4) impairment of platelet aggregation and inhibition of vitamin K leading to prolonged bleeding. Initially, uncoupling of oxidative phosphorylation results in increased carbon dioxide production, oxygen consumption, and heat production. Hypoglycemia may occur from increased peripheral use of glucose or interference with gluconeogenesis. Furthermore, salicylic acid may interfere with brain glucose metabolism. Conversely, increased blood glucose levels may reflect the effect of epinephrine release secondary to stimulation of the central nervous system by salicylic acid. Noncardiogenic pulmonary edema often occurs during the first 24 hours after salicylic overdose.[35]

Hyperventilation is characteristic of salicylic acid overdose. This response is due to increased carbon dioxide production and direct stimulation of the respiratory center. Resulting respiratory alkalosis favors extracellular distribution of salicylic acid. For example, nearly all salicylic acid is in ionized and water soluble forms at physiologic pH. Therefore, respiratory alkalosis serves to maintain or even increase ionized fractions of salicylic acid in the circulation. Presence of ionized salicylic acid in the circulation favors renal elimination of this substance. Furthermore, alkalinization of the urine also facilitates excretion of salicylic acid.

Metabolic acidosis may accompany salicylic acid overdose. This is hazardous, since reductions in systemic pH to 7.2 doubles the fraction of nonionized and lipid soluble drug in the circulation. Lipid soluble fractions of salicylic acid can leave the blood and enter tissues, including the brain, where toxic effects are produced. Therefore, proper management of salicylic acid overdose requires monitoring of the arterial pH, to allow early recognition of the onset of metabolic acidosis. Sodium bicarbonate administration may be necessary to maintain arterial pH at or above 7.4. Controlled ventilation of the lungs via a tube in the trachea is indicated if central nervous system depression and alveolar hypoventilation are prominent. Dehydration and electrolyte disturbances may require treatment. Other manifestations of salicylic acid overdose include tinnitus, vomiting, hyperthermia, seizures, and unconsciousness.

There is a correlation between the severity of salicylic acid overdose and salicylate blood levels. Usually, plasma salicylate concentrations above 85 mg·dl^{-1} indicate severe overdose. Decreasing plasma salicylate levels may reflect urinary excretion of salicylic acid, or undesirable cellular penetration of this substance secondary to metabolic acidosis. Hemodialysis is indicated when potentially lethal plasma concentrations of salicylate are present (above 100 mg·dl^{-1}) or there is an inability to alkalinize the urine.

Acetaminophen Overdose

Acetaminophen overdose (greater than 150 mg·kg^{-1}) manifests as vomiting and abdominal pain within 12 hours to 48 hours after ingestion.[31] Hepatic damage is indicated by the appearance of elevated plasma transaminase enzyme concentrations. Centrilobular hepatic necrosis leads to hepatic failure in 1 percent to 2 percent of patients. Hepatic failure is most likely due to consumption of glutathione by reactive intermediary metabolites of acetaminophen. Normally, these metabolites are rendered harmless by conjugation with glutathione. Depletion of glutathione by acetaminophen permits these metabolites to bind to and destroy hepatocytes.

Initial treatment of acetaminophen overdose consists of clearing residual drug from the gastrointestinal tract by induced emesis or gastric lavage and administration of cathartics. The most reliable predictor of hepatotoxicity is the blood level of acetaminophen (Fig. 33-4).[36] If there is a high probability of liver damage based on elevated acetaminophen blood levels, the administration of oral methionine or oral or intravenous acetylcysteine is indicated. Both of these compounds are sulfhydryl donors (i.e., glutathione precursors) and are able to bind reactive intermediate breakdown products of acetaminophen, thus lessening the severity of liver damage. Hepatic damage is most likely to be attenuated if these substances are given within 10 hours of acetaminophen overdose.[37]

Tricyclic Antidepressant Overdose

Deliberate self-administration of overdoses of tricyclic antidepressant drugs is the most common cause of death from drug ingestion.[38] Since the usual indication for their use is mental depression, it is not surprising that deliberate overdose is a problem (see Chapter 32). Potentially lethal doses of these drugs are only five times to ten times the therapeutic daily doses. An overdose primarily affects the parasympathetic nervous system, central ner-

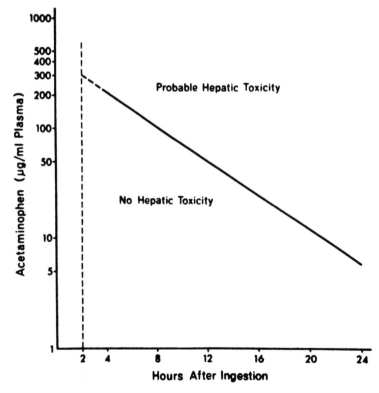

FIG. 33-4. Semilogarithmic plot of plasma acetaminophen concentrations with time and the likelihood of associated hepatic toxicity. (Rumack BH, Matthew H. Acetaminophen poisoning and toxicity. Pediatrics 1975;55:871–6. Reproduced by permission of Pediatrics.)

vous system, and cardiovascular system (see Chapter 32). Progression from being alert with mild symptoms to life-threatening changes (seizures, hypoventilation, hypotension, coma) may be extremely rapid. Striking signs of anticholinergic effects include tachycardia, mydriasis, flushed dry skin, delayed gastric emptying, and urinary retention. Cardiovascular toxicity with intractable myocardial depression, ventricular tachycardia, or ventricular fibrillation are the most common causes of death. The likelihood of seizures and cardiac dysrhythmias is increased when the duration of QRS complexes on the electrocardiogram exceeds 100 msec.[39] Conversely, plasma concentrations of tricyclic antidepressant drugs do not correlate with the likely occurrence of seizures or cardiac dysrhythmias.[39] The comatose phase of tricyclic antidepressant overdose lasts 24 hours to 72 hours. Even after this phase passes, the risk of life-threatening cardiac dysrhythmias persists for up to 10 days, necessitating continued monitoring of the electrocardiogram in these patients.[40]

Treatment of tricyclic antidepressant overdose in the presence of protective upper airway reflexes is initially with induced emesis and/or gastric lavage, even if as long as 12 hours have elapsed since drug ingestion, emphasizing the likely presence of drug-induced delays in gastric emptying. Depression of ventilation and/or coma may require intubation of the trachea and mechanical support of ventilation. Coma usually resolves within 24 hours. Alkalinization of the plasma, either by administration of intravenous sodium bicarbonate or hyperventilation of the lungs, to a pH above 7.45 can temporarily attenuate drug-induced cardiotoxicity, including suppression of cardiac dysrhythmias.[10] Lidocaine is also effective in treatment of cardiac dysrhythmias. Patients remaining hypotensive after volume expansion and alkalinization may require vasopressor or inotropic support as guided by measurement of cardiac filling pressures and cardiac output.

Diazepam may be useful to control seizures. Physostigmine often reverses central nervous system effects of tricyclic antidepressant overdose, although this is a nonspecific and somewhat unpredictable effect. It must likewise be remembered that the duration of action of physostigmine is only 1 hour to 2 hours and repeated doses of this drug may be necessary owing to longer elimination half-times of most tricyclic antidepressant drugs. Hemodialysis and forced diuresis are not effective since the high lipid solubility of tricyclic antidepressant drugs results in a fixed and slow rate of excretion.

Ethyl Alcohol Overdose

Clinical manifestations of acute ethyl alcohol overdose depend on the amount of alcohol consumed, rate and duration of consumption, rate of hepatic oxidation, and presence of central nervous system tolerance. The critical aspect of treatment is maintenance of ventilation. Hypoglycemia may be profound, if heavy alcohol consumption is associated with food deprivation. It must be appreciated that other central nervous system depressant drugs are often ingested simultaneously with ethyl alcohol.

Methyl Alcohol Ingestion

Methyl alcohol ingestion is associated with metabolic acidosis. This reflects metabolism of methyl alcohol to formaldehyde and formic acid. These acids are presumed to be responsible for the toxic effects that manifest at the optic nerve (blindness) and brain. Severe abdominal pain, which may mimic a surgical emergency or ureteral colic, may also accompany ingestion of methyl alcohol.

Treatment of methyl alcohol ingestion is with intravenous administration of sodium bicarbonate, as guided by arterial pH determinations. Administration of intravenous or oral ethyl alcohol may prevent dangerous accumulations of acid metabolites of methyl alcohol. The effectiveness of ethyl alcohol is due to its affinity for the enzyme system responsible for the breakdown of methyl alcohol. As a result, less metabolism of methyl alcohol can occur. Hemodialysis is also an effective treatment for removing methyl alcohol and prevention of visual and cerebral damage.[41]

Ethylene Glycol Ingestion

Metabolites of ethylene glycol, especially oxalate, are highly cytotoxic. Hypocalcemia due to oxalate chelation of calcium may also occur. Central nervous system depression is followed by cardiac, respiratory, and renal failure. Metabolic acidosis reflects accumulation of acid metabolites.

Ethyl alcohol is a competitive inhibitor of ethylene glycol metabolism and, as with methyl alcohol ingestion, may be administered to reduce the accumulation of toxic metabolites.[42] Intravenous administration of sodium bicarbonate and replacement of calcium are often necessary. Hemodialysis is the most effective treatment available, as it removes both ethylene glycol and oxalate.

Pretroleum Product Ingestion

Morbidity associated with ingestion of petroleum products (gasoline, kerosene, lighter fluid, furniture polish) is usually secondary to pulmonary aspiration during spontaneous vomiting or after induced emesis and not from absorption from the gastrointestinal tract. Symptoms of hydrocarbon pneumonitis arise only if aspiration occurs and range from coughing and dyspnea with tachypnea to life-threatening adult respiratory distress syndrome.[43] Of those patients who develop hydrocarbon pneumonitis, nearly all manifest radiographic changes within 12 hours of ingestion.[43] Pneumonitis is presumably due to hydrocarbon-induced alterations in physical properties of pulmonary surfactant leading to atelectasis and airway closure. Gastrointestinal symptoms of

ingestion of petroleum products include burning of the mouth and throat, nausea, vomiting, and diarrhea. Central nervous system symptoms are mild. Indeed, unconsciousness or seizures generally only occur as a result of arterial hypoxemia secondary to aspiration. Renal function is not uniquely altered by petroleum product ingestion.

Since the principal hazard of petroleum product ingestion is pulmonary aspiration, induced emesis is not indicated. Intubation of the trachea solely for gastric lavage is not indicated since the seal provided by the cuff on the tube is not a guarantee against aspiration of these low density liquids. Activated charcoal and cathartics are not beneficial. The course and severity of hydrocarbon pneumonitis is not altered by administration of corticosteroids. Broad spectrum antibiotics should be used only if bacterial infection can be documented.

Gasoline and glue sniffing have been implicated as causes of sudden and often fatal cardiac dysrhythmias. This may reflect sensitization of the myocardium to endogenous catecholamines.[44]

Organophosphate Overdose

Organophosphate overdose is produced by anticholinesterase insecticides. These compounds may be ingested, inhaled, or absorbed through the skin resulting in excess acetylcholine accumulation manifesting as muscarinic effects (miosis, lacrimation, diaphoresis, salivation, bradycardia, vomiting, diarrhea, and bladder evacuation) and nicotinic effects (respiratory paralysis).[31,45] Hyperthermia and seizures can also occur.

Diagnosis of organophosphate overdose may be confirmed by decreased erythrocyte or plasma cholinesterase enzyme activity. Muscarinic effects may be controlled by intravenous administration of atropine (0.05 $mg \cdot kg^{-1}$), whereas breathing and blood pressure are supported. Seizures may be controlled with administration of benzodiazepines.

Phosphorylation of cholinesterase enzyme

by organophosphates is reversible within the first 24 hours after ingestion by administration of pralidoxime, which acts as a cholinesterase inhibitor antagonist. Destruction of accumulated acetylcholine can then proceed, and neuromuscular junctions will again function, normally relieving the paralysis of respiratory muscles. Atropine is usually required concomitantly to block effects of accumulated acetylcholine in the central nervous system.

Organophosphate overdose may be followed by delayed peripheral neuropathy involving the distal muscles of the extremities.[45] This neuropathy appears 2 weeks to 5 weeks after the overdose. Skeletal muscle weakness developing 1 day to 4 days after organophosphate overdose involves primarily proximal limb muscles, flexors of the neck, certain cranial nerves, and muscles of respiration. Weakness of the muscles of respiration may require urgent support of ventilation.

Carbon Monoxide

Carbon monoxide intoxication is the most frequent immediate cause of death from fire. This colorless, odorless gas exerts its adverse effects by decreasing oxygen delivery to tissues, by virtue of its greater affinity for hemoglobin. Specifically, the affinity of carbon monoxide for oxygen binding sites on hemoglobin is 240 times greater than that of oxygen for the same sites. Because of this affinity, inspired carbon monoxide concentrations of 0.1 percent in room air produce equal blood concentrations of oxyhemoglobin and carboxyhemoglobin and result in 50 percent reductions in the oxygen-carrying capacity of the blood. Carbon monoxide also produces tissue hypoxia by shifting the oxyhemoglobin dissociation curve to the left (Fig. 33-5).[46]

Diagnosis of carbon monoxide intoxica-

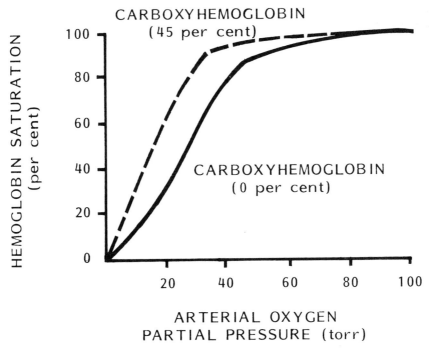

FIG. 33-5. Severe carbon monoxide poisoning producing carboxyhemoglobin levels of 45 percent or greater shifts the oxyhemoglobin dissociation curve to the left. This shift means that oxygen is more tightly bound to hemoglobin such that release of oxygen to tissues at given arterial partial pressures of oxygen (torr or mmHg) is reduced.

tion is suggested by low oxygen saturations of hemoglobin in the presence of normal arterial oxygen partial pressures. Measurement of carboxyhemoglobin concentrations in the blood confirms the diagnosis. It is important to recognize that the presence of high plasma concentrations of carboxyhemoglobin can cause the pulse oximeter to overestimate the true percent of hemoglobin saturation with oxygen.[47] Carbon monoxide intoxication is considered to be severe when blood concentrations of carboxyhemoglobin exceed 40 percent. Despite marked reductions in oxygen-carrying capacity of the blood, minute ventilation is typically unchanged, since the carotid bodies respond principally to changes in arterial oxygen partial pressures, which are likely to be normal in the presence of carbon monoxide intoxication. Therefore, increased minute ventilation may not occur until lactic acidosis develops from tissue hypoxia.

Treatment of carbon monoxide intoxication is with inhalation of oxygen, so as to displace carbon monoxide from hemoglobin. For example, if patients are breathing room air, half-times for elimination of carboxyhemoglobin are 250 minutes. Administration of 100 percent oxygen increases the dissociation of carbon monoxide from hemoglobin and reduces these times to about 50 minutes.[46] Inhalation of oxygen in hyperbaric chambers is reasonable if facilities for this method of treatment are readily available. It is prudent to administer oxygen initially to all persons who may have been exposed to carbon monoxide, especially if inhalation of smoke associated with a fire has occurred.

REFERENCES

1. Jenkins LC. Anaesthetic problems due to drug abuse and dependence. Can Anaesth Soc J 1972;19:461–77
2. McGoldrick KE. Anesthetic implications of drug abuse. Anesthesiology Review 1980;7:12–7
3. Jaffe JH. Drug addiction and drug abuse. In: Gilman AG, Goodman L, eds. The Pharmacologic Basis of Therapeutics. New York. MacMillan. 1985:532–581
4. Blachly PH. Management of the opiate abstinence syndrome. Am J Psychiatry 1966;122:742–59
5. Gold MS, Pottash AC, Sweeney DR, Kleber HD. Opiate withdrawal using clonidine: A safe, effective, and rapid nonopiate treatment. JAMA 1980;243:343–6
6. Giuffrida JG, Bizzarri DV, Saure AC, Sharoff RL. Anesthetic management of drug abusers. Anesth Analg 1970;49:273–82
7. Weintraub SJ, Naulty JS. Acute abstinence syndrome after epidural injection of butorphanol. Anesth Analg 1985;64:452–3
8. Marck LC. Hypotension during anesthesia in narcotic addicts. NY State J Med 1966;66:2685–97
9. Berkowitz BA, Finck AD, Hynes MD, Ngai SH. Tolerance to N₂O anesthesia in rats and mice. Anesthesiology 1979;51:309–14
10. Allgulander C. Dependence on sedative and hypnotic drugs. Acta Psychiatr Scand 1978;270:1–120
11. Wikler A. Diagnosis and treatment of drug dependence of the barbiturate type. Amer J Psychiatry 1968;125:759–66
12. Hubbard TF, Goldbaum LR. The mechanism of tolerance of thiopental in mice. J Pharmacol 1949;97:488–94
13. Lee PKY, Cho MH, Dobkin AB. Effects of alcoholism, morphinism, and barbiturate resistance on induction and maintenance of general anesthesia. Can Anaesth Soc J 1974;11:366–71
14. Kramer JC, Fichman VS, Littlefield DC. Amphetamine abuse. JAMA 1967;201:89–99
15. Citron HP, Halpern M, McCann M, et al. Necrotizing angiitis associated with drug abuse. N Engl J Med 1970;283:1103–7
16. Johnston RR, Way WL, Miller RD. Alteration of anesthetic requirements by amphetamine. Anesthesiology 1972;36:357–63
17. Cregler LL, Mark H. Medical complications of cocaine abuse. N Engl J Med 1986;315:1495–1500
18. Pollin W. The danger of cocaine. JAMA 1985;254:98
19. Kossowsky WA, Lyon AF, Chou AY. Cocaine and ischemic heart disease. Practical Cardiology 1986;12:164–78
20. Koehntop DE, Kiao JC, Van Bergen FH. Effects of pharmacologic alteration of adrenergic mechanisms by cocaine, tropolone, aminophylline, and ketamine on epinephrine-induced arrhythmias during halothane-nitrous oxide anesthesia. Anesthesiology 1977;46:83–9
21. Stoelting RK, Creasser CW, Martz RC. Effect of cocaine administration of halothane MAC in dogs. Anesth Analg 1975;54:422–4

22. Barash P, Kopriva CJ, Langou R, et al. Is cocaine a sympathetic stimulant during general anesthesia? JAMA 1980;243:1437–41

23. Freedman DX. The psychopharmacology of hallucinogenic agents. Annu Rev Med 1969;20:409–22

24. Zsigmond EK, Foldes FF, Foldes VM. The inhibitory effect of psilocybin and related compounds on human cholinesterases. Fed Proc 1961;20:393–8

25. Johnstone RC, Lief PL, Kulp RA, Smith TC. Combination of delta-9-tetrahydrocannabinol with oxymorphone or pentobarbital. Anesthesiology 1975;42:674–9

26. Siemons AJ, Kalant H, Khanna JM. Effect of cannabis on pentobarbital-induced sleeping time and pentobarbital metabolism in the rat. Biochem Pharmacol 1974;23:447–53

27. Sofia RD, Knoblock LC. The effect of delta-9-tetrahydrocannabinol pretreatment on ketamine, thiopental, or CT-1341-induced loss of righting reflex in mice. Arch Int Pharmacodyn Ther 1974;207:270–9

28. Vitez TS, Way WL, Miller RD, Eger EI. Effects of delta-9-tetrahydrocannibinol on cyclopropane MAC in the rat. Anesthesiology 1973;38:525–7

29. Stoelting RK, Martz RC, Garnter J, et al. Effects of delta-9-tetrahydrocannibinol on halothane MAC in dogs. Anesthesiology 1973;38:521–4

30. Poster DS, Penta JS, Bruno S, Macdonald JS. Tetrahydrocannibinol in clinical oncology. JAMA 1981;245:2047–51

31. Nicholson DP. The immediate management of overdose. Med Clin North Am 1983;67:1279–93

32. Vale JA. The immediate care of cases of poisoning. Anaesthesia 1977;32:483–93

33. Khnatzian EJ, McKenna GJ. Acute toxic and withdrawal reactions associated with drug use and abuse. Ann Inter Med 1979;90:361–72

34. Jonsson S, O'Meara M, Young JB. Acute cocaine poisoning. Am J Med 1983;75:1061–4

35. Hoymachea E, Carlson RW, Rogove H, et al. Hypovolemia, pulmonary edema and protein changes in severe salicylate poisoning. Am J Med 1979;66:1046–50

36. Rumack BH, Matthew H. Acetaminophen poisoning and toxicity. Pediatrics 1975;55:871–6

37. Prescott LF, Sutherland GR, Park J et al. Cysteamine, methionine and penicillamine in the treatment of paracetamal poisoning. Lancet 1976;2:109–13

38. Frommer DA, Kulig KW, Marx JA, Rumack B. Tricyclic antidepressant overdose. A review. JAMA 1987;257:521–6

39. Boehnert MT, Lovejoy FH. Value of the QRS duration versus the serum drug level in predicting seizures and ventricular arrhythmias after an acute overdose of tricyclic antidepressants. N Engl J Med 1985;313:474–9

40. Vohra J, Burrows GD. Cardiovascular complications of tricyclic antidepressant overdosage. Drugs 1974;8:432–7

41. Keyvan-Larijarni H, Tannenberg AM. Methanol intoxication. Arch Intern Med 1974;134:293–6

42. Peterson CD, Collins AJ, Himes JM, et al. Ethylene glycol poisoning. N Engl J Med 1981;304:21–3

43. Mayhew JF. Hydrocarbon ingestion. Anesthesiology Review 1980;7:48–50

44. Bass M. Death from sniffing gasoline (letter). N Engl J Med 1978;299:203

45. Davies JE. Changing profile of pesticide poisoning. N Engl J Med 1987;316:807–8

46. Jackson DL. Accidental carbon monoxide poisoning. JAMA 1980;772–4

47. Barker SJ, Tremper KK. The effect of carbon monoxide inhalation on pulse oximetry and transcutaneous PO_2. Anesthesiology 1987;66:677–9

34

Pregnant Patients

PHYSIOLOGIC CHANGES IN PREGNANCY

Pregnancy and subsequent labor and delivery are accompanied by predictable physiologic changes in the cardiovascular, respiratory, central nervous, and gastrointestinal systems. Furthermore, alterations in hepatic and renal function occur. Understanding these changes and appreciating their implications as they relate to responses to anesthesia is essential for safe management of the parturient and fetus.

Cardiovascular System

Changes in the cardiovascular system during pregnancy provide for the needs of the developing fetus and prepare the mother for events that will occur during labor and delivery. Specifically, important alterations occur in intravascular fluid volume and its constituents, in cardiac output, and in the peripheral circulation (Table 34-1). It is also important to understand the pathophysiology of the supine hypotension syndrome.

INTRAVASCULAR FLUID VOLUME

Increases in maternal intravascular fluid volume begin in the first trimester and at term result in an average expansion of about 1,000

ml (Fig. 34-1). Plasma volume increases about 45 percent and red blood cell volume about 20 percent. This disproportionate increase in plasma volume accounts for the relative anemia of pregnancy. Maternal hemoglobin concentrations below $11 \text{ g} \cdot \text{dl}^{-1}$ (hematocrit 33 percent) usually reflect an iron deficiency anemia.

Increased intravascular fluid volume is accommodated by the enlarged capacity of the uterine, mammary, renal, skeletal muscle, and cutaneous vascular systems. Furthermore, this increased intravascular fluid volume offsets the 400 ml to 600 ml blood loss that accompanies vaginal delivery and the average 1,000 ml blood loss that accompanies cesarean section. Indeed, transfusion of blood is usually not necessary unless maternal blood loss exceeds

TABLE 34-1. Changes in the Cardiovascular System

	Average Change from Nonpregnant Value (%)
Intravascular fluid volume	+35
Plasma volume	+45
Erythrocyte volume	+20
Cardiac output	+40
Stroke volume	+30
Heart rate	+15
Peripheral circulation	
Systolic blood pressure	No change
Systemic vascular resistance	−15
Diastolic blood pressure	−15
Central venous pressure	No change
Femoral venous pressure	+15

749

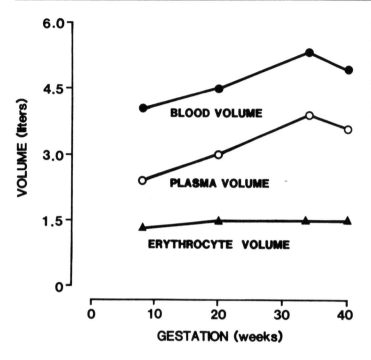

FIG. 34-1. Changes in intravascular fluid volume (blood volume), plasma volume, and erythrocyte volume during progression of normal pregnancy. The disproportionate increase in plasma volume accounts for the relative anemia of pregnancy.

1,500 ml. The normal nonpregnant intravascular fluid volume is usually reestablished 7 days to 14 days postpartum.

Total plasma protein concentrations are reduced to below 6 g·dl^{-1} at term, reflecting the dilutional effect of the expanded blood volume. Decreased plasma albumin concentrations explain the decrease in colloid oncotic pressure that accompanies pregnancy. Protein binding of drugs such as thiopental, however, is not affected by reductions in plasma concentrations of albumin.[1]

CARDIAC OUTPUT

Cardiac output is increased about 40 percent above nonpregnant levels by the 10th week of gestation and maintained at this level throughout the second and third trimesters. Augmentation of cardiac output is due to an elevated stroke volume (30 percent) and heart rate (15 percent). It is likely that placental and ovarian steroids are important in producing and sustaining this increase. Earlier studies suggesting that cardiac output decreased during the third trimester were in error. Instead, this decrease reflected reduced venous return

due to obstruction of the inferior vena cava by the gravid uterus.

Onset of labor is associated with additional increases in cardiac output. For example, compared with prelabor values, cardiac output increases about 15 percent during the latent phase, 30 percent during the active phase, and as much as 45 percent during the expulsive stage of labor. Furthermore, each uterine contraction can increase cardiac output an additional 20 percent. The greatest increase occurs immediately after delivery, when output is elevated as much as 60 percent above prelabor values. Cardiac output returns to nonpregnant values by 2 weeks postpartum.

Changes in cardiac output during gestation impose increased workloads on the heart. Cardiac reserve in the healthy parturient enables her to meet these demands. Conversely, parturients with co-existing heart disease may not be able to increase cardiac output during labor, delivery, and the immediate postpartum period. Regional anesthesia has been shown to be capable of attenuating increases in cardiac output during labor and, therefore, may be an useful way of protecting compromised cardiovascular systems during the peripartum period.[2]

PERIPHERAL CIRCULATION

Systolic blood pressure never increases above nonpregnant levels during an uncomplicated pregnancy. Since cardiac output is elevated, systemic vascular resistance must decrease for the blood pressure to remain normal. Indeed, diastolic blood pressure is usually decreased about 15 percent during pregnancy, reflecting such a decrease. There is no change in the central venous pressure during pregnancy. In contrast, femoral venous pressure is increased about 15 percent, presumably reflecting compression of the inferior vena cava by the enlarging uterus.

Peripheral venous distensibility is increased during pregnancy. This results in sluggish venous blood flow, which could lead to delayed absorption of drugs injected subcutaneously or intramuscularly. Conceivably, this slowed venous blood flow could also contribute to an increased incidence of thromboembolism.

SUPINE HYPOTENSION SYNDROME

Reductions in maternal blood pressure associated with the supine position occur in nearly 10 percent of parturients near term. Diaphoresis, nausea, vomiting, and changes in cerebration may accompany this hypotension. This symptom complex is termed the supine hypotension syndrome.

The mechanism for this syndrome is decreased venous return due to obstruction of the inferior vena cava by the gravid uterus when the parturient assumes the supine position. Decreased venous return leads to reductions in left ventricular cardiac output and decreases in blood pressure. Compression of the inferior vena cava is most common late in pregnancy, before the presenting part becomes fixed in the pelvis. Fortunately, the majority of parturients are able to initiate compensatory responses that offset the potential adverse hemodynamic sequelae of this phenomenon. For example, increased venous pressure below the level of the inferior vena cava obstruction serves to divert venous blood from the lower one-half of the body via the paravertebral venous plexuses to the azygos vein. Flow from the azygos vein enters the superior vena cava and right heart to maintain venous return, cardiac output, and blood pressure. This compensatory response means that inadvertent intravascular injection of local anesthetics during an attempted lumbar epidural block can result in bolus delivery of drugs to the heart. As a result, cardiac depression may be profound. An additional compensatory response that offsets obstruction of the inferior vena cava is an increase in sympathetic nervous system activity and subsequent elevation of systemic vascular resistance, which permits blood pressure to be maintained despite a diminished cardiac output. It is important to appreciate that compensatory increases in systemic vascular resistance are impaired by regional anesthetic techniques. Indeed, arterial hypotension is more common and profound during regional anesthetics administered to parturients, compared to nonpregnant patients. Nevertheless, this impairment of compensatory vasoconstriction by regional anesthetics may be less ominous than pain-induced changes, which result in vasoconstriction that includes the uterine vasculature.

In addition to impairment of blood flow through the inferior vena cava, angiographic studies have demonstrated compression of the lower abdominal aorta by the gravid uterus when parturients assume the supine position.[3] This compression leads to arterial hypotension in the lower extremities and decreased uterine blood flow. In contrast to compression of the inferior vena cava, obstruction to flow through the abdominal aorta is not associated with maternal symptoms or reductions in blood pressure, as measured in the arm.

Aortocaval compression results in uteroplacental insufficiency and fetal asphyxia due to decreased uterine blood flow. Even in the presence of healthy uteroplacental units, reductions in maternal systolic blood pressure to less than 100 mmHg that persist for longer than 10 minutes to 15 minutes may be associated with progressive fetal acidosis and bradycardia.[4] This emphasizes that uterine and, therefore, placental blood flow varies directly with maternal blood pressure.

The incidence of the supine hypotension syndrome can be minimized by nursing par-

TABLE 34-2.   Changes in the Respiratory System

	Average Change from Nonpregnant Value
Minute ventilation	+50%
Tidal volume	+40%
Respiratory rate	+10%
Arterial PO_2	+10 mmHg
Arterial CO_2	−10 mmHg
Arterial pH	No change
Total lung capacity	No change
Vital capacity	No change
Functional residual capacity	−20%
Expiratory reserve volume	−20%
Residual volume	−20%
Airway resistance	−35%
Oxygen consumption	+20%

turients in the lateral position. Measures to increase maternal blood pressure should be instituted whenever (1) systolic blood pressure decreases below 100 mmHg in previously normotensive parturients, (2) there is a 20 percent to 30 percent reduction in blood pressure in previously hypertensive parturients, or (3) there are fetal heart rate changes suggestive of uteroplacental insufficiency. Therapeutic measures include intravenous administration of fluids, left uterine displacement, and intravenous administration of ephedrine. Left uterine displacement is effective by moving the gravid uterus off the inferior vena cava or aorta. Displacement of the uterus to the left can be accomplished manually by lifting and displacing the uterus to the left. Alternatively, parturients can be positioned by rotating the delivery table 15 degrees to the left or by elevation of the right buttock 10 cm to 15 cm with a blanket or foam rubber wedge.

Respiratory System

Changes in the respiratory system during pregnancy are manifest as alterations in the upper airway, minute ventilation, lung volumes, and arterial oxygenation (Table 34-2) (Fig. 34-2). These changes can influence selection of tracheal tube sizes and rate of induction of and emergence from anesthesia.

UPPER AIRWAY

Capillary engorgement of the mucosal lining of the upper respiratory tract can result in difficult nasal breathing and a propensity to develop nose bleeds. Symptoms can be exacerbated by even a mild upper respiratory tract infection or edema associated with toxemia of pregnancy. These changes emphasize the need for gentleness during instrumentation of the upper airway. Vigorous oropharyngeal suctioning, placement of nasal or oral airways, or trauma during direct laryngoscopy can result in hemorrhage and further edema. It is prudent to select smaller sizes of cuffed tracheal tubes (6.5 mm to 7.0 mm I.D.) since the false vocal cords and arytenoids are often edematous.

MINUTE VENTILATION

An increase in minute ventilation is one of the earliest and most dramatic changes in respiratory function during pregnancy. Minute ventilation is increased about 50 percent above nonpregnant levels during the first trimester and maintained at this elevated level for the remainder of pregnancy. Increased circulating levels of progesterone are presumed to be the stimulus for increased minute ventilation. Mechanically, elevations in minute ventilation are achieved by an increased tidal volume; the respiratory rate is not greatly altered.

Resting maternal arterial carbon dioxide partial pressures decrease from 40 mmHg to about 30 mmHg during the first trimester as a reflection of increased minute ventilation. Arterial oxygen partial pressures increase a similar amount. Arterial pH remains near normal because of increased renal excretion of sodium bicarbonate, resulting in about a 4 mEq·L^{-1} decrease in plasma bicarbonate concentrations. Pain associated with labor and delivery results in further hyperventilation, which can be attenuated by epidural analgesia.[5] Indeed, hyperventilation of the lungs can result in arterial partial pressures of carbon dioxide as low as 10 mmHg.

LUNG VOLUMES

In contrast to the early appearance of increased minute ventilation, lung volumes do not begin to change until about the fifth month

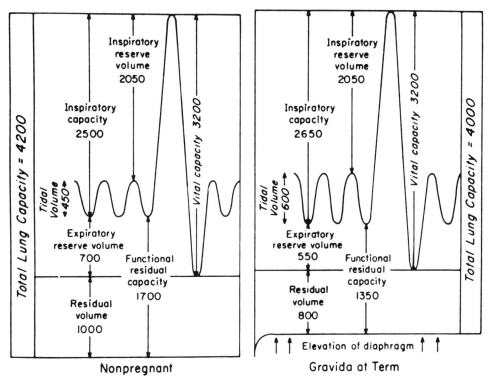

FIG. 34-2. Comparison of lung volumes and capacities in the nonpregnant patient and the gravida at term. (Bonica JJ. Principles and Practice of Obstetric Analgesia and Anesthesia. Philadelphia. FA Davis, 1976)

of gestation. With increasing enlargement of the uterus, the diaphragm is forced to assume a more cephalad position. This change is largely responsible for the 20 percent reductions in expiratory reserve volumes and residual volumes present at term (Fig. 34-2). As a result of these changes, functional residual capacity is decreased to a similar degree. Other lung volumes and capacities, including vital capacity, are not significantly changed during pregnancy.

The combination of increased minute ventilation and decreased functional residual capacity speeds the rate at which changes in alveolar concentrations of inhaled anesthetic drugs can be achieved. Induction of anesthesia, emergence from anesthesia, and changes in the depth of anesthesia are notably faster in parturients. This occurs in spite of an elevated cardiac output, emphasizing that ventilatory changes are more important than circulatory

alterations in determining alveolar concentrations of inhaled anesthetics. In addition, dose requirements for volatile anesthetic drugs are likely to be reduced during pregnancy (Fig. 34-3).[6] This combination of accelerated onset and decreased anesthetic requirements makes parturients susceptible to anesthetic overdoses. For example, low concentrations of inhaled anesthetics may result in loss of protective upper airway reflexes during delivery of inspired concentrations of anesthetics that are usually considered safe.

ARTERIAL OXYGENATION

Induction of general anesthesia in parturients may be associated with marked reductions in arterial oxygen partial pressures, if apnea is prolonged, as during intubation of the trachea. This tendency for rapid decreases in

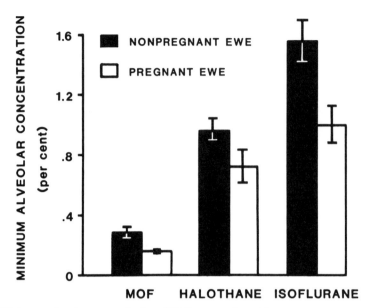

FIG. 34-3. Minimum alveolar concentration (MAC) was reduced in pregnant as compared with non-pregnant ewes. (Data adapted from Palahniuk RJ, Shnider SM, Eger II EI. Pregnancy decreases the requirements for inhaled anesthetic agents. Anesthesiology 1974;41:82–3)

arterial oxygenation reflects decreased oxygen reserves secondary to reductions in functional residual capacity. The nearly 20 percent increase in oxygen consumption present near term also contributes to a decreased oxygen reserve. These changes emphasize the importance of preoxygenation before any anticipated period of apnea in parturients. In order to maximize fetal benefits of preoxygenation, the maternal inhalation of oxygen may need to be continued for about 6 minutes, since this is the estimated time required for maternal to fetal equilibration.[7] A mean increase in the umbilical vein oxygen partial pressure from 22 mmHg to 28 mmHg can be expected in fetuses of parturients breathing pure oxygen for this period of time.

Maternal arterial oxygen partial pressures while breathing room air often exceed 100 mmHg, reflecting the presence of chronic hyperventilation. It is important to appreciate that arterial oxygenation can be influenced by changing from the sitting or semirecumbent to the supine position. For example, about 25 percent of parturinets near term will develop re-

ductions in arterial oxygen partial pressures upon assuming the supine position,[8] most likely reflecting reductions in cardiac output due to aortocaval compression. Furthermore, small airways closure may contribute to perfusion of unventilated alveoli. Since it is not possible to predict the susceptibility of parturients to such reductions, it would seem prudent to provide routinely left uterine displacement and to administer supplemental oxygen when regional anesthesia is used.

Nervous System Changes

Anesthetic requirements for methoxyflurane, halothane, and isoflurane are reduced 25 percent to 40 percent in gravid animals at term (Fig. 34-3).[6] It is presumed, but not documented, that similar changes occur for nitrous oxide requirements. Conceivably, sedative effects produced by progesterone could be responsible for decreases in anesthetic requirements. Nevertheless, in animals, anesthetic requirements return to nonpregnant values within 5 days postpartum, while plasma concentrations of progesterone remain elevated, suggesting that the mechanism for reduction cannot be attributed entirely to progesterone.[9] Regardless of the mechanism, the important clinical implication is that alveolar concentrations of inhaled drugs that would not produce unconsciousness in nonpregnant patients may approximate anesthetizing concentrations in parturients. This degree of central nervous system depression may also impair protective upper airway reflexes and subject parturients to hazards of pulmonary aspiration.

Increased intra-abdominal pressure as pregnancy progresses, plus shunting of blood via paravertebral venous plexuses due to compression of the inferior vena cava, results in engorgement of epidural veins. This engorgement decreases the size of the epidural space and by compression may also reduce the volume of cerebrospinal fluid in the subarachnoid space. These engorged veins also exert a pumping-like effect, resulting in spread of local anesthetics placed in the epidural space over more segments than would normally be expected. Furthermore, high pressures in the epidural space may facilitate transfer of local anesthetics into the cerebrospinal fluid and favor the action of the drug directly on the spinal cord. In addition, each spinal nerve root is accompanied by an epidural vein as it passes out the intervetebral foramina. If this vein is swollen, it may decrease the size of the foramina and reduce the escape of drugs that have been injected into the epidural space. Even exaggerated lumbar lordosis of pregnancy may contribute to cephalad spread of local anesthetics. These changes are consistent with the 30 percent to 50 percent reductions in dose requirements of local anesthetics necessary for epidural or subarachnoid anesthesia at term, as compared with nonpregnant patients.[10] The observation that exaggerated spread of local anesthetics placed in the epidural space as early as the first trimester suggests a role of biochemical and mechanical changes.[11] For example, reduced plasma concentrations of bicarbonate in compensation for hyperventilation could reduce buffer capacity and contribute to enhanced actions of local anes-

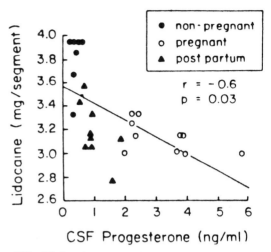

FIG. 34-4. Correlation between lidocaine dose requirements (mg per segment) and cerebrospinal fluid progesterone concentrations (ng·ml⁻¹) in nonpregnant, pregnant and postpartum patients. (Datta S, Hurley RJ, Naulty JS, et al. Plasma and cerebrospinal fluid progesterone concentrations in pregnant and nonpregnant women. Anesth Analg 1986;65:950–4 Reprinted with permission from IARS)

thetics. Likewise, increased plasma and cerebrospinal fluid concentrations of progesterone parallel the augmented dermatomal spread of local anesthetics placed in the subarachnoid space (Fig. 34-4).[12] Despite these observations, there are also data that do not demonstrate a difference in the level of sensory anesthesia achieved when equal volumes of local anesthetic are injected into the epidural space of pregnant and nonpregnant patients if care is exercised to prevent aortocaval compression in parturients.[13]

Renal Changes

Renal blood flow and glomerular filtration rate are increased about 50 percent by the fourth month of gestation. During the third trimester, these values slowly return toward nonpregnant levels. As a reflection of these changes, normal upper limits of blood urea nitrogen concentrations and plasma creatinine concentrations are reduced about 50 percent.

Hepatic Changes

Plasma bilirubin concentrations and hepatic blood flow are not changed during pregnancy, although the majority of parturients have abnormal bromsulphalein excretion tests.[14] In addition, plasma protein concentrations and plasma cholinesterase activity are decreased. For example, plasma cholinesterase activity is decreased about 25 percent from the 10th week of gestation to 2 weeks to 6 weeks postpartum.[15] This decreased activity is unlikely to be associated with prolongation of the neuromuscular blocking effects of succinycholine, although occasional unexpected prolonged responses have been observed.[16,17] For unknown reasons, plasma transaminase concentrations and the circulating levels of alkaline phosphatase are often elevated during pregnancy.

Acute fatty liver of pregnancy is a rare but potentially fatal disorder, which typically manifests in the 35th week of gestation.[18] Jaundice and hepatic encephalopathy occur late in the disease. Plasma transaminase levels are usually modestly elevated in contrast to marked elevations characteristic of viral hepatitis. Hepatic dysfunction may also accompany toxemia of pregnancy, but plasma transaminase levels are usually only minimally elevated. Treatment is supportive plus rapid termination of pregnancy.

Gastrointestinal Changes

Gastrointestinal changes during pregnancy make parturients vulnerable to regurgitation of gastric contents and to the development of acid pneumonitis should pulmonary aspiration occur. For example, the enlarged uterus displaces the pylorus upward and backward, which retards gastric emptying. Furthermore, progesterone decreases gastroin-testinal motility. As a result, gastric emptying time is prolonged and gastric fluid volume tends to be elevated, even in fasting states. In addition, gastrin, which is secreted by the placenta, stimulates gastric hydrogen ion secretion, such that pH of gastric fluid is predictably low in parturients. Finally, the enlarging uterus changes the angle of the gastroesophageal junction, leading to relative incompetence of the physiologic sphincter mechanism. Indeed, lower esophageal sphincter pressure is less and gastric pressure greater in pregnant as compared with nonpregnant patients.[19] As a result, gastric fluid reflux into the esophagus and esophagitis are common in parturients. These changes emphasize that parturients are prone to silent regurgitation, even in the absence of sedative drugs or general anesthesia.

Onset of labor may introduce additional hazards for parturients. Regardless of the time interval since ingestion of food, parturients in labor must be treated as having full stomachs. It is estimated that 30 percent to 50 percent of maternal deaths associated with anesthesia are due to pulmonary aspiration of gastric contents. Pain, anxiety, and drugs (opioids, anticholinergics) can significantly retard gastric emptying times beyond already prolonged transit times. Dehydration and starvation ketosis also slow gastric emptying times and can stimulate gastric secretion of hydrogen ions. Excessive use of opioids may be associated with vomiting in parturients with potentially attenuated protective airway reflexes. Hypotension resulting from aortocaval compression or peripheral sympathetic nervous system blockade, as accompanies regional anesthetics, can result in nausea, vomiting, and impairment of consciousness from cerebral hypoxia.

Increased risk to parturients for pulmonary aspiration of gastric contents is the reason for recommending placement of a cuffed tube in the trachea of every parturient who is going to be rendered unconscious with central nervous system depressant drugs. Only in rare situations, when intubation of the trachea is technically impossible and there is fetal distress necessitating early delivery, should general anesthesia in the absence of a cuffed tube in the trachea be considered acceptable. In this situation, sustained cricoid pressure should be employed to reduce the possibility of passively regurgitated material entering the hypopharynx. Furthermore, cricoid pressure should prevent excessive gastric distention.

Recognition that pH of inhaled gastric fluid is important in production and severity of acid pneumonitis is the basis for the administration of oral antacids to parturients during labor and before delivery.[20,21] There is no doubt that oral antacids are effective in elevating the pH of gastric fluid. Nevertheless, it is difficult to confirm benefits of routine use of oral antacids.[22,23] Inhalation of antacids containing particulate matter can produce adverse pulmonary changes.[24,25] In attempts to obviate hazards of inhalation of particulate matter, use of nonparticulate antacids, such as sodium citrate, has been recommended.[26] It is of interest that administration of opioids to provide analgesia during labor slows gastric emptying and prolongs the duration of action of antacids.[27] Frequent antacid administration to patients also receiving opioids could result in accumulating gastric fluid volume. For this reason, when antacids are administered as prophylaxis before general anesthesia they should be administered just before the induction of anesthesia. Considering the potential accumulation of antacids in the stomach and the possible rebound hypersecretion of gastric hydrogen ions, especially when calcium containing antacids are administered, there seems little reason to recommend routine use of antacids at regular intervals during labor.[27]

Additional drugs for increasing gastric fluid pH and decreasing the gastric fluid volume can be considered. For example, anticholinergic drugs, by interfering with parasympathetic nervous system innervation of the stomach, result in dose-related decreases in secretion of gastric hydrogen ions. Any theoretical advantage that anticholinergic drugs might exert on secretion of hydrogen ions by the stomach is reduced by the fact these drugs decrease the tone of the lower esophageal sphincter. Therefore, these drugs could increase the likelihood of gastric fluid reflux into the esophagus. In contrast, metoclopramide increases lower esophageal sphincter tone and speeds gastric emptying of patients in active labor.[28] Of special interest is the fact that metoclopramide, crosses the blood-brain barrier and the placenta. In view of its beneficial effects, metoclopramide may be a useful drug to administer to parturients at high risk for elevated gastric fluid volumes (apprehension, opioid analgesia, recent food ingestion, obesity, heartburn indicative of lower esophageal dysfunction, and gastric hypomotility) and requiring general anesthesia. Metoclopramide, however, may not reverse gastric hypomotility due to opioids. In the absence of active labor and elevated gastric fluid volumes, metoclopramide has not been shown to result in significant differences in gastric fluid volumes compared with untreated parturients.[29] For this reason, routine administration of metoclopramide to parturients before elective cesarean section may not be useful.

Histamine H-2 receptor antagonists, such as cimetidine 300 mg administered intramuscularly, predictably elevate gastric fluid pH in parturients when administered 1 hour to 3 hours preoperatively.[30] Cimetidine crosses the placenta but has no detectable effects on neonates. Intravenous administration of cimetidine may be associated with reductions in heart rate and blood pressure.

PHYSIOLOGY OF UTEROPLACENTAL CIRCULATION

The placenta provides for the union of the maternal and fetal circulations for the purpose of physiologic exchange. Maternal blood is delivered to the placenta by the uterine arteries, and fetal blood arrives via two umbilical arteries. Nutrient-rich and waste-free blood is delivered to the fetus via a single umbilical vein. The most important determinants of placental function are uterine blood flow and the placental area available for exchange of nutrients. An acute decrease in placental function interferes with the passage of oxygen to and carbon dioxide from the fetus, resulting in fetal hypoxemia and acidosis. A chronic decrease in placental function is associated with delayed fetal growth, reflecting absence of necessary nutrient factors.

Uterine Blood Flow

Uterine blood flow at term is 500 ml·min^{-1} to 700 ml·min^{-1}, which represents about 10 percent of the maternal cardiac output. About 80 percent of this blood flow is to the placenta, and the remainder supplies the myometrium. Uterine blood flow is not auto-regulated. Therefore, uterine blood flow and subsequently placental blood flow is directly proportional to mean perfusion pressure (uterine arterial pressure minus uterine venous pressure) and inversely proportional to uterine vascular resistance.

Maintenance of uterine blood flow is critical, as this flow determines the adequacy of placental circulation, and ultimately fetal well-being. Uterine blood flow is reduced by drugs or events that decrease perfusion pressure or increase uterine vascular resistance. For ex-

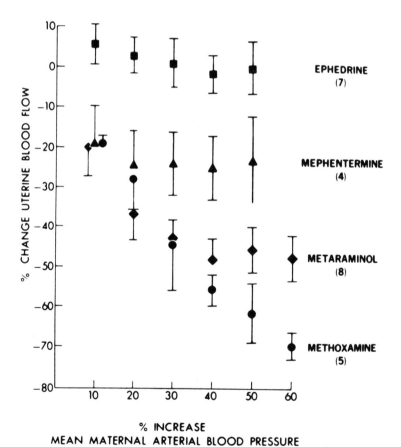

FIG. 34-5. Uterine blood flow was measured in pregnant ewes before and after increases in maternal arterial blood pressure produced by intravenous administration of sympathomimetic drugs. With the exception of ephedrine, these drugs decreased uterine blood flow, despite increasing mean arterial pressure. All values are Mean ± SE, the number of animals studied for each drug is in parentheses. (Ralston DH, Shnider SM, deLorimer AA. Effects of equipotent ephedrine, metaraminol, mephentermine, and methoxamine on uterine blood flow in the pregnant ewe. Anesthesiology 1974;40:354–70)

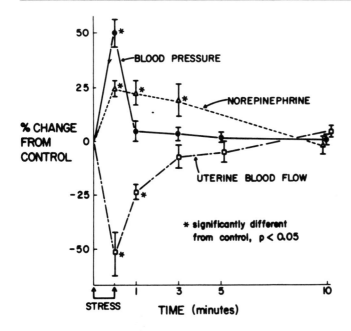

FIG. 34-6. Electrically-induced stress in pregnant ewes lasting 30 seconds to 60 seconds resulted in increased maternal blood pressure and plasma norepinephrine concentrations (Mean ± SE). Uterine blood flow was reduced about 50 percent at the time of maximum blood pressure and catecholamine elevation. (Shnider SM, Wright RG, Levinson G, et al. Uterine blood flow and plasma norepinephrine changes during maternal stress in the pregnant ewe. Anesthesiology 1979;50:524–7)

ample, maternal hypotension or excessive uterine activity are the events most likely to reduce acutely uterine blood flow. In the presence of a normal placenta, it is estimated that uterine blood flow can decrease about 50 percent before fetal distress, as reflected by acidosis, is detectable.[31]

HYPOTENSION

Hypotension due to aortocaval compression or peripheral sympathetic nervous system blockade decreases uterine blood flow by reductions in perfusion pressure. Conversely, uterine contractions reduce uterine blood flow secondary to elevated uterine venous pressure. Finally, because uterine vessels are richly supplied by the sympathetic nervous system, alpha-adrenergic stimulation reduces uterine blood flow by increasing uterine vascular resistance. Indeed, alpha-adrenergic drugs such as methoxamine and metaraminol can produce uterine vascular constriction that results in decreased uterine blood flow and development of fetal acidosis (Fig. 34-5).[32] Conversely, ephedrine does not decrease uterine blood flow, despite substantial increases in maternal arterial pressure (Fig. 34-5).[32]

UTERINE VASCULAR RESISTANCE

Increased uterine vascular resistance, with reductions in uterine blood flow, can result from maternal stress or pain that stimulates endogenous release of catecholamines (Fig. 34-6).[33] This response suggests that adequate regional or general anesthesia may be protective to the fetus.

HYPOCAPNIA

Occurrence of maternal hypocapnia is frequent during labor and delivery. Nevertheless, effects of low maternal arterial carbon dioxide partial pressures on uterine blood flow are controversial. In one report, hyperventilation of the lungs to arterial carbon dioxide partial pressures of 17 mmHg was associated with decreased uterine blood flow.[34] Conversely, others have not shown adverse effects on uterine blood flow at similar degrees of hypocarbia. Indeed, during controlled ventilation of the lungs decreases in uterine blood flow may be due to mechanical effects of positive pressure and not maternal carbon dioxide partial pressures (Fig. 34-7).[35]

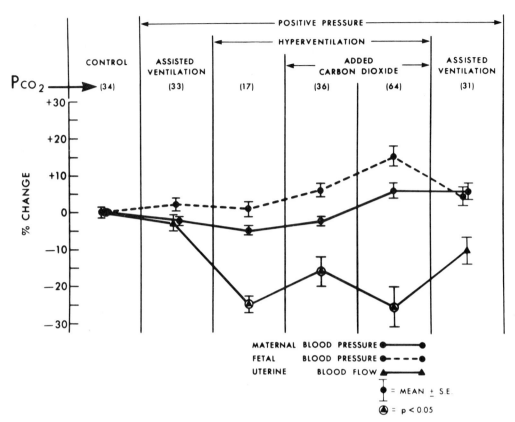

FIG. 34-7. Mean maternal blood pressure, fetal blood pressure, and uterine blood flow were determined during positive pressure ventilation of the lungs at varying maternal arterial carbon dioxide partial pressures (PCO_2). Reductions in uterine blood flow were unrelated to maternal arterial PCO_2, suggesting that mechanical effects of positive pressure ventilation of the lungs were responsible. (Levinson G, Shnider SM, deLorimer AA, Steffenson JL. Effects of maternal hyperventilation on uterine blood flow and fetal oxygenation and acid-base status. Anesthesiology 1974;40:340–7)

DRUGS

Drugs administered to parturients to produce analgesia and anesthesia during labor and delivery may produce profound effects on uterine blood flow and, therefore, fetal well-being. These effects are most likely due to drug-induced changes in maternal blood pressure, rather than to direct effects of anesthetics on uterine tone or vasculature. Data on the effects of anesthetics on uterine blood flow are almost exclusively from animal models, most often the pregnant ewe.

When inspired concentrations of halothane are less than 1 percent, fetal acid-base status is not adversely affected, suggesting that uterine blood flow is not significantly reduced.[36] Higher inspired concentrations of halothane are associated with maternal hypotension and fetal acidosis. Isoflurane and, by inference, enflurane, when administered at concentrations comparable to those studied for halothane, have similar effects on uterine blood flow.[37]

Short-acting barbiturates, such as thiopental, decrease uterine blood flow in proportion to drug-induced reductions in blood pressure. Ketamine, in doses up to 1 mg·kg^{-1}, is unlikely to alter uterine blood flow.[38] Higher doses of ketamine may produce increases in uterine tone that are associated with reductions in uterine blood flow despite normal to increased maternal blood pressures (Fig. 34-8).[38] Epidural anesthesia with chloroprocaine[39] or bupivacaine[40] does not alter uterine blood flow, if maternal hypotension is avoided. Furthermore, addition of epinephrine to local anesthetic solutions does not seem to influence uterine blood flow.

Placenta Exchange

Passive diffusion is the principal mechanism for transfer of substances across the placenta, from the maternal circulation to the fetus and vice versa. Diffusion of substances across the placenta depends on maternal-to-fetal concentration gradients, molecular weight, lipid solubility, and degree of ionization. Interaction of these factors is described by Fick's equation of passive diffusion (Table 34-3). Minimizing maternal blood concentrations of drugs is the most important method for limiting the amount of drugs that ultimately reach the fetus. Furthermore, transfer of drugs to the fetus can be decreased by intravenous injection of drugs just before uterine contractions, since maternal blood flow to the placenta

is markedly decreased during contractions. Finally, in addition to simple diffusion, materials may cross the placenta by active transport, facilitated transport, transfer through pores, and pinocytosis.

PERINATAL PHARMACOLOGY

Maternally administered drugs reach the fetus after traversing the placenta. The amount of drug transferred to the fetus depends on uterine blood flow to the intervillous space of the placenta and the amount of diffusable drug in the maternal intervillous space. Eventual fetal concentrations depend on fetal uptake and distribution of drugs.

Uterine Blood Flow to the Intervillous Space

Maternal drug delivery to the placental exchange site depends on the fraction of total uterine blood flow that perfuses intervillous

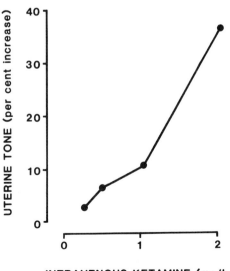

FIG. 34-8. Intravenous administration of ketamine produces dose-related (cumulative dose) increases in mean uterine tone, as measured in five parturients at term. (Data adapted from Galloon S. Ketamine for obstetric delivery. Anesthesiology 1976;44:522–4)

TABLE 34-3. Fick's Equation for Passive Diffusion

$$\frac{Q}{t} = K\frac{A(C_m - C_f)}{D}$$

$\dfrac{Q}{t}$ = quantity transferred per unit time

  K = diffusion constant (determined by lipid solubility, molecular weight, and ionization of the substance or drug)

  A = surface area available for diffusion

C_m = maternal blood concentration

C_f = fetal blood concentration

  D = thickness of the placenta

spaces. In addition, the amount of drug present in this blood will depend on when the drug was injected relative to uterine contractions. For example, drugs injected as a bolus during uterine contractions, when uterine arterial perfusion ceases, would theoretically be unable to reach the placenta, at least during the first maternal circulation time. Conversely, the same drugs injected at the onset or decline of uterine contractions, when only uterine venous outflow was impeded, might be sequestered in the placenta, with potentially greater transfer to the fetus. Furthermore, aortocaval compression could alter drug delivery of drugs to intervillous spaces.

Diffusible Drug in the Maternal Intervillous Space

The amount of drug in maternal intervillous spaces that is available for diffusion to the fetus is dependent on the physical and chemical characteristics of the drugs (Table 34-4). These characteristics include maternal protein

TABLE 34-4. Determinants of Diffusion Across the Placenta

	Rapid Diffusion	Slow Diffusion
Maternal protein binding	Low	High
Molecular weight	500	1000
Lipid solubility	High	Low
Ionization	Minimal	Maximum

binding, molecular weight, lipid solubility, and the maternal pH relative to the pK of the drugs. Placental transfer of drugs to the fetus is facilitated by minimal binding to maternal proteins, low molecular weight, high lipid solubility, and minimal ionization at the pH of maternal blood.

MATERNAL PROTEIN BINDING

Maternal protein binding of local anesthetics is important, since that portion of drug not bound to protein is available for diffusion across the placenta. Maternal protein binding of local anesthetics varies with individual drugs and their plasma concentrations (Fig. 34-9).[41] At typical clinical concentrations, 50 percent to 70 percent of lidocaine is bound to protein, compared with 95 percent for bupivacaine. The greater degree of protein binding for bupivacaine could impair placental transfer by reducing the amount of free drug available for diffusion. This is consistent with the observation that the ratio of umbilical vein-to-uterine artery concentrations of bupivacaine is lower than the ratio measured for lidocaine. Nevertheless, dissociation of local anesthetic from protein is rapid, and it is questionable whether protein binding of drugs significantly impairs diffusion across the placenta. Decreased protein binding, as plasma concentrations of local anesthetics increase, presumably reflects saturation of available sites for binding. As a result, high plasma concentrations of local anesthetics, as follow accidental intravascular injections, are associated with an increased fraction of pharmacologically active unbound drug.

MOLECULAR WEIGHT AND LIPID SOLUBILITY

Large molecular weight and poor lipid solubility of nondepolarizing muscle relaxants are consistent with the fact that these drugs cross the placenta only to limited extents. Succinylcholine has a low molecular weight but is highly ionized and, therefore, does not readily cross the placenta. Conversely, placental transfer of thiobarbiturates, local anesthetics,

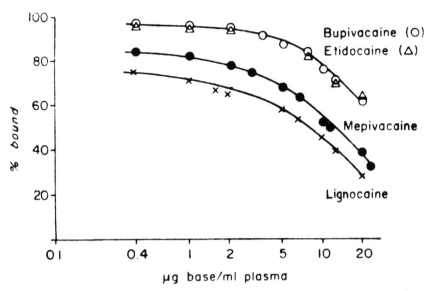

FIG. 34-9. Maternal plasma protein binding (percent bound) of local anesthetics depends on the drug and on the plasma concentration (μg base per ml plasma) of that drug. As plasma concentrations of local anesthetics increase, the percent bound to protein decreases. As a result, pharmacologically active unbound fractions increase. (Tucker GT, Mather LE. Pharmacokinetics of local anesthetic agents. Br J Anaesth 1975;47:213–24)

and opioids is facilitated by the relatively low molecular weights of these substances. Furthermore, a large fraction of these drugs exist in lipid-soluble, nonionized forms at the pH of maternal blood.

Fetal Uptake

Fetal uptake of drugs from intervillous spaces is determined by solubility of drugs in fetal blood and distribution of fetal blood flow to the intervillous spaces. Fetal blood is more acidic (0.1 pH unit lower) than maternal blood. The lower fetal pH means that weakly basic drugs, such as local anesthetics and opioids, which cross the placenta in nonionized forms will become ionized in the fetal circulation. Since ionized drugs cannot readily cross the placenta back to the maternal circulation, it follows that these drugs will accumulate in fetal blood against a concentration gradient. This phenomenon is known as ion trapping and may explain higher concentrations of lidocaine found in the fetus when acidosis due to fetal distress is present (Fig. 34-10).[42] Furthermore, conversion of lidocaine to the ionized fraction maintains concentration gradients from mother to fetus for continued passage of nonionized lidocaine to the fetus. Another consideration is the ability of the fetus and newborn to metabolize local anesthetics in the liver. Despite reduced activity, compared with an adult, fetal hepatic enzyme systems are adequately developed to metabolize most drugs, including local anesthetics. An important exception is the limited ability of the fetus to either metabolize mepivacaine or excrete this local anesthetic via the kidneys.[43]

Fetal Distribution

Unique characteristics of the fetal circulation influence the distribution of drugs in the fetus. For example, about 75 percent of the um-

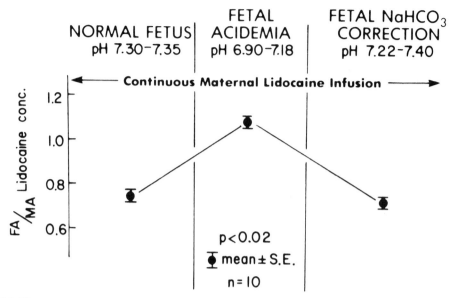

FIG. 34-10. Fetal-to-maternal arterial (FA/MA) lidocaine ratios were higher during fetal acidemia than during control (normal fetus), or during pH correction with sodium bicarbonate. Presumably, acidosis in the fetus favors the existence of lidocaine in the ionized fraction. Since ionized forms of drugs cannot easily cross lipid barriers, such as the placenta, it is predictable that this form of lidocaine will be trapped (ion trapping) in the fetus. Furthermore, conversion of lidocaine to the ionized fraction maintains the gradient from mother to fetus for continued passage of the nonionized fraction of lidocaine to the fetus. (Biehl D, Shnider SM, Levinson G, Callender K. Placental transfer of lidocaine: Effects of fetal acidosis. Anesthesiology 1978;48:409–12)

bilical venous blood flows through the liver; the remainder of this blood passes through the ductus venosus into the inferior vena cava. As a result of hepatic perfusion, a significant amount of drug can be metabolized. Indeed, hepatic metabolism reduces the concentrations of drugs that are eventually delivered by the fetal arterial circulation to vital organs such as the brain and heart. Furthermore, drugs in that portion of the umbilical venous blood that enters the inferior vena cava via the ductus venosus will be diluted by drug-free blood returning from the lower extremities and pelvic viscera of the fetus. Therefore, it is likely that drug concentrations measured in umbilical vein blood will be substantially higher than concentrations delivered to fetal tissues by the arterial circulation. This is consistent with the observation that maternal depression produced by drugs, such as thiopental or inhaled anesthetics, is not paralleled by similar degrees of fetal central nervous system depression. In-

deed, the unique anatomy of the fetal circulation serves to protect the vital organs of the fetus from exposure to high concentrations of drugs that may be present in the umbilical venous blood, secondary to diffusion of these drugs from the maternal circulation. Nevertheless, fetal acidosis is associated with increased myocardial blood flow and cerebral blood flow, with a resulting increased delivery of drugs to these organs during fetal distress.

MATERNAL MEDICATION DURING LABOR

Despite increasing use of epidural analgesia for pain relief during labor, there are still occasional roles for systemic medications to relieve pain and anxiety. There is no ideal drug, as all systemic medications cross the placenta to some extent, and produce depressant effects on the fetus. The amount of fetal depression depends primarily on the dose of drug and route and time of administration before delivery. Drugs likely to be administered as systemic medications are benzodiazepines, opioids, and dissociative drugs. Barbiturates or scopolamine are no longer popular.

Benzodiazepines

Benzodiazepines rapidly cross the placenta. When the maternal dose of diazepam exceeds 30 mg, there is associated fetal hypotonia, decreased feeding, and hypothermia.[44] Beat-to-beat variability of fetal heart rate is decreased with small intravenous doses of diazepam (5 mg to 10 mg), but there are no detectable adverse effects on the fetus. Therefore, small intravenous doses of diazepam (2.5 mg to 10 mg) or midazolam (1 mg to 5 mg) are acceptable for relieving anxiety, as during cesarean section performed with epidural anesthesia.

A theoretical problem is the use of sodium benzoate as a buffer for diazepam. Sodium benzoate is a bilirubin-albumin uncoupler and might increase susceptibility of infants to kernicterus, though this is an unlikely problem when small doses of diazepam are used.[45] Furthermore, the maternal liver should rapidly metabolize sodium benzoate.

Opioids

Opioids are the most effective systemic medications for the relief of pain. Maternal side-effects of opioids include (1) orthostatic hypotension; (2) stimulation of the chemoreceptor trigger zone in the medulla, producing nausea and vomiting; (3) delayed gastric emptying; and (4) decreased uterine activity, with impaired progress of labor if administered during the latent or early stages of labor. All opioids rapidly cross the placenta and are capable of decreasing beat-to-beat variability of fetal heart rate. In addition, residual effects of opioids may manifest as neonatal ventilatory depression and alterations in the neurobehavioral status.

Meperidine is a popular opioid for administration to parturients. Morphine is rarely used; one reason is the apparent greater sensitivity of the respiratory center of the newborn to morphine, as compared with meperidine.[46] It should be appreciated that the incidence of neonatal depression associated with maternal administration of intramuscular meperidine (50 mg to 100 mg) is greatest in neonates born 2 hours to 4 hours after injection of the opioid.[47] Depression of neonates is less when delivery occurs within 1 hour or more than 4 hours after injection. The reason for the apparent safe period with intramuscular meperidine is not known. Finally, meperidine can displace bupivacaine from protein binding sites and thus increase the level of unbound and pharmacologically active bupivacaine in maternal plasma.[48]

When opioid depressant effects on neonates are anticipated, an opioid antagonist, such as naloxone, may be administered to parturients 10 minutes to 15 minutes before delivery or to neonates immediately after delivery. A theoretical but undocumented concern as to the safety of naloxone is related to the possible role of endorphins as neurotransmitters. Conceivably, blocking the effects of endorphins could interfere with responses of neonates to stress. Finally, naloxone should not be administered to opioid addicts or their neonates, since acute withdrawal symptoms could be precipitated.

Dissociative Drugs

Intermittent intravenous doses of ketamine (10 mg to 15 mg) can be titrated to produce intense analgesia in parturients, without resulting in loss of consciousness.[49] The onset of action is within 1 minute, and the duration is 5 minutes to 15 minutes. The dose of ketamine should not exceed 100 mg in 30 minutes, or a total dose of 3 $mg \cdot kg^{-1}$. This low-dose approach is particularly useful for parturients in whom vaginal delivery is imminent or when regional analgesia is incomplete. Ketamine readily crosses the placenta but in low doses does not cause neonatal depression. Large doses of ketamine can cause obtundation of maternal laryngeal reflexes. It must be recognized that adverse psychological changes may accompany even low doses of ketamine.

PROGRESS OF LABOR

Progress of labor refers to increasing cervical dilation, effacement, and descent of the presenting fetal part with time (Fig. 34-11).[50] This progress is divided into the first and second stages of labor, depending on the dilation of the cervix. The first stage is further subdivided into a latent and an active phase. The active phase consists of an acceleration phase, phase of maximum slope, and deceleration phase. The onset of regular contractions signals the beginning of the first stage of labor. This stage lasts 7 hours to 13 hours in primigravidas, and 4 hours to 5 hours in multigravidas. The second stage of labor begins with complete dilation of the cervix.

Progress of labor is unpredictable because it is influenced by many variables, including maternal pain, parity, size and presentation of the fetus, and drugs and techniques used to provide analgesia or anesthesia. Abnormal progress of labor can be classified as slow latent phase, active phase arrest, and arrest of descent (Table 34-5). Excessive sedation or anesthesia is the most common cause for prolongation of the latent phase. The mechanism is decreased uterine activity secondary to depressant drugs. During the active phase, the most likely causes of delayed progress of labor

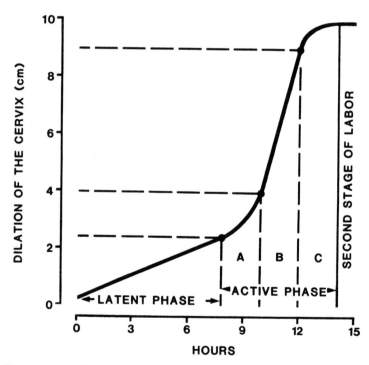

FIG. 34-11. The progress of labor is divided into first and second stages, depending on the dilation of the cervix. The first stage is further subdivided into a latent and an active phase. The active phase consists of the accelerated phase (A), the phase of maximum slope (B), and the deceleration phase (C). (Graph adapted from Friedman EA. Primigravid labor. A graphicostatistical analysis. Obstet Gynecol 1955;6:567–89. Reprinted with permission from the American College of Obstetricians and Gynecologists)

TABLE 34-5. Abnormal Progress of Labor

	Slow Latent Phase	Active Phase Arrest	Arrest of Descent
Primigravida	20 hours	No dilation of cervix for 2 hours	No descent for 1 hour
Multigravida	14 hours	As above	As above

are cephalopelvic disproportion, fetal malposition, and fetal malpresentation.

Anesthetic techniques affect uterine activity and progress of labor. It is taught that regional anesthesia administered early in the course of labor will slow progress.[51] This admonition is difficult to confirm, since early progress of labor is so variable. Indeed, labor can slow during the latent phase in the absence of anesthesia. Furthermore, catecholamines released in response to pain can inhibit coordinated and effective uterine contractions such that analgesia provided by appropriate regional anesthetic techniques may actually enhance early progress of labor. The impact of anesthesia on progress of labor is more predictable after labor has become active. For example, during the active phase of the first stage, a T-10 sensory level produced by a subarachnoid block[52] or a lumbar epidural block[53] has no significant effect on uterine activity or the progress of labor, provided fetal malposition or malpresentation is absent and hypotension is avoided. Regional anesthesia, however, by removing the reflex urge of parturients to bear down, may prolong the second stage of labor. Nevertheless, there is no evidence that labor prolonged by regional anesthesia is harmful to the fetus.

An increased incidence of midforceps deliveries may occur when regional anesthesia is administered.[54] Furthermore, relaxation of pelvic musculature interferes with flexion and internal rotation of the fetus, which may predispose to persistent occiput posterior presentations. These problems can be minimized by using low concentrations of local anesthetics for epidural analgesia, so as to preserve skeletal muscle function, and withholding perineal doses of local anesthetics until descent and rotation of the fetus has occurred.

Volatile anesthetics produce dose-related decreases in uterine activity. Indeed, the most reliable way of rapidly producing uterine relaxation is with general anesthesia. Equipotent doses of halothane, enflurane, and isoflurane produce similar degrees of uterine relaxation.[55] Nevertheless, inhalation analgesia with low inspired concentrations of halothane (0.5 percent) or enflurane (1 percent) during vaginal delivery or cesarean section does not decrease uterine activity, prolong labor, increase postpartum blood flow, or interfere with uterine responses to oxytocin. Halothane (1 percent inspired) or enflurane (2 percent inspired) and presumably isoflurane will relax the uterus but not block responses to oxytocin.

REGIONAL ANALGESIA FOR LABOR AND VAGINAL DELIVERY

Compared with analgesia produced by inhaled or parenteral drugs, use of regional analgesia for labor and vaginal delivery reduces the likelihood of fetal drug depression and maternal pulmonary aspiration. Rational use of regional anesthetic techniques requires an understanding of the pathways responsible for the transmission of pain during labor and vaginal delivery (Fig. 34-12). For example, pain of labor arises primarily from receptors in uterine and perineal structures. Afferent pain impulses from the cervix and uterus travel in nerves that accompany sympathetic nervous system fibers and enter the spinal cord at T10-12 and L1. Pain pathways from the perineum travel to S2-4 via the pudendal nerve. Pain during the first stage of labor results from dilation of the cervix, contraction of the uterus, and traction on the round ligament. Pain during this first stage of labor is visceral and is referred to dermatomes supplied by spinal cord seg-

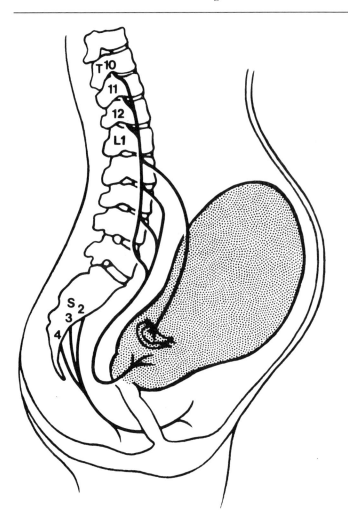

FIG. 34-12. Schematic diagram of pain pathways during parturition. Afferent pain impulses from the cervix and uterus are carried by nerves that accompany sympathetic fibers and enter the spinal cord at T10-L1. Pain pathways from the perineum travel to S2-4 via the pudendal nerves.

ments T10-L1. In the second stage of labor, pain is produced by distention of the perineum and stretching of fascia, skin, and subcutaneous tissues. This pain is typically somatic.

The afferent sensory component of pain during labor and vaginal delivery can be interrupted by paracervical block, lumbar epidural block, caudal block, subarachnoid (saddle) block, and pudendal nerve block (Table 34-6). Blocks effective during the first stage of labor include paracervical, lumbar epidural, and caudal. Selective spinal analgesia using intrathecal or epidural opioids has also been evaluated for relief of pain during the first stage of labor. Pain during the second stage of labor is relieved by lumbar epidural, caudal, subarachnoid, or pudendal nerve blocks.

Paracervical Block

Injection of local anesthetics into the fornix of the vagina lateral to the cervix (3 and 9 positions) anesthetizes sensory fibers from the uterus, cervix, and upper vagina. Maternal hypotension does not result, since sympathetic nervous system blockade does not occur. Sensory fibers from the perineum are not blocked; therefore, paracervical block is effective only during the first stage of labor.

The major disadvantage of a paracervical block is the 8 percent to 40 percent incidence of fetal bradycardia that develops 2 minutes to 10 minutes after injection of local anesthetics.[56] The cause is not clear but is probably

TABLE 34-6. Regional Analgesia for Labor and Vaginal Delivery

Technique	Area of Anesthesia
Paracervical block	Blocks pain impulses that travel via T10 to L1
Lumbar epidural block	
Segmental	T10–L1
Standard	T10–S5
Caudal block	T10–S5
Subarachnoid block	
Saddle	S1–S5
Standard	T10–S5
Pudendal block	S2–S4

related to decreased uterine blood flow secondary to uterine vasoconstriction from local anesthetics applied in close proximity to the uterine artery, plus direct cardiac toxicity due to high fetal blood levels of local anesthetics. Because the paracervical area is highly vascular, there is rapid systemic absorption of local anesthetics, which then readily cross the placenta to the fetus. In addition, bradycardia produced by a paracervical block is often associated with fetal acidosis. It would seem prudent to avoid this block in parturients with uteroplacental insufficiency or when there is co-existing fetal distress. Certainly, continuous monitoring of fetal heart rate is indicated whenever a paracervical block is administered.

Intrathecal or Epidural Opioids

The efficacy of subarachnoid or epidural injection of opioids for the relief of visceral pain during the first stage of labor is not well defined. The response may depend on the site of drug placement, as well as the dose administered. For example, 1 mg to 2 mg of morphine placed in the subarachnoid space during the first stage of labor provided complete analgesia within 15 minutes to 60 minutes, which lasted 8 hours to 11 hours.[57] Conversely, epidural morphine (2 mg and 5 mg) was not effective in providing adequate analgesia during the first stage of labor, whereas 7.5 mg was effective in some but not all parturients.[58] Maternal side effects associated with intrathecal or epidural opioids include a high incidence of pruritus, somnolence, and vomiting. Neonatal depression does not seem to occur. During the second stage of labor and in the presence of somatic pain, it is necessary to supplement opioids with local anesthetics placed in the subarachnoid or epidural spaces.

Lumbar Epidural Block

Institution of a continuous lumbar epidural block is appropriate when the first stage of labor is well established, as evidenced by dilation of the cervix (6 cm to 8 cm in a nullipara or 4 cm to 6 cm in a multipara) and the presence of strong and regular uterine contractions. Advantages of this block include the (1) ability to achieve segmental bands of analgesia (T10-12) during the first stage of labor, when total anesthesia is not required; (2) minimal local anesthetic requirements; and (3) maintenance of pelvic muscle tone, so that rotation of the fetal head is more easily accomplished. Pain of the first stage of labor can be relieved by injection of 6 ml to 8 ml of 0.25 percent bupivacaine into the lumbar epidural space. This low dose of local anesthetic produces a sensory band of analgesia that is unlikely to produce sufficient peripheral sympathetic nervous system blockade to result in maternal hypotension. Nevertheless, parturients should be encouraged to remain in the lateral position. Alternatively, addition of small doses of opioids (50 µg to 150 µg of fentanyl) to dilute (subanesthetic) solutions of local anesthetics (0.125 percent bupivacaine) may accelerate onset of analgesia with minimal skeletal muscle weakness. Addition of fentanyl to higher concentrations of bupivacaine has not been shown to improve analgesia beyond that achieved with the local anesthetic alone.[59] Additional local anesthetic is injected to provide perineal analgesia as labor progresses. Furthermore, a lumbar epidural block can be supplemented to provide adequate anesthesia should a cesarean section become necessary.

It is a clinical notion that injection of local anesthetics into the epidural space during uterine contractions may produce a higher level of anesthesia than occurs if drugs are injected between uterine contractions. Nevertheless, a controlled study failed to document a difference in sensory level whether local anesthetics are injected during or between uterine contractions.[60] This suggests uterine contractions do not influence spread of local anesthetics in the epidural space.

Caudal Block

After placement of a catheter into the sacral epidural space, analgesia is produced by injection of 10 ml to 12 ml of 0.25 percent bupivacaine. Advantages of this approach, compared with a continuous lumbar epidural technique, include a lower incidence of inadvertent dural puncture and more profound perineal analgesia. Disadvantages of this technique include (1) difficulty in keeping the sacral area clean; (2) technical difficulties in about 10 percent of patients, most often reflecting variations in sacral anatomy; (3) extensive peripheral sympathetic nervous system blockade during the first stage of labor; (4) a high incidence of malrotation of the fetal head; (5) possibility of toxic reactions due to vascular absorption of the local anesthetic; and (6) accidental injection into the fetal head. Finally, it may not be possible to produce a sufficient level of anesthesia with this technique should a cesarean section become necessary.

Subarachnoid Block (Saddle Block)

Subarachnoid block is administered immediately before vaginal delivery by injecting small doses of hyperbaric tetracaine (3 mg to 5 mg) or lidocaine (25 mg to 30 mg) into the lumbar subarachnoid space, with parturients in the sitting position. The sitting position is maintained for 60 seconds to 90 seconds to assure that only perineal analgesia (area of the body that would be in contact with a saddle)

occurs. A true saddle block does not produce complete pain relief, as afferent fibers from the uterus are not blocked. In reality, a true saddle block is rarely achieved. The more likely result is sensory blockade that extends to about T10, which prevents pain from contractions of the uterus.

Subarachnoid block is technically easy to perform and provides a rapid and reliable onset of anesthesia. When the sensory level is kept below T10, a spinal block does not involve significant peripheral sympathetic nervous system blockade and the likelihood of hypotension is reduced. The major disadvantage is the occasional occurrence of a postspinal headache. Typically, this headache is accentuated by sitting up and relieved by assuming the supine position. Presumably, the cause of headache is cerebrospinal fluid hypotension due to loss of fluid through the hole in the dura produced during performance of the block. Compared with nonpregnant patients, parturients are twice as likely to experience such a headache. The incidence of postspinal headache can be minimized (incidence 1 percent or less) by using small bore spinal needles (25 gauge). It should be recognized that accidental dural puncture occurs in 1 percent to 2 percent of attempted epidural blocks. In this event the dura is punctured with a large bore needle (17-gauge to 18-gauge) and over one half of these patients develop severe headaches. If headaches persist despite bed rest and hydration, the recommended approach is epidural injection of autologous blood (blood patch). Finally, there is an increased need for forceps delivery when abdominal muscle relaxation accompanies a subarachnoid block.

Complaints of backache may follow performance of an epidural or subarachnoid block administered for vaginal delivery. Backache is a frequent complaint in parturients, and the incidence is similar after general anesthesia and regional anesthetic techniques. Backache most likely reflects ligamentous strain from lordosis of pregnancy. In extreme cases, the muscular efforts of labor may give rise to a prolapsed intervertebral disc, with subsequent nerve root compression, typically manifested as back pain and numbness in the affected segmental area.

The most common type of nerve damage

in the postpartum period is caused by compression of the lumbosacral trunk between the descending fetal head and the sacrum. Lumbosacral trunk injuries are characterized by foot drop combined with sensory loss. In addition, compression of the femoral nerve (L2-4) or lateral femoral cutaneous nerve can occur at the inguinal ligament, resulting in sensory loss over the lateral aspect of the thigh and leg. This compression usually occurs from a prolonged posture in the lithotomy position. The sciatic nerve (L4-S3) divides into the common peroneal nerve and tibial nerve. The common peroneal nerve is superficial as it extends laterally around the head of the fibula and is subject to damage at this area due to compression from improper positioning in stirrups during vaginal delivery (see Chapter 18). Such damage is manifest by an inability to dorsiflex the great toe, foot drop, and sensory loss over the lateral aspect of the leg and the anterior portion of the foot. When neurologic deficits develop in the postpartum period, particularly after a lumbar epidural or subarachnoid block, it is important to establish whether the lesion is within the spinal canal or distal to the intervertebral foramen.

The incidence of paresthesias and motor dysfunction after labor and vaginal delivery is about 1.9 percent per 1,000 deliveries.[61] These symptoms resolve within 72 hours with supportive therapy, and the incidence is not influenced by the use of regional anesthesia.

Vascular anomalies of the spinal cord are usually associated with a history of leg weakness before the onset of labor. Rarely, puncture of an epidural vein during performance of a lumbar epidural block will result in an epidural hematoma. This potential complication is most likely to occur in patients with co-existing clotting abnormalities.

Pudendal Nerve Block

A pudendal nerve block is typically administered transvaginally by the obstetrician just before delivery. Bilateral pudendal nerve blocks using local anesthetics such as lidocaine (10 ml of 1 percent) provide satisfactory perineal analgesia for normal vaginal delivery but not for application of forceps. This block is not associated with peripheral sympathetic nervous system blockade, and labor is not prolonged. Unfortunately, even in experienced hands, a successful bilateral pudendal nerve block is achieved in only about 60 percent of attempts.

INHALATION ANALGESIA FOR VAGINAL DELIVERY

The goal of inhalation analgesia is to maintain parturients in awake and cooperative states with intact laryngeal reflexes for the first and second stages of labor. The major risk is the loss of protective airway reflexes due to inadvertent overdoses of inhaled anesthetics made most likely by the reduced functional residual capacity and decreased anesthetic requirements that accompany pregnancy.

Placental transfer of inhaled anesthetics occurs rapidly, as these drugs are lipid soluble and possess a low molecular weight. The degree of neonatal depression is directly proportional to the maternal inspired concentrations and duration of administration. Analgesic concentrations of inhaled anesthetics, however, are free from excessive depressant effects on the fetus, even if continued for a prolonged period.[62]

Nitrous oxide must be inhaled for about 50 seconds before effective analgesic concentrations are reached; less than satisfactory analgesia results when nitrous oxide is administered only during uterine contractions. Therefore, more effective inhalation analgesia is obtained by the continuous administration of 30 percent to 40 percent nitrous oxide. After delivery, rapid passage of nitrous oxide from blood into alveoli can cause diffusion hypoxia in the newborn infant. Therefore, infants born during administration of nitrous oxide analgesia may benefit from supplemental oxygen for 30 seconds to 60 seconds after delivery.

Intermittent inhalation of methoxyflurane (0.1 percent to 0.3 percent inspired) is an alternative to continuous administration of nitrous oxide. Analgesic concentrations of methoxyflurane do not dangerously depress maternal larygneal reflexes, and neonates are not sedated. Both maternal and neonatal serum fluoride levels, however, are increased in a dose-related manner after administration of methoxyflurane.[63,64] Nevertheless, there is no evidence of renal dysfunction in either parturients or neonates. Enflurane (0.5 percent inspired) provides analgesia during the second stage of labor similar to that achieved with nitrous oxide (30 percent to 40 percent).[65] Halothane is not popular for inhalation analgesia during labor because unconsciousness may occur before development of adequate maternal analgesia.

ANESTHESIA FOR CESAREAN SECTION

Common indications for cesarean section include a previous cesarean section, cephalopelvic disproportion, failure of labor to progress, maternal hemorrhage, and fetal distress. The dictum that a previous cesarean section mandated the same route of delivery for all subsequent pregnancies is undergoing modification. In selected patients (prior low segment transverse uterine incision and cephalic presentation), it is acceptable to allow vaginal delivery despite prior cesarean section.[66] Cesarean section may be selected to avoid the potential trauma of a difficult vaginal delivery, as with breech presentations. The use of electronic and biochemical monitoring of the fetus has increased the number of fetuses judged to be in jeopardy and in need of rapid delivery by cesarean section. Indeed, assuming a cesarean section rate of 15 percent, one can estimate that this operation is performed over 500,000 times yearly in the United States, making it one of the most frequent of all surgical procedures.[67]

The decision to select general or regional anesthesia to provide analgesia for cesarean section depends on the desires of the patient and the presence or absence of fetal distress. When fetal distress is present, general anes-

thesia may be preferable, since anesthesia can be established quickly and maternal hypotension is less likely. Regional anesthesia is more often chosen for elective cesarean section, particularly when maternal awareness is desirable. Furthermore, regional anesthesia minimizes the likelihood of maternal pulmonary aspiration and avoids fetal depression.

General Anesthesia

Preoperative medication may include pharmacologic attempts to increase gastric fluid pH (see the section Gastrointestinal Changes). Antacids are widely used for this purpose. It is common practice to administer antacids such as sodium citrate before the induction of anesthesia. An H-2 receptor antagonist, such as cimetidine, is also effective in increasing gastric fluid pH; but the time required for this drug, unlike antacids, precludes its use when induction of anesthesia is imminent.[30] Furthermore, cimetidine, unlike antacids, has no effect on pH of gastric fluid present in the stomach at the time the drug is administered. Clearly, antacids are the logical choice to increase gastric fluid pH when an emergency cesarean section is planned. Metoclopramide could be administered to facilitate gastric emptying before the induction of anesthesia, although the usefulness of this drug in parturients undergoing elective cesarean section has not been confirmed (see the section Gastrointestinal Changes). If anticholinergic drugs are judged to be necessary, glycopyrrolate is useful, since its quaternary ammonium structure prevents significant transfer across lipid barriers such as the placenta. Finally, if the cesarean section is elective and the parturient is extremely apprehensive, a benzodiazepine can be administered for the purpose of allaying anxiety.

Following preoxygenation, induction of general anesthesia is usually accomplished with intravenous administration of thiopental (3 mg·kg^{-1} to 4 mg·kg^{-1}) plus succinylcholine to facilitate intubation of the trachea. Cricoid pressure should be applied until the trachea is protected with a cuffed endotracheal tube. The importance of preoxygenation is emphasized by the rapid reduction in maternal arterial oxygenation that can occur during apnea, as associated with direct laryngoscopy for intubation of the trachea. This vulnerability to arterial hypoxemia reflects reductions in functional residual capacity and increased metabolic oxygen requirements associated with pregnancy. Use of small doses of nondepolarizing muscle relaxants to prevent fasciculations produced by the subsequent administration of succinylcholine is often included in the induction sequence.

Thiopental rapidly crosses the placenta, and peak concentrations are present in the umbilical venous blood in 1 minute. Nevertheless, the fetal brain will not be exposed to high concentrations of the drug if the maternal dose does not exceed 4 mg·kg^{-1},[68] as clearance by the fetal liver and dilution by blood from the viscera and extremities exposes the brain to reduced concentrations. Clearly there is no advantage to delaying delivery until thiopental has been redistributed in the mother or fetus.

Maintenance of anesthesia until delivery of the fetus is often with nitrous oxide (50 percent to 60 percent inspired) in oxygen plus succinylcholine for skeletal muscle paralysis. Maternal alveolar concentrations of nitrous oxide approach inspired concentrations rapidly, reflecting the reduced functional residual capacity that accompanies pregnancy. It must also be remembered that nitrous oxide is rapidly transferred across the placenta. Nevertheless, concentrations of nitrous oxide delivered to the fetal central nervous system are reduced by tissue uptake and dilution in blood returning from the lower extremities. As a result, fetal central nervous system depression from nitrous oxide is minimal. Finally, nitrous oxide does not produce significant uterine relaxation.

The major disadvantage of using only nitrous oxide until delivery of the infant is patient awareness during the operation. The reported incidence of awareness is 2 percent to 26 percent.[69] Maternal amnesia can be assured by the administration of low inspired concentrations of volatile anesthetics (halothane 0.5 percent, enflurane 1.0 percent, isoflurane 0.75 percent) with nitrous oxide.[70] These low doses of volatile drugs do not increase maternal blood loss, alter the response of the uterus to

oxytocin, or produce neonatal depression. An additional advantage of using volatile anesthetics is a reduction in the inspired concentrations of nitrous oxide. As a result, fetal oxygenation can be improved by increasing inspired maternal oxygen concentrations. Finally, nitrous oxide supplemented with volatile anesthetics is associated with reduced sympathetic nervous system responses to surgical stimulation and a better maintenance of uterine blood flow[33] thought to reflect inhibition of endogenous norepinephrine secretion by volatile anesthetics.

Ventilation of the lungs is controlled; excessive hyperventilation must be avoided, as effects of positive pressure can reduce uterine blood flow. Furthermore, respiratory alkalosis will increase affinity of maternal hemoglobin for oxygen and thus decrease placental transfer of oxygen to the fetus.

Succinylcholine can be used to provide skeletal muscle relaxation during the operative procedure. Although plasma cholinesterase activity is decreased at term, clinical responses to succinylcholine do not seem to be altered (see the section Hepatic Changes).[16] Administration of succinylcholine to parturients with unsuspected atypical cholinesterase enzyme, however, will cause prolonged apnea in neonates who are also homozygotes for the atypical enzyme.[71] Alternatives to succinylcholine for maintenance of skeletal muscle relaxation are the intermediate-acting drugs, atracurium or vecuronium.

Succinylcholine and nondepolarizing muscle relaxants, when administered in appropriate clinical doses, do not cross the placenta in amounts sufficient to produce effects on the fetus. Detection of iodide in the fetal plasma, after maternal administration of gallamine triethiodide, led to the suggestion that this muscle relaxant crossed the placenta in significant amounts. This finding most likely reflects placental passage of iodide independent of gallamine, and it can be assumed that this muscle relaxant, like others, crosses the placenta in only small amounts.

There is controversy regarding the optimal time for delivery when general anesthesia is used for cesarean section. In the absence of maternal hypotension, a time from induction of anesthesia to delivery that approaches 30 minutes is not associated with acidosis in the neonate.[72] More important is a short time to delivery after incision into the uterus has been made. Indeed, Apgar scores are often decreased when the uterine incision to delivery time exceeds 90 seconds. Adverse responses associated with a prolonged time to delivery after uterine incision may reflect impaired uteroplacental blood flow and/or reduced umbilical vein blood flow due to manipulation of the uterus. All factors considered, it seems prudent to minimize the times from both induction of anesthesia and uterine incision to delivery, so as to assure optimal conditions in neonates.

After delivery, anesthesia can be supplemented with additional volatile drugs or opioids. It would seem reasonable to pass an oral tube into the stomach to evacuate gastric fluid before the conclusion of surgery. The cuffed tube should not be removed from the trachea until it is assured that maternal laryngeal reflexes have returned. Finally, it may be important to administer oxygen to neonates for 30 seconds to 60 seconds to prevent development of arterial hypoxemia due to the rapid elimination of nitrous oxide from the fetal circulation into the lungs.

Regional Anesthesia

Subarachnoid or epidural block is often selected for an elective cesarean section. This form of anesthesia permits the mother to be awake, minimizes the likelihood of maternal pulmonary aspiration, avoids drug depression from general anesthetics, and permits administration of high inspired concentrations of oxygen to the mother. Selection of subarachnoid or lumbar epidural techniques is based on the relative advantages and disadvantages of each as they relate to individual parturients. Administration of supplemental oxygen to the parturients during regional anesthesia improves fetal oxygen stores during cesarean section.

SUBARACHNOID BLOCK

Advantages of subarachnoid block include its technical ease and high success rate. Fetal depression from local anesthetics does not occur, since small doses are used and absorption of local anesthetics from the subarachnoid space is minimal. Disadvantages of this technique include (1) difficulty in controlling the sensory level; (2) a high incidence of hypotension, reflecting the abrupt onset of peripheral sympathetic nervous system blockade; (3) nausea and vomiting; and (4) postoperative headache.

Parturients are particularly prone to hypotension after completion of a subarachnoid block. The incidence of hypotension is less in the presence of active labor, compared with patients who are not in labor. A possible explanation may be the autotransfusion of about 300 ml of blood, which occurs with each uterine contraction. Hypotension is hazardous, since decreases in maternal blood pressure are associated with comparable falls in uterine blood flow and placental perfusion, leading to fetal hypoxemia and acidosis. The incidence and magnitude of hypotension may be minimized by continuous left uterine displacement, intravenous hydration with 500 ml to 1000 ml of lactated Ringer's solution administered 15 minutes to 30 minutes before performing the block, and the intramuscular injection of 25 mg to 50 mg of ephedrine approximately 15 minutes before performing the block.[73] If hypotension occurs (systolic blood pressure below 100 mmHg in normotensive parturients or a 30 percent decrease in a previously hypertensive parturient) despite the above measures, additional intravenous doses of ephedrine (2.5 mg to 10 mg) are indicated. Onset of nausea after a subarachnoid block should immediately suggest the presence of hypotension leading to reductions in cerebral blood flow. In the absence of hypotension, nausea may be due to traction on the peritoneum, or an imbalance of autonomic nervous system activity due to blockade of the sympathetic nervous system fibers in the presence of intact vagal innervation. If excessive parasympathetic nervous system activity is the cause of nausea intravenous administration of anticholinergic drugs may be considered. Although glycopyrrolate is less likely than atropine to cross the placenta, fetal heart rate was not significantly altered by either drug administered intravenously.[74]

Technically, the lumbar subarachnoid

TABLE 34-7. Dose of Local Anesthetic for Subarachnoid Block Prior to Cesarean Section

Height (cm)	Tetracaine (mg)	Lidocaine (mg)	Bupivacaine (mg)
155	7	50	7
155–170	8	60	8
170	9	70	9

space is entered with a 25-gauge needle. A convenient guide for judging the appropriate dose of local anesthetic (tetracaine or lidocaine) to be injected into the subarachnoid space is based on the height of the parturient (Table 34-7). A sensory level of T4-6 is necessary to assure adequate anesthesia for performance of the cesarean section. After injection of local anesthetics into the subarachnoid space, parturients are placed supine, with the right hip elevated to minimize aortocaval compression. Maternal blood pressure must be monitored frequently until delivery of the neonate.

LUMBAR EPIDURAL BLOCK

Compared with subarachnoid blocks, the sensory level is more controllable and hypotension less precipitous with lumbar epidural blocks. Presumably, the slower onset of peripheral sympathetic nervous system blockade is responsible for the more gradual decrease in blood pressure. Unlike subarachnoid block, anesthesia provided with an epidural block requires doses of local anesthetics associated with significant systemic absorption of the drugs. Absorbed local anesthetics, particularly lidocaine or mepivacaine, can cross the placenta and produce detectable effects on the fetus. Nevertheless, infants whose mothers receive epidural anesthesia with bupivacaine do not demonstrate measurable differences from infants born after subarachnoid anesthetics. Technically, lumbar epidural blocks are more difficult to perform than subarachnoid blocks. Postoperative headache does not occur, since the dura is not punctured.

Bupivacaine concentrations injected into the epidural space must be at least 0.5 percent to ensure adequate anesthesia for the surgical stimulus associated with the performance of cesarean sections. This contrasts with the degree of analgesia acceptable for vaginal delivery produced using 0.25 percent bupivacaine. Limitation of the concentration of bupivacaine to 0.5 percent is recommended to minimize the likelihood of cardiotoxicity should this local anesthetic be accidentally injected intravenously. When local anesthetics are injected into the epidural space, it is mandatory to administer a test dose to detect unrecognized placement of the epidural catheter in a vein or subarachnoid space. Administration of 3 ml of local anesthetic containing 1:200,000 epinephrine (15 μg) usually produces transient maternal tachycardia if the drug goes intravenously and signs of subarachnoid block if the solution enters the subarachnoid space. Assuming a negative test dose response and absence of subarachnoid block following the test dose, an additional amount of bupivacaine is injected through the lumbar epidural catheter, so as to produce a T4-6 sensory level of anesthesia. When rapid onset of analgesia is necessary, 3 percent 2-chloroprocaine-CE can be used. When chloroprocaine is used, it is imperative that subarachnoid injections be avoided, since permanent neurologic damage has been reported after accidental subarachnoid injections of large volumes of this local anesthetic.[75,76] Local anesthetics, such as bupivacaine, administered after placement of chloroprocaine in the epidural space, may be less effective. An alternative to chloroprocaine when a rapid onset of analgesia would be desirable is the use of the amide local anesthetic prilocaine, 1 percent to 3 percent. Methemoglobinemia after systemic absorption and metabolism of prilocaine is not likely if the total dose of drug placed in the epidural space does not exceed 600 mg. In the past, lidocaine has not been a popular drug because of neurobehavioral changes detectable in neonates of mothers who received this local anesthetic during epidural analgesia or anesthesia. Nevertheless, there is no convincing evidence that these neurobehavioral changes are hazardous nor have these observations been reproducible.[77] Therefore, lidocaine would seem to be an appropriate alternative to either bupivacaine or chloroprocaine.

Postoperative analgesia after cesarean section may be provided by epidural administration of opioids. For example, morphine 5 mg and 7.5 mg, placed in the epidural space, provided analgesia for about 24 hours without cardiopulmonary side effects (Fig. 34-13).[78] Nausea and pruritus were frequent but usually mild. In the same study, intramuscular morphine 7.5 mg or epidural morphine 2.0 mg provided short duration and minimal pain relief.

ABNORMAL PRESENTATIONS AND MULTIPLE BIRTHS

Presentation of the fetus is determined by the presenting part and that aspect of the fetus felt by manual examination through the cervix. Description of fetal position is based on the relationship of the fetal occiput, chin, or sacrum to the left or right side of the parturient. Approximately 90 percent of deliveries are cephalic presentations in either occiput transverse or occiput anterior positions. All other presentations and positions are considered abnormal.

Persistent Occiput Posterior

During active labor the occiput undergoes internal rotation to the occiput anterior position. If this rotation does not occur, the persistent occiput posterior position results, and labor becomes prolonged and painful. For example, severe back pain reflects pressure on the posterior sacral nerves by the fetal occiput. Spontaneous delivery requires more uterine and abdominal work. The incidence of cervical and perineal lacerations and postpartum bleeding is increased. Although spontaneous delivery may occur, it is more likely that manual or forceps rotation and extraction will be necessary. A prolonged second stage of labor or difficult midforceps rotation is associated with increased birth trauma, intracranial hemorrhage, and birth asphyxia in the neonate.

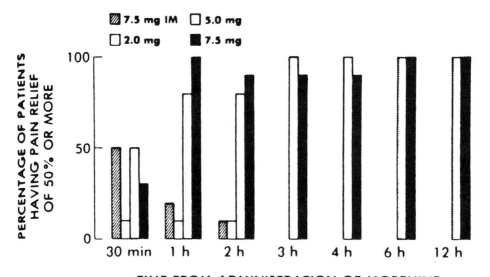

FIG. 34-13. Pain relief produced by intramuscular morphine (IM) or morphine placed in the epidural space was determined in parturients after cesarean section. Prolonged analgesia was provided by 2 mg or 5 mg placed in the epidural space. (Rosen MA, Hughes SC, Shnider SM, et al. Epidural morphine for the relief of postoperative pain after cesarean delivery. Anesth Analg 1983;62:666–72 Reprinted with permission from IARS)

Regional anesthetic techniques that relax maternal perineal muscles are best avoided until spontaneous internal rotation of the fetal head occurs. Analgesia can be provided with a segmental (T10-L1) lumbar epidural block. If back pain persists, analgesia may be extended to the sacral areas by injecting dilute concentrations of bupivacaine (0.125 percent to 0.25 percent), which should not paralyze the skeletal muscles necessary for internal rotation of the fetal head. Complete analgesia and perineal relaxation is appropriate when midforceps rotation is planned.

Breech Presentations

Breech rather than cephalic presentations characterize about 3.5 percent of pregnancies. Breech presentations are classified as (1) frank (feet are against the face), (2) complete (buttocks with feet along side them present at the cervix), and (3) incomplete or footling (one or both present at the cervix). Frank breech is present in about 60 percent of breech deliveries, complete breech in about 10 percent, and incomplete breech in about 30 percent.

Causes of breech presentations are not known. However, conditions that seem to predispose to this presentation include prematurity, placenta previa, multiple gestations, and uterine anomalies. Fetal abnormalities, including hydrocephalus and polyhydramnios, are associated with breech presentations.

Breech deliveries result in an increased maternal morbidity. Compared to cephalic presentations, there is a greater likelihood of cervical lacerations, perineal injury, retained placenta, and shock due to hemorrhage. Neonatal morbidity and mortality are increased. These infants are more likely to experience arterial hypoxemia and acidosis during delivery, due to umbilical cord compression. Prolapse of the umbilical cord occurs in about 10 percent of complete or incomplete breech presentations, compared with an incidence of 0.5 percent for cephalic and frank breech presentations, and is thought to reflect failure of the presenting part to fill the lower uterine segment. Finally, there are increased chances of fetal intracranial

hemorrhage due to head trauma during breech deliveries.

Delivery by Cesarean Section

There is a growing trend to deliver breech presentations by elective cesarean section. If cesarean section is planned, either regional or general anesthesia may be selected. It should be appreciated that during regional anesthesia, there may be difficulty in extracting the infant through the uterine incision. If uterine hypertonus is the cause, it will be necessary to produce general anesthesia rapidly. After intubation of the trachea, administration of volatile anesthetics such as halothane will relax the uterus.

VAGINAL DELIVERY

For vaginal delivery of breech presentations, parturients must be able to expel the fetus until the umbilicus is visible. The obstetrician then completes the delivery, either manually or with the application of forceps. Analgesia during labor is often provided with intramuscular or intravenous medications, followed by perineal infiltration of local anesthetics or performance of a pudendal block. Inhalation analgesia may also be administered. Rapid induction of general anesthesia, with intubation of the trachea, may be necessary, if perineal muscle relaxation is inadequate for delivery of the aftercoming fetal head, or if the lower uterine segment contracts and traps the head. An alternative to infiltration and inhalation analgesia is use of lumbar epidural block. For example, continuous lumbar epidural block provides analgesia and maximal perineal relaxation for delivery of the fetal head. Furthermore, abilities of parturients to push during the delivery can be preserved by using minimal concentrations of local anesthetics (0.25 percent bupivacaine) and providing constant maternal encouragement. Indeed, the incidence of complete breech extraction is not increased in the presence of epidural analgesia.[79] If uterine relaxation is required for facilitation of a breech extraction during vaginal delivery, it will be necessary to produce general anesthesia.

Multiple Gestations

The incidence of twin gestations is approximately 1 in 90 births. Preeclampsia, eclampsia, anemia, premature labor, breech presentations, and hemorrhage are more common in multiple gestations. Approximately 60 percent of twins are premature. The large uterus associated with multiple gestations produces more aortocaval compression, predisposing parturients to a higher incidence of severe supine hypotension. This hypotension may be even further exaggerated if sympathetic nervous system blockade is produced by a subarachnoid or epidural block. Blood loss during twin delivery is twice that of a single gestation, and manual extraction of the placenta is required twice as often. It must be appreciated that the second twin is more likely to be depressed, presumably reflecting a period of fetal arterial hypoxemia and acidosis due to contraction of the uterus or to premature separation of the placenta after the first neonate is delivered.

Considerations for the choice of anesthesia in the presence of multiple gestations relate to the frequent occurrence of prematurity and breech presentations. Preparations must be made for the possibility of providing anesthesia for version, extraction, breech delivery, cesarean section, or midforceps delivery. Pudendal block with or without inhalation analgesia introduces minimal depression to the fetus, but maternal analgesia is incomplete and relaxation of the perineal muscles is absent. Continuous lumbar epidural block provides good analgesia and eliminates the need for administration of opioids to the parturient, which is particularly important for avoiding depression in premature neonates. Segmental lumbar epidural block with bupivacaine (0.25 percent) provides adequate analgesia and preserves sufficient abdominal muscle strength so that the

mother may assist in delivery. In addition, forceps deliveries, likely with multiple gestations, are more easily accomplished in the presence of perineal muscle relaxation provided by epidural block. Intravenous infusion of fluids and left uterine displacement are important in minimizing aortocaval compression when peripheral sympathetic nervous system blockade is produced.

PREGNANCY AND HEART DISEASE

Maternal heart disease is estimated to be present in about 1.6 percent of all pregnancies. The two most common causes are congenital malformations and acquired abnormalities due to rheumatic fever. Management of anesthesia requires an appreciation of the pathophysiology of heart disease (see Chapters 2 and 3).

Many of the signs and symptoms of normal pregnancy can mimic those of cardiac disease. For example, dyspnea associated with interstitial pulmonary edema due to left ventricular failure may be difficult to distinguish from labored breathing typical of normal pregnancy. Leg edema from congestive heart failure can be mistaken for venous stasis due to aortocaval compression. Presence of congestive heart failure is suggested by hepatomegaly and jugular venous distention, as these changes do not accompany a normal pregnancy. It may be difficult to differentiate heart murmurs due to organic lesions from those due to increased blood flow. Finally, rotation of the maternal heart, which occurs from elevation of the diaphragm as pregnancy progresses, can be mistaken for cardiac hypertrophy.

Pregnancy and labor result in circulatory changes that may have adverse effects on the already diseased cardiovascular system. For example, cardiac output is increased about 40 percent during gestation and can be increased an additional 30 percent to 45 percent above prelabor values during labor and delivery. After delivery, relief of aortocaval obstruction contributes to increased venous return and central blood volume, resulting in even further increases in cardiac output above prelabor values. These increases, well tolerated by the normal heart, may result in congestive heart failure in the presence of co-existing heart disease. Indeed, 30 percent to 50 percent of patients with symptoms of heart disease during minimal activity or at rest develop congestive heart failure during pregnancy.

Detection and evaluation of heart disease is crucial for planning management of anesthesia during labor and delivery. For most types of heart disease, no one anesthetic technique is specifically indicated or contraindicated. Nevertheless, analgesia produced by a continuous lumbar epidural block can minimize adverse effects of increased cardiac output due to pain or anxiety. Inhalation analgesia or anesthesia is usually selected when sudden reductions in blood pressure would be detrimental.

Invasive monitoring during labor and delivery is probably not necessary in the absence of cardiac symptoms due to co-existing heart disease. Exceptions are parturients with pulmonary hypertension, right-to-left intracardiac shunts, or coarctation of the aorta. In these patients the ability to measure cardiac output and cardiac filling pressures, as well as to calculate systemic and pulmonary vascular resistance, is helpful. Since hemodynamic changes seen during labor and delivery can persist into the postpartum period, it is logical to continue invasive cardiac monitoring for several hours after delivery.

Mitral Stenosis

Mitral stenosis is the most common type of cardiac valvular defect present during pregnancy. Parturients with mitral stenosis have an increased incidence of pulmonary edema, atrial fibrillation, and paroxysmal atrial tachycardia. A continuous lumbar epidural block producing segmental analgesia is useful for labor and vaginal delivery, as this approach minimizes undesirable effects produced by pain on heart rate and cardiac output. Perineal analgesia prevents the parturient's urge to push and eliminates deleterious effects of Valsalva

maneuvers on venous return. General or regional anesthesia can be provided for cesarean section. If general anesthesia is selected, drugs that produce tachycardia and events that increase pulmonary vascular resistance (arterial hypoxemia, hypoventilation) must be avoided (see Chapter 2).

Mitral Regurgitation

Mitral regurgitation is the second most common cardiac valvular defect present during pregnancy. In contrast to parturients with mitral stenosis, these patients usually tolerate pregnancy well. Indeed, clinical symptoms related to mitral regurgitation do not usually develop until after the age of childbearing.

Continuous lumbar epidural analgesia is recommended for labor and vaginal delivery, as this technique reduces peripheral vasoconstriction associated with pain and thus helps to maintain forward left ventricular stroke volume. Regional techniques, however, will also increase venous capacitance, such that intravenous fluids may be required to maintain filling volumes of the left ventricle. General anesthesia is acceptable when cesarean section is planned (see Chapter 2).

Aortic Regurgitation

Complications of aortic regurgitation, like those of mitral regurgitation, usually develop after the age of childbearing. Therefore, these patients usually have an uneventful pregnancy, although a small percentage may develop congestive heart failure. Decreases in systemic vascular resistance and increases in heart rate that occur during pregnancy may reduce both the regurgitant flow and the intensity of the cardiac murmur associated with aortic regurgitation. Conversely, increases in systemic vascular resistance associated with pain during labor and vaginal delivery can lead to reduced forward left ventricular stroke volume. As with mitral regurgitation, a continuous lumbar epidural block is recommended for analgesia during labor and vaginal delivery. General anesthesia is acceptable when cesarean section is planned (see Chapter 2).

Aortic Stenosis

Rarity of aortic stenosis during pregnancy reflects the typical 35 year to 40 year latent period between acute rheumatic fever and symptoms of aortic stenosis. Asymptomatic parturients are not at increased risk during labor and delivery. The fixed orifice valve lesion, however, means that these parturients are vulnerable to decreased stroke volume and hypotension should systemic vascular resistance be abruptly decreased. Therefore, if a regional block is selected, a gradual onset of analgesia produced by a continuous lumbar epidural block is useful. In view of the hazards of hypotension, techniques using systemic medication, pudendal block, and inhalation analgesia are often used for labor and vaginal delivery. General anesthesia is acceptable when cesarean section is planned (see Chapter 2).

Atrial or Ventricular Septal Defect

These types of cardiac defects, when present in adults, are most often small and associated with minimal left-to-right intracardiac shunts. Therefore, pulmonary hypertension is unlikely. Pregnancy is usually uneventful but can be complicated by infective endocarditis or congestive heart failure. For labor and vaginal delivery or cesarean section, a continuous lumbar epidural block minimizes the likelihood of increases in systemic vascular resistance, which could accentuate the magnitude of the shunt.

Patent Ductus Arteriosus

Very few pregnant patients present with this defect, since most defects are surgically closed in childhood. When a patent ductus arteriosus persists, a continuous lumbar epidural block prevents undesirable increases in systemic vascular resistance. Therefore, this type of anesthesia is useful for vaginal delivery or cesarean section.

Tetralogy of Fallot

Pregnancy increases morbidity and mortality associated with tetralogy of Fallot. For example, pain during labor and vaginal delivery may elevate pulmonary vascular resistance and lead to increases in the right-to-left intracardiac shunts with reductions in pulmonary blood flow and accentuation of arterial hypoxemia. In addition, normal decreases in systemic vascular resistance that accompany pregnancy can also increase right-to-left shunts and accentuate arterial hypoxemia. Indeed, most cardiac complications develop immediately postpartum, when systemic vascular resistance is lowest.

Analgesia for labor and vaginal delivery is best provided with pudendal block. Regional anesthesia must be used with caution because of hazards of decreased blood pressure due to peripheral sympathetic nervous system blockade. Therefore, general anesthesia is usually selected for cesarean section (see Chapter 3). Invasive monitoring, including continuous measurement of arterial and cardiac filling pressures, is helpful. Easy access to arterial blood facilitates determination of arterial oxygen partial pressures and early detection of increased arterial hypoxemia, which can occur if the magnitude of right-to-left shunts is accentuated by decreases in systemic blood pressure. Pulse oximetry will also reflect changes in arterial oxygenation.

Eisenmenger's Syndrome

Eisenmenger's syndrome consists of obliterative pulmonary vascular disease with resultant pulmonary hypertension, right-to-left or bidirectional intracardiac shunts, and arterial hypoxemia. This combination of problems is not amenable to surgical correction, and pregnancy is not well tolerated. Indeed, maternal mortality can approach 30 percent, with the highest comparable mortality being around 4 percent in parturients with coarctation of the aorta or tetralogy of Fallot.[80]

HAZARDS INTRODUCED BY PREGNANCY

Major hazards facing parturients with Eisenmenger's syndrome are decreases in systemic vascular resistance, which lead to increases in the magnitude of right-to-left intracardiac shunts, and thromboembolism, which may interfere with an already decreased pulmonary blood flow. Indeed, the magnitude of intracardiac shunts can be accentuated by normal decreases in systemic vascular resistance that accompany pregnancy or the widespread pulmonary vasoconstriction that accompanies even small pulmonary emboli. The greatest risk to these patients occurs during delivery and immediately postpartum.

MANAGEMENT OF ANALGESIA FOR LABOR AND DELIVERY

The principle of any technique of analgesia chosen for patients with Eisenmenger's syndrome is to avoid decreases in systemic vascular resistance or reductions in cardiac output. Likewise, events that could further increase pulmonary vascular resistance (hypercarbia, increased arterial hypoxemia) must be avoided. Finally, meticulous attention is required to prevent infusion of air through tubing used to deliver intravenous fluids, since the possibility of paradoxical air embolism is great.

Vaginal delivery is an acceptable goal. Analgesia provided with a continuous lumbar epidural block avoids the stress of an exhausting and painful labor. If epidural analgesia is selected, however, it is crucial that reductions in systemic vascular resistance be minimized. Epinephrine probably should not be added to local anesthetics, since reductions in systemic vascular resistance can be accentuated by peripheral beta-adrenergic effects of epinephrine absorbed from the epidural space. Analgesia for vaginal delivery may also be provided with inhaled drugs.

Delivery by cesarean section is most often accomplished using general anesthesia. Extensive peripheral sympathetic nervous system blockade is the major disadvantage of an epidural or subarachnoid block. Nevertheless, epidural block has been successfully used to provide anesthesia for elective cesarean section.[80] Regardless of the anesthetic technique selected, antibiotics should be given in the perioperative period as protection against infective endocarditis. It should be recognized that the arm-to-brain circulation time is rapid due to the right-to-left intracardiac shunt. Therefore, drugs given intravenously will have a rapid onset of action. Ketamine has theoretical advantages over barbiturates in these patients, since it does not reduce systemic vascular resistance, although increases in pulmonary vascular resistance are theoretically possible. In contrast to parenteral drugs, the rate of rise of arterial concentrations of inhaled drugs is slow due to decreased pulmonary blood flow. Despite the slow onset of effects, myocardial depressant and vasodilating actions of volatile drugs emphasize the potential hazards of using these anesthetics in patients with Eisenmenger's syndrome. Even nitrous oxide can have adverse effects, as this drug has been shown to increase pulmonary vascular resistance.[81] It must be appreciated that increased airway pressures, as associated with positive pressure ventilation of the lungs, can decrease pulmonary blood flow. Invasive monitoring of arterial and cardiac filling pressures is helpful. Since the right ventricle is at greater risk than the left ventricle for dysfunction, measurements of right atrial pressure are a uniquely useful determinations. The value of pulmonary artery catheters in these patients has been questioned.[82]

Coarctation of the Aorta

Coarctation of the aorta, like aortic stenosis, represents a fixed obstruction to the forward ejection of the left ventricular stroke volume. Increases in cardiac output can be achieved primarily by increases in heart rate. During periods of high demand, as during labor or acute increases in intravascular fluid volume produced by uterine contraction, the heart rate may not be able to increase to the extent necessary to maintain an adequate stroke volume. This sequence of events may result in acute left ventricular failure. Another hazard during labor and vaginal delivery is damage to the vascular wall of the aorta. Specifically, with the increased heart rate and myocardial contractility that accompany the pain of labor, the rate of ejection of blood from the left ventricle will increase and may lead to dissection of the aorta.

Maintenance of heart rate, myocardial contractility, and systemic vascular resistance are important considerations in the management of anesthesia. As with aortic stenosis, analgesia for labor and vaginal delivery is often provided with systemic medications or inhalation analgesia and pudendal block. Likewise, general anesthesia is recommended for cesarean section. Invasive monitoring of arterial and cardiac filling pressures is helpful.

Congenital Pulmonary Stenosis

Parturients with congenital pulmonary stenosis usually experience an uneventful pregnancy. Right ventricular failure, however, can be precipitated by increased intravascular fluid volume or heart rate. Furthermore, decreased systemic vascular resistance may adversely influence a low right ventricular output. Analgesia for labor and vaginal delivery is often provided with systemic or inhalation analgesia and pudendal block. General anesthesia is useful for cesarean section.

Primary Pulmonary Hypertension

Primary pulmonary hypertension is a disease that predominates in young women. Maternal mortality is over 50 percent, with most

deaths occurring during labor and the early postpartum period. Monitoring pressures in the systemic and pulmonary circulations is indicated. Pulmonary hypertension is considered to be present when pulmonary artery pressures exceed 30/15 mmHg or mean pressures are greater than 25 mmHg (see Chapter 9). Subtle but progressive increases in right atrial pressure may signal right ventricular failure.

Pain during labor and vaginal delivery is especially detrimental because it may further increase pulmonary vascular resistance. Analgesia for labor and vaginal delivery is often provided with systemic medications or inhalation analgesia plus pudendal block. If a continuous lumbar epidural block is selected, careful titration of local anesthetics is essential to minimize reductions in systemic vascular resistance. General anesthesia is recommended for cesarean section.

Cardiomyopathy of Pregnancy

Left ventricular failure late in the course of pregnancy or during the first 6 weeks postpartum has been termed cardiomyopathy of pregnancy. If such failure persists despite diuretics and digitalis, it is recommended that analgesia for labor and vaginal delivery be provided with continuous lumbar epidural blocks. Acute increases in systemic vascular resistance should be avoided. In about one-half of these parturients, heart failure is transient and recurs only during subsequent pregnancies. In the remaining parturients, idiopathic congestive cardiomyopathy persists and death is likely, especially if another pregnancy is allowed to progress to term.

Dissecting Aneurysm of the Aorta

There is a recognized association between pregnancy and dissecting aneurysm of the aorta. Indeed, nearly 50 percent of such aneurysms in women less than 40 years of age occur in association with pregnancy. Continuous lumbar epidural blocks are recommended to maintain a pain-free state and a normal to slightly decreased blood pressure in parturients known to have developed this disorder.

Hypertrophic Cardiomyopathy

Left ventricular outflow obstruction associated with hypertrophic cardiomyopathy is exacerbated by increased myocardial contractility, tachycardia, and decreased systemic vascular resistance (see Chapter 8). Conversely, increased intravascular fluid volume causes distention of the left ventricle, leading to decreases in the magnitude of outflow obstruction. Anesthesia for labor and vaginal delivery is often provided with systemic medications or inhalation analgesia plus pudendal block. Epidural or subarachnoid blocks may decrease systemic vascular resistance and accentuate left ventricular outflow obstruction. General anesthesia is useful for cesarean section. Indeed, volatile anesthetics may be used to decrease myocardial contractility and thus reduce left ventricular outflow obstruction (see Chapter 8).

Previous Mitral or Aortic Valve Replacement

After mitral valve replacement, cardiac output often remains low, and some element of cardiac dysfunction and pulmonary hypertension may persist (see Chapter 2). Pregnancy aggravates these abnormalities because of associated increases in intravascular fluid volume and elevated myocardial oxygen requirements. Furthermore, thromboembolism is a risk, and these patients are usually anticoagulated. Typically, coumarin anticoagulants are replaced during pregnancy with heparin, which does not cross the placenta. Anticoag-

ulation limits use of epidural or subarachnoid blocks in these patients.

Patients with prosthetic aortic valves have a lower incidence of complications than those with artificial mitral valves. Cardiac output is better maintained and ventricular function is not likely to be compromised. The risk of thromboembolism is low, and residual pulmonary hypertension is unlikely. Therefore, these patients would not seem to be at an increased risk during pregnancy.

Cardiac Treatments and the Fetus

Lidocaine, propranolol, and digoxin readily cross the placenta. Maternal lidocaine blood levels above 5 $\mu g \cdot ml^{-1}$ are associated with neonatal depression. Propranolol may produce fetal bradycardia and hypoglycemia. Elimination half-time of digoxin is likely to be significantly longer in the fetus. Finally, electrical cardioversion, as used to treat paroxysmal atrial tachycardia, has no adverse fetal effects.[83]

TOXEMIA OF PREGNANCY

Toxemia of pregnancy refers to either preeclampsia or eclampsia. Preeclampsia is a syndrome manifesting after the 20th week of gestation, characterized by hypertension, proteinuria, and generalized edema. Symptoms and signs of preeclampsia usually abate within 48 hours after delivery. Blood pressures above 140/90 mmHg, with urine protein losses greater than 2 $g \cdot day^{-1}$ is sufficient evidence for the diagnosis. Severe preeclampsia is indicated by blood pressures above 160/110 mmHg; urine protein losses greater than 5 $g \cdot day^{-1}$; and complaints of headache, visual disturbances, and epigastric pain. Eclampsia is present when convulsions are superimposed on preeclampsia. Eclampsia occurs in 5 percent of parturients with preeclampsia and is associated with a maternal mortality of about 10 percent. Causes of maternal mortality from eclampsia include congestive heart failure and intracranial hemorrhage. Toxemia of pregnancy has a higher incidence in economically underprivileged women; in primigravidas; and in the presence of multiple gestations, diabetes mellitus, and polyhydramnios.

Hypertension that occurs during pregnancy may be unrelated to toxemia of pregnancy. For example, chronic hypertension is considered to be present when blood pressure elevations manifest before the 20th week of gestation and persist for more than 6 weeks postpartum. Gestational hypertension is characterized by the onset of hypertension, without proteinuria or edema, during the last few weeks of gestation or in the immediate postpartum period.

Pathophysiology

The etiology of toxemia of pregnancy has not been confirmed. One possible mechanism is an antigen-antibody reaction between fetal and maternal tissues in the first trimester that initiates placental vasculitis. This vasculitis subsequently leads to tissue hypoxia and release into the maternal circulation of vasoactive substances responsible for the clinical manifestations of toxemia. The pathophysiology involves nearly every organ system.[84]

CENTRAL NERVOUS SYSTEM

The central nervous system is hyperirritable, reflecting cerebral edema due to increased intracellular fluid volume of the brain cells. Grand mal seizures can occur spontaneously or secondary to additional increases in maternal blood pressure. Coma, in association with increased intracranial pressure, may follow. Cerebral hemorrhage accounts for 30 percent to 40 percent of deaths in these patients.[84]

CARDIOVASCULAR SYSTEM

The peripheral vasculature in the presence of toxemia of pregnancy exhibits increased sensitivity to catecholamines, sympathomimetic drugs, and the oxytocics. There is generalized arteriolar vasoconstriction consistent with elevations of maternal blood pressure. Increased afterload can lead to left ventricular failure and pulmonary edema.

RESPIRATORY SYSTEM

Reductions of colloid oncotic pressure can result in interstitial accumulation of fluid in the lungs. Indeed, reductions of arterial oxygen partial pressures are a frequent occurrence in the presence of toxemia of pregnancy. Edema of the upper airway and larynx, which accompanies normal gestation, is exaggerated in these parturients. This change may influence the size of tube chosen for intubation of the trachea.

HEPATORENAL

Hepatic dysfunction is associated with decreased hepatic blood flow and conceivably decreased plasma cholinesterase activity. In addition progressive decreases in renal blood flow and glomerular filtration rate may culminate in oliguric renal failure. Increased renal loss of protein leads to reductions of colloid oncotic pressure.

INTRAVASCULAR FLUID VOLUME

Intravascular fluid volume is often decreased below nonpregnant levels in the presence of toxemia of pregnancy. This hypovolemia results in an increased hematocrit which may obscure the presence of anemia.

COAGULATION

Abnormalities of the coagulation system may progress to disseminated intravascular coagulation, as manifested by increased plasma concentrations of fibrin degradation products. Platelet counts are also frequently reduced in parturients with toxemia of pregnancy, presumably reflecting increased platelet consumption.

UTEROPLACENTAL CIRCULATION

Perfusion of the uterus and placenta is reduced in the presence of toxemia of pregnancy. Decreased uterine blood flow predisposes to a hyperactive uterus, and premature labor is common. The fetus is at increased risk due to marginal placental function. Neonates are often premature and small for gestational age. As a result, these infants are vulnerable to depression from drugs used to provide maternal analgesia. Finally meconium aspiration is a common problem in neonates born from these mothers.

Treatment

Definitive treatment of toxemia of pregnancy is delivery of the fetus and placenta. Until delivery is possible, therapy is directed at treating major organ dysfunction. For example, intravenous infusion of fluids is guided by atrial filling pressures and urine output. Approximately one-third of the fluid infused should consist of 5 percent albumin to correct decreased osmotic pressure. Digitalis and a renal tubular diuretic are indicated if pulmonary edema and congestive heart failure accompany toxemia. Cerebral edema may be managed with osmotic diuretics, such as mannitol. Bed rest in the lateral position, so as to minimize aortocaval compression, is important. Sodium restriction is not recommended, as this may lead to sodium depletion and activation of the renin-angiotensin-aldosterone system. Magnesium and antihypertensive drugs are frequently used in the treatment of toxemia of pregnancy.

MAGNESIUM

Magnesium is administered to parturients with toxemia of pregnancy in attempts to decrease irritability of the central nervous system. Magnesium also decreases hyperactivity at the neuromuscular junction. The mechanism for these effects is the ability of magnesium to decrease the presynaptic release of acetylcholine, as well as to reduce sensitivity of the postjunctional membranes to acetylcholine. In addition, magnesium has mild relaxant effects on vascular and uterine smooth muscle. Uterine relaxation is beneficial, since uterine blood flow is improved.

Clinically, therapeutic effects of magnesium therapy are estimated in terms of its effects on deep tendon reflexes. Marked depression of patellar reflexes is an indication of impending magnesium toxicity. Periodic determination of plasma magnesium levels is also helpful in adjusting supplemental doses of magnesium, so as to keep plasma concentrations in therapeutic ranges of 4 mEq·L^{-1} to 6 mEq·L^{-1}. Commonly, parturients receive an intravenous loading dose of magnesium 4 g in a 20 percent solution infused over 5 minutes. Therapeutic plasma concentrations are maintained by continuous infusion of 1 g·hr^{-1} to 2 g·hr^{-1}. Plasma magnesium levels in excess of the therapeutic range can lead to severe skeletal muscle weakness, with ventilatory failure and cardiac arrest. Administration of intravenous calcium counteracts adverse effects of magnesium. Magnesium is excreted by the kidneys and must be used with caution when renal function is impaired.

Potentiation of both depolarizing and nondepolarizing muscle relaxants by magnesium is clinically significant. This potentiation introduces the need for careful titration of the dose of muscle relaxants and for monitoring the effects produced at the neuromuscular junction. Toxemia of pregnancy may be associated with reductions in plasma cholineserase activity that are greater than those normally associated with pregnancy resulting in potentiation of the effects of succinylcholine independent of magnesium therapy.[85] Doses of sedatives and opioids should be reduced, as magnesium can potentiate their effects. Since magnesium readily crosses the placenta, it seems possible that neonatal skeletal muscle tone could be decreased at birth. Nevertheless, deleterious effects of maternal magnesium therapy do not occur in nonasphyxiated full-term neonates, suggesting that depression of ventilation previously attributed to magnesium was due to asphyxia and/or prematurity.[86] Conversely, hypomagnesemia may cause postpartum neurologic dysfunction, which is erroneously attributed to regional anesthetic techniques used during labor and delivery.[87]

ANTIHYPERTENSIVE DRUGS

It is appropriate to initiate therapy with antihypertensive drugs when diastolic blood pressures remain above 110 mmHg. Hydralazine (5 mg to 10 mg) is frequently selected because of its rapid onset (15 minutes) when given intravenously. Additional doses of hydralazine are administered as necessary to maintain diastolic blood pressures near 90 mmHg. Hydralazine often increases cardiac output, uteroplacental circulation, and renal blood flow. Alpha-methyldopa has the disadvantage of a slow onset and the potential for producing hepatic dysfunction.

Continuous intravenous infusions of trimethaphan (0.01 percent) may be lifesaving for treatment of a hypertensive crisis in parturients with toxemia of pregnancy. The goal is to reduce maternal diastolic blood pressures to around 100 mmHg; one must remember that sudden drops in blood pressure may jeopardize uteroplacental circulation and lead to fetal distress. Fetal heart rate should be continuously monitored during pharmacologic treatment of a maternal hypertensive crises to insure an early warning if blood pressure lowering is compromising uteroplacental circulation. Diazoxide is not popular in these patients because of the unpredictable magnitude of blood pressure reduction produced by this drug.

Nitroprusside is not recommended for treatment of hypertensive crises in parturients. This recommendation is based on the knowledge that cyanide readily crosses the placenta, introducing the possibility of fetal cyanide toxicity. Indeed, the fetus has less thiosulfate substrate for rhodanase detoxification of cyanide than the adult and, therefore, may be uniquely vulnerable to development of cyanide toxicity from sodium nitroprusside infusions.[87] Nevertheless, deliberate hypotension with sodium nitroprusside has been used to facilitate surgery for control of intracranial aneurysms in

parturients, with no apparent adverse effects on the fetuses.[88] Indeed, a 20 percent reduction in blood pressure for 1 hour, produced with an average dose of nitroprusside of 1 $\mu g \cdot kg^{-1} \cdot min^{-1}$ administered to an animal model, had no adverse effects on the fetuses.[87] Conversely, similar reductions in blood pressure in animals requiring average doses of nitroprusside of 25 $\mu g \cdot kg^{-1} \cdot min^{-1}$ produced cyanide toxicity and in utero fetal death. Perhaps short-term use of nitroprusside in low doses is acceptable for treatment of hypertensive parturients.

Management of Anesthesia

Vaginal delivery in the presence of toxemia of pregnancy and in the absence of fetal distress is acceptable. Continuous lumbar epidural block is a useful method of analgesia for labor and vaginal delivery for volume repleted preeclamptic patients under good medical control. Epidural analgesia negates the need for maternal opioids and thus their possible adverse effects on a preterm fetus. The absence of maternal pushing reduces the likelihood of associated blood pressure increases. Furthermore, vasodilating effects produced by the epidural block improve placental blood flow and could conceivably increase renal blood flow.[89]

Before continuous lumbar epidural block is instituted, patients should be hydrated with intravenous fluids (1 L to 2 L of lactated Ringer's solution), as guided by central venous pressure monitoring. Furthermore, coagulation studies should be performed before placement of lumbar epidural catheters, particularly if the preeclampsia is severe. Initially, a segmental band of anesthesia (T10-L1) will provide analgesia for uterine contractions. As the second stage of labor is entered, the lumbar epidural block can be extended to provide perineal analgesia. Because of hypersensitivity of the maternal vasculature to catecholamines, it would seem prudent not to add epinephrine to local anesthetics used for the epidural blocks. Nevertheless, use of epinephrine containing local anesthesia solutions has not produced adverse circulatory responses in these patients.[90]

If vaginal delivery is imminent, a subarachnoid block limited to the sacral area is an acceptable approach. As with lumbar epidural techniques, institution of intravenous hydration before performance of subarachnoid blocks is desirable. The disadvantage of subarachnoid blocks is the possible rapid onset of peripheral sympathetic nervous system blockade and hypotension should the sensory level extend above T10. Should systolic blood pressures decrease more than 30 percent from the preblock value, treatment is with left uterine displacement and increased rates of fluid infusion. If hypotension persists, small doses of ephedrine (2.5 mg) administered intravenously are appropriate.

Cesarean section is often necessary in parturients with toxemia of pregnancy. The indication for cesarean section is fetal distress, reflecting progressive deterioration of the uteroplacental circulation. General anesthesia is usually preferred when an emergency cesarean section is necessary. Extensive peripheral sympathetic nervous system blockade that would accompany epidural or subarachnoid blocks could make management of blood pressure difficult in these patients during cesarean section. Before induction of anesthesia, an attempt must be made to restore intravascular fluid volume. Continuous monitoring of intra-arterial pressure, cardiac filling pressures, urine output, and fetal heart rate is useful. Induction of anesthesia is often with thiopental (3 $mg \cdot kg^{-1}$ to 4 $mg \cdot kg^{-1}$) plus succinylcholine (1 $mg \cdot kg^{-1}$ to 1.5 $mg \cdot kg^{-1}$), to facilitate placement of a cuffed tube in the trachea. Cricoid pressure is provided by an assistant until the trachea is protected by a cuffed tube. Use of defasciculating doses of nondepolarizing muscle relaxants before administration of succinylcholine may not be necessary, since magnesium therapy is likely to attenuate fasciculations produced by succinylcholine. Exaggerated edema of the upper airway structures may interfere with visualization of the glottic opening (swollen tongue and epiglottis), and laryngeal swelling may result in the need to insert a smaller endotracheal tube than anticipated. In patients with impaired coagulation, laryngoscopy may evoke profuse bleeding. Blood pressure increases that predictably accompany direct laryngoscopy and intubation of the trachea might be exaggerated in these parturients, increasing

the likelihood of cerebral hemorrhage or pulmonary edema. A short duration of laryngoscopy is helpful for minimizing the magnitude and duration of blood pressure increases. Hydralazine (5 mg to 10 mg), administered intravenously 10 minutes to 15 minutes before the induction of anesthesia, or intravenous nitroglycerin (1 $\mu g \cdot kg^{-1}$ to 2 $\mu g \cdot kg^{-1}$), just before starting direct laryngoscopy, has also been recommended for attenuating these blood pressure responses.[91] Volatile anesthetics (0.5 MAC) can be used before intubation of the trachea and during anesthetic maintenance to both attenuate and treat hypertension. Potentiation of muscle relaxants by magnesium must be remembered, and a peripheral nerve stimulator used to monitor activity of the neuromuscular junction. Removal of the cuffed tube from the trachea should be considered only after return of the upper airway reflexes. Use of synthetic oxytocics to treat uterine atony after delivery must be done cautiously in view of the hypersensitive peripheral vasculature predictably present in these parturients.

PREGNANCY AND DIABETES MELLITUS

Insulin requirements in parturients with diabetes mellitus change markedly during pregnancy. For example, less insulin is needed in the first trimester and more in the second trimester. Maternal insulin requirements drop precipitously in the postpartum period. Insulin does not cross the placenta. Conversely, oral hypoglycemic drugs readily cross the placenta and can induce hypoglycemia in the neonate.

Glucose levels during pregnancy in nondiabetic parturients are lower than nonpregnant levels. Therefore, blood glucose concentrations are often maintained at lower than normal levels in parturients with diabetes mellitus. Accomplishment of this goal may require multiple injections of insulin and rigid adherence to diet. Diabetic parturients are at increased risk for development of ketoacidosis during the second and third trimesters. Toxemia of pregnancy is also more common in the presence of diabetes mellitus. Neonates born from diabetic mothers are often large for gestational age and have increased risks for developing respiratory distress syndrome.

The goal is to insure continuation of pregnancy to near term, so as to allow maximal fetal lung maturation. Elective cesarean section is often performed in an attempt to avoid the high incidence of fetal death that occurs late in the third trimester, presumably due to placental insufficiency. The best choice of anesthesia is not defined. Fetal acidosis following cesarean section has been reported with epidural or subarachnoid blocks that were complicated by maternal hypotension.[92,93] Indeed, there is a suggestion that fetal outcome is better after cesarean section performed under general anesthesia.[93] Nevertheless, regional anesthetic techniques in diabetic parturients provide the advantages of (1) avoiding hyperglycemic responses to surgery, (2) monitoring the central nervous system status of the mother, and (3) providing anesthesia without added drug depression should operative delivery be difficult and prolonged. Regardless of the technique selected for anesthesia, blood glucose concentrations should be checked in the early neonatal period of infants born to diabetic parturients.

MYASTHENIA GRAVIS AND PREGNANCY

The course of myasthenia gravis during gestation is highly variable and unpredictable.[94] Exacerbations are most likely to take place during the first trimester or in the first 10 days of the postpartum period. Anticholinesterase drugs should be continued during pregnancy and labor. Theoretically, these drugs would increase uterine contractility, but an increased incidence of spontaneous abortion or premature labor does not occur.

Myasthenia gravis does not affect the course of labor. The use of sedative drugs should be avoided in view of the limited margin of reserve in these patients. A continuous lumbar epidural block is acceptable for labor

and vaginal delivery. Outlet forceps are frequently used to shorten the second stage of labor and thereby minimize skeletal muscle fatigue associated with expulsive efforts. Regional anesthesia can be used safely for cesarean section, but it must be appreciated that coexisting skeletal muscle weakness may lead to hypoventilation in the presence of high sensory levels.

Neonatal myasthenia gravis can occur transiently in 20 percent to 30 percent of babies born to mothers with this disorder. Manifestations usually occur within 24 hours of birth and are characterized by generalized skeletal muscle weakness and an expressionless face. When respiratory efforts are inadequate, a tube should be placed in the trachea and ventilation of the lungs should be mechanically supported. Anticholinesterase therapy is usually necessary for about 21 days after birth.

HEMORRHAGE IN THE OBSTETRIC PATIENT

Hemorrhage remains the leading cause of maternal mortality. Although bleeding can occur at any time during pregnancy, third trimester hemorrhage is most threatening to maternal and fetal well-being (Table 34-8).[95] Placenta previa and abruptio placentae are the major causes of bleeding during the third trimester. Uterine rupture can be responsible for uncontrolled hemorrhage that manifests during active labor. Postpartum hemorrhage occurs after 3 percent to 5 percent of all vaginal deliveries and is typically due to retained placenta, uterine atony, or cervical or vaginal lacerations.

Placenta Previa

Placenta previa is the abnormally low implantation of the placenta in the uterus, which occurs in up to 1 percent of full-term pregnancies (Table 34-8).[95] The cause is not known, although there is an association with advancing age of the parturient and with high parity.

TABLE 34-8. Causes of Third Trimester Bleeding

	Placenta Previa	Abruptio Placentae	Uterine Rupture

Clinical features	Painless bleeding	Abdominal pain
		Bleeding partially or
		  wholly concealed
		Uterine irritability
		Shock
		Coagulopathy
		Acute renal failure
		Fetal distress
			Severe abdominal pain
			Shock
			Disappearance of fetal
			  heart tones

Predisposing conditions	Advanced age
	High parity
		High parity
		Uterine anomalies
		Compression of inferior
		  vena cava
		Chronic hypertension
			Previous uterine incision
			Rapid spontaneous
			  delivery
			Excessive uterine
			  stimulation
			Cephalopelvic
			  disproportion
			High parity
			Polyhydramnios
			Spontaneous

Incidence	0.1–1%	0.2–2.4%	0.08–0.1%
Maternal mortality	<1%	0–3.1%	About 5%
Fetal mortality	About 20%	30–55%	About 50%

(Data from Gatt SP. Anaesthetic management of the obstetric patient with antepartum or intrapartum haemorrhage. Clin Anaesthesiol 1986;4:233–46)

Placenta previa is classified as (1) complete, in which the entire internal cervical os is covered by placental tissue; (2) partial, in which the internal cervical os is covered by placental tissue when closed, but not when fully dilated; and (3) marginal, in which placental tissue encroaches on or extends to the margin of the internal cervical os. Nearly 50 percent of patients with placenta previa have marginal implantations.

The cardinal symptom of placenta previa is painless vaginal bleeding, which usually stops spontaneously. Bleeding typically manifests around week 32, when the lower uterine segment is beginning to form. When this diagnosis is suspected, the position of the placenta should be confirmed by ultrasonography or radioisotope scan. If these tests are not conclusive and vaginal bleeding persists, the diagnosis is made by direct examination of the cervical os. This examination should be done in the delivery room, only after preparations have been taken to replace acute blood loss and to proceed with an emergency cesarean section. The combination of direct examination of the cervical os in a patient who is surgically prepared for an immediate cesarean section is known as a "double set-up." When manual ex-

amination of the cervical os triggers hemorrhage, it is likely that bleeding will persist until the placenta can be removed. Ketamine is a useful drug for induction of anesthesia in the presence of acute hemorrhage due to placenta previa. It should be remembered, however, that doses of ketamine in excess of 1 mg·kg⁻¹ are associated with increased uterine tone.[38] Theoretically, such increases could further decrease an already compromised uteroplacental circulation. Maintenance of anesthesia before delivery is determined by the hemodynamic status of the mother. Often, anesthesia is maintained with 50 percent nitrous oxide plus succinylcholine, to produce skeletal muscle relaxation. Neonates delivered from parturients in hemorrhagic shock are likely to be severely acidotic and hypovolemic. Treatment of placenta previa not accompanied by hemorrhage is bed rest followed by elective cesarean section.

Abruptio Placentae

Abruptio placentae is separation of a normally implanted placenta after 20 weeks of gestation (Table 34-8).[95] The cause is not known, but the incidence is increased with high parity, uterine anomalies, compression of the inferior vena cava, and occurrence of hypertension during pregnancy. Abruptio placentae accounts for about one-third of third trimester hemorrhages.

Clinical manifestations of abruptio placentae depend on the site and extent of the placental separation but abdominal pain is almost always present. When the separation involves only placental margins, the escaping blood can appear as vaginal bleeding. Alternatively, large volumes of blood loss can remain entirely concealed in the uterus. Severe blood loss from abruptio placentae manifests as maternal hypotension, uterine irritability and hypertonia, plus fetal distress or even demise. Clotting abnormalities, due to unknown causes but resembling disseminated intravascular coagulation, can occur. Therefore, measurements of coagulation status must be obtained in these patients. The classic hematologic picture includes thrombocytopenia, depletion of fibrinogen, and prolonged plasma thromboplastin times.[95] Acute renal failure may accompany disseminated intravascular coagulation, reflecting fibrin deposition in renal arterioles. Fetal distress reflects loss of functioning placenta and decreased uteroplacental perfusion because of maternal hypotension.

Definitive treatment of abruptio placentae is to empty the uterus. If there are no signs of maternal hypovolemia, if clotting studies are normal, and if there is no evidence of uteroplacental insufficiency, the use of a continuous lumbar epidural block is useful to provide analgesia for labor and vaginal delivery. When the magnitude of placental separation and resulting hemorrhage is severe, an emergency cesarean section is necessary, using general anesthesia. Ketamine is a useful drug for induction of anesthesia, followed by addition of 50 percent nitrous oxide until the fetus is delivered. It is predictable that neonates born under these circumstances will be acidotic and hypovolemic.

It is not uncommon for blood to dissect between layers of the myometrium following premature separation of the placenta. As a result, the uterus is unable to contract adequately after delivery, and postpartum hemorrhage oc-curs. Uncontrolled hemorrhage may require an emergency hysterectomy. Finally, bleeding may be exaggerated by a coagulopathy, in which case infusion of fresh frozen plasma and platelets should replace deficient clotting factors. Clotting parameters usually revert to normal within a few hours after delivery of the neonate.

Uterine Rupture

Uterine rupture occurs in up to 0.1 percent of full-term pregnancies and my be associated with separation of a previous uterine scar, rapid spontaneous delivery, excessive oxytocin stimulation, or multigravidas with cephalopelvic disproportion or unrecognized transverse presentations.[95] Overall, however, more than 80 percent of uterine ruptures are spontaneous without an obvious explanation.[95] Furthermore, uterine rupture and dehiscence represent a spectrum ranging from incomplete ruptures or gradual scar dehiscences with minimal pain to explosive rupture with intraperitoneal extrusion of uterine contents. Manifestations may include (1) severe abdominal pain, often referred to the shoulder due to subdiaphragmatic irritation by intra-abdominal blood; (2) maternal hypotension; and (3) disappearance of fetal heart tones. Occasionally, parturients with previous cesarean sections are allowed to deliver vaginally. In these patients, continuous lumbar epidural analgesia has been questioned, since this form of analgesia could mask abdominal pain, which may be the first indication of impending or actual uterine rupture. Nevertheless, this theoretical concern has not been confirmed by clinical experience and with the proper precautions (continuous fetal monitoring, avoidance of oxytocic stimulation of the uterus), epidural analgesia produced by dilute concentrations of local anesthetics may be safely used in parturients with a previous cesarean section.[95,96]

Retained Placenta

Retained placenta occurs in about 1 percent of all vaginal deliveries and usually necessitates manual exploration of the uterus. If epidural or subarachnoid blocks are not used for vaginal delivery, manual removal of the placenta may be first attempted under continuous inhalation analgesia. General anesthesia, including administration of volatile drugs to provide uterine relaxation, will be necessary if the uterus remains firmly contracted around the placenta. Intubation of the trachea is necessary when general anesthesia is used to relax the uterus. Ketamine, in doses exceeding 1 mg· kg^{-1}, is not recommended in view of dose-related increases in uterine tone produced by this drug.[38]

Uterine Atony

Uterine atony following vaginal delivery is an important cause of postpartum bleeding and is a potential cause of maternal mortality. A completely atonic uterus may result in a 2,000 ml blood loss in 5 minutes. Conditions associated with uterine atony include high parity, multiple births, polyhydramnios, large fetuses, and retained placenta. Uterine atony may occur immediately after delivery or manifest several hours later. Treatment is with intravenous oxytocin to cause contraction of the uterus. In rare instances, it may be necessary to perform an emergency hysterectomy.

AMNIOTIC FLUID EMBOLISM

Amniotic fluid embolism, which is estimated to occur once in every 20,000 to 30,000 deliveries, is signalled by the sudden onset of respiratory distress, profound hypotension, and arterial hypoxemia.[97] Entry of amniotic fluid into the pulmonary circulation results in (1) pulmonary vascular obstruction, with consequent reductions in cardiac output and hypotension; (2) pulmonary hypertension, with acute cor pulmonale; and (3) ventilation-perfusion inequality, producing severe arterial hypoxemia. In some instances, grand mal seizures precede the appearance of cardiorespiratory symptoms. Excessive bleeding is usu-

ally not present initially but develops later in nearly every affected parturient. Hemorrhage is attributed to disseminated intravascular coagulation.

There is no specific treatment for amniotic fluid embolism, other than that directed toward cardiopulmonary resuscitation and replacement of intravascular fluid volume. Arterial hypoxemia is severe, and supplemental oxygen plus intubation of the trachea and controlled ventilation of the lungs will usually be necessary. Positive end-expiratory pressure may be instituted if arterial hypoxemia persists. Corticosteroids have been used but do not seem to be of demonstrable benefit. Mortality from a massive amniotic fluid embolism is over 80 percent.

Multiparous parturients who experience a tumultuous labor are most likely to experience amniotic fluid embolism. Definitive diagnosis is made by demonstrating amniotic fluid material in maternal blood, which has been aspirated from a central venous catheter.[98] Indeed, examination of a blood smear should be performed in every parturient suspected of having amniotic fluid embolism. Conditions that can mimic amniotic fluid embolism include inhalation of gastric contents, pulmonary embolism, air embolism, and reactions to local anesthetics. Pulmonary aspiration is more likely when bronchospasm accompanies the clinical picture. Indeed, bronchospasm is rare in parturients who experience amniotic fluid embolism. Pulmonary embolism is usually accompanied by chest pain.

ANESTHESIA FOR OPERATIONS DURING PREGNANCY

It is estimated that about 50,000 pregnant women a year in the United States undergo an operative procedure requiring anesthesia.[99] The most frequent nonobstetrical procedure is excision of an ovarian cyst. Appendicitis is the second most frequent indication for operative intervention. Treatment of an incompetent cervix (cervical cerclage) requires anesthesia early in pregnancy. Finally, there is always the possibility that anesthesia may be unknowingly administered in early undiagnosed pregnancy. The objectives for management of anesthesia in pregnant patients undergoing nonobstetric operative procedures are avoidance of teratogenic drugs, avoidance of intrauterine fetal hypoxia and acidosis, and prevention of premature labor.[100,101]

Avoidance of Teratogenic Drugs

Almost all commonly used medications, including drugs used for anesthesia, have been demonstrated to be teratogenic in at least one animal species. For a drug to be teratogenic, it must be given to a susceptible species in an appropriate dose and during a specific period of organ development. Each organ system undergoes a critical stage of development, during which vulnerability to teratogens is greatest. In humans, the critical period of organogenesis is between 15 days and 56 days of gestation; however, surveys of women who had received inhalation anesthesia for operations during pregnancy have failed to demonstrate that any anesthetic is a teratogen or induces abortions.[101,102] Nevertheless, sufficient circumstantial evidence of the harmful nature of nitrous oxide exists to suggest caution in administration of this drug to women during early pregnancy.[101]

There is concern that subteratogenic doses of some psychoactive drugs, such as anesthetics, could produce behavioral and learning defects without causing gross morphologic changes. This concern is based on the fact that development of the central nervous system is not complete even at birth. Therefore, it has been proposed that drugs administered to parturients, including those used for anesthesia during labor and delivery, might produce permanent organ dysfunction. Indeed, short duration administration of halothane to pregnant rats resulted in learning deficits in offspring of those animals who were exposed during the first and second but not third trimesters.[103] Nevertheless, at present, there is no evidence

establishing the validity of the assertion that anesthesia administered to a parturient adversely affects later mental and neurologic development of the offspring.[104] Finally, there is no evidence that any anesthetic drug is carcinogenic to the fetus.

Avoidance of Intrauterine Fetal Hypoxia and Acidosis

Intrauterine fetal hypoxia and acidosis are prevented by avoiding maternal hypotension, arterial hypoxemia, and excessive changes in arterial carbon dioxide partial pressures. It must be appreciated that uterine blood flow and thus placental perfusion is pressure-dependent. Hazards to the fetus from decreased maternal oxygenation are obvious. Conversely, maternal hyperoxia does not produce uterine artery vasoconstriction. Furthermore, high maternal arterial oxygen partial pressures rarely produce fetal arterial oxygen partial pressures above 45 mmHg. This reflects the high oxygen consumption of the placenta and uneven distribution of maternal and fetal blood flow in the placenta. For this reason, maternal hyperoxia does not produce in utero retrolental fibroplasia or premature closure of the ductus arteriosus. Maternal hyperventilation should be avoided intraoperatively, as positive airway pressures may reduce uterine blood flow and metabolic alkalosis increases maternal hemoglobin affinity for oxygen, resulting in release of less oxygen to the fetus at the placenta.

Prevention of Premature Labor

There is no evidence that specific anesthetic drugs or techniques are associated with a higher or lower incidence of premature delivery.[102] Indeed, it is the underlying pathology necessitating the operative intervention that determines the onset of premature labor. For example, premature labor occurs in 28 percent to 40 percent of patients undergoing a cervical cerclage, whereas orthopedic, neurosurgical, or plastic surgical procedures were not associated with premature labor. After successful completion of an operative procedure, it is advisable to continue intensive monitoring of the mother and fetus in the recovery period. Specifically, continuous monitoring of the fetal heart rate and maternal uterine activity is important.

Premature labor can be treated with selective beta-2-adrenergic agonist drugs such as terbutaline or ritordine. These drugs relax uterine smooth muscle, resulting in inhibition of uterine contractions. Relaxation of the uterus also contributes to improved uteroplacental blood flow and fetal well-being. It is important to realize that significant maternal side effects, including pulmonary edema, cardiac dysrhythmias, and hypokalemia, can accompany the use of these drugs.[105,106] These drugs cross the placenta and can cause fetal tachycardia and hypoglycemia. The mechanism for alterations in maternal plasma potassium concentrations is not established. It is thought that beta-2-agonist drugs stimulate both glycolysis and insulin release, resulting in shifts of potassium into intracellular spaces. It is important to be aware that hypokalemia observed during administration of beta-2-agonist drugs persists despite potassium chloride supplementation. Plasma potassium concentrations will return to preinfusion levels about 30 minutes after drug infusion is discontinued. Therefore, it may be prudent to discontinue beta-agonist infusions about 30 minutes before administration of an anesthetic for delivery.[106] Continuous monitoring of the electrocardiogram and avoidance of intraoperative hyperventilation of the lungs are important principles for management of anesthesia. Intravenous alcohol has also been used to stop premature labor. Maternal and neonatal central nervous system depression are undesirable side effects of this treatment.

trimester. Emergency surgery in the first trimester is often performed with lumbar epidural or subarachnoid blocks. Subarachnoid anesthesia is useful, as this technique minimizes fetal drug exposure. Nevertheless, there is no evidence that inhaled anesthetics cause adverse responses when administered to parturients undergoing nonobstetric surgery.[102] Continuous intraoperative monitoring of fetal heart rate after the 16th week of gestation is helpful in providing early warning of fetal hypoxia and acidosis due to impaired uteroplacental perfusion (see the section Diagnosis and Management of Fetal Distress). When inhalation anesthesia is chosen, it should be appreciated that low concentrations of volatile drugs are not associated with significant reductions in uterine blood flow because of concomitant decreases in uterine vascular resistance. Although controversial, it may be prudent to avoid administration of nitrous oxide to women in early pregnancy.[101] Regardless of the anesthetic techniques selected, inspired concentrations of oxygen should be maintained at about 50 percent.

DIAGNOSIS AND MANAGEMENT OF FETAL DISTRESS

Fetal distress due to intrauterine hypoxia and acidosis is most likely to occur when uterine blood flow decreases with each uterine contraction. Indeed, a placenta with borderline function before the onset of labor may not be able to maintain fetal well-being when gas transfer across the placenta is further compromised by decreases in uterine blood flow associated with vigorous contractions of the uterus.

Management of Anesthesia

Elective surgery should be deferred until after delivery. When surgery is urgent, it is best to delay the operation until the second or third

Electronic Fetal Monitoring

Electronic fetal monitoring allows evaluation of fetal well-being by following changes in fetal heart rate as recorded using an external monitor (Doppler) or fetal scalp electrode. The basic principle of electronic fetal monitoring is to correlate changes in fetal heart rate with fetal movement and uterine contractions. For example, fetal well-being is evaluated by determination of beat-to-beat variability of fetal heart rate, as computed from the R-R intervals on the fetal electrocardiogram.[107,108] Another method is evaluation of fetal heart rate decelerations associated with contractions of the uterus.[108,109] The three major types of fetal heart rate decelerations are classified as early, late, and variable. Fetal scalp sampling is indicated when abnormal fetal heart rate patterns occur. It has been observed that the fetus is usually depressed when one or more fetal scalp pH values are below 7.20.

BEAT-TO-BEAT VARIABILITY

Fetal heart rate varies 5 beats·min^{-1} to 20 beats·min^{-1}, with normal heart rates ranging between 120 beats·min^{-1} to 160 beats·min^{-1}. This normal heart rate variability is thought to reflect integrity of neural pathways from the fetal cerebral cortex through the medulla, vagus nerve, and cardiac conduction system.

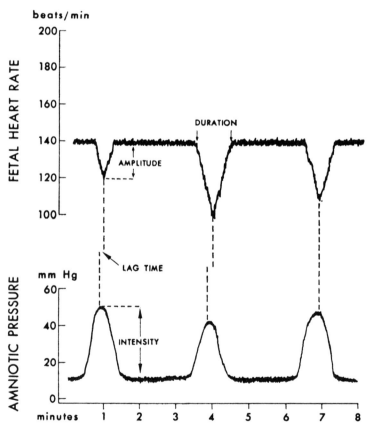

FIG. 34-14. Early decelerations of the fetal heart rate are characterized by a short lag time between the onset of uterine contractions and the beginning of fetal heart rate slowing. Maximum slowing is usually less than 20 beats·min^{-1} and occurs at the peak intensity of the contractions. Heart rate has returned to normal by the time the contractions have ceased. The most likely explanation for this pattern is a vagal reflex due to compression of the fetal head. (Shnider SM. Diagnosis of fetal distress: Fetal heart rate. In: Shnider SM, ed. Obstetrical Anesthesia: Current Concepts and Practice. Baltimore. Williams & Wilkins Co. 1970: 197–203)

Fetal well-being is assured when beat-to-beat variability is present. Conversely, fetal distress, due to arterial hypoxemia, acidosis, or central nervous system damage, is associated with minimal to absent beat-to-beat variability.

Drugs administered to the parturient may eliminate fetal heart rate variability, even in the absence of fetal distress. Those drugs most frequently associated with loss of beat-to-beat variability are benzodiazepines, opioids, barbiturates, anticholinergics, and local anesthetics, as used for continuous lumbar epidural analgesia. These drug-induced effects do not appear to be deleterious but may cause difficulty in interpretation of fetal heart rate monitoring. In addition, absence of heart rate variability may be normally present in the premature fetus and during fetal sleep cycles.

EARLY DECELERATIONS

Early decelerations are characterized by slowing of fetal heart rate that begins with the onset of uterine contractions (Fig. 34-14). Slowing becomes maximum at the peak of contractions, returning to near baseline at their termination. Decreases in heart rate are usually not greater than 20 beats·min^{-1} or below an absolute rate of 100 beats·min^{-1}. This deceleration pattern is thought to be caused by vagal stimulation secondary to compression of the fetal head. Early decelerations are not prevented by increasing fetal oxygenation but are blocked by the administration of atropine. Most important, this fetal heart rate pattern is not associated with fetal distress.

LATE DECELERATIONS

Late decelerations are characterized by slowing of fetal heart rate that begins 10 seconds to 30 seconds after the onset of uterine contractions. Maximum slowing occurs after the peak intensity of the contractions (Fig. 34-15). A mild late deceleration is classified as a decrease in heart rate less than 20 beats·min^{-1}; profound slowing is considered present when reductions are more than 40 beats·min^{-1}. Late decelerations are associated with fetal distress, most likely reflecting myocardial hypoxia sec-

ondary to uteroplacental insufficiency. Primary factors contributing to the appearance of late decelerations include maternal hypotension, uterine hyperactivity, and chronic uteroplacental insufficiency, as may be due to diabetes mellitus or hypertension. When this pattern persists, there is a predictable correlation with the development of fetal acidosis.[108,109] Late decelerations can be corrected by improving fetal oxygenation. Finally, when beat-to-beat variability of fetal heart rate persists despite late decelerations, the fetus is still likely to be born vigorous.

VARIABLE DECELERATIONS

Variable decelerations are the most common pattern of fetal heart rate changes observed in the intrapartum period. As the term indicates, these decelerations are variable in magnitude, duration, and time of onset relative to uterine contractions (Fig. 34-16). For example, this pattern may begin before, with, or after the onset of uterine contractions. Characteristically, deceleration patterns are abrupt in onset and cessation. Fetal heart rate almost invariably falls below 100 beats·min^{-1}. Variable decelerations are thought to be caused by umbilical cord compression. Atropine diminishes the severity of variable decelerations, but administration of oxygen to the mother is without effect. If deceleration patterns are not severe and repetitive, there are usually only minimal alterations in the fetal acid-base status. Severe variable deceleration patterns that persist 15 minutes to 30 minutes are associated with fetal acidosis.

EVALUATION OF THE FETUS

It is important to identify intrauterine growth retardation (lower weight than would be expected for gestational age) and prematurity (born less than 37 weeks after the last menstrual period). Infants small for gestational age are more likely to develop hypoglycemia and sepsis, and congenital abnormalities occur more frequently. It is postulated that the nu-

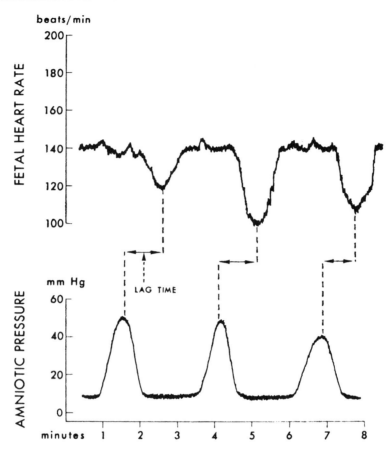

FIG. 34-15. Late decelerations of the fetal heart rate are characterized by a long lag time between the onset of uterine contractions and the beginning of fetal heart rate slowing. The heart rate does not return to normal until after the contractions have ceased. A mild late deceleration pattern is present when slowing is less than 20 beats·min^{-1}; profound slowing is present when fetal heart rate slows more than 40 beats·min^{-1}. Late decelerations indicate uteroplacental insufficiency. (Shnider SM. Diagnosis of fetal distress: Fetal heart rate. In: Shnider SM, ed. Obstetrical Anesthesia: Current Concepts and Practice. Baltimore. Williams & Wilkins Co. 1970: 197–203)

tritional deficiency or chronic arterial hypoxemia that results in low birth weight is also responsible for poor neurologic development. Premature neonates have an increased incidence of fetal distress, respiratory distress syndrome, hypovolemia, hypoglycemia, sepsis, intracranial hemorrhage, and temperature instability; they are also susceptible to the development of retrolental fibroplasia (see Chapter 35).

A number of laboratory studies can be used to assess fetal function and maturity. These tests include measurement of maternal urinary estriol excretion and plasma placental lactogen concentrations, analysis of amniotic fluid for lecithin and sphingomyelin levels, and assessment of fetal biparietal diameter by ultrasonography.

Maternal Urinary Estriol

Determination of estriol excretion in the maternal urine has been used as a test of fetal well-being before the onset of labor.[107] This

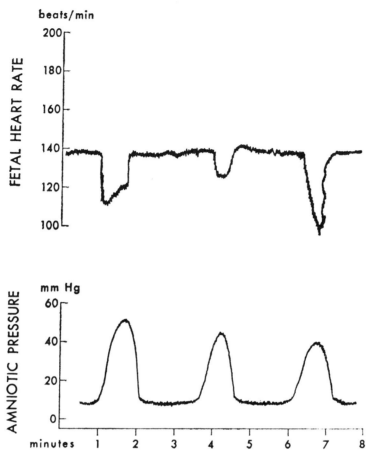

FIG. 34-16. Variable decelerations of the fetal heart rate are characterized by reductions in the heart rate of varying magnitude and duration. Furthermore, these slowings do not show consistent relationships to uterine contractions. This pattern of fetal heart rate slowing is associated with umbilical cord compression. (Shnider SM. Diagnosis of fetal distress: Fetal heart rate. In: Shnider SM, ed. Obstetrical Anesthesia: Current Concepts and Practice. Baltimore. Williams & Wilkins Co. 1970: 197–203)

hormone is synthesized by the placenta from androgen precursors originating in the fetal adrenal gland and the liver. Estriol passes from the fetus into the maternal circulation and is excreted by the kidneys. Maternal urinary estriol excretion increases with gestational age.

A breakdown at any point in the production or transport of estriol can lead to reductions of maternal urinary excretion of this hormone. A downward trend or precipitous fall in estriol levels is suggestive of fetal deterioration. Indeed, decreasing estriol excretion has been observed before fetal demise in pregnancies complicated by diabetes mellitus, hyper-

tension, or toxemia of pregnancy. Other causes of low estriol values include fetal anencephaly, fetal liver dysfunction, and maternal renal disease.

Human Placental Lactogen

Human placental lactogen is a protein hormone produced by the placenta. Maternal plasma levels of this hormone correlate with placental and fetal weight. For example, elevation of human placental lactogen levels, in association with multiple gestations or diabetes mellitus, reflects increased placental mass. Likewise, levels are likely to be reduced in the presence of intrauterine growth retardation.

Amniotic Fluid Analysis

An index of fetal lung maturity is often obtained before elective cesarean section is performed or induction of labor is undertaken. For example, amniotic fluid, as obtained by abdominal amniocentesis, can be used to as-

sess fetal lung maturity. With maturation of the appropriate enzyme system at about 35 weeks of gestation, there is an abrupt rise of the lecithin concentration in the amniotic fluid (Fig. 34-17).[110] A ratio of lecithin to sphingomyelin greater than 2 to 3.5, as determined by thin layer chromatography, confirms adequate pulmonary surfactant activity and virtually assures that the neonate will not develop respiratory distress syndrome. Surfactant activity, as an index of fetal lung maturity, can also be measured by using the amniotic fluid foam test.[111] The foam test is based on the ability of lecithin to stabilize foam produced by mechanical agitation of a solution of amniotic fluid and alcohol. Advantages of the foam test are its rapidity and simplicity.

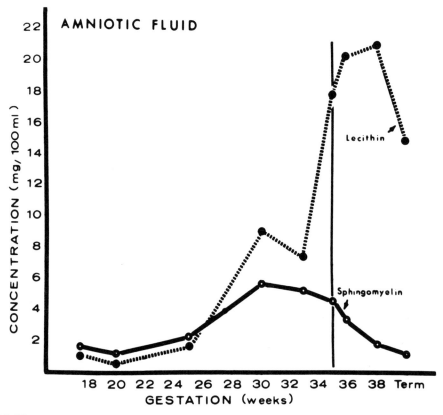

FIG. 34-17. Concentrations of lecithin and sphingomyelin in amniotic fluid increase as gestation progresses. An abrupt increase in concentrations of lecithin at about 35 weeks of gestation parallels fetal lung maturity. (Gluck L, Kulovich MV, Borer RC, et al. The diagnosis of the respiratory distress syndrome (RDS) by amniocentesis. Am J Obstet Gynecol 1971;109:440–5)

Ultrasonography

Fetal biparietal diameter, as measured by ultrasound, relates precisely to fetal age. Therefore, ultrasound is frequently used to confirm fetal maturity before elective cesarean section and to diagnose intrauterine growth retardation. Ultrasound is also useful in detecting hydramnios, hydrocephaly, anencephaly, and anomalies of the fetal spine.

EVALUATION OF THE NEONATE

The importance of assessment immediately after birth is to identify promptly depressed infants who require active resuscitation. As a guide to identifying and treating depressed neonates, the Apgar score has not been surpassed.

Apgar Score

The Apgar score assigns a numerical value to five vital signs measured or observed in neonates 1 minute and 5 minutes after delivery (Table 34-9). Of the five criteria, heart rate and the quality of the respiratory effort are the most important, and color the least informative, in identifying distressed newborns. Heart rates less than 100 beats·min^{-1} usually signify arterial hypoxemia. Disappearance of cyanosis is usually rapid when ventilation and circulation are normal. Nevertheless, many healthy infants still have cyanosis at 1 minute, due to peripheral vasoconstriction in response to cold ambient temperatures in delivery rooms. Acidosis and pulmonary vasoconstriction are the most likely causes of persistent cyanosis.

Apgar scores correlate well with acid-base measurements performed immediately after birth. When scores are above 7, neonates are either normal or have a mild respiratory acidosis. Infants with scores of 4 to 6 are moderately depressed; those with scores of 3 or below have combined metabolic and respiratory acidosis. Mild to moderately depressed infants (scores 3 to 7) frequently improve in response to oxygen administered by face mask, with or without positive pressure ventilation of the lungs. Intubation of the trachea and perhaps external cardiac massage are indicated when Apgar scores are less than 3. Apgar scores are not sufficiently sensitive to detect reliably drug-related changes or to provide data necessary to evaluate subtle effects of obstetric anesthetic techniques on neonates (see the section Neurobehavioral Testing).

Time-to-Sustained Respiration

The time interval between delivery and the establishment of sustained respiration has been used to identify depressed neonates. A time-to-sustained respiration greater than 90 seconds indicates a depressed neonate and correlates with Apgar scores of 6 or less. Routine determination of the time-to-sustained respiration is not recommended, since this time would be better used by ventilating the neonate's lungs with oxygen.

TABLE 34-9. Evaluation of Neonates Using the Apgar Score

Score	Heart Rate (beats·min^{-1})	Respiratory Effort	Reflex Irritability	Muscle Tone	Color
0	Absent	Absent	No response	Limp	Pale Cyanotic
1	<100	Slow Irregular	Grimace	Flexion of extremities	Body pink Extremities cyanotic
2	>100	Crying	Cry	Active	Pink

Neurobehavioral Testing

Neurobehavioral testing (early neonatal neurobehavioral scale) is able to detect subtle or delayed effects of drugs administered during labor and delivery, which are not appreciated by Apgar scores.[112,113] This testing evaluates the neonate's state of wakefulness, reflex responses, skeletal muscle tone, and responses to sound. Ability of neonates to decrease their responses to stimuli is known as habituation and probably represents the earliest example of processing of information by the cerebral cortex. Habituation has been shown to be impaired by anesthetic drugs administered as maternal systemic medication during labor and delivery. Data demonstrating that neonates born from mothers who received epidural anesthesia with lidocaine or mepivacaine had lower scores on tests of skeletal muscle strength and tone ("floppy") than did neonates born from mothers receiving epidural anesthesia with bupivacaine have not been reproducible.[112,113] Indeed, more recent data have failed to show any difference between these local anesthetics and lidocaine has regained acceptance as a local anesthetic for obstetric anesthesia.[113] Compared with subarachnoid blocks, the use of general anesthesia for elective cesarean sections resulted in infants who exhibited generalized depression of neurobehavioral testing, despite similar Apgar scores in both groups. Despite the documented decrease in neurobehavioral performance, there is no evidence of prolonged adverse effects on the infant.[113]

Alternatives to neurobehavioral testing to determine the impact of drugs administered to the mother during labor on the neonate are the use of the neurologic and adaptive capacity scores.[114] In contrast to neurobehavioral testing, this score places more emphasis on skeletal muscle tone, avoids the use of noxious stimuli, and provides a single numerical value that identifies depressed or vigorous neonates. It is recommended that the neurologic and adaptive capacity be performed initially in the delivery room approximately 15 minutes after birth and repeated 2 hours later. If abnormalities are present, the examination should be repeated at 24 hours.

IMMEDIATE NEONATAL PERIOD

Immediately after delivery, major changes in the neonatal cardiovascular system and respiratory system must occur. For example, with clamping of the umbilical cord at birth, systemic vascular resistance increases, left atrial pressure rises, and flow through the foramen ovale ceases. Expansion of the lungs reduces pulmonary vascular resistance, and the entire right ventricular output is diverted to the lungs. In normal newborns, increases in arterial oxygen partial pressures to above 60 mmHg causes vasoconstriction and functional closure of the ductus arteriosus. When adequate oxygenation and ventilation are not established after delivery, a fetal circulation pattern persists, characterized by increased pulmonary vascular resistance and decreased pulmonary blood flow. Furthermore, the ductus arteriosus and foramen ovale remain open, resulting in large right-to-left intracardiac shunts, with associated arterial hypoxemia and acidosis.

A high index of suspicion must be maintained for serious abnormalities, which can be present at birth or manifest shortly after delivery. These include meconium aspiration, choanal stenosis and atresia, diaphragmatic hernia, hypovolemia, hypoglycemia, tracheoesophageal fistula, laryngeal anomalies, and Pierre Robin syndrome. (see Chapter 35).

Meconium Aspiration

Meconium is the breakdown product of swallowed amniotic fluid, gastrointestinal cells, and secretions. It is seldom present before 34 weeks of gestation. After about 34 weeks, intrauterine arterial hypoxemia can result in increased gut motility and defecation. Gasping associated with arterial hypoxemia causes the fetus to inhale amniotic fluid and debris into the lungs. If delivery is delayed, meconium will be broken down and excreted from the lung. If birth occurs within 24 hours after aspiration, meconium will still be present in the major airways and will be distributed to the lung periphery with the onset of breathing. Obstruction of small airways causes mismatching of ventilation and perfusion. The respiratory rate may be over 100 breaths·min^{-1}, and lung compliance decreases to levels seen in infants with respiratory distress syndrome. In severe cases, pulmonary hypertension and right-to-left shunting through the patent foramen ovale and ductus arteriosus (persistent fetal circulation) lead to severe arterial hypoxemia. Pneumothorax is also a common problem in the presence of meconium aspiration.

Treatment of meconium aspiration is placement of a tube in the trachea immediately after delivery. Suction is applied to the tube by the attendant's mouth and the tube is removed. If meconium is present in the tube, the trachea is again intubated and suction once more applied. This procedure is repeated until the tube no longer contains meconium. Gentle ventilation of the lungs with oxygen may be necessary between tracheal intubations.

Choanal Stenosis and Atresia

Nasal obstruction should be suspected in any neonate who has good respiratory efforts but in whom air entry is absent. Cyanosis develops if these infants are forced to breathe with their mouths closed. Diagnosis of unilateral or bilateral choanal stenosis is made by failing to pass a small catheter through each naris; such failure may reflect congenital (anatomic) obstruction or more commonly functional atresia due to blood, mucus, or meconium. The congenital form of choanal atresia must be treated surgically in the neonatal period. An oral airway may be necessary until surgical correction can be accomplished. Functional choanal atresia is treated by nasal suctioning. Opioids such as heroin often cause congestion of the nasal mucosa and obstruction. Such congestion can be treated with phenylephrine nose drops.

Diaphragmatic Hernia

Severe respiratory distress at birth, associated with cyanosis and a scaphoid abdomen, suggests the diagnosis of diaphragmatic hernia (see Chapter 35). A persistent fetal circulation pattern is present, with right-to-left shunting at the ductus arteriosus. A radiograph of the chest reveals abdominal contents in the thorax. Initial treatment in the delivery room includes intubation of the trachea and ventilation of the lungs with oxygen. A pneumothorax on the side opposite the hernia is likely, if attempts are made to expand the ipsilateral lung.

Hypovolemia

Newborns with mean arterial pressures below 50 mmHg at birth are likely to be hypovolemic. Poor capillary refill, tachycardia, and tachypnea are present. Hypovolemia frequently follows intrauterine fetal distress, during which greater than normal portions of fetal blood are shunted to the placenta and remain there after delivery and clamping of the umbilical cord. Umbilical cord compression is also frequently associated with hypovolemia.

Hypoglycemia

Hypoglycemia can manifest as hypotension, tremors, and seizures. Infants with intrauterine growth retardation and those born from diabetic mothers or after severe intrauterine fetal distress, are vulnerable to hypoglycemia.

Tracheoesophageal Fistula

Tracheoesophageal fistula should always be suspected when polyhydramnios is present (see Chapter 35). An initial diagnosis in the delivery room is suggested when a catheter inserted into the esophagus cannot be passed into the stomach. Copious amounts of oropharyngeal secretions are usually present. A radiograph of the chest with the catheter in place will confirm the diagnosis.

Laryngeal Anomalies

Stridor is present at birth as a manifestation of both laryngeal anomalies and subglottic stenosis. Insertion of a tube into the trachea beyond the obstruction alleviates the symptoms. Vascular rings are anomalies of the aorta, which may compress the trachea, producing both inspiratory and expiratory obstruction (see Chapter 3). It may be difficult to advance a tracheal tube beyond the obstruction produced by a vascular ring.

Pierre Robin Syndrome

Pierre Robin syndrome is characterized by glossoptosis and micrognathia in all patients and the presence of cleft palate in over one-half of patients. Respiratory obstruction occurs when the tongue is sucked against the posterior pharyngeal wall by negative intrapharyngeal pressure. Initial treatment in the delivery room is establishment of a patent airway, either by inserting an oral airway or by pulling the tongue anterior with a clamp. The prone position also helps displace the tongue away from the posterior pharyngeal wall. A small tube passed through the naris into the posterior pharynx may be required to vent negative intraoral pressures. Under no circumstances should these infants be given muscle relaxants, as paralysis may make ventilation of the lungs impossible.

POSTPARTUM TUBAL LIGATION

Postpartum tubal ligation is the most common type of surgery performed in the early postpartum period.[115] The problem of the risk of aspiration and timing of surgery is resolved to a great extent if the surgery has been anticipated and continuous epidural analgesia or spinal block is used for delivery. Residual anesthesia from delivery is used to perform the intra-abdominal procedure, which necessitates a T5 level to assure patient comfort. When epidural or spinal blocks have not been used for delivery, it is common practice to wait 8 hours to 12 hours postpartum before inducing anesthesia for tubal ligation. This time interval is useful to allow the parturient to reach cardiovascular stability and increase the likelihood of gastric emptying. Nevertheless, there is no demonstrable difference in gastric fluid volume and pH when parturients are studied 1 hour to 8 hours after vaginal delivery.[115] If general anesthesia is selected, many recommend administration of antacids or H-2 antagonists before induction of anesthesia and subsequent placement of a cuffed tube in the trachea.

Spinal anesthesia provides a rapid onset of surgical anesthesia compared with epidural blocks and is also technically easier to accomplish. The incidence and severity of hypotension and occurrence of nausea and vomiting are less after postpartum tubal ligation than cesarean section, reflecting the decreased size of the uterus. Avoiding spinal block in preference for epidural block based on a concern that headache may follow the former is questionable considering the low incidence of this side effect when small gauge needles are used to puncture the dura and the likely occurrence of a severe headache if the dura is accidently punctured during performance of an epidural block with a large bore needle.[115]

REFERENCES

1. Morgan DJ, Blackman GL, Paull JD, Wolfe LJ. Pharmacokinetics and plasma binding of thiopental. II. Studies at cesarean section. Anesthesiology 1981;54:474–80
2. Ueland K, Hansen JM. Maternal cardiovascular dynamics. III. Labor and delivery under local and caudal analgesia. Am J Obstet Gynecol 1969;103:8–18
3. Eckstein K-L, Marx GF. Aortocaval compression

and uterine displacement. Anesthesiology 1974;40:92–6

4. Zilanti SM. Fetal heart rate and pH of fetal capillary blood during epidural analgesia in labor. Obstet Gynecol 1970;36:881–6

5. Fisher A, Prys-Roberts C. Maternal pulmonary gas exchange. A study during normal labor and extradural blockade. Anaesthesia 1968;23:350–6

6. Palahniuk RJ, Shnider SM, Eger II EI. Pregnancy decreases the requirement of inhaled anesthetic agents. Anesthesiology 1974;41:82–3

7. Gare DJ, Shime J, Paul WM, Hoskins M. Oxygen administration during labor. Am J Obstet Gynecol 1969;105:954–61

8. Ang CK, Tan TH, Walters WA, Wood C. Postural influence on maternal capillary oxygen and carbon dioxide tension. Br Med J 1969;4:201–3

9. Strout DD, Nahrwold ML. Halothane requirement during pregnancy and lactation in rats. Anesthesiology 1981;55:322–3

10. Bromage PR. Spread of analgesic solutions in the epidural space and their site of action: A statistical study. Br J Anaesth 1962;34:161–78

11. Fagraeus L, Urban BJ, Bromage PR. Spread of epidural analgesia in early pregnancy. Anesthesiology 1983;58:184–7

12. Datta S, Hurley RJ, Naulty JS, et al. Plasma and cerebrospinal fluid progesterone concentrations in pregnant and nonpregnant women. Anesth Analg 1986;65:950–4

13. Grundy EM, Zamora AM, Winnie AP. Comparison of spread of epidural anesthesia in pregnant and nonpregnant women. Anesth Analg 1979;57:544–6

14. Smith BE, Moya F, Shnider SM. The effects of anesthesia on liver function during labor. Anesth Analg 1962;41:24–31

15. Whittaker M. Plasma cholinesterase variants and the anaesthetist. Anaesthesia 1980;35:174–97

16. Blitt CD, Petty WC, Alberternst EE, Wright BJ. Correlation of plasma cholinesterase and duration of action of succinylcholine during pregnancy. Anesth Analg 1977;56:78–81

17. Weissman DB, Ehrenwerth J. Prlonged neuromuscular blockade in a parturient associated with succinylcholine. Anesth Analg 1983;62:444–6

18. Kaplan MM. Acute fatty liver of pregnancy. N Engl J Med 1985;313:367–70

19. Brock-Utne JB, Dow TGB, Dimopoulos GE, et al. Gastric and lower oesophageal sphincter (LOS) pressures in early pregnancy. Br J Anaesth 1981;53:381–4

20. Taylor G, Pryse-Davies J. The prophylactic use of antacids in the prevention of the acid-pulmonary aspiration syndrome (Mendelson's syndrome). Lancet 1966;1:288–91

21. Roberts RB, Shirley MA. Reducing the risk of acid aspiration during cesarean section. Anesth Analg 1974;53:859–68

22. Scott DB. Mendelson's syndrome (editorial). Br J Anaesth 1978;50:977–8

23. Hutchinson BR. Acid aspiration syndrome (correspondence). Br J Anaesth 1979;51:75

24. Gibbs CP, Schwartz MD, Wynne JW, et al. Antacid pulmonary aspiration in the dog. Anesthesiology 1979;51:380–5

25. Bond VK, Stoelting RK, Gupta CD. Pulmonary aspiration syndrome after inhalation of gastric fluid containing antacids. Anesthesiology 1979;51:452–3

26. Viegas OJ, Ravindran RS, Shumacker CA. Gastric fluid pH in patients receiving sodium citrate. Anesth Analg 1981;60:521–3

27. O'Sullivan GM, Bullingham RE. Noninvasive assignment by radiotelemetry of antacid effect during labor. Anesth Analg 1985;64:95–100

28. Howard FA, Sharp DS. Effect of metoclopramide on gastric emptying during labour. Br Med J 1973;1:446–8

29. Cohen SE, Jasson J, Talafre M-L, et al. Does metoclopramide decrease the volume of gastric contents in patients undergoing cesarean section? Anesthesiology 1984;61:604–7

30. Hodgkinson R, Glassenberg R, Joyce TH, et al. Comparison of cimetidine (Tagamet) with antacid for safety and effectiveness in reducing gastric acidity before elective cesarean section. Anesthesiology 1983;59:86–90

31. Parer JT, Behrman RE. The influence of uterine blood flow on the acid base status of the rhesus monkey. Am J Obstet Gynecol 1970;107:1241–9

32. Ralston DH, Shnider SM, deLorimier AA. Effects of equipotent ephedrine, metaraminol, mephentermine, and methoxamine on uterine blood flow on the pregnant ewe. Anesthesiology 1974;40:354–70

33. Shnider SM, Wright RG, Levinson G, et al. Uterine blood flow and plasma norepinephrine changes during maternal stress in the pregnant ewe. Anesthesiology 1979;50:524–7

34. Motoyama EK, Rward G, Acheson F, Cook CD. Adverse effect of maternal hyperventilation on the foetus. Lancet 1966;1:286–8

35. Levinson G, Shnider SM, deLorimier AA, Steffenson JL. Effects of maternal hyperventilation on uterine blood flow and fetal oxygenation and acid-base status. Anesthesiology 1974;40:340–7

36. Cosmi EV, Marx GF. The effect of anesthesia on

the acid-base status of the fetus. Anesthesiology 1969;30:238–42

37. Palahniuk RJ, Shnider SM. Maternal and fetal cardiovascular and acid-base changes during halothane and isoflurane anesthesia in the pregnant ewe. Anesthesiology 1974;41:462–72

38. Galloon S. Ketamine for obstetric delivery. Anesthesiology 1976;44:522–4

39. Wallis KL, Shnider SM, Hicks JS, Spivey HT. Epidural anesthesia in the normotensive pregnant ewe: Effects on uterine blood flow and fetal acid-base status. Anesthesiology 1976;44:481–7

40. Jouppila R, Jouppila P, Hollmen A, Kuikka J. Effect of segmental extradural analgesia on placental blood flow during normal labour. Br J Anaesth 1978;50:563–7

41. Tucker GT, Mather LE. Pharmacokinetics of local anesthetic agents. Br J Anaesth 1975;47:213–24

42. Biehl D, Shnider SM, Levinson G, Callender K. Placental transfer of lidocaine. Effects of fetal acidosis. Anesthesiology 1978;48:409–12

43. Brown WU, Bell GC, Lurie AO, et al. Newborn blood levels of lidocaine and mepivacaine in the first postnatal day following maternal epidural anesthesia. Anesthesiology 1975;42:698–707

44. Cree IE, Meyer J, Hailey DM. Diazepam in labour: Its metabolism and effect on the clinical condition and thermogenesis of the newborn. Br Med J 1973;4:251–5

45. Nathenson G, Cohen MI, McNamara H. The effect of sodium benzoate on serum bilirubin of the gunn rat. J Pediatr 1975;86:799–803

46. Way WL, Costley EC, Way EL. Respiratory sensitivity of the newborn infant to meperidine and morphine. Clin Pharmacol Ther 1965;6:454–61

47. Shnider SM, Moya F. Effects of meperidine on the newborn infant. Am J Obstet Gynecol 1964;89:1009–15

48. Ghoneim MM, Pandya H. Plasma protein binding of bupivacaine and its interaction with other drugs in man. Br J Anaesth 1974;46:435–8

49. Akamatsu TJ, Bonica JJ, Rhemet R, et al. Experiences with the use of ketamine for parturition. I. Primary anesthetic for vaginal delivery. Anesth Analg 1974;53:284–6

50. Friedman EA. Primigravid labor. A graphicostatistical analysis. Obstet Gynecol 1955;6:567–89

51. Friedman EA, Sachtleben MR. Caudal anesthesia. The factors that influence its effect on labor. Obstet Gynecol 1959;13:442–50

52. Johnson WL, Winter WW, Eng M, et al. Effect of pudendal, spinal, and peridural block anesthesia on the second stage of labor. Am J Obstet Gynecol 1972;113:166–75

53. Vasicka A, Kretchmer H. Effect of conduction and inhalation anesthesia on uterine contractions. Am J Obstet Gynecol 1961;82:600–11

54. Hoult IJ, MacLenna AH, Carrie LES. Lumbar epidural analgesia in labour: Relation to fetal malposition and instrumental delivery. Br Med J 1977;1:14–6

55. Coleman AJ, Downing JW. Enflurane anesthesia for cesarean section. Anesthesiology 1975;43:354–7

56. Paul RH, Freeman RK. Fetal cardiac response to paracervical block anesthesia. Am J Obstet Gynecol 1972;113:592–7

57. Baraka A, Noueihid R, Hajj S. Intrathecal injection of morphine for obstetric analgesia. Anesthesiology 1981;54:136–40

58. Hughes SC, Rosen MA, Shnider SM, et al. Maternal and neonatal effects of epidural morphine for labor and delivery. Anesth Analg 1984;63:319–24

59. Cohen SE, Tan S, Albright GA, Halpern J. Epidural fentanyl/bupivacaine mixtures for obstetric analgesia. Anesthesiology 1987;67:403–7

60. Sivakumaran C, Ramanthan S, Chalon J, Turndorf H. Uterine contractions and the spread of local anesthetics in the epidural space. Anesth Analg 1982;61:127–9

61. Ong BY, Cohen MM, Esmail A, et al. Paresthesias and motor dysfunction after labor and delivery. Anesth Analg 1987;66:18–22

62. Clark RB, Cooper JO, Brown WE, Greifenstein FE. The effect of methoxyflurane on the foetus. Br J Anaesth 1970;42:286–94

63. Creasser CW, Stoelting RK, Krishna G, Peterson C. Methoxyflurane metabolism and renal function after methoxyflurane analgesia during labor and delivery. Anesthesiology 1974;41:62–6

64. Clark RB, Beard AG, Thompson DS. Renal function in newborns and mothers exposed to methoxyflurane analgesia for labor and delivery. Anesthesiology 1979;51:464–7

65. Abbound TK, Shnider SM, Wright RG, et al. Enflurane analgesia in obstetrics. Anesth Analg 1981;60:133–7

66. Gellman E, Goldstein MS, Kaplan S, Shapiro WJ. Vaginal delivery after cesarean section. JAMA 1983;249:2935–7

67. Datta S, Alper MH. Anesthesia for cesarean section. Anesthesiology 1980;53:142–60

68. Kosaka Y, Takahashi T, Mark LC. Intravenous thiobarbiturate anesthesia for cesarean section. Anesthesiology 1969;31:489–506

69. Crawford JS. Awareness during operative ob-

stetrics under general anesthesia. Br J Anaesth 1971;43:179–82

70. Warren TM, Datta S, Ostheimer GW, et al. Comparison of the maternal and neonatal effects of halothane, enflurane, and isoflurane for cesarean delivery. Anesth Analg 1983;62:516–20

71. Baraka A, Haroun S, Bassili M. Response of the newborn to succinylcholine injection in homozygotic atypical mothers. Anesthesiology 1975;43:115–6

72. Crawford JS, James FM, Crawley M. A further study of general anaesthesia for cesarean section. Br J Anaesth 1976;48:661–7

73. Gutsche BB. Prophylactic ephedrine preceding spinal analgesia for cesarean section. Anesthesiology 1976;45:462–5

74. Abboud T, Raya J, Sadri S, et al. Fetal and maternal cardiovascular effects of atropine and glycopyrrolate. Anesth Analg 1983;62:426–30

75. Reisner LS, Hochman BN, Plumer MH. Persistent neurologic deficit and adhesive arachnoiditis following intrathecal 2-chloroprocaine injection. Anesth Analg 1980;59:452–4

76. Ravindran RS, Bond VK, Tasch MD, et al. Prolonged neural blockade following regional analgesia with 2-chloroprocaine. Anesth Analg 1980;59:447–51

77. Kuhnert BR, Harrison MJ, Lin PL, Kuhmert PM. Effects of maternal epidural anesthesia on neonatal behavior. Anesth Analg 1984;63:301–8

78. Rosen MA, Hughes SC, Shnider SM, et al. Epidural morphine for the relief of postoperative pain after cesarean delivery. Anesth Analg 1983;62:666–72

79. Crawford JS. An appraisal of lumbar epidural blockade in patients with singleton fetus presenting by the breech. Br J Obstet Gynaecol 1974;81:867–72

80. Spinnato JA, Kraynack BJ, Cooper MW. Eisenmenger's syndrome in pregnancy: Epidural anesthesia for elective cesarean section. N Engl J Med 1981;304:1215–6

81. Hilgenberg JC, McCammon RL, Stoelting RK. Pulmonary and systemic vascular responses to nitrous oxide in patients with mitral stenosis and pulmonary hypertension. Anesth Analg 1980;59:323–6

82. Robinson S. Pulmonary artery catheters in Eisenmenger's syndrome: Many risks, few benefits. Anesthesiology 1983;58:588–9

83. Schroeder JS, Harrison DC. Repeated cardioversion during pregnancy. Treatment of refractory paroxysmal tachycardia during three successive pregnancies. Am J Cardiol 1971;27:445–6

84. Wright JP. Anesthetic considerations in preeclampsia-eclampsia. Anesth Analg 1983;63:590–61

85. Kambam JR, Mouton S, Entman S, Sastry, Smith BE. Effect of pre-eclampsia on plasma cholinesterase activity. Can J Anaesth 1987;34:509–11

86. Green KW, Key TC, Coen R et al. The effects of maternally administered magnesium sulfate on the neonate. Am J Obstet Gynecol 1983;146:29–33

87. Ravindran RS, Carrelli A. Neurologic dysfunction of postpartum patients caused by hypomagnesemia. Anesthesiology 1987;66:391–2

88. Rigg D, McDonagh A. Use of sodium nitroprusside for deliberate hypotension during pregnancy. Br J Anaesth 1981;53:985–7

89. Jouppila P, Jouppila R, Hollmen A et al. Lumbar epidural analgesia to improve intervillous blood flow during labor in severe preeclampsia. Obstet Gynecol 1982;59:158–61

90. Heller PJ, Goodman C. Use of local anesthetics with epinephrine for epidural anesthesia in preeclampsia. Anesthesiology 1986;65:224–6

91. Snyder SW, Wheeler AS, James FM. The use of nitroglycerin to control severe hypertension of pregnancy during cesarean section. Anesthesiology 1979;51:563–4

92. Datta S, Brown WU, Ostheimer GW, et al. Epidural anesthesia for cesarean section in diabetic parturients: Maternal and neonatal acid-base status and bupivacaine concentration. Anesth Analg 1981;60:574–8

93. Datta S, Brown WU. Acid-base status in diabetic mothers and their infants following general or spinal anesthesia for cesarean section. Anesthesiology 1977;47:272–6

94. Rolbin SH, Levinson G, Shnider SM, Wright RG. Anesthetic considerations for myasthenia gravis and pregnancy. Anesth Analg 1978;57:441–7

95. Gatt SP. Anaesthetic management of the obstetric patient with antepartum or intrapartum haemorrhage. p. 233 In: Ostheimer GW (ed): Clinics in Anesthesiology. Vol. 4. WB Saunders Co., London, 1986

96. Carlsson C, Nybell-Lindahl G, Ingemarsson I. Extradural block in patients who had previously undergone caesarean section. Br J Anaesth 1980;52:827–30

97. Sperry K. Amniotic fluid embolism. To understand an enigma. JAMA 1986;255:2183–6

98. Schaerf RHM, deCampo T, Civetta JA. Hemodynamic alterations and rapid diagnosis in a case of amniotic fluid embolus. Anesthesiology 1977;46:155–7

99. Brodsky JB, Cohen EN, Brown BW, et al. Surgery during pregnancy and fetal outcome. Am J Obstet Gynecol 1980;138:1165–7

100. Pedersen H, Finster M. Anesthetic risk in the pregnant surgical patient. Anesthesiology 1979;51:439–51

101. Davis AG, Moir DD. Anaesthesia during pregnancy. p. 233 In: Ostheimer GW (ed): Clinics in Anesthesiology. Vol. 4 WB Saunders Co., London, 1986

102. Duncan PG, Pope WDB, Cohen MM, Greer N. Fetal risk of anesthesia and surgery during pregnancy. Anesthesiology 1986;64:790–4

103. Smith RF, Bowman RE, Katz J. Behavioral effects of exposure to halothane during early development in the rat. Sensitive period during pregnancy. Anesthesiology 1978;49:319–23

104. Committee on Drugs of the American Academy of Pediatrics and the Committee on Obstetrics (Maternal and Fetal Medicine) of the American College of Obstetricians and Gynecologists: Effect of medication during labor and delivery on infant outcome. Pediatrics 1978;62:402–3

105. Ravindran R, Viegas OJ, Padilla LM, LaBlonde P. Anesthetic considerations in pregnant patients receiving terbutaline therapy. Anesth Analg 1980;59:391–2

106. Moravec MA, Hurlbert BJ. Hypokalemia associated with terbutaline administration in obstetrical patients. Anesth Analg 1980;59:917–20

107. Finster M, Petrie RH. Monitoring of the fetus. Anesthesiology 1976;45:198–215

108. Sachs BP, Friedman EA. Antepartum and in-trapartum assessment of the fetus: Current status and does it influence outcome? p. 53 In: Ostheimer GW (ed): Clinics in Anesthesiology. Vol. 4 WB Saunders Co., London, 1986

109. Paul RH, Suidan AK, Yeh SY, et al. Clinical fetal monitoring. VII. The evaluation and significance of intrapartum baseline FHR variability. Am J Obstet Gynecol 1975;123:206–10

110. Gluck L, Kulovich MV, Barer RC, et al. The diagnosis of the respiratory distress syndrome (RDS) by amniocentesis. Am J Obstet Gynecol 1971;109:440–5

111. Clements JA, Platzker ACG, Tierney DF, et al. Assessment of the risk of the respiratory distress syndrome by a rapid test for surfactant in amniotic fluid. N Engl J Med 1972;286:1077–81

112. Scanlon JW, Brown WU, Weiss JB, Alper MH. Neurobehavioral responses of newborn infants after maternal epidural anesthesia. Anesthesiology 1974;40:121–8

113. Corke BC. Neonatal neurobehavior. II. Current clinical status. In: Ostheimer GW, ed. Clinics in Anaesthesiology. London. WB Saunders Co. 1986;4:219–27

114. Amiel-Tison C, Barrier G, Shnider SM, et al. A new neurologic and adaptive capacity scoring system for evaluating obstetric medications in full-term newborns. Anesthesiology 1982;56:340–50

115. Abouleish E. Anaesthesia for postpartum surgery. Clin Anaesthesiol 1986;4:419–28

35

Pediatric Patients

Traditionally, the risk of complications related to the administration of anesthesia has been considered to be higher for pediatric patients than adult patients. For example, studies published in the 1960s suggested that anesthetic-related mortality in children less than 15 years of age was several times greater than that observed for adults.[1,2] Often, anesthetic-related mortality occurred in otherwise healthy children. Nevertheless, it is now felt that pediatric patients are not inherently at a higher risk for anesthetic complications. Indeed, there are series consisting of large numbers of pediatric surgical cases with admirably low mortality rates. For example, in one series, the mortality rate attributed to anesthesia was 0.6 per 10,000 for 62,678 anesthetics.[3] In another report, anesthesia mortality was 0.2 per 10,000 for 50,000 anesthetics.[4]

Pediatric patients differ anatomically, physiologically, and pharmacologically from adult patients. An understanding of these differences and the availability of accurate monitoring devices permits safe administration of anesthesia to pediatric patients. It must be appreciated that neonates (up to 28 days of age) and infants (up to 14 months of age) are the age groups in which differences from adult patients are most marked.

ANATOMY OF THE AIRWAY

The large head and tongue, mobile epiglottis, and anterior position of the larynx characteristic of neonates makes intubation of the trachea easier with the head in a neutral or slightly flexed position than with the head hyperextended (Fig. 35-1).[5] Since the infant's larynx is higher in the neck than the adult's, the infant's tongue more easily obstructs the airway. The cricoid cartilage is the narrowest portion of the larynx in pediatric patients and necessitates selection of tracheal tubes that minimize the risk of trauma to the airway and the subsequent development of subglottic edema. For example, a 3.0 mm internal diameter tracheal tube is recommended for term neonates. As in adults, angulation of the right main stem bronchus favors a right endobronchial intubation if the tracheal tube is inserted too far.[6] To prevent endobronchial intubation of the neonate's trachea, a convenient guideline for depth of insertion from the lips is a distance of 7 cm for 1 kg neonates and an additional centimeter of depth for each kilogram increase in body weight, to a maximum depth of 10 cm for term neonates.[7] Ultimately, tracheal tube diameter and depth of insertion to

807

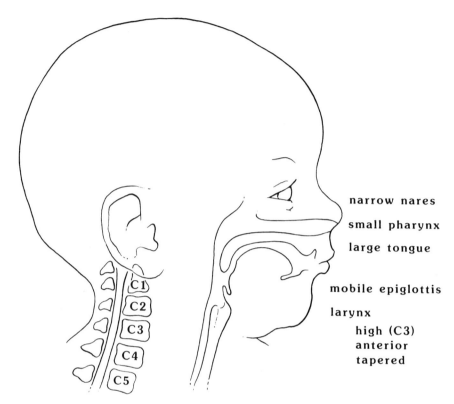

narrow nares

small pharynx

large tongue

mobile epiglottis

larynx

   high (C3)

   anterior

   tapered

FIG. 35-1. Schematic depiction of the anatomic characteristics of the neonate, which may influence the ease of intubation of the trachea during direct laryngoscopy.

TABLE 35-1. Endotracheal Tube Size

Weight or Age	Internal Diameter* (mm)	Distance of Tube Insertion from Lips to Result in a Midtrachea Position (cm)
1 kg	2.5 uncuffed	7
1.5 kg	3.0 uncuffed	7.5
2 kg	3.0 uncuffed	8
3 kg (preterm)	3.0 uncuffed	9
3 kg (term)	3.0 uncuffed	10
6–12 months	3.5 uncuffed	11
12–18 months	3.5 uncuffed	12
18–36 months	4.0 uncuffed	13
3–5 years	4.5 uncuffed	14
5–6 years	5.0 cuffed	15
6–8 years	5.5 cuffed	16
8–10 years	6.0 cuffed	18
10–12 years	6.5 cuffed	18

* Endotracheal tube size should result in a fit in the trachea that allows an audible air leak when positive airway pressure equivalent to 25 cmH_2O is applied.

result in a midtrachea position of the distal end of the tube are based on age (Table 35-1).

PHYSIOLOGY

Physiologic differences between pediatric and adult patients are an important determinant in the development of working concepts when administering anesthesia to children. The dynamic physiology of neonates necessitates an understanding of the potential effects of anesthesia on homeostatic mechanisms present in this age group.

RESPIRATORY SYSTEM

Respiratory immaturity of preterm neonates is well known. Development of the fetal lung begins during the fourth week of gestation.[8] By 16 weeks, conducting airways are formed, although further differentiation subsequently occurs. From the 24th week until term, the terminal air sacs are formed. At term, neonates have a primitive alveolar structure. Indeed, alveolar maturation is not complete until 8 years to 10 years of age. Of paramount important to normal lung function is the production and secretion of surfactant. Adequate respiratory function after birth is critically dependent on adequate amounts of surfactant in the lungs. Surfactant is a complex of surface active phospholipids produced exclusively by type II pneumocytes. Although type II pneumocytes begin to differentiate at 24 weeks gestation, a marked synthesis of surfactant does not begin until 34 weeks to 36 weeks of gestation. Surfactant serves as both an antiatelectasis factor and as a waterproofing agent for alveolar membranes.

The single most important difference that physiologically separates pediatric from the adult patients is oxygen consumption. Oxygen consumption of neonates is greater than 6 ml·kg^{-1}·min^{-1}, which is about twice that of adults on a weight basis (Table 35-2). To satisfy this increased demand, minute alveolar ventilation is doubled compared to adults. Carbon dioxide production is also increased in neonates, but elevated alveolar ventilation results in maintenance of near normal arterial partial pressures of carbon dioxide. Since tidal volume on a weight basis is the same for both infants and adults, increased alveolar ventilation is achieved by increasing the respiratory rate. Indeed, the relatively large abdomen, weak intercostal muscles, and horizontal rib placement characteristic of infants make it more efficient to increase respiratory rate rather than tidal volume. The shape of the rib cage and angle of insertion of the diaphragm make contraction of this muscle less efficient in neonates. Finally, the diaphragm of neonates is composed of a decreased number of high oxidative muscle fibers capable of sustained work. As a result, the diaphragm of neonates is prone to fatigue with resultant apnea.[9] Arterial partial pressures of oxygen increase rapidly after birth, but several days are required to achieve levels comparable to older children. Initially low arterial partial pressures of oxygen are secondary to a decreased functional residual capacity and perfusion of fluid-filled alveoli. Although methods of measuring functional residual capacity in newborns are not always reproducible, most evidence demonstrates a rapid increase in this lung capacity after birth. For example, functional residual capacity at 10 minutes of age is 17 ml·kg^{-1}, and by 30 minutes is 25 ml·kg^{-1} to 30 ml·kg^{-1}. Functional residual capacity reaches adult levels (about 30 ml·kg^{-1}) by 4 days of age (Table 35-2).

Control of ventilation requires complex interactions of central ventilatory centers, peripheral chemoreceptors, and peripheral skeletal muscle sensors. It is well known that control of ventilation is immature in neonates. The response of older children and adults to hypoxemia and hypercarbia is sustained hyperventilation. Both preterm and term neonates, when challenged with hypoxic inspired gas mixtures, have an initial 1 minute to 2 minute period of hyperventilation, followed by sustained hypoventilation. As age increases, hyperventilation becomes sustained, but this response develops more slowly in preterm than term neonates. Hypercarbia, a potent stimulus to ventilation in children and adults, is not as potent a stimulus to neonates and may

TABLE 35-2. Mean Pulmonary Function Values

	Neonate (3 kg)	Adult (70 kg)
Oxygen consumption (ml·kg^{-1}·min^{-1})	6.4	3.5
Alveolar ventilation (ml·kg^{-1}·min^{-1})	130	60
Carbon dioxide production (ml·kg^{-1}·min^{-1})	6	3
Tidal volume (ml·kg^{-1})	6	6
Respiratory rate (breaths·min^{-1})	35	15
Vital capacity (ml·kg^{-1})	35	70
Functional residual capacity (ml·kg^{-1})	30	35
Tracheal length (cm)	5.5	12
PaO$_2$ (F$_I$O$_2$ .21, mmHg)	65–85	85–95
PaCO$_2$ (mmHg)	30–36	36–44
pH	7.34–7.40	7.36–7.44

be a respiratory depressant to preterm neonates.[10] Conceivably, the combination of ventilatory depression from residual anesthetic drugs plus immature control of ventilation of neonates could result in hypoventilation during the postoperative period.

Cardiovascular System

Birth and the beginning of spontaneous ventilation initiate circulatory changes, which permit neonates to survive in an extrauterine environment.[11] Fetal circulation is characterized by high pulmonary vascular resistance, low systemic vascular resistance (placenta), and right-to-left shunting of blood via the foramen ovale and ductus arteriosus. Onset of spontaneous ventilation at birth is associated with decreases in the pulmonary vascular resistance and increases in pulmonary blood flow. As left atrial blood flow and pressures increase, the foramen ovale functionally closes. Anatomic closure of the foramen ovale occurs between 3 months and 1 year of age, although 20 percent to 30 percent of adults have probe patent foramen ovales.[12] Functional closure of the ductus arteriosus normally occurs 10 hours to 15 hours after birth, with anatomic closure taking place in 4 weeks to 6 weeks. Constriction of the ductus arteriosus occurs in response to increased arterial partial pressures of oxygen that develop after birth. Nevertheless, the ductus arteriosus may reopen during periods of arterial hypoxemia. In addition, certain conditions, such as diaphragmatic hernia,

meconium aspiration, pulmonary infection, and polycythemia, are associated with high pulmonary vascular resistance and persistence of fetal circulatory patterns.[13] Presumably, high pulmonary vascular resistance results in shunting of desaturated pulmonary arterial blood into the systemic circulation through the ductus arteriosus. The diagnosis of persistent fetal circulation can be confirmed by measurement of the arterial partial pressures of oxygen in blood obtained simultaneously from preductal (right radial) and postductal (umbilical, posterior tibial, dorsalis pedis) arteries (Fig. 35-2). A difference of greater than 20 mmHg verifies the diagnosis.[13]

Cardiovascular responses of neonates differ from those of adults. For example, cardiac muscle in neonates is less compliant. Decreased cardiac compliance is secondary to increased amounts of noncontractile tissue in fetal myocardium. On a weight basis 30 percent of neonatal cardiac tissue is contractile, as opposed to 60 percent in adults. As a result, for a given myocardial fiber length, neonatal cardiac muscle develops less isometric tension. The compliance difference is reflected in comparison of pressure-volume relations of fetal, neonatal, and adult hearts. The respective right and left ventricular compliance curves form a spectrum from fetal life to adult life. In the fetus, pressure-volume and wall tension-radius relationships are comparable for both the left and right ventricles. Soon after birth the neonatal ventricle develops a pressure-volume relationship intermediate between the fetus and adult. It has also been observed that filling one ventricle reduces distensibly of the opposite ventricle. Lack of distensibility of the left ven-

FIG. 35-2. Schematic depiction of sites for sampling of arterial blood relative to the ductus arteriosus.

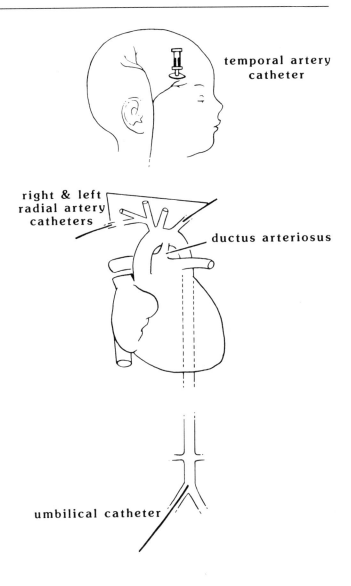

temporal artery catheter

right & left radial artery catheters

ductus arteriosus

umbilical catheter

tricle limits diastolic filling and limits the significance of increasing the stroke volume as a means of increasing cardiac output. Nevertheless, neonatal hearts are capable of increasing contractility and significant improvements in cardiac function do occur during the first year of life.[14,15] Reductions in heart rate significantly decrease the neonate's cardiac output. It must also be remembered that blood pressure in neonates varies significantly with gestational age and weight (Table 35-3).

The developing myocardium has immature sympathetic nervous system innervation and consequently may manifest altered responses to vasoactive drugs. For example, when compared to adult myocardium, neonatal cardiac muscle is more sensitive to norepinephrine, but equally sensitive to isoproterenol. Dopamine depends in part upon release of endogenous norepinephrine to produce its inotropic effects. The neonatal myocardium, deficient in sympathetic nervous system innervation, is less responsive to dopamine.[16] Vasoconstrictive responses of neonates to hemorrhage are less than that of adults. For example, 10 percent reductions in

TABLE 35-3. Mean Circulatory Values for the Neonate

	Weight (kg)				
	0.75	1	2	3	>3
Systolic blood pressure (mmHg)	44	49	54	62	66
Mean arterial pressure (mmHg)	33	34	41	46	50
Heart rate (beats·min^{-1})				120	
Cardiac index (L/min^{-1}·m^{-2})				4.1	

intravascular fluid volume cause 15 percent to 30 percent decreases in mean arterial blood pressure in neonates.[17] Decreased vasoconstrictive responses may reflect immaturity of alpha-adrenergic receptors and reduced sensitivity of baroreceptor reflexes. Indeed, responses to direct-acting vasopressors are less in neonates than adults.[18] Furthermore, baroreceptor responses are attenuated by halothane to greater degrees in young animals than in their adult counterparts.[19] This latter finding, if applicable to humans, emphasizes that neonates could have limited ability to compensate for hypotension and decreased cardiac output when anesthetized because cardiac output in infants is, to a large extent, heart rate-dependent. Animals studies have also shown that halothane, isoflurane, and enflurane are more depressant to neonatal than adult hearts.[20] In older children (ages 2 years to 7 years), isoflurane produces less myocardial depression than halothane.[21]

Hypotension that accompanies administration of volatile anesthetics to premature neonates is more likely due to decreased intravascular fluid volume and/or anesthetic overdose than immaturity of the autonomic nervous system.[22] For example, systolic blood pressure decreases similar amounts in premature neonates, full-term neonates, and infants up to 6 months of age when equivalent MAC doses of volatile anesthetics are administered (see the section Anesthetic Requirements). In premature neonates intravascular fluid volume may be reduced owing to fluid restriction and diuretic-induced diuresis in attempts to reduce excess lung water.

Distribution of Body Water

Total body water content and extracellular fluid volume are proportionally increased in neonates. Extracellular fluid volume is equivalent to about 40 percent of the body weight of neonates compared to about 20 percent in adults. By 18 months to 24 months of age, the proportion of extracellular fluid volume relative to body weight is similar to adults.

Increased metabolic rate characteristic of neonates results in accelerated turnover of extracellular fluid and dictates meticulous attention to intraoperative fluid replacement. Intraoperative fluid replacement may be considered as maintenance fluids and replacement fluids (Table 35-4). Recommended fluids often contain glucose although the clinical impression that pediatric patients are more prone than adults to hypoglycemia during fasting has been challenged.[23,24] Maintenance fluids are best correlated with metabolic rate: replacement fluid requirements should be based on the underlying pathologic process, extent of surgery, and anticipated fluid translocation. Third space translocation of fluids is similar for neonates and adults. Maintenance fluid requirements for the first 24 hours of life are approximately 75 ml·kg^{-1} to 80 ml·kg^{-1}. Preterm neonates have greater fluid requirements in the first 24 hours equivalent to 100 ml·kg^{-1}. Insensible fluid losses vary greatly. Fever, radiant warmers, phototherapy, increased ambient temperature, and decreased humidity all increase insensible fluid losses. Small neo-

TABLE 35-4. Intraoperative Fluid Therapy for Infants

	5% Dextrose in Lactated Ringer's Solution (ml·kg^{-1}·hr^{-1})		
	Maintenance	Replacement	Total
Minor surgery (herniorrhaphy)	4	2	6
Moderate surgery (pyloromyotomy)	4	4	8
Extensive surgery (bowel resection)	4	6	10

nates require more radiant energy to maintain a neutral thermal environment, such that there is a greater insensible fluid loss in these patients.

Renal Function

Nephrogenesis is generally complete by 36 weeks of gestation. There are several aspects of renal function not fully developed in neonates that are particularly important to management of anesthesia. For example, glomerular filtration rate of term neonates is approximately 20 ml·min^{-1}·1.7 m^{-2} at birth (Table 35-5).[25] By 3 weeks to 5 weeks of age, glomerular filtration rate is increased threefold. Preterm neonates show delayed increases in glomerular filtration rate. The ability of developing kidneys to control sodium balance is also decreased. In addition, distal renal tubules of neonates are relatively unresponsive to aldosterone, which further impairs control of sodium reabsorption. Clinical consequences of these findings are that neonates are less able to compensate for extremes of fluid balance. At one end of the spectrum, neonates are obligate sodium losers and cannot concentrate urine as effectively as adults. Therefore, adequate exogenous sodium and water must be supplied during the perioperative period. Conversely, it must also be appreciated that neonates excrete volume loads more slowly than adults and, therefore, are more susceptible to fluid overload. Decreased renal function can also delay excretion of drugs dependent upon renal clearance for elimination.

TABLE 35-5. Mean Glomerular Filtration Rate (GFR)

Age	GFR (ml·min^{-1}·1.7 m^{-2})
Preterm neonate	16
Term neonate	20
3–5 weeks	60
1 year	80
Adult	120

Hematology

Certain features of fetal hemoglobin influence oxygen transport. For example, fetal hemoglobin has a P$_{50}$ of 19 mmHg, compared to 26 mmHg for adult hemoglobin. The decreased P$_{50}$ for fetal hemoglobin causes a shift of the oxyhemoglobin dissociation curve to the left. The resulting increased affinity of hemoglobin for oxygen manifests as decreased release of oxygen to peripheral tissues. This decreased release of oxygen to tissues is offset by increased oxygen delivery provided by elevated hemoglobin concentrations characteristic of neonates (Table 35-6). By 2 months to 3 months of age, however, physiologic anemia occurs. After 3 months, there are progressive increases in erythrocyte mass and hematocrit. By 4 months to 6 months, oxyhemoglobin dissociation curves approximate those of adults.

Shifts to the left of the oxyhemoglobin dissociation curve, plus decreased cardiovascular reserves of neonates, are the reasons that hematocrits of neonates should be maintained near 40 percent, rather than the 30 percent acceptable for older children. Calculation of estimated erythrocyte mass and acceptable erythrocyte loss provides a useful guide for intraoperative blood replacement (Table 35-7).[26]

Coagulation tests, with the exception of bleeding time, are usually abnormal in neonates. Concentrations of vitamin K dependent factors (II, VII, IX, X) are decreased, leading to prolonged prothrombin times. Partial thromboplastin times are also prolonged. Fibrinogen and factor V concentrations are the same as for adults. Despite these laboratory abnormalities, blood of term neonates coagulates normally or at increased rates because of deficiencies of naturally occurring anticoagulants.[27] Acutely ill neonates, however, may have a bleeding diathesis, on the basis of thrombocytopenia or vitamin K-dependent factor deficiencies.

Colloid osmotic pressure is a readily measured parameter obtainable for neonates. This pressure in healthy neonates is lower than that of adults (16 mmHg to 19 mmHg for neonates

TABLE 35-6. Normal Hemogram Values

Age	Hemoglobin (g·dl⁻¹)	Hematocrit (%)	Leukocytes (mm³)
1 day	19.0	61	18,000
2 weeks	17.3	54	12,000
1 month	14.2	43	
2 months	10.7	31	
6 months	12.3	36	10,000
1 year	11.6	35	
6 years	12.7	38	
10–12 years	13.0	39	8,000

TABLE 35-7. Estimation of Acceptable Erythrocyte Loss

A 3.2 kg term infant is scheduled for intra-abdominal surgery. The preoperative hematocrit is 50 percent. What is the acceptable intraoperative blood loss to maintain the hematocrit at 40 percent?

Calculations*

Estimated blood volume	85 ml·kg⁻¹ × 3.2 kg = 272 ml
Estimated erythrocyte mass	272 ml × 0.5 = 136 ml
Estimated erythrocyte mass to maintain hematocrit at 40%	272 ml × 0.4 = 109 ml
Acceptable intraoperative erythrocyte loss	136 ml − 109 ml = 27 ml
Acceptable intraoperative blood loss to maintain hematocrit at 40%	27 × 2† = 54 ml

* These calculations are only a guideline. They do not consider the potential impact of intravenous infusion of crystalloid or colloid solutions on the hematocrit.
† Factor to correct for original hematocrit of 50%.

and 25 mmHg for adults) and increases with increasing birth weight and gestational age.[28,29]

Thermoregulation

Neonates and infants are particularly vulnerable to hypothermia during the perioperative period. This age group loses body heat more rapidly than older children or adults because of its large body surface area relative to body weight, thin layer of insulating subcutaneous fat, and decreased ability to produce heat. Shivering is of little significance for heat production in neonates, whose primary mechanism is nonshivering thermogenesis mediated by brown fat. Brown fat is specialized adipose tissue located in the posterior neck, interscapular and vertebral areas, and surrounding the kidneys and adrenal glands. Metabolism in brown fat is stimulated by norepinephrine and results in triglyceride hydrolysis and thermogenesis.

An important mechanism for loss of body heat in the operating room is radiation. To minimize oxygen consumption, neonates must be in a neutral thermal environment. Neutral temperature is defined as the ambient temperature that results in the least oxygen consumption (Table 35-8). Critical temperature is that ambient temperature below which an unclothed, unanesthetized individual cannot maintain a normal core body temperature (Table 35-8). Most operating rooms are below the critical temperature of even term neonates, and it is imperative that heat loss be minimized. Steps that can decrease loss of body heat include transporting neonates in heated modules, increasing ambient temperature of operating rooms, humidifying and warming inspired

TABLE 35-8. Neutral and Critical Temperatures

	Neutral Temperature (Celsius)	Critical Temperature (Celsius)
Preterm neonate	34	28
Term neonate	32	23
Adult	28	1

gases, using warm solutions to cleanse the skin, warming infused blood and intravenous solutions, and using heating mattresses and radiant warmers. Use of plastic drapes during transport of neonates and during surgery will also significantly reduce heat loss.

PHARMACOLOGY

Pharmacologic responses produced by drugs may differ in pediatric patients compared to adult patients. Specifically, there may be differences in anesthetic requirements, responses to muscle relaxants, and altered pharmacokinetics of drugs.

Anesthetic Requirements

Fetal animals demonstrate reduced anesthetic requirements. Human fullterm neonates require lower concentrations of volatile anesthetics than infants 1 month to 6 months of age. For example, minimum alveolar concentration (MAC) has been shown to be about 25 percent less in neonates as compared to infants (Fig. 35-3).[30,31] Furthermore, MAC in preterm neonates less than 32 weeks gestational age is less than MAC in preterm neonates 32 weeks to 37 weeks gestational age and both of these age groups are less than MAC in full-term neonates.[32] Low anesthetic requirements of newborns may be related to immaturity of the central nervous system and elevated levels of progesterone and beta endorphins.[30] MAC steadily increases until 2 months to 3 months of age. After 3 months of age MAC steadily declines with aging, although there are slight increases at the time of puberty.

Uptake of inhaled anesthetics is more rapid in infants than older children or adults (Fig. 35-4).[33–35] Infants have a high alveolar ventilation relative to functional residual capacity which may explain this accelerated uptake. Volatile anesthetics are potent negative inotropes when administered to neonates (see the section Cardiovascular System). Indeed,

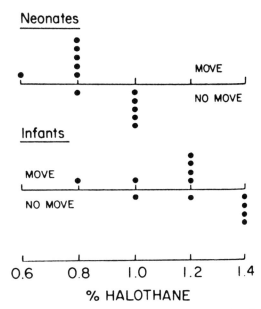

FIG. 35-3. Solid circles represent individual end-tidal halothane concentrations immediately before skin incision, and position of the symbol above (move) or below (no move) the horizontal line depicts patients' responses to skin incision. Anesthetic requirements to prevent movement in response to a painful stimulus (i.e., MAC) are less in neonates (less than 1 month of age, 0.87 percent) than infants (1 month to 6 months of age, 1.20 percent). (Lerman J, Robinson S, Willis MM, Gregory GA. Anesthetic requirements for halothane in young children 0–1 month and 1–6 months of age. Anesthesiology 1983;59:421–4)

neonates and infants are more likely to develop hypotension during the administration of volatile anesthetics.[36,37] Considering these factors, a reduced margin of safety when volatile anesthetics are administered to infants is predictable.

Barbiturates and Opioids

An immature blood-brain barrier and decreased ability to metabolize drugs could increase the sensitivity of neonates to effects of barbiturates and opioids. As a result, neonates might require lower doses of barbiturates for

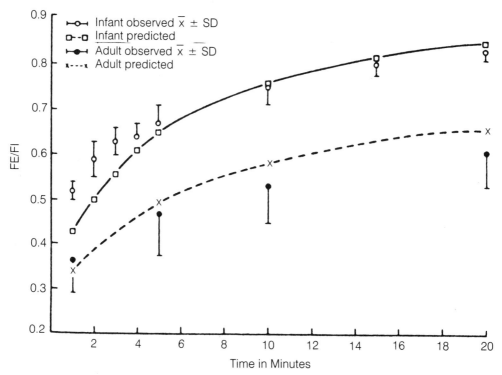

FIG. 35-4. The predicted and observed rates at which end-tidal halothane concentrations approach the inspired (FE/FI) is more rapid in infants than in adults. (Brandon DW, Brandom RB, Cook DR. Uptake and distribution of halothane in infants: In vivo measurements and computer simulations. Anesth Analg 1983;62:404–10. Reprinted with permission from IARS)

induction of anesthesia. Nevertheless, children between the ages of 5 years and 15 years require somewhat higher doses of thiopental (6 mg·kg^{-1}) and methohexital (2 mg·kg^{-1}) than adults for induction of anesthesia (Fig. 35-5).[38]

Opioids such as fentanyl and sufentanil are being used with increasing frequency for pediatric anesthesia. Fentanyl (50 μg·kg^{-1} to 75 μg·kg^{-1}) and sufentanil (5 μg·kg^{-1} to 10 μg·kg^{-1}) produce minimal hemodynamic changes even in preterm infants.[39,40] In contrast to the negative hemodynamic effects of halothane, fentanyl (50 μg·kg^{-1}) produces few hemodynamic changes in newborn piglets.[41] The efficacy of fentanyal and sufentanil is particularly apparent for infants undergoing cardiac surgery, although substantial respiratory depression occurs and postoperative ventilatory support may be required.

Nondepolarizing Muscle Relaxants

It is known that morphologic and functional maturation of the neuromuscular junction is not complete until about 2 months of age.[42] The implications of this immaturity on the pharmacodynamics or muscle relaxants is not clear. Neuromuscular transmission in preterm infants is even less mature than in term neonates. Responses of pediatric patients, especially neonates and infants, to nondepolarizing muscle relaxants has been the subject of conflicting reports. Early studies suggested that neonates require lower doses of muscle relaxants than adults when these drugs are administered according to body weight. Clinical experience seemed to support this concept. Nevertheless, data from the mid-1970s sug-

FIG. 35-5. Dose response curves for loss of various reflex responses 60 seconds after intravenous administration of thiopental to unpremedicated patients 5 years to 15 years of age. (Cote CJ, Goudsouzian NG, Liu LMP, et al. The dose response of intravenous thiopental for the induction of general anesthesia in unpremedicated children. Anesthesiology 1981;55:703–5)

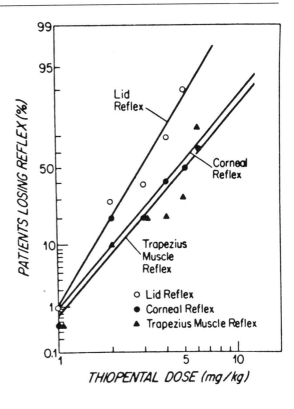

gested that pediatric dose requirements for d-tubocurarine are similar over a wide range of ages (Table 35-9).[43] In patients ranging from newborn to 10 days of age, however, there is wide individual variability of dose requirements for d-tubocurarine, which could account for differing clinical impressions as to the responses evoked by this drug. To further complicate this issue, there is convincing data demonstrating that infants are more sensitive to d-tubocurarine.[44] Because of the relatively large volume of distribution, however, initial doses of d-tubocurarine calculated on a body weight basis for infants are not different from adults (Fig. 35-6).[44] Because of this increased sensitivity and reduced elimination of d-tubocurarine subsequent doses must be reduced. As with d-tubocurarine, initial doses of metocurine and pancuronium necessary to produce 95 percent depression of twitch response are similar in pediatric and adult patients.[45] In many cases pancuronium is useful for infants because heart rate is maintained or increased by this drug.

Atracurium and vecuronium are both well suited for use in infants and children as well

TABLE 35-9. Age and Response to d-Tubocurarine

Age	Mean Dose and Range to Depress Twitch 95% (mg·kg⁻¹)	Mean Time for Recovery from 25 to 50% of Control Twitch Height (minutes)
Newborn–10 days	0.34 (0.15–0.62)	15.2
11–60 days	0.34 (0.25–0.47)	16.4
2–12 months	0.29 (0.25–0.32)	13.1
1–7 years	0.32 (0.26–0.38)	16.0

(Data from Goudsouzian NG, Donlon JV, Savarese JJ, Ryan JF. Re-evaluation of dosage and duration of action of d-tubocurarine in the pediatric age group. Anesthesiology 1975;43:416–25)

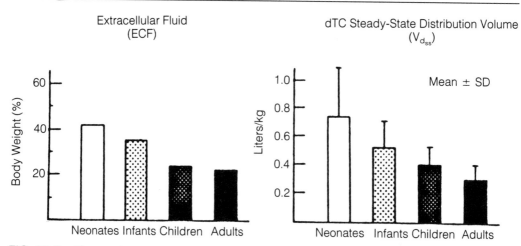

FIG. 35-6. The steady state distribution volume (Vdss) for d-tubocurarine (dTC) parallels extracellular fluid volume in neonates (0–2 months), infants (2 months–12 months), children (1 year–12 years) and adults (12 years–30 years). This increased dilutional volume in neonates and infants masks an increased sensitivity of these age groups to dTC. (Fisher DM, O'Keefe C, Stanski DR, et al. Pharmacokinetics and pharmacodynamics of d-tubocurarine in infants, children and adults. Anesthesiology 1982;57:203–8)

as adults. As is true for d-tubocurarine, infants are more sensitive to atracurium but because of the relatively larger volume of distribution initial doses calculated on a body weight basis are not different from adult doses.[46] Interestingly, recovery time from atracurium is more rapid in infants as compared to adults. Atracurium has little effect on blood pressure or heart rate and this drug is also suitable for administration by continuous infusion in children.[47] Vecuronium can be used in doses similar to adult doses but recovery from neuromuscular blockade may be delayed in infants when compared to older children and adults.[48] This delayed recovery may be a result of reduced liver metabolism caused by immaturity of hepatic enzyme systems.

On the basis of clinical impression, it has been suggested that infants require larger doses of neostigmine than adults for antagonism of neuromuscular blockade. It has been shown, however, that infants actually require less neostigmine for reversal of d-tubocurarine-induced neuromuscular blockade (Fig. 35-7).[49]

Succinylcholine

Neonates and infants require more succinylcholine on a body weight basis than older children to produce neuromuscular blockade (Table 35-10).[50] This reflects the increased ex-

TABLE 35-10. Age and Response to Succinylcholine

Age	Mean Depression of Twitch Response Following Intravenous Administration of Succinylcholine (%)		Time to 90% Recovery of Twitch Response (minutes)	
	0.5 mg·kg^{-1}	1 mg·kg^{-1}	0.5 mg·kg^{-1}	1.0 mg·kg^{-1}
1–10 weeks	69	85	2.3	4.0
5–7 years	84	100	3.0	4.8

(Data from Cook DR, Fischer CG. Neuromuscular blocking effects of succinylcholine in infants and children. Anesthesiology 1975;42:662–5)

FIG. 35-7. Dose-response curves demonstrate that infants and children require less neostigmine than adults to antagonize nondepolarizing neuromuscular blockade produced by d-tubocurarine. (Fisher DM, Cronnelly R, Miller RD, Sharma M. The neuromuscular pharmacology of neostigmine in infants and children. Anesthesiology 1983;59:220–5)

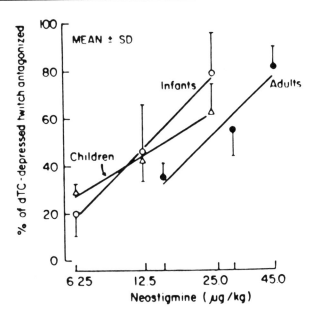

tracellular fluid volume characteristic of these patients. Consequently, there is a greater volume of distribution for succinylcholine. As a result, pediatric patients require 2 mg·kg^{-1} of succinylcholine administered intravenously to provide conditions for intubation of the trachea, that are similar to those produced with 1 mg·kg^{-1} administered to adults. Intramuscular administration of succinylcholine may be required when intravenous routes are not available. Intramuscular administration of succinylcholine 4 mg·kg^{-1} produces satisfactory conditions for intubation of the trachea in most children within 3 minutes to 4 minutes.[51] Intralingual succinylcholine, 1 mg·kg^{-1}, has a more rapid onset of action than intramuscular administration. Potential risks of an intralingual hematoma and cardiac dysrhythmias, however, detract from use of this route.

Effects of succinylcholine at sites other than the neuromuscular junction need to be considered. Succinylcholine often produces an initial bradycardia, followed by tachycardia. Rarely, transient cardiac asystole may occur. Pretreatment with atropine administered intravenously will block or significantly attenuate succinylcholine-induced heart rate slowing.[52] Succinylcholine produces only small changes in intragastric pressure in children.[53] Therefore, pretreatment with nondepolarizing mus-

cle relaxants to prevent initial contraction of abdominal muscles in response to succinylcholine is not necessary as prophylaxis against regurgitation. Nevertheless, use of cricoid pressure during rapid sequence inductions of anesthesia is recommended to prevent passive regurgitation. Other undesirable effects of succinylcholine include an increased incidence of myoglobinemia in children and an increase in intraocular pressure. Succinylcholine should also be avoided in children with recent thermal injury and spinal cord transection. The development of pulmonary edema after the intramuscular injection of succinylcholine has been described.[54] Availability of intermediate-acting muscle relaxants, such as atracurium and vecuronium, may eliminate the need for succinylcholine in many pediatric patients.

PHARMACOKINETICS

Pharmacokinetics differ in neonates and infants as compared to adults. Diminished hepatic and renal clearance of drugs which is characteristic of neonates, can produce prolonged drug effects. For many drugs, including theophylline, phenytoin, phenobarbital, and diazepam, clearance during the neonatal period is decreased. Clearance rates increase to adult levels by 5 to 6 months of age, and during later childhood may even exceed adult rates. Protein binding of many drugs is decreased in infants which can result in higher plasma levels of unbound and active drug, leading to increased pharmacologic effects.

MONITORING DURING THE PERIOPERATIVE PERIOD

As in adults, monitoring of pediatric patients is directed toward early detection of unacceptable deviations from accepted norms. Since neonates and infants have decreased physiologic reserves, early detection of adverse effects of anesthesia and surgery assumes a major role. On the other hand, use of monitoring devices and techniques must reflect an appreciation of the risk-benefit ratio for each monitor. The amount and type of monitoring used depends on the physiologic status of the patient and the extent of the surgical procedure. Monitoring of neonates and infants during the perioperative period often includes continuous display of the electrocardiogram, measurement of blood pressure, measurement of body temperature, use of a precordial or esophageal stethoscope, and monitoring of systemic oxygenation (transcutaneous oxygen electrode or pulse oximeter).

Electrocardiogram

The advantage of a continuous display of the electrocardiogram is the rapid identification of cardiac dysrhythmias. Indeed, changes on the electrocardiogram occurring in pediatric patients are usually related to cardiac rhythm rather than myocardial ischemia. As a result, lead II, and not a precordial lead, is the most useful lead to monitor.

Blood Pressure

Decreased cardiovascular reserve, altered anesthetic requirements, and exaggerated hypotensive response during general anesthesia make monitoring of the blood pressure of neonates and infants mandatory. Noninvasive blood pressure monitors are dependent on use of an inflatable cuff, which must be appropriately sized for the arm of each patient. A cuff that is too small will produce an artificially elevated blood pressure: one which is too large will produce a falsely low reading. There are several methods for detecting return of blood flow after cuff inflation. The classic method, using the audible detection of Korotkoff sounds, is applicable only for older children. Alternatively, the Doppler transducer is an accurate method of noninvasive blood pressure monitoring and has the additional advantage of continuous monitoring of arterial blood flow. Consequently, it serves as a monitor of cardiac rhythm and to a limited extent can reflect output of the heart during cardiac dysrhythmias. The oscillometric method of noninvasive blood pressure monitoring, as represented by the Dinamapp, is also reliable for pediatric patients.

A catheter placed in a peripheral artery can be a useful monitor. Specifically, the presence of an arterial catheter provides moment-to-moment assessment of blood pressure and permits intermittent sampling of blood for measurement of blood gases, electrolytes, pH, glucose, and colloid osmotic pressure. The peripheral artery selected for percutaneous placement of the catheter is particularly important in neonates. For example, blood sampled from an artery that arises distal to the ductus arteriosus (left radial artery, umbilical artery, posterior tibial artery) may not accurately reflect arterial partial pressures of oxygen being delivered to the retina or brain in the presence of a patent ductus arteriosus (Fig. 35-2). If retinopathy of the newborn is a consideration, a preductal artery, such as the right radial artery, should be cannulated. The temporal artey is also a potential preductal site. This artery, however, has the disadvantage of a risk of embolization of cerebral vasculature by the retrograde flushing of microemboli.

Body Temperature

Monitoring of body temperature is essential during the perioperative period for the detection of hypothermia and to facilitate recognition of malignant hyperthermia. Hypothermia, as is likely to occur in neonates or infants during anesthesia, results in increased total body oxygen consumption, depression of ventilation, bradycardia, metabolic acidosis, and hypoglycemia. Sites available for monitoring body temperature include the nasopharynx, esophagus, and rectum. Care must be taken if a rectal probe is placed to avoid rectal perforation. On a routine basis, use of nasopharyngeal or esophageal temperature probes is recommended for patients who have a tracheal tube in place.

Stethoscope

A precordial or esophageal stethoscope permits assessment of ventilation, heart rate, and cardiac rhythm. The initial placement of the stethoscope is precordial during manual ventilation of the lungs via a face mask. Subsequent placement of an esophageal stethoscope after tracheal intubation provides a more reliable monitor. Contraindications to placement of an esophageal stethoscope include a hemorrhagic diathesis, endoscopic or intraoral procedures, esophageal malformations, and vascular rings.

Transcutaneous Oxygen Monitor

The transcutaneous oxygen monitor provides a noninvasive monitor of arterial oxygenation.[55] Indeed, transcutaneous partial pressures of oxygen correlate well with the arterial partial pressures, especially in neonates and infants. Nevertheless, for transcutaneous partial pressures of oxygen to approximate the arterial partial pressures, cutaneous blood flow must be adequate. During periods of reduced cutaneous blood flow, such as hypovolemia, transcutaneous partial pressures of oxygen will be less than the arterial partial pressures of oxygen. Interestingly, the cutaneous vascular bed is quite dynamic and transcutaneous oxygen monitors are effective monitors of reductions in cardiac output and hypovolemia.[56]

Anesthetic gases can interfere with transcutaneous oxygen measurements, although modifications of the membrane covering the oxygen electrode have minimized this interference.[57] In addition, there is evidence that transcutaneous oxygen monitors may provide falsely low indications of arterial oxygenation when the arterial partial pressures are greater than 100 mmHg to 150 mmHg.[55] Another disadvantage of transcutaneous oxygen monitors is the time delay between changes in the arterial partial pressures of oxygen and the subsequent changes in the transcutaneous partial pressures of oxygen.

Pulse Oximeter

The pulse oximeter is a rapid and reliable noninvasive monitor of saturation of hemoglobin with oxygen and thus serves as an early warning of the development of arterial hypoxemia.[58] The pulse oximeter, however, may overestimate hemoglobin saturation with oxygen in children with cyanotic heart disease, especially when saturation is less than 75 percent.[59] Unlike older oximeters, the pulse oximeter employs two selected wavelengths of light and is keyed to arterial pulsation. This technology eliminates light absorption by nonpulsatile tissues. Very low saturations of hemoglobin with oxygen, especially below 70 percent, may not be accurately reflected by older design pulse oximeters.

End-tidal Carbon Dioxide Monitor

End-tidal carbon dioxide monitoring has a wide range of clinical applications. For example, appearance of a carbon dioxide wave form and/or presence of carbon dioxide in exhaled gases sampled from a tube placed in the trachea serves to confirm a tracheal placement of the tube. End-tidal carbon dioxide measurements in adults have been shown to be accurate reflections of arterial carbon dioxide partial pressures. End-tidal carbon dioxide monitoring is also reliable in children, although there are some limitations in neonates and infants. For example, because of the small tidal volumes and large inspired gas flows, there may be dilution of exhaled carbon dioxide. This would produce false low end-tidal partial pressures of carbon dioxide.[60] Large gas leaks around the tracheal tube will also produce false low end-tidal carbon dioxide partial pressures. If these limitations are considered, the end-tidal carbon dioxide monitor remains as useful for children as for adults.

Central Venous Pressure

The central venous circulation of pediatric patients can be cannulated via the subclavian or jugular veins, as in adults. Successful placement of catheters, however, is not as frequent, and the complication rate is higher.

NEONATAL MEDICAL DISEASES

Significant technologic and medical advances have resulted in improved survival of large numbers of low birth weight preterm neonates. Perioperative care of preterm and term neonates requires a thorough knowledge of those diseases unique to this age group. Neonatal medical diseases include respiratory distress syndrome, bronchopulmonary dysplasia, intracranial hemorrhage, retinopathy of prematurity, apnea spells, kernicterus, hypoglycemia, hypocalemia, and sepsis.

Respiratory Distress Syndrome (Hyaline Membrane Disease)

Respiratory distress syndrome is responsible for 50 percent to 75 percent of deaths that occur in preterm neonates. This syndrome is caused by a deficiency in the alveoli of surface active phospholipids known as surfactant. The function of surfactant is to maintain alveolar stability. Without surfactant, alveoli collapse, leading to right-to-left intrapulmonary shunting, arterial hypoxemia, and metabolic acidosis. Surfactant is produced by type II alveolar cells. Before 26 weeks gestation, however, there are not enough type II cells to produce adequate amounts of surfactant. By 35 weeks, there are large numbers of type II cells capable of sufficient surfactant synthesis. Until adequate surfactant can be produced, arterial oxygenation must be maintained using supplemental oxygen, with or without mechanical ventilation of the lungs. In certain circumstances, antenatal steroids administered to the mother may accelerate maturation of the lungs and prevent development of respiratory distress syndrome in preterm infants. Limited, but promising success has been achieved with tracheal administration of human surfactant to preterm infants.[61]

During anesthesia in the presence of respiratory distress syndrome, the arterial partial pressures of oxygen should be maintained at preoperative levels. It should be remembered that volatile anesthetics can alter arterial oxygenation by depressing cardiac output and by inhibiting regional hypoxic pulmonary vasoconstriction. Ideally, the arterial partial pressures of oxygen should be monitored from blood obtained from catheters placed in preductal arteries (Fig. 35-2) (see the section Monitoring During the Perioperative Period). For short procedures or when arterial cannulation is not feasible, a transcutaneous oxygen monitor or pulse oximeter is satisfactory. The degree of pulmonary dysfunction in individual neonates with respiratory distress syndrome is highly variable. The least afflicted neonates may require only supplemental oxygen for short periods of time. Severely afflicted neonates can require mechanical ventilation of the lungs with high inspired oxygen concentrations and positive end-expiratory pressure. Pneumothorax is an ever present danger and should be considered if oxygenation deteriorates abruptly in neonates being treated for respiratory distress syndrome. An alternative to mechanical ventilation of the lungs of these neonates may be high frequency ventilation.[62] Hypotension is a frequently encountered problem during anesthesia. Intravenous administration of albumin 1 g·kg^{-1} to preterm neonates with respiratory distress syndrome has been shown to increase blood volume and the glomerular filtration rate. The hematocrit of neonates should be maintained at 40 percent to optimize tissue oxygen delivery. Fluid administration must be meticulously monitored because excess hydration may reopen the ductus arteriosus.

Bronchopulmonary Dysplasia

Bronchopulmonary dysplasia is a chronic pulmonary disorder, which usually afflicts children with a previous history of respiratory distress syndrome.[63] Although the exact mechanism is not known, certain risk factors have been identified. For example, increased inspired oxygen concentrations and positive pressure ventilation of the lungs, as used for treatment of the respiratory distress syndrome, may be etiologic factors. Indeed, 11 percent to 21 percent of neonates with respiratory distress syndrome requiring supplemental oxygen for more than 24 hours develop bronchopulmonary dysplasia.[63] Clinically, infants with bronchopulmonary dysplasia are ones with respiratory distress syndrome who enter a chronic phase. The more severe the respiratory distress syndrome the greater the degree of bronchopulmonary dysplasia.

Bronchopulmonary dysplasia is characterized by increased airway resistance, decreased pulmonary compliance, mismatch of ventilation to perfusion, decreased arterial oxygenation, and tachypnea. Oxygen consumption is increased by as much as 25 percent. It should

be assumed that children with prior histories of respiratory distress syndrome requiring supplemental oxygen and mechanical ventilation of the lungs probably have some degree of residual pulmonary disease. Survivors of the respiratory distress syndrome who develop bronchopulmonary dysplasia have an increased incidence of pulmonary infections, especially during the first year of life. Nevertheless, the prognosis for children surviving the first year of life is good, and pulmonary function gradually improves. Increased airway resistance, however, may persist until 9 years of age.

The choice of drugs for anesthesia in patients with bronchopulmonary dysplasia is not as important as management of the airway. For example, management of anesthesia in these children includes intubation of the trachea, delivery of increased inspired concentrations of oxygen, and mechanical ventilation of the lungs. Although these children may appear well clinically, pulmonary compliance is usually decreased. It should be appreciated, however, that pulmonary dysfunction in these patients will be most marked in the first year of life.

Intracranial Hemorrhage

The four types of intracranial hemorrhage in the neonatal period are subdural, primary subarachnoid, periventricular-intraventricular, and intercellular. The most frequent and important type is periventricular-intraventricular hemorrhage.

The incidence of periventricular-intraventricular hemorrhage is 40 percent to 45 percent in neonates less than 35 weeks of gestational age. Newborn immaturity is the single most important risk factor for intracranial hemorrhage.[64] Other factors that predispose preterm neonates to such hemorrhage are impaired autoregulation of cerebral blood flow, increased central venous pressure, and immaturity of neonatal cerebral capillary beds. Severe respiratory complications and infections are also associated with intracranial hemorrhage. The degree of autoregulation of cerebral blood flow in normal neonates is unknown, although impaired autoregulation of cerebral blood flow has been demonstrated in stressed neonates.[65] When autoregulation is impaired, an elevation of blood pressure will cause increased cerebral blood flow, which may result in periventricular-intraventricular hemorrhage. Arterial hypoxemia and hypercapnia that occur during asphyxia associated with delivery can also result in such hemorrhage.

Diagnosis of periventricular-intraventricular hemorrhage can be made by maintaining a high index of suspicion in susceptible neonates and by clinical and radiologic features. Clinical features can range from subtle and not easily elicited neurologic aberrations to catastrophic deterioration with rapid onset of coma. Ultrasound scanning and computed tomography provide useful modes for identifying such hemorrhage. Administration of phenobarbital to preterm infants has been suggested for prophylaxis against intraventricular hemorrhage, although data concerning the efficacy of this thearapy are conflicting.[66]

Although effects of anesthesia on cerebral blood flow in neonates are not known, certain recommendations can be made concerning management of anesthesia. Certainly, factors known to precipitate periventricular-intraventricular hemorrhage, such as arterial hypoxemia and hypercapnia, should be avoided. In view of altered autoregulation of cerebral blood flow, systolic blood pressure should be maintained in the normal range to reduce risks of cerebral overperfusion. To accomplish these goals, careful monitoring of arterial blood gases and blood pressure is required.

Retinopathy of Prematurity (Retrolental Fibroplasia)

Retinopathy of prematurity is probably due to multiple interacting events. The most significant risk factor is prematurity. The risk of retinopathy is inversely related to birth weight with significant risk occurring in infants less than 1,500 grams.[67] Retinal development and maturation is a complicated process. Our understanding of the process and factors that may alter development of retinal vasculature is poor. Under normal circumstances, retinal vasculature develops from the optic disc toward the periphery of the retina. During arterial hyperoxia, retinal vasoconstriction occurs, and normal retinal development is disturbed. When normoxic conditions return, vascularization of the retina resumes in an abnormal fashion, with resultant neovascularization and scarring. Although 80 percent to 90 percent of retinal changes will regress spontaneously, 10 percent to 20 percent of children will be left with some visual impairment. There are many unanswered questions concerning retinopathy. It is not known what magnitude or duration of arterial hyperoxia produces adverse effects on retinal vasculature. Although retinopathy may be a result of the interaction between vasoconstriction and an immature retina, it is also possible that direct effects of oxygen may produce retinal damage. Retinopathy has even occurred in preterm infants who did not receive supplemental oxygen and infants with cyanotic congenital heart disease. Clearly, arterial hyperoxia is an important risk factor in development of retinopathy but prematurity must also be present. The risk of developing retinopathy is negligible after 44 weeks postconception. Therefore, preterm infants born after 36 weeks of gestation remain at risk for retinopathy until after 8 weeks of age.

Management of anesthesia in these patients introduces the dilemma of trying to minimize oxygen administration to a group of patients that is also prone to arterial hypoxemia. To reduce the risk of retinopathy in susceptible infants, it is recommended that arterial oxygen partial pressures by maintained between 60 mmHg and 80 mmHg.[67] During anesthesia, it is important to dilute inspired concentrations of oxygen using nitrous oxide or air. Delivered concentrations of oxygen should be confirmed by an oxygen analyzer. Although it is desirable to monitor arterial oxygenation in blood sampled from preductal arteries (Fig. 35-2) (see the section Monitoring During the Perioperative Period), the use of transcutaneous oxygen monitors is acceptable if cutaneous blood flow is normal. It should also be appreciated that arterial hypoxemia is a significant threat to neonates. Certainly, attempts to prevent arterial hyperoxia must be tempered with the realization that unrecognized arterial hypoxemia can result in irreversible brain damage.

Apnea Spells

Apnea spells are defined as cessation of breathing that lasts for at least 20 seconds and produce cyanosis and bradycardia. It is estimated that 20 percent to 30 percent of preterm infants experience apnea spells during the first month of life.[68] The more premature the infant the greater the likelihood of developing apnea spells. Preterm infants may also have respiratory distress syndrome and bronchopulmonary dysplasia in addition to apnea spells. Inguinal hernias and incarceration of inguinal hernias are quite common in preterm infants. Consequently, many preterm infants require inguinal hernia repair. Despite the fact that infant inguinal hernia repair is a minor surgical procedure, up to 33 percent of such preterm infants have respiratory complications during the perioperative period.[69] Apnea spells and atelectasis are the most frequent respiratory complications. In this regard, it is important to review carefully the respiratory history of infants during the preoperative visit. Specifically, a history of prematurity and respiratory distress syndrome should be sought.

Since all anesthetics, both inhaled and intravenous, affect control of breathing, it is likely that the risk of apnea spells will be increased during the postoperative period, especially in preterm infants less than 60 weeks postconception age.[70] Consequently, preterm infants with a history of apnea spells are not suitable candidates for outpatient surgery. It is recommended that these patients be monitored in the hospital for at least 12 hours after surgery.[70,71] The risk of postoperative apnea spells seems to be reduced beyond 60 weeks postconception leading some to favoring postponement of nonessential surgery in preterm infants to after this age.

Kernicterus

Kernicterus is the term applied to a syndrome caused by toxic effects of unconjugated bilirubin on the central nervous system. The gross clinical features of kernicterus include hypertonicity, opisthotonos, and spasticity. It is also evident that bilirubin encephalopathy can produce more subtle changes, such as dyslexia, hyperactivity, and decreased intellectual development.

Bilirubin is not lipophilic and does not readily cross the blood-brain barrier. Nevertheless, the blood-brain barrier of neonates, especially preterm neonates, is immature, which may explain the ability of bilirubin to enter the brain and produce cell damage.[72] In addition, alterations in the blood-brain barrier by arterial hypoxemia, hypercapnia, or acidosis may facilitate passage of bilirubin into the central nervous system. Rapid changes in cerebral blood flow, such as may occur during exchange transfusion or rapid blood transfusion, may also disrupt the blood-brain barrier and permit entry of both bound and unbound bilirubin into the central nervous system. Neonates with other diseases, such as respiratory distress syndrome and sepsis, have decreased bilirubin-binding capacity, and an increased risk of kernicterus. In addition, drugs may affect bilirubin clearance, either by displacing bilirubin from albumin binding sites or by altering hepatocyte function and diminishing conjugation of bilirubin (Table 35-11).

Treatment of hyperbilirubinemia includes phototherapy, exchange blood transfusions, and drugs. Phototherapy converts bilirubin to photobilirubin. Photobilirubin is water soluble and does not bind to albumin. Although exchange blood transfusions are usually performed when plasma bilirubin concentrations are greater than 18 mg·dl^{-1}, other risk factors,

TABLE 35-11. Drugs That Interfere with Bilirubin Binding to Protein

Cephalothin	Furosemide
Diazepam	Phenylbutazone
Digoxin	Salicylate
Ethacrynic acid	Sulfonamide

such as low birth weight, decreased plasma albumin concentrations, acidosis, arterial hypoxemia, and hypothermia, must also be considered and may necessitate exchange blood transfusions at lower plasma bilirubin concentrations.

There are no data concerning effects of anesthesia on plasma concentrations of bilirubin in preterm infants. Although undocumented, it is conceivable that anesthetic drugs could alter bilirubin binding and/or bilirubin conjugation.

Hypoglycemia

Neonates in contrast to adults have poorly developed systems for maintenance of adequate plasma glucose concentrations and, therefore, are susceptible to development of hypoglycemia. By definition, hypoglycemia is a plasma glucose concentration less than 25 mg·dl^{-1} for preterm neonates and less than 35 mg·dl^{-1} for term neonates less than 3 days of age. Plasma glucose concentrations at 3 days of age should be greater than 45 mg·dl^{-1} for term neonates.

Signs of hypoglycemia in neonates include irritability, seizures, bradycardia, hypotension, and apnea. Many of the signs are nonspecific, and a high index of suspicion must be maintained. Manifestations of hypoglycemia are attenuated by anesthesia. Intraoperatively, plasma glucose concentrations can be measured by use of a variety of devices. Maintenance of adequate plasma glucose concentrations in neonates requires intravenous infusion of solutions containing glucose. The immediate treatment of hypoglycemia is intravenous infusion of glucose 0.5 g·kg^{-1} to 1 g·kg^{-1} or continuous infusion at 8 mg·kg^{-1}·min^{-1}. Hyperglycemia must also be avoided as plasma glucose concentrations in excess of 125 mg·dl^{-1} can produce osmotic diuresis with resultant dehydration. Neonates can also develop hyperglycemia when preoperative glucose infusion rates are maintained during surgery.[73]

Hypocalcemia

Fetal calcium stores are largely achieved during the last trimester of gestation. Preterm neonates, therefore, are prone to develop hypocalcemia. Hypocalcemia in neonates is defined as plasma calcium concentrations less than 3.5 mEq·L^{-1} or plasma ionized calcium concentration less than 1.5 mEq·L^{-1}. It should be remembered that total plasma calcium concentrations do not reliably reflect ionized plasma calcium concentrations. For example, ionized plasma calcium concentrations may be decreased, whereas total plasma calcium concentrations are normal. Signs of hypocalcemia are nonspecific and include irritability, hypotension, and seizures. Neonates with hypocalcemia exhibit increased skeletal muscle tone and twitching, in contrast to skeletal muscle hypotonia associated with hypoglycemia.

Hypocalcemia can occur with rapid intraoperative infusion of citrate, as may occur during exchange transfusions or infusions of citrated blood or fresh frozen plasma. Hypotensive effects of hypocalcemia during rapid blood transfusions can be minimized by administration of 1 mg to 2 mg of calcium gluconate·ml^{-1} of blood transfused.

Sepsis

Sepsis in neonates is associated with a mortality that approaches 50 percent.[74] Presumably this high mortality reflects the immature immune system of neonates. The clinical presentation of neonatal sepsis is nonspecific. Consequently, the evaluation for sepsis has become an integral part of neonatal intensive care. Suggestive signs include lethargy, skeletal muscle hypotonia, hypoglycemia, and ventilatory distress. In contrast to adults, increases in body temperature or leukocytosis may be absent in neonates. Positive blood cultures are considered the critical diagnostic feature. Common sequelae of untreated neonatal sepsis include meningitis and disseminated intravascular coagulation.

Most neonates presenting for surgery are already receiving antibiotics, as risks of sepsis are great. Nevertheless, occurrence of pulmonary dysfunction in the postoperative period should arouse suspicion as to the possible presence of sepsis.

NEONATAL SURGICAL DISEASE

Surgery performed in the first days of life is invariably of an urgent nature. In addition to the physiologic aberrations produced by the disease process, incomplete adaptation to the extrauterine environment may further complicate perioperative management. Neonatal surgical diseases include diaphragmatic hernia, tracheoesophageal fistula, omphalocele, gastroschisis, pyloric stenosis, lobar emphysema, and necrotizing enterocolitis.[75]

Diaphragmatic Hernia

Diaphragmatic hernia results from incomplete embryologic closure of the diaphragm.[76] The incidence is about 1 in every 5,000 live births. Although herniation of abdominal contents into the thorax can occur at several sites, the most common diaphragmatic defect occurs through the left posterolateral pleuroperitoneal canal (foramen of Bochdalek) (Fig. 35-8). Herniation of abdominal contents into the thorax during gestation interferes with normal fetal lung maturation, resulting in varying degrees of pulmonary hypoplasia. Despite significant progress in pediatric surgery and anesthesia, perioperative mortality is high (33 percent to 66 percent) and has remained relatively constant during the past 25 years.[77] This relatively constant mortality rate may reflect better resuscitation of infants who would have died before surgery in past years.

EMBRYOLOGY

Embryologic development of the diaphragm, gastrointestinal tract, heart, and lungs occur simultaneously. As a result, abnormal development of one organ system affects the development of others. Under normal circumstances, separate pleural and peritoneal cavities are formed by the diaphragm at 8 weeks to 10 weeks of gestation. At the same time, the gastrointestinal tract herniates into the umbil-

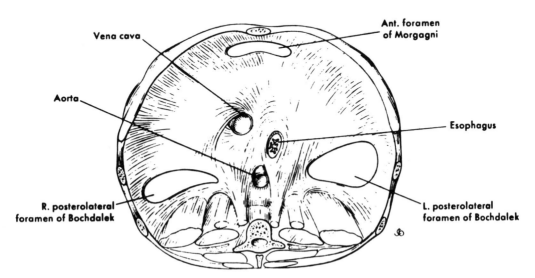

FIG. 35-8. Diaphragmatic hernia with passage of abdominal viscera into the thorax most commonly occurs through the left posterolateral pleuroperitoneal canal (foramen of Bochdalek). (Smith RM. Anesthesia for Infants and Children. 4th Ed. St. Louis. CV Mosby 1980)

ical stalk but eventually returns to the abdominal cavity. The pleuroperitoneal canals progressively narrow and are finally obliterated by the 10th week of gestation. Diaphragmatic hernia may result from either the early return of the midgut to the abdominal cavity or delayed closure of the pleuroperitoneal canal. The degree of pulmonary hypoplasia associated with diaphragmatic hernia is related to the timing of the herniation of abdominal contents into the thorax. Early diaphragmatic herniation will cause more pulmonary hypoplasia, resulting in a less favorable prognosis. Hypoplasia of the left ventricle may also occur, contributing to postnatal cardiac insufficiency.[78]

SIGNS AND SYMPTOMS

Signs and symptoms of diaphragmatic hernia evident soon after birth include scaphoid abdomen, barrel-shaped chest, detection of bowel sounds during auscultation of the chest, and profound arterial hypoxemia. Radiographs of the chest show loops of intestine in the thorax and a shift of the mediastinum to the opposite side (Fig. 35-9).[75] Arterial hypoxemia reflects the presence of right-to-left shunting through the ductus arteriosus as a manifestation of persistent fetal circulation. Indeed, pulmonary arterioles from lungs of infants with diaphragmatic hernia are characterized by significant increases in smooth muscle mass, as compared to normal arterioles. Increased pulmonary vascular resistance due to these thickened arterioles is further aggravated by arterial hypoxemia, hypercapnia, and acidosis, insuring that the ductus arteriosus will remain patent and a fetal pattern of circulation will persist. Finally, there is a high incidence of congenital heart disease and intestinal malrotation in neonates with diaphragmatic hernia.

TREATMENT

Immediate treatment of neonates with suspected diaphragmatic hernias should include decompression of the stomach with an orogastric or nasogastric tube and administration of supplemental oxygen. Positive pressure ventilation by mask should be avoided, as passage of gas into the esophagus may increase stomach volume and further compromise pulmonary function. Indeed, awake intubation of the trachea should be performed if the need for mechanical ventilation of the lungs is anticipated for any sustained period of time. After intubation of the trachea, positive airway pressure during mechanical ventilation of the lungs should not exceed 25 cmH$_2$0 to 30 cmH$_2$0, since excessive airway pressures can result in damage to the normal lung, manifesting as pneumothorax.

MANAGEMENT OF ANESTHESIA

Management of anesthesia for neonates with diaphragmatic hernias consists of awake intubation of the trachea after preoxygenation. In addition to routine monitors, the right radial or temporal artery (i.e., preductal arteries) should be cannulated for monitoring of blood pressure, blood gases, and pH. Anesthesia can be induced and maintained with low concentrations of volatile drugs. Nitrous oxide should be avoided, as its diffusion into loops of intestine present in the chest may result in distention of these loops and subsequent compression of functioning lung tissue. If the level of arterial oxygenation permits, excessive inspired concentrations of oxygen can be prevented by adding air to the oxygen until desired delivered concentrations of oxygen, as reflected by an oxygen analyzer, are attained. Since prolonged postoperative ventilation of the lungs is required by almost all infants with diaphragmatic hernia, an alternative approach to inhaled drugs for anesthesia is an opioid such as fentanyl plus a muscle relaxant, often pancuronium.[79] This regimen can also be continued during the postoperative period. The advantage of this technique is that hormonal responses to stress can be minimized postoperatively. Mechanical ventilation of the lungs is recommended, but airway pressures should be monitored and maintained below 25 cmH$_2$0 to 30 cmH$_2$0 to minimize risks of pneumothorax. Reduction of the diaphragmatic hernia is accomplished through an abdominal surgical approach. After reduction of the hernia, attempts to inflate the hypoplastic lung are not recommended, as it is unlikely to expand, and damage to the normal lung can occur from excessive positive airway pressures. In addition

FIG. 35-9. Radiograph of the chest in a newborn with a diaphragmatic hernia, as evidenced by the loops of intestine in the left thorax, displacement of the mediastinum to the right, and compression of the right lung. Notice the dilated stomach contributing to mediastinal displacement.

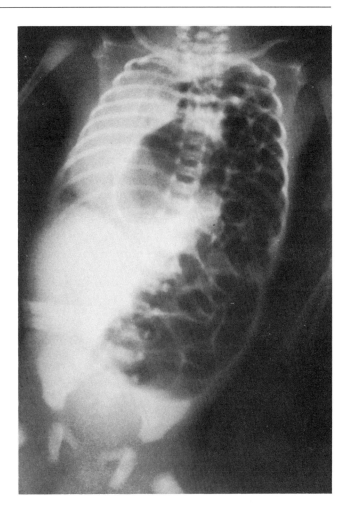

to a hypoplastic lung, these neonates are likely to have an underdeveloped abdominal cavity, such that a tight surgical abdominal closure will cause increased intra-abdominal pressure, with cephalad displacement of the diaphragm, a reduced functional residual capacity, and compression of the inferior vena cava. To prevent an excessively tight closure, it is often necessary to create a ventral hernia, which can be repaired later.

POSTOPERATIVE MANAGEMENT

Postoperative management of infants with diaphragmatic hernias presents significant challenges. Prognosis of these infants is ultimately determined by the degree of pulmonary hypoplasia. There is no effective treatment for pulmonary hypoplasia, other than keeping the infant alive with the hope that lung maturation will occur. Extracorporeal membrane oxygenation has been used successfully for this purpose in these patients.[80]

The postoperative course, after surgical reduction of diaphragmatic hernias is often characterized by rapid improvement, followed by sudden deterioration, with profound arterial hypoxemia, hypercapnia, and acidosis, resulting in death. The mechanism for this deterioration is the reappearance of fetal patterns of circulation, with right-to-left shunting through the foramen ovale and ductus arteriosus. If shunting occurs through the ductus arteriosus, a presumptive diagnosis of persistent fetal circulation can be made if there is a 20 mmHg or greater difference in the arterial partial pressure of oxygen measured in samples obtained simultaneously from a preductal and postductal artery. If shunting is occurring predominantly through the foramen ovale, then no such gradient will exist.

Infants with postoperative alveolar-to-arterial oxygen partial pressure differences that exceed 400 mmHg, when breathing 100 percent oxygen, are likely to need aggressive postoperative care.[81] Various drugs, including morphine, chlorpromazine, tolazoline, and isoproterenol, have been used with some success to decrease pulmonary vascular resistance. Logical use of these types of drugs requires the presence of a pulmonary artery catheter to monitor changes in pulmonary artery pressures.

Tracheoesophageal Fistula

Survival of neonates with tracheoesophageal fistula and no associated defects approaches 100 percent.[82] Nevertheless, about 20 percent of neonates with tracheoesophageal fistula have a major co-existing cardiovascular anomaly (ventricular septal defect, tetralogy of Fallot, coarctation of the aorta, atrial septal defect), and 30 percent to 40 percent are born preterm. Survival in those infants with other anomalies is reduced. Five types of tracheoesophageal fistula are associated with esophageal atresia (Fig. 35-10). The most common defect consists of a blind upper esophageal pouch and a fistula between the lower esophagus and trachea.

SIGNS AND SYMPTOMS

Diagnosis of tracheoesophageal fistula is usually made soon after birth, when an oral catheter cannot be passed into the stomach, or when infants develop cyanosis and coughing during oral feedings.[83] Pulmonary aspiration is likely to occur. After the diagnosis is suspected, the blind upper pouch must be decompressed, and infants are placed in head-up positions. Gastric distention can be of sufficient magnitude to impair diaphragmatic excursion.

TREATMENT

Treatment of newborns with tracheoesophageal fistula is initiated by performing a gastrostomy as soon as possible after birth, during local anesthesia. The gastrostomy provides a vent for excess gas that may enter the stomach through the tracheoesophageal fistula, during mechanical ventilation of the lungs. Thoracot-

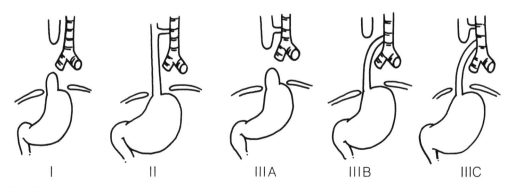

FIG. 35-10. The five types of tracheoesophageal fistula are classified as I, II, IIIA, IIIB, and IIIC, depending on the anatomic characteristics of the trachea and esophagus. A blind upper esophageal pouch and a fistula connecting the stomach to the trachea (IIIB) is the most common type of tracheoesophageal fistula. (Dierdorf SF, Krishna G. Anesthetic management of neonatal surgical emergencies. Anesth Analg 1981;60:204–15. Reprinted with permission from IARS)

omy for definitive repair of the lesion is delayed for 48 hours to 72 hours, to permit adequate hydration and assessment of cardiopulmonary function.

MANAGEMENT OF ANESTHESIA

Proper placement of the tracheal tube is critical; it should be above the carina but below the tracheoesophageal fistula. By placing the gastrostomy tube into a beaker of water and applying positive airway pressure, one can determine the position of the tracheal tube (Fig. 35-11).[75] For example, absence of bubbling in the beaker during positive airway pressure confirms that the distal end of the tracheal tube is beyond the fistula. Likewise, it is critical that the tracheal tube be above the carina, as the right lung is compressed during the thoracot-

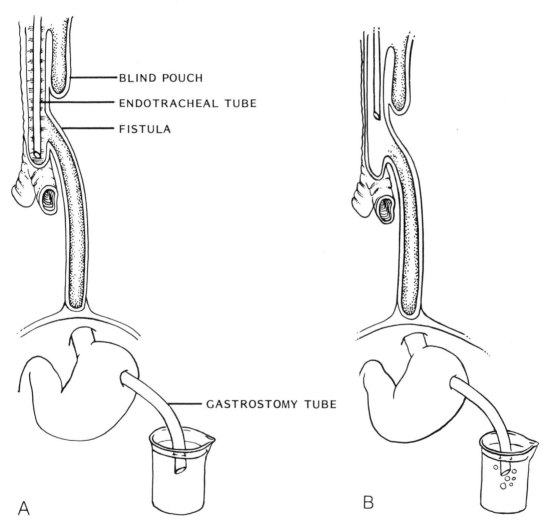

BLIND POUCH

ENDOTRACHEAL TUBE

FISTULA

GASTROSTOMY TUBE

A

B

FIG. 35-11. (A) Application of positive airway pressure via a tube correctly positioned in the trachea distal to the tracheoesophageal fistula will not produce bubbling in the beaker of water in which the gastrostomy tube is placed. (B) Incorrect placement of the tube in the trachea proximal to the tracheoesophageal fistula is detected by the presence of bubbling in the beaker containing the gastrostomy tube when positive airway pressure is applied. (Dierdorf SF, Krishna G. Anesthetic management of neonatal surgical emergencies. Anesth Analg 1981;60:204–15. Reprinted with permission from IARS)

omy. Accidental intubation of the right main stem bronchus will result in precipitous decreases in arterial oxygenation.

Selection of anesthetic drugs for administration during surgical correction of tracheoesophageal fistula depends on the physiologic status of the neonates. Volatile anesthetics may be used if neonates are adequately hydrated. Nitrous oxide should be used with caution in neonates without a gastrostomy, as diffusion of this gas into the distended stomach would be undesirable. If nitrous oxide is not administered, it will be necessary to dilute inspired concentrations of oxygen with air to avoid arterial hyperoxia and the risk of retinopathy of prematurity. In addition to routine monitors, a catheter placed in a peripheral artery will permit continuous monitoring of blood pressure and measurement of blood gases and pH. A transcutaneous oxygen monitor or pulse oximeter is a useful monitor for detecting rapid changes in arterial oxygenation.[84]

A consistent pathologic finding in neonates with tracheoesophageal fistula is a reduced amount of tracheal cartilage. This reduced support can result in tracheal collapse after extubation and require immediate reintubation of the trachea. On the other hand, some neonates develop symptomatic tracheal compression several months after tracheoesophageal fistula repair. Chronic gastroesophageal reflux and aspiration pneumonitis can follow corrective surgery, necessitating antireflux surgical procedures.

Omphalocele and Gastroschisis

Omphalocele and gastroschisis are congenital defects of the anterior abdominal wall, which permit external herniation of abdominal viscera.[85]

OMPHALOCELE

Omphalocele is associated with external herniation of abdominal viscera through the base of the umbilical cord (Fig. 35-12).[75] The incidence is about 1 in every 5,000 to 10,000 live births, with a male predominance. Omphalocele is associated with a 75 percent incidence of other congenital defects, including cardiac anomalies, trisomy-21, and Beckwith syndrome (omphalocele, organomegaly, macroglossia, and hypoglycemia). About 33 percent of neonates with omphalocele are preterm. Cardiac defects and prematurity are major causes of the 30 percent mortality in newborns with omphaloceles.

GASTROSCHISIS

Gastroschisis is characterized by external herniation of abdominal viscera through a 2 cm to 5 cm defect in the anterior abdominal wall, lateral to the normally inserted umbilical cord (Fig. 35-13).[75] Unlike omphalocele, a hernia sac does not cover the herniated abdominal viscera. Gastroschisis is rarely associated with other congenital anomalies. The incidence of preterm birth, however, is higher than in neonates with an omphalocele.

PREOPERATIVE PREPARATION

Considerations in preoperative preparation of neonates with omphalocele or gastroschisis are prevention of infection and minimization of fluid and heat loss from exposed abdominal viscera. Covering exposed viscera with moist dressings and a plastic bowel bag and maintaining a neutral thermal environment are effective methods for decreasing fluid and heat loss. The stomach should be decompressed with an orogastric tube to decrease the risk of regurgitation and pulmonary aspiration. Adequate hydration in the preoperative period is essential. Initial fluid requirements in these neonates are increased, ranging from 6 ml·kg^{-1}·hr^{-1} to 12 ml·kg^{-1}·hr^{-1}. These neonates experience considerable protein loss and third space translocation. Hypovolemia is evidenced by hemoconcentration and metabolic acidosis. Plasma albumin concentrations and colloid oncotic pressures are reduced. To maintain normal oncotic pressures, protein-containing solutions should constitute 25 percent of the resuscitation fluids. Sodium bicarbonate ad-

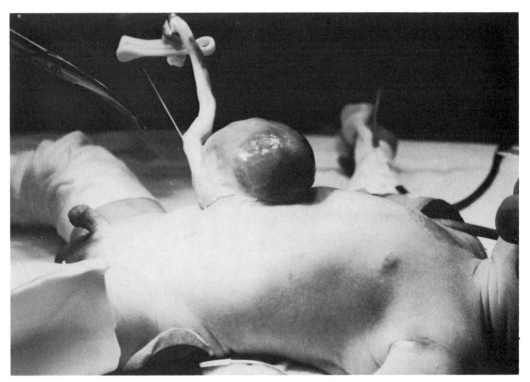

FIG. 35-12. Omphalocele is the herniation of abdominal viscera through the base of the umbilical cord. An intact hernia sac covers the abdominal contents. (Dierdorf SF, Krishna G. Anesthetic management of neonatal surgical emergencies. Anesth Analg 1981;60:204–15. Reprinted with permission from IARS)

ministration to correct metabolic acidosis should be guided by arterial pH measurements.

MANAGEMENT OF ANESTHESIA

Important aspects of management of anesthesia for surgical treatment of omphalocele and gastroschisis include maintenance of body temperature and continuation of fluid resuscitation. Awake intubation of the trachea, after decompression of the stomach and preoxygenation, is indicated. Opioids such as fentanyl or sufentanil or volatile anesthetics may be used. Because of co-existing hypovolemia, anesthetics must be carefully titrated to avoid hypotension. Use of nitrous oxide may be questioned, since this gas could diffuse into the intestinal tract and interfere with the ease of returning exposed and distended loops of bowel back into the abdomen. If nitrous oxide

is not used, inspired concentrations of oxygen are adjusted by dilution with air, a necessity because these often preterm neonates are vulnerable to the development of retinopathy of prematurity. Muscle relaxants must be administered judiciously, as excessive skeletal muscle paralysis may make it difficult to determine whether primary surgical abdominal wall closure is feasible. It must be remembered that these neonates have an underdeveloped abdominal cavity; a tight surgical abdominal closure can result in reduction of diaphragmatic excursion and compression of the inferior vena cava. Monitoring airway pressures is helpful for detecting changes in pulmonary compliance due to abdominal closure. If primary surgical abdominal closure is not possible, temporary coverage with a Dacron reinforced silastic silo is performed. The hernia is then gradually reduced over 1 week to 2 weeks.

Intensive intraoperative and postoperative

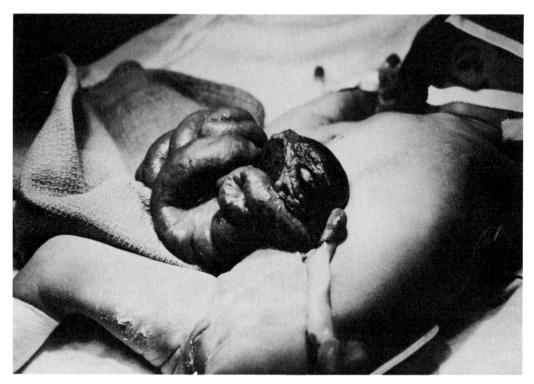

FIG. 35-13. Gastroschisis is the herniation of abdominal viscera through a defect in the abdominal wall lateral to the normally inserted umbilical cord. A hernia sac to cover the abdominal viscera is absent. (Dierdorf SF, Krishna G. Anesthetic management of neonatal surgical emergencies. Anesth Analg 1981;60:204–15. Reprinted with permission from IARS)

monitoring is recommended. Direct monitoring of arterial blood gases and pH is valuable for guiding fluid therapy, minimizing the risk of development of retinopathy of prematurity, and recognizing previously undiagnosed cardiac anomalies. Elective mechanical ventilation of the lungs is indicated for 24 hours to 48 hours for most neonates with omphalocele or gastroschisis.[83] Refinement of techniques of postoperative mechanical ventilation of the lungs and availability of total parenteral nutrition have increased survival of infants with omphalocele to about 75 percent.[86]

Pyloric Stenosis

Pyloric stenosis occurs in about 1 of every 500 live births, and usually manifests at 2 weeks to 5 weeks of age. Pyloric stenosis is as common in preterm as term neonates. Although the etiology of pyloric stenosis is unknown, autonomic nervous system imbalance and humoral disorders have been suggested as causative factors.

SIGNS AND SYMPTOMS

Pyloric stenosis is characterized by persistent vomiting, resulting in the loss of hydrogen ions from the stomach. As hydrogen ions are lost, the kidneys secrete potassium in exchange for hydrogen ions, in an effort to maintain a normal arterial pH. In addition, the kidneys begin exchanging potassium and hydrogen ions for sodium ions, as the infant becomes sodium depleted from vomiting. The result is a dehydrated infant with a hypokalemic, hypochloremic metabolic alkalosis. Measurement of plasma electrolyte concentrations, arterial blood gases, and pH will help quantitate the degree of metabolic abnormality. Severe cases of pyloric stenosis can manifest as metabolic acidosis secondary to severe dehydration and hypoperfusion.

TREATMENT

Surgical treatment of pyloric stenosis is not an emergency. Patients with pyloric stenosis should be treated initially with intravenous fluids containing sodium and potassium chloride. Surgery is performed electively after 24 hours to 48 hours of intravenous fluid therapy.

MANAGEMENT OF ANESTHESIA

Pulmonary aspiration of gastric fluid is a definite risk in infants with pyloric stenosis. This risk is further enhanced if these infants have had radiographic examinations of the upper gastrointestinal tract using barium. Therefore, the stomach should be emptied as completely as possible with a large bore catheter before induction of anesthesia. Awake intubation of the trachea is indicated for less vigorous infants. Rapid sequence induction of anesthesia, with the intravenous administration of barbiturates followed by succinylcholine and during continuous cricoid pressure, can be used for more vigorous infants. Maintenance of anesthesia with volatile drugs, with or without nitrous oxide, is acceptable. Skeletal muscle relaxation, as provided by muscle relaxants, is usually not needed during the maintenance of anesthesia. Mechanical ventilation of the lungs is recommended during the operation.

POSTOPERATIVE MANAGEMENT

Postoperative depression of ventilation often occurs in infants with pyloric stenosis. The cause is not known but may be related to cerebrospinal fluid alkalosis and intraoperative hyperventilation of the lungs. For this reason, infants should be fully awake and should manifest acceptable patterns of ventilation before extubation of the trachea is considered.

Hypoglycemia may occur 2 hours to 3 hours after surgical correction of pyloric stenosis.

Lobar Emphysema

Lobar emphysema is a cause of varying degrees of respiratory distress in neonates. Pathologic causes of congenital lobar emphysema include collapse of bronchi from hypoplasia of supporting cartilage, bronchial stenosis, mucous plugs, obstructing cysts, and vascular compression of bronchi. Acquired lobar emphysema may be a result of bronchopulmonary dysplasia. The right upper and right middle lobes are most commonly affected by lobar emphysema.

SIGNS AND SYMPTOMS

Regardless of the cause of lobar emphysema, the end result is an overdistended lobe, which produces compression atelectasis of normal lung tissue, mediastinal shift, and impaired venous blood return, with subsequent arterial hypoxemia and hypotension. About one-half of patients will develop significant findings during the first month of life. Signs of lobar emphysema include tachypnea, tachycardia, cyanosis, wheezing, and assymetric breath sounds. A radiograph of the chest will reveal a hyperinflated lobe with mediastinal shift.

MANAGEMENT OF ANESTHESIA

Management of anesthesia in the presence of lobar emphysema must consider cardiovascular and pulmonary changes that can occur with mechanical ventilation of the lungs.[87] For example, an obstructed bronchus can act as a one-way valve, permitting gas entry into the affected lobe, but not allowing gas egress. Nitrous oxide should not be used, as its diffusion into the diseased lobe can cause further distention. Severely decompensated infants may require emergency needle aspiration or thoracotomy for decompression of the affected lobe.

Necrotizing Enterocolitis

Necrotizing enterocolitis is primarily a disease of small preterm neonates, resulting in substantial perinatal morbidity and mortality.[88] Neonates at greatest risk are less than 32 weeks gestation and weigh less than 1,500 grams. Survivors of necrotizing enterocolitis have significant long-term nutritional and developmental problems.[89]

ETIOLOGY

The etiology of necrotizing enterocolitis is multifactoral. Perinatal asphyxia, infection, umbilical artery catheterization, exchange blood transfusions, hyperosmolar feedings, and cyanotic congenital heart disease have all been implicated. The common feature of this disease is hypoperfusion of the gastrointestinal tract, with subsequent mucosal and bowel wall ischemia. Initial mucosal ischemia may make the bowel more susceptible to bacterial damage and the effects of hyperosmolar feedings.

SIGNS AND SYMPTOMS

The most common initial signs of necrotizing enterocolitis are abdominal distention and bloody feces. Apnea spells, lethargy, and thermal instability also occur. Hypovolemic shock and metabolic acidosis may occur secondary to generalized peritonitis from multiple bowel perforations. A hemorrhagic diathesis secondary to thrombocytopenia is often present. Bowel gas frequently penetrates the damaged mucosa and enters the submucosal region; as a result, gas may gain access to mesenteric veins and the portal venous system. Gas in the intestinal submucosa results in the classic *pneumatosis intestinalis* seen on radiographs of the abdomen. Respiratory distress syndrome requiring mechanical ventilation of the lungs frequently co-exists.

TREATMENT

Medical treatment, consisting of gastric decompression, intravenous fluids, and antibiotics, is often successful in the management of neonates with necrotizing enterocolitis.[90] Surgery is reserved for those neonates in whom medical treatment has failed, as evidenced by peritonitis, bowel perforation, and progressive metabolic acidosis.

MANAGEMENT OF ANESTHESIA

Neonates with necrotizing enterocolitis are frequently hypovolemic and require vigorous fluid resuscitation with crystalloid and colloid solutions before induction of anesthesia. Blood and platelet transfusions are often necessary. Adequate monitoring of fluid resuscitation is critical. Catheters placed in peripheral arteries provide the ability to measure blood pressure continuously, as well as to monitor arterial blood gases, pH, hematocrit, and electrolytes. Transcutaneous oxygen monitors reflect not only skin oxygen partial pressures but also skin blood flow and, therefore, are helpful not only for monitoring oxygenation but also for monitoring hydration status. It must be appreciated that rapid fluid administration to preterm neonates may cause intracranial hemorrhage or the reopening of the ductus arteriosus.[91]

Volatile anesthetics can produce significant hypotension in these neonates, particularly if hypovolemia is present. Therefore, reduced doses of ketamine, fentanyl, or sufentanil plus nondepolarizing muscle relaxants are useful for the maintenance of anesthesia. Nitrous oxide should be avoided, as it may increase the size of gas bubbles in mesenteric veins and the portal venous system. Gas embolism can also occur if portal venous gas bubbles traverse the ductus venosus and enter the inferior vena cava.[92] Postoperative mechanical ventilation of the lungs is usually required because of abdominal distention and co-existing respiratory distress syndrome.

NERVOUS SYSTEM

Diseases of the nervous system that afflict pediatric patients include cerebral palsy, hydrocephalus, myelomeningocele, craniostenosis, seizure disorders, trisomy-21, neurofibromatosis, and Reye's syndrome. Management of these patients in the perioperative period is optimized by understanding the pathophysiology of their diseases.

Cerebral Palsy

Cerebral palsy includes a group of nonprogressive disorders characterized by central motor deficits resulting from hypoxic or anoxic cerebral damage. Etiologic factors include genetic abnormalities, metabolic defects, or injury to the brain, which may occur in the perinatal period. In addition, mechanical birth trauma, congenital cerebrovascular malformations, intrauterine and neonatal infections, toxins, prematurity, kernicterus, and hypoglycemia are known causes of cerebral palsy. Finally, cerebral palsy can be due to anatomic disorders, with localized or diffuse atrophy of the cerebral cortex, basal ganglia, and subcortical white matter. Despite the seeming association between a multitude of factors and cerebral palsy, the cause of most cases of cerebral palsy is unknown.[93]

SIGNS AND SYMPTOMS

Cerebral palsy is classified as spastic, extrapyramidal, atonic, and mixed. The most common manifestation is skeletal muscle spasticity. Extrapyramidal cerebral palsy is associated with choreoathetosis and dystonia. Cerebellar ataxia is characteristic of atonic cerebral palsy. Varying degrees of mental retardation and speech defects can accompany cerebral palsy. Seizure disorders can co-exist with cerebral palsy.

Children with cerebral palsy may have varying degrees of spasticity of different skeletal muscle groups, resulting in contractures and fixed deformities of several joints of both upper and lower extremities. These include fixed flexion and internal rotation deformities of the hip joint due to involved adductor and flexor muscles and plantar flexion of the ankles due to involvement of the Achilles tendon.

These children often undergo elective orthopedic corrective procedures, such as Achilles tendon lengthening, hip adductor and iliopsoas release, and derotational osteotomy of the femur. Stereotactic surgery may be performed in attempts to reduce skeletal muscle rigidity, spasticity, and dyskinesia. Dental restorations requiring general anesthesia are frequently necessary in patients with cerebral palsy. Gastroesophageal reflux is common in children with central nervous system disorders, and antireflux operations are often performed.

Children with cerebral palsy are frequently receiving phenobarbital and phenytoin for control of seizures, and dantrolene for relief of skeletal muscle spasticity. Phenytoin may lead to gingival hyperplasia and megaloblastic anemia. Phenobarbital stimulates hepatic microsomal enzyme activity, and may result in altered responses to drugs that undergo metabolism in the liver.

MANAGEMENT OF ANESTHESIA

Management of anesthesia in patients with cerebral palsy includes intubation of the trachea because of the propensity for gastroesophageal reflux and poor function of laryngeal and pharyngeal reflexes. Although patients with cerebral palsy have skeletal muscle spasticity, succinylcholine does not produce abnormal potassium release.[94] Body temperature should be monitored, as these patients are susceptible to the development of hypothermia during the intraoperative period. Emergence from anesthesia may be quite slow because of the cerebral damage from cerebral palsy and the presence of hypothermia. Extubation of the trachea should be delayed until these children are fully awake and body temperature has returned to normal. Postoperatively, these children have a high incidence of pulmonary complications.

Hydrocephalus

Hydrocephalus in infants and children is due to an increase in cerebrospinal fluid volume, resulting in enlarged cerebral ventricles and increased intracranial pressure. Hydrocephalus due to overproduction or abnormal absorption of cerebrospinal fluid is classified as nonobstructive or communicating hydrocephalus, as there is no obstruction to the flow of cerebrospinal fluid. Obstructive hydrocephalus is present when there is obstruction to the flow of cerebrospinal fluid between the sites of production and its absorption from the subarachnoid space. This obstruction can be due to congenital, neoplastic, post-traumatic, or postinflammatory lesions. Congenital causes of obstructive hydrocephlus include (1) Arnold-Chiari malformation, in which the basilar subarachnoid pathways are underdeveloped; (2) aqueductal stenosis between the third and fourth ventricles; and (3) Dandy-Walker syndrome, with occlusion at the outlet of the fourth ventricle by a congenital membrane. Ventricular dilation commonly follows periventricular-intraventricular hemorrhage that occurs in the preterm infants.

SIGNS AND SYMPTOMS

Signs and symptoms depend on the age of the child and the rapidity with which hydrocephalus occurs. For example, the prominent feature of congenital hydrocephalus is an abnormal enlargement of the head, which may present at birth or may occur soon after birth. Enlargement of the head is usually prominent in the frontal area of the skull. The cranial vault transilluminates in affected areas, and cranial sutures are separated. Percussion of the skull produces a resonant note. The eyes are often deviated inferiorly. Scalp veins are dilated, and the skin is thin and shiny. Optic atrophy due to compression of the optic nerve can occur in chronic and untreated cases of hydrocephalus. Late onset hydrocephalus may not result in an enlarged head but instead may cause significant increases in intracranial pressure. Hydrocephalus due to Arnold-Chiari malformation or aqueductal stenosis can lead to medullary and lower cranial nerve dysfunction, resulting in swallowing abnormalities, stridor, and atrophy of the tongue. Hydrocephalic children may have varying degrees of intellectual dysfunction; the dysfunction does not correlate with the size of the ventricles or

the thinness of the cortical mantle. Serial measurement of head circumference, radiographs of the skull, and computed tomography will confirm the diagnosis.

TREATMENT

Treatment depends on the mechanism responsible for hydrocephalus. Operative excision of the lesion responsible for obstruction to flow of cerebrospinal fluid is performed if feasible. A shunting procedure is necessary if the obstruction cannot be relieved surgically. The shunt system employs a one-way valve, which directs flow of cerebrospinal fluid away from the ventricles. Shunting procedures include ventriculocisternotomy (Torkildsen's procedure), and ventriculoatrial and ventriculoperitoneal shunts. Less common are ventriculocholecystostomy, ventriculoureterostomy, and ventriculospinal shunts.

The ventriculoatrial shunt is performed for either nonobstructive or obstructive hydrocephalus. The distal end of the catheter is placed in the right atrium, as indicated by monitoring changes in venous pressure wave patterns, as the catheter is advanced into the atrium from the superior vena cava. Complications from atrial catheters include thrombosis of the internal jugular vein or superior vena cava, septicemia, meningitis, pleural effusion, pulmonary embolism, and pulmonary hypertension. Furthermore, growth of these children will displace cardiac ends of catheters into the superior vena cava, necessitating revision of shunts or their conversion to ventriculoperitoneal shunts. Erosion of a ventriculoperitoneal catheter into a bronchus, with development of a ventriculobronchial fistula, has been described.[95]

MANAGEMENT OF ANESTHESIA

Operative procedures in children with hydrocephalus are likely to be necessary for placement, revision, or removal of shunts. Some of these children will have increased intracranial pressure, and precautions for control of such pressure during anesthesia should be taken. This is particularly important if these children are having shunts inserted before craniotomy for excision of intracranial tumors. For infants and children with normal intracranial pressure, induction of anesthesia with thiopental plus succinylcholine or intermediate-acting muscle relaxants to facilitate intubation of the trachea, followed by maintenance of anesthesia with volatile anesthetics or opioids plus nitrous oxide, is acceptable. In the presence of co-existing intracranial hypertension, it may be important to consider the potential for further increases in intracranial pressure to occur in association with administration of succinylcholine.[96] It should be appreciated that sudden hypotension sometimes occurs when tensely distended cerebral ventricles are decompressed. Furthermore, venous air embolism and increased blood loss can occur when large neck veins are opened for placement of atrial catheters. Postoperatively, these patients are maintained in slight head-up positions, to allow free drainage of cerebrospinal fluid.

During surgery in children with a ventriculoperitoneal shunts, excessive pressure on the skin of the scalp overlying the shunt should be avoided by rotating the head to the side opposite the shunt. Pressure over the ventricular reservoir can produce skin necrosis and possibly cause shunt malfunction.

Myelomeningocele

The neural tube of the embryo is formed from the ectodermal neural crest. The neural crest deepens to form the neural groove, the margins of which fuse to form the neural tube. Failure of closure of the caudal end of the neural tube can result in (1) spina bifida, characterized by defects of the vertebral arches; (2) meningocele, characterized by a sac that contains meninges; and (3) myelomeningocele, characterized by a sac that contains neural elements.

SIGNS AND SYMPTOMS

Children with a meningocele are usually born without neurologic deficits; those with myelomeningocele are likely to manifest varying degrees of motor and sensory deficit. For example, children with lumbosacral myelomeningoceles manifest flaccid paraplegia; loss of sensation to pin prick; and loss of anal, urethral, and vesical sphincter tone. Associated congenital anomalies include club foot, hydrocephalus, dislocation of the hips, extrophy of the bladder, prolapsed uterus, Klippel-Feil syndrome, and congenital cardiac defects.

These children may develop severe dilation of the upper urinary tract, necessitating urinary diversion procedures, such as vesicostomy, cutaneous ureterostomies, and ileal or colon conduits. They are likely to experience recurrent urinary tract infections, which may be complicated by gram-negative sepsis. The need for corrective orthopedic procedures on the lower extremities is predictable. As these patients mature, they have a tendency to develop varying degrees of scoliosis, often requiring posterior spinal fusion. Finally, there is frequent need for replacement or revision of ventriculoperitoneal or ventriculoatrial shunts because of infection of the shunt or its malfunction due to malposition of the distal end of the catheter, reflecting normal patient growth.

MANAGEMENT OF ANESTHESIA

Absence of skin covering a myelomeningocele introduces the risk of infection, necessitating surgical closure within a few hours of birth. Closure is performed during local or general anesthesia. If general anesthesia is selected, awake tracheal intubation may be performed in the lateral decubitus position to avoid pressure on the meningeal sac. Anesthesia may also be induced in the supine position if the sac is protected by elevation of the infant on a doughnut-shaped support. Maintenance of anesthesia is with inhaled anesthetics, delivered using mechanical ventilation of the lungs. The operative procedures is performed with these patients in the prone position. Although succinylcholine may be used to facilitate tracheal intubation, longer-acting muscle relaxants should be avoided, as the surgeon may need to use a nerve stimulator to identify functional neural elements. Surgical closure of the myelomeningocele sac must be tight enough to prevent leakage of cerebrospinal fluid, as confirmed by raising pressures in the sac with positive airway pressure. Postoperatively, neonates should be kept in the prone position and a high index of suspicion maintained for the development of increased intracranial pressure.

Older children with myelomeningoceles require numerous corrective procedures, primarily involving the urologic and musculoskeletal systems. Although myelomeningoceles produce both upper and lower motor neuron dysfunction, succinylcholine does not produce excessive increases in potassium levels.[97] Inhaled anesthetics or opioids may be used for maintenance of anesthesia. Myelomeningocele patients, however, may have abnormal ventilatory responses to hypoxia and hypercarbia.[98] These patients often have gastroesophageal reflux and abnormal vocal cord motility, emphasizing the need to take precautions against the occurrence of aspiration.

Craniostenosis (Craniosynostosis)

Craniostenosis is a congenital disorder resulting in a variety of deformities due to premature closure of one or more cranial sutures. Premature closure of the sagittal suture is the most common. The incidence of craniostenosis is 1 in every 1,000 live births.

SIGNS AND SYMPTOMS

Craniostenosis results in deformity of the skull, which may lead to exophthalmus, optic atrophy, blindness, increased intracranial pressure, seizures, and mental retardation. Congenital cardiac defects and hydrocephalus may also be associated with craniostenosis. The shape of the deformed skull depends on the location of the suture that closes prematurely, since the cranial vault can compensate and grow only in areas with patent sutures. Radiographs of the skull and computed tomography will confirm the diagnosis.

TREATMENT

Craniectomy is the surgical procedure effective for treatment of craniostenosis. This operation is usually performed as soon as the diagnosis is confirmed, since prompt correction has fewer complications and better cosmetic results. When multiple cranial sutures are involved, craniectomy is performed as a staged procedure. Craniectomy involves removing linear strips of bone on either side of the involved sutures and extending them across the adjoining normal cranial sutures. The adjacent periosteum is stripped widely to retard new bone formation.

MANAGEMENT OF ANESTHESIA

The possibility of increased intracranial pressure must be considered in children with craniostenosis. Nevertheless, most of these children have normal intracranial pressures, and induction of anesthesia with intravenous administration of thiopental, followed by succinylcholine or intermediate-acting muscle relaxants to facilitate intubation of the trachea, is an acceptable approach. Selection of drugs for maintenance of anesthesia should consider the likelihood that the surgeon will infiltrate the incision area with local anesthetic solutions containing epinephrine so as to minimize blood loss associated with skin incision. Continuous monitoring of arterial blood pressure via a catheter in a peripheral artery is useful. Sudden and rapidly exsanguinating blood loss from the longitudinal sinus is possible during craniectomy. Most of the blood loss, however, occurs during bone stripping and is gradual. Since most of these patients are positioned prone, care should be taken to prevent pressure damage to the face and eyes. Patients are often tilted into slight head-up positions to minimize blood loss from venous oozing. Depending on the degree of tilt and area of surgery, intraoperative venous air embolism is a distinct possibility; and precautions should be taken to prevent, recognize, and acutely treat such episodes.

Postoperatively, blood is likely to ooze into the wound, and these patients often need additional transfusion of blood. They should be closely monitored for the onset of hypotension or localizing neurologic signs indicative of epidural hematomas.

Seizure Disorders (Epilepsy)

Seizure disorders are characterized by recurrent, but usually transient, episodes of disturbed central nervous system function (see Chapter 18). Causes of seizure disorders in children are often unknown but known causes include metabolic disorders (phenylketonuria, hypoglycemia, kernicterus, tuberous sclerosis) and organic cerebral disorders (brain tumor, cerebral injury).

Seizure disorders can be classified as generalized and partial. Generalized seizure disorders are subdivided into grand mal and focal cortical. Petit mal, akinetic, myoclonic, and psychomotor are examples of partial seizure disorders. Treatment is with drugs proven effective for suppressing seizure activity for the specific type of disorder (see Tables 18-3 and 18-4).

GRAND MAL SEIZURES

Grand mal seizures are characterized by tonic-clonic motor activity, usually preceded by sensory or motor aura. An abrupt onset of tonic skeletal muscle spasm parallels the loss of consciousness. Anal and bladder sphincter tone is lost. All respiratory activity is arrested, resulting in arterial hypoxemia. The tonic phase lasts 20 seconds to 40 seconds and is followed by a clonic phase lasting for a variable period of time. In the postictal period, patients may sleep or enter into a confused state, performing automatic acts. Treatment is directed toward maintaining arterial oxygenation and stopping excess skeletal muscle activity (see Chapter 18).

FOCAL CORTICAL SEIZURES

Focal cortical seizures are also known as Jacksonian epilepsy. Manifestations can be motor or sensory, depending on the site of neu-

ronal discharge in the central nervous system. There is no loss of consciousness. Localized sensory attacks are rare in children. Focal cortical seizure activity may spread to adjoining areas in the central nervous system, culminating in grand mal seizures.

PETIT MAL SEIZURES

Petit mal seizures are characterized by brief losses of awareness, which may be associated with such additional manifestations as staring, blinking, or rolling of the eyes. These seizures usually last less than 30 seconds and rarely are associated with loss of postural motor tone. Clinical evidence of petit mal seizure disorders rarely appears before 3 years of age and frequently disappears by puberty.

AKINETIC SEIZURES

Akinetic seizures are characterized by sudden brief losses of consciousness and absence of postural muscle tone.

MYOCLONIC SEIZURES

Myoclonic seizures often manifest as isolated clonic jerks in response to sensory stimuli. Sudden drooping of the head and flexion of the arms is characteristic. Usually a single group of skeletal muscles is involved. Infantile myoclonic seizure disorders typically afflict children less than 2 years of age and may involve more than one group of skeletal muscles. This disorder is often associated with degenerative and metabolic brain diseases.

PSYCHOMOTOR SEIZURES

Psychomotor seizures are characterized by impairment of consciousness, inappropriate but purposeful motor acts, hallucinations, illusions, sudden feelings of fear, amnestic episodes, and bizarre visceral sensations. These types of seizure disorders are often preceded by an aura. During psychomotor seizures, these children may gradually lose postural tone, without the occurrence of clonic or tonic movements.

Trisomy-21
(Down's Syndrome)

Trisomy-21 occurs in about 0.15 percent of live births. About 80 percent of conceptions with trisomy-21 terminate in spontaneous abortion. The abnormality in these patients is due to the presence of an extra (trisomy) 21st chromosome. The risk of having a child with trisomy-21 increases with maternal age. For example, the 20-year-old mother has a risk of about 1 in 2,000, but the risk increases to about 1 in 400 by age 35, and to 1 in 40 in mothers over 45.

SIGNS AND SYMPTOMS

Children with trisomy-21 are readily recognized by their characteristic flat facies with oblique palpebral fissures (hence the old term "mongolism"), single palmar crease (simian crease), and dysplastic middle phalanx of the fifth finger. Several features alter the upper airway in these children. For example, the nasopharynx is narrow, and the tonsils and adenoids unusually large. The tongue is normal at birth but later becomes enlarged due to hypertrophy of the papillae. To compensate for their restricted airways, these children habitually hold their mouths open, with their tongues slightly protruding. Chronic upper airway obstruction, which may lead to arterial hypoxemia, is a result of airway changes characteristic of trisomy-21.

Congenital heart disease occurs in about 40 percent of patients with trisomy-21. Endocardial cushion defects account for about one-half of the total, and ventricular septal defects occur in about one-fourth of these patients. Other abnormalities include tetralogy of Fallot, patent ductus arteriosus, and atrial septal defect of the secundum type. Surgical correction of congenital heart disease in children with

trisomy-21 is associated with increased morbidity (postoperative atelectasis and pneumonia) and mortality, presumably due to increased susceptibility to recurrent infections, and an increased incidence of co-existing pulmonary hypertension. It has been suggested that impaired development of alveoli and the pulmonary vasculature, combined with arterial hypoxemia due to chronic upper airway obstruction, predispose patients with trisomy-21 to preoperative pulmonary hypertension and postoperative pulmonary complications.[99]

Congenital duodenal atresia occurs 300 times more frequently in patients with trisomy-21. Microcephaly and small brain mass are present. Mental retardation in noninstitutionalized patients tends to be mild to moderate, and measurements of social and vocational adjustment tend to be in the low-normal range. Behavioral traits are subject to great individual variability, but infants with trisomy-21 are most often described as being good babies. Later, they are often characterized as content, good-natured, and affectionate. They may also be noted for their extreme stubborness.

Oblique palpebral fissures and the presence of Brushfield spots (light-colored, slightly elevated spots near the periphery of the iris) are characteristic of the eyes in trisomy-21. There is a high incidence of cataracts and strabismus, often necessitating surgical correction. Otitis media and hearing loss are common, necessitating frequent ear examinations and myringotomies.

The skin appears too large for the skeleton, especially at the wrists and ankles. Furthermore, these patients are frequently obese. Both of these factors tend to make venous cannulation more difficult than in average pediatric patients.

Numerous musculoskeletal changes are noted in patients with trisomy-21. For example, about 20 percent of these patients have an asymptomatic dislocation of the atlas on the axis. Although spinal cord compression is rare, this potential hazard must be remembered if the head and neck are forcefully manipulated during intubation of the trachea.[100] Screening for atlanto-axial instability includes lateral radiographs of the neck in flexed, extended, and neutral positions. If the distance between the anterior arch of the atlas and the adjacent odontoid process exceeds 5 mm, the diagnosis of atlanto-axial instability is likely.[100] Posterior cervical spine fusion is required for any patient who is symptomatic from this subluxation.

Most hematologic parameters are within normal limits, although polycythemia has been observed. Leukemia occurs in 1 percent of patients, but an increased incidence of other malignancies is not observed. Plasma concentrations of dopamine-B-hydroxylase, the enzyme that converts dopamine to norepinephrine, are reduced. Plasma concentrations of norepinephrine are not lowered, and the sympathetic nervous system responds normally to stress. Pharmacologic responses to atropine are unusual in that mydriasis occurs more rapidly in these patients, although the degree and duration of pupillary dilation is normal. Furthermore, cardiovascular responses to atropine are not altered. Thyroid function is normal in these patients.

MANAGEMENT OF ANESTHESIA

Preoperative medication of patients with trisomy-21 may include anticholinergic drugs, such as atropine or glycopyrrolate, to reduce upper airway secretions. As with other patients with mental retardation, responses to sedatives are unpredictable. Occasionally, small doses of ketamine injected intramuscularly will facilitate preparation for induction of anesthesia in obstinate patients. Patency of the upper airway may be difficult to maintain after the patient loses consciousness, reflecting the short neck, small mouth, narrow nasopharynx, and large tongue characteristic of these patients. Nevertheless, tracheal intubation is usually not difficult if one remembers that asymptomatic dislocation of the atlas on the axis is present in about 20 percent of these patients. In the absence of congenital heart disease, most commonly used inhalation or intravenous techniques of general anesthesia are acceptable. Otherwise, selection of anesthetic drugs is determined by the pathophysiology of the congenital cardiac lesion (see Chapter 3).

Neurofibromatosis

Neurofibromatosis is a congenital and progressive disease of supportive tissues of the nervous system, with an incidence of 1 in every 3,000 live births (see Chapter 18). Inheritance is an autosomal dominant trait with variable penetrance, although spontaneous cases also occur. It is estimated that 40 percent of children with an affected parent will develop neurofibromatosis.

SIGNS AND SYMPTOMS

Café-au-lait spots are the classic skin lesion associated with neurofibromatosis. These spots are macular brown pigmented areas of skin with definite circumscribed geographic borders. Five or more café-au-lait spots greater than 0.5 cm in diameter are diagnostic. Like many of the signs and symptoms of neurofibromatosis, café-au-lait spots are often absent or minimally present at birth. Axillary freckling is also diagnostic. In older patients, benign cutaneous and subcutaneous neurofibromas, ranging in size from a few millimeters to several centimeters in size, may be scattered over the entire surface of the body.

Benign neurofibromas arise from cells that comprise the sheaths of peripheral, cranial, or autonomic nerves. These tumors may be pendulous or plexiform. Their mass frequently results in cosmetic, neurologic, or obstructive problems, which necessitate radical surgical excision. Plexiform neurofibromas have a propensity for malignant degeneration. Indeed, nearly 30 percent of adults with neurofibromatosis eventually develop peripheral nerve sarcomas. Sarcomatous degeneration, however, rarely occurs in children. In addition to sarcomas, patients with neurofibromatosis also have an increased incidence of epithelial cancers, particularly malignant melanoma and carcinoma of the breast.

Neurofibromas may develop in almost any part of the central nervous system, including the cranial nerves. In children, the most common intracranial tumor is an optic glioma; in adults acoustic neuroma is most common. Mental retardation occurs in 8 percent of patients. The mental defect dates from birth and does not usually progress with age. Seizure disorders are present in about 10 percent of patients, and nearly 50 percent of these patients have associated intracranial tumors.

Neurofibromatosis can involve the upper airway, including the larynx.[101] For example, macroglossia or the presence of intraoral neurofibromas may make direct laryngoscopy for intubation of the trachea difficult. Cranial nerve involvement may impair swallowing and gag reflexes. Large mediastinal tumors can compress the lungs and lead to pulmonary insufficiency. Pulmonary parenchyma may be primarily involved, with obliteration of alveoli and blood vessels by a process referred to as fibrosing alveolitis. Pulmonary hypertension may be present in advanced stages.

Disorders of bone growth are noted in at least one-half of patients with neurofibromatosis. Scoliosis and cranial deformities are the most frequent and serious of the skeletal defects. Surgical correction of scoliosis is often necessary in children with neurofibromatosis. Patients with scoliosis may also have an associated defect in the cervical spine, such that inadvertent cervical cord damage can result while positioning these patients for corrective orthopedic surgery.

Involvement of blood vessels occurs frequently in children with neurofibromatosis. Vascular lesions can lead to arterial stenosis or obstruction. Children usually present either with diminished or absent peripheral pulses, or with renal hypertension resulting from coarctation of the aorta or renal artery stenosis.

Neurofibromas may arise from Auerbach's plexus anywhere in the gastrointestinal tract. These patients may present with an asymptomatic mass, gastrointestinal obstruction, or bleeding. Genitalia are rarely involved in the cutaneous manifestations of neurofibromatosis.

Pheochromocytoma occurs in about 1 percent of patients with neurofibromatosis. Indeed, deaths occurring during or after administration of anesthesia have been reported in patients with neurofibromatosis and unsuspected pheochromocytoma.[102] The two most common solid tumors of childhood, neuroblastoma and nephroblastoma (Wilms' tumor), have also been linked to neurofibromatosis.

MANAGEMENT OF ANESTHESIA

Airway obstruction occurring after induction of anesthesia in patients with neurofibromatosis can reflect the presence of oral, laryngeal, neck, or thoracic masses.[103] In older patients, fibrosing alveolitis, resulting in ventilation-perfusion mismatch, decreased pulmonary compliance, and pulmonary hypertension may impair ventilatory reserve. The occurrence of hypertension or cardiac dysrhythmias during the perioperative period may relate to renal hypertension or unrecognized pheochromocytoma.[102] Patients with neurofibromatosis and scoliosis are also likely to have cervical spine defects, which must be recognized before positioning for operative procedures. Responses to muscle relaxants must be monitored carefully, since these patients have been reported to be both sensitive and resistant to succinylcholine and sensitive to nondepolarizing muscle relaxants.[104] Nevertheless, the true incidence or clinical significance of altered responses to muscle relaxants in these patients has not been confirmed.

Reye's Syndrome

Reye's syndrome, or acute encephalopathy with fatty infiltration of the viscera, causes death via diffuse cerebral edema, resulting ultimately in brain infarction and herniation. Management of patients with Reye's syndrome is directed toward monitoring and control of intracranial pressure, until natural resolution of the disease process occurs.[105]

SIGNS AND SYMPTOMS

Most cases of Reye's syndrome develop in preteen children, after a 3 day to 7 day prodromal viral illness involving the respiratory and/or gastrointestinal tracts. Protracted vomiting or neurologic signs associated with increased intracranial pressure herald the onset of Reye's syndrome. The initial physical examination reveals a mild fever, tachycardia, tachypnea, and hepatomegaly. Neurologic examination may reveal either a lethargic individual or a combative one, with hyperactive tendon reflexes. Serial neurologic examinations may reveal rapid deterioration in neurologic status.

Laboratory abnormalities include elevated plasma concentrations of liver transaminase enzymes and ammonia. Prothrombin and partial thromboplastin times are prolonged. Plasma glucose concentrations are often decreased. Respiratory alkalosis is a frequent finding on measurement of the arterial blood gases and pH. Examination of cerebrospinal fluid typically reveals no cellular or protein abnormalities, and glucose concentrations parallel plasma glucose levels.

PATHOPHYSIOLOGY

The brain and the liver are the principal organs affected in Reye's syndrome, although the kidneys, pancreas, and skeletal muscles may also be involved. Clinical symptoms and biochemical derangements indicate that both liver and brain are already injured by the time the patient is first examined. Signs of injury to these organs progress for 3 days to 6 days and then resolve rapidly if cerebral edema does not result in death.

On pathologic examination, all hepatocytes and cortical neurons appear to have been damaged. Light microscopy of liver specimens reveals a panlobular fatty liver with abundant and small fat droplets in hepatocytes. Similar microvescicular fatty infiltrates are seen in renal, pancreatic, and myocardial cells. Electron microscopy reveals mitochondrial de-rangement in liver, skeletal muscle, and cortical neuron tissues, which reverts to normal with recovery. The generalized mitochondrial injury is thought to result in derangements in metabolic pathways of the urea and Kreb cycles, resulting in elevated plasma concentrations of ammonia and free fatty acids. In addition, there is depletion of glycogen stores, leading to hypoglycemia.

ETIOLOGY

Reye's syndrome is predominantly found in patients under the age of 10 years.[106] Almost all cases are associated with a prodromal viral illness. Influenza A and B and varicella are the most frequently associated viral infections, but more than a dozen others have also been implicated. There is a striking association between the use of salicylates during these viral illnesses and development of Reye's syndrome.[107] Since discovery of this association and appropriate warnings about use of salicylates, there has been a steady decline in the incidence of Reye's syndrome. In fact, in 1985 the incidence of Reye's syndrome was the lowest since epidemiologic surveillance was instituted in 1973. Cases associated with influenza tend to be clustered in midwinter. In contrast, varicella-associated cases tend to be sporadic and occur throughout the year. Retrospective studies of autopsies indicate that this may be a relatively new disease, as very few cases compatible with this diagnosis can be found before 1950.

TREATMENT

Treatment of mild cases of Reye's syndrome (plasma ammonia concentrations less than 100 μM·L^{-1}) is directed toward reversing associated metabolic derangements. For example, management of these patients includes administration of intravenous fluids, vitamin K if the prothrombin time is prolonged, oral neomycin, and lactulose.

Treatment of severe Reye's syndrome (plasma ammonia concentrations greater than

100 μM·L^{-1}) is similar to treatment of patients with increased intracranial pressure. Therapeutic and monitoring measures include intubation of the trachea, mechanical ventilation of the lungs, placement of an intracranial pressure monitor, insertion of a central venous or pulmonary artery catheter, and introduction of a catheter into a peripheral artery. These measures are initiated in the operating room. Intubation of the trachea is performed after intravenous administration of thiopental and muscle relaxants (succinylcholine questionable in view of its ability to transiently elevate intracranial pressure) plus hyperventilation of the lungs to lower the arterial partial pressures of carbon dioxide to 20 mmHg to 25 mmHg. After tracheal intubation, a burr hold is created for placement of a transducer to monitor intracranial pressure. This transducer must be accurate and reliable, since therapeutic interventions are highly dependent on measurements of intracranial pressure. The goal is to maintain intracranial pressure below 15 mmHg and cerebral perfusion pressure above 50 mmHg. Transducers used to measure arterial blood pressure must be placed at the level of the circle of Willis to assure accurate calculation of cerebral perfusion pressure. Placement of the central venous or pulmonary artery catheter is often accomplished through the basilic vein of the arm, so as to circumvent the need for the head-down position, which would be necessitated by use of the subclavian or internal jugular veins. It must be appreciated that even transient head-down positioning may result in sustained increases in intracranial pressure. Cerebral perfusion pressure can usually be maintained above 50 mmHg if intravascular fluid volume is optimized by administering colloid and crystalloid solutions, so as to maintain central venous pressures between 5 mmHg and 10 mmHg.

Cerebral water content in patients with severe Reye's syndrome is thought to be increased, secondary to swelling of glial structures that follows mitochondrial damage. In addition, computed tomography has suggested that cerebral blood volume is increased in patients with Reye's syndrome. The volume of the intracranial contents can be decreased by several mechanisms. For example, cerebral

water content can be decreased by administration of osmotic diuretics such as mannitol. Cerebral blood volume can be decreased by (1) placement of patients in 30 degree head-up positions to eliminate the contribution of venous pressure to cerebral blood volume; (2) hyperventilation of the lungs to decrease cerebral blood flow via vasoconstriction; and (3) administration of large doses of barbiturates to decrease cerebral blood flow via vasoconstriction. Barbiturates are useful if intracranial pressure cannot be maintained below 15 mmHg using maximal doses of mannitol. Barbiturate coma is induced with large doses of pentobarbital (5 mg·kg^{-1} to 20 mg·kg^{-1} loading dose and 2 mg·kg^{-1}·hr^{-1} to 3.5 mg·kg^{-1}·hr^{-1}).[105] Plasma concentrations of pentobarbital are maintained between 25 μg·ml^{-1} to 45 μg·ml^{-1} by adjusting the rate of barbiturate infusion. Intravenous dexamethasone (1.0 mg·kg^{-1}·day^{-1}) is also given, although this drug is of unproven value for management of patients with Reye's syndrome. Bifrontal craniectomy is used as a final method to maintain cerebral blood flow should intracranial pressure remain elevated despite maximum medical therapy. Management of anesthesia for craniectomy is directed solely toward maintaining cerebral perfusion pressure, as these patients are likely to have already received large doses of barbiturates.

Cerebral perfusion pressures may become inadequate because of decreases in mean arterial blood pressure. The differential diagnosis includes decreased intravascular fluid volume, myocardial depression from barbiturates, vasodilation from septic shock, and vasodilation from barbiturates. In this situation, measurement of thermodilution cardiac outputs and cardiac filling pressures by means of a pulmonary artery catheter is of value in making the correct diagnosis and instituting proper therapy. For example, continuous infusions of catecholamines, such as dopamine or dobutamine, may be necessary to improve cardiac output and restore mean arterial blood pressure to acceptable levels.

Treatment for severe Reye's syndrome can be gradually withdrawn when intracranial pressure remains below 15 mmHg for 36 hours to 48 hours. Intensive treatment of patients with Reye's syndrome, including barbiturate coma and occasionally bifrontal craniectomy, appears to have substantially reduced the mortality associated with this disease. Patients who survive Reye's syndrome are likely to recover completely, with no permanent metabolic or neurologic sequelae.

CRANIOFACIAL ABNORMALITIES

Craniofacial abnormalities are of consequence to patients because of cosmetic appearance. Indeed, these patients will often present for major reconstructive surgical procedures. In addition, these abnormalities are important because they may be associated with airway obstruction. Craniofacial abnormalities likely to require surgical correction include (1) cleft lip and palate; (2) mandibular hypoplasia as associated with Pierre Robin, Treacher Collins', and Goldenhar syndromes; and (3) hypertelorism.[108]

Cleft Lip and Palate

Cleft lip and palate, considered together, constitute the third most common congenital anomaly requiring surgical correction at an early age. About 50 percent of patients have both cleft lip and palate, and 14 percent of patients with cleft lip (with or without cleft palate) and 33 percent with cleft palate have associated congenital anomalies, which may include congenital heart disease. Infants with cleft lip and palate have problems with deglutition and frequently experience pulmonary aspiration. Furthermore, the incidence of upper respiratory tract infections is increased, resulting in chronic otitis media. Anemia is often present, reflecting poor nutrition due to feeding problems.

TREATMENT

Surgical treatment of cleft lip (cheiloplasty) is based on variations of a Z-plasty. Treatment for cleft palate (platoplasty) is per-formed by midline closure of the cleft, after adequate mobilization of the tissues of the hard and soft palate with bilateral relaxing incisions. Pushback palatoplasty is a procedure performed to add length to the soft palate with a local soft tissue flap. Posterior pharyngeal flap is another procedure, wherein a flap of mucosa and muscle is raised from the posterior pharyngeal wall and attached to the posterior aspect of the soft palate. Cheiloplasty is usually performed when infants are 2 weeks to 3 months of age, but palatoplasty is delayed until about 18 months of age.

MANAGEMENT OF ANESTHESIA

Induction of anesthesia for children with cleft lip and/or palate depends on the degree of airway abnormality. For example, induction of anesthesia for patients with no other airway anomalies can be safety accomplished by intravenous administration of barbiturates followed by muscle relaxants to facilitate intubation of the trachea. Conversely, volatile anesthetics and intubation of the trachea during spontaneous ventilation are recommended for children with associated anomalies such as Pierre Robin syndrome. In infants with large cavernous defects of the palate, intubation of the trachea may be difficult if the blade of the laryngoscope slips into the cleft, making it difficult to manipulate the blade. Inserting a small piece of sponge or dental roll to fill the gap will reduce the likelihood of this problem. Tracheal tubes should be taped to the lower lip in the midline, so as to minimize distortion of facial anatomy. Use of preformed (RAE) tracheal tubes reduces the likelihood of tracheal tube occlusion by the palate retractor during palatoplasty.

Maintenance of anesthesia is most often with volatile anesthetics plus nitrous oxide. The presence of associated congenital heart disease may influence selection of anesthetic drugs and muscle relaxants, as well as the management of ventilation. In addition, selection of volatile anesthetics should consider the likelihood that the surgical site will be infiltrated with local anesthetic solutions containing epinephrine. Nevertheless, in contrast to adults, children tolerate high doses of epinephrine without development of cardiac dysrhythmias during general anesthesia.[108,109] A high index of suspicion for accidental dislodgement of the tube from the trachea must be maintained during the operative procedure. Indeed, breath sounds should be constantly monitored with a precordial stethoscope. An end-tidal carbon dioxide monitor is also a useful monitor for continued tracheal placement of the tube during intraoral surgery. Conjunctivitis and corneal abrasions are possible hazards, such that the eyes should be lubricated with ophthalmic ointment and protected with eye covers. Blood loss requiring transfusion is uncommon during cheiloplasty or palatoplasty.

Postoperative airway problems are common after palatoplasty. For this reason, a suture is usually placed through the middle of the tongue and taped to the cheek. In case of airway obstruction, the tongue can be pulled forward with the suture and patency of the upper airway reestablished. Children with other anomalies associated with small oral cavities may have significant postoperative airway obstruction because of surgical edema. Tracheal intubation for 48 hours to 72 hours after surgery may be necessary.

Mandibular Hypoplasia

Mandibular hypoplasia is a prominent feature of Pierre Robin, Treacher Collins, and Goldenhar syndromes. In these syndromes, the small mandible leaves little room for the tongue and makes the larynx appear to be anterior. Therefore, upper airway obstruction and difficult intubation of the trachea are likely to result.

Pierre Robin Syndrome

Pierre Robin syndrome consists of micrognathia, which is usually accompanied by glossoptosis (posterior displacement of the tongue) and cleft palate. Mandibular hypoplasia may be responsible for displacement of the tongue

into the pharynx, which subsequently prevents fusion of the palate. Acute upper airway obstruction can occur in neonates or infants with Pierre Robin syndrome. Feeding problems, failure to thrive, and cyanotic episodes are other early complications of this syndrome. Associated congenital heart disease is frequent. Fortunately, sufficient mandibular growth during early childhood markedly reduces the degree of airway problems in later years.

Treacher Collins Syndrome

Treacher Collins syndrome is the most common of the mandibulofacial dysotoses. Inheritance of this syndrome is as an autosomal dominant trait with variable expression. A lethal prenatal defect occurs frequently, as fetal wastage is common in affected families.

Micrognathia results in early airway problems similar to those experienced by infants with Pierre Robin syndrome. About 30 percent of children with Treacher Collins syndrome have an associated cleft palate. Congenital heart disease, particularly ventricular septal defects, frequently accompanies this syndrome. Other features include malar hypoplasia, colobomas (notching of the lower eyelids), and an antimongoloid slant of the palpebral fissures. Ear tags and gross deformities of the external ear canals and ossicular chain are common. Mental retardation is not a primary feature of Treacher Collins syndrome but may result from hearing loss. Intubation of the trachea, as in infants with Pierre Robin syndrome, is difficult and sometimes impossible. Tracheal intubation of the older child with Treacher Collins syndrome may be extremely difficult once full dentition has been achieved. Patients with Treacher Collins syndrome may present for upper airway management, palatoplasty, treatment of chronic otitis media, and correction of congenital heart defects. In addition, some patients with Treacher Collins syndrome will undergo extensive craniofacial osteotomies for correction of cosmetic deformities (see the section Hypertelorism).

Goldenhar Syndrome

Goldenhar syndrome is characterized by unilateral mandibular hypoplasia. Associated anomalies include eye, ear, and vertebral abnormalities on the affected side. Ease of tracheal intubation is highly variable. Some patients present little difficulty for intubation of the trachea, whereas for other patients intubation is extremely difficult.

MANAGEMENT OF ANESTHESIA

Management of anesthesia for patients with Pierre Robin, Treacher Collins, or Goldenhar syndromes begins with evaluation of the upper airway and formulation of a plan for intubation of the trachea. In addition, preoperative assessment should focus on the cardiovascular system and the level of hemoglobin. Some patients with chronic airway obstruction become hypoxemic and develop pulmonary hypertension.

Inclusion of anticholinergic drugs in the preoperative medication is recommended to reduce upper airway secretions. Opioids and other ventilatory depressants are often avoided for preoperative medication. Oral administration of cimetidine or ranitidine may be logical additions to the preoperative regimen in infants and children at risk for aspiration during induction of anesthesia and intubation of the trachea.[110] Several approaches to intubation of the trachea may be considered, but alternative methods must be immediately available, including facilities for emergency bronchoscopy, cricothyrotomy, or tracheostomy.[111] Attempts at direct laryngoscopy may be preceded by intravenous administration of atropine to minimize the likelihood of vagal stimulation and resultant bradycardia. Preoxygenation before initiating direct laryngoscopy is recommended. Administration of muscle relaxants to these patients is not recommended until mechanical ventilation of the lungs via a tracheal tube is established. Awake intubation of the trachea can sometimes be accomplished by either the oral or nasal routes after adequate topical anesthesia has been achieved. Awake intubation of the trachea may produce undue trauma to the upper airway and does not eliminate the risk of pulmonary aspiration. More often, intubation of the trachea is accomplished after induction of anesthesia with volatile anesthetics, provided that a patent upper airway can be maintained until an adequate depth of anesthesia is attained. Spontaneous ventilation is desirable during induction of anesthesia, so as to assure continuous airway control and to avoid inflating the child's stomach with air. Direct laryngoscopy should not be attempted until a sufficient depth of anesthesia has been established. Transtracheal injection of lidocaine 4 mg·dl^{-1} will reduce the risk of laryngospasm during laryngoscopy. Forward traction on the tongue may facilitate maintenance of a patent upper airway until a sufficient depth of anesthesia can be obtained. Blind nasal intubation of the trachea may also be performed. Tracheal intubation with the aid of a fiberoptic laryngoscope is an alternative technique for tracheal intubation of older children. Tracheostomy during local anesthesia may be required when all other attempts to intubate the trachea have failed. Tracheostomy in these children, however, may be technically difficult and prone to immediate and delayed complications. Certainly, risks of pneumothorax, bleeding, air embolism, and poor positioning of the tracheostomy site are increased in a struggling child.

Extubation of the trachea after surgery should be delayed until these patients are fully awake and alert. In addition, equipment for reintubation must be immediately available.

Hypertelorism

Hypertelorism is an increased distance between the eyes and is associated with many craniofacial anomalies, such as Crouzon's disease and Apert's syndrome. Crouzon's disease consists of hypertelorism, craniostenosis, shallow orbits with marked proptosis, and midface hypoplasia. Apert's syndrome is characterized by essentially the same features, with the addition of syndactyly of all extremities. Other anomalies associated with hypertelorism are cleft palate, synostosis of the cervical spine, hearing loss, and mental retardation. In actuality, hypertelorism is representative of many craniofacial disorders that are amenable to facial reconstructive surgery.

TREATMENT

Correction of major craniofacial deformities may involve mandibular osteotomies, craniotomy with wide exposure of the frontal lobes, maxillary osteotomies with forward displacement of the maxilla, medial displacement of the orbits, and multiple rib grafts. Such complex operations may require 24 hours for completion and involve more than a hundred separate surgical steps.[112] Surgical correction is often performed in infancy before ossification of the facial bones occurs.

MANAGEMENT OF ANESTHESIA

Management of anesthesia for craniofacial surgery in children with hypertelorism is a complex undertaking, that begins with meticulous preoperative assessment and preparation and extends into the postoperative period for several days.[113] Craniofacial surgery should be attempted only by a qualified team of physicians under ideal circumstances. There are many potential problems and anesthetic considerations.

Airway. Management of the patient's airway must not interfere with exposure required to perform the corrective surgery. Predictably, intubation of the trachea may be difficult. Intraoperatively, tracheal tubes may become dislodged or kinked during maxillary advancement, mandibular osteotomy, or repositioning of the head and neck. In addition, the tube may be displaced into a mainstem bronchus when the neck is flexed, or may be inadvertently cut by the osteotome. Improperly humidified inspired gases are likely to lead to mucous plugs in the tracheal tube during these long operations, especially if a small diameter tube is required.

Establishment of a tracheostomy 3 days before operation is an attractive alternative to translaryngeal intubation of the trachea for some patients. Advantages include reliable control of the airway during and after the operative procedure. In addition, reinstitution of anesthesia is easily accomplished should it be necessary. Furthermore, performance of the tracheostomy 3 days earlier reduces the likelihood of complications (bleeding, penumothorax, and subcutaneous emphysema) on the day of the corrective surgery.

Blood Loss. Blood loss generally occurs in a steady ooze from multiple osteotomies and bone graft donor sites, averaging about 1.2 blood volumes. Quantitation of blood loss is difficult because of diffuse oozing. Measurement of serial hematocrits, central venous pressure, and urine output are helpful for estimating blood loss and guiding intravenous fluid replacement. Availability of appropriate amounts of whole blood (1.5 times the expected blood loss), platelets, and fresh frozen plasma should be confirmed before surgery. Intravenous catheters must be of sufficient number and diameter to permit rapid transfusion of blood.

Blood loss may be reduced by positioning patients in 15 degree to 20 degree head-up positions. In addition, controlled hypotension, using nitroprusside during phases of surgery when major hemorrhage is anticipated, is useful. Mean arterial blood pressure, as measured at the level of the circle of Willis, should not decrease below 50 mmHg during controlled hypotension. Blood must be filtered; warmed; and, if given rapidly to small children, accompanied by calcium gluconate (1 mg to 2 mg for every milliliter of blood infused), to prevent the possibility of citrate intoxication.

LENGTH OF PROCEDURE

Complex craniofacial reconstructions average 14 hours.[113] Hypothermia during these lengthy operations can be prevented by placing patients on warming blankets; warming intravenous fluids and blood; and using warmed, humidified inspired gases. Pressure necrosis and nerve injuries can be avoided by careful positioning and padding with emphasis on avoiding traction on the patient's brachial plexus. Venous stasis can be minimized by wrapping the legs with elastic bandages.

INTRACRANIAL PRESSURE

Hyperventilation of the lungs to maintain the arterial partial pressures of carbon dioxide between 30 mmHg to 35 mmHg; maintenance of the head-up position; and administration of furosemide, mannitol, and corticosteroids are used to minimize brain swelling. Free water is limited by administering 5 percent dextrose in lactated Ringer's solution, at a rate of 4 ml· $kg^{-1} \cdot hr^{-1}$. Anesthetic techniques that minimize brain blood volume (nitrous oxide plus opioids) are useful. Intraoperative brain swelling can be minimized by continuous drainage of lumbar cerebrospinal fluid. Many reconstructive procedures are extracranial, and cerebral edema is not a consideration.

Ocular. Corneal abrasions are likely in patients where ocular proptosis is pronounced. Therefore, eye ointment should be used and the eyelids sutured closed. In addition, ocular or orbital manipulations can evoke the oculocardiac reflex. Release of pressure on the orbits, or administration of small doses of atropine, will rapidly block the reflex.

Monitors. In addition to routine monitors, a catheter placed in a peripheral artery for continuous measurement of blood pressure is mandatory. Blood from the arterial catheter also permits determination of blood gases, pH, hematocrit, and plasma osmolarity. A central venous pressure catheter and a Foley catheter are helpful for evaluation of the adequacy of intravenous fluid replacement. An end-tidal carbon dioxide monitor is useful for following the adequacy of ventilation and early recognition of dislodgement of the tube from the trachea.

Postoperative Management. Postoperatively, the entire head may be wrapped in a pressure dressing, through which only the tracheal tube protrudes. It is likely that the jaws will be wired shut. Pharyngeal bleeding, laryngeal edema, and increased intracranial pressure may be present. Therefore, no attempt

need be made to reverse opioid or muscle relaxant effects at the end of the operation. Indeed, mechanical ventilation of the lungs should be maintained for at least the first night, and often for several days postoperatively.

DISORDERS OF THE UPPER AIRWAY

Numerous pathologic processes may involve the upper airway and respiratory tract of pediatric patients. Specific disorders include epiglottitis, laryngotracheobronchitis, post-intubation laryngeal edema, foreign body aspiration, laryngeal papillomatosis, and lung abscess.

Epiglottitis (Supraglottitis)

Epiglottitis usually presents with characteristic signs and symptoms (Table 35-12).[114] At times, however, classic signs and symptoms are not present, and it may be difficult to differentiate epiglottitis from laryngotracheobronchitis.

SIGNS AND SYMPTOMS

Classically, children with epiglottitis are 2 years to 6 years old and present with histories of acute difficulty swallowing, high fever, and inspiratory stridor. These signs and symptoms have usually developed over a period of less than 24 hours. In addition, there may be excessive drooling, a muffled voice, leukocytosis, and the characteristic posture of sitting upright and leaning forward. In fact, a change in this posture may cause more airway obstruction. A lateral radiograph of the neck may demonstrate swelling of the epiglottis and aryepiglottic folds. Nevertheless, time to perform the radiograph should not be taken if these children are in respiratory distress or if the clinical diagnosis is evident. Definitive diagnosis of epig-

TABLE 35-12.   Clinical Features of Epiglottitis and Laryngotracheobronchitis

	Epiglottitis	Laryngotracheobronchitis
Age group affected	2–6 years	2 years or less
Incidence	Accounts for 5% of children with stridor	Accounts for about 80% of children with stridor
Etiologic agent	Bacterial (*H. influenzae*)	Viral
Onset of symptoms	Rapid over 24 hours	Gradual over 24–72 hours
Signs and symptoms	Inspiratory stridor	Inspiratory stridor
	Pharyngitis	Croupy cough
	Drooling	Rhinorrhea
	Fever (often >39 degrees Celsius)	Fever (rarely >39 degrees Celsius)
	Lethargic to restless	
	Insists on sitting up and leaning forward	
	Tachypnea	
	Cyanosis	
Laboratory	Neutrophilia	Lymphocytosis
Lateral radiograph of the neck	Swollen epiglottis	Narrowing of subglottic area
Treatment	Oxygen	Oxygen
	Urgent intubation of the trachea or tracheostomy during general anesthesia	Aerosolized racemic epinephrine
	Fluids	Fluids
	Antibiotics	Humidity
	Corticosteroids (?)	Corticosteroids
		Intubation of the trachea for severe airway obstruction

lottitis is made in the operating room during direct laryngoscopy for intubation of the trachea. The etiologic agent of epiglottitis is most often *Hemophilus influenzae*.

TREATMENT

It is mandatory that children with suspected epiglottitis be admitted to the hospital. The history can be quickly obtained and the child examined for signs of upper airway obstruction. An attempt to visualize the epiglottitis should not be undertaken until these children are in the operating room and preparations are completed for intubation of the trachea and possible emergency tracheostomy. It should be remembered that total upper airway obstruction can occur in children with epiglottitis at any time, especially with instrumentation of the upper airway, perhaps reflecting glottic obstruction by the edematous epiglottis, laryngospasm from aspirated saliva, and respiratory muscle fatigue. A physician skilled in intubation of the trachea and positive pressure ventilation of the lungs with a face mask should accompany these children at all times.

Definitive treatment of epiglottitis includes appropriate antibiotics and a secured airway, until inflammation of the epiglottis subsides. Ampicillin is the antibiotic of choice, although chloramphenicol is required for ampicillin-resistant Hemophilus strains. Translaryngeal intubation of the trachea during general anesthesia is the recommended approach for securing the airway.[114] Although epiglottitis is primarily a disease of children, there are an increasing number of reports of epiglottitis in adults. A difference between adult and pediatric epiglottitis may be the appearance of the tissues on physical examination. For example, most children with *H. influenzae* epiglottitis manifest a striking erythematous ("cherry red") swelling, whereas adults often have only a mild erythema or even a pale watery edema. It has been recommended that adult patients be managed in the same manner as children with epiglottitis.[115,116]

MANAGEMENT OF ANESTHESIA

Induction and maintenance of anesthesia for intubation of the trachea is with volatile anesthetics, most often halothane, in oxygen.

High inspired concentrations of oxygen permitted by the use of volatile anesthetics facilitates optimal oxygenation in these patients. Before induction of anesthesia, preparations are made for an emergency tracheostomy, which may be required if airway obstruction occurs and translaryngeal intubation of the trachea is not possible. A catheter should be placed in a peripheral vein before induction of anesthesia, and administration of atropine (6 $\mu g \cdot kg^{-1}$ to 10 $\mu g \cdot kg^{-1}$) or glycopyrrolate (3 $\mu g \cdot kg^{-1}$ to 5 $\mu g \cdot kg^{-1}$) may be useful.

Induction of anesthesia with volatile anesthetics is begun with these children in the sitting position. After the onset of drowsiness, these children are placed supine, and ventilation of the lungs is assisted as necessary. When an adequate depth of anesthesia has been established, direct laryngoscopy is performed, and a tube placed in the trachea. After successful intubation of the trachea, a thorough direct laryngoscopy is performed to confirm the diagnosis of epiglottitis. The next step is replacement of the orotracheal tube with a nasotracheal tube under direct vision. A nasotracheal tube is preferred, as it is easier to secure and is more comfortable for awake children. After nasotracheal intubation is accomplished, these children are allowed to awaken from the anesthetic. Usually, intubation of the trachea is required for 48 hours to 96 hours, although one report has indicated that 8 hours to 12 hours may be adequate.[117] In some cases, pulmonary edema, pericarditis, meningitis, or septic arthritis may accompany epiglottitis.[114]

RECOVERY FROM EPIGLOTTITIS

Extubation of the trachea may be considered when body temperature is no longer elevated and other signs such as decreases in leukocyte counts have occurred. A clinical sign of the resolution of the swelling of the epiglottis is the development of an air leak around the tracheal tube. Regardless of the clinical impression, it is best to take these children to the operating room and perform direct laryngoscopy during general anesthesia to confirm that inflammation of the epiglottis has resolved before extubation of the trachea.

Epiglottitis is a short-lived disease, and prognosis is excellent if the airway is secured

and appropriate antibiotic therapy is prescribed. Epiglottitis can be fatal if airway obstruction and arterial hypoxemia develop. Success of an epiglottitis treatment protocol depends on cooperation between physicians and multiple specialty disciplines so as to assure rapid diagnosis and treatment.

Laryngotracheobronchitis (Croup, Subglottic Infection)

Laryngotracheobronchitis is a viral infection of the upper respiratory tract that typically afflicts children less than 2 years of age (Table 35-12).[114] The etiology is usually viral. Parainfluenza, adenoviruses, myxoviruses, and influenza A viruses have been implicated as causative agents. Laryngotracheobronchitis and epiglottitis share certain clinical features and at times are confused with each other (Table 35-12).[114]

SIGNS AND SYMPTOMS

Laryngotracheobronchitis, in contrast to epiglottitis, has a gradual onset over 24 hours to 72 hours. There are signs of upper respiratory tract infection, such as rhinorrhea and low-grade fever. Leukocyte counts are normal or only slightly elevated with a lymphocytosis. The cough has a characteristic "barking" or "brassy" quality.

TREATMENT

Treatment of laryngotracheobronchitis includes supplemental oxygen, humidification of inspired gases, and aerosolized racemic epinephrine. For example, hourly treatments with aerosolized racemic epinephrine have been shown to alleviate airway obstruction secondary to laryngotracheobronchitis effectively and thus reduce the need for intubation of the trachea.[118] Corticosteroids (dexamethasone 0.5 $mg \cdot kg^{-1}$ to 1.0 $mg \cdot kg^{-1}$ administered intravenously) remain controversial therapy. Tracheal intubation is required if physical exhaustion occurs, as evidenced by increased arterial partial pressures of carbon dioxide. If tracheal intubation is required, a smaller than normal tracheal tube should be used to minimize edema from intubation. Should a smaller than normal tracheal tube fit too tightly in the subglottic area, a tracheostomy may be required. Although laryngotracheobronchitis is generally a short-lived disease, there is evidence that patients with a history of this disease have hyperreactive airways.[119]

Postintubation Laryngeal Edema

Postintubation laryngeal edema is a potential complication of intubation of the trachea in all children, although the incidence is greatest in children between the ages of 1 year and 4 years. Studies to delineate the etiology of postintubation laryngeal edema are lacking, but certain predisposing factors seem predictable. For example, mechanical trauma to the airway during intubation of the trachea and placement of a tube that produces a tight fit are possible causes.[120] Significant postintubation laryngeal edema is usually avoidable if the size of the tube in the trachea is such that an audible air leak occurs around it during positive airway pressures equivalent of 15 cmH_2O to 25 cmH_2O.

Treatment of postintubation laryngeal edema is with humidification of inspired gases and aerosolized racemic epinephrine, administered hourly until symptoms subside. The dose of racemic epinephrine is $0.05 \ ml \cdot kg^{-1}$ (maximum of 0.5 ml) in 2.0 ml saline. For most cases of postintubation laryngeal edema, one or two treatments will produce significant improvement. Reintubation of the trachea or tracheostomy should be required only rarely. Although intravenous administration of dexamethasone ($0.1 \ mg \cdot kg^{-1}$ to $0.2 \ mg \cdot kg^{-1}$) as a single dose has been used for the prevention and treatment of this edema, its efficacy for this condition is undocumented.

Foreign Body Aspiration

Foreign body aspiration into the airway, with its resultant airway obstruction, can produce a wide range of responses. For example, complete obstruction at the level of the larynx or trachea can result in death from asphyxiation. At the opposite end of the spectrum, passage of foreign bodies into distal airways may elicit only mild symptoms, which may go unnoticed for years. Children 1 year to 3 years of age, because of their curiosity and newfound abilities of locomotion, are most prone to such aspiration.

SIGNS AND SYMPTOMS

Common clinical features of foreign body aspiration are cough, wheezing, and decreased air entry into the affected lung. The most frequent site of aspiration is the right bronchus. Foreign body aspiration often presents with the misdiagnosis of upper respiratory tract infection, asthma, or pneumonia. Radiographic evaluation provides direct evidence if the aspirated object is radiopaque. If the aspirated object is radiolucent, indirect evidence can be obtained by demonstrating hyperinflation of the affected lung with atelectasis distal to the foreign body. Radiographs of the chest during exhalation may accentuate the hyperinflation. Measurement of the arterial partial pressures of oxygen is helpful for evaluating the degree of right-to-left intrapulmonary shunting due to airway obstruction.

The type of foreign body aspirated can influence the clinical course. For example, nuts and certain vegetable materials are very irritating to the bronchial tree. Nuts also tend to result in multiple site aspiration. Inert substances, such as plastics, are relatively nonirritating, and produce minimal inflammatory reaction.

TREATMENT

Treatment for an aspirated foreign body is endoscopic removal.[121] The improved technology of pediatric bronchoscopic equipment has increased the efficacy and safety of this procedure. It is best to remove the foreign body within 24 hours after aspiration. Risks of leaving the foreign body in the airway for longer than 24 hours include migration of the aspirated material, pneumonia, and residual pulmonary disease.

MANAGEMENT OF ANESTHESIA

Few types of cases demand as much flexibility of the anesthesiologist as do children with an aspirated foreign body. Each case mandates individualization of the technique to fit the clinical situation. Techniques for induction of anesthesia will depend on the severity of airway obstruction. When airway obstruction is present, induction of anesthesia, using only volatile anesthetics in oxygen, is useful. Induction of anesthesia with barbiturates, followed by inhalation of volatile anesthetics, is acceptable if the airway is less tenuous. After an adequate depth of anesthesia has been attained, direct laryngoscopy is performed, and the larynx is sprayed with lidocaine (2 mg·kg^{-1} to 4 mg·kg^{-1}). Topical anesthesia is effective in preventing laryngospasm when endoscopic manipulation is performed. Intravenous administration of atropine (6 μg·kg^{-1} to 10 μg·kg^{-1}) or glycopyrrolate (3 μg·kg^{-1} to 5 μg·kg^{-1}) is useful to reduce the likelihood of bradycardia from vagal stimulation during endoscopy. Muscle relaxants are best avoided during bronchoscopy, as spontaneous ventilation is desirable, providing greater flexibility and additional time for the endoscopist. Furthermore, positive airway pressure could contribute to distal migration of the foreign body, thereby complicating its extraction. In addition, if the foreign body has produced a ball-valve phenomenon, use of positive pressure ventilation of the lungs could contribute to hyperinflation and possibly pneumothorax. During bronchoscopy, anesthesia is maintained with volatile anesthetics in oxygen. Ventilation through the bronchoscope can be difficult because of the high resistance to gas flow imposed by the narrow bronchoscope and the large gas leak, which often occurs around the bronchoscope. Therefore, maintenance of spontaneous ventilation is again desirable.

Skeletal muscle paralysis produced with succinylcholine may be required for removal of the bronchoscope and foreign body if the object is too large to pass through the moving vocal cords.

Complications that may occur during bronchoscopy include airway obstruction, fragmentation of the foreign body, arterial hypoxemia, and hypercapnia. Trauma to the tracheobronchial tree from the foreign body and instrumentation can result in subglottic edema. After bronchoscopy, inhalation of aerosolized racemic epinephrine and intravenous administration of dexamethasone may reduce subglottic edema. Radiographs of the chest should be obtained after bronchoscopy for detection of atelectasis or pneumothorax. Postural drainage and chest percussion will enhance clearance of secretions and reduce the subsequent risk of infection.

Laryngeal Papillomatosis

Laryngeal papillomatosis is the most common benign laryngeal tumor of childhood.[122] The likely cause is a tissue response to a virus. Malignant degeneration of juvenile papillomas is rare but can occur in older patients. A change in the character of the voice is the most common symptom of papillomatosis. Most children with papillomatosis present with symptoms before the age of 7 years. Some degree of airway obstruction is present in over 40 percent of patients. Papillomas usually regress spontaneously at puberty.

TREATMENT

Various forms of treatment for laryngeal papillomatosis have been used, including surgical excision, cryosurgery, topical 5-fluorouracil, exogenous interferon, and laser ablation. Since the disease is ultimately self-limiting, complications of therapy must be avoided. For example, seeding of the distal airways can occur after tracheostomy. Surgical therapy with laser coagulation has been useful. Because papillomas recur, frequent laser coagulation is required until spontaneous remission occurs.

MANAGEMENT OF ANESTHESIA

Management of anesthesia for removal of laryngeal papillomas depends upon the severity of airway obstruction. Awake intubation of the trachea is recommended for severe airway obstruction. Certainly, children with severe airway obstruction should not receive muscle relaxants in attempts to facilitate intubation of the trachea. Indeed, in some patients the glottic opening can be identified only with the child breathing spontaneously. A rigid broncho-scope should be readily available, as this may be the only means of securing an airway in some children. It should be appreciated that the degree of airway obstruction can vary greatly in the same patient between surgical procedures.

Induction and maintenance of anesthesia is best achieved with volatile anesthetics delivered in high inspired concentrations of oxygen. Surgical therapy for papillomatosis, either laser coagulation or forceps excision, is usually done as a microlaryngoscopic procedure. During microlaryngoscopy, the vocal cords must be quiescent. Skeletal muscle paralysis or deep anesthesia, therefore, is required to produce acceptable operating conditions. Intermediate-acting muscle relaxants, such as vecuronium or atracurium, are useful for this purpose. Intravenous administration of procaine ($1 \ mg \cdot kg^{-1} \cdot min^{-1}$) has been used in conjunction with inhalation anesthesia to provide satisfactory operating conditions.[123] A cuffed tracheal tube of a smaller than predicted diameter should be employed for intubation of the trachea. This will improve visualization of the glottis by the endoscopist. In some instances apneic oxygenation techniques with temporary removal of the tracheal tube are required. For laser ablation of papillomas, the usual safety precautions concerning laser use should be observed. These precautions may include wrapping the tracheal tube with metallic tape, inflation of the tracheal tube cuff with saline, and protection of the patient's face and eyes. After resection of papillomas, the tracheal tube should be removed only when these children are fully awake and laryngeal bleeding has ceased. After extubation of the trachea, inhalation of aerosolized racemic epinephrine and intravenous administration of dexamethasone may reduce subglottic edema.

Lung Abscess

Lung abscess in children is most likely the result of inhalation of secretions containing disease-producing bacteria. In addition, bronchial obstruction by tumor may result in a lung abscess distal to the airway obstruction.

Surgical excision of the abscess cavity is indicated for those cases that do not respond to antibiotic therapy. Nevertheless, surgical intervention introduces the risk of rupture of the lung abscess and flooding of the tracheobronchial tree with large amounts of purulent material. Flooding of the lungs can acutely impair ventilation and oxygenation and lead to abscess formation in previously uncontaminated portions of the lung. Isolation of the affected lobe or lung is desirable to minimize this risk. Appropriately sized double-lumen tracheal tubes or bronchial blockers, however, are not reliably available for use in children.[124] The affected lobe can be effectively blocked with a Fogarty catheter, passed under direct vision through a ventilating bronchoscope.[125] After the Fogarty catheter balloon is inflated, a tracheal tube is positioned in the mainstem bronchus of the normal lung. This procedure results in protection of the normal lung and isolation of the affected lobe of the diseased lung. High inspired concentrations of oxygen are necessary, as one-lung anesthesia produces an increase in the magnitude of right-to-left intrapulmonary shunting, resulting in decreases in the arterial partial pressures of oxygen. Arterial partial pressures of carbon dioxide are not influenced by one-lung anesthesia if minute ventilation is maintained.

JEUNE SYNDROME

Jeune syndrome is an inherited autosomal recessive disorder that occurs in a neonatal form (asphyxiating thoracic dystrophy) and in a childhood form (diffuse interstitial fibrosis of the kidneys). In its neonatal form, the deformity of the thoracic wall prevents normal intercostal respiratory movement and respiratory failure ensues. Lung volumes are predictably decreased. Pulmonary hypoplasia and persistent pulmonary hypertension may be present. Even if normoxic at rest, these infants are prone to profound arterial hypoxemia when stimulated because of asynchronous rib and abdominal movements. Cor pulmonale is a sequela of chronic arterial hypoxemia. Hepatic fibrosis and myocardial dysfunction have also been observed.

These children may require anesthesia for thoracoplasty, renal transplantation, bronchoscopy and tracheostomy.[126] Older children undergoing renal transplantation also have the typical thoracic deformity, although it is less severe than in neonates. During the intraoperative period, peak airway pressures should be minimized to reduce the likelihood of barotrauma. Choice of drugs for anesthesia should consider their impact on pulmonary, cardiovascular, and renal function. Infants undergoing thoracoplasty will require prolonged mechanical support of ventilation.

MALIGNANT HYPERTHERMIA

Malignant hyperthermia is a classic example of a pharmacogenetic disease.[127] Susceptible patients possess a genetic predisposition for development of this disease, which is not manifested until they are exposed to triggering agents, such as drugs or stressful environmental factors. Malignant hyperthermia was initially thought to be transmitted as a nonsex-linked autosomal dominant trait with reduced penetrance and variable expressivity. It is currently thought that the mode of transmission is polygenic and that the inheritance pattern can be recessive or dominant. This concept is supported by the variable susceptibility of individuals to the development of this disease. Susceptible patients should be thoroughly educated with respect to potential hazards and implications of malignant hyperthermia. Malignant hyperthermia

has an estimated incidence of 1 in 12,000 pediatric anesthetics and 1 in 40,000 adult anesthetics.[128] The incidence is higher when succinylcholine is used with other trigger agents.[129] The incidence has an apparent geographic variation, as it is more prevalent in certain areas of the United States. Malignant hyperthermia usually occurs in children and young adults but has been reported at the extremes of age ranging from 2 months to 70 years. Two-thirds of susceptible patients manifest this syndrome during their first anesthetic and the remaining one-third during subsequent anesthetics.

Pathophysiology

The pathophysiology of malignant hyperthermia has not been conclusively elucidated. The defect, however, appears to be in the excitation-contraction coupling of skeletal muscles and the concentration of calcium in myoplasm. For example, during normal skeletal muscle contractions, calcium is released into the myoplasm from the sarcolemma and sarcoplasmic reticulum. This increase in calcium inhibits the inhibitor protein troponin. Inhibition of troponin permits the actin and myosin filaments to interact and skeletal muscle contractions occur. Contractions then cease as calcium concentrations in the myoplasm decrease due to reuptake of calcium by the sarcoplasmic reticulum. In malignant hyperthermia, exposure to triggering agents leads to decreased reuptake of calcium. As a result, calcium concentrations in the myoplasm remain elevated and skeletal muscle contractions are sustained. These sustained contractions are associated with evidence of accelerated metabolism, which includes acidosis and heat production. In addition dysfunction of the sarcolemma occurs, allowing leakage of intracellular constituents out of skeletal muscle cells.

Signs and Symptoms

Malignant hyperthermia is characterized by signs and symptoms of hypermetabolism (up to ten times normal). Clinical features of this disorder are nonspecific, and include tachycardia, tachypnea, arterial hypoxemia, hypercarbia, metabolic and respiratory acidosis, hyperkalemia, cardiac dysrhythmias, hypotension, skeletal muscle rigidity (trismus or masseter spasm) after the administration of succinylcholine and elevations in body temperature.

The earliest signs of malignant hyperthermia are those related to enormous increases in metabolic rate. Increases in carbon dioxide production occur early, emphasizing the value of monitoring end-tidal carbon dioxide concentrations by capnography or mass spectrometry.[130] Tachycardia is also an early sign of the onset of malignant hyperthermia. Tachycardia reflects release of epinephrine and norepinephrine, as well as metabolic and respiratory acidosis. Cardiac dysrhythmias, such as ventricular bigeminy, multifocal premature ventricular beats, and ventricular tachycardia, may also occur, especially when hyperkalemia is associated with this syndrome. Skin signs may vary from flushing, caused by vasodilation, to blanching, secondary to intense vasoconstriction.

Susceptible patients may develop spasm of the masseter muscles after administration of succinylcholine. This skeletal muscle spasm may be so severe that it is impossible to open the mouth to perform direct laryngoscopy for intubation of the trachea. Conversely, in other patients, drug-induced skeletal muscle spasms are mild and transient or even absent. Nevertheless, onset of skeletal muscle rigidity after administration of succinylcholine should be regarded as a sign of impending development of malignant hyperthermia. Patients who develop masseter spasm have a 50 percent incidence of muscle biopsies positive for susceptibility to malignant hyperthermia.[131] Generalized skeletal muscle rigidity during an anesthetic that includes halothane and/or succinylcholine may be a more specific predictor of malignant hyperthermia susceptibility than is masseter spasm after administration of succinylcholine.[132] Skeletal muscle biopsies are positive for malignant hyperthermia susceptibility in all patients in whom plasma creatine kinase concentrations exceed 20,000 $IU \cdot L^{-1}$ after succinylcholine-induced masseter spasm.[131]

Body temperature elevations are often late manifestations of malignant hyperthermia. Indeed, diagnosis of malignant hyperthermia should not depend on rises in body temperature. Nevertheless, increases in body temperature may be precipitous, increasing at rates of 0.5 degrees Celsius every 15 minutes, and reaching levels as high as 46 degrees.

Analysis of arterial and central venous blood will reveal arterial hypoxemia, hypercarbia (100 mmHg to 200 mmHg), respiratory and metabolic acidosis (pH 7.15 to 6.80), and marked central venous oxygen desaturation. Hyperkalemia may occur early in the course of the disease, but after normothermia returns, plasma potassium concentrations may drop rapidly. Plasma concentrations of transaminase enzymes and creatine kinase will be markedly elevated, although peak levels may not occur for 12 hours to 24 hours after acute episodes. Plasma and urine myoglobin concentrations (gives urine a color similar to hemoglobin) are also elevated, reflecting massive rhabdomyolysis. Late complications of untreated malignant hyperthermia include disseminated intravascular coagulation, pulmonary edema, and acute renal failure. Central nervous system damage may manifest as blindness, seizures, coma, or paralysis.

Treatment

Successful treatment of malignant hyperthermia depends on early recognition of the diagnosis and institution of a preplanned therapeutic regimen. Maintenance of appropriate equipment and drugs in a central location within the operating room area will save valuable time. Treatment of malignant hyperthermia can be divided into etiologic and symptomatic. Etiologic treatment is directed at correction of the underlying causative mechanism. Symptomatic therapy is directed toward maintenance of renal function and correction of hyperthermia, acidosis, and arterial hypoxemia.

ETIOLOGIC TREATMENT

Dantrolene, administered intravenously, is the only drug that is reliably effective for the treatment of malignant hyperthermia.[127,133]

Availability of intravenous dantrolene preparations has reduced mortality from malignant hyperthermia from over 70 percent to about 10 percent.[129] The site of action of dantrolene is not clear, but it acts distal to the motor nerve. Dantrolene is believed to inhibit excitation-contraction of skeletal muscles by inhibiting calcium release from sarcoplasmic reticulum or by increasing calcium uptake by sarcoplasmic reticulum. Dantrolene does not affect skeletal muscle membrane potentials, electrical excitability of skeletal muscles, or neuromuscular transmission. The mean plasma half-time of dantrolene is 5 hours when given intravenously. Dantrolene is slowly metabolized in the liver, and metabolites are excreted in the urine.

Treatment of acute episodes of malignant hyperthermia is with 1 $mg \cdot kg^{-1}$ to 2 $mg \cdot kg^{-1}$ of dantrolene mixed with sterile distilled water and administered rapidly intravenously. This dose is repeated every 5 minutes to 10 minutes to a maximum dose of 10 $mg \cdot kg^{-1}$ depending on the patient's temperature response. Typically, 2 $mg \cdot kg^{-1}$ to 5 $mg \cdot kg^{-1}$ of dantrolene is required for treatment of acute episodes. In addition, dantrolene should be continued in the postoperative period to prevent possible recrudescences of malignant hyperthermia. One approach is to administer dantrolene intravenously 1 $mg \cdot kg^{-1}$ to 2 $mg \cdot kg^{-1}$ every 4 hours to 6 hours for at least 24 hours after resolution of the acute episode. An alternate regimen is administration of oral dantrolene 4 $mg \cdot kg^{-1}$ daily for 2 days to 4 days.

SYMPTOMATIC TREATMENT

Symptomatic treatment for malignant hyperthermia includes immediate termination of the administration of inhaled anesthetics and the surgical procedure. Under no circumstances should the administration of volatile anesthetics be continued with the false hope that anesthetic-induced vasodilation would aid cooling or that high concentrations of these drugs would reduce metabolic rate. The patient's lungs should be hyperventilated with 100 percent oxygen and active cooling initiated. Active cooling may be done with surface cooling and intracavitary lavage of the stomach

and bladder with cold crystalloid solutions. Intravenous solutions infused through peripheral intravenous catheters should also be cooled. Although rarely practical, cooling via extracorporeal circulation with a heat exchanger has been used.[134] Cooling is discontinued when body temperature reaches 38 degrees. Other symptomatic therapy includes intravenous infusion of sodium bicarbonate to correct metabolic acidosis, hydration with normal saline, and maintenance of urine output at 1 $ml \cdot kg^{-1} \cdot hr^{-1}$ to 2 $ml \cdot kg^{-1} \cdot hr^{-1}$ with osmotic or tubular diuretics. Administration of glucose with regular insulin provides an exogenous energy source to replace depleted cerebral metabolic substrates. Failure to maintain diuresis may result in acute renal failure due to deposition of myoglobin in the renal tubules. Procainamide (15 $mg \cdot kg^{-1}$) can be used for the treatment of ventricular dysrhythmias, which may occur during malignant hyperthermia.

After recovery from acute episodes of malignant hyperthermia, patients should be closely monitored in an intensive care unit for 24 hours to 48 hours. Urine output, arterial blood gases, pH, and serum electrolyte concentrations should be determined frequently. It must be appreciated that malignant hyperthermia may recur in the intensive care unit, in the absence of obvious triggering events.[135]

Identification of Malignant Hyperthermia Susceptible Patients

Advantages of detecting malignant hyperthermia susceptible patients before anesthesia are obvious. A detailed medical and family history, with particular reference to previous anesthetic experiences, should be obtained. Prior uneventful anesthetics do not necessarily indicate that individuals are not susceptible. Environmental stresses, a consistent trigger of malignant hyperthermia in animals, have also been reported in humans.[136] Therefore, a history of the patient's response to physical exertion may be helpful. Physical examination should focus on the musculoskeletal and cardiac systems. Two distinct myopathic syndromes result in increased risks of malignant hyperthermia. The first type of myopathy features wasting of the distal ends of the vastus muscles and hypertrophy of the proximal femoris muscles of the thigh. The second myopathy features cryptorchidism, pectus carinatum, kyphosis, lordosis, ptosis, and hypoplastic mandible. The incidence of malignant hyperthermia is increased in patients with Duchenne muscular dystrophy (see Chapter 28). Malignant hyperthermia has also been reported in patients with Burkitt lymphoma, osteogenesis imperfecta, myotonia congenita, neuroleptic malignant syndrome, and myelomeningocele.[137,138] There is also evidence of cardiac muscle involvement in patients who are susceptible to malignant hyperthermia. Cardiac findings include ventricular dysrhythmias and abnormal myocardial imaging with radionuclides.

Creatine kinase should be measured in patients being evaluated for susceptibility to malignant hyperthermia. About 70 percent of malignant hyperthermia susceptible patients have elevations of resting plasma concentrations of creatine kinase. On the other hand, individuals from some families with susceptibility to malignant hyperthermia have normal creatine kinase levels.[139] Other conditions, such as muscular dystrophy and skeletal muscle trauma, also produce elevations of creatine kinase levels. For these reasons, measurements of creatine kinase levels are not definitive screening tests for malignant hyperthermia. Electromyographic changes are seen in 50 percent of malignant hyperthermia susceptible patients.[127] These findings include an increased incidence of polyphasic action potentials and fibrillation potentials.

Skeletal muscle biopsies with in vitro isometric contracture testing are the definitive tests for confirming malignant hyperthermia susceptibility.[127] Skeletal muscle biopsies are typically taken from the vastus muscles of the thigh, with the patient under local or regional anesthesia. Histologic changes in skeletal muscles from malignant hyperthermia susceptible patients are not diagnostic. Instead, skeletal muscle specimens must be subjected to isometric contracture testing under the influence of caffeine, halothane, or both. Caffeine and halothane produce exaggerated contractures of skeletal muscles from individuals susceptible to malignant hyperthermia. Since there is some overlap between normal and susceptible individuals, an established laboratory should be employed.

Management of Anesthesia

No anesthetic regimens have been shown to be reliably safe for patients who are susceptible to malignant hyperthermia. Nevertheless, certain guidelines should be followed in the management of these patients. Dantrolene in doses of 2.5 mg·kg^{-1} should be administered over a 15 minute to 30 minute period shortly before induction of anesthesia.[140] Oral dantrolene prophylaxis is probably not necessary, as this approach does not always prevent malignant hyperthermia and associated side effects (sedation, skeletal muscle weakness, nausea) are undesirable in awake patients.[141,142] In the absence of signs of malignant hyperthermia intraoperatively, it is probably not necessary to continue administration of dantrolene into the postoperative period.

Malignant hyperthermia susceptible patients should be well sedated before induction of anesthesia. Use of phenothiazines, however, should be avoided, as these drugs may stimulate release of calcium from sarcoplasmic reticulum. Preoperative medication should not include anticholinergic drugs, so as to avoid confusion regarding heart rate changes or possible interference with normal body heat loss. All preparations for treatment of malignant hyperthermia must be made before induction of anesthesia (see the section Treatment). Drugs which may trigger malignant hyperthermia include volatile anesthetics, succinylcholine, and d-tubocurarine (Table 35-13). Other drugs

TABLE 35-13. Drugs That May Trigger Malignant Hyperthermia

Halothane	Succinylcholine
Enflurane	d-Tubocurarine
Isoflurane	Gallamine (?)

TABLE 35-14. Drugs Considered Safe for Administration to Malignant Hyperthermia Susceptible Patients

Barbiturates	Pancuronium
Opioids	Atracurium
Benzodiazepines	Vecuronium
Ketamine	Anticholinesterases
Droperidol	Anticholinergics
Nitrous Oxide	Sympathomimetics
	Local Anesthetics

to be avoided include calcium and potassium. Drugs considered safe for these patients include barbiturates, opioids, benzodiazepines, ketamine, droperidol, pancuronium, and intermediate-acting muscle relaxants (Table 35-14). Nitrous oxide is probably a safe drug to administer to these patients, although its use has been implicated in the occurrence of malignant hyperthermia.[141] Conceivably, nitrous oxide could influence the course of malignant hyperthermia indirectly through its capacity to stimulate the sympathetic nervous system. Reversal of nondepolarizing muscle relaxants has not been shown to trigger malignant hyperthermia in susceptible patients. Vasopressors, digitalis and methylxanthines are acceptable drugs when specific indications for their use are present. No studies confirm that malignant hyperthermia can be triggered by residual concentrations of volatile anesthetics, especially halothane, delivered from previously used anesthesia machines. Nevertheless, some have advocated a dedicated machine, which has never been used, to administer volatile anesthetics in these patients. A more practical and acceptable alternative would be to use a conventional anesthesia machine with (1) a disposable anesthesia breathing circuit; (2) new carbon dioxide absorbent; (3) vaporizers removed; and (4) continuous flow of oxygen at 3 L·min^{-1} to 5 L·min^{-1} for 12 hours preceding use of the machine.

Regional anesthesia is an attractive and acceptable selection for anesthesia for malignant hyperthermia susceptible patients. In the past, avoidance of amide local anesthetics was recommended, as it was felt that these drugs could trigger malignant hyperthermia in susceptible patients. This opinion, however, seems to be changing; and ester, as well as amide local anesthetics, are considered to be acceptable for production of regional or local anesthesia, as may be necessary for performance of skeletal muscle biopsies in these patients.[143,144] It must be appreciated that regional anesthesia may not protect susceptible patients from triggering of malignant hyperthermia due to stress. Therefore, anxiety should be alleviated by sedating these patients during regional anesthesia.

FAMILIAL DYSAUTONOMIA

Familial dysautonomia (Riley-Day syndrome) is a rare inherited disorder found almost exclusively in children of Eastern European Jewish ancestry (see Chapter 18). Among North American Jews, approximately 1 in 50 are heterozygous carriers, resulting in an incidence of this disease of about 1 in 10,000 live births. Approximately 50 percent of these children die by the age of 4 years, usually as a result of respiratory complications. Nevertheless, as a result of a better understanding of this disease and its treatment, many afflicted children have now survived to adulthood.

Signs and Symptoms

Dysfunction of the autonomic nervous system is the most apparent manifestation of familial dysautonomia. Excessive drooling, feeding difficulties, and recurrent aspiration in infants of Jewish extraction should suggest the possibility of this disease. Presenting symptoms in older children may include retarded growth, delayed motor development, cyclical vomiting episodes, indifference to pain, emotional lability, and erratic temperature control. The tongue is smooth, due to the absence of fungiform papillae. Pain sensation is dramatically lacking. For example, a history of painless injury, such as a fracture or burn, is common. Split thickness skin grafts have been harvested from these patients without anesthesia. Corneal anesthesia and the absence of tears predispose to corneal ulcerations. Taste and thermal discrimination are invariably defective. For example, the patient cannot distinguish tap water from ice water.

Vasomotor instability is characterized by labile hypertension and postural hypotension associated with syncope. Orthostatic hypotension may reflect defective baroreceptor reflex activity and/or deficient release of norepinephrine. Indeed, measurement of urinary metabolites of norepinephrine and epinephrine suggests a deficiency of the endogenous production of catecholamines, with shunting of precursors to homovanillic acid. Conversely, older children may become hypertensive, hyperthermic, and vasoconstricted, in response to emotional stresses, presumably reflecting exaggerated responses to endogenous catecholamines. Indeed, exogenous infusion of norepinephrine results in an exaggerated degree of blood pressure increase, accompanied by tachycardia. Absence of reflex bradycardia most likely reflects attenuated activity of the parasympathetic nervous system in these patients.

Neurologic dysfunction in patients with familial dysautonomia is evidenced by poor coordination and absent deep tendon reflexes. Speech is dysarthric. The gag reflex and esophageal motility are markedly impaired, predisposing to recurrent pulmonary aspiration. Kyphoscoliosis occurs in nearly 90 percent of these children, reflecting neuromuscular imbalance. Severe kyphoscoliosis may result in restrictive pulmonary disease, culminating in mismatch of ventilation to perfusion and pulmonary hypertension. About 40 percent of patients have histories of seizure disorders. Of these, 60 percent are febrile seizures. Indeed, ventilatory responses to arterial hypoxemia and hypercarbia are greatly impaired in these patients. Emotional lability and immature, dependent behavior are characteristic. Mild mental retardation may be secondary to chronic illness, motor incoordination, and sensory deprivation, rather than being a primary feature of the disease.

Vomiting crises, common reasons for hospitalization of children with familial dysautonomia, are characterized by convulsive retching, which occurs as often as every 15 minutes to 20 minutes over a period of 1 day to 5 days and are accompanied by hypertension and diaphoresis. Dehydration and pulmonary aspiration of vomitus may occur during these crises. Hematemesis complicates 25 percent of these crises and surgical intervention is occasionally required. Intramuscular chlorpromazine (0.5 mg·kg^{-1} to 1 mg·kg^{-1}) is effective for reducing anxiety and blood pressure, while also acting as an antiemetic.

Temperature control in children with familial dysautonomia is erratic. Early morning temperature may be 35 degrees Celsius or lower. Conversely, mild infections may trigger marked elevations in body temperatures and appearance of febrile seizures. In contrast, major infections may not be accompanied by febrile responses.

Management of Anesthesia

Administration of anesthesia to children with familial dysautonomia is not associated with prohibitive risks.[145] Preoperative assessment should focus on pulmonary function. Measurement of blood gases and performance of pulmonary function tests are particularly important for preparation of patients for surgical correction of kyphoscoliosis. Fluid and electrolyte status must be carefully assessed, especially in children experiencing vomiting crises.

Intramuscular administration of chlorpromazine (0.5 mg·kg^{-1} to 1.0 mg·kg^{-1}) has been used extensively for preoperative medication in children with familial dysautonomia. Alpha-adrenergic blockade produced by chlorpromazine, however, may contribute to hypotension during induction of anesthesia. Promethazine, which is also a potent tranquilizer and antiemetic with antihistaminic properties, would seem a logical alternative. Atropine has been used preoperatively but may thicken secretions. In addition, atropine, administered as intramuscular preoperative medication, will not prevent bradycardia or hypotension during induction of anesthesia for these patients. Nevertheless, intravenous administration of atropine produces a normal increase of heart rate. Use of opioids as preoperative medication is not recommended, since children with familial dysautonomia are relatively insensitive to pain. Furthermore, opioids may serve to depress further already blunted ventilatory responses to arterial hypoxemia and hypercarbia.

Continuous monitoring of blood pressure, cardiac rhythm, and body temperature is essential. A central venous or pulmonary artery catheter is helpful during major operations, particularly when pulmonary function is already marginal.

Induction of anesthesia with titrated doses of barbiturates is acceptable for patients with familial dysautonomia. Succinylcholine and nondepolarizing muscle relaxants have been used without adverse effects. Furthermore, muscle relaxants have been uneventfully antagonized with neostigmine combined with atropine. Nitrous oxide plus muscle relaxants are often sufficient for maintenance of anesthesia, since these patients are relatively insensitive to pain. Addition of volatile anesthetics or opioids is acceptable, but it must be appreciated that precipitous drops in blood pressure and heart rate may occur. Blood pressure is critically dependent on blood volume in these patients. Therefore, hypovolemia must be scrupulously avoided and blood pressure carefully monitored during positional changes. Hypotension is treated with intravenous infusions of crystalloid solutions or administration of small doses of direct-acting vasopressors such as phenylephrine. Hypertensive episodes are best treated by increasing the depth of anesthesia. Mechanical ventilation of the lungs during the operative procedure is recommended. Particular care should be taken to avoid corneal abrasions, as these patients often have corneal anesthesia, and tear production is deficient.

Postoperative Management

Complications in the postoperative period include persistent vomiting, pulmonary aspiration, hyperpyrexia, labile blood pressure, arterial hypoxemia, hypoventilation, and seizure disorders. Increased inspired concentrations of oxygen should be routinely administered to these patients. Measurement of arterial blood gases and pH is indicated if there is any question regarding the adequacy of oxygenation or ventilation. The need for opioids to produce analgesia is unlikely, as these patients have decreased sensory perception. Chlorpromazine has been a useful drug for controlling nausea, hyperthermia, and elevated blood pressure in the postoperative period.

SOLID TUMORS

Solid tumors that develop in infants and children may be intra-abdominal or retroperitoneal in origin. Nearly 60 percent of intra-abdominal tumors in children reflect leukemia involving the liver and spleen.[146] Conversely, most intra-abdominal tumors in infants are benign and of renal origin. Retroperitoneal solid tumors are also likely to be of renal origin. Two-thirds of these renal masses are cystic lesions such as hydronephrosis, whereas the remainder are nephroblastomas (Wilms' tumors). Neuroblastoma is another example of a solid tumor that tends to occur in the retroperitoneal space.

Neuroblastoma

Neuroblastoma results from malignant proliferation of sympathetic ganglion cell precursors. These tumors may arise anywhere along the sympathetic ganglion chain, but 60 percent to 75 percent occur in the adrenal medulla and the retroperitoneal area. Neuroblastoma has an incidence of about 1 in every 10,000 live births. It is estimated that 10 percent to 20 percent of solid tumors in children are neuroblastomas. Neuroblastomas most often manifest in children less than 1 year of age.

SIGNS AND SYMPTOMS

Children with neuroblastomas typically present with protruberant abdomens, often discovered by a parent. On clinical examination, a neuroblastoma is a large, firm, nodular, sometimes painful flank mass, which is usually fixed to surrounding structures. Ptosis and periorbital ecchymosis secondary to periorbital metastases may be present. Some children present with pulmonary metastases. Paraspinal neuroblastoma may extend through the neural foramina into the epidural space producing paralysis. Enlarged peripheral lymph nodes, Horner's syndrome, complete to partial absence of the iris, and metastatic enlargement of the liver may also be present.

Neuroblastomas may secrete vasoactive intestinal peptides, which are responsible for persistent watery diarrhea, with loss of fluid and electrolytes. These tumors also synthesize catecholamines, but the incidence of hypertension is low.

DIAGNOSIS

Ultrasonography and computed tomography are the primary diagnostic procedures for evaluation of abdominal masses in children. Arteriography is helpful in delineating the extent of involvement of the great vessels by the tumor and its resectability. In some cases, the great vessels are entrapped by the tumor, such that attempts at complete resection would risk major blood loss. An inferior vena cavagram may be necessary to reveal the extent of involvement of this vessel by the tumor. Urinary excretion of vanillylmandelic acid is increased in the majority of children with neuroblastomas, reflecting metabolism of catecholamines produced by these tumors.

Neuroblastomas are divided into four stages, depending on their growth and involvement of other tissues. Stage I is a localized tumor. Stage II is a tumor with extension to regional lymph nodes. Stage III is a large tumor that crosses the midline. Stage IV refers to tumor with distant metastases. Unfortunately, stage IV tumor is present in 50 percent of children at the time of diagnosis. Indeed, the overall survival rate in children with neuroblastomas is only 30 percent.

TREATMENT

Treatment of neuroblastoma is surgical removal, including local metastases and involved lymph nodes. If these tumors cannot be resected completely, it is removed by morcellation. An alternative is to treat with chemotherapy or radiation before surgical resection. Children presenting with signs of spinal cord compression and varying degrees of paralysis may require performance of a myelogram during general anesthesia, followed by emergency laminectomy for removal of the tumor that has extended into the epidural space. Radiation therapy can be given either as palliative or as a therapeutic measure. Drugs used for chemotherapy, in varied combinations, include cyclophosphamide, vincristine, and doxorubicin. Possible adverse effects of chemotherapy must be considered in the preoperative evaluation of these patients (see Chapter 30 and Table 30-3). For example, cyclophosphamide produces bone marrow depression, and toxic metabolites that are excreted in the urine may cause microscopic hematuria or exsanguinating hemorrhage due to bladder irritation. Vincristine has little or no bone marrow suppressive effects but rather causes neurotoxicity, with loss of deep tendon reflexes. Doxorubicin produces suppression of all bone marrow elements. This drug is also cardiotoxic, as manifested by changes on the electrocardiogram, characterized by nonspecific ST-T wave changes and cardiac dysrhythmias. Cardiomyopathy with congestive heart failure may result from severe cases of adriamycin-induced toxicity (see Chapter 30).

Although aggressive treatment of children with other solid tumors has increased survival, the survival rate from neuroblastomas has changed little in the past 20 years.

MANAGEMENT OF ANESTHESIA

Management of anesthesia for resection of neuroblastomas is as described for children with nephroblastomas.

Nephroblastoma (Wilms' Tumor)

Nephroblastomas account for about 10 percent of solid tumors in children. One-third of these tumors occur in children less than 1 year of age, and three-fourths are diagnosed by 4 years of age.[146] The incidence is about 1 in every 13,500 live births.

SIGNS AND SYMPTOMS

Nephroblastomas typically present as asymptomatic flank masses in otherwise healthy children. The mass is usually accidentally discovered by the parents or the physician during routine physical examinations. Nephroblastomas vary in size and are usually firm, nontender, and free from surrounding structures. Pain, fever, and hematuria are usually late manifestations. These children may manifest malaise, weight loss, anemia, disturbances of micturition, and symptoms such as vomiting or constipation, due to compression of adjacent portions of the gastrointestinal tract by these tumors. Hypertension may be a manifestation of nephroblastomas, particularly if these tumors involve both kidneys. Increases in blood pressure are usually mild, but on rare occasions, hypertension may be so severe that encephalopathy and congestive heart failure develop. Hypertension may reflect renin production by these tumors or indirect stimulation of renin release due to compression of renal vasculature. Secondary hyperaldosteronism and hypokalemia may be present. Hypertension usually disappears after nephrectomy but may recur if metastases develop.

DIAGNOSIS

Radiographs of the abdomen reveal a renal mass and occasional calcification. Intravenous pyelography reveals distortion of the renal collecting system and occasionally absence of excretion by the involved kidney. This diagnostic test also provides an assessment of the function of the contralateral kidney. An inferior vena cavagram may reveal tumor invasion of this blood vessel. Arteriograms will reveal the extent of the tumor and involvement of the contralateral kidney. Radiographs of the chest or liver scans may reveal metastatic disease.

Nephroblastomas are divided into four stages. Stage I is a tumor limited to the kidneys. Stage II tumor is characterized by renal vein, perirenal tissue, or local lymph node involvement. A stage III lesion has peritoneal implants; and a stage IV tumor is characterized by metastases to lungs, liver, brain, bones, or distant lymph nodes.

TREATMENT

Treatment of nephroblastomas is nephrectomy, with or without subsequent radiation and chemotherapy, depending on the stage of involvement. For example, treatment of stage II tumors and beyond includes radiation therapy and chemotherapy, after surgical resection. Combined treatment of nephroblastomas is associated with a survival rate that approaches 80 percent.

Extensive tumors may necessitate radical enblock resections, including portions of the inferior vena cava, pancreas, spleen, and diaphragm. The presence of metastases may require multiple surgical procedures. If the tumor is inoperable on initial exploration or if the patient is in poor clinical condition, radiation therapy is given initially to shrink the tumor, and the patient is then reexplored. Prior radiation therapy may produce radiation nephritis of the normal kidney, especially when given in association with chemotherapy.

Bilateral nephroblastomas occur in 3 percent to 10 percent of patients. Two-thirds of these manifest at the same time; in the remainder, involvement of the contralateral kidney occurs at a later date. Depending on the magnitude of tumor involvement, surgical treatment can be bilateral partial nephrectomy or bilateral total nephrectomy followed by dialysis and eventually renal transplantation.

MANAGEMENT OF ANESTHESIA

Infants and children scheduled for exploration and resection of neuroblastomas or nephroblastomas will be in varying degrees of general health. For example, if tumors are diagnosed at a late stage, it is likely that anemia will be severe. In addition, adverse effects related to chemotherapy must be considered (see Chapter 30 and Table 30-3).

Anemia should be corrected to a minimum concentration of $10 \text{ g} \cdot \text{dl}^{-1}$. Children scheduled for surgery after radiation and chemotherapy may have low platelet counts, requiring the transfusion of platelets before induction of anesthesia. An adequate amount of blood should be crossmatched preoperatively, since resection of neuroblastomas or nephroblastomas may be associated with excessive blood loss. These children need to be well hydrated preoperatively and have electrolyte and acid-base imbalance corrected, especially if these children have lost excessive fluid and electrolytes due to diarrhea, as may be associated with neuroblastomas. Children receiving chemotherapy with doxorubicin need to be evaluated for the presence of cardiomyopathy and congestive heart failure (see Chapter 30). Conceivably, myocardial depressant drugs should be avoided in these patients.

In addition to routine monitoring, a catheter placed in a peripheral artery is recommended to allow constant monitoring of blood pressure plus frequent determination of arterial blood gases and pH. Intraoperative hypotension is not uncommon due to the sudden blood loss most likely to occur during dissection of these tumors from around major blood vessels. Catheters for infusion of intravenous fluids should be placed in the upper extremity or in the external jugular vein. Lower extremity veins should be avoided, since it may be necessary to ligate or partially resect the inferior vena cava. Measurement of central venous pressure is helpful for evaluating intravascular fluid volume and the adequacy of fluid replacement. Likewise, a Foley catheter for monitoring urine output will aid in maintaining an optical intravascular fluid volume.

Precautions need to be taken during induction of anesthesia to prevent pulmonary aspiration, particularly if these tumors are producing compression of the gastrointestinal tract. Children in poor general condition may develop sudden hypotension during induction of anesthesia, particularly if intravascular fluid volume has not been restored with preoperative infusion of crystalloid and colloid solutions. Hypertension, as present in some of these children, must be considered and measures taken for preventing excessive increases in blood pressure during intubation of the trachea. Although this is usually not a troublesome feature in these patients, as compared to patients with pheochromocytomas, it is conceivable that catecholamine-secreting neuroblastomas could cause hypertension similar to that produced by pheochromocytomas. In addition, hypertension may reflect manipulation of the adrenal medulla during resection of these tumors. Manipulation of the inferior vena cava containing metastatic tumor can result in tumor embolism to the heart or pulmonary artery.[147,148] This may result in varying degrees of obstruction to blood flow at the level of the right atrium or produce signs characteristic of pulmonary embolism, including precipitous hypotension, cardiac dysrhythmias, and cardiac arrest.

Maintenance of anesthesia is acceptably provided with nitrous oxide plus volatile anesthetics or opioids. Muscle relaxants are necessary to optimize surgical exposure. The stomach should be continuously decompressed via a nasogastric tube connected to low suction.

THERMAL (BURN) INJURIES

About 70,000 persons are hospitalized annually in the United States for thermal injuries, and one-half of these are children. Of the thermal related deaths, one-third are children less than 15 years of age. Survival after thermal injury depends on the age of the patient and the percentage of body area burned (Fig. 35-14).[149] Extent of thermal injury is estimated by determining the percent of the body surface area affected by the burn. Relative contributions of various portions of the body-to-body surface area varies with age (Fig. 35-15).[150]

Pathophysiology

Thermal injuries produce predictable pathophysiologic responses. These responses must be considered when formulating management of anesthesia for burned patients.

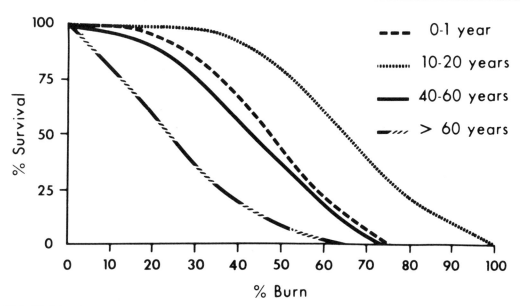

FIG. 35-14. Survival after thermal injury is influenced by the age of the patient and the percentage of the body surface area involved by the burn. (Stein ED, Stein JM. Anesthesia for the burn patient. Weekly anesthesiology update. Princeton: Weekly Anesthesiology Update, 1977;1:1)

CARDIAC OUTPUT

Cardiac output falls dramatically in the immediate postburn period. This initial fall precedes any measurable loss of intravascular fluid volume and may reflect the presence of a circulating low molecular weight myocardial depressant factor.[151] Subsequently, cardiac output is even more profoundly depressed by acute hypovolemia, which occurs as third-space fluid shifts result in decreases in intravascular fluid volume. Although prompt fluid resuscitation results in return of urine flow within 3 hours, cardiac output remains depressed until the beginning of the second postburn day. Intense vasoconstriction, increased metabolic demands, and hemolysis of red blood cells further strain the myocardium. Sudden circulatory decompensation may occur at this time if depressant effects of volatile anesthetics are superimposed.

After the initial 24 hours of fluid resuscitation, the circulatory system enters a hyperdynamic state, which will persist well into the postburn period. Blood pressure and heart rate are elevated, and cardiac output stabilizes at about twice normal. A high ejection fraction and rapid rate of myocardial fiber shortening are indicative of excessive myocardial activity. Pulmonary artery occlusion pressures will be in low-normal ranges, unless high output congestive heart failure supervenes. Pulmonary edema is rare during the initial few days of fluid resuscitation but is encountered later during the first postburn week, when edema fluid is being reabsorbed and intravascular fluid volume is maximally increased.

HYPERTENSION

Approximately 30 percent of children with extensive thermal injuries become hypertensive during the postburn period.[152] Onset of hypertension is usually within the first 2 weeks. Boys less than 10 years of age are at greatest risk for developing hypertension. Hypertension is usually transient but on occasion may persist for several weeks. Indeed, about 10 percent of these children, if untreated, will develop hypertensive encephalopathy, characterized by irritability and headache, with or without seizures. Etiology of this hypertension is unknown but may be related to

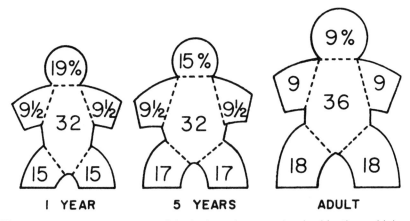

FIG. 35-15. In determining the percent of the body surface area involved by thermal injury, one must consider the age of the patient. (Smith El. Acute management of thermal burns in children. Surg Clin North Am 1970;50:807–14)

INTRAVASCULAR FLUID VOLUME

Intravascular fluid volume deficits after thermal injuries are roughly proportional to the extent and depth of the burn. In the first postburn day, the vascular compartment becomes permeable to plasma proteins, including fibrinogen. This increased permeability exists throughout the vascular system but is most pronounced in the area of the burn. Extravasated plasma proteins exert an osmotic pressure that can hold large volumes of fluid in an extravascular third space. During this period, administration of colloids would be of no benefit and could actually exacerbate third-space losses. Loss of fluid from the vascular compartment during the first postburn day is about 4 ml·kg^{-1} for each percent of body surface burned. For example, in a 40 kg child with a 50 percent burn, fluids needed for the first 24 hours would be 8,000 ml. The most effective restoration of intravascular fluid volume occurs when two-thirds of this fluid is given during the first 8 hours postburn.[153]

During the second postburn day, capillary integrity is largely restored, and fluid and plasma protein losses are markedly reduced. Decreasing amounts of fluid are required to maintain intravascular fluid volume. Further rapid administration of electrolyte solutions at this time results in edema in excess of any gain in circulatory dynamics. Therefore, infusion of crystalloid solutions are sharply reduced after the first postburn day, and colloid solutions are administered.

AIRWAY

Direct thermal injuries to the airways, with the exception of steam inhalation, do not occur below the level of the vocal cords, reflecting the low thermal capacity of air and the efficient cooling ability of the upper air passages.[154] Thermal and/or chemical injuries of the upper airways, however, can cause severe edema. Hoarseness, stridor, and tachypnea demand prompt airway evaluation, since swelling of supraglottic tissues can result in sudden, complete upper airway obstruction hours after the original thermal injury. The airway should be secured before respiratory decompensation occurs, since translaryngeal intubation of the trachea after edema of the airway has progressed is likely to be difficult. The small caliber of the pediatric airway accentuates the impact of airway edema on resistance to breathing. If in-

Patients with elevated plasma concentrations of catecholamines and/or activation of the renin-angiotensin system. Treatment with antihypertensive drugs, such as hydralazine or nitroprusside, is indicated in some children.

tubation of the trachea is required for children, nasotracheal tubes are preferred, as nasal tubes are more comfortable and more easily secured than oral tubes.

Tracheostomy should be reserved for patients who develop late pulmonary complications that will require prolonged ventilatory support. Performance of a tracheostomy in a burned child with swelling of the face and neck is a formidable surgical challenge. Early complications of tracheostomy in burn patients include hemorrhage, pneumothorax, and malposition of the tracheostomy tube; late complications are related to mechanical factors (displacement of the cannula) and to tracheal erosion with massive bacterial invasion.

SMOKE INHALATION

Inhalation of suspended particles (smoke) and toxic products of incomplete combustion results in chemical pneumonitis similar to that resulting from aspiration of acidic gastric fluid.[154] Most patients with smoke inhalation will have associated face and neck burns or a history of being trapped in closed spaces. As in other forms of respiratory distress syndrome, smoke inhalation victims often experience an asymptomatic period, lasting for as long as 48 hours before respiratory distress becomes overt. An initial radiograph of the chest may be clear, but arterial partial pressures of oxygen while the patient is breathing room air are consistently decreased. Production of carbonaceous sputum and detection of wheezes and rales during auscultation of the chest herald impending respiratory failure.

Treatment of respiratory distress syndrome related to smoke inhalation is symptomatic. Administration of warm, humidified oxygen and bronchodilators is indicated. Early institution of positive pressure ventilation of the lungs with positive end-expiratory pressure should be considered if the arterial oxygen partial pressures are less than 60 mmHg breathing room air. Prophylactic antibiotic administration is not beneficial, and the value of corticosteroids is controversial. Extracorporeal membrane oxygenation has been attempted, but the results have not been encouraging. A catheter placed in a peripheral artery is essen-

tial for monitoring patients with symptomatic smoke inhalation injury. Presence of cardiac dysfunction in association with respiratory distress is often the indication to place a pulmonary artery catheter.

CARBON MONOXIDE

Carbon monoxide poisoning often complicates burns that occur in closed spaces and is the most common immediate cause of death from fire. Carbon monoxide has a high affinity for hemoglobin (210 times the affinity of oxygen) and, therefore, displaces oxygen to form carboxyhemoglobin. In addition to reducing oxygen transport by displacing oxygen, carbon monoxide shifts the oxyhemoglobin dissociation curve to the left, thereby hindering release of oxygen from hemoglobin to tissues. Symptoms of carbon monoxide poisoning reflect arterial hypoxemia and include headache, nausea, restlessness, and confusion. Carboxyhemoglobin concentrations in excess of 40 percent are associated with coma. The classic cherry-red appearance of these patients is usually not present when concentrations of carboxyhemoglobin are less than 40 percent. Treatment of carbon monoxide poisoning is with administration of pure oxygen. For example, one-half of the carbon monoxide in blood will be eliminated every 4 hours during spontaneous breathing with room air; with pure oxygen, this same reduction can be accomplished in 40 minutes. Severe poisoning with carbon monoxide is best treated with intubation of the trachea, followed by mechanical ventilation of the lungs with pure oxygen.

RESTRICTIVE THERMAL INJURY

Mechanical factors resulting from thermal injury may interfere with pulmonary function. For example, circumferential burns of the chest and upper abdomen can lead to restriction of chest wall motion, as the eschar contracts and hardens. This restriction is further aggravated by ileus and abdominal distention. Escharotomies may be necessary to relieve the restriction.

THERMOREGULATION AND METABOLISM

An increase in metabolic rate will occur in proportion to the extent of thermal injury. Metabolic rate can be more than doubled in patients with thermal injuries that involve 50 percent of the body surface area. Total parenteral nutrition may be required to meet these increased metabolic requirements. Accompanying this hypermetabolic response, the metabolic thermostat is reset upward, so that burn patients tend to increase their skin and core temperatures somewhat above normal, regardless of environmental temperatures.

Thermoregulatory functions of the skin, including vasoactivity, sweating, piloerection, and insulation, are abolished or diminished by thermal injuries. In addition, skin no longer functions as an effective water vapor barrier, resulting in loss of ion-free water. It is estimated that daily evaporative water loss is equivalent to 4,000 ml·m^{-2} of burn surface in children, compared to 2,500 ml in adults.[152] Assuming that 0.58 calories are lost for each milliliter of evaporative water loss, a 4,000 ml water loss would represent a daily energy loss of about 2,400 calories. Failure of occlusive dressings or increases in ambient temperatures to lower substantially the metabolic rate confirms that the hypermetabolism of burn patients does not relate exclusively to loss of water and heat through the area of thermal injuries. In children, intense vasoconstriction in the nonburned areas of skin can result in increases in body temperature sufficient to cause febrile convulsions. Conversely, when metabolism and peripheral vasoconstriction are depressed, as during general anesthesia, children with thermal injuries may experience rapid falls in body temperature.

GASTROINTESTINAL TRACT

Adynamic ileus is virtually universal after thermal injuries of greater than 20 percent of the body surface area. Therefore, early decompression of the stomach via a nasogastric tube is indicated. Acute ulceration of the stomach or duodenum, known as Curling's ulcer, is the most frequent life-threatening gastrointestinal complication. The precise etiology of Curling's ulcer is unknown; however, the ulcers are most frequent in patients with sepsis and/or extensive burns. Duodenal ulcers occur twice as frequently in children with thermal injuries as in adults (14 percent versus 7 percent).[151] Most patients with Curling's ulcer can be managed conservatively with antacids or H-2 antagonist drugs, but occasional patients may require vagotomy, with or without partial gastrectomy.

Acalculous cholecystitis may occur during the second or third postburn week. Immediate cholecystectomy is indicated for treatment of this complication. Superior mesenteric artery syndrome may occur at the time of maximum weight loss in burn patients. If conservative therapy fails, duodenojejunostomy or other intra-abdominal surgery may be required.

RENAL FUNCTION

Immediately after thermal injuries occur, cardiac output and intravascular fluid volumes decrease, and plasma catecholamine concentrations increase, resulting in falls in renal blood flow and glomerular filtration rate. Diminished renal blood flow activates the renin-angiotension-aldosterone system and stimulates the release of antidiuretic hormone. The net effect on renal function is retention of sodium and water and exaggerated losses of potassium, calcium, and magnesium. Later, after adequate fluid resuscitation, renal blood flow and glomerular filtration may rise dramatically.

Hourly urine output remains the most readily available and reliable guide to adequacy of fluid resuscitation. For example, urine output should be about 1.0 ml·kg^{-1}·hr^{-1} in adequately resuscitated children. Renal failure is rare in children who have received adequate fluid resuscitation, unless there are extensive electrical burns or massive thermal injuries of skeletal muscles. In the latter circumstance, hemochromogens may be released into the circulation and precipitate in renal tubules, leading to acute tubular necrosis.

ELECTROLYTES

An increase in plasma concentrations of potassium due to tissue necrosis and hemolysis is common during the first 2 postburn days. This is followed over the next several days by marked hypokalemia, due to accentuated renal losses of potassium. Diarrhea and gastric suction will further exaggerate potassium losses. Iatrogenic cardiac dysrhythmias may occur in hypokalemic patients who receive drugs that promote intracellular movement of potassium (insulin, glucose, sodium bicarbonate) or drugs that oppose myocardial conduction effects of potassium (calcium salts). Digitalis administration is particularly hazardous in these patients and should not be used prophylactically.

Plasma concentrations of ionized calcium may be reduced in the postburn period. Since children are more sensitive than adults to effects of citrate and/or potassium in stored blood, children with extensive thermal injuries who are receiving large volumes of rapidly infused whole blood should receive calcium gluconate, 1 mg to 2 mg for every milliliter of infused blood.

ENDOCRINE RESPONSES

Endocrine responses to thermal injuries are characterized by massive outpourings of adrenocorticotrophic hormone, antidiuretic hormone, renin, angiotensin, aldosterone, glucagon, and catecholamines. Plasma concentrations of insulin may be increased or decreased. Nevertheless, plasma glucose concentrations will be elevated, due to increased concentrations of glucagon and catecholamine-induced glycogenolysis in liver and skeletal muscles. Indeed, glycosuria occurs frequently in nondiabetic burn patients. Burn patients may be particularly susceptible to development of nonketotic hyperosmolar coma, especially if total parenteral nutrition is being utilized.

Maximum increases in plasma concentrations of norepinephrine occur 3 days to 4 days postburn and may remain elevated for several days. Peak plasma concentrations of norepinephrine may be 26 times normal.[152] These markedly elevated concentrations produce intense vasoconstriction of skin and splanchnic vessels. Increased plasma concentrations of norepinephrine have been implicated as causative factors in many of the adverse manifestations of thermal injuries in children, including ischemia of the gastrointestinal tract, liver dysfunction, Curling's ulcer, oliguria, disseminated intravascular coagulation, cardiac dysfunction, hypertensive crises, and elevations of body temperature. Occasionally, peripheral vasodilators, including phentolamine or hydralazine, have been infused in the early postburn period to offset vasoconstriction and improve tissue perfusion.

RHEOLOGY

Blood viscosity increases acutely after thermal injuries and remains elevated for several days postburn, even after the hematocrit has returned to normal. After a transient depression, elevations of plasma concentrations of fibrinogen and factors V and VIII persist for several weeks. This hypercoagulable state may give rise to disseminated intravascular coagulation. Diagnosis of disseminated intravascular coagulation is difficult, since plasma concentrations of fibrin split products are almost invariably elevated after thermal injuries.

Hemolysis of erythrocytes in response to thermal injuries is not extensive. Therefore, early transfusion of whole blood or erythrocytes, in the absence of other injuries, is rarely necessary. Nevertheless, generalized suppression of erythrocyte production and reduction of erythrocyte survival time follow thermal injuries and may persist well into the postburn period. Therefore, transfusion of erythrocytes is often needed by about the fifth postburn day to maintain hemoglobin concentrations above 10 g·dl^{-1}.

IMMUNOLOGY

Leukocyte function is depressed and levels of immunoglobulin G and M are low following thermal injuries. Sepsis is the most common cause of death in children with thermal injuries. Gram-negative bacteremia produces a significantly increased mortality. Pneumonia, suppurative thrombophlebitis, and bacterial invasion of the burn eschar are likely explanations for sepsis. Clearly, aseptic techniques must be strictly observed by all persons participating in the care of burned children.

LIVER FUNCTION

Liver function tests are frequently abnormal in burn patients, even when areas of thermal injuries are small. Overt liver failure, however, is uncommon, unless the postburn course is complicated by hypotension, sepsis, or multiple transfusions of blood. Halothane-associated liver dysfunction in burn patients has not been described.

Management of Anesthesia

Historic information regarding the time and type of burn injuries is pertinent for the management of acutely burned children.[155,156] For example, time of injury is important, as initial fluid requirements are based on time elapsed since the burn occurred. Children who were trapped in closed spaces are likely to have suffered smoke inhalation injury. Electrical burns may produce far more tissue destruction than the surface burns would indicate (see the section Electrical Burns).

Physical examination should focus on the status of the airway. Head and neck burns, singed nasal hairs, and hoarseness are signs that supraglottic edema may develop or is already present. Carbonaceous sputum, wheezes, or diminished breath sounds suggest presence of smoke inhalation injuries. Abdominal distention may indicate paralytic ileus, warranting special precautions during induction of anesthesia, so as to reduce hazards of pulmonary aspiration. A careful search should be made during the preoperative evaluation for sites suitable for placement of intravenous catheters and monitoring devices.

Measurement of arterial blood gases and pH and evaluation of radiographs of the chest are indicated in patients suspected of having experienced smoke inhalation. Carboxyhemoglobin levels are helpful only for the first few hours after thermal injuries. In the presence of carboxyhemoglobin, the pulse oximeter may overestimate saturation of hemoglobin with oxygen, emphasizing the need for caution in relying on this monitor in patients with recent carbon monoxide exposure.[157] Conversely, transcutaneous partial pressures of oxygen decline in a linear fashion, as plasma concentrations of carboxyhemoglobin increase. Plasma glucose concentrations and osmolarity should be determined, particularly if patients are receiving total parenteral nutrition. Measures of renal function are indicated after extensive electrical burns. Adequacy of fluid replacement can be best judged by urine output, which should be about 1 $ml \cdot kg^{-1} \cdot hr^{-1}$. Coagulation profiles should be obtained in patients where extensive intraoperative blood loss is anticipated.

Establishment of intravenous infusion lines may be difficult in severely burned children. In some instances, it may become necessary to use veins in areas that escaped thermal injuries, such as the axilla, the scalp, or the web spaces between the digits. Reliable intravenous catheters of sufficient caliber are essential for patients undergoing excision of burn eschar, as large amounts of blood can be lost in a short time. Even split thickness skin grafts are associated with about 80 ml of blood loss for each 100 cm^2 of skin harvested.[151]

Children with extensive thermal injuries may need intensive monitoring, yet not have an unburned limb available for a blood pressure cuff. Catheters placed into peripheral arteries will occasionally have to be inserted through burn eschar. Septic complications are likely, such that catheters placed through the eschar should be removed as soon as possible. Venous cannulation sites are likewise vulnerable to septic complications. Reductions in body temperature are exaggerated during the intraoperative period, reflecting loss of insulating properties of the skin, evaporative loss of water from the eschar, and depression of metabolic rate by general anesthesia. Routine measures for reducing heat loss include use of warming blankets and radiant overhead warmers. Inspired gases should be warmed and humidified and intravenous fluids administered through a warmer. Ambient temperature of the operating rooms should be maintained near 25 degrees Celsius. Plastic or paper drapes will reduce evaporative and convective heat losses.

PHARMACOLOGY

A number of pathophysiologic alterations produced by burn trauma affect drug disposition.[157] Immediately after burn injury, there are decreases in organ and tissue blood flow caused by hypovolemia, depressed myocardial function, and release of vasoactive substances. Drugs administered by any route other than intravenously will have predictably delayed absorptions. Intravenous and inhaled drugs may have increased effects on the brain and heart because of relative increases in blood flow to these critical organs. After adequate fluid resuscitation, the hypermetabolic phase begins 48 hours after injury. During this time oxygen and glucose consumptions are markedly increased. Plasma albumin concentrations are decreased after burn trauma, so that albumin-bound drugs (benzodiazepines, anticonvulsant drugs) will have an increased free fraction. Conversely, plasma concentrations of alpha-1 acid glycoprotein are increased, so that drugs bound to this protein (muscle relaxants, tricyclic antidepressant drugs) will have a decreased free fraction.

Pharmacokinetics after burn injuries are further complicated by superimposed effects of sepsis, co-existing systemic diseases, and renal dysfunction. Cimetidine is used extensively for the prevention of stress ulcers in burn patients. Since cimetidine also reduces hepatic blood flow, it may alter disposition of drugs dependent on hepatic clearance. Although burn patients have an increased tolerance to

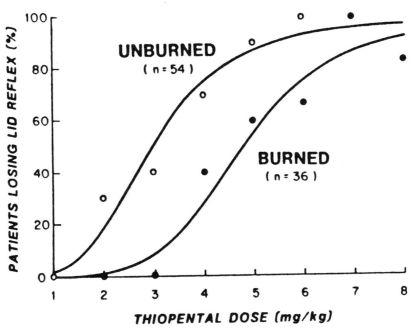

FIG. 35-16. Doses of thiopental administered intravenously to produce loss of the lid reflex were greater in burned children (greater than 15 percent burn and more than 1 year after injury) than in unburned children. (Cote CJ, Petkau AJ. Thiopental requirements may be increased in children reanesthetized at least 1 year after recovery from extensive thermal injury. Anesth Analg 1985;64:1156–60. Reprinted with permission from IARS)

diazepam, repeated administration of diazepam may produce significant accumulation when coadministered with cimetidine.[158]

Pharmacologic alterations may persist after recovery from burn injuries. It has been shown that thiopental requirements are increased in children for more than a year after burn injuries (Fig. 35-16).[159] Opioid requirements may also be increased in burn patients.

Of all the classes of drugs, the effects of burn injuries on muscle relaxants have been the most extensively studied. The hyperkalemic response to succinylcholine is well known. The risk of hyperkalemia is probably related to the severity of the burn and the time from injury to succinylcholine administration. The greatest risk, appears to be between 10 days and 50 days after injury.[160] Nevertheless, these zones are very poorly defined, and the safest recommendation may be avoidance of succinylcholine. Several studies have shown that burned patients develop marked resistance (up to threefold increases in dose requirements) to nondepolarizing muscle relaxants (Fig. 35-17).[156,161–164] Altered pharmacokinetics and increased plasma protein binding of muscle relaxants contribute little to the increased dose requirements for these drugs in burn injury patients. Instead, increased dose requirements for muscle relaxants most likely reflect a pharmacodynamic mechanism due to proliferation of extrajunctional cholinergic receptors, which are responsive to acetylcholine. Evidence for this pharmacodynamic mechanism is the nearly fivefold increase in plasma concentrations of d-tubocurarine required to produce the same degree of neuromuscular blockade in burn injury patients compared to normal patients (Fig. 35-18).[165] Resistance to neuromuscular blocking effects of metocurine has been observed as long as 463 days after a 35 percent third-degree burn (Fig. 35-19).[166] This prolonged duration of resistance is presumed to reflect an increased number of cholinergic receptors and has implications for use of succinylcholine in burn patients, since it is also presumed that hyperkalemia after administration of this drug reflects an increased number of cholinergic receptors for potassium exchange to occur during succinylcholine-induced depolarization.

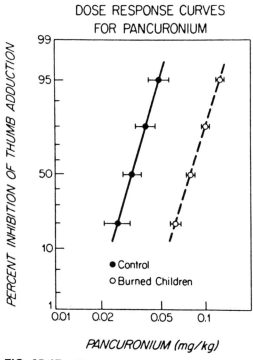

FIG. 35-17. The dose of pancuronium administered intravenously to produce inhibition of thumb adduction is greater in burned children (body surface area burn 4 percent to 85 percent studied 34 ± 7.9 (SE) days after injury) compared to control children. (Martyn JAJ, Liu LMP, Szyfelbein SK, et al. The neuromuscular effects of pancuronium in burned children. Anesthesiology 1983;59:561–4)

Ketamine has been used for many years as an anesthetic for burn injury patients, especially for dressing changes and escharotomies.[167] This drug can be administered either intravenously or intramuscularly with good effect. Administration of ketamine should be preceded by anticholinergic drugs, as excessive salivation is likely. A single intravenous dose of ketamine 2 mg·kg^{-1} to 4 mg·kg^{-1} provides excellent somatic analgesia for 15 minutes to 20 minutes. Recovery of consciousness from single intravenous injections of ketamine is usually rapid, allowing early return to oral nutritional support. Nitrous oxide can be administered to reduce random motion of the limbs, which often accompanies ketamine anesthesia. The incidence of postoperative de-

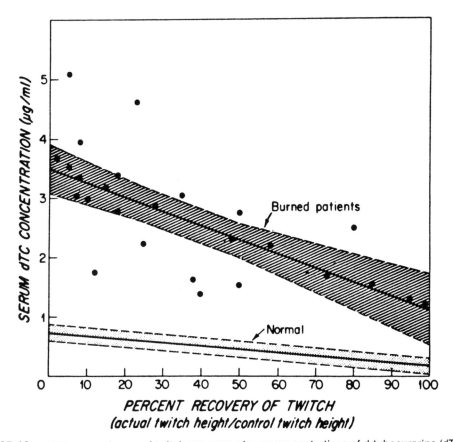

FIG. 35-18. At the same degree of twitch recovery, plasma concentrations of d-tubocurarine (dTC) are greater in burned patients than in normal patients. (Martyn JAJ, Szyfelbein SK, Ali HH, et al. Increased d-tubocurarine requirement following major thermal injury. Anesthesiology 1980;52:352–5)

lirium after administration of ketamine to pediatric patients has been minimal. Nevertheless, central effects of ketamine, if they occur, can be at least partially reversed by intravenous administration of physostigmine (30 µg·kg⁻¹).[168] Excessive movement during emergence from anesthesia may dislodge skin grafts or promote hemorrhage, resulting in early graft loss. Halothane is the most frequently used inhaled drug for anesthesia in children with thermal injuries. This volatile anesthetic permits maintenance of spontaneous ventilation and allows administration of high concentrations of oxygen if necessary. Depth of anesthesia can be adjusted for the surgical stimulus, such that increased inspired concentrations of halothane can be administered during high intensity

stimulation associated with harvesting skin grafts. Application of skin grafts is essentially painless, and concentrations of halothane are reduced during this period. Halothane associated hepatic dysfunction has not been observed in burn injury patients, despite repeated exposures to the drug.[155] Enflurane and isoflurane are acceptable alternatives to halothane, particularly in older patients who require multiple anesthetics.

It is evident that physiologic alterations produced by burn injuries can markedly affect responses to drugs. Altered responses are highly dependent on the time from injury and the degree of resuscitation. Many of these problems may persist for months to years after recovery from burn injuries. Therefore, careful

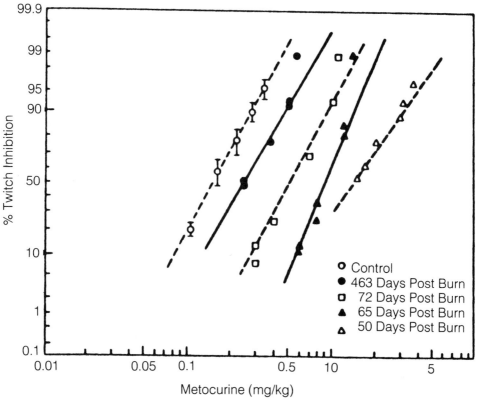

FIG. 35-19. The dose-response curve for metocurine administered intravenously to a burned patient is displaced to the right of unburned patients (control) between 50 days and 463 days postburn. (Martyn JAJ, Matteo RS, Szyfelbein SK, Kaplan RF. Unprecedented resistance to neuromuscular blocking effects of metocurine with persistence after complete recovery in a burned patient. Anesth Analg 1982;61:614–6. Reprinted with permission from IARS)

monitoring of drug responses is indicated when administering anesthesia to burn injury patients.

ELECTRICAL BURNS

High-voltage electrical currents cause tissue damage by conversion to thermal energy.[169] The amount of thermal energy transferred to tissues depends on the voltage of the electrical source, skin resistance of the victim, and the duration of the contact with the source of electrical currents. Tissue damage will be greatest where electrical currents are most con-

centrated, as occurs at points of entry and exit, and where the involved extremities are narrowest. Visceral injuries due to electrical currents are unlikely.

Deep tissue destruction produced by electrical burns is often extensive, since these tissues cannot dissipate thermal energy as rapidly as more superficial tissues. This makes the extent of damage produced by electrical currents difficult to judge from the extent of superficial injuries. Fasciotomies, multiple debridements of wounds, and arteriograms to define the level of viability of affected limbs may be necessary.

At the time of initial electrical injuries, cardiopulmonary arrest requiring cardiopulmonary resuscitation may have occurred. Indeed, cardiac dysrhythmias occur in 1 out of every 6 patients who experience electrical burns.[170] These patients should be monitored by continuous displays of the electrocardiogram for at least the first 48 hours postburn.

Renal failure may accompany electrical burns, reflecting precipitation of myoglobin from injured skeletal muscles in renal tubules. Furthermore, the extent of superficial tissue damage may result in underestimation of the initial fluid requirements. Nevertheless, with recognition of the deep tissue injuries accompanying electrical burns and concurrent administration of fluids and diuretics to maintain urine output near $1 \text{ ml} \cdot \text{kg}^{-1} \cdot \text{hr}^{-1}$, renal failure has become uncommon.

The development of neurologic complications after electrical burns are common. Peripheral nerve deficits or spinal cord deficits can occur early, reflecting direct injuries of nerves, or later, as a result of perineural scarring or neural ischemia. Neuropathies may involve nerves far removed from points of electrical contact and may progress for several years after injuries. Cataract formation is another late sequela.

A common type of electrical burn in children occurs when the child bites through an electrical cord. The resulting burn usually involves the oral commissure. Subsequent scar formation can narrow the oral opening, leading to difficulty in maintaining the upper airway or accomplishing intubation of the trachea during corrective surgery.

Injury due to lightning represents a special form of electrical burns.[171] Lightning tends to flow around the exterior of its victims, resulting in superficial flash burns rather than deep tissue thermal injuries, as is characteristic of electrical burns. Transient neurologic deficits and cardiac dysrhythmias are common after injuries due to lightning. Most of the deaths associated with lightning are due to cardiopulmonary arrest at the time of the initial injuries.

SEPARATION OF CONJOINED TWINS

Surgical separation of conjoined twins requires thorough preoperative preparation and discussion among surgeons, pediatricians, and anesthesiologists.[172-176] A detailed rehearsal of the entire procedure, beginning with transportation to the operating room, serves to emphasize the needs and responsibilities of all involved. Preoperative evaluation demonstrates shared organ systems. Management of anesthesia requires two teams and separate anesthetic machines, delivery systems and ventilators, and monitoring systems. Ultimately, a second operating table will be required.

Awake intubation of the trachea before the administration of muscle relaxants is often recommended but not mandatory.[174] Monitoring must be extensive and invasive (central venous pressure, intra-arterial) to facilitate replacement of blood loss and provide indicators of ventilation. Maintenance of body temperature is important. Monitoring of plasma concentrations of ionized calcium and appropriate replacement is useful for maintaining myocardial contractility and optimizing coagulation.[175] Color coding of all vascular lines, monitors, apparatus, records, and personnel is useful.[173] Presence of cross-circulation means drugs administered to one infant are likely to produce detectable effects in the other infant. The magnitude of cross-circulation may vary from minute to minute, making prediction of drug effects even more difficult. Aggressive efforts are required to maintain normothermia. Metabolic acidosis may be prominent and require treatment with sodium bicarbonate. The need for continued support of ventilation of the lungs in the postoperative period is likely.

REFERENCES

1. Graff TD, Phillips OC, Benson DW, Kelley E. Baltimore anesthesia study committee: Factors in pediatric anesthesia mortality. Anesth Analg 1964;43:407–14
2. Rackow H, Salnitre E, Green LT. Frequency of cardiac arrest associated with anesthesia in infants and children. Pediatrics 1961;28:697–704
3. Smith RM. Anesthesia for Infants and Children. 3rd Ed. St. Louis. CV Mosby 1986
4. Downes JJ, Raphaely RC. Anesthesia and intensive care. In: Ravitch MM, Kelch KJ, Benson CD,

eds. Pediatric Surgery. Chicago. Year Book Medical Publishers 1979:12–38

5. Eckenhoff JE. Some anatomic considerations of the infant larynx influencing endotracheal anesthesia. Anesthesiology 1951;12:401–10

6. Kubota Y, Toyoda Y, Nagata N, et al. Tracheobronchial angles in infants and children. Anesthesiology 1986;64:374–6

7. Tochen ML. Orotracheal intubation in the newborn infant: A method of determining depth of tube insertion. J Pediatr 1979;95:1050–1

8. Inselman LS, Mellins RB. Growth and development of the lungs. J Pediatr 1981;98:1–15

9. Muller N, Gulston G, Cade D, et al. Diaphragmatic muscle fatigue in the newborn. J Appl Physiol 1979;46:688–95

10. Rigatto H. Ventilatory response to hypercapnia. Semin Perinatol 1977;1:363–7

11. Pang LM, Mellins RB. Neonatal cardiorespiratory physiology. Anesthesiology 1975;43:171–96

12. Hagen PT, Scholz DG, Edwards WD. Incidence and size of patent foramen ovale during the first 10 decades of life on autopsy study of 965 normal hearts. Mayo Clin Proc 1984;59:17–20

13. Levin DL, Heymann MA, Kitterman JA, et al. Persistent pulmonary hypertension of the newborn infant. J Pediatr 1976;89:626–30

14. Baylen BG, Ogata H, Ikegami M, et al. Left ventricular performance and contractility before and after volume infusion: A comparative study of preterm and full-term newborn lambs. Circulation 1986;73:1042–9

15. Crone RK. The cardiovascular effects of isoproterenol in the preterm newborn lamb. Crit Care Med 1984;12:33–5

16. Kliegman R, Fanaroff AA. Caution in the use of dopamine in the neonate. J Pediatr 1978;93:540–1

17. Young M. Responses of the systemic circulation of the newborn infant. Br Med Bull 1966;22:70–2

18. Manders WT, Pagani M, Vatner SF. Depressed responsiveness to vasoconstrictor and dilator agents and baroreflex sensitivity in conscious newborn lambs. Circulation 1979;60:945–55

19. Wear R, Robinson S, Gregory GA. The effects of the baroresponse of adult and baby rabbits. Anesthesiology 1982;56:188–91

20. Rao CC, Boyer MS, Krishna G, Paradise RR. Increased sensitivity of the isometric contraction of the neonatal isolated rat atria to halothane, isoflurane, and enflurane. Anesthesiology 1986;64:13–8

21. Wolf WJ, Neal MB, Peterson MD. The hemodynamic and cardiovascular effects of isoflurane and halothane anesthesia in children. Anesthesiology 1986;64:328–33

22. Berry GA, Gregory GA. Do premature infants require anesthesia for surgery. Anesthesiology 1987;67:291–3

23. Welborn LG, Hannallah RS, McGill WA, et al. Glucose concentrations for routine intravenous infusion in pediatric outpatient surgery. Anesthesiology 1987;67:427–30

24. Sieber FE, Smith DS, Traystman FJ, Wollman H. Glucose: A reevaluation for its intraoperative use. Anesthesiology 1987;67:72–81

25. Aperia A, Broberger O, Elinder G, et al. Postnatal development of renal function in pre-term and full-term infants. Acta Paediatr Scand 1981;70:183–7

26. Furman EB, Roman DG, Lemmer LAS, et al. Specific therapy in water, electrolyte, and blood volume replacement during pediatric surgery. Anesthesiology 1975;42:187–93

27. Hathaway WE. The bleeding newborn. Semin Hematol 1975;12:175–88

28. Sola A, Gregory GA. Colloid osmotic pressure of normal newborns and premature infants. Crit Care Med 1981;9:568–72

29. Wu PYK, Rockwell G, Chan L, et al. Colloid osmotic pressure in newborn infants: Variations with birth weight, gestational age, total serum solids, and mean arterial pressure. Pediatrics 1981;68:814–9

30. Lerman J, Robinson S, Willis MM, Gregory GA: Anesthetic requirement for halothane in young children 0–1 month and 1–6 months of age. Anesthesiology 1983;59:421–4

31. Cameron CB, Robinson S, Gregory GA. The minimum anesthetic requirement of isoflurane in children. Anesth Analg 1984;63:418–20

32. LeDez KM, Lerman J. The minimum alveolar concntration (MAC) of isoflurane in preterm neonates. Anesthesiology 1987;67:301–7

33. Cook DR. Newborn anesthesia; pharmacological considerations. Can Anaesth Soc J 1986;33:38–42

34. Steward DJ, Creighton RE. The uptake and excretion of nitrous oxide in the newborn. Can Anaesth Soc J 1978;25:215–7

35. Brandon BW, Brandon RB, Cook DR. Uptake and distribution of halothane in infants: In vivo measurements and computer simulations. Anesth Analg 1983;62:404–10

36. Boudreaux JP, Schieber RA, Cook DR. Hemodynamic effects of halothane in the newborn piglet. Anesth Analg 1984;63:731–7

37. Friesen RH, Lichtor JL. Cardiovascular effects of inhalation induction with isoflurane in infants. Anesth Analg 1983;62:411–4

38. Cote CJ, Foudsouzian NG, Liu LMP, et al. The

dose response of intravenous thiopental for the induction of general anesthesia in unpremedicated children. Anesthesiology 1981;55:703–5

39. Robinson S, Gregory GA. Fentanyl-air-oxygen anesthesia for ligation of patent ductus arteriosus in preterm infants. Anesth Analg 1981;60:331–34

40. Hickey PR, Hansen DD. Fentanyl and sufentanil-oxygen-pancuronium anesthesia for cardiac surgery in infants. Anesth Analg 1984;63:117–24

41. Schieber RA, Stiller RL, Cook DR. Cardiovascular and pharmacodynamic effects of high-dose fentanyl in newborn piglets. Anesthesiology 1985;63:166–171

42. Goudsouzian NG. Maturation of neuromuscular transmission in the infant. Br J Anaesth 1980;50:205–13

43. Goudsouzian NG, Donlon JV, Savarese JJ, Ryan JF. Re-evaluation of dosage and duration of action of d-tubocurarine in the pediatric age group. Anesthesiology 1975;43:416–25

44. Fisher DM, O'Keeffe C, Stanski DR, et al. Pharmacokinetics and pharmacodynamics of d-tubocurarine in infants, children, and adults. Anesthesiology 1982;57:203–8

45. Goudsouzian NG, Liu LMP, Cote CJ. Comparison of equipotent doses of non-depolarizing muscle relaxants in children. Anesth Analg 1981;60:862–6

46. Brandom BW, Woelfel SK, Cook DR, et al. Clinical pharmacology of atracurium in infants. Anesth Analg 1984;63:309–12

47. Cook DR, Brandom BW, Woelfel SK, et al. Atracurium infusion in children during fentanyl, halothane, and isoflurane anesthesia. Anesth Analg 1984;63:201

48. Fisher DM, Miller RD. Neuromuscular effects of vecuronium (ORG NC45) in infants and children during N_2O halothane anesthesia. Anesthesiology 1983;58:519–23

49. Fisher DM, Cronnelly R, Miller RD, Sharma M. The neuromuscular pharmacology of neostigmine in infants and children. Anesthesiology 1983;59:220–25

50. Cook DR, Fischer CG. Neuromuscular blocking effects of succinylcholine in infants and children. Anesthesiology 1975;42:662–5

51. Liu LMP, DeCook TH, Goudsouzian NG, et al. Dose response to succinylcholine in children. Anesthesiology 1981;55:599–602

52. Cook DR. Muscle relaxants in infants and children. Anesth Analg 1981;60:335–43

53. Salem MR, Wong AY, Lin YH. The effect of suxamethonium on the intragastric pressure in infants and children. Br J Anaesth 1972;44:166–9

54. Cook DR, Westman HR, Rosenfeld L, Hendershot RJ. Pulmonary edema in infants: Possible association with intramuscular succinylcholine. Anesth Analg 1981;60:220–3

55. Venus B, Patel KC, Pratap SK, et al. Transcutaneous PO_2 monitoring during pediatric surgery. Crit Care Med 1981;9:714–6

56. Reed RL, Maier RV, Landicho D, et al. Correlation of hemodynamic variables with transcutaneous PO_2 measurements in critically ill adult patients. J Trauma 1985;25:1045–53

57. Eberhard P, Mindt W. Interference of anesthetic gases at skin surface sensors for oxygen and carbon dioxide. Crit Care Med 1981;9:717–20

58. Fait CD, Wetzel RC, Dean JM, et al. Pulse oximetry in critically ill children. J Clin Monit 1985;1:232–35

59. Chapman KR, Liu FLW, Watson RM, Rebuck AS. Range of accuracy of two wavelength oximetry. Chest 1986;89:540–42

60. Sasse FJ. Can we trust end-tidal carbon dioxide measurements in infants? J Clin Monit 1985;1:147–8

61. Merritt TA, Hallman M, Blown BT, et al. Prophylactic treatment of very premature infants with human surfactant. N Engl J Med 1986;315:785–90

62. Froese AB, Butler PO, Fletcher WA, Byford LJ. High-frequency oscillatory ventilation in premature infants with respiratory failure: A preliminary report. Anesth Analg 1987;66:814–8

63. Bancalari E, Gerhardt T. Bronchopulmonary dysplasia. Pediatr Clin N Amer 1986;33:1–23

64. Low JA, Galbraith RS, Sauerbrei EE, et al. Maternal, fetal, and newborn complications associated with newborn intracranial hemorrhage. Am J Obstet Gynecol 1986;154:345–51

65. Roberts MC, Nugent SK, Traystman RJ. Control of cerebral circulation in the neonate and infant. Crit Care Med 1980;8:570–4

66. Kuban KC, Leviton A, Krishnamoorthy KS, et al. Neonatal intracranial hemorrhage and phenobarbital. Pediatrics 1986;77:443–50

67. Flynn JT. Oxygen and retrolental fibroplasia: Update and challenge. Anesthesiology 1984;60:397–99

68. Gregory GA, Steward DJ. Life-threatening perioperative apnea in the ex-"premie". Anesthesiology 1983;59:495–98

69. Steward DJ. Preterm infants are more prone to complications following minor surgery than are term infants. Anesthesiology 1982;56:304–6

70. Kurth CD, Spitzer AR, Broennle AM, Downes JJ. Postoperative apnea in preterm infants. Anesthesiology 1987;66:483–8

71. Liu LMP, Cote CJ, Goudsouzian NG, et al. Life-

threatening apnea in infants recovering from anesthesia. Anesthesiology 1983;59:506–10

72. Hansen TWR, Bratlid D. Bilirubin and brain toxicity. Acta Paediatr Scand 1986;75:513–22

73. Srinivasan G, Jain R, Pildes RS, Kannan CR. Glucose homeostasis during anesthesia and surgery in infants. J Pediatr Surg 1986;21:718–21

74. Marks MI, Welch DF. Diagnosis of bacterial infections of the newborn infant. Clin Perinatol 1981;8:537–58

75. Dierdorf SF, Krishna G. Anesthetic management of neonatal surgical emergencies. Anesth Analg 1981;60:204–15

76. Harrison MR, deLorimer AA. Congenital diaphragmatic hernia. Surg Clin North Am 1981;61:1023–35

77. Adleman S, Benson CD. Bochdalek hernia in infants: Factors determining mortality. J Pediatr Surg 1976;11:569–73

78. Siebert JR, Haas JE, Beckwith JB. Left ventricular hypoplasia in congenital diaphragmatic hernia. J Pediatr Surg 1984;19:567–71

79. Vacanti JP, Crone RK, Murphy JD, et al. The pulmonary hemodynamic response to perioperative anesthesia in the treatment of high-risk patients with congenital diaphragmatic hernia. J Pediatr Surg 1984;19:672–9

80. Bartlett RH, Toomasian J, Roloff D, et al. Extracorporeal membrane oxygenation (ECMO) in neonatal respiratory failure. 100 cases. Ann Surg 1986;204:236–45

81. Harrington J, Raphaely RC, Downes JJ. Relationship of alveolar-arterial oxygen tension difference in diaphragmatic hernia of the newborn. Anesthesiology 1982;56:473–6

82. Grosfeld JL, Ballantine TVN. Esophageal atresia and tracheoesophageal fistula: Effect of delayed thoracotomy on survival. Surgery 1978;84:394–402

83. Holder TM, Ashcraft RW. Developments in the care of patients with esophageal atresia and tracheoesophageal fistula. Surg Clin North Am 1981;61:1051–61

84. Bautista MJ, Kuwahara BS, Henderson CU. Transcutaneous oxygen monitoring in an infant undergoing tracheoesophageal fistula repair. Can Anaesth Soc J 1986;33:505–8

85. Grosfeld JL, Dawes L, Weber TR. Congenital abdominal wall defects: Current management and survival. Surg Clin North Am 1981;15:1037–49

86. Yazbeck S, Ndoye M, Khan AH. Omphalocele: A 25-year experience. J Pediatr Surg 1986;21:761–3

87. Cote CJ. The anesthetic management of congenital lobar emphysema. Anesthesiology 1978;49:296–8

88. O'Neill JA. Neonatal necrotizing enterocolitis. Surg Clin North Am 1981;61:1013–22

89. Cikrit D, West KW, Schreiner R, Grosfeld JL. Long-term follow-up after surgical management of necrotizing enterocolitis: Sixty-three cases. J Pediatr Surg 1986;21:533–35

90. Walsh MC, Kliegman RM. Necrotizing enterocolitis: Treatment based on staging criteria. Pediatr Clin North Am 1986;33:179–201

91. Goldberg RN, Chung D, Goldman SL, Bancalari E. The association of rapid volume expansion and intraventricular hemorrhage in the preterm infant. J Pediatr 1980;96:1060–3

92. Haselby KA, Dierdorf SF, Krishna G, et al. Anaesthetic implications of neonatal necrotizing enterocolitis. Can Anaesth Soc J 1982;29:255–9

93. Nelson KB, Ellenberg JH. Antecedents of cerebral palsy. N Engl J Med 1986;315:81–6

94. Dierdorf SF, McNiece WL, Rao CC, et al. Effect of succinylcholine on plasma potassium in children with cerebral palsy. Anesthesiology 1985;62:88–90

95. Rao CC, Krishna G, Haselby K, et al. Ventriculobronchial fistula complicating a ventriculoperitoneal shunt. Anesthesiology 1977;47:388–90

96. Minton MD, Grosslight K, Stirt JA, Bedford RF. Increases in intracranial pressure from succinylcholine: Prevention by prior nondepolarizing blockade. Anesthesiology 1986;65:165–9

97. Dierdorf SF, McNiece WL, Rao CC, et al. Failure of succinylcholine to alter plasma potassium in children with myelomeningocele. Anesthesiology 1986;64:272–73

98. Davidson-Ward SL, Nickerson BG, vanderHal A, et al. Absent hypoxic and hypercapneic arousal responses in children with myelomeningocele and apnea. Pediatrics 1986;78:44–50

99. Morray JP, MacGillivray R, Duker G. Increased perioperative risk following repair of congenital heart disease in Down's syndrome. Anesthesiology 1986;65:221–24

100. Williams JP, Somerville GM, Miner ME, Reilly D. Atlanto-axial subluxation and trisomy-21: Another perioperative complication. Anesthesiology 1987;67:253–4

101. Williams JP, Somerville GM, Miner ME, Reilly D. Atlanto-axial subluxation and trisomy-21: Another perioperative complication. Anesthesiology 1987;67:253–4

102. Krishna G. Neurofibromatosis, renal hypertension, and cardiac dysrhythmias. Anesth Analg 1975;54:542–5

103. Yamashita M, Matsuki A, Oyama R. Anesthetic considerations on von Recklinghausen's dis-

ease (multiple neurofibromatosis). Anaesthetist 1977;26:117–8

104. Baraka A. Myasthenic response to muscle relaxants in von Recklinghausen's disease. Br J Anaesth 1974;46:701–3

105. Hubert CH. Critical care and anesthetic management of Reye's syndrome. South Med J 1979;72:684–9

106. Barrett MJ, Hurwitz ES, Schonberger LB, Rogers MF. Changing epidemiology of Reye's syndrome in the United States. Pediatrics 1986;77:598–602

107. Hurwitz ES, Barrett MJ, Bergman D, et al. Public health service study of Reye's syndrome and medications. Report of the main study. JAMA 1987;257:1905–11

108. Steward RE. Craniofacial malformations—clinical and genetic considerations. Pediatr Clin North Am 1978;25:485–515

109. Karl HW, Swedlow DB, Lee KW, Downes JJ. Epinephrine-halothane interactions in children. Anesthesiology 1983;58:142–5

110. Goudsouzian N, Cote CJ, Liu LMP, Dedrick DF. The dose response effects of oral cimetidine on gastric pH and volume in children. Anesthesiology 1981;55:533–6

111. Sklar GS, King BD. Endotracheal intubation and Treacher-Collins syndrome. Anesthesiology 1976;44:247–9

112. Converse JM, Woodsmith D. Report on a series of 50 craniofacial operations. Plast Reconstr Surg 1975;55:283–93

113. Davies DW, Munro IR. The anesthetic management and intraoperative care of patients undergoing major facial osteotomies. Plast Reconstr Surg 1975;55:50–5

114. Diaz JH. Croup and epiglottitis in children. Anesth Analg 1985;64:621–33

115. Mayo-Smith MF, Hirsch PJ, Wodzinski SF, Schiffman FJ. Acute epiglottitis in adults. N Engl J Med 1986;314:1133–9

116. Muller BJ, Fliegel JE. Acute epiglottitis in a 79-year-old-man. Can Anaesth Soc J 1985;32:415–17

117. Phelan PD, Mullins GC, Laundau LI, Duncan AW. The period of nasotracheal intubation in acute epiglottitis. Anaesth Intensive Care 1980;8:402–3

118. Adair JC, Ring WH, Jordan WS, Elwyn RA. Ten-year experience with IPPB in the treatment of acute laryngotracheobronchitis. Anesth Analg 1971;50:649–55

119. Loughlin GM, Taussig LM. Pulmonary function in children with a history of laryngotracheobronchitis. J Pediatr 1979;94:365–9

120. Koka BV, Jeon IS, Andre JM, et al. Postintubation croup in children. Anesth Analg 1977;56:501–5

121. Baraka A. Bronchoscopic removal of inhaled foreign bodies in children. Br J Anaesth 1974;46:124–6

122. Cohen SR, Gelelr KA, Seltzer S, Thompson JW. Papilloma of the larynx and tracheobronchial tree in children. Ann Otolaryngol 1980;89:497–503

123. Lawson NW, Rogers D, Seifen A, et al. Intravenous procaine as a supplement to general anesthesia for carbon dioxide laser resection of laryngeal papillomas in children. Anesth Analg 1979;58:492–6

124. Baskoff JD, Stevenson RL. Endobronchial intubation in children. Anesthesiology Review 1981;8:29–31

125. Rao CC, Krishna G, Grosfeld JL, Weber TL. One-lung pediatric anesthesia. Anesth Analg 1981;60:450–2

126. Borland LM. Anesthesia for children with Jeune's syndrome (asphyxiating thoracic dystrophy). Anesthesiology 1987;66:86–8

127. Gronert GA. Malignant hyperthermia. Anesthesiology 1980;53:395–423

128. Sessler DI. Malignant hyperthermia. J Pediatr 1986;109:9–14

129. Ording H. Incidence of malignant hyperthermia in Denmark. Anesth Analg 1985;64:700–4

130. Newbauer KR, Kaufman RD. Another use for mass spectrometry: Detection and monitoring of malignant hyperthermia. Anesth Analg 1985;64:837–9

131. Rosenberg H, Fletcher JE. Masseter muscle rigidity and malignant hyperthermia susceptibility. Anesth Analg 1986;65:161–4

132. Larach MG, Rosenberg H, Larach DR, Broennle AM. Prediction of malignant hyperthermia susceptibility by clinical signs. Anesthesiology 1987;66:547–50

133. Britt BA. Dantrolene. Can Anesth Soc 1984;31:61–75

134. Ryan JF, Donlon JV, Malt RA, et al. Cardiopulmonary bypass in the treatment of malignant hyperthermia. N Engl J Med 1974;290:1121–2

135. Mathieu A, Bogosain AJ, Ryan JF, et al. Recrudescence after survival of an initial episode of malignant hyperthermia. Anesthesiology 1979;51:454–5

136. Gronert GA, Thompson RL, Onofrio BM. Human malignant hyperthermia: Awake episodes and correction by dantrolene. Anesth Analg 1980;59:377–8

137. Lees DE, Gadde PL, Macnamara TE. Malignant hyperthermia in association with Burkitt's lymphoma: Report of a third case. Anesth Analg 1980;59:514–5

138. Anderson TE, Drummond DS, Breed AL, Taylor CA. Malignant hyperthermia in myelomeningocele: A previously unreported association. J Pediatr Orthop 1981;1:401–3

139. Paasuke RT, Brownell AKW. Serum creatine kinase level as a screening test for susceptibility to malignant hyperthermia. JAMA 1986;255:769–71

140. Flewellen EH, Nelson TE, Jones WP, et al. Dantrolene dose response in awake man: Implications for management of malignant hyperthermia. Anesthesiology 1983;59:275–80

141. Ruhland G, Hinkle AJ. Malignant hyperthermia after oral and intravenous pretreatment with dantrolene in a patient susceptible to malignant hyperthermia. Anesthesiology 1984;60:159–60

142. Fitzgibbons DC. Malignant hyperthermia following preoperative oral administration of dantrolene. Anesthesiology 1981;54:73–5

143. Berkowitz A, Rosenberg H. Femoral block with mepivacaine for muscle biopsy in malignant hyperthemia patients. Anesthesiology 1985;62:651–2

144. Gielen M, Viering W. 3-in-1 lumbar plexus block for muscle biopsy in malignant hyperthemia patients. Amide local anaesthetics may be used safely. Acta Anaesthesiol Scand 1986;30:581–3

145. Inkster JS. Anaesthesia for a patient suffering from familial dysautonomia (Riley-Day syndrome). Br J Anaesth 1971;43:509–11

146. Grosfeld JL, Ballantine TVN, Baehner RL. Current management of childhood solid tumors. Surg Clin North Am 1976;56:513–35

147. Milne B, Cervenko FW, Morales A, Salerno TA. Massive intraoperative pulmonary tumor embolus from renal cell carcinoma. Anesthesiology 1981;54:253–5

148. Akyon MG, Arslan G. Pulmonary embolism during surgery for Wilm's tumor (nephroblastoma). Br J Anaesth 1981;53:903–5

149. Stein ED, Stein JM. Anesthesia for the burn patient. Weekly Anesthesiology Update. Princeton: Weekly anesthesiology Update, 1977:1

150. Smith EI. Acute management of thermal burns in children. Surg Clin North Am 1970;50:807–14

151. Moncrief JA. Burns. N Engl J Med 1973;288–444–54

152. Popp MB, Friedberg DL, MacMillan BG. Clinical characteristics of hypertension in burned children. Ann Surg 1980;191:473–8

153. Pruitt BA. Fluid and electrolyte replacement in the burned patient. Surg Clin North Am 1978;58:1291–1312

154. Fein A, Leff A, Hopewell PC. Pathophysiology and management of the complications resulting from fire and the inhaled products of combustion: A review of the literature. Crit Care Med 1980;8:94–8

155. Boswick JA, Thompson JD, Kershner CJ. Critical care of the burned patient. Anesthesiology 1977;47:164–70

156. Martyn J. Clinical pharmacology and drug therapy in the burned patient. Anesthesiology 1986;65:67–75

157. Barker SJ, Tremper KK. The effect of carbon monoxide inhalation on pulse oximetry and transcutaneous PO_2. Anesthesiology 1987;66:677–9

158. Martyn JAJ, Greenblatt DJ, Quinby WC. Diazepam kinetics in patients with severe burns. Anesth Analg 1983;62:293–7

159. Cote CJ, Petkau AJ. Thiopental requirements may be increased in children reanesthetized at less than one year after recovery from extensive thermal injury. Anesth Analg 1985;64:1156–60

160. Katz RL, Katz LE. Complications associated with the use of muscle relaxants. In: Orkin FK, Cooperman LH, eds. Complications in Anesthesiology. J.B. Philadelphia. Lippincott 1983;557–9

161. Martyn JAJ, Matteo RS, Grenblatt DJ, et al. Pharmacokinetics of d-tubocurarine in patients with thermal injury. Anesth Analg 1982;61:241–6

162. Martyn JAJ, Liu MLP, Szyfelbein SK, et al. The neuromuscular effects of pancuronium in burned children. Anesthesiology 1983;59:561–4

163. Martyn JAJ, Goudsouzian NG, Matteo RS, et al. Metocurine requirements and plasma concentrations in burned pediatric patients. Br J Anaesth 1983;55:263–8

164. Dwersteg JF, Pavlin EG, Heimbach DM. Patients with burns are resistant to atracurium. Anesthesiology 1986;65:517–20

165. Martyn JAJ, Szyfelbein SK, Ali HH, et al. Increased d-tubocurarine requirement following major thermal injury. Anesthesiology 1980;52:352–5

166. Martyn JAJ, Matteo RS, Szyfelbein SK, Kaplan RF. Unprecedented resistance to neuromuscular blocking effects of metocurine with persistence after complete recovery in a burned patient. Anesth Analg 1982;61:614–7

167. Demling RH, Ellerbe S, Jarrett F. Ketamine anesthesia for tangential excision of burn eschar: A burn unit procedure. J Trauma 1978;18:269–70

168. Toro-Mates A, Rendon-Platas AM, Avila-Valdez E, Villarrel-Guzman RA. Physostigmine antagonizes ketamine. Anesth Analg 1980;59:764–7

169. Hunt JL, Mason AD, Masterson TS, Pruitt BA. The pathophysiology of acute electric injuries. J Trauma 1976;16:335–40

170. Solem L, Fischer RP, Strate RC. The nature of electrical injury. J Trauma 1977;17:487–92

171. Cooper MA. Lightning injuries: Prognostic signs for death. Ann Emerg Med 1980;9:134–8

172. Block EC, Karis JH. Cardiopagus in neonatal thoracopagus twins: Anesthetic management. Anesth Analg 1980;59:304–7

173. Furman EB, Roman DG, Hairabet J, et al. Management of anesthesia for surgical separation of newborn conjoined twins. Anesthesiology 1971;34:95–101

174. Hoshima H, Tanaka O, Obara H, Iwai S. Thoracopagus conjoined twins: Management of anesthetic induction and postoperative chest wall defect. Anesthesiology 1987;66:424–6

175. Georges LS, Smith KW, Wong KC. Anesthetic challenges in separation of craniopagus twins. Anesth Analg 1987;66:783–7

176. Diaz JH, Furman ER. Perioperative management of cojoined twins. Anesthesiology 1987;67:965–73

36

Geriatric Patients

Geriatric patients are arbitrarily defined as those individuals over 65 years of age, although it is recognized that there is not necessarily a correlation between chronologic and biologic age.[1] Individuals 65 years or older comprise about 11 percent of the population in the United States and represent the fastest growing segment of our society. Indeed, 5,000 Americans reach age 65 years every day and more than 50 percent of these individuals reach 75 years of age. Thirty percent of drug prescriptions are written for geriatric patients.[2] It is estimated that one-half of patients who reach 65 will require surgery before they die. The five most frequently performed surgical procedures in geriatric age patients are cataract extraction, transurethral resection of the prostate, herniorrhaphy, cholecystectomy, and reduction of a fractured hip. Of those who live to the age of 90, an estimated one-third of women and one-sixth of men will experience a hip fracture.[3] Morbidity and mortality are increased in geriatric patients undergoing surgery, especially if the operation is an emergency. Nevertheless, advanced age alone cannot be considered a contraindication to surgery.

Undoubtedly, improved medical care has contributed to prolonged life expectancy, which currently is approximately 74 years for men and 78 years for women. Continued increases in longevity, however, based on new medical discoveries may be minimal. For example, it is estimated that cure of cardiovascular and renal disease would add only 7.5 years to the life expectancy and cure of cancer only 1.5 years.[4] The real problem limiting longevity is the aging process itself. To date, causes of aging and senescence have eluded discovery. It seems likely that aging is a complex process involving genetics, development, and environment.

Care of geriatric patients in the perioperative period must consider changes in major organ function and altered responses to drugs that predictably accompany aging. Changes in organ function manifest as a decreased margin of reserve; in fact, old age can be characterized as a continuation of life with decreasing capacities for adaptation (Fig. 36-1).[5] Reduced function can often be demonstrated only by stress testing. For example, cardiac function sufficient for a sedentary life may become inadequate during the perioperative period should anemia or infection occur.

NERVOUS SYSTEM

Aging is associated with progressive declines in central nervous system activity and loss of neurons, particularly in the cerebral cortex. Explanations for decreased central nervous system activity include decreased neuronal

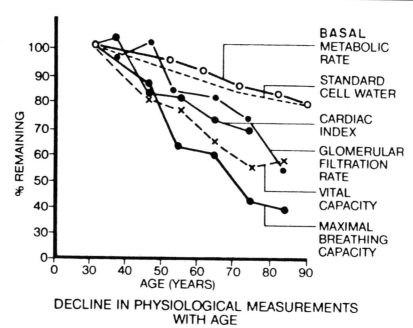

DECLINE IN PHYSIOLOGICAL MEASUREMENTS
WITH AGE

FIG. 36-1.   Aging is associated with progressive reductions in function (1 percent to 1.5 percent annually) of major organ systems. (Evans TI. The physiological basis of geriatric general anesthesia. Anaesth Intensive Care 1973;1:319–28)

density, decreased cerebral metabolic oxygen consumption, decreased cerebral blood flow, reduced number of receptor sites for neurotransmitter action, and decreased rate of synthesis of neurotransmitters. Conduction velocity in peripheral nerves gradually slows with advancing age, and there may be a reduced number of fibers in spinal cord tracts. Conceivably, these changes could increase susceptibility of geriatric patients to drugs that act on the peripheral and central nervous systems. Indeed, requirements for local anesthetics and volatile drugs are known to decrease with aging.[6–8] For example, dose requirements for epidural anesthesia may decrease in a linear manner after the age of 18.5 years and theoretically would reach zero at age 137 years (Fig. 36-2)[6,7] (see the section Epidural Anesthesia). Likewise, the minimum alveolar concentration (MAC) for volatile anesthetics decreases with aging (Fig. 36-3).[8] Global impairment of cognitive function (Alzheimer's disease) increases in frequency after 65 years of age (see Chapter 18).

CARDIOVASCULAR SYSTEM

Cardiovascular system changes, which accompany aging, often reflect decreased responsiveness to stimulation from the autonomic nervous system, with associated reductions in the ability of the heart to compensate for stress.[9]

Cardiac Output

Cardiac output declines about 1 percent·yr^{-1} after 30 years of age. Cerebral, coronary, and skeletal muscle blood flow are relatively maintained despite this decline in cardiac output, so that these organs receive a greater percentage of cardiac output in geriatric patients. The overall reduction in cardiac output parallels reductions in oxygen requirements of

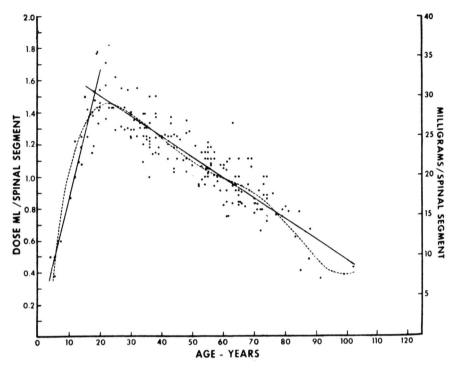

FIG. 36-2. The relationship between age and the dose of local anesthetic (ml or mg necessary to block a spinal segment) was measured in 201 patients between 4 and 102 years of age. Dose requirements increased in a linear manner from age 4 and reached a maximum at 18.5 years. After 18.5 years of age, requirements declined progressively with increasing age. Computer linear (-) and curvilinear (−) regression lines have been drawn through the data points. (Bromage PR. Ageing and epidural dose requirements. Segmental spread and predictability of epidural analgesia in youth and extreme age. Br J Anaesth 1969;41:1016–22)

aged tissue. The notion that cardiac output declines with aging may not be true for all geriatric patients. Specifically, those individuals who maintain physical fitness may sustain relatively unchanged cardiac outputs from approximately age 30 to age 60, at which point cardiac output may decline rapidly.[9]

Although resting stroke volume remains relatively unaffected by aging, the normal response to stress may be impaired. For example, the aged heart is less able to increase its cardiac output in response to stress, and vulnerability to drug-induced reductions in myocardial contractility may be increased. Indeed, inotropic responses to catecholamines are diminished in aged cardiac muscle, despite an absence of change in beta-adrenergic receptor density.[10] Decreases in beta receptor responsiveness without changes in receptor density suggests functional alterations in receptor affinity or uncoupling of the beta receptor-adenylate cyclase system. These changes are also consistent with resistance of aged hearts to chronotropic responses evoked by catecholamines, especially isoproterenol (see the section, Heart Rate). Further evidence for decreased beta receptor responsiveness is the presence of increased plasma concentrations of norepinephrine, presumably reflecting an attempt by the autonomic nervous system to compensate for reduced beta receptor activity.

Left ventricular hypertrophy accompanies aging. This change is most likely related to chronic increases in afterload to left ventricular ejection imposed by elevations of peripheral vascular resistance. Stroke volume is prob-

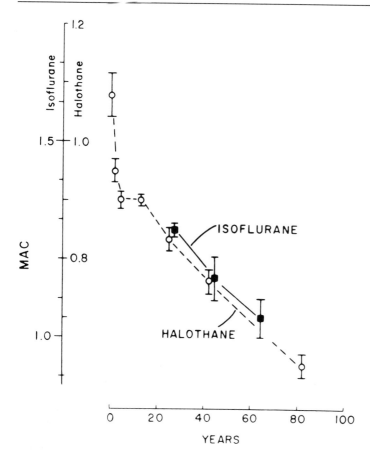

FIG. 36-3. Minimal alveolar concentration (MAC) for isoflurane and halothane decreases with increasing age. (Quasha AL, Eger EI, Tinker JH. Determination and applications of MAC. Anesthesiology 1980;53: 315–34)

ably decreased by aging, although ejection fractions are reported to be normal in geriatric patients.[11] Prolonged circulation time can delay onset of drug effects after their intravenous administration. This may manifest as a prolonged induction of anesthesia or delayed onset of skeletal muscle paralysis.

Heart Rate

Heart rate decreases with advancing age, suggesting an increase in activity of the parasympathetic nervous system. For example, compared with that of young adults, resting heart rate decreases by about 20 percent by 80 years of age.[10] Degenerative changes secondary to aging can involve the sinus node and/or cardiac conduction systems, resulting in atrioventricular heart block and manifesting as bradycardia. Maximum heart rate increases in response to exercise, isoproterenol, atropine, arterial hypoxemia, and hypercarbia are diminished in geriatric patients. Conversely, geriatric patients may be resistant to the heart rate effects of beta-adrenergic antagonists. Aging causes significant reductions in the heart rate response to hypotension, reflecting diminished activity of carotid sinus reflex responses.

Blood Pressure

Blood pressure increases with aging, reflecting development of thickened elastic fibers in walls of large arteries. As a result, blood vessels are poorly compliant and systolic blood pressure increases. Pulse pressure is also increased in geriatric patients.

PULMONARY SYSTEM

Mechanical ventilatory function and the efficiency of gas exchange deteriorate with aging.[1] At rest, geriatric patients may not have symptoms of pulmonary dysfunction; but pulmonary changes produced by surgery, superimposed upon the already present changes of aging, can result in severe symptomatology because of the decreased margin of reserve in these patients.

Mechanical Ventilatory Function

Mechanical ventilatory function is impaired because of decreased elasticity of the lungs and reduced maximal movement of the thorax. These changes reflect progressive destruction of pulmonary parenchyma and calcification of costochondral cartilages. Age-associated pulmonary parenchymal changes are characterized by loss of alveolar septae with expansion of alveolar spaces, thus mimicking emphysema. Furthermore, muscles of breathing have decreased strength and fatigue easily.

LUNG VOLUMES

Total lung capacity declines about 10 percent by 70 years of age, reflecting loss of height due to deterioration of intervertebral discs. Increased stiffness of the thoracic cage is accompanied by progressive dorsal kyphosis, with upward and anterior rotation of the ribs and sternum leading to increases in the anterior-to-posterior diameter of the chest and restricted chest expansion. Despite these changes, residual volume and functional residual capacity are increased. For example, residual volume is increased about 20 percent at 60 years of age,

compared to the volume at 20 years of age. The ratio of residual volume to total lung capacity is increased from a normal of 20 percent to nearly 40 percent. Vital capacity decreases with aging. Finally, the volume of the lungs at which small airways begin to close increases with aging, such that at rest in the supine position, closing volume will begin to exceed the functional residual capacity at about 45 years of age.[12] Closure of small airways during exhalation is made likely by loss of alveolar septa that normally exert a supportive (tethering) effect on terminal bronchioles.

FLOW RATES

Forced exhaled volume in 1 second and the forced vital capacity decrease progressively with aging. For example, the ratio of forced exhaled volume in 1 second to forced vital capacity decreases from greater than 80 percent in young adults to less than 70 percent in patients 70 years of age.[1] This change occurs in the absence of smoking and most likely reflects a loss of elastic tissue surrounding alveoli and alveolar ducts, an increased anterior-to-posterior diameter of the chest, and a weakening of the muscles of breathing. Maximum breathing capacity is reduced at least 50 percent at 70 years of age, compared with the value present at 30 years of age. Static lung compliance and airway resistance do not change greatly with increasing age.[1]

Efficiency of Gas Exchange

Efficiency of gas exchange is reduced by increasing age, as emphasized by progressive reductions in arterial partial pressures of oxygen. As a guideline, arterial partial pressures of oxygen decrease about 0.5 mmHg·yr^{-1} after the age of 20 years (Fig. 36-4).[13] Likewise, alveolar-to-arterial differences for oxygen increase from about 8 mmHg at 20 years of age to more than 20 mmHg at 70 years of age. This decreased efficiency of arterial oxygenation is thought to reflect increased airway closure and decreased cardiac output, leading to mis-

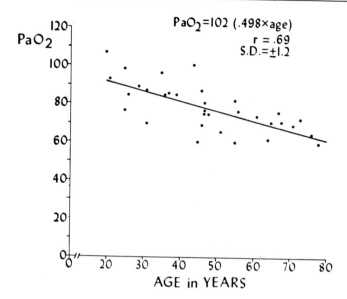

$$PaO_2 = 102 \, (.498 \times age)$$
$$r = .69$$
$$S.D. = \pm 1.2$$

FIG. 36-4. Arterial partial pressures of oxygen (PaO_2) were measured in patients between 20 years and 78 years of age. There was a significant inverse relationship between PaO_2 and increasing age. Note that the formula for PaO_2 should indicate that the product of .498 × age is subtracted from 102. (Wahba WM. Body build and preoperative arterial oxygen tensions. Can Anaesth Soc J 1975;22:653–8)

matches of ventilation to perfusion. Arterial oxygenation is also compromised by a decreased surface area for gas exchange due to degenerative changes and loss of alveolar septae.

Arterial-to-alveolar differences for carbon dioxide are likely to be increased in geriatric patients, as compared with young adults. This reflects an increased physiologic dead space, which accompanies aging. Indeed, pulmonary vasculature undergoes fibrosis with aging, increasing the likelihood of ventilation of unperfused alveoli. Nevertheless, arterial partial pressures of carbon dioxide are not altered by aging alone.

RENAL SYSTEM

Advancing age is associated with progressive declines in renal blood flow and renal function, as manifested by decreases in glomerular filtration rate and urine concentrating ability.[14] Combinations of decreased renal and cardiac function make geriatric patients more vulnerable to fluid overload. In addition, renal elimination of drugs may be impaired in these patients (see the section Pharmacokinetics).[15]

Renal Blood Flow

Declines in renal blood flow are due to decreases in cardiac output that accompany aging, plus reductions in the size of the renal vascular bed. It is estimated that renal blood flow decreases progressively by 1 percent·yr^{-1} to 2 percent·yr^{-1}, resulting in a 40 percent to 50 percent decrease between 25 years and 65 years of age.[14]

Glomerular Filtration Rate

Glomerular filtration rate decreases in parallel with decreases in renal blood flow. Despite this reduction in filtration rate, plasma creatinine concentrations do not increase, reflecting the decreased production of creatinine, which results from reduced skeletal muscle mass that accompanies aging. Therefore, increased plasma concentrations of creatinine in geriatric patients emphasize the presence of severe renal dysfunction. Creatinine clearance, which is based on 24 hour urinary excretion, as well as on plasma creatinine concentrations, is a more reliable indicator of renal function. Creatinine clearance remains unchanged until about 35 years of age, when a linear decrease of about 1 ml·min^{-1}·yr^{-1} begins. For drugs depending on renal excretion, it may be useful to adjust the dose to parallel reductions in creatinine clearance.

Concentrating Ability

Decreased urine concentrating ability in geriatric patients reflects degeneration of renal cortical vasculature, with relative sparing of the vasculature in the renal medulla. As a result, distal renal tubular function is impaired, but proximal renal tubular function remains essentially unchanged. Therefore, geriatric patients are less able to concentrate urine after water deprivation, and the ability to secrete an acid load is reduced. For example, maximum urine concentrating ability in response to vasopressin is reduced 30 percent at 80 years of age, compared with age 30. Furthermore, a greater urinary volume is necessary to excrete an olbigatory solute load, emphasizing the need to maintain urine output at about 1 ml· kg^{-1}·hr^{-1} during the perioperative period.

Adaptive Mechanisms

Adaptive mechanisms responsible for maintaining the volume and composition of the extracellular fluid are impaired in geriatric patients. For example, ability to conserve sodium is reduced, making this age group vulnerable to reductions in total body concentrations of sodium, particularly when acute illness leads to diminished oral intake of sodium. Renin activity and plasma concentrations of aldosterone decrease 30 percent to 50 percent in geriatric patients, leading to an increased vulnerability to the development of hyperkalemia. In addition, associated reductions in glomerular filtration rate make geriatric patients at risk for the development of hyperkalemia during intravenous infusion of solutions containing potassium.

HEPATOBILIARY SYSTEM

Hepatic blood flow decreases with age, paralleling reductions in cardiac output. Evidence for age-related decreases in activity of hepatic microsomal enzymes is suggested by reduced plasma clearance of drugs known to be extensively metabolized in the liver (see the section Pharmacokinetics). Decreased hepatic blood flow, rather than microsomal enzyme activity, however, is often the major determinant of total clearance of drugs. Production of albumin by the liver decreases with aging, but the impact of this change, if any, on responses to drugs has not been defined. Although not documented, it seems likely that geriatric patients would be more susceptible than young patients to hepatic damage from drugs or arterial hypoxemia. Plasma concentrations of bilirubin and transaminase enzymes show little change with aging. There are age-related increases in plasma retention of bromsulphalein, but this change may reflect decreased cell storage of dye rather than reduced clearance. Reductions in hepatic vein blood flow may also be responsible for reduced hepatobiliary function in geriatric patients.

GASTROINTESTINAL SYSTEM

Changes in function of the gastrointestinal tract associated with aging include decreased gastric cell function leading to impaired acid secretion and elevation of gastric fluid pH. Decreased rates of gastric emptying also accompany aging. Since drug absorption is minimal in the gastric portion of the gastrointestinal tract, age-dependent alterations in the stomach are unlikely to influence absorption of drugs.[15] Furthermore, progressive involution of the mucosa of the small intestine has not been documented to alter absorption of drugs. Reduced perfusion of the gastrointestinal tract with increasing age parallels decreases in cardiac output. This decreased perfusion could delay absorption of orally administered drugs, particularly those with high lipid solubilities.

ENDOCRINE SYSTEM

Pancreatic function declines during aging. Indeed, the incidence of diabetes mellitus increases with age, becoming greatest at 60 years to 70 years. Glucose intolerance often accompanies aging, even in the presence of normal plasma concentrations of insulin, implying either reduced hormonal effects or receptor site insensitivity to insulin's effect.

Subclinical hypothyroidism manifested solely by elevated plasma concentrations of thyroid stimulating hormone is present in 13.2 percent of healthy geriatric patients, particularly women[14] (see Chapter 18). Chronic thyroiditis (Hashimoto's thyroiditis) is the most likely cause of impaired thyroid function. In the absence of clinical symptoms of hypothyroidism (dry skin, cold intolerance, fatigue) and normal plasma concentrations of thyroxine, it is probably not necessary to treat these patients.

PHARMACOKINETICS

Pharmacokinetics depicts absorption, distribution, metabolism and elimination of drugs. Age-related changes in pharmacokinetics most often manifest as prolongation of elimination (beta) half-times of drugs (Fig 36-5). Increases in elimination half-times of drugs can reflect decreased clearance or increases in the volume of distribution. Events that lead to prolonged elimination half-times also make geriatric patients vulnerable to cumulative drug effects, which occur with repeated doses. Therefore, monitoring plasma concentrations of drugs has added significance when caring for these patients. Furthermore, because of age-related alterations in the pharmacokinetics of drugs, geriatric patients are at increased risk for the occurrence of adverse drug interactions.

Reductions in Rate of Clearance

Reductions in rate of clearance of drugs most often reflect decreased renal elimination or reduced hepatic metabolism.

RENAL ELIMINATION

With advancing age, there is considerable decline in renal clearance of drugs including digoxin, cimetidine, lithium and most of the commonly used antibiotics. Indeed, impaired renal clearance is probably the factor most responsible for increased plasma drug concentrations in geriatric patients. Presumably, declines in clearance are due to marked reductions in renal blood flow and associated decreases in glomerular filtration rate, which occur with aging. In addition, efficiency of renal tubular transport systems may decline with aging.

Numerous examples of alterations in elimination half-times of drugs can be attributed to impairment of renal function, which accompanies aging. For example, extended elimination half-times of digoxin are most likely related to reduced renal clearance. Penicillin, which is eliminated largely via renal tubular transport mechanisms, also exhibits prolonged elimination half-times in geriatric patients. The possible impact of decreased renal elimination of long-acting nondepolarizing muscle relaxants is a consideration in geriatric patients. Indeed, slowed rates of clearance of pancuronium from the plasma of geriatric patients reflects principally age-related reductions in renal function (Fig. 36-6).[16] This delayed renal clearance is associated with prolonged times for recovery from the neuromuscular effects of pancuronium when administered to geriatric patients (Table 36-1).[17] Reduced renal function also prolongs the duration of action of d-tubocurarine and metocurine in geriatric patients.[18]

HEPATIC METABOLISM

Reduced hepatic metabolism, leading to prolongation of the elimination half-times of drugs administered to geriatric patients, reflects decreased hepatic blood flow and/or reduced hepatic microsomal enzyme activity. For example, decreased hepatic blood flow, resulting in a reduced hepatic first pass effect, is presumed to be responsible for the nearly five-fold greater plasma concentrations of propranolol in geriatric as compared with younger pa-

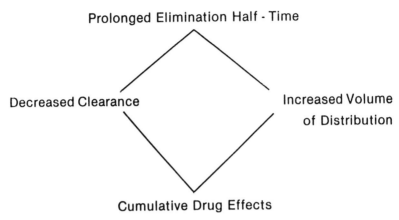

Prolonged Elimination Half - Time

Decreased Clearance

Increased Volume
of Distribution

Cumulative Drug Effects

FIG. 36-5. Age-related changes in pharmacokinetics most often manifest as a prolonged elimination half-time due to decreased clearance or increased volume of distribution of drugs. Cumulative drug effects are likely to occur with repeated doses.

FIG. 36-6. Clearance of pancuronium from the plasma (V) decreases with progressive increases in age. It is presumed that age-related reductions in renal function are more responsible than decreased hepatic metabolism for delayed clearance. Data are plotted with a least squares regression line and 95 percent confidence limits for the regression estimate. (McLeod K, Hull CJ, Watson MJ. Effects of aging on the pharmacokinetics of pancuronium. Br J Anaesth 1979;51:435–8)

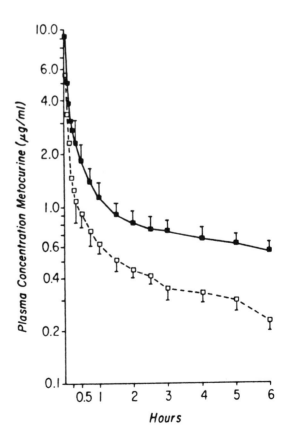

TABLE 36-1. Duration of Action of Pancuronium (Mean ± SD)

	Control Patients	Elderly Patients
Injection to return of twitch height to 25 percent of control (minutes)	44 ± 10	73 ± 22*
Recovery of twitch height from 25 to 75 percent of control (minutes)	39 ± 13	62 ± 30†

* P < 0.001 vs. control patients
† P < 0.01 vs. control patients
(Duvaldestin P, Saada J, Berger JL. Pharmacokinetics, pharmacodynamics, and dose-response relationships of pancuronium in control and elderly subjects. Anesthesiology 1982;56:36–40)

tients.[19] Presumably, similar responses would be present after administration of lidocaine, which, like propranolol, is highly dependent on hepatic extraction for its hepatic metabolism.

Increases in Volume of Distribution

Increases in volume of distribution of drugs result in increased tissue distribution of those drugs, manifesting as prolonged elimination half-times from the plasma. Volume of distribution of drugs may be influenced by total body fat content, total body water content, and protein binding. Therefore, it is important to appreciate that aging is associated with an increased total body fat content, decreased total body water content, and reduced protein binding of drugs.

TOTAL BODY FAT CONTENT

The fraction of total body weight composed of adipose tissue may increase with age from approximately 18 percent to 36 percent in men and from 33 percent to 48 percent in women.[15] This increase will extend the retention time of drugs and prolong their elimination half-times, particularly if the compounds are lipid soluble. Conversely, increased distribution of drugs into fat will reduce plasma concentrations of those drugs and thus decrease the likelihood of systemic toxicity.

Diazepam is an example of a lipid soluble drug characterized by age-dependent increases in volume of distribution and prolongation of elimination half-times from the plasma. For example, elimination half-times of diazepam are 20 hours at 20 years of age and 90 hours at 80 years of age (Fig. 36-7).[20] This observation is consistent with the increased incidence of drowsiness that follows administration of a diazepam to geriatric as compared with young patients.[21] Furthermore, doses of diazepam administered intravenously to produce conditions acceptable for elective cardioversion are less in geriatric patients. Elimination half-times of midazolam are also increased in geriatric patients.[22]

TOTAL BODY WATER CONTENT

Total body water content is reduced 10 percent to 15 percent during aging, leading to decreases in the volume of distribution of drugs that are restricted to extracellular fluid. Plasma concentrations of nondepolarizing muscle relaxants present in geriatric patients could be increased by this mechanism, as well as by decreased renal clearance. Decreases in total body water content are predictable, considering the anhydrous characteristic of adipose tissue.

PROTEIN BINDING

Decreased binding of drugs to protein, such as albumin, results in increased volumes of distribution, as well as increased plasma concentrations, of pharmacologically active

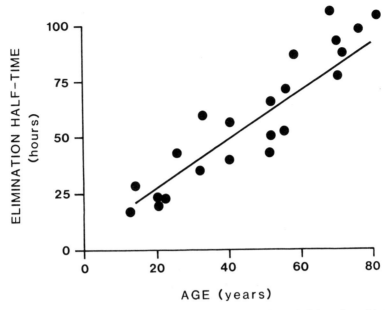

FIG. 36-7. Elimination half-times of diazepam were measured after administration of intravenous (0.1 mg·kg^{-1}) or oral (10 mg) diazepam to normal volunteers between 15 years and 82 years of age. There was a linear increase in elimination half-times of diazepam with increasing age. (Data from Klotz U, Avant GR, Hoyumpa A, et al. The effects of age and liver disease on the disposition and elimination of diazepam in adult man. J Clin Invest 1975;55:347–59)

unbound drugs. Aging is associated with about a 20 percent decline in the plasma concentration of albumin, presumably reflecting decreased hepatic production of this protein. There appears to be a positive correlation between age-related decreases in plasma concentrations of albumin and declines in plasma protein binding of certain drugs. A striking example of protein binding and aging is the decrease in the fraction of meperidine bound to protein in geriatric patients. For example, the bound fraction of meperidine is about 75 percent at 35 years of age and only 35 percent at 75 years of age (Fig. 36-8).[23] Such increased amounts of unbound drug in geriatric patients could contribute to exaggerated and prolonged responses. The impact of decreased protein binding of drugs, however, is theoretically offset by increased availability of the unbound drug fraction for hepatic metabolism and clearance.

PHARMACODYNAMICS

Pharmacodynamics depicts the responsiveness of receptors to drugs, as reflected by pharmacologic responses elicited.[24] The number of receptors present in a given tissue is often speculated to decrease with aging. Nevertheless, density of beta-adrenergic receptors does not change with aging but the affinity of these receptors for adrenergic agonists declines with aging (see the section Cardiovascular System).[10]

Confirmation of pharmacodynamic changes is demonstration of increases or decreases in plasma concentrations of drugs required to produce specific pharmacologic effects. For example, age-related decreases in MAC requirements for inhaled anesthetics reflects pharmacodynamic changes, although the mechanism is not documented. Conversely,

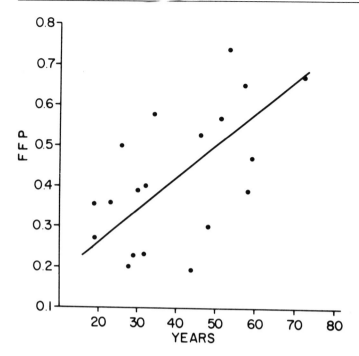

FIG. 36-8. The fraction of meperidine unbound in plasma (FFP) was measured in patients between 18 years and 73 years of age. The unbound fraction of meperidine increases progressively with age. (Mather LE, Tucker GT, Pflug AE, et al. Meperidine kinetics in man. Intravenous injection in surgical patients and volunteers. Clin Pharmacol Ther 1975;17:21–30)

plasma concentrations of long-acting nondepolarizing muscle relaxants necessary to produce specific degrees of twitch depression are not altered by increased age, suggesting that changes in the neuromuscular junction do not occur in geriatric patients (Fig. 36-9).[18]

Preoperative Evaluation

Preoperative evaluation of geriatric patients must consider the likely presence of co-existing diseases of major organ systems independent of the reason for surgery. Therefore, it is mandatory to appreciate changes in major organ function that accompany aging. Preoperative baseline evaluation of nervous system, cardiac, pulmonary, renal, and hepatic function is essential. A recent change in mental function should not be attributed to progressive aging until cardiac or pulmonary disease has been eliminated as an etiology. Co-existing diseases that frequently accompany aging and influence management in the perioperative period include essential hypertension, coronary artery disease, chronic pulmonary disease, diabetes mellitus, rheumatoid arthritis and osteoarthritis. Hazards of co-existing diseases are emphasized by increases in postoperative mortality in geriatric patients especially when emergency surgery is necessary. Nevertheless, surgery should not be denied solely on the basis of increased risks related to aging. For example, perioperative mortality after an elective cholecystectomy is less than 5 percent in patients 75 years to 94 years of age. Craniotomy is associated with the highest perioperative mortality in patients over 75 years of age.

Drug Interactions

The likelihood of adverse drug interactions is increased by alterations in pharmacokinetics and pharmacodynamics characteristic of aging (see the sections Pharmacokinetics and Pharmadodynamics). Furthermore, geriatric patients are likely to be taking several different drugs, which can result in adverse effects or drug interactions (Table 36-2). Indeed,

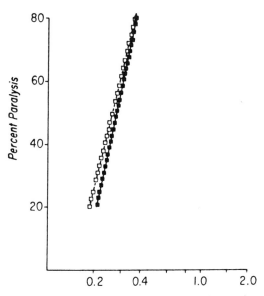

FIG. 36-9. Plasma concentrations of metocurine necessary to produce specific degrees of twitch depression are similar in geriatric patients (solid symbols) and younger controls (clear symbols) suggesting that changes in the neuromuscular junction do not occur with aging. (Matteo RS, Backus WW, McDaniel DD, Brotherton WP, Abraham R, Diaz J. Pharmacokinetics and pharmacodynamics of d-tubocurarine and metocurine in the elderly. Anesth Analg 1985;64:23–9. Reprinted with permission from IARS)

the incidence of drug interactions increases from 11.9 percent at 50 years of age to 24.9 percent after the age of 80.[15]

Intravascular Fluid Volume

Reduced intravascular fluid volume and anemia are common preoperative findings in geriatric patients. Orthostatic hypotension associated with increases in heart rate is suggestive of decreased intravascular fluid volume. Conversely, orthostatic hypotension not accompanied by increases in heart rate is suggestive of a sympathetic nervous system that is not functioning properly. Ideally, deficits of intravascular fluid volume and/or hemoglobin concentration are corrected slowly to permit adequate time for compensatory changes to occur in the circulation. Selection of crystalloid solutions, colloid solutions, or blood products to increase intravascular fluid volume is often a matter of personal preference. Monitoring cardiac filling pressures and urine output are helpful for guiding the rate of intravenous fluid infusion. Inadequate preoperative fluid replacement will often manifest as hypotension during induction of anesthesia.

Airway

Preoperative evaluation of the airway should consider the presence of changes characteristic of aging. For example, the potential existence of vertebrobasilar arterial insufficiency mandates evaluation of the effect of extension and rotation of the head on mental status. Poor dentition or the presence of dentures must be confirmed. Approximately 50 percent of patients over 65 years of age are edentulous. It must be appreciated that maintenance of a patent upper airway may be difficult when edentulous patients are rendered unconscious. If maintenance of anesthesia by mask is anticipated, it is acceptable to ask edentulous patients to wear their dentures to the operating room. Cervical osteoarthritis or rheumatoid arthritis may interfere with visualization of the glottic opening by direct laryngoscopy. Presence of hoarseness in the preoperative period can reflect involvement of the larynx by rheumatoid arthritis. Weakening of the posterior membranous portion of the trachea that accompanies aging can increase the likelihood of damage from the tube placed in the trachea. This possibility should be appreciated when considering the use of a stylet to facilitate placement of a tube in the trachea.

Skin Damage

Senile atrophy, with collagen loss and decreases in elasticity, makes the skin more sensitive to injury from adhesive tape and moni-

TABLE 36-2. Drugs Commonly Prescribed for Geriatric Patients

	Adverse Effects or Drug Interactions
Diuretics	Hypokalemia
	Hypovolemia
Digitalis	Cardiac dysrhythmias and conduction disturbances
Beta-adrenergic antagonists	Bradycardia
	Congestive heart failure
	Bronchospasm
	Attenuation of autonomic nervous system activity
Centrally acting antihypertensive drugs	Attenuation of autonomic nervous system activity
	Decreased anesthetic requirements
Tricyclic antidepressants	Anticholinergic effects
	Cardiac conduction disturbances
	Cardiac dysrhythmias with pancuronium and halothane or reversal with anticholinesterase drugs
	Increased anesthetic requirements
Lithium	Cardiac dysrhythmias
	Prolongation of muscle relaxants
Antidysrhythmics	Prolongation of muscle relaxants
Antibiotics	Prolongation of muscle relaxants

toring electrodes, as used for recording of the electrocardiogram or eliciting the response to a peripheral nerve stimulator. Geriatric patients are prone to injury from warming blankets, particularly if they have peripheral vascular disease. Likewise, pressure points must be avoided during positioning for surgery. Arthritic changes in peripheral joints should be appreciated in anticipation of the position required by the operative procedure. For example, the lithotomy position may be particularly uncomfortable because of arthritic changes in the lumbosacral hip joints.

PREOPERATIVE MEDICATION

Preoperative medication for geriatric patients is best achieved by detailed explanations of events that are going to occur in the perioperative period. If additional anxiety relief is desired, oral doses of benzodiazepines should be considered. Administration of anticholinergic drugs is probably not necessary. Atropine or scopolamine can exert undesirable central nervous system effects. Glycopyrrolate, which does not cross the blood-brain barrier in significant amounts, is an appropriate choice if anticholinergic effects without central nervous system manifestations are desired.

Preoperative administration of prophylactic digitalis to elderly patients in the absence of congestive heart failure is controversial. The potential for digitalis toxicity in the perioperative period detracts from routine prophylactic administration of this drug.

MANAGEMENT OF ANESTHESIA

Selection of drugs and techniques for the management of anesthesia in geriatric patients must consider major organ function changes that accompany aging, likely altered responses to drugs because of changes associated with aging, and potential interactions of drugs administered intraoperatively with medications taken preoperatively (Table 36-2). For example, geriatric patients are likely to be vulnerable to drug-induced hypotension, because of reduced activity of the sympathetic nervous system and decreased intravascular fluid volume. Decreased cardiac output and delayed clearance of drugs emphasize the likely delayed onset of effects produced by drugs administered intravenously. Furthermore, this delayed onset is likely to be followed by prolonged pharmacologic effects. The prudent approach is to reduce the dose and rate of administration of drugs administered intravenously, until individual responses of geriatric patients can be confirmed. In addition, a reduced cardiac output combined with decreased anesthetic requirements increases the hazards of a drug overdose with volatile anesthetics. Postoperative confusion and impairment of memory may also contribute to morbidity in geriatric patients.

Regional Anesthesia

Regional anesthesia is an appropriate selection for geriatric patients undergoing transurethral resection of the prostate, gynecologic procedures, inguinal herniorrhaphy, and repair of hip fractures. A T8 sensory level is desirable for these operative procedures. A prerequisite for selecting regional techniques is an alert and cooperative patient. In selected patients, regional anesthesia may be associated with less postoperative confusion compared with patients receiving general anesthesia.[25]

Maintenance of consciousness during surgery permits rapid recognition of acute changes in cerebral function or the onset of angina pectoris. Apprehension despite adequate anesthesia may require intravenous supplementation of regional techniques. Small doses of diazepam (2.5 mg to 5 mg), or midazolam (1 mg to 2.5 mg) are useful for reducing apprehension in awake patients.

SPINAL ANESTHESIA

Spinal anesthesia using hypobaric solutions may be used for procedures on the hip performed with patients in the lateral position. This allows positioning of patients before performance of the subarachnoid injection of local anesthetics.

It should be appreciated that geriatric patients may be more sensitive to spinal anesthesia than their younger counterparts. Although unconfirmed by objective measurements, a prolonged duration of spinal anesthesia is thought to reflect decreased vascular absorption of local anesthetics due to decreased blood flow to vessels surrounding the subarachnoid space in arteriosclerotic geriatric patients. Furthermore, geriatric patients are likely to develop greater reductions in blood pressure than young adults, despite equal sensory levels. In the presence of an adequate intravascular fluid volume, this lesser blood pressure reduction in young patients most likely reflects a higher residual inherent vascular tone that persists after sympathetic denervation, as well as more active compensatory reflexes. Although a controversial practice, some administer prophylactic intramuscular ephedrine 25 mg to 50 mg 5 minutes to 10 minutes before institution of the block, in an attempt to attenuate hypotensive effects of spinal anesthesia in geriatric patients.

EPIDURAL ANESTHESIA

Epidural anesthesia is an acceptable alternative to spinal anesthesia. A possible advantage of epidural anesthesia in geriatric patients is a more gradual onset of reductions in blood pressure, in contrast to the often abrupt hypotension that accompanies spinal anesthesia. Doses of local anesthetics required to achieve given sensory levels during epidural anesthesia decrease with aging, although not all reports describe strong linear relationships between dose and age (Fig. 36-2).[6,26,27] It is suggested that decreased dose requirements in geriatric patients are due, in part, to anatomic changes in the epidural space, characterized by progressive occlusion of intervertebral foramina with connective tissue. As a result, less local anesthetic escapes through the intervertebral foramina and there is increased spread in the epidural space. This change would also result in an increased surface area for absorption of local anesthetic from the epidural space, which is consistent with higher peak plasma concentrations of lidocaine observed after epidural placement in geriatric patients compared with young adults.[26] Exaggerated spread of epidural analgesia in patients with arteriosclerosis apparently does not occur (Fig. 36-10).[28]

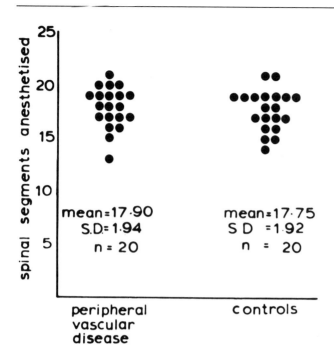

FIG. 36-10. The number of spinal segments anesthetized after injection of 10 ml of 0.75 percent bupivacaine into the epidural space was measured in patients with peripheral vascular disease and in normal individuals (controls) of similar age and weight (about 66 years of age and 66 kg). There was no significant difference between the number of segments anesthetized in the 20 patients with peripheral vascular disease (17.9 segments) and in the 20 normal patients (17.75 segments). (Sharrock NE. Lack of exaggerated spread of epidural anesthesia in patients with arteriosclerosis. Anesthesiology 1977;47:307–8)

General Anesthesia

General anesthesia is as acceptable as regional anesthesia for geriatric patients. Furthermore, expansion of collapsed alveoli with positive airway pressure plus the ability to remove tracheobronchial secretions during general anesthesia may improve postoperative oxygenation.[29]

INDUCTION OF ANESTHESIA

Induction of anesthesia is acceptably accomplished by the intravenous administration of barbiturates, benzodiazepines or etomidate. Doses and rates of administration of these drugs should be reduced, compared with younger patients, as compensatory reflexes via the autonomic nervous system in response to drug-induced vasodilation are attenuated in geriatric patients. Furthermore, doses of thiopental and etomidate required to produce specific pharmacologic effects are reduced in geriatric patients due to decreases in the initial volume of distribution of these drugs (Fig. 36-

11).[30,31] The onset of sedative effects may be delayed due to a reduced cardiac output. This delayed onset should not be interpreted as an inadequate initial dose; indeed, administration of an additional dose can lead to a drug overdose.

Progressive decreases in reactivity of protective upper airway reflexes with aging (Fig. 36-12)[32] plus the high incidence of hiatal hernia in geriatric patients emphasizes the importance of protecting the lungs from aspiration by placement of a cuffed tube in the trachea. Intubation of the trachea is typically facilitated by administration of muscle relaxants.

MAINTENANCE OF ANESTHESIA

Injected or inhaled drugs are probably equally acceptable for maintenance of anesthesia for geriatric patients. As with all drugs, it must be appreciated that geriatric patients require lower doses and are more susceptible to depressant effects. The combination of decreased cardiac output and reduced anesthetic requirements will contribute to rapid achievement of anesthetizing partial pressures of in-

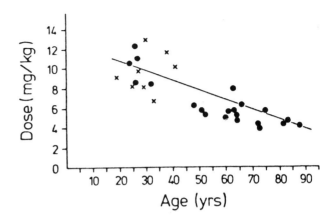

FIG. 36-11. Doses of thiopental administered as continuous intravenous infusions to produce early burst suppression on the electroencephalogram decrease (solid line) with age. Solid circles represent surgical patients who underwent arterial sampling, and X symbols represent volunteer subjects who underwent venous blood sampling. (Homer TD, Stanski DR. The effect of increasing age on thiopental disposition and anesthetic requirements. Anesthesiology 1985;62:714–24)

haled drugs in the arterial blood. An increased functional residual capacity, characteristic of aging, may offset the impact of a reduced cardiac output. The importance of this increased lung volume, however, in slowing achievement of partial pressures of inhaled drugs in arterial blood is probably minimal. Furthermore, controlled ventilation of the lungs negates this factor, while possibly contributing to even further reductions in cardiac output. In addition to predictable reductions in anes-

thetic requirements associated with aging, it must be appreciated that drugs taken by patients preoperatively may further reduce anesthetic requirements (Table 36-2).

Drug Selection. There is no evidence that specific inhaled or injected drugs are preferable for maintenance of anesthesia for geriatric patients. Age-related declines in renal and hepatic function, however, should be considered when selecting enflurane or halothane.

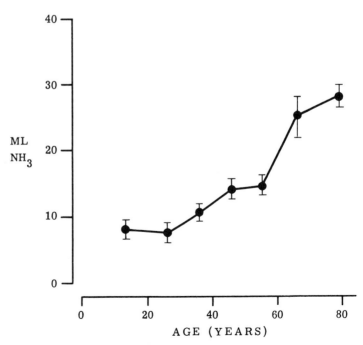

FIG. 36-12. The threshold of the protective airway reflexes was determined in 103 subjects by using ammonia as an irritant gas. The dose of ammonia gas (ml of NH_3) necessary to cause momentary closure of the glottis and a brief pause in inspiration was found to be increased in geriatric patients, suggesting decreased sensitivity of airway reflexes with advancing age. The greatest reduction in sensitivity occurred between 50 years and 70 years of age and is consistent with the increased incidence of pulmonary aspiration that occurs in geriatric patients. (Data from Pontoppidan H, Beecher HK. Progressive loss of protective reflexes in the airway with the advance of age. JAMA 1960;174:2209–13)

Increases in heart rate associated with administration of isoflurane are less likely to occur in geriatric compared with younger patients.[1] The possible delayed metabolism of drugs such as opioids must be appreciated and doses adjusted appropriately. Indeed, elimination half-times of fentanyl 10 $\mu g \cdot kg^{-1}$ are prolonged in geriatric compared with younger patients, presumably reflecting decreased hepatic metabolism in older individuals (Fig. 36-13).[33] This delayed clearance of fentanyl from the plasma would likely result in longer durations of drug effects in geriatric patients. Recurrence of fentanyl-induced depression of ventilation after apparent awakening has been observed and would seem to be particularly important in geriatric patients.[34] Direct myocardial depression due to volatile drugs may be exaggerated in geriatric patients, emphasizing the need to minimize doses of these drugs.

Ventilation. Mechanical ventilation of the lungs with supplemental oxygen is useful during the intraoperative period. Hyperventilation and associated hypokalemia must be avoided, particularly if geriatric patients are receiving diuretics and/or digitalis preparations preoperatively.

Muscle Relaxant. The intensity of neuromuscular blockade after administration of long-acting nondepolarizing muscle relaxants is likely to be exaggerated in geriatric patients.[17] This is predictable, considering reductions of skeletal muscle mass, extracellular fluid volume, and renal function that accompany aging. As with anesthetic drugs, initial doses of muscle relaxants should be reduced and responses produced at the neuromuscular junction observed using a peripheral nerve stimulator. In contrast to long-acting muscle relaxants, intermediate-acting drugs are less dependent on renal or hepatic clearance mechanisms and thus less likely to be influenced by age-related changes in cardiac output. For example, clearance of atracurium is independent of renal or hepatic function, and thus its duration of action is not influenced by aging (Fig.

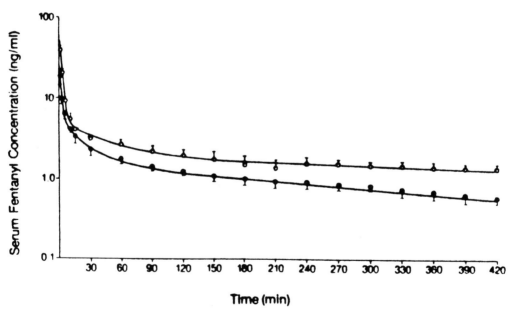

FIG. 36-13. Elimination half-times of fentanyl, as depicted by the rate of decline in plasma concentrations after intravenous administration of 10 $\mu g \cdot kg^{-1}$, are prolonged in geriatric patients (clear symbols, greater than 60 years of age) compared with younger controls (solid symbols, less than 50 years of age). Mean ± SE. (Bentley JB, Borel JD, Nenad RE, Gillespie TJ. Age and fentanyl pharmacokinetics. Anesth Analg 1982;61:968–71. Reprinted with permission from IARS)

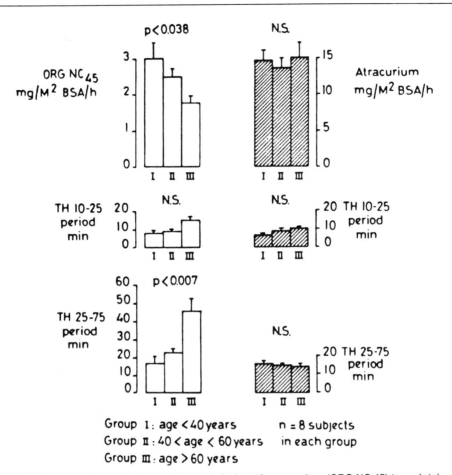

FIG. 36-14. Dose requirements for continuous infusion of vecuronium (ORG NC 45) to maintain steady states of neuromuscular blockade decrease with aging, and times for twitch to recover from 10 percent to 25 percent of control (TH 10-25) and 25 percent to 75 percent of control (TH 25-75) after discontinuation of the infusion increase with aging. Aging does not influence the dose requirements or rate of recovery from atracurium. Mean ± SE. (D'Hollander AA, Luyckx C, Barvais L, DeVille A. Clinical evaluation of atracurium besylate requirements for a stable muscle relaxation during surgery: Lack of age related effects. Anesthesiology 1983;59:237–40)

36-14).[35] Vecuronium shows detectable but modest prolongation of duration of action in older compared with younger patients (Fig. 36-14).[35]

Pancuronium, because of its sympathomimetic effects, may be a useful drug for production of skeletal muscle paralysis in geriatric patients. It should be appreciated, however, that the incidence of cardiac dysrhythmias may be increased during halothane anesthesia when pancuronium is administered to patients who were receiving tricyclic antidepressants preoperatively.[36] Reversal of nondepolarizing neuromuscular blockade with anticholinesterase drugs does not seem to introduce any unique risks in geriatric patients.

Monitoring. Monitoring of geriatric patients does not introduce unique considerations, other than an appreciation that the margin of reserve is reduced in these patients. Therefore, appropriate use of monitors is essential. Likewise, complications of invasive monitors may be increased in geriatric patients. For example, complications from insertion of catheters into peripheral arteries may be greater in geriatric patients with co-existing arteriosclerosis. This potential complication emphasizes the logic of confirming the adequacy of collateral circulation before insertion. Nevertheless, there is no evidence that performance of arterial catheterization in the presence of an abnormal Allen's test increases the likelihood of subsequent arterial insufficiency.[37] Monitoring of cardiac filling pressures may be necessary to guide fluid replacement and to monitor cardiac function. Pulmonary artery catheters are often used for operations associated with the likelihood of massive blood loss and the need to administer large volumes of fluid. Measurements of urine output are an acceptable method for following the adequacy of intravascular fluid replacement during most operations. Detection of myocardial ischemia is facilitated by monitoring a precordial lead of the electrocardiogram. Body temperature should be monitored to provide early detection of spontaneous hypothermia, which can occur rapidly in geriatric patients anesthetized in cold operating rooms.

Controlled Hypotension. Sensitivity to nitroprusside increases with advancing age (Fig. 36-15).[38] This increased sensitivity might reflect diminished activity of carotid sinus reflex responses and/or decreased responsiveness of cardiac beta receptors to catecholamine

stimulation. Indeed, heart rate responses evoked by nitroprusside-induced reductions in blood pressure are less in geriatric compared with younger patients.

POSTOPERATIVE CARE

Complications after surgery in geriatric patients are most often related to cardiac, pulmonary, renal, or hepatic dysfunction. Therefore, constant attention, especially in monitoring these four organ systems, is essential throughout the postoperative period. The need for intensive support of ventilation of the lungs after major surgery is to be expected. Pulse oximetry may provide early recognition of marginal arterial oxygenation in the early postoperative period. Supplemental oxygen is indicated to offset the impact of mismatch of ventilation to perfusion. The electrocardiogram should be monitored continuously in the early postoperative period when the possibility of myocardial ischemia is a consideration. Opioids to provide postoperative analgesia are best administered intravenously and in reduced doses. Early ambulation is particularly important in geriatric patients to decrease the likelihood of pulmonary infections or the development of thrombus in the deep veins of the legs. Other measures that may min-

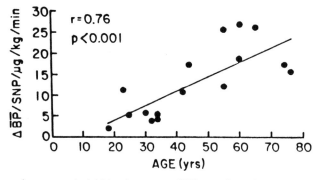

FIG. 36-15. Changes in mean arterial blood pressure (BP) per given dose of nitroprusside (SNP) show significant (P < 0.001) correlations with age demonstrating that sensitivity to SNP is increased in geriatric patients compared with younger patients. (Wood M, Hyman S, Wood AJJ. A clinical study of sensitivity to sodium nitroprusside during controlled hypotensive anesthesia in young and elderly patients. Anesth Analg 1987;66:132–6. Reprinted with permission from IARS)

imize the possibility of thromboembolic disease include the use of elastic support stockings, elevation of the legs, and administration of anticoagulants. Finally, careful attention to fluid and electrolyte balance is essential in geriatric patients.

PROGERIA (HUTCHINSON-GILFORD SYNDROME)

Progeria is a syndrome characterized by premature aging.[39,40] This disease is inherited as an autosomal recessive disorder, with clinical manifestations becoming apparent after about 6 months of age. These patients develop all the diseases of old age during the first or second decades of life. For example, coronary artery disease, hypertension, cerebral vascular disease, osteoarthritis, and diabetes mellitus are common. The cause of progeria is not known, and there is no effective treatment. Mean survival age is 13 years, with death usually occurring by age 25 from congestive heart failure or myocardial infarction.

Management of anesthesia for patients with progeria must consider changes in major organ system function that accompany normal aging.[40] In addition, the presence of mandibular hypoplasia and micrognathia may lead to difficulty in management of the airway and intubation of the trachea. Presence of a narrow glottic opening and need for a small tracheal tube is suggested by the typical high-pitched voice characteristic of these patients. Even minimal laryngeal edema can compromise the patency of the airway. Careful movement and positioning of patients with progeria are necessary to avoid injury to the thin and fragile extremities.

REFERENCES

1. McLeskey CH. Anesthesia for the geriatric patient. In: Stoelting RK, Barash PG, Gallagher TJ (eds). Advances in Anesthesia. Chicago. Year Book Medical Publishers 1985:31–68

2. Thompson TL, Moran MG, Nies AS. Psychotropic drug use in the elderly. N Engl J Med 1983;308:136–41

3. Kelsey JL, Hoffman S. Risk factors for hip fracture. N Engl J Med 1987;316:404–6

4. Burch GE. People live no longer anymore. Am Heart J 1972;83:285–6

5. Evans TI. The physiological basis of geriatric general anesthesia. Anaesth Intensive Care 1973;1:319–28

6. Bromage PR. Ageing and epidural dose requirements. Segmental spread and predictability of epidural analgesia in youth and extreme age. Br J Anaesth 1969;41:1016–22

7. Sharrock NE. Epidural anesthetic dose responses in patients 20 to 80 years old. Anesthesiology 1978;49:425–8

8. Quasha AL, Eger EI, Tinker JH. Determination and applications of MAC. Anesthesiology 1980;53:315–34

9. Craig DB, McLeskey CH, Mitenko PA, et al. Geriatric anaesthesia. Can J Anaesth 1987;34:156–67

10. Feldman RD, Limbird LE, Nadeau J, et al. Alterations in leukocyte beta-receptor affinity with aging: A potential explanation for altered beta-adrenergic sensitivity in the elderly. N Engl J Med 1984;310:815–9

11. Latour J, DeLaFuente R, Caird FI. Measurement of ejection fraction in the elderly. Age Ageing 1980;9:157–64

12. Don H. Measurement of gas trapped in the lungs at FRC and effects of posture. Anesthesiology 1971;35:582–90

13. Wahba W. Body build and preoperative arterial oxygen tension. Can Anaesth Soc J 1975;22:653–8

14. Cooper DS. Subclinical hypothyroidism. JAMA 1987;258:246–7

15. Greenblatt DJ, Sellers EM, Shader RI. Drug disposition in old age. N Engl J Med 1982;306:1081–8

16. McLeod K, Hull CJ, Watson MJ. Effects of ageing on the pharmacokinetics of pancuronium. Br J Anaesth 1979;51:435–8

17. Duvaldestin P, Saada J, Berger JL. Pharmacokinetics, pharmacodynamics, and dose-response relationships of pancuronium in control and elderly subjects. Anesthesiology 1982;56:36–40

18. Matteo RS, Backus WW, McDaniel DD, et al. Pharmacokinetics and pharmacodynamics of d-tubocurarine and metocurine in the elderly. Anesth Analg 1985;64:23–9

19. Castleden CM, Kaye CM, Parsons RL. The effect of age on plasma levels of propranolol and practolol in man. Br J Clin Pharmacol 1975;2:303–6

20. Klotz U, Avant GR, Hoyumpa A, et al. The effects

of age and liver disease on the disposition and elimination of diazepam in adult man. J Clin Invest 1975;55:347–59

21. Boston Collaborative Surveillance Program. N Engl J Med 1973;288:277–80

22. Greenblatt DJ, Abernathy DR, Locniskar A, et al. Effect of age, gender, and obesity on midazolam kinetics. Anesthesiology 1984;61:27–35

23. Mather LE, Tucker GT, Pflug AE, et al. Meperidine kinetics in man: Intravenous injection in surgical patients and volunteers. Clin Pharmacol Ther 1975;17:21–30

24. Bender AD. Pharmacodynamic principles of drug therapy in the aged. J Am Geriatr Soc 1974;22:296–303

25. Chung F, Meier R, Lautenschlager E, Carmichael FJ, Chung A. General or spinal anesthesia: Which is better in the elderly? Anesthesiology 1987;67:422–7

26. Finucane BT, Hammonds WD, Welch MB. Influence of age on vascular absorption of lidocaine from the epidural space. Anesth Analg 1987;66:843–6

27. Park WY, Hagins FM, Rivat EL, Macnamara TE. Age and epidural dose response in adult men. Anesthesiology 1982;56:318–20

28. Sharrock NE. Lack of exaggerated spread of epidural anesthesia in patients with arteriosclerosis. Anesthesiology 1977;47:307–8

29. Hamilton WK, Sokoll MD. Choice of anesthetic technique in patients with acute pulmonary disease. JAMA 1966;197:135–6

30. Homer TD, Stanski DR. The effect of increasing age on thiopental disposition and anesthetic requirement. Anesthesiology 1985;62:714–24

31. Arden JR, Holley FO, Stanski DR. Increased sensitivity to etomidate in the elderly: Initial distribution versus altered brain response. Anesthesiology 1986;65:19–27

32. Pontoppidan H, Beecher HK. Progressive loss of protective reflexes in the airway with the advance of age. JAMA 1960;174:2209–13

33. Bentley JB, Borel JD, Nenad RE, Gillespie TJ. Age and fentanyl pharmacokinetics. Anesth Analg 1982;61:968–71

34. Becker LD, Paulson BA, Miller RD, et al. Biphasic respiratory depression after fentanyl-droperidol of fentanyl alone used to supplement nitrous oxide anesthesia. Anesthesiology 1976;44:291–6

35. D'Hollander AA, Luyckx C, Barvais L, DeVille A. Clinical evaluation of atracurium besylate requirement for a stable muscle relaxation during surgery: Lack of age-related effects. Anesthesiology 1983;59:237–40

36. Edwards RP, Miller RD, Roizen MF, et al. Cardiac responses to imipramine and pancuronium during anesthesia with halothane or enflurane. Anesthesiology 1979;50:421–5

37. Slogoff S, Keats AS, Arlund C. On the safety of radial artery cannulation. Anesthesiology 1983;59:42–7

38. Wood M, Hyman S, Wood AJJ. A clinical study of sensitivity to sodium nitroprusside during controlled hypotension anesthesia in young and elderly patients. Anesth Analg 1987;66:132–6

39. Debusk FL. The Hutchinson-Gilford progeria syndrome. J Pediatr 1972;80:696–724

40. Chapin JW, Kahre J. Progeria and anesthesia. Anesth Analg 1979;58:424–5

Index

Page numbers followed by t denote tables; those followed by f denote figures.